CLINICAL METHODS
Second Edition

THE HISTORY, PHYSICAL AND LABORATORY EXAMINATIONS

EDITORS

H. Kenneth Walker, MD, FACP
Professor of Medicine
Emory University School of Medicine
Atlanta, Georgia

W. Dallas Hall, MD, FACP
Professor of Medicine
Emory University School of Medicine
Atlanta, Georgia

J. Willis Hurst, MD, MACP, FACC
Professor of Medicine (Cardiology)
Chairman of the Department of Medicine
Emory University School of Medicine
Atlanta, Georgia

With the assistance of
Rosalind Washington Jackson
and the editorial assistance of
Terri Langston

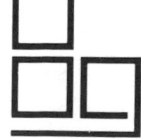 BUTTERWORTH PUBLISHERS INC.
Boston   London   Toronto
Durban   Sydney   Singapore

This book is dedicated to the Patients and Staff of
GRADY MEMORIAL HOSPITAL
ATLANTA, GEORGIA
and to
J. WILLIAM PINKSTON, JR.
EXECUTIVE DIRECTOR
whose leadership, wisdom, and
devotion inspire all of us

Library of Congress Cataloging in Publication Data
Main entry under title:

Clinical methods

   Includes bibliographies and index.
   1. Diagnosis. I. Walker, Henry Kenneth, 1936–
II. Hall, Wilbur Dallas, 1938–   III. Hurst, John
Willis, 1920–   (DNLM: 1. Diagnosis. 2. Diagnosis,
Laboratory. WB141 C638).
RC71.C63 1980   616.07'5   80–18835
ISBN 0–409–95190–0 (Hardcover)
ISBN 0–409–90013–3 (Paperback)

Butterworth Publishers
80 Montvale Avenue
Stoneham, MA 02180

10 9 8 7 6 5 4

Printed in the United States of America.

Contributors

Claudia R. Adkison, PhD, Associate Professor of Anatomy, Emory University School of Medicine

J. Galt Allee, MD, Clinical Assistant Professor of Medicine, Emory University School of Medicine; Internal Medicine and Cardiology Practice, Tallahassee, Florida

J. Richard Amerson, MD, Professor of Surgery, Emory University School of Medicine

John C. Ammons, MD, Associate Professor of Neurology, Emory University School of Medicine; Chief, Neurology Section, Veterans Administration Medical Center (Atlanta)

J. Thomas Apgar, MD, Clinical Assistant Professor of Dermatology, Emory University School of Medicine

Albert N. Badre, PhD, Associate Professor of Information and Computer Science, Associate Professor of Psychology, Georgia Institute of Technology

Frank C. Bell, MD, Associate Professor of Ophthalmology, Emory University School of Medicine

Algie C. Brown, MD, Clinical Associate Professor of Medicine, Emory University School of Medicine; Director, Dermatopathology Laboratory, Atlanta Skin and Cancer Clinic

Henry Camp, BA, Clinical Instructor in Medicine, Emory University School of Medicine

David D. Clark, OTR, Chief Therapist, Occupational Therapy, Grady Memorial Hospital

Stephen D. Clements, Jr., MD, Associate Professor of Medicine (Cardiology), Emory University School of Medicine

Robert B. Copeland, MD, Clinical Professor of Medicine, Emory University School of Medicine, Director, Georgia Heart Clinic, LaGrange, Georgia

I. Sylvia Crawley, MD, Associate Professor of Medicine (Cardiology), Emory University School of Medicine; Chief, Cardiology Section, Veterans Administration Medical Center (Atlanta)

James C. Crutcher, MD, Professor of Medicine, Emory University School of Medicine

John R. Darsee, MD, Research Fellow in Cardiology, Harvard Medical School and Peter Bent Brigham Hospital, Boston, Massachusetts

Joseph Z. Davids, MD, Assistant in Medicine, Chief of Cardiology, Good Samaritan Hospital, Baltimore, Maryland

Eugene Davidson, MD, Assistant Professor of Surgery, Emory University School of Medicine; Assistant Chief of Surgery, Veterans Administration Medical Center (Atlanta)

John K. Davidson, MD, Professor of Medicine (Endocrinology), Director, Diabetes Unit, Emory University School of Medicine

Harry K. Delcher, MD, Assistant Professor of Medicine (Endocrinology), Emory University School of Medicine

Steven P. Dewees, MD, Assistant Professor of Medicine, Medical University of South Carolina; Director, Emergency Room, Charleston County Hospital, Charleston, South Carolina

Mario DiGirolamo, MD, Professor of Medicine (Endocrinology), Associate Professor of Physiology, Co-Director, Division of Endocrinology, Emory University School of Medicine

Constantine Droulias, MD, Athens, Greece

Louis J. Elsas II, MD, Professor of Pediatrics, Director, Division of Medical Genetics; Assistant Professor of Medicine, Emory University School of Medicine

Joel M. Felner, MD, Associate Professor of Medicine (Cardiology), Emory University School of Medicine

Susan K. Fellner, MD, Associate Professor of Medicine (Nephrology), Emory University School of Medicine

Robert M. Fine, MD, Clinical Professor of Dermatology, Emory University School of Medicine and Veterans Administration Medical Center (Atlanta)

J. Donald Fite, MD, Clinical Assistant Professor of Ophthalmology, Emory University School of Medicine

Alan S. Fleischer, MD, Associate Professor of Surgery, Division of Neurological Surgery, Emory University School of Medicine

P. Bailey Francis, MD, Associate Professor of Medicine (Pulmonary Diseases), Emory University School of Medicine; Chief, Pulmonary Diseases Section, Veterans Administration Medical Center (Atlanta)

Malcolm G. Freeman, MD, Professor of Gynecology and Obstetrics, Emory University School of Medicine

John T. Galambos, MD, Professor of Medicine (Digestive Diseases), Director, Division of Digestive Diseases, Emory University School of Medicine

Donna L. Gibbas, MD, Assistant Professor of Pediatrics, Emory University School of Medicine

Charles A. Gilbert, MD, Clinical Professor of Medicine, Emory University School of Medicine

John A. Goldman, MD, Associate Professor of Medicine, Emory University School of Medicine

John B. Griffin, MD, Associate Professor of Psychiatry, Emory University School of Medicine

Patrick A. Griffith, MD, Assistant Professor of Neurology, Emory University School of Medicine

Joseph E. Hardison, MD, Professor of Medicine (Hematology and Oncology), Emory University School of Medicine; Chief, Medical Service, Veterans Administration Medical Center (Atlanta)

Robert A. Hatcher, MD, Associate Professor of Gynecology and Obstetrics, Director of Family Planning, Emory University School of Medicine

Theodore Hersh, MD, Professor of Medicine (Digestive Diseases), Co-Director, Division of Digestive Diseases, Emory University School of Medicine

Richard P. Holm, MD, Assistant Professor of Medicine (General Medicine), Emory University School of Medicine

Charles M. Huguley, MD, Professor of Medicine (Hematology and Oncology), Director, Division of Hematology and Oncology, Emory University School of Medicine

Zafar H. Israili, MS, PhD, Associate Professor of Medicine (Clinical Pharmacology), Emory University School of Medicine

Norman Jacobs, MD, Clinical Assistant Professor of Medicine, Emory University School of Medicine

Julian Jacobs, MD, Professor of Medicine (Hematology), Emory University School of Medicine; Chief, Hematology Section, Veterans Administration Medical Center (Atlanta)

Horacio Jinich, MD, Attending Physician, American British Hospital, Mexico City, Mexico

Henry Earl Jones, MD, Professor and Chairman, Department of Dermatology, Emory University School of Medicine

Herbert E. Kann, Jr., MD, Clinical Associate Professor of Medicine (Hematology and Oncology), Emory University School of Medicine

James W. Keller, MD, Associate Professor of Medicine (Hematology and Oncology), Emory University School of Medicine

Pearon G. Lang, MD, Assistant Professor of Dermatology, Emory University School of Medicine

Michael F. Lubin, MD, Assistant Professor of Medicine (General Medicine), Emory University School of Medicine

John E. McGowan, Jr., MD, Associate Professor of Medicine (Infectious Diseases), Emory University School of Medicine

Stephen B. Miller, MD, Assistant Professor of Medicine (Rheumatology-Immunology), Emory University School of Medicine

William J. Millikan, MD, Assistant Professor of Surgery, Emory University School of Medicine

Melvin R. Moore, MD, Associate Professor of Medicine (Hematology and Oncology), Emory University School of Medicine

Douglas C. Morris, MD, Associate Professor of Medicine (Cardiology), Emory University School of Medicine

Sidney Olansky, MD, Professor of Dermatology, Emory University School of Medicine

David P. O'Brien, MD, Assistant Professor of Surgery, Emory University School of Medicine

Nettleton S. Payne, MD, Clinical Neurosurgery, Atlanta, Georgia

John H. Per-Lee, MD, Associate Professor of Surgery, Emory University School of Medicine

R. Waldo Powell, MD, Associate Professor of Surgery, Emory University School of Medicine

John R. K. Preedy, MD, Professor of Medicine (Endocrinology), Director, Division of Endocrinology, Emory University School of Medicine

E. Stephen Purdom, MD, Internal Medicine Practice, Columbus, Georgia

Albert P. Rauber, MD, Professor of Pediatrics, Emory University School of Medicine

Michael Rein, MD, Assistant Professor of Medicine (Infectious Diseases), University of Virginia School of Medicine

Stewart T. Roberts, Jr., MD, Associate Professor of Radiology, Assistant Professor of Medicine, Emory University School of Medicine

Ms. Cheryl Rock, RD, MMSc, Research Dietitian, Department of Medicine, Emory University School of Medicine

Barry J. Rosenbaum, MD, Clinical Assistant Professor of Medicine, Emory University School of Medicine, Director, Atlanta Nephrology Referral Center

David Schlossberg, MD, Director, Department of Internal Medicine, Chief, Division of Infectious Medicine, Polyclinic Hospital, Harrisburg, Pennsylvania

Jonas A. Shulman, MD, Professor of Medicine (Infectious Diseases), Director, Division of Infectious Diseases, Emory University School of Medicine

Barry D. Silverman, MD, Clinical Assistant Professor of Medicine (Cardiology), Emory University School of Medicine and Northside Hospital

Mark E. Silverman, MD, Professor of Medicine (Cardiology), Emory University School of Medicine and Piedmont Hospital

Vladimir Slamecka, DLS, Professor of Information and Computer Sciences, Georgia Institute of Technology, Clinical Professor of Medicine, Emory University School of Medicine

Robert B. Smith III, MD, Professor of Surgery, Emory University School of Medicine; Chief, Surgical Service, Veterans Administration Medical Center (Atlanta)

Hiram M. Sturm, MD, Clinical Professor of Dermatology, Emory University School of Medicine

John D. Thompson III, MD, Professor and Chairman, Gynecology and Obstetrics, Emory University School of Medicine

Sumner E. Thompson III, MD, Assistant Professor of Medicine (Infectious Diseases), Emory University School of Medicine; Chief, Clinical Studies Section of Venereal Disease Control Division, Atlanta Center for Disease Control

John S. Turner, Jr., MD, Professor of Surgery, Chief, Division of Otolaryngology, Emory University School of Medicine

Elbert P. Tuttle, Jr., MD, Professor of Medicine (Nephrology), Director, Division of Nephrology, Emory University School of Medicine

Gerald W. Vogel, MD, Professor of Psychiatry, Emory University School of Medicine; Director, Sleep Laboratory, Georgia Mental Health Institute

David H. Vroon, MD, Assistant Professor of Pathology, Emory University School of Medicine; Director, Clinical Laboratories, Grady Memorial Hospital

William B. Walker, DDS, Practice of Oral and Maxillofacial Surgery, Brunswick, Georgia

Kenneth N. Walton, MD, Professor of Surgery (Urology), Chief, Division of Urology, Emory University School of Medicine

John A. Ward, MD, Professor of Medicine (Endocrinology), Emory University School of Medicine; Chief, Endocrinology Section, Veterans Administration Medical Center (Atlanta)

James O. Wells, MD, Associate Professor of Medicine (Nephrology), Emory University School of Medicine

Nanette K. Wenger, MD, Professor of Medicine (Cardiology), Emory University School of Medicine

Ms. Lydia W. Whatley, ACSW, Assistant Professor of Medicine, Emory University School of Medicine

Charles W. Wickliffe, MD, Clinical Assistant Professor of Medicine, Emory University School of Medicine

Colon H. Wilson, Jr., MD, Professor of Medicine (Rheumatology-Immunology), Director, Division of Rheumatology-Immunology, Associate Professor of Rehabilitation Medicine, Emory University School of Medicine

Gary L. Wollam, MD, Assistant Professor of Medicine (Hypertension), Emory University School of Medicine

W. Dallas Hall, Jr., MD, Professor of Medicine, Director, Division of Hypertension, Emory University School of Medicine

J. Willis Hurst, MD, Professor of Medicine (Cardiology), Chairman, Department of Medicine, Emory University School of Medicine

H. Kenneth Walker, MD, Professor of Medicine, Emory University School of Medicine

Stuart G. Yeoman, MD, ENT Department, Emory University School of Medicine

Contents

Preface   xxiii

Part One   THE INTRODUCTION   1

Chapter One   CLINICAL METHODS   2
               H. Kenneth Walker
Chapter Two   THE MEDICAL RECORD   4
               W. Dallas Hall
Chapter Three TEACHING AND LEARNING CLINICAL
               METHODS   13
               J. Willis Hurst
Chapter Four   A STYLE FOR PATIENT PRESENTATION   21
               H. Kenneth Walker, W. Dallas Hall, and
               J. Willis Hurst

Part Two   THE HISTORY   25

Chapter Five   THE HISTORY   26
               Introduction to the History   26
               Robert B. Copeland and H. Kenneth Walker
            1 Chief Complaint and Present Illness   28
               H. Kenneth Walker

GENERAL   33
            2 Weight Change   33
               Melvin R. Moore and W. Dallas Hall
            3 Fever and Chills   38
               Jonas A. Shulman and David Schlossberg
            4 Night Sweats   41
               W. Dallas Hall

5 Dizziness 44
H. Kenneth Walker and W. Dallas Hall

ENDOCRINE SYSTEM 52
6 Heat or Cold Intolerance 52
John A. Ward
7 Thyroid Problems 54
John A. Ward
8 Neck Surgery or Irradiation to the Neck 59
John A. Ward
9 Diabetes and Diabetic Indicators 62
John K. Davidson and Harry Delcher

EYE 64
10 Visual Dysfunction 64
Frank C. Bell

EAR, NOSE, THROAT 67
11 Difficulty Hearing or Deaf 67
John H. Per-Lee
12 Tinnitus 71
Michael F. Lubin
13 Epistaxis 76
John H. Per-Lee
14 Hoarseness 78
John S. Turner
15 Sinusitis 80
John H. Per-Lee
16 Vertigo 84
Stuart G. Yeoman

GASTROINTESTINAL SYSTEM 89
17 Nausea and Retching 89
Horacio Jinich and Theodore Hersh
18 Vomiting 91
Theodore Hersh and Horacio Jinich
19 Hematemesis 94
Horacio Jinich and Theodore Hersh
20 Melena 97
H. Kenneth Walker
21 Dysphagia 99
Theodore Hersh and Horacio Jinich
22 Indigestion 102
Theodore Hersh and Horacio Jinich
23 Heartburn 106
Theodore Hersh and Horacio Jinich
24 Abdominal Pain 109
Horacio Jinich and Theodore Hersh
25 Abdominal Swelling 116
Theodore Hersh and Horacio Jinich

26 Jaundice   119
    Horacio Jinich and Theodore Hersh
27 Hematochezia   123
    Theodore Hersh and Horacio Jinich
28 Diarrhea   125
    Theodore Hersh and Horacio Jinich
29 Constipation   131
    Theodore Hersh and Horacio Jinich
30 Hernia   134
    Theodore Hersh and Horacio Jinich
31 Hemorrhoids   136
    Theodore Hersh and Horacio Jinich
32 History of Peptic Ulcer Disease   138
    Theodore Hersh and Horacio Jinich
33 History of Gallbladder Disease   141
    Theodore Hersh and Horacio Jinich
34 History of Pancreatitis   143
    Theodore Hersh and Horacio Jinich
35 History of Gastrointestinal Surgery   146
    Theodore Hersh and Horacio Jinich
36 History of Alcoholic Intake   148
    Horacio Jinich and Theodore Hersh

PULMONARY SYSTEM   152
37 Dyspnea, Breathlessness, and Shortness of Breath   152
    P. Bailey Francis
38 Cough and Sputum Production   155
    P. Bailey Francis
39 Hemoptysis   158
    P. Bailey Francis
40 Wheezing and Asthma   161
    P. Bailey Francis
41 Tuberculosis or Exposure to Tuberculosis   164
    John E. McGowan, Jr.
42 PPD Test   166
    John E. McGowan, Jr.
43 Previous Chest Radiograph   168
    P. Bailey Francis
44 Respiratory Infections and Pneumonia   170
    P. Bailey Francis
45 Smoking History   173
    P. Bailey Francis
46 Environmental Inhalation   175
    P. Bailey Francis

CARDIOVASCULAR SYSTEM   178
47 Exercise Level   178
    Charles A. Gilbert
48 Orthopnea and Paroxysmal Nocturnal Dyspnea   182
    Douglas C. Morris

49 Chest Discomfort or Pain 185
Mark E. Silverman
50 Palpitation 192
Barry Silverman
51 Syncope 194
Nanette K. Wenger
52 Edema 199
see section 164
53 Phlebitis 199
see section 165
54 Claudication 200
Robert B. Smith III
55 Hypertension 203
Elbert P. Tuttle, Jr.
56 Rheumatic Fever 206
Donna Gibbas
57 Past Heart Disease 211
Mark E. Silverman
58 Family History of Heart Disease 214
Mark E. Silverman

GENITOURINARY SYSTEM 220
59 Urinary Frequency, Urgency, and Dysuria 220
Kenneth N. Walton and David P. O'Brien
60 Urinary Tract Infection 223
Susan K. Fellner
61 Flank Pain 225
Kenneth N. Walton
62 Nocturia 227
Susan K. Fellner
63 Hematuria 229
Kenneth N. Walton
64 Past Stones 231
James O. Wells, Jr.
65 Urinary Stream Flow Abnormality: Hesitancy,
Intermittency, and Incontinence 234
David P. O'Brien
66 Urethral Discharge 237
Norman F. Jacobs, Jr.
67 Syphilis or Positive Serology 239
Sumner E. Thompson III
68 Male Genital Lesions 243
Sidney Olansky
69 Testicular Mass or Pain 245
Kenneth N. Walton
70 Impotence 246
W. Dallas Hall
71 Family History of Renal Disease 250
W. Dallas Hall

BIRTH CONTROL   253
   72 Birth Control   253
       Robert A. Hatcher

FEMALE GENITALIA   259
       Introduction to the Gynecologic History   259
       John D. Thompson
   73 Pelvic Pain   260
       John D. Thompson
   74 Vaginal Discharge   263
       Sumner E. Thompson III and Michael Rein
   75 Abnormal Vaginal Bleeding   269
       John D. Thompson and John R. K. Preedy
   76 Pelvic Mass   275
       John D. Thompson

SEXUAL DIFFICULTIES   276
   77 Introduction to the Sexual History   276
       Malcolm G. Freeman
       Frequency of Intercourse   287
       Malcolm G. Freeman
       Masturbation   290
       Malcolm G. Freeman
       Premature Ejaculation   294
       Malcolm G. Freeman
       Ejaculatory Incompetence   297
       Malcolm G. Freeman
       Erective Difficulty   299
       Malcolm G. Freeman
       Frigidity   303
       Malcolm G. Freeman
       Anorgasmia   306
       Malcolm G. Freeman
       Dyspareunia and Vaginismus   310
       Malcolm G. Freeman

BREAST   314
   78 Breast Lump   314
       R. Waldo Powell and Constantine Droulias
   79 Breast Pain   316
       R. Waldo Powell and Constantine Droulias
   80 Nipple Discharge   319
       R. Waldo Powell and Constantine Droulias

SKIN   321
   81 The Dermatological History   321
       Pearon G. Lang
   82 Itching   325
       Hiram M. Sturm

83   Change in Mole   327
      J. Thomas Apgar
84   Skin Cancer   332
      J. Thomas Apgar

NEUROLOGICAL SYSTEM   336
85   Headaches   336
      Patrick A. Griffith and H. Kenneth Walker
86   Epileptic Seizures   340
      H. Kenneth Walker
87   Episodic Neurological Symptoms   348
      H. Kenneth Walker
88   Pain and Sensory Perversions   351
      Nettleton S. Payne
89   Weakness   357
      H. Kenneth Walker
90   Head Trauma   360
      Alan S. Fleischer
91   Muscle Cramps   362
      Claudia R. Adkison and H. Kenneth Walker
92   Stroke   369
      H. Kenneth Walker
93   Sleep Disorders   378
      Gerald W. Vogel

HEMATOPOIETIC SYSTEM   385
94   Excessive Bleeding or Bruising   385
      Julian Jacobs
95   Anemia   390
      Julian Jacobs
96   Pica   393
      Julian Jacobs
97   Family History of Sickle Cell Gene Inheritance   396
      Julian Jacobs

MUSCULOSKELETAL SYSTEMS   401
98   Joint Stiffness   401
      Colon Wilson and John A. Goldman
99   Joint Pain   403
      Colon Wilson and John A. Goldman
100   Joint Swelling   406
      Colon Wilson and John A. Goldman
101   Family History of Musculoskeletal Disease   410
      Colon Wilson and John A. Goldman

PSYCHIATRIC HISTORY   413
102   Previous Psychiatric Problems   413
      John B. Griffin, Jr.
103   Interpersonal Relationships   416
      John B. Griffin, Jr.

104 Anxiety 422
John B. Griffin, Jr.
105 Depression 425
John B. Griffin, Jr.
106 Loss of Control 430
John B. Griffin, Jr.
107 Psychological Disturbances of Vegetative Function 433
John B. Griffin, Jr.
108 Substance Abuse 437
John B. Griffin, Jr.

ALLERGIES 441
109 Drug Allergy 441
Robert M. Fine

IMMUNIZATIONS 445
110 Past Immunizations 445
Sumner E. Thompson III

FAMILY HISTORY 450
111 Family Pedigree and Heritable Disease Potential 450
Louis J. Elsas II

HOSPITALIZATIONS AND MEDICATIONS 456
112 Past Hospitalizations 456
Stephen D. Clements
113 Current and Past Medications 457
Stephen D. Clements and Zafar H. Israili

Part Three THE PATIENT PROFILE 467

Chapter Six THE PATIENT PROFILE 468
114 Occupation 468
Lydia W. Whatley
115 Usual Day's Activities 472
David D. Clark
116 Hobbies and Special Interests 474
J. Galt Allee
117 Nutritional History 477
Cheryl L. Rock and Richard P. Holm
118 Education 486
Lydia W. Whatley
119 Finances 489
Lydia W. Whatley

Part Four THE PHYSICAL EXAMINATION 495

Chapter Seven THE PHYSICAL EXAMINATION 496
W. Dallas Hall

GENERAL   499
   120 General Appearance   499
         W. Dallas Hall
   121 Temperature   502
         see section 3
   122 Respiratory Rate and Rhythm   502
         James C. Crutcher
   123 Pulse Rate and Rhythm   507
         I. Sylvia Crawley
   124 Blood Pressure   513
         Gary L. Wollam and Elbert P. Tuttle
   125 Body Size: Height and Weight   521
         Cheryl L. Rock, Richard P. Holm, and W. Dallas Hall
   126 Body Habitus   528
         John R. Preedy
   127 Hair   532
         Algie C. Brown
   128 Physical Examination of the Skin   536
         Henry E. Jones
   129 Nails   541
         John A. Ward

HEAD, EARS, NOSE   548
   130 Cranial and Orbital Bruits   548
         Joseph E. Hardison
   131 Pinnae, Canals, and Drums   552
         John S. Turner
   132 The Nose   558
         John S. Turner

EYES   563
   133 External Eye Examination   563
         Frank C. Bell
   134 The Fundus Examination   571
         Frank C. Bell
   135 The Pupil   577
         J. Donald Fite and H. Kenneth Walker

ORAL CAVITY AND ASSOCIATED STRUCTURES   585
   136 Teeth, Gums, and Oral Mucosa   585
         William B. Walker
   137 Tongue   596
         Charles Huguley
   138 Tonsils and Pharynx   599
         John S. Turner
   139 Parotid Enlargement   605
         Mark E. Silverman and W. Dallas Hall

NECK   609
   140 Neck Inspection   609
         John A. Ward

141 Carotid Bruits   612
    Joseph Hardison
142 The Cervical Venous Hum   614
    Joseph Hardison
143 Thyroid Examination   617
    John A. Ward

NODES   621
144 Lymphadenopathy   621
    James W. Keller

CHEST   628
145 Chest Structure   628
    James C. Crutcher
146 Chest Motion   631
    James C. Crutcher
147 Chest Auscultation   634
    James C. Crutcher
148 Chest Percussion   639
    James C. Crutcher

BREAST   641
149 Breast Mass   641
    R. Waldo Powell and Constantine Droulias
150 Nipple and Areola   651
    R. Waldo Powell and Constantine Droulias

CARDIOVASCULAR SYSTEM   653
151 Jugular Venous Pressure   653
    Joseph Z. Davids
152 Jugular Venous Pulsations   656
    Joseph Z. Davids
153 Carotid Pulse   663
    Joseph Z. Davids
154 Apex Impulse   669
    Joseph Z. Davids
155 Parasternal Impulse   677
    Joseph Z. Davids
156 Pulmonary Artery Pulsation   679
    Joseph Z. Davids
157 The First Heart Sound   681
    Joel M. Felner
158 The Second Heart Sound   688
    Joel M. Felner
159 The Third Heart Sound   695
    Joel M. Felner
160 The Fourth Heart Sound   700
    Joel M. Felner
161 Clicks   705
    Charles W. Wickliffe

162   Systolic Murmurs   708
      I. Sylvia Crawley
163   Diastolic Murmurs   719
      I. Sylvia Crawley
164   Edema   723
      Elbert P. Tuttle, Jr.
165   Thrombophlebitis   726
      W. Dallas Hall
166   Clubbing (Acropachy)   730
      P. Bailey Francis
167   Cyanosis   733
      P. Bailey Francis
168   Pulsus Alternans   735
      Joel M. Felner
169   Peripheral Pulses and Bruits   740
      Robert B. Smith III

ABDOMEN   748
170   Inspection   748
      J. Richard Amerson and William J. Millikan
171   Auscultation: Bowel Sounds, Bruits, and Rubs   753
      J. Richard Amerson and William J. Millikan
172   Palpation: Pain and Tenderness, Masses   756
      William J. Millikan and J. Richard Amerson
173   Ascites   762
      Theodore Hersh and Horacio Jinich
174   Liver: Auscultation   766
      Joseph E. Hardison
175   Liver: Size and Shape   769
      Horacio Jinich and Theodore Hersh
176   Spleen   772
      Joseph E. Hardison
177   Inguinal Canal   776
      J. Richard Amerson and Eugene Davidson

MALE GENITALIA   779
178   External Male Genitalia   779
      David P. O'Brien III

FEMALE GENITALIA   781
179   Pelvic Examination   781
      John D. Thompson

RECTAL   788
180   Rectal Examination   788
      Horacio Jinich and Theodore Hersh
181   Prostate   790
      David P. O'Brien III
182   Stool Guaiac   793
      Theodore Hersh and Horacio Jinich

MUSCULOSKELETAL 796

  183 The Musculoskeletal Examination 796
      Colon Wilson and Stephen B. Miller

NEUROLOGICAL AND PSYCHIATRIC 810

     Introduction to the Mental Status Examination 810
     H. Kenneth Walker
  184 Appearance, Affect, and Motor Behavior 812
     John B. Griffin, Jr.
  185 General Intellectual Function 817
     John B. Griffin, Jr.
  186 Attention Span 820
     John B. Griffin, Jr.
  187 Judgment 822
     John B. Griffin, Jr.
  188 Abstraction 825
     John B. Griffin, Jr.
  189 Delusions, Hallucinations, and Illusions 828
     John B. Griffin, Jr.
  190 Associations of Thought 831
     John B. Griffin, Jr.
  191 Orientation 834
     E. Stephen Purdom
  192 Memory 837
     H. Kenneth Walker
  193 Level of Consciousness 844
     H. Kenneth Walker
  194 Speech and Other Lateralizing Cortical Functions 853
     H. Kenneth Walker
  195 Cranial Nerve I: Olfactory Nerve 878
     H. Kenneth Walker
  196 Cranial Nerve II: Optic Nerve 882
     A. Visual Acuity 882
        J. Donald Fite and H. Kenneth Walker
     B. Visual Fields 888
        H. Kenneth Walker and J. Donald Fite
  197 Cranial Nerves III, IV, and VI: Oculomotor,
     Trochlear, and Abducens Nerves 897
     A. Conjugate Gaze 897
        H. Kenneth Walker and J. Donald Fite
     B. Brainstem Nuclei and Peripheral Nerves 906
        J. Donald Fite and H. Kenneth Walker
  198 Cranial Nerve V: The Trigeminal Nerve 915
     H. Kenneth Walker
  199 Cranial Nerve VII: The Facial Nerve and Taste 923
     H. Kenneth Walker
  200 Cranial Nerve VIII: The Acoustic Nerve 930
     John Turner

201 Cranial Nerves IX and X: The Glossopharyngeal
     and Vagus Nerves   934
     H. Kenneth Walker
202 Cranial Nerve XI: The Spinal Accessory Nerve   938
     H. Kenneth Walker
203 Cranial Nerve XII: The Hypoglossal Nerve   941
     H. Kenneth Walker
204 Sensation   942
     H. Kenneth Walker
205 The Motor System   955
     H. Kenneth Walker
206 The Cerebellum   969
     H. Kenneth Walker
207 Involuntary Movements: Tremor, Chorea, Athetosis,
     Myoclonus, Asterixis   975
     H. Kenneth Walker
208 Suck, Snout, and Grasp Reflexes   981
     H. Kenneth Walker
209 Deep Tendon Reflexes   983
     H. Kenneth Walker
210 The Plantar Reflex   992
     H. Kenneth Walker

Chapter Eight   CLINICAL METHODS FOR THE
                PEDIATRIC PATIENT   997
                Albert Rauber

Part Five   THE LABORATORY   1003

Chapter Nine   INTRODUCTION TO THE LABORATORY   1004
               David H. Vroon and W. Dallas Hall
211 Hematocrit   1011
     Herbert Kann
212 White Blood Cell Count   1014
     Herbert Kann
213 White Blood Cell Differential   1016
     Herbert Kann
214 Platelets   1020
     Herbert Kann
215 Red Blood Cell Morphology   1022
     Herbert Kann
216 Urinalysis: Color and Odor   1027
     Barry J. Rosenbaum
217 Urinalysis: Specific Gravity   1030
     Barry J. Rosenbaum
218 Proteinuria   1033
     W. Dallas Hall

219 Glucosuria and Ketonuria   1035
John K. Davidson, Harry K. Delcher, and W. Dallas Hall

220 Urine Sediment   1040
W. Dallas Hall

221 Blood Urea Nitrogen   1044
W. Dallas Hall and David H. Vroon

222 Plasma Glucose   1048
John K. Davidson, Harry K. Delcher, and W. Dallas Hall

223 Serum Sodium   1054
W. Dallas Hall and David H. Vroon

224 Serum Potassium   1058
W. Dallas Hall and David H. Vroon

225 Serum Chloride   1062
W. Dallas Hall and David H. Vroon

226 Serum Total CO_2 Content   1065
W. Dallas Hall

227 Serum Glutamate-Oxaloacetate Transaminase   1070
W. Dallas Hall and David H. Vroon

228 Lactate Dehydrogenase   1073
David H. Vroon and W. Dallas Hall

229 Alkaline Phosphatase   1077
David H. Vroon

230 Serum Bilirubin   1081
David H. Vroon and W. Dallas Hall

231 Uric Acid   1084
W. Dallas Hall and David H. Vroon

232 Serum Creatinine   1089
W. Dallas Hall and David H. Vroon

233 Serum Calcium   1093
James O. Wells, Jr., W. Dallas Hall, and David H. Vroon

234 Serum Inorganic Phosphate   1100
W. Dallas Hall and David H. Vroon

235 Cholesterol   1104
Mario DiGirolamo

236 Serum Total Protein: Albumin and Globulin   1111
W. Dallas Hall and David H. Vroon

237 PPD Tuberculin Skin Test   1115
John E. McGowan, Jr.

238 Serologic Testing for Syphilis   1118
Sumner E. Thompson III

ECG   1122

239 The Electrocardiogram   1122
John R. Darsee and J. Willis Hurst

X-RAY   1162

240 The Chest X-Ray   1162
Stewart R. Roberts, Jr.

241   Approach to the Radiographic Examination
of the Abdomen   1176
Stewart R. Roberts, Jr.

Appendix   MARI: THE MEDICAL AGGREGATE RECORD
INQUIRY SYSTEM   1183
V. Slamecka, H.N. Camp, A.N. Badre, W.D. Hall

Index   1198

Preface

The goal of this second edition of CLINICAL METHODS is provision of the most up-to-date clinical methods to clinicians and students. Readers' suggestions over the past three years have guided us in adding new sections and expanding or deleting others. The content is based upon the sixth revision of the *Defined Data Base* in use on the Medical Service of Emory University School of Medicine at Grady Memorial Hospital in Atlanta. This Data Base responds to the needs of our patient population and aids our teaching program and curriculum for house officers and students. We believe it is universal enough to be used generally as the basis for learning and teaching clinical methods.

The contributors to this book are our colleagues at Emory University School of Medicine. The editors take pleasure in making the clinical and teaching skills of their colleagues available to a larger audience.

We are indebted to the thousands of patients who have presented with both rare and usual findings of diseases which provided our contributors with clinical experience peculiar to a given symptom, sign or laboratory abnormality.

We also wish to thank Larry Weed and his associates Harold Cross and Charles Burger. The structure and philosophy of this book was greatly influenced by exposure to them.

We wish to express our appreciation to Ms. Linda Garr Markwell of the Emory Medical Library; Ms. Patsy Bryan, Mr. Grover Hogan, Mr. Eddie Jackson and Ms. Martha Tarrant of the Emory Department of Medical Illustrations; and Ms. Sadie Owens and Mr. Walter Harris. The patience, support and skill of Ms. Susan M. Gay and Ms. Pauline Dishmon of Butterworth's are appreciated.

> *H. Kenneth Walker, MD*
> *W. Dallas Hall, MD*
> *J. Willis Hurst, MD*
> Emory University School of Medicine
> Atlanta, Georgia

PART ONE

The Introduction

CHAPTER ONE

Clinical Methods

H. KENNETH WALKER, MD

Mastering the art and skill of history taking and physical diagnosis is a student's most pleasurable task. The threshold is crossed and the journey begun the very first time the student faces another human being with the goal of discovering abnormality. Who among us will ever forget the unique emotion evoked during this very first encounter? It marks the symbolic beginning of becoming a clinician in a fashion never equaled by the study of books or cadavers. Ensuing mastery requires only a few ingredients: a good book, a teacher, a subject, and lots of practice.

This book is our attempt to provide the first ingredient. It contains the most modern clinical examination techniques in a usable and accessible format. It covers 231 history, patient profile, physical, and laboratory items. *Each item stands alone:* the reader does not have to refer to different texts of anatomy, physiology, and medicine to know how to begin collecting patient information. The information is presented in a way which capitalizes on an already existing fund of basic science knowledge. Each item has five components:

Definition. An explanatory statement or a definition of the item. We have tried to make these definitions as usable, applicable, and practical as possible.

Technique. The *how* of collecting the item.

Background Information. The basic information from anatomy, physiology, biochemistry, and behavioral and social fields as related to the specific item under discussion. The background information provides a bridge connecting basic science and clinical medicine.

Clinical Significance. Presents the significance of abnormal findings.

Selected References. The references cite in-depth discussions on each topic.

The contents of the book progress as follows:

Chapter 2 outlines the structure for data collection upon which the book rests. The clinical process is presented in a visible and therefore "learnable" structure. The problem-oriented method helps organize the learning and practice of medicine.

Chapter 3 provides the background for teaching faculty to optimally use the text and for students to maximize their learning skills.

Chapter 4 summarizes a style for presenting data to other clinicians, predicated on the setting and purpose of the patient presentation.

Chapters 5–8 contain more than 200 sections representing each item on the Defined Data Base. Sections are categorized into history, patient profile, physical, and laboratory examinations.

Chapter 9 summarizes important variations for the history and physical examination of the pediatric patient.

Chapter 10 covers 29 specific laboratory tests that are commonly employed. Also included are discussions of the techniques and significance of electrocardiograms, chest x-rays and various radiographic abdominal procedures.

The book ends with a section describing the applications of modern computer technology to the processing of medical information and knowledge.

This second edition of *Clinical Methods* adds significant basic science and clinical information to that contained in the 1976 edition. In addition, we have also now assembled a set of 15 videotapes made by many of the same contributors who have written sections of this text. These tapes illustrate visually the textual material.

The book and the tapes originate from many clinicians who evaluate patients daily with skill, respect, and pleasure. We hope these qualities prove transmissible to both students and clinicians.

Reference

1. Walker HK, producer: *Clinical Methods Videotape Series.* Atlanta, Ga, Emory Medical Television Network, 1978.

CHAPTER TWO

The Medical Record

W. DALLAS HALL, MD

In the 1960s Dr. Lawrence Weed described an approach to the medical record that can be the organizing principle behind the study and practice of medicine. This is known as the Problem Oriented Medical Record (POMR). There are four components to the POMR:

    I.   The Defined Data Base
   II.   The Complete Problem List
  III.   The Initial Plans
  IV.   The Progress Notes

The differences between the POMR and the classic or source-oriented medical record can be understood by considering an encounter between a clinician and a patient. The patient may come to the clinician with the complaint of a headache. On physical examination the clinician discovers an enlarged thyroid gland, and a laboratory report reveals anemia. The clinician collects various data in the history, physical, and laboratory examinations related to each of these three problems, then analyzes the facts related to each problem and makes specific plans for that problem. The patient returns as these plans are carried out, and again the clinician analyzes each problem individually and notes the progress toward the solution of each problem.

Consider how the information collected by the clinician and other members of the health care team is entered in the classic medical record. Information is entered according to the *source* from which it originated. Each source has a territory in the chart: doctors' progress notes, nurses' notes, x-ray reports, laboratory reports, and so forth. In the example given above, each territory will have a mixture of facts related to each problem. The only common denominator is that each fact was derived from the source in whose territory it was placed.

The method of organization suggested by Weed links information in a medical record to problems. Every entry is problem oriented, that is, placed under the heading of a specific problem. This principle is combined with a Complete Problem List that appears at the beginning of the record and serves as an index or table of contents for the record. Information present in the POMR is readily accessible and the logical pathways are preserved.

I. THE DEFINED DATA BASE

The specific content of the history, patient profile, and physical and laboratory portions of this book draws on the concept of a Defined Data Base. Weed developed the concept in response to this question: What exact information can be collected most productively and economically on each patient who enters medical care? For example, should every adult patient have an electrocardiogram? Should every patient have a thorough physical examination? If not, then which patients should have one?

The universe of information concerning each patient is potentially infinite. As such, thousands of items can be included in a data base. Such indiscriminate data collection is impractical, uneconomical, and unnecessary. An otherwise healthy 20 year old with a bacterial pharyngitis does not need febrile agglutinins and serum immunoelectrophoresis. Yet what does this patient need? The process of making finite the universe of data is termed "defining the data base."

Different types of Defined Data Bases are appropriate for the goals of different types of encounters between clinician and patient.

1. A Comprehensive Care Data Base is the type of data base represented in this book. It identifies most of the existing and potential problems in a specific patient population. A primary physician such as an internist or family practitioner usually collects this type of data base.

2. A Specialty Data Base may be appropriate for a specialist who has decided to limit his type of practice. The content usually includes both general and specific data. The former reveals problems relating to the general health of the patient; the latter, problems that characteristically pertain to the scope of the specialty. An example would be the Defined Data Base an otolaryngologist might collect on patients hospitalized for a tonsillectomy.

3. A Problem-specific Data Base deals only with problems such as diabetes, hypertension, or upper respiratory infections. Each data base contains relevant items from the history, physical, and laboratory examinations. Problem-specific Data Base styles are appropriate for areas such as emergency clinics.

There exists no "complete" data base. We would all agree that a complete patient profile, history, physical, and laboratory examination could potentially require weeks or months at an incredible time and economic cost to the patient and health care team. The key word is "defined," not "complete."

A prerequisite in selecting a Defined Data Base is to determine the practical objectives and goals of patient care in the setting at hand. The Defined Data Base may thus represent an initial complete or annual examination in a group practice, an evaluation format for all hospitalized patients, or a relatively brief number of items to be collected on all patients seen with walk-in, intermittent, or emergency problems. Definition of a data base is useful in each of these settings.

Individual physicians do not usually find preformed data bases very satisfactory. This is due to the wide spectrum of practice goals, the individuality of patient populations, and the variation in available facilities. We therefore recommend that each health care facility consider developing a Defined Data Base tailored to its specific practice goals. The following considerations can guide this effort.

I. Practice goals
    A.   Type of practice
        1.   Comprehensive care
        2.   Specialty-consultative
        3.   Relatively problem-specific
    B.   Patient groups included or excluded: eg, children, elderly
    C.   Type of health care delivered
        1.   Preventive
        2.   Acute illness
        3.   Chronic illness
    D.   Place(s) care given
        1.   Outpatient
        2.   Hospital
        3.   Limited care facility
II. Patient population
    A.   Demography: age, sex, race, ethnic distribution
    B.   Occupation
    C.   Geography
    D.   Permanency versus transiency of patients
    E.   Reasons why patients most often seek care
III. Logistics
    A.   Time constraint per patients
    B.   Personnel availability
    C.   Laboratory facilities
    D.   Patient finances
    E.   Yield of abnormality for each data base item considered
    F.   Capacity to proceed with action on each abnormal data item found

G.   Cost of conversion to a predefined format
IV.   Feedback loops
    A.   Analysis of positive yield of data base over time
    B.   Follow-up of patients and detection of problems by complaint
    C.   Autopsy results
    D.   Audit of clinician performance

The data base used in this text was developed for medical patients seen at Grady Memorial Hospital in Atlanta. It screens the complex, multiple problems of a large number of male and female patients who are over 16 years of age; who live in crowded city conditions; who are known to have a high prevalence of acute and chronic illnesses; and who seek help at an Emory University Medical School facility where medical students, allied health personnel, house officers, advanced trainees, and senior staff are engaged in patient care, education, and research. The content helps detect and resolve common patient problems based on a review of the presenting symptoms and outcome of patients hospitalized on the medical service in the preceding year. Designed in 1969, the original data base has required significant annual alterations.

Those who are to develop a Defined Data Base should recognize that the one reproduced in this text may require modification since the population of patients, availability of personnel, and practice objectives may differ.

A crucial principle is that the Defined Data Base document generates the Complete Problem List.

II. THE COMPLETE PROBLEM LIST

The Complete Problem List forms the first page of each record and serves as the index or table of contents for the record. A problem is any abnormality that is discovered in the Defined Data Base and which interferes with the quality of life as perceived by the patient. A problem may or may not be a diagnosis and can come from any area: history (symptom), physical finding (sign), laboratory value, or social disturbance. The following points should be noted about a Complete Problem List (Fig 1):

1.   Date problem entered. This instantly lets anyone know where to look in a chronologically arranged record to find the first complete statement about the problem.
2.   Number of problem. This number stays constantly with the particular cluster of patient data. The problem nomenclature may change (eg, from abdominal mass to pseudocyst of the pancreas) as the problem is resolved. However, the original number con-

COMPLETE PROBLEM LIST
Permanent Part of Medical Record
GRADY MEMORIAL HOSPITAL
Atlanta, Georgia

Date Problem Entered	ACTIVE	INACTIVE
2/27/76	#1 CORONARY ATHEROSCLEROTIC HEART DISEASE	
	a) ANGINA PECTORIS, STABLE	
2/27/76	#2* ANEMIA ⟶ 2/28/76 HYPOCHROMIC MICROCYTIC ANEMIA ⟶	3/5/76 CARCINOMA OF COLON
2/27/76	#3 RIGHT PLEURAL EFFUSION ⟶	
2/27/76	#4 DIABETES MELLITUS	
	a) ARTERIOPATHY	
	b) NEUROPATHY	
2/27/76	#5	PNEUMOCOCCAL PNEUMONIA 1966
2/27/76	#6 ALLERGY TO PENICILLIN	

* Reason for Admission

Figure 1. The problem list document.

tinues to identify the cluster of data related to abdominal mass

3. Problem formulation. This is the statement of the problem at the highest level of resolution possible when the problem list is written. The specific formulation is predicated upon the available evidence plus the experience and ability of the clinician. The formulation should never reflect guesswork or speculation but instead what the clinician is absolutely confident about at that

point in time. Rule-outs do not go on the Complete Problem List but belong in the Initial Plans.

4.   Arrow. This is placed after each problem that requires further diagnostic resolution. Abdominal mass or jaundice would have an arrow, but diabetes or hiatal hernia might not.
5.   Date problem resolved. The date placed by or above the arrow indicates the place in the record where there are data concerning the evidence and reasoning used by the clinician to resolve the problem.
6.   Inactive problems. These are problems that do not require current medical attention. When space is a factor, they are often signaled by the description, "status post" (S/P).

In addition to serving as the chart index, the Complete Problem List helps to quickly remind the clinician of all the patient's problems. A specialist can better handle a particular problem in context of all the patient's problems.

III. INITIAL PLANS

A plan written for each active problem begins with the problem number and title (Fig 2). Each plan contains the following components:

1.   Diagnostic: the rule-outs. Specific tests or procedures follow each rule-out.
2.   Therapeutic. The specific drugs, dosages, and therapeutic procedures, including plans for monitoring results or side effects of the therapy.
3.   Patient education. What the patient and family have been told about this problem. Also includes future educational plans.

IV. PROGRESS NOTES

After citation of problem number and title, each narrative Progress Note follows the structure (Fig 3):

Subjective   symptoms
Objective   physical and laboratory data
Assessment   interpretation of above data
Plans   one or more of the following as appropriate:
                  diagnostic
                  therapeutic
                  patient education

INITIAL PLANS

GRADY MEMORIAL HOSPITAL
ATLANTA, GEORGIA

PATIENT IDENTIFICATION

INITIAL PLANS

 # 3 PLEURAL EFFUSION

DX: RULE OUT TUBERCULOSIS : SKIN TEST, SPUTUM CULTURE
AND STAIN, THORACENTESIS.

RULE OUT MALIGNANCY: SPUTUM CYTOLOGY, THORACENTESIS
WITH CYTOLOGY.

RULE OUT CHYLOUS EFFUSION: CHARACTER OF
THORACENTESIS FLUID.

RX: NONE UNTIL DIAGNOSIS ESTABLISHED.

PT. EDUC.: PATIENT TOLD SHE HAS AN ACCUMULATION OF
FLUID IN HER CHEST: CAUSE UNKNOWN. WE WILL HAVE
TO DO A SPECIAL TEST (DESCRIBED AND PERMISSION
OBTAINED) TO HELP US TRY TO DISCOVER THE CAUSE.

(Initial Plans are listed for each problem identified on admission, according to Problem Title and Number.
Each plan contains three elements: Diagnostic Plans, Therapeutic Plans, Patient Education Plans.)

Figure 2. The initial plans document.

Summary progress notes such as discharge and death notes have a similar structure. All information entered in the chart is problem oriented and is in chronological sequence.

The careful construction of a Complete Problem List helps ensure that all of the patient's known problems are conveniently identified on a

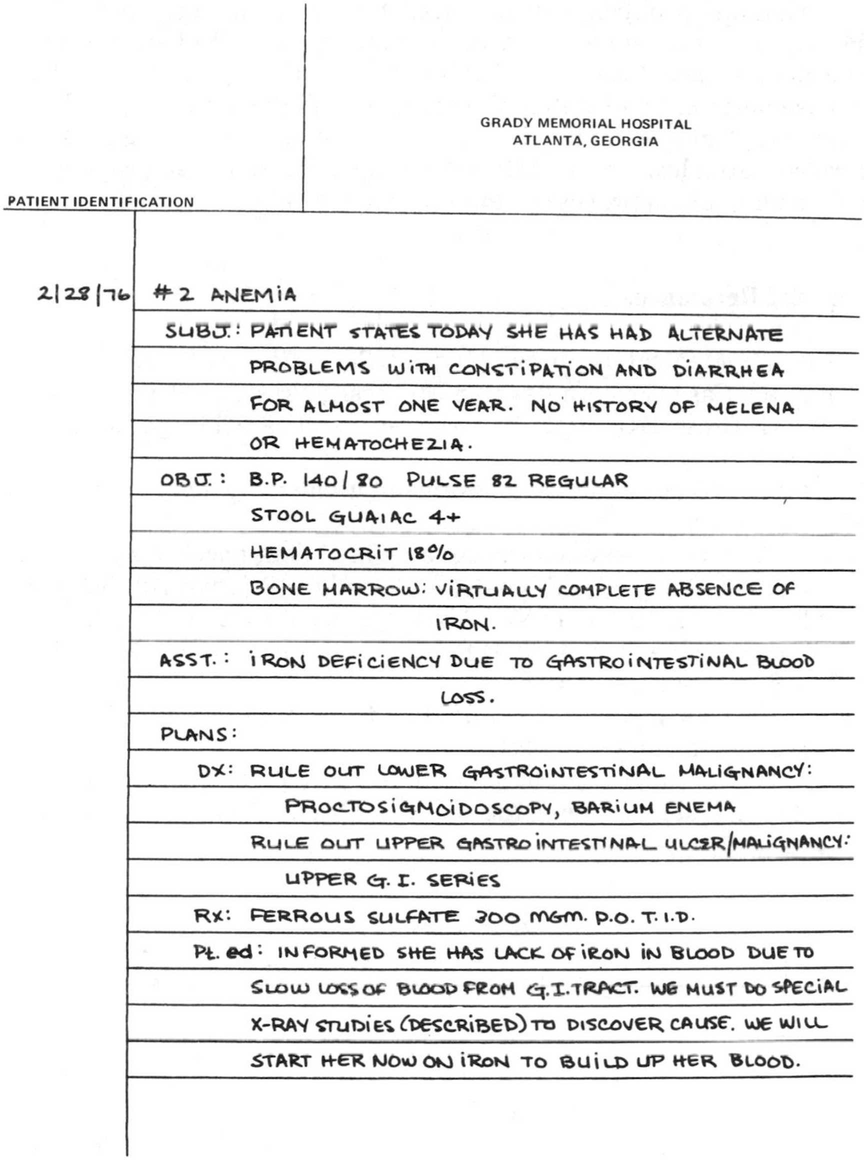

GRADY MEMORIAL HOSPITAL
ATLANTA, GEORGIA

PATIENT IDENTIFICATION

2/28/76	#2 ANEMIA
	SUBJ.: PATIENT STATES TODAY SHE HAS HAD ALTERNATE
	PROBLEMS WITH CONSTIPATION AND DIARRHEA
	FOR ALMOST ONE YEAR. NO HISTORY OF MELENA
	OR HEMATOCHEZIA.
	OBJ.: B.P. 140/80 PULSE 82 REGULAR
	STOOL GUAIAC 4+
	HEMATOCRIT 18%
	BONE MARROW: VIRTUALLY COMPLETE ABSENCE OF
	IRON.
	ASST.: IRON DEFICIENCY DUE TO GASTROINTESTINAL BLOOD
	LOSS.
	PLANS:
	DX: RULE OUT LOWER GASTROINTESTINAL MALIGNANCY:
	PROCTOSIGMOIDOSCOPY, BARIUM ENEMA
	RULE OUT UPPER GASTROINTESTINAL ULCER/MALIGNANCY:
	UPPER G.I. SERIES
	RX: FERROUS SULFATE 300 MGM. P.O. T.I.D.
	Pt. ed: INFORMED SHE HAS LACK OF IRON IN BLOOD DUE TO
	SLOW LOSS OF BLOOD FROM G.I. TRACT. WE MUST DO SPECIAL
	X-RAY STUDIES (DESCRIBED) TO DISCOVER CAUSE. WE WILL
	START HER NOW ON IRON TO BUILD UP HER BLOOD.

Figure 3. Narrative progress note.

single page, prominently located within the record. The clinician may then see the whole patient more clearly as he moves from data collection to problem formulation and then to Initial Plans and Progress Notes. On occasion it may be useful for the patient to receive a copy of the record.

A specialist can give care within the framework of total health care. The surgeon who might be primarily responsible for a patient can decide which nonsurgical problem will be cared for by consultants and which ones he will be responsible for. A consultant can see all of the patient's problems in one place, locate detailed information about any one problem, and exercise judgment and skill in the context of all the patient's problems.

Much problem solving in clinical medicine involves missing data and uncontrolled variables. The POMR helps reflect the stepwise progression of this decision-making process as the solution unfolds.

Selected References

1.   Weed LL: *Medical Records, Medical Education and Patient Care.* Cleveland, Case Western Reserve University Press, 1969, pp 15–24.
2.   Bjorn JC, Cross HD: *Problem-Oriented Practice.* Chicago, McGraw-Hill, 1970.
3.   Hurst JW, Walker HK: *The Problem-Oriented System.* New York, Medcom, 1972.
4.   Hurst JW: How does one develop a defined data base? Who collects the data? in Walker HK, Hurst JW, Woody MF (eds): *Applying the Problem-Oriented System.* New York, Medcom, 1973, pp 25–27.
5.   Hurst JW, Walker HK, Hall WD: More reasons why Weed is right. *N Engl J Med* 288:629–630, 1973.
6.   Weed LL: *Your Health Care and How to Manage It.* Essex Junction, Vt, Essex Publishing Co., 1975.
7.   Hall WD: A defined laboratory data base, in Walker HK, Hurst JW, Woody MF (eds): *Applying the Problem-Oriented System.* New York, Medcom, 1973, pp 407–411.

CHAPTER THREE

Teaching and Learning Clinical Methods

J. WILLIS HURST, MD

The Old Method

The type of information to be collected from a patient and the technique of collecting it has changed drastically over the years. In the beginning of medicine people learned that if patients bled from a wound they might die. More experienced people learned that if an individual developed a yellow color of the skin that continued and became more intense the subject might die. This introduced the Hippocratic era.

Later Corvisart and Laennec and many other physicians clarified the meaning of symptoms and developed the physical examination as a method of collecting information from patients. More recently Sir William Osler and those who followed him have brought us to the modern era. Along the way it became clear that a great deal of information could be learned about the patient from the information obtained by the history. The system of the body that was diseased could frequently be identified by this method alone. Over the years the physical examination has been refined because the meaning of physical signs has been clarified by modern techniques. Finally, in addition to the information gained from the history and physical examination, the abnormalities found by laboratory means have been added to the data collection process. First, urinalysis was performed, then "routine" blood work was added, still later chest x-ray and electrocardiogram were added, and now numerous chemical tests on the blood and urine are done on patients. (In the beginning physicians did too little because they knew little to do. Now they run the risk of doing too much because they know a great deal more.)

During the last 50 years sophomore medical students have been taught clinical methods in the following way. The course was called "physical diagnosis" even though history taking was also taught. The course was usually taught with a textbook entitled "Physical Diagnosis" that was reviewed in the lectures. Patients were interviewed and examined. The objective, as a rule, was to complete a form given to the student by the instructor. The form consisted of a series of "headings" that, over the years, had stood the test of time as being useful. The origin of the form was not discussed. Physical examination was emphasized. The laboratory examination was often left out (or was allocated to a separate course). The objective of the exercise was seldom stated with clarity. It was assumed by the instructor that the areas selected and emphasized were important and that the student would profit from the exercise.

The student did profit because he knew nothing at the beginning of the course and knew more at the end of the course. The student learned many skills. One could defend such an approach since it was student oriented and was very valuable for the student. But—the following began to happen. The sophomore became a junior student and he filled out another long form on the patient he "worked up." The origin of this form, which was often different from the form he used as a sophomore, was rarely discussed. Teaching sessions consisted of discussing (or reciting from memory) the contents of the form. The discrimination of data was rarely emphasized. In a session of 20 students one remained awake while he recited and 19 students and the instructor "slept." The same prevailed as a senior student. The intern was permitted to write a shorter note. The resident was permitted to write an even shorter note. The guidelines for writing the short notes were never discussed by instructors. What was left out was never discussed. The principles of practice were never considered. No emphasis was placed on what should be done and what should not be done in the data collection process during the training of a house officer even though three separate notes were often written by different people on the same patient. (The notes were rarely checked by an instructor.) What was done and what was left out was determined by the individual. The individual did not know whether or not the data collected actually screened the patient for illness.

Later, in practice, two groups of physicians emerged. Some created beautiful, concise notes about their patients. They obviously collected the proper information from their patients. They discriminated and analyzed data wisely. Another group continued to leave out information about their patients until their records became meaningless. Dictating equipment helped those who had a clear objective in their efforts to create an excellent record. Dictating equipment deterred those who did not have a clear objective in their effort to create an excellent record. The record in the latter instance was often very long and looked beautiful but key information was left out. The discrimination of data and the analysis of data are not automatically assured by mechanical equipment. A long note about a patient does not assure quality. The following discussion emphasizes a different approach to this important problem.

The New Approach

The following approach to clinical methods has been created in an effort to retain the best of the old and to add a few new concepts that have been created by the progress of medicine. I have worked with sophomore medical students at Emory University School of Medicine for several years in an effort to perfect the views expressed here. The discussion that follows moves in an orderly fashion through the logic of the system—from theory to practice—in an effort to bridge the gap between talking (writing) and doing.

The course in clinical methods taught at Emory University School of Medicine is not a course in history taking only, or physical examination only, or laboratory medicine only. *The course deals with the collection of information from patients using the history, physical examination, and laboratory, and stresses the integration of the data.* This is accomplished by indicating to the students that they are to consider themselves primary physicians who intend to give comprehensive, continuous care to their patients.

The objective of the course is not to emphasize that the items the instructor determines on his own are useful but to learn to collect the information from a patient that will screen the patient for illnesses. This is accomplished by emphasizing the collection of a Defined Data Base; the identification of abnormalities in the data collected, synthesizing them, and formulating a Complete Problem List (placed at the front of the chart); creating Initial Plans for each problem; and following the problems up and writing a carefully designed Progress Note. The entire system is taught to the sophomore, but the first item, the collection of a Defined Data Base, is emphasized throughout the course. Problem formulation is emphasized during the last portion of the course. The collection of the Defined Data Base, Problem Formulation, writing Initial Plans, and the proper follow-up of problems (Progress Notes) are emphasized during the junior and senior year of medical school and during each house staff and fellowship year. During the sophomore year the Defined Data Base for a given hospital—Grady Memorial Hospital—is used as a model. This serves as a guide for the sophomore and the instructors. It is the same data base that the student will use later as a junior student assigned to the ward service at Grady Memorial Hospital. Only one Defined Data Base is filled out by the combined efforts of the student and first-year house officer. It is checked by the second-year house officer and attending physician. The old system which included the first-year resident writing a brief note of arbitrary content and the second-year house officer doing the same is eliminated. The entire effort is to determine if the proper data is collected properly, if the problems are formulated wisely, if acceptable plans are written, and if the proper items are being followed. The new method of teaching clinical methods requires that the start made by the sophomore be organized so that he may be able to continue his efforts to perfect the system.

The guideline for the sophomore is the Defined Data Base. It is therefore important to restate the definition of a Defined Data Base. A Defined Data Base is a carefully planned scientific document and differs greatly from the arbitrarily contrived history and physical examination of the past. The Defined Data Base makes it possible to use such terms as "complete work-up" and "thorough work-up" as realistic goals rather than noble clichés. By defining what should be done in the initial data-gathering process one is not complete or thorough to the extent the prescribed data base is not completed. (Of course, there are many proper reasons why a Defined Data Base is not completed initially. For example, if the patient is in coma, it is not possible to complete the data base. Under such circumstances, problem number one—incomplete data base—is written on the problem sheet.)

The creation of a Defined Data Base involves the following principles. The goal of the endeavor must be clearly perceived. For the sophomore, junior, senior, first-year and second-year house officers, the goal is to give comprehensive care to adults. Accordingly, the Defined Data Base created for the medical service at one particular hospital, Grady Memorial, is used as a model. The exact data base should not be transferred to another hospital or office since the items in the data base were developed to screen the population of patients who go to Grady Memorial Hospital, and certain items needed to screen a patient for illness may be needed there and not elsewhere.

The Defined Data Base for the medical wards at Grady Memorial Hospital was created in the following manner. Seven years ago when one of the editors (W.D.H.) was chief resident, he kept a list of the problems found on each patient admitted to the medical service. After considering the problems the patients actually had, a Defined Data Base was developed so that comprehensive care could be given and the problems the patients actually had would more likely be discovered. Low-yield activity, such as percussion of the heart, was left out. Other items included could be defended since they assisted in the early discovery of serious problems. Several years ago we checked all of the autopsy results in order to determine if an abnormality was missed because it was not on the Defined Data Base. No abnormality was found at autopsy that could have been discovered by performing the acts listed in the Defined Data Base. Items that were missed, were missed because of lack of skill, but not by ignoring them.

The Defined Data Base must be created with the understanding that it will be completed on all patients. This makes it possible to emphasize what must be done every time. If the problem can be formulated at a high level of understanding without other data, then such should be the case. If, based on initial data, the problem is still poorly resolved, then a clear statement of what is needed next and for what reason should be shown in the initial plans and orders, and these must be numbered and titled to match the problem list. The point is, do not place any item in the Defined Data Base that is not done every time. Some complain that the Defined Data Base is too long. This always signifies a lack of understanding. Never make a Defined Data Base so long that it is impossible to complete it. The length of a Defined Data Base is determined by the prevalence of illness known to exist in the population but also considers the number of patients to be screened and the number of health professionals who are assigned to collect the data. When one physician attempts to see 100 patients in one day a Defined Data Base must be created very carefully with consideration of what data is left out and why. Obviously, under such circumstances, comprehensive care cannot be given and cannot be the goal. In such a case, the Defined Data Base should be created to discover the most prevalent diseases and the most serious diseases, but not all diseases.

The Defined Data Base reproduced in this book represents the sixth generation of a Defined Data Base. We have constantly improved the document from a scientific point of view and have made it more convenient to use. It is not too long for our purposes, and we have sufficient personnel to complete it; but other situations will require a different Defined Data Base. The sophomores are instructed regarding the creation of a Defined Data Base and actually use the one reprinted here as a model.

As stated earlier, the sophomore develops his skills by learning to complete the Defined Data Base, and toward the end of the course he begins to formulate problems. This textbook evolved because of our efforts to define a given abnormality, demonstrate the technique for discovering the abnormality, highlight the background information needed to understand the abnormality, and state the clinical significance of the abnormality that can be discovered by completing the Defined Data Base. This was created so that comprehensive care can be given to the population of patients who come to the medical service of Grady Memorial Hospital.

PRACTICAL CONSIDERATIONS REGARDING
THE IMPLEMENTATION OF THE COURSE

The course in clinical methods at Emory University School of Medicine is divided into four parts.

Part I.   The Defined Data Base is used as the guide. The student is asked to complete a Defined Data Base on himself during the summer before the sophomore year begins. In doing so the student is asked to assume that the physical examination and laboratory data are normal. The objective of this exercise is to have the student become familiar with the Defined Data Base and to sense the task that is ahead. (The medical dictionary should be used freely.) Part I of the course in clinical methods meets twice a week for 22 sessions. The course meets from 1–4 PM on Tuesday afternoons. The first hour is designated as "library time"; 2–4 PM is allocated to patient demonstrations, lectures, and discussions of specifically designated units of the course.

The course is divided into 22 units, and the early units consist of discussions regarding the nature of a Defined Data Base, problem formulation, Initial Plans, and Progress Notes. The remaining sessions deal with the items in the Defined Data Base. A schedule of activity for each unit is prepared. Accordingly, the student receives a booklet of the 22 units with each page giving specific instructions regarding what to do on a particular day. Each session is concerned with specific items in the history, physical examination, and laboratory data. For example, the student might begin with the items in the history and physical examination that are listed under general examination. At another session the student may be concerned with the items of history, physical examination, and laboratory data related to the endocrine system. Special sessions are held on the examination of the blood and urine.

Each Tuesday session is organized in advance. It is hoped that this book will assist the student in his efforts to learn the definition, technique of performing, background information, and clinical significance of a given item in the history, physical examination, and laboratory examination. Instructors are requested to adhere to the plan and to discuss the assignment as specified on the "unit" schedule. The instructor must refrain from teaching the student items that are not done on every patient. Instructors have an enormous desire to teach a skill that is not used on every patient and to ignore items that should be done on every patient. One value of the Defined Data Base is to instruct the instructors as to the exact content of the course. The instructors come, for the most part, from the Department of Medicine, but certain instructors come from psychiatry, surgery, obstetrics and gynecology, and physical medicine. A series of videotapes has been developed to assist the student in learning clinical methods. The videotapes have been carefully designed to demonstrate the act of data acquisition and should be viewed by the student before the student examines a patient.

Thursday afternoon is devoted to work with patients. Each student in a class of 110 is assigned a patient. This is accomplished by utilizing Grady Memorial Hospital, Emory University Hospital, The Atlanta Veterans Administration Hospital, Crawford W. Long Hospital, Piedmont Hospital, Georgia Baptist Hospital, and Northside Hospital. Each hospital has a designated person as a hospital coordinator. The student works at one hospital for 11 weeks (or units) and then shifts to another hospital. The students are met by the hospital coordinator each Thursday at 1:30 PM. The hospital coordinator reviews the material that was discussed the previous Tuesday and answers any questions that may arise. The student begins work with his patient at 2 PM. The objective is to deal with the assignment as discussed on the previous Tuesday. An instructor is assigned to two students, and they meet at 4 PM for discussion. The instructor observes the student perform certain tasks and advises him as the need arises. All instructors come from the Department of Medicine.

Each week a little more of the Defined Data Base is covered. The assignment is small in the beginning, but the student is expected to start at the beginning each time he examines a patient so that toward the last quarter of Part I he has performed several complete examinations. (Complete in the sense that the prescribed amount of work, indicated in the Defined Data Base, is completed.)

In summary, the Defined Data Base serves as a guide for Part I. It is divided into 22 units. One unit is covered each week. The items in each unit are studied in this book. Tuesday afternoon is devoted to lectures and demonstrations. Pertinent videotapes are viewed by the student whenever it is convenient to do so. Thursday afternoon is devoted to patient examination. Each student is assigned one patient and is expected to emphasize the material covered on Tuesday. One instructor is assigned to two students. The amount of work assigned to the student grows each Thursday by the increment that was discussed on the previous Tuesday.

The student is asked to begin in his effort to formulate problems by unit 16. In addition to this, the student is urged to look up new material encountered on Thursday in a standard textbook of medicine. These two activities prepare the student for more intense work in Part III of the course.

Part II. Part II of the course is given in the spring quarter. About one-half of the spring quarter curriculum is assigned to clinical methods. The class is divided into sixths and students are assigned to more specialized areas. Remember that most of Part I was taught by members of the Department of Medicine. During Part II the students rotate through Neurology, Cardiology, Obstetrics and Gynecology, Pediatrics, Dermatology, Surgery, Rheumatology, Psychiatry, Ophthalmology, and Otolaryngology. The members of the faculty are advised to check the students on the material contained in the Defined Data Base. This must be done before expecting the student to learn skills he will rarely use. In certain instances, for example Pediatrics, a New Defined Data Base is taught since the data to be collected on children is different from that which is collected on adults.

Throughout Part I and Part II of the course the students give frequent evaluations of the faculty, and the faculty evaluate the students emphasizing whether or not the student was thorough (did the student complete the prescribed work); whether or not the student was reliable; whether or not the student was efficient; and whether or not there was evidence of the development of an analytical sense obtained by simply asking what a given abnormality might signify.

Part III.   Part III of clinical methods occurs during the junior year. Two things happen during the junior year. The student is assigned 2–3 patients each week for the two months he is assigned to the medical service. The student completes the same Defined Data Base that he worked on as a sophomore on each patient. The student is expected to refine the skills demanded by this effort and is checked by the second-year house officer and attending physician. The student must now develop his ability to create a superb problem list on each patient and begin to consider the plans for each problem and how to follow up each problem. In addition to this, which is a refinement and extension of Part I, a special course is given several afternoons each week in advanced clinical methods. The objective of this course is to go beyond the Defined Data Base. Remember the Defined Data Base must be completed on every new patient. Advanced clinical methods is concerned with those things that are not done on every patient. The point is, if a certain test is valuable and it is not done on every patient, then we are obligated to state exactly when it is to be done. This holds for items in the history, physical examination, or laboratory. Accordingly, such sessions are given by members of the Department of Medicine in Advanced Clinical Methods. Each session is devoted to "tests" that are commonly done on patients but are not done on every patient.

Part IV.   Part IV of clinical methods involves the further refinement of the skills required to collect data from a patient. This occurs during the senior year and during residency and fellowship. It takes a long time to develop the skills necessary to be a physician. Part IV is symbolic of that fact. All students, house officers, and fellows are encouraged to remember that good patient care depends upon the identification of a set of problems or conditions that represent how the patient's health has gone astray. If you don't find the problems, you can't plan the care of the patient. It is patently obvious that the problem list must emerge from a Defined Data Base and that the collection of data depends upon the skill of the individual. This is why so much time and effort must be devoted to clinical methods.

CHAPTER FOUR

A Style for Patient Presentation

H. KENNETH WALKER, MD
W. DALLAS HALL, MD
J. WILLIS HURST, MD

The ability to present a patient clearly and concisely is the corner-stone of communication with peers and is one of the principal means by which professional skills are evaluated. There are many ways in which to do this, and no one way is "right." What follows are suggestions about how to present patients in a problem-oriented fashion. The length of the presentation and the content will vary according to the goal of the particular presentation: eg, a presentation at morning report will be quite brief compared to one at attending rounds. However, the *structure* of the presentation is the same in both cases (Table 1).

Table 1. Summary of presentation.

1. Obtain patient's permission ahead of time
2. Introductions
3. Patient's age and other descriptive data (*not* disease)
4. Chief complaint and day of admission
5. Pertinent problems from Complete Problem List
6. Major Problem
    Subjective
    Objective
    Assessment
    Plans
7. Other problems

1. Prior to the presentation explain to the patient what is going to happen and request the patient's permission. Begin the presentation by introducing the patient and members of the group to each other. Then start with the name, age, and occupation or similar descriptive phrase of the patient. There is no point in giving gender if you use Mr. or Ms. Do not include race unless it is pertinent to the problems. Generally avoid using disease appellations such as "Ms. Smith is a 36-year-old diabetic." This is not the proper place to insert such information, since doing so implies you are presenting a disease rather than presenting a patient.
2. State the chief complaint and day of admission to the hospital.
3. Enumerate those problems (from the Complete Problem List) which your audience needs to know in order to have an overall picture of the patient: "The problem list includes the following active problems..." The introductory material given up to this point forms the broad clinical picture of the patient. Move now to the details of the major problem to be presented. Your audience can fit these details into the perspective you have just given of the patient's overall clinical picture.
4. Select from the data base the relevant positive and negative facts which relate to the major problem requiring admission. Begin with the subjective (history) data from the present illness. Confine yourself to the facts relevant to this problem. Do not give facts related to other problems unless they are clearly relevant.
5. Proceed to those portions of the physical examination only as they relate to the admitting problem. Avoid components of the examination that are relevant to other problems, but not to the one under discussion.
6. Next, give the laboratory data relevant to the admitting problem, and no other data.
7. State your assessment of the problem.
8. Give the Initial Plans for the problem in the following sequence:
    a. Goal
    b. Diagnostic: R/O A with ...
                 R/O B with ...
    c. Therapeutic
    d. Patient education
9. Now give the next problem you wish to present: "The next active problem is ..." The sequence is just as above:
    a. Subjective data (history)
    b. Objective data (physical examination and laboratory data)
    c. Assessment

     d.   Plan
         Goal
         Diagnostic
         Therapeutic
         Patient education
10.   Proceed in a similar fashion with any other active problem(s)

The social history, occupational history, and other components of the patient profile can be presented separately or incorporated into specific problems when relevant.

A concise and informative patient presentation requires considerable preliminary planning by the presenter. First, determine the objectives of the presentation and whether the information is to be conveyed in 2 or 15 minutes. Carefully select the subjective (history) and objective (physical and laboratory) data that pertain to each active problem. Present only information that you can defend as clearly relevant to the problem being presented. Make every effort to have key materials (patient chart, x-ray, ECG, and so forth) readily available for critical review by the individual or group to whom the presentation is directed. Consider your assessment in detail, including the major differential diagnoses and the relative likelihood of each; include comorbidity and prognosis in making the assessment for a given problem. Decide on the initial plans which are most appropriate and cost-effective in confirming the diagnosis or resolving the differential diagnoses. Do not list or present future diagnostic test possibilities which are not actually to be performed as part of the initial evaluation. If several initial diagnostic tests are deemed necessary, list them in the sequence of anticipated performance; ic, intravenous pyelogram, then barium enema, then upper gastrointestinal series with gallbladder series. End the initial plans presentation with a statement concerning the patient's knowledge of his illness and of the projected diagnostic tests.

In many circumstances the setting of the presentation (on the ward, at a group conference) and the information involved is such that one must determine the wisdom of presenting in front of the patient. The bedside is appropriate in certain cases, and the conference room in others.

The following is an example of a presentation:

Mr. Jones is a 52-year-old car mechanic admitted two days ago with a chief complaint of cough. The major problems which we have identified on the Complete Problem List are:

    1.   Right pleural effusion ⟶
    3.   Chronic tobacco abuse ⟶
    4.   Hypercalcemia ⟶
    7.   Elevated alkaline phosphatase ⟶

Problem 1, Right Pleural Effusion. Mr. Jones has smoked at least one pack of cigarettes daily for 10 years, but had only a minimal nonproductive cough until two months ago. He has had no hemoptysis, but has noted wheezing at night. There is no contact history for tuberculosis and he denies fever, chills, or night sweats. In the past three months he has had anorexia and has lost 23 pounds.

On physical examination he was afebrile. Cervical nodes were not palpable. Breath sounds were decreased in the lower half of the right lung where percussion was dull. The liver was not palpable. There was evidence of muscle wasting and generalized weakness which was neither specifically proximal nor distal.

The white count was normal with 6% monocytes and 2% bands; the platelet estimate was not high. Electrolytes and other chemistries were within normal limits except for a calcium of 11.1 and an alkaline phosphatase of 181. The chest x-ray revealed a large right pleural effusion with no visible mass or bone lesions.

Our assessment was that lung cancer and tuberculous pleural effusion were the two leading diagnostic possibilities. We favor malignancy because of the lack of fever or night sweats, the extent of weight loss in such a short interval, and the elevated levels of serum calcium and alkaline phosphatase.

The goal of our initial plans is to make the correct diagnosis and implement appropriate therapy. To help rule out lung cancer, we have ordered three morning sputum specimens for cytology and performed a limited thoracentesis with cytology and chemistries. To help rule out tuberculosis, we have placed a PPD and are obtaining sputum AFB smears and cultures.

We have held any initial therapy until the diagnosis can be obtained. This and the planned procedures have been explained to the patient.

The second active problem is 4, Hypercalcemia . . .

This type of patient presentation can be accomplished in minutes. The listeners can assess the validity of the patient diagnosis and the rationale for special diagnostic tests. The presentation provides insight into the ability of the presenter to synthesize fundamental data as collected in the history and physical and laboratory examinations. The patient's major problems are placed in the perspective of the total patient. This type of presentation helps avoid the garble of a clinician trying to convey how he has integrated over 200 bits of data into 4 or more conclusions with 8 or 10 separate plans for each. The teacher is provided with insight into specific areas in which the student and house officer can be assisted with integration of data and planning of diagnostic and therapeutic strategies.

Selected Reference

1.   Hurst JW: The art and science of presenting a patient's problems. *Arch Intern Med* 128:463–465, 1971.

Department of Medicine
Emory University School of Medicine
Grady Memorial Hospital

Defined Data Base*

Date_____

Name_____ Initial Data Base? ☐

(check one)

Age_____ Sex_____ Interval Data Base? ☐

See Data Base of

Source_____ Reliability_____

| Month | Day | Year |

Patient's Major Physician or Pre-admission Clinic Area (Enter "none" if none)

THE HISTORY

1   Chief Complaint and Present Illness:

Continue on Reverse

*(The section numbers in the Defined Data Base Form correspond to the section numbers given in the table of contents for *Clinical Methods,* 2nd Edition, H.K. Walker, W.D. Hall, J.W. Hurst. Woburn: Butterworths, 1980.)

Defined Data Base Forms may be ordered from:
**Department of Medicine, Emory University School
of Medicine, 69 Butler St. S.E., Atlanta, GA 30303.**

1

Present Illness (cont'd):

INSTRUCTIONS

Check **no** or **yes** for the history; check **normal** or **abnormal** for the physical. Leave blank if not asked or not done. Write **NA** if not applicable. Write **NK** if unknown by the patient or examiner. Give narrative description in space on right for all **yes** answers.

	No		Yes

No   **Yes**

General

2	☐	Weight change	☐
3	☐	Fever/chills	☐
4	☐	Night sweats	☐
5	☐	Dizziness	☐
	☐	Other	☐

Endocrine System

6	☐	Heat/cold intolerance	☐
7	☐	Thyroid problems	☐
8	☐	Neck surgery/irradiation	☐
9	☐	Diabetes/diabetic indicators	☐

Eye

10	☐	Visual dysfunction	☐
	☐	Other	☐

Ear, Nose, Throat

11	☐	Difficulty hearing/deaf	☐
12	☐	Tinnitus	☐
13	☐	Epistaxis	☐
14	☐	Hoarseness	☐
15	☐	Sinusitis	☐
16	☐	Vertigo	☐
	☐	Other	☐

Gastrointestinal System

17	☐	Nausea/retching	☐
18	☐	Vomiting	☐
19	☐	Hematemesis	☐
20	☐	Melena	☐
21	☐	Dysphagia	☐
22	☐	Indigestion	☐
23	☐	Heartburn	☐
24	☐	Abdominal pain	☐
25	☐	Abdominal swelling	☐
26	☐	Jaundice	☐
27	☐	Hematochezia	☐
28	☐	Diarrhea	☐
29	☐	Constipation	☐
30	☐	Hernia	☐
31	☐	Hemorrhoids	☐
32	☐	Peptic ulcer disease	☐
33	☐	Gallbladder disease	☐
34	☐	Pancreatitis	☐
35	☐	GI surgery	☐

	No		Yes
36	☐	Alcohol intake	☐
	☐	Other	☐

Pulmonary System

37	☐	Dyspnea/breathlessness/shortness of breath	☐
38	☐	Cough/sputum production	☐
39	☐	Hemoptysis	☐
40	☐	Wheezing/asthma	☐
41	☐	Tuberculosis/tbc exposure	☐
42	☐	Past PPD	☐
43	☐	Previous chest	☐
44	☐	Respiratory infections/pneumonia	☐
45	☐	Smoking history	☐
46	☐	Environmental inhalation	☐
	☐	Other	☐

Cardiovascular System

47	☐	Inadequate exercise level	☐
48	☐	Orthopnea/paroxysmal nocturnal dyspnea	☐
49	☐	Chest discomfort/pain	☐
50	☐	Palpitations	☐
51	☐	Syncope	☐
52	☐	Edema	☐
53	☐	Phlebitis	☐
54	☐	Claudication	☐
55	☐	Hypertension	☐
56	☐	Rheumatic	☐
57	☐	Past heart disease	☐
58	☐	Family history heart disease	☐
	☐	Other	☐

Genitourinary System

59	☐	Urinary frequency/urgency/dysuria	☐
60	☐	Urinary tract infection	☐
61	☐	Flank pain	☐
62	☐	Nocturia	☐
63	☐	Hematuria	☐
64	☐	Past stones	☐
65	☐	Urinary stream flow abnormality	☐
66	☐	Urethral discharge	☐
67	☐	Syphilis/positive serology	☐
68	☐	Male genital lesions	☐
69	☐	Testicular mass/pain	☐
70	☐	Impotence	☐
71	☐	Family history renal disease	☐
	☐	Other	☐

Birth Control

72	☐	Birth Control method	☐

Gynecologic System

73	☐	Pelvic pain	☐
74	☐	Vaginal discharge	☐

	No		Yes
75	☐	Abnormal vaginal bleeding	☐

      a. Menarche: Age _____ yr.
      b. Menopause: Age _____ yr.
      c. Menstrual flow, interval: _____ days
      d. Menstrual flow, duration: _____ days
      e. Menstrual flow, amount: _____
      f. Date last menstrual period: _____
      g. Postcoital bleeding
      h. Postmenopausal bleeding

| 76 | ☐ | Pelvic Mass | ☐ |
| | ☐ | Other | ☐ |

Sexual History

| 77 | ☐ | Sexual difficulties | ☐ |

Breast

78	☐	Breast lump	☐
79	☐	Breast pain	☐
80	☐	Nipple discharge	☐
	☐	Other	☐

Skin

81	☐	Skin disorder	☐
82	☐	Itching	☐
83	☐	Mole(s)	☐
84	☐	Skin cancer	☐
	☐	Other	☐

Neurological System

85	☐	Headaches	☐
86	☐	Epileptic seizures	☐
87	☐	Episodic neurological symptoms	☐
88	☐	Pain/sensory perversions	☐
89	☐	Weakness	☐
90	☐	Head trauma	☐
91	☐	Muscle cramps	☐
92	☐	Stroke	☐
93	☐	Sleep disorder	☐
	☐	Other	☐

Hematopoietic System

94	☐	Excessive bleeding/bruising	☐
95	☐	Anemia	☐
96	☐	Pica	☐
97	☐	Family history sickle cell	☐
	☐	Other	☐

Musculoskeletal System

98	☐	Joint stiffness	☐
99	☐	Joint pain	☐
100	☐	Joint swelling	☐

	No		Yes
101	☐	Family history musculoskeletal disease	☐
	☐	Other	☐

Psychiatric

	No		Yes
102	☐	Previous psychiatric problems or hospitalizations	☐
103	☐	Interpersonal relationship difficulties	☐
104	☐	Anxiety	☐
105	☐	Depression	☐
106	☐	Loss of control/violence potential	☐
107	☐	Disturbances of vegetative function	☐
108	☐	Substance abuse	☐
	☐	Other	☐

Allergies

	No		Yes
109	☐	Drug allergies	☐
	☐	Other	☐

Immunizations

	No		Yes
110	☐	Past immunizations	☐

Family History

	No		Yes
111	☐	Heritable disease potential	☐

Hospitalizations and Medications

	No		Yes			
112	☐	Past hospitalizations	☐	Date	Location	Reason

	No		Yes
113	☐	Current/recent medications	☐

Drug (current)	Dose	Frequency		Drug (current)	Dose	Frequency
1.			6			
2.			7.			
3.			8.			
4.			9.			
5.			10.			

6

☐   Other history data not included in   ☐
       Data Base Items 1-113

THE PATIENT PROFILE

114 Occupation: _____

_____

_____

_____

115 Usual day's activities:

Morning: _____

Afternoon: _____

Evening: _____

116 Hobbies/interests:

_____

_____

_____

_____

117 Nutritional history:

_____

_____

_____

_____

118 Education:

_____

_____

_____

_____

119 Financial difficulties:

_____

_____

_____

_____

_____

THE PHYSICAL EXAMINATION

Normal*   **Abnormal***

General

120	☐	General appearance	☐
121	☐	Temperature (oral ☐ rectal ☐), ____C°	☐
122	☐	Respiratory	☐

    a. Rate: ____/min.
    b. Rhythm: ____

123	☐	Pulse	☐

    a. Rate: ____/min.
    b. Rhythm: ____

124	☐	Blood Pressure: ____/____ mm Hg If abnormal:	☐

    a. Leg: ____/____ mm Hg
    b. Standing: ____/____ mm Hg

125	☐	Body size	
125a	☐	Height ____ (cm ☐ in ☐)	☐
125b	☐	Weight ____ (kg ☐ lb ☐)	☐

    a. ideal body weight: ____
    b. % of ideal body weight: ____%

126	☐	Body habitus	☐
127	☐	Hair	☐
128	☐	Skin	☐
129	☐	Nails	☐
	☐	Other	☐

Head, Ears, Nose

130	☐	Cranial/orbital bruit	☐
131	☐	Pinnae/canals/drums	☐
132	☐	Nose	☐
	☐	Other	☐

Eyes

133	☐	External eye	☐
134	☐	Fundi	☐
135	☐	Pupil	☐
	☐	Other	☐

R   **Figure 1**   L

*Occasionally normal/abnormal does not apply as well as absent/present. Item 139, Parotid enlargement, is an example. If present mark abnormal. If absent mark normal.

9

	Normal		Abnormal

Oral Cavity

136	☐	Teeth/gums/oral mucosa	☐
137	☐	Tongue	☐
138	☐	Tonsils/pharynx	☐
139	☐	Parotid enlargement	☐
	☐	Other	☐

Neck

140	☐	Inspection	☐
141	☐	Carotid bruit (R) (L)	☐
142	☐	Venous hum	☐
143	☐	Thyroid	☐
	☐	Other	☐

Nodes

| 144 | ☐ | Lymphadenopathy | ☐ |

If present indicate location:

	R	L
Cervical	a	b
Epitrochlear	c	d
Axillary	e	f
Inguinal	g	h
Other	i	j

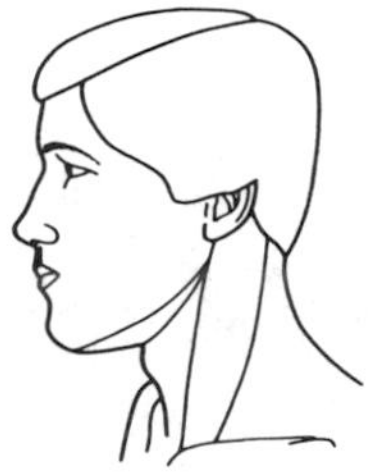

Figure 2

Chest

145	☐	Chest structure	☐
146	☐	Chest motion	☐
147	☐	Chest auscultation	☐
148	☐	Chest percussion	☐
	☐	Other	☐

Breast

149	☐	Mass	☐
150	☐	Nipple/areola	☐
	☐	Other	☐

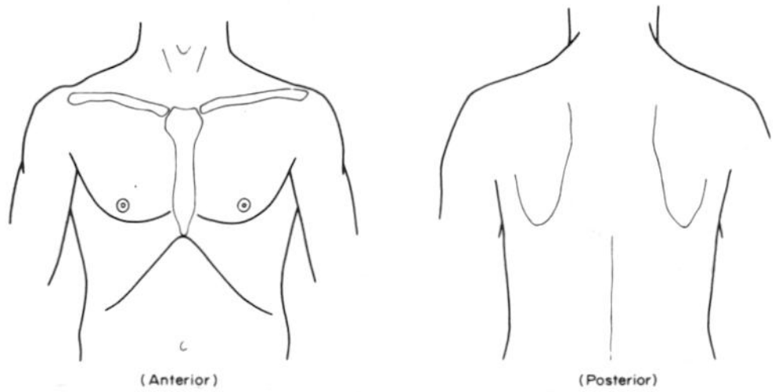

(Anterior)   (Posterior)

Figure 3

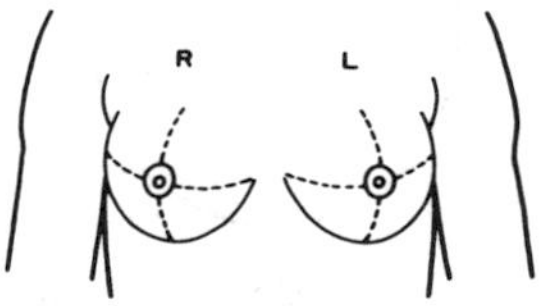

Figure 4

Normal		Abnormal

Cardiovascular System

151	☐	Jugular venous pressure: _____ cm at _____°	☐
152	☐	Jugular venous pulsations	☐
153	☐	Carotid pulse	☐
154	☐	Apex impulse	☐
155	☐	Parasternal impulse	☐
156	☐	Pulmonary artery pulsation	☐
157	☐	First heart sound	☐
158	☐	Second heart sound	☐
159	☐	Third heart sound	☐
160	☐	Fourth heart sound	☐
161	☐	Click	☐
162	☐	Systolic murmur	☐
163	☐	Diastolic murmur	☐
164	☐	Edema:	☐

Right leg 1 2 3 4
Left leg 1 2 3 4

165	☐	Thrombophlebitis	☐
166	☐	Clubbing	☐
167	☐	Cyanosis	☐
168	☐	Pulsus alternans	☐
	☐	Other	☐

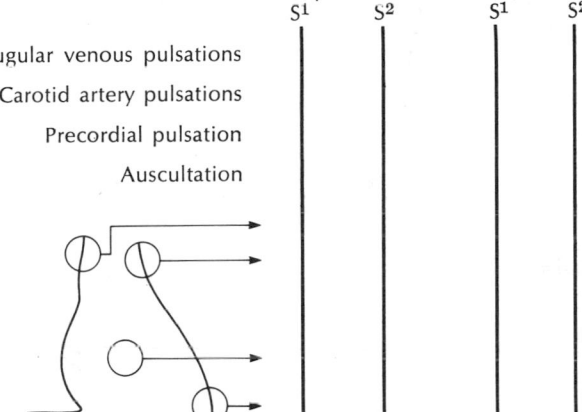

Inspiration S¹ S²   Expiration S¹ S²

Jugular venous pulsations

Carotid artery pulsations

Precordial pulsation

Auscultation

Figure 5

169   ☐   Peripheral pulses/bruits   ☐

Complete chart. Scale pulses 0-4 (normal = 3) and circle if bruit present.

	Carotid	Brachial	Radial	Aorta	Femoral	Popliteal	PT	DP
Right	a	c	e		h	j	l	n
Left	b	d	f	g	i	k	m	o

	Normal		Abnormal

Abdomen

170	☐	Inspection	☐
171	☐	Auscultation: bowel sounds/bruits/rubs	☐
172	☐	Palpation: pain/tenderness	☐
173	☐	Ascites	☐
174	☐	Liver: auscultation	☐
175	☐	Liver: shape/size	☐
176	☐	Spleen	☐
177	☐	Inguinal canal	☐
	☐	Other	☐

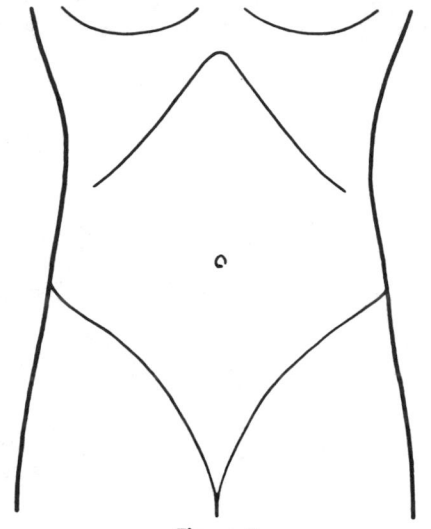

Figure 6

Male Genitalia

| 178 | ☐ | External male genitalia | ☐ |

Female Genitalia

| 179 | ☐ | Pelvic exam:
Indicate site(s) of abnormality | ☐ |

a. External genitalia
b. Vagina
c. Cervix
d. Uterus
e. Adnexa
f. Pap test: done ☐   not done ☐

| | ☐ | Other | ☐ |

Rectal Examination

180	☐	Rectal: inspection/tone/hemorrhoids	☐
181	☐	Prostate	☐
182	☐	Stool occult blood: _____	☐

Normal					Abnormal

Musculoskeletal

183 ☐ Musculoskeletal exam: ☐

	R	L
Hands and wrists	a	b
Elbow	c	d
Shoulder	e	f
TMJ	g	h
Cervical spine	i	
Thoracic and lumbar spine	j	
Hip	k	l
Knee	m	n
Foot and ankle	o	p

    ☐ Other ☐

Neurological and Psychiatric

184	☐	Appearance/affect/motor behavior	☐
185	☐	General intellectual functions	☐
186	☐	Attention span	☐
187	☐	Judgment	☐
188	☐	Abstraction	☐
189	☐	Delusions/hallucinations/illusions	☐
190	☐	Associations of thought	☐
191	☐	Orientation	☐
192	☐	Memory	☐
193	☐	Level of consciousness	☐
194	☐	Speech and other lateralizing cortical functions	☐

Cranial Nerves:

195	☐	I. Olfactory nerve	☐
196	☐	II. Optic nerve	☐

    a. Visual acuity
    b. Visual fields

197	☐	III., IV., VI. Oculomotor, Trochlear and Abducens nerves	☐
198	☐	V. Trigeminal nerve	☐
199	☐	VII. Facial nerve	☐
200	☐	VIII. Acoustic nerve Weber/Rinne tuning fork test	☐
201	☐	IX., X. Glossopharyngeal and Vagus nerves	☐
202	☐	XI. Spinal accessory nerve	☐
203	☐	XII. Hypoglossal nerve	☐
204	☐	Sensation: (specify modalities tested)	☐

Upper extremities:

Lower extremities:

13

	Normal		Abnormal

205 ☐ Motor system (strength, atrophy, ☐
    fasciculations, drift, fine movements)
   Upper extremities:

   Lower extremities:

   Gait:

206 ☐ Cerebellum ☐
207 ☐ Involuntary Movements ☐

   a. Tremor ☐
   b. Chorea ☐
   c. Athetosis ☐
   d. Myoclonus ☐
   e. Asterixis ☐

208 ☐ Suck/snout, grasp reflexes ☐
209 ☐ Deep tendon reflexes ☐
210 ☐ Plantar reflex ☐

Grade 0-4 where 4 = repeating clonus; plantar reflex ↑, ↓ or →

	BICEPS (C 5-6)	BR-RAD (C 5-6)	TRICEPS (C 5-7)	FJ (C^{8}T^1)	KNEEJERK (L 3-4)	ANKLEJERK (S 1-2)	Plantar Reflex
Right	a	c	e	g	i	k	210a
Left	b	d	f	h	j	l	210b

  ☐ Other ☐

  ☐ Other physical examination data not ☐
   included in Data Base Items 120-210

Hematology

211 ☐ Hematocrit ___ vol % ☐
212 ☐ White blood cell count ___/mm^3 ☐
213 ☐ Differential:___S,___L,___M,___E,___B ☐
214 ☐ Platelets ___/hpf or ___/mm^3 ☐
215 ☐ RBC morphology ☐

	Normal		Abnormal

Urinalysis

	Normal			Abnormal
216	☐	Urine color/odor		☐
217	☐	Urine specific gravity 1.0 ___ ___		☐
218	☐	Proteinuria Neg Tr 1 2 3 4		☐
219	☐	Glucosuria/Ketonuria G: Neg Tr 1 2 3 4		☐
		K: Neg Tr 1 2 3 4		
220	☐	Urine sediment: ___ wbc/hpf; ___ rbc/hpf		☐
		Other: _____		

Chemistries

	Normal			Abnormal
221	☐	BUN	___mg/dl	☐
222	☐	Glucose: (serum ☐ plasma ☐)	___mg/dl	☐
223	☐	Serum sodium (Na)	___meq/L	☐
224	☐	Serum potassium (K)	___meq/L	☐
225	☐	Serum chloride (Cl)	___meq/L	☐
226	☐	Serum total CO_2 Content (CO_2)	___meq/L	☐
227	☐	SGOT	___Iu/L	☐
228	☐	LDH	___Iu/L	☐
229	☐	Alkaline phosphatase	___Iu/L	☐
230	☐	Total bilirubin	___mg/dl	☐
231	☐	Uric acid	___mg/dl	☐
232	☐	Creatinine	___mg/dl	☐
233	☐	Calcium	___mg/dl	☐
234	☐	Serum inorganic phosphorus	___mg/dl	☐
235	☐	Cholesterol	___mg/dl	☐
236	☐	Total protein:	___gm/dl	☐
	☐	Albumin/globulin	___/ ___gm/dl	☐

Miscellaneous

	Normal			Abnormal
237	☐	Intermediate PPD: ___mm induration		☐
238	☐	VDRL/RPR		☐

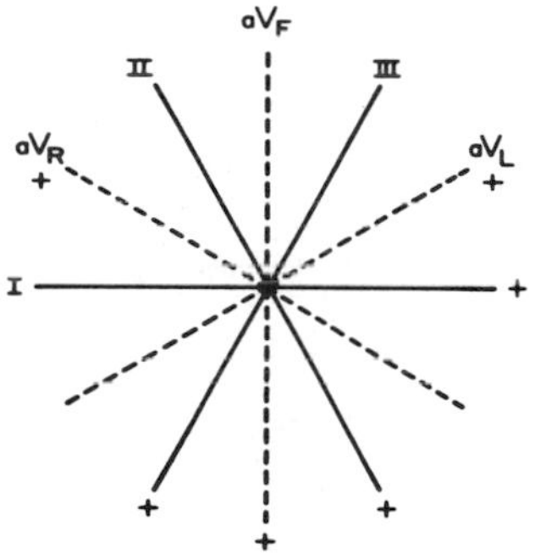

Figure 7

Electrocardiogram

	Normal		Abnormal
239	☐	EKG	☐

a. Rate: ___/min. b. Rhythm: _____
Intervals: c. PQ ___; d. QRS _____;
e. QT ___;
f. Interpretation: _____

_____

_____

15

	Normal			Abnormal

Chest X-Ray

240 ☐   Chest X-Ray   ☐
         Interpretation:_____

_____

_____

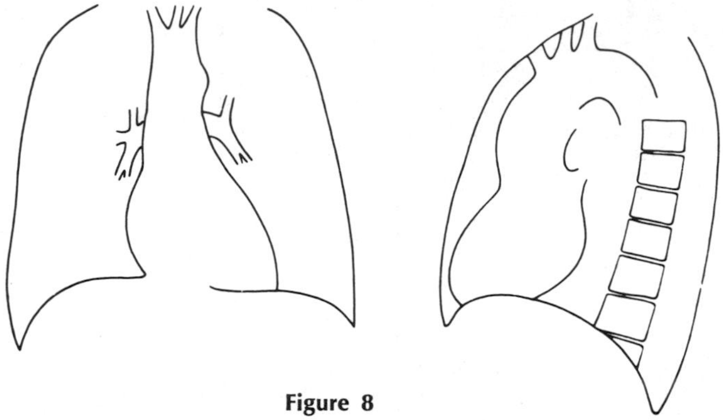

Figure 8

☐   Other laboratory data not included in   ☐
     Data Base Items 211-240.

Signatures indicate agreement with   Signed:_____
    Data Base content. Exceptions   Student
    and additions should be noted,
    initialed, and dated on the Data   _____
    Base.   Houseofficer

                                   _____
                                  Subspecialty Fellow

                                   _____
                                  Attending Physician

PART TWO

The History

CHAPTER FIVE

The History

Introduction to the History

ROBERT B. COPELAND, MD
H. KENNETH WALKER, MD

It is better to rely on an assistant's physical examination than on his history taking, if both cannot be accomplished by oneself.
—Paul Dudley White, MD

The mastery of history taking from patients is not easily or quickly learned. It involves many intangible psychological aspects in relating to patients, as well as requiring sound scientific medical knowledge and effective problem-solving capability.

The essentials in relating to patients include emotional maturity, sensitivity, and genuine care. At the initial interview excellent physicians are able to establish a rapport assuring the patient that he is recognized and respected as a unique individual whose problems are meaningful and for whom all will be done that can be done. Such rapport is the cornerstone of a satisfactory relationship between physician and patient.

The initial interview is composed of three components: emotional, factual, and therapeutic.

The emotional components of the clinical interview include the attitudes and opinion-making features of any interrelationship between two human beings. In the clinical interview, however, the physician or clinical student must effectively discover, characterize, and help solve the problems of the patient. He must do this well despite the almost ubiquitous sense of fear that patients have regarding illness; and despite other factors such as denial, skepticism, hostility, exhaustion, and occasional attempts for secondary gain.

It is necessary to be well aware of the initial reactions of the patient and the clinician relative to what each perceives the other to be. Previous experience with physicians, the health delivery system, and dependency affect the patient's relationship to every physician. Characteristics such as sex, race, age, ethnic group, appearance, and speech all influence how each looks upon the other. Initial opinions can be far from correct, and the results can greatly modify the quality of information obtained.

It is good to remind students that the most difficult or offensive patients may have remarkable medical problems that have been previously overlooked because of difficulties in relating to other physicians. "Let me see in the sufferer the man alone.... Let me be intent on one thing, O Father of Mercy, to be always merciful to Thy suffering children" (Maimonides).

The factual component of the interview relates to information obtained about the problems of the patient such as particular symptoms and their chronology. Diagnostic hypotheses are created from these. By further questioning, attempts are made to corroborate or discredit these hypotheses and to define problems and diagnoses. Only recently have objective studies of clinical problem-solving processes been reported.

It is worthwhile for the clinical student to take the history as well as he can, then give himself adequate time to reflect on the correlations of the symptoms to basic science and clinical knowledge. Strongly recommended is reading basic textbook material concerning the apparent problems, then taking the history a second time before final formulation of the data.

The third component of the clinical interview is therapy. This begins at the initial contact of physician and patient. Future compliance by the patient with the regimen suggested by the physician may be profoundly influenced by impressions made at the time of initial contact. A quiet sense of self-confidence is both reassuring and motivating to the patient. It is critical that the patient see the physician as compassionate, respectful, and competent.

Selected References

1. Morgan WL, Engel GL: *The Clinical Approach to the Patient.* Philadelphia, WB Saunders, 1969.
2. Kassirer JP, Gorry GA: Clinical problem solving: A behavioral analysis. *Ann Intern Med* 89:245–255, 1978.
3. Elstein AS, Shulman LS, Sprafka SA: *Medical Problem Solving. An Analysis of Clinical Reasoning.* Cambridge, Harvard University Press, 1978.

1. Chief Complaint and Present Illness
H. KENNETH WALKER, MD

Definition

The major problem for which the patient has sought medical attention (chief complaint) and a characterization of the details of the patient's current problem(s) (present illness).

Technique

The phases of this portion of the medical interview are:

1. Introduction of the interviewer and, if appropriate, an explanation of the relationship of the interviewer to the patient.
2. Inquiry into the comfort of the patient.
3. Establishment of the problem for which the patient has sought help (chief complaint) and other problems as seen by the patient.
4. A detailed characterization of each problem. Initially the patient spontaneously describes the problem with minimal guidance from the interviewer. Then the interviewer asks specific questions in order to more fully characterize each problem.

Begin by introducing yourself to the patient. If appropriate, define your role: I am the student doctor assigned to you, Mrs. Jones; I am the blood specialist.

Then inquire about the comfort of the patient: Are you in any pain? Is there anything I can do for you before I ask some questions? You thereby apprise the patient of your direct personal interest, your desire to help, and your respect for the patient as an equal human being, and the patient can begin to relate to you in an appropriate fashion. By the end of this phase the patient should feel at ease and be well on the way to feeling secure in the relationship with the interviewer. This phase should be of whatever length necessary to achieve these goals. The beginning interviewer should always pause at the end of this phase and silently ask himself or herself the question: Have I achieved my goals for this phase of the interview? Do not proceed until the answer is yes.

Now establish why the patient is seeking medical help: What brought you to the hospital? What is the thing bothering you most? Or ask whatever similar question the patient understands best. The patient will then state the chief complaint or major problem: I had a severe pain in my stomach. Most patients then stop and wait for the interviewer to indicate how they should proceed. At this point do not ask specific questions about the major problem. Your goal is to get the patient to tell you *all* the problems. When the patient stops, use whatever device is necessary to get the patient to proceed: "And what else is bothering you?" "and?" "uh-huh?" or nonverbal techniques such as silence, or leaning forward slightly with an anticipatory look on your face. Patients will frequently describe a series of symptoms in temporal sequence in answer to this question. Often it is useful to get them to recount this sequence several times: each time new facts or problems emerge. Recounting the tale more than once is useful because the first time patients are intent upon getting across what they feel are the main points. Other points are frequently bypassed or forgotten as this main thrust is occurring. After the initial presentation, the patients relax. During the repeat telling of the story, the patients can be more thoughtful and bring up additional facts now that you have been told all the "important" facts.

At the end of this phase of interviewing, you should feel content that the patient has told you the exigent problems. However, for various reasons such as current stress, forgetfulness, denial, not trusting you totally yet, or modesty, other problems will likely come out later.

At this point often you have two different sets of problems: (1) those related to the chief complaint and present illness, eg, abdominal pain followed sequentially by vomiting blood, syncope, and shock; and (2) other problems, some of which are clearly unrelated to (1) such as operations in the past; and some of which are possibly related to (1) such as severe problems with employer or a recent tragedy in the family.

The interviewer needs to carefully consider all the problems and decide the rank order in which to fully explore or characterize each problem. Usually the best decision is to take the cluster of problems related to the present illness and explore them one by one in chronological sequence, beginning with when the patient was last in the usual state of health.

After ranking the problems, approach each as follows:

Begin by saying to the patient, "Now tell me about . . ." eg, "your stomach pain" or "your headaches." The goal again is to get the patient to give spontaneously as much information as possible. Use any technique that will get the patient to talk freely about that particular problem. Be as nondirective as possible until you feel the patient has exhausted his spontaneous information about that particular problem. Then ask whatever specific questions you deem necessary in order to characterize that problem to your satisfaction. Well-chosen directive questions are indispensable. However, they must be interjected at the right time in a particular line of questioning and with very careful phrasing. The use of directive or leading questions should probably be directly proportional to the experience of the interviewer.

By the time your questioning has ended you should have gathered information on each of the following seven points (taken from Morgan and Engel):

1. Chronology: beginning and course the problem has followed
2. Body location: where the problem is located, including radiation
3. Quality
4. Quantity
5. Setting: under what circumstances it occurs
6. Aggravating and alleviating factors
7. Associated manifestations

Approach each problem in the above fashion. Be careful to avoid leading questions. Ask, "Have you had any difficulties with your bowels?" not "Has your stool turned black?" Ask the most specific question only after the patient has had an opportunity to answer the more general one. When possible ask a question that will provoke a denial. For example, when questioning a patient who has manifestly lost weight, do not ask: You have lost weight, haven't you? Instead put the question like this: I take it you have been gaining weight? The denial evoked by the latter question gives a validity to the answer not possessed by a flat yes.

Remember the interviewer must *observe* as well as *listen*. The patient's body language is often at least as revealing as his words.

Background Information

The interviewing technique described above can be summarized as follows:

1. The interviewer uses a nondirective open-ended approach to get the patient to spontaneously state all problems.
2. The interviewer takes the problems one by one and starts with an open-ended approach: "Tell me about your headaches"; then progressively uses more specific questions in order to fully characterize each problem. The interviewer ends with very specific questions: Does coughing change your headache in any way?

Enelow and Swisher pointed out that physicians engaged in dealing with organic disease have traditionally used the "direct-interrogative" or inquisitory approach: the physician has a long list of specific yes-or-no questions that are put to the patient one by one: Do you have trouble swallowing? Do you have indigestion? A major difficulty with this as the sole interview technique is that the patient must respond to literally hundreds of questions before the physician can be confident that all potential problems have come forth. This takes much time and never allows any expression of the patient's concerns. The mental health disciplines have emphasized the nondirective approach, with emphasis on patient-interviewer communication and the establishment of rapport.

The approach outlined here combines these alternative approaches and has the advantages of each. In addition, the combined method turns out to be the best way to gather data rapidly, in that spontaneous information given by the patient is more likely to provide a larger amount of relevant data in a shorter time than a long list of questions.

One good guideline for this type of interviewing is that the patient should say more than the interviewer: a decent estimate would be 75% of the talking should be done by the patient, with the interviewer exerting guidance or control only when necessary.

It is difficult for beginning interviewers to know techniques that keep the patient talking. Some useful devices are:

1.   Silence
2.   Nonverbal signals of close attention such as leaning forward in anticipation
3.   Short verbal indicators of expectation: yes? and? un-huh
4.   Repeating an important phrase used by the patient: And your head hurts only on the left side?
5.   "Recycling": asking the patient to go over previously covered territory

The goal is to get the patient to speak in paragraphs, not monosyllables (yes, no) or sentences.

Clinical Significance

The history consists of emotional, therapeutic, and factual components. The emotional information lets the clinician know the kind of person being dealt with. The patient's compliance with the therapeutic regimen begins with the rapport established between the patient and clinician.

The factual information, when correlated with data gathered during the physical and laboratory examinations, becomes the basis for clinical decision making. Of this triad, history-physical-laboratory, the history is *primus inter pares* (first among equals). The historical data often leads the clinician rapidly and surely to awareness of deranged anatomy and physiology.

An important factor to remember is that the history represents what the *patient* feels to be wrong. Even if it turns out that the clinician finds a more severe problem that is asymptomatic, eg, in a patient complaining of hemorrhoids the clinician discovers cervical carcinoma, the patient's complaints merit careful attention.

The skill of the interviewer relates ultimately to the quality of his clinical decision making. The medical interview in many respects is a much more difficult skill to acquire than the ability to do a good physical examination. Each episode of history taking should reflect a conscious effort on the part of the clinician to do better than last time. Try phrasing one particular question in many different ways and learn for yourself the best way to phrase it to get the most reliable data.

Do not content yourself with taking the "chief complaint" and "present illness" only once, especially in a hospitalized patient. Each day say to the patient, "Now tell me again about the chest pain you had." Important data will frequently be remembered by the patient.

A beginning student should allow several hours for history taking. In especially difficult cases even vastly experienced practitioners will take one hour or longer to carefully acquire the history.

In the selected references, the book by Morgan and Engel is the classic book in this field. Enelow and Swisher give valuable insight into many aspects of the techniques of the interview.

Selected References

1.   Enelow AJ, Swisher SN: *Interviewing and Patient Care.* New York, Oxford University Press, 1972.
2.   Morgan WL, Engel GL: *The Clinical Approach to the Patient.* Philadelphia, WB Saunders, 1969.

2. Weight Change

MELVIN R. MOORE, MD
W. DALLAS HALL, MD

Definition

Weight change in adults is a gain or loss of more than 7% of body weight within one year. This implies abnormality for a 7-, 10-, or 14-lb weight change in adults with baseline weights of 100, 150, and 200 lb, respectively. This definition is not entirely satisfactory since there are no readily available data to validate the clinical significance of these proposed ranges of weight change over a one-year interval. One kilogram is equivalent to approximately 2.2 pounds.

Technique

Weight change is a major area of concern in our society. Information regarding weight will often be spontaneously provided by the patient. Accurate determination of the presence of weight change is facilitated by asking when and where the patient has most recently been weighed. Then proceed with such questions as: How often do you check your weight? What is the most you have ever weighed? the least? How much do you usually weigh? Do you think you have either gained or lost weight in the past year? Do you know how much you weighed last month, or last summer? When patients are unable to provide answers to the above questions, indirect evidence of weight change should be sought: Do your clothes fit you any differently in recent months or in the past year? Has your belt size or dress size changed? Have your family and friends commented on any recent change in your appearance? When possible, family members and friends should also be questioned.

When weight change, particularly weight loss, is present, the following information should be obtained:

1. Amount and duration of weight change
2. Presence or absence of associated constitutional signs or symptoms (fever, fatigue, malaise)

3. Nutritional history
4. Presence or absence of gastrointestinal symptomatology (particularly abdominal pain, nausea, vomiting and change in bowel habits)
5. Presence or absence of endocrine symptomatology
6. Complete medication history
7. Presence or absence of psychiatric, social, or economic problems

Questions regarding anorexia should be as specific as possible: Are there certain times of the day when your appetite is poor? Are there certain foods that you used to like but no longer like? Does the way that certain foods taste, smell or look make you lose your appetite? Questions regarding nutrition should also be specific: What did you eat for breakfast this morning? for lunch and supper yesterday? Did you eat everything that was served? Are these meals characteristic of what you usually eat? Ask for and listen to the patient's explanation for a recent change in weight.

Record the data specifically, ie, "10 pounds lost in the last 2.5 months," rather than "recent weight loss" or "10-pound weight loss."

Background Information

Weight loss and weight gain are not opposite ends of a single continuum, but represent entirely different physiologic and pathologic problems. Weight loss associated with malnutrition is usually the result of abnormalities in obtaining, assimilating, and metabolizing nutrients. It may lead to deficiency states and generalized debility. Weight gain is more often concerned with central and peripheral mechanisms governing hunger and satiety. Excessive weight gain is associated with increased morbidity from cardiovascular disease and an increased prevalence of clinical diabetes mellitus. Both weight loss and weight gain are common and nonspecific complaints that require the integration of basic and clinical data for full comprehension.

The body is composed of four major compartments: protoplasm, adipose tissue, extracellular fluid, and bone. Body weight represents the sum of the mass contained in these compartments. The average adult is 50% protoplasm, 25% extracellular fluid, 18% adipose tissue, and 7% bone.

Weight change is most often caused by changes in protoplasm and adipose tissue. Loss of protoplasm and adipose tissue are manifested chemically by negative nitrogen, potassium, and phosphate balances. Clinical signs may include a wasted appearance with muscle atrophy and loss of subcutaneous tissue in the triceps, deltoid, and other skinfolds.

More subtle signs include concavity of the temporalis muscles, or of the medial thigh just above the knee when the leg is extended. Increased adipose tissue and protoplasm are characterized chemically by a decrease in bone density with unchanged or positive nitrogen, potassium, and phosphate balances. These patients are characterized by obesity, particularly as measured by increased skinfold thickness.

Changes in extracellular fluid are often unrelated to changes in protoplasm and adipose tissue and may confuse the evaluation of weight change. Rapid changes in body weight occurring within hours or a few days are often due to changes in extracellular fluid. Weight loss due to loss of extracellular fluid is characterized chemically by a negative balance of sodium, chloride, and water. Clinical signs include poor skin turgor, orthostatic hypotension, tachycardia, and no visible jugular neck veins in the supine position. Weight gain due to an increase in extracellular fluid will usually be associated with a positive balance of sodium, chloride, and water. Clinical manifestations will depend on the presence of adequate plasma oncotic pressure. With normal plasma oncotic pressure, expansion of both the intravascular and interstitial compartments will occur, leading to jugular venous distention, edema, hypertension, cardiomegaly, atrial and ventricular gallops, hepatomegaly, and effusions. When plasma oncotic pressure is low, as in severe liver disease or nephrotic syndrome, the clinical findings may be those of extracellular fluid depletion despite the presence of edema, ascites, and pleural effusions. Loss of protoplasm and adipose tissue may be masked by the presence of extracellular fluid expansion. Pathologic mechanisms may thus result in a stable or increasing weight. Recall that 1 liter of water weighs 2.2 lb (1 kg) and that 2 to 5 liters of fluid can easily be contained within the pleural, peritoneal, or subcutaneous fluid spaces. Consider the malnourished and cachectic cirrhotic patient who has gained weight during accumulation of massive ascites.

The mechanisms of loss of protoplasm and adipose tissue differ greatly with individual disease states and will be discussed under Clinical Significance.

The mechanisms of weight gain resulting in obesity are highly speculative. Hunger may be stimulated by a central excitatory neural system involving neurons containing the catecholamine neurotransmitters norepinephrine and dopamine, arising in the pons and mesencephalon and having diverse connections throughout the brain. The stimulus for excitation of this system is unknown but seems to begin with the recruitment of stored fuels. Feeding results in increased levels of insulin that bring about an elevation in brain serotonin that may reciprocally inhibit the noradrenergic neurons involved in the stimulus for hunger and other arousal behaviors. Obesity may result from a primary dysfunction involving lipogenic enzymes and insulin secretion, in which case hunger is an appropriate response to the increased disposal of ingested nutrients.

Obesity may also result from an abnormality in the general level of activation, where hunger is part of a nonspecific neural mechanism to increase arousal or calming behaviors.

Clinical Significance

It is axiomatic that failure to identify a clinical problem will result in failure to define and solve that problem. Weight loss, even in the presence of an obvious underlying disease such as malignancy, should be noted as a problem since specific diagnostic and therapeutic plans may greatly benefit the patient. When the diagnosis and therapy of underlying disease is not sufficient to reverse a significant weight loss, specific nutritional therapy including vitamin supplements, and enteral or parenteral hyperalimentation techniques may be indicated to decrease the generalized weakness, fatigue, myopathy, and skin and mucous membrane changes that accompany clinical malnutrition.

Pathologic loss of protoplasm and adipose tissue will usually eventuate in protein-calorie malnutrition as defined by abnormalities in creatinine-to-height excretion ratios, mid-arm muscle circumference, anthropomorphic measurements of skinfold thickness, and clinical debility. The differential diagnosis of protein-calorie malnutrition may be simplified by considering five broad categories of inadequate nutrition.

1. The patient is unable to obtain nutrients. The single largest cause of protein-calorie malnutrition worldwide is the lack of availability of an adequate diet for economic, social, political, or cultural reasons. An interesting subset of patients suffering from iatrogenic protein-calorie malnutrition consists of hospitalized patients subsisting on parenteral fluid therapy for prolonged periods.

2. The patient is unable to ingest nutrients. Included in this group are patients with anorexia due to malignancy (particularly pancreatic adenocarcinoma, gastric adenocarcinoma, bronchogenic carcinoma, colon adenocarcinoma, hypernephroma, and Hodgkin's disease), uremia, liver disease, chronic or acute infections (particularly tuberculosis), active inflammatory disease, inflammatory bowel disease or other diarrheal illness, Addison's disease, drug toxicity (particularly digitalis), psychiatric illness including depression, anxiety, and anorexia nervosa. Also in this group are nonanorectic patients with mechanical disorders such as ill-fitting dentures or dental and periodontal disease, stomatitis (eg, candidiasis secondary to antibiotics), and dysphagia secondary to tumors of the head and neck or esophagus, and dysphagia secondary to esophageal stricture.

3. The patient is unable to absorb nutrients. This group includes inflammatory bowel disease and other diarrheal illness and malabsorptive states (eg, nontropical sprue, diabetes mellitus, small-bowel lymphoma,

short bowel, and blind loop syndrome). Illnesses and drugs causing increased gastrointestinal motility (nausea, vomiting and diarrhea) and bowel obstruction will also result in a failure to absorb nutrients.

4. The patient has increased metabolic requirements. Hyperthyroidism, pheochromocytoma, advanced malignancy, major surgery, active infection, and inflammatory diseases may all be associated with weight loss secondary to increased metabolic demands. An increased appetite and weight loss are observed in diabetes mellitus, hyperthyroidism, and certain types of malabsorption.

5. The patient has an increased loss of nutrients. This group overlaps with the malabsorptive states included in the third category, but also includes patients with blood loss, nephrotic syndrome, and advanced malignancy with large tumor masses or malignant effusions.

In many of the disease states above, treatment of the underlying illness will result in a rapid reversal of weight loss and its sequelae. When such treatment is not feasible, specific nutritional support should be considered.

Weight gain caused by an expansion of the extracellular fluid compartment may occur with congestive heart failure, cirrhosis, nephrotic syndrome, and certain malignancies. Weight gain on a hormonal basis is seen in hypothyroidism, pituitary disorders, and in patients on corticosteroid or progestogen therapy. As discussed above, obesity may be viewed as primary (caused by abnormal lipogenic enzymes and insulin secretion) or as secondary (with hyperphagia often associated with an inappropriate level of general activity). Patients with primary obesity should have intense hunger when fasted; they respond poorly to diet therapy. Patients with secondary obesity should tolerate fasting and may respond to behavioral or pharmacologic dietary intervention.

Selected References

1. Stricker EM: Hyperphagia. N Engl J Med 298:1010–1013, 1978.
2. Rudman D, Millikan WJ, Richardson TJ, et al: Elemental balances during intravenous hyperalimentation of underweight adult subjects. J Clin Invest 55:94–104, 1975.
3. DeWys WD: Anorexia in cancer patients. Cancer Res 37:2354–2358, 1977.
4. Theologides A: Anorexia-producing intermediary metabolites. Am J Clin Nutr 29:552–558, 1976.
5. Keys A, Grande F: Body weight, body composition and calorie status, in Goodhart RS, Shils ME (eds): Modern Nutrition in Health and Disease. Philadelphia, Lea and Febiger, 1973.

3.   Fever and Chills

JONAS A. SHULMAN, MD
DAVID SCHLOSSBERG, MD

Definition

Fever is an elevation of body temperature above the normal daily variations. Chills are sensations of chilliness usually preceding or accompanying rapid changes in body temperature. The formula for converting Fahrenheit to Centigrade is: $^{\circ}C = (^{\circ}F - 32) \times 0.555$. The formula for converting Centigrade to Fahrenheit is: $^{\circ}F = (^{\circ}C \times 1.8) + 32$.

Technique

Many patients present a history of fever and have actually recorded their temperature with an oral or rectal thermometer. Patients who have not recorded their temperature need to be carefully questioned as to whether they have had hot or chilly feelings. Fatigue, night sweats, headache, or myalgias are common accompaniments of fever. Chilly sensations may dominate the history and may be of such severity that the patient will describe bed-shaking or teeth-chattering.

When symptoms of fever are present, acquire detailed information concerning the onset, the pattern (eg, afternoon spikes or low sustained fever), the presence or absence of chills, and the influence of antipyretic agents. Since fever may be induced by many drugs, a careful history of drug ingestion should be taken.

Background Information

Disease states such as infection, neoplasms, and autoimmune disorders may cause a rise in temperature. The final common pathway in the production of fever is probably the production of "endogenous pyrogen" from polymorphonuclear leukocytes, monocytes, and tissue cells during the process of inflammation. This pyrogen in turn acts on the thermoregulatory centers of the hypothalamus.

The normal variation of the human body temperature is considerable. A temperature of 98.6°F (37°C) is considered normal, but patients' peak daily temperature may range from a low of 97°F to a high of 99.6°F. In addition to this variability in the peak temperatures among normal patients, there is also a diurnal variation of about 1°F in each individual. The highest daily temperature is usually present in the late afternoon or early evening, and the nadir is about 4 AM. This variation is exaggerated with fever; it may be reversed in old age, miliary tuberculosis, and during salicylate intake. The rectal temperature is usually about 1°F higher than the oral. The oral temperature is about 1°F higher than the axillary. Physiologic states that can cause slight rises in temperature include digestion, exercise, ovulation, pregnancy, warm environment, and emotion.

Clinical Significance

Infection is the most frequent and important pathologic cause of fever. Early detection of infection may indicate specific treatment. Several variations in the ability of the host to respond to tissue injury or infection with fever must be considered. For example, the very young may have an exaggerated febrile response to infection. Infants often announce infection by a febrile convulsion, related to a rapid and pronounced rise in temperature. Fevers of 40.5–41.7°C are not particularly uncommon in the young. In contrast, adults rarely have extreme elevation in temperature (41.7–42.2°C) except with heatstroke, cerebral infarction, or the postoperative complication of malignant hyperpyrexia secondary to administration of certain muscle relaxants and anesthetics. Elderly patients tend to have a diminished temperature response to infection. They may become disoriented when febrile.

Classically, observers have described four patterns of fever in an attempt to associate specific diseases with the fever pattern. These four patterns are intermittent, remittent, sustained, and relapsing. Intermittent refers to high spikes with returns to normal. Remittent is like intermittent, but the temperature never returns to normal. Sustained is like remittent, but with less marked swings of temperature. Relapsing refers to several days of fever alternating with periods of normal temperature.

Unfortunately, these types of fever patterns are not very helpful since there are many exceptions. Many factors affect the temperature response and may change the fever pattern in an individual patient. For example, a history of chills suggests extreme swings of temperature, but if the patient is taking antipyretics, the chills may be caused by the rapid defervescence induced by the antipyretics. Chills may also result from cooling of the skin. However, a few fever patterns are suggestive of specific diseases. For example, typhoid fever classically manifests a sustained temperature elevation, while fever from an abscess is typically remittent.

A relapsing fever is particularly helpful since it may indicate malaria, rat-bite fever, cholangitis, or infection with *Borrelia recurrentis*. Important noninfectious causes of relapsing fever include Hodgkin's disease and intermittent obstruction of the common bile duct.

Occasionally there is reason to doubt the veracity of a patient's illness. One way of simulating organic illness is for the patient to contrive a temperature elevation. Some physiologic clues to "factitious fever" include a temperature greater than 41°C, a rapid fall in temperature without concomitant diaphoresis, a lack of diurnal variation in the temperature curve, a lack of rise in heart and respiratory rate with the fever, and a disparity between the measured rectal temperature and the temperature of a freshly voided urine sample. Heart rate usually increases about 10 beats per minute per −17°C temperature increase. Absence of this expected febrile acceleration of heart rate is referred to as "relative bradycardia" and occurs most notably in infections such as typhoid fever, mycoplasma pneumonia, and psittacosis.

Fevers that occur in the nonhospitalized population and that are short-lived (less than 1 week) are usually caused by self-limited viral illnesses. Common bacterial causes of short-term fever are infection of the throat, ear, paranasal sinuses, bronchi, or urinary tract. Patients who remain febrile for more than 1–2 weeks require more intensive investigation. This clinical setting has been conventionally called "fever of undetermined origin" (FUO).

Infection is a very important cause of the treatable FUOs. The most frequent systemic infections responsible for FUO are tuberculosis (usually miliary) and subacute bacterial endocarditis. Tumors, especially hematologic or lymphatic, collagen vascular diseases, hypersensitivity diseases, inflammatory bowel states, and pulmonary emboli are additional important causes. Localized infections may also cause FUO. These are frequently present in the abdomen and pelvis, rendering their detection difficult. In the abdomen, an obscure abscess may be found in the right upper quadrant, within the liver, or in the subphrenic or subhepatic location. Intermittent obstruction of the biliary tree may produce cholangitis with Charcot's intermittent biliary fever.

The evaluation of FUO becomes increasingly invasive as the etiology remains obscure. Serologic investigation may reveal such noninfectious causes as systemic lupus or rheumatoid arthritis. The patient may manifest a pathologic skin lesion or enlarged lymph node accessible to biopsy. Marrow biopsy may also be useful. The most productive biopsy site is the liver, even in the absence of hepatomegaly or derangement of liver tests. Appropriate smears and cultures should be performed on biopsy specimens and body fluids, including techniques to detect aerobes, anaerobes, tubercle bacilli, and fungi. Radiographic studies of the gastrointestinal, urinary, and biliary tract are often necessary. Neoplastic disorders may be unmasked during this phase of the evaluation. For example, a marrow biopsy may show tumor infiltration, or an intravenous pyelogram (IVP) may be consistent with hypernephroma. Modern scanning techniques are sometimes useful to delineate an abscess or tumor in organs such as liver, pancreas, and bone. Ultrasound is another noninvasive technique useful in delineating masses and in distinguishing solid from cystic mass lesions. Angiography may outline an abscess or tumor or show characteristic vascular changes such as seen in polyarteritis nodosa. Finally, laparotomy may on occasion establish the diagnosis, but this is an extreme measure and should be employed only after careful deliberation. It is most helpful in finding a small abscess, especially in the right upper quadrant and in the pelvis.

Selected References

1. Bennett IL Jr, Hook EW: Fever of unknown origin. *DM*, pp 1–48, 1957.
2. Petersdorf RG, Beeson PB: Fever of unexplained origin: Report on 100 cases. *Medicine* 40:1–30, 1961.
3. Molavi A, Weinstein L: Persistent perplexing pyrexia: Some comments on etiology and diagnosis. *Med Clin N Am* 54:379–396, 1970.
4. Bodel P: Tumors and fever. *Ann NY Acad Sci* 230:6–13, 1974.
5. Atkins E, Bodel P: Fever, in Zweifach BW, Grant L, McCluskey RT (eds): *The Inflammatory Process*, ed 2. New York, Academic Press, 1973.
6. Hellon RF: Monoamines, pyrogens and cations: Their actions on central control of body temperature. *Pharmacol Rev* 26:289–321, 1974.
7. Dinarello CA, Wolff SM: Pathogenesis of fever in man. *N Engl J Med* 298:607–612, 1978.

4. Night Sweats

W. DALLAS HALL, MD

Definition

Night sweating is a normal occurrence which goes unnoticed by most individuals. Night sweats are abnormal when they become noticeable to the patient and are not accounted for by environmental heat.

Technique

Begin with an open-ended question such as: Are you a person who tends to sweat a lot? If the answer is yes, ask additional questions: Has this been true all of your life? When did it start? Does it occur more during the day or night?

Inquire about the environmental thermal conditions at the time of night sweats: Do you have air conditioning or a fan in your room at night? Where do you usually set your thermostat?

Ask: Does anything else happen exactly at the same time as the sweating? Patients may then describe simultaneous fever, chills, pain, headaches, palpitations, flushing, hunger, confusion, or nightmares.

Background Information

Human sweat glands are of two types: apocrine and eccrine. Large apocrine glands are located primarily in the axillary and anogenital area. These glands, like those of the palms and soles, respond to sympathetic stimuli. Emotional stress or a cold environment may thus be associated with axillary, anogenital, or palmar sweating. Smaller eccrine sweat glands relate more to body temperature regulation. These glands respond mainly to parasympathetic stimulation, mediated by release of acetylcholine. Belladonna alkaloids such as atropine and scopolamine reduce eccrine sweat production and may produce fever. Sympathetic stimulation also activates eccrine sweat glands. The rate of sweating increases with a rise in the temperature of either the skin or circulating blood. The anterior hypothalamus interacts to regulate sweat production independent of skin temperature.

Normal individuals have an increase in sweat production within 30 minutes of falling asleep. This corresponds with a nocturnal fall in rectal temperature, and the majority of sweating occurs before the lowest rectal temperature at 3:30 AM (range 2:10–4:30 AM). The nocturnal drop in rectal temperature averages approximately 0.6°C. Rectal temperature usually begins to rise by 5:30 AM such that night sweating at this time would be less likely due to diurnal temperature extremes than other conditions such as hypoglycemia. The higher the initial rectal temperature, the greater the nocturnal temperature drop and magnitude of night sweating. In a normal individual, nocturnal sweating increases about threefold and is unnoticed. Increments of threefold to fivefold are usually apparent to the patient, and eightfold increments are typically manifest by wet bed clothing or pillow cases. Both normal and abnormal nocturnal sweating tends to occur in bursts such that the patient may complain of drenching night sweats. Environmental factors must be considered since the magnitude of temperature fall (and therefore sweating) is related to room temperature. Patients in warmer rooms have higher baseline temperatures but less temperature fall and related sweating than patients in cooler rooms. In addition, factors other than nocturnal temperature drop are associated with sweating during sleep. For instance, normal individuals also sweat with afternoon naps, a time when there is no decrease in rectal temperature. Male patients and black patients tend to sweat more and at lower temperature thresholds than their respective counterparts.

Pilocarpine stimulates sweat glands in the absence of innervation. Acetylcholine injection (usually intradermal) stimulates sweating only when postganglionic fibers are intact.

Clinical Significance

Nocturnal sweating usually results from an exaggeration of the normal diurnal temperature variation. Night sweats are thus most prominent in patients who have elevated nocturnal temperatures. Classic examples include tuberculosis, Hodgkin's disease, brucellosis, lung abscess, and bacterial endocarditis. Any etiology of fever may be an etiology of night sweats.

Night sweats have acquired special significance for the diagnosis of tuberculosis. This is probably because the fever is low-grade, superimposed on the usual diurnal pattern, and often unnoticed by the patient. The same clinical significance should be attached to any disease process with similar pyrogenic features. In contrast, higher temperatures and shaking chills are often more prominent clinical signs in inflammatory diseases such as bacterial pneumonia, pyelonephritis, cholecystitis, or localized abscesses. Night sweats occasionally occur in noninflammatory disease states. Examples include the hypothermia associated with nocturnal hypoglycemia and the anginal pain induced by nightmares. Nocturnal sweating may also be a symptom of congestive heart failure, particularly in children.

Of note are a few relatively rare, but interesting clinical disorders of sweating. Patients with pheochromocytoma manifest a classic symptom triad of headache, palpitations, and sweating; episodic bursts of sweating may dominate the clinical picture. Excessive localized sweating may accompany the pain or paresthesias of peripheral nerve lesions; in contrast, nerve section usually causes loss of sweating in the distribution of the affected nerve. Horner's syndrome usually has a loss of sweating on the side of the face with the smaller pupil.

Patients with familial dysautonomia (Riley-Day syndrome) tend to sweat excessively, a sign often noted by the mother in early infancy. Normal persons may complain of excessive sweating of the face and neck after ingestion of spicy foods or excessive tyramine. This is known as gustatory sweating and may be prominent following parotid gland injury

(Frey's syndrome) or in diabetic patients with autonomic neuropathy. Widespread autonomic neuropathy such as with diabetes or idiopathic orthostatic hypotension is associated more frequently with a generalized decrease in sweating.

Selected References

1. Geschickler EH, Andrews PA, Bullard RW: Nocturnal body temperature regulation in man: A rationale for sweating in sleep. *J Appl Physiol* 21:623–630, 1966.
2. Nadel ER, Bullard RW, Stolwijk JAJ: Importance of skin temperature in the regulation of sweating. *J. Appl Physiol* 31:80–87, 1971.
3. Randall WC, Kimura KK: The pharmacology of sweating. *Pharm Rev* 7:365–397, 1955.
4. Gibson TE, Shelley WB: Sexual and racial differences in the response of sweat glands to acetylcholine and pilocarpine. *J Invest Derm* 11:137–142, 1948.
5. Allen JA, Roddie IC: Sweat production during catecholamine infusion in man. *J Physiol* 222:70–71, 1972.
6. Watkins PJ: Facial sweating after food: a new sign of diabetic autonomic neuropathy. *Br Med J* 1:583–587, 1973.
7. Johnson RH, Spalding JMK: *Disorders of the Autonomic Nervous System.* Philadelphia, FA Davis, 1974, pp 179–198.
8. Stuart DD: Diabetic gustatory sweating. *Ann Intern Med* 89:223–224, 1978.

---

5.   Dizziness

H. KENNETH WALKER, MD
W. DALLAS HALL, MD

Definition

This term is applied by patients to an immense variety of sensations such as spinning of self and/or environment, light-headedness, swimming and fuzziness of the head, faintness, seasickness, drunkenness, staggering, unsteadiness, and giddiness. Vertigo is preferred whenever there is a sensation of rotation or movement. In the discussion to follow, dizziness refers to nonvertiginous sensations.

Technique

Many physicians feel faint themselves when a patient offers the word "dizzy" as a complaint. The frequent inability of patients to expand upon their meaning creates additional frustration. But the term is clinically important, not only because it represents a common complaint, but also because many diseases first announce themselves by the symptomatology that, for want of a better word, patients express as dizziness.

The history in a patient with dizziness is often far more revealing than the physical examination. Begin by allowing a spontaneous description from the patient. Have the patient repeat and detail the occurrences. Then focus the patient's attention upon potential associated symptoms that may have been omitted from the initial description. Suggest analogies if the patient has difficulty putting the sensation into words, eg: Is the sensation one of being about to faint or one like that accompanying merry-go-round rides, spinning in a circle, or overindulging in alcohol? Determine if there is a sense of rotation or movement of self or surroundings. The latter is defined as vertigo, which may be considered a distinct category of dizziness.

Sensations of faintness, dimness of vision, and partial or actual loss of consciousness are especially valuable clues since they may indicate etiologies such as epilepsy or impaired cardiac output. Determine the relation of the onset of dizziness to posture. Does it occur while recumbent? Just after standing? Especially on arising in the morning ("matutinal" dizziness)? While or just after walking? Precipitating factors such as onset with sudden motion, sudden head turning, or bending over often point to abnormalities of the peripheral vestibular apparatus.

Ascertain the temporal characteristics of the dizziness. Is the onset abrupt? What is the duration? Is the dizziness episodic or constant? Ask about gait. Is it abnormal during the attacks? Does turning when walking precipitate the dizziness? Does the dizziness cause the patient to cease activities such as walking or driving?

Always ask about all current medications since a large number can produce orthostatic hypotension with dizziness (see section 123, Current and Past Medication).

Associated symptoms are often the key to localizing the anatomical system responsible for the dizziness. The neurological system is implicated by associated symptoms of brainstem dysfunction including diplopia, dysarthria, limb weakness, occipital headache, numbness of the face and/or limbs, and drop attacks. Nausea and vomiting may also accompany dizziness from brainstem lesions. Epilepsy can have dizziness as the aura.

Psychiatric disorders, such as anxiety and depression, can be accompanied by a complaint of dizziness. If your questions up to now have been unrevealing, ask about feelings of panic, fright, detachment, loss of initiative, and difficulties with attention and concentration. Patients with hyperventilation complain of dizziness, usually in conjunction with circumoral and digital paresthesias, carpopedal muscle spasms, and rapid respiration. Note any other symptoms or diseases such as diabetes, hypertension, cardiovascular disease, or evidence of blood loss such as melena. A list of important points in the history taking from patients complaining of dizziness follows:

1. Spontaneous description
2. Analogies
3. Rotation, movement (vertigo)
4. Faintness, loss of consciousness
5. Position and precipitating factors
6. Temporal characteristics
7. Gait
8. Medications
9. Neurological symptoms
10. Psychiatric symptoms
11. Other diseases and symptoms

Background Information

Sensory impulses from a variety of receptors are integrated in the brainstem, cerebellum, and cortex to produce proper perception of the position of the body in relation to its surroundings. The principal impulses originate in the labyrinth, proprioceptors of the joints and muscles, and the retina. These vestibular, proprioceptive, and visual data are integrated in the brainstem (vestibular, oculomotor, and red nuclei especially) and in the cerebellum. The cortex finally receives this information and integrates it to produce a body schema that in turn is related to the surroundings or environmental schema. Dysfunction arises chiefly from problems with the neural centers or from lack of perfusion of these centers due to cardiovascular, cerebrovascular, or autonomic nervous system dysfunction.

The labyrinth conveys information about the position of the head or changes in the position of the head. It is composed of three semicircular canals, a utricle, and a saccule. The semicircular canals are stimulated by rotatory movements; the utricle is stimulated by gravitational forces and linear acceleration. These receptors are innervated by the vestibular ganglion in the internal auditory meatus. Fibers from this ganglion course centrally with the acoustic (eighth) nerve through the cerebellopontine angle to the four vestibular nuclei in the floor of the fourth ventricle and to the cerebellum. Fibers arising in the vestibular nuclei then project to the cerebellum, to all spinal levels, to the medial longitudinal fasciculus, and to the pontine reticular formation. Vestibular fibers in the medial longitudinal fasciculus project to nuclei of the third, fourth, and sixth cranial nerves, thereby stimulating reflex conjugate eye movements as the position of the head changes. Fibers descending to the spinal level affect the axial and limb muscles and are chiefly concerned with muscle tone and spinal reflexes.

Afferent proprioceptive impulses from muscles and tendons ascend to the cerebellum by various spinal cord tracts, chiefly the dorsal and ventral spinocerebellar tracts. Joint-position and vibratory impulses first ascend in the dorsal colums to the nucleus gracilis and nucleus cuneatus, then in the medial lemniscus to the VPL (Ventral Posterolateral Nucleus) of the thalamus, and finally project to the cortex. Visual impulses project from the retina to the occipital lobe. Visual information is integrated with proprioceptive and vestibular information in ways that are incompletely understood.

There is no clear agreement on the "cortical vestibular area," ie, the area of the cortex where the vestibular nuclei project. Dizziness or vertigo have been reported with stimulation of the following areas: a circle in the region of the junction of the temporal, occipital, and parietal lobes; the superior temporal convolution; the midtemporal convolution; and the supramarginal and angular gyri. One study (Frederickson et al) has located the cortical vestibular area in a small region close to the face subdivision of the first somatosensory area in area 2 of Brodmann—an area known to be involved in the reception of sensations from tissues such as joints (Brodal, p 387). The cortical projection is contralateral. A reasonable assumption would be that the cortical area concerned with the perception of the relationship of the body to the surroundings would have input from vestibular, proprioceptive, and visual areas. It may be that the chief cortical area for orientation is in the nondominant hemisphere, which is known to be closely associated with spatial orientation.

Dizziness or vertigo can probably be produced by decreased vascular perfusion of any of the central areas noted above. However, the "main vascular theater of dizziness" is the region of confluence of the vertebral arteries that form the basilar artery (Fisher). The internal auditory artery, which arises from either the anterior inferior cerebellar artery (AICA) or from the basilar artery, supplies the peripheral apparatus of the vestibular system. The vestibular nuclei are supported by penetrating branches of the AICA and vertebral arteries. This blood supply explains why occlusion or transient ischemic attacks of the posterior circulation are prominent causes of dizziness or vertigo.

Maintenance of blood pressure in the standing position is primarily a function of short-term regulation by the autonomic nervous system. Normally, upon standing there is a slight fall in systolic blood pressure and a slight rise in diastolic blood pressure, resulting in a minimal change in the mean arterial blood pressure available for organ perfusion. The venous pooling and decreased venous return associated with standing would result in shock were it not for compensatory mechanisms. Standing induces release of norepinephrine, renin, and angiotensin II, providing arteriolar wall constriction to help maintain peripheral resistance. The baroreceptor reflex (primarily in the carotid sinus) senses a transient fall in intracarotid pressure and forwards afferent signals to the vasomotor center in the brainstem. These impulses are integrated to inhibit alpha-adrenergic CNS receptors such that sympathetic outflow tracts from the brain are stimulated (note the opposite effects of alpha adrenergic stimulation in the brain versus periphery). Interference or dysfunction of any of the autonomic regulatory functions (neurologic disorders, diabetes, drugs) may block the usual mechanisms for maintenance of blood pressure in the standing position. Patients may thus experience orthostatic dizziness, faintness, or syncope.

Clinical Significance

Drachman and Hart, in a study that is a model of its kind, carefully studied 104 patients who had a chief complaint of "dizziness" (Table 2).

Peripheral vestibular disorders accounted for the largest number. They included benign positional vertigo, peripheral vestibulopathy, "vestibular neuronitis," Meniere's disease and chronic labyrinthine imbalance. The typical patient had unmistakable rotational vertigo with nausea and vomiting, without other brainstem deficits. The symptoms were repro-

Table 2   Etiologies of dizziness in 104 patients

Etiology	Percentage
Peripheral vestibular disorders	38
Hyperventilation syndrome	23
Multiple sensory deficits	13
Psychiatric disorders	9
Uncertain diagnosis	9
Brainstem cerebrovascular accident	5
Other neurological disorders	4
Cardiovascular disorders	4
Other	6

From Drachman DA, Hart CW: An approach to the dizzy patient. *Neurology* 22:323–334, 1972. Used with permission.

duced by rotational or caloric tests. Benign positional vertigo, in which the vertigo occurred only on change of position, was twice as frequent as other vestibular disorders.

The hyperventilation syndrome produced dizziness in 23%. The complaint of dizziness in these patients was precisely reproduced with hyperventilation.

Thirteen percent of the patients had what was characterized as multiple sensory deficits. These patients were often elderly and diabetic. Their sensory deficits included two or more of the following: uncorrectible visual impairment, neuropathy, vestibular deficits, cervical spondylosis, and orthopedic disorders interfering with walking. The dizziness or light-headedness usually occurred when walking, especially when turning. Touching the examiner's finger often provided enough additional sensory input to relieve the dizzy sensation. Hence, when there are deficits in the visual, proprioceptive, and tactile systems, the patient may become disoriented in the purest sense of the word—with the sensation being described as "dizziness."

Fisher has discussed the occurrence of dizziness or vertigo in his experience with cerebrovascular disease. The following is a summary of dizziness encountered with various lesions:

1. Internal carotid artery and middle cerebral artery disease. Of 140 patients, 8% complained of dizziness, which always occurred with other cerebral signs and was never identified as an isolated symptom of cerebrovascular disease. The best examples of dizziness occurred with disease of the nondominant hemisphere, ie, the hemisphere having the most to do with spatial orientation.

2. Posterior cerebral artery. Of 50 patients with infarction in the distribution of this artery, 24% complained of dizziness. In 8 patients it occurred as prodromal TIAs (Transient Ischemic Attacks) preceding the stroke; in 4 patients it occurred as part of the stroke.

3. Basilar artery. Of 112 patients with basilar artery occlusion, 77% had dizziness. In one-fourth of these patients it was the initial manifestation and was not accompanied initially by any other symptoms. The occurrence of dizziness as the initial symptom and completion of the stroke were usually within six weeks of each other, although in a few cases the dizziness lasted some months before the stroke. The second most common symptom of basilar artery occlusion was dysarthria, followed by numbness of the face, hemiparesis, headache, and diplopia.

4. Anterior inferior cerebellar artery and internal auditory artery. Fisher had 10 cases of sudden onset of unilateral deafness, pointing to occlusion of one of these two arteries. Nine of these cases

complained of dizziness. In 3 of the 10, it was an isolated first sign.

5. Lateral medullary syndrome and vertebral artery. Out of 36 patients, 29 had dizziness; the other 7 had a disturbance of balance but not a feeling of dizziness. Dizziness was an isolated first sign in 7 of the 29 patients and was accompanied by other symptoms in 17 patients. TIAs preceding the stroke usually lasted a day or two, and three weeks at the most.

6. Cerebellar hemorrhage. Acute dizziness, vomiting, and inability to stand or walk may be the initial manifestations of cerebellar hemorrhage.

The generalizations that apply to cerebrovascular disease and dizziness may be summarized as follows (Fisher):

1. Rotatory sensations (vertigo) are more common in peripheral vestibular disorders than in cerebrovascular accidents. Of 86 patients who had dizziness with basilar artery occlusion, only 22% expressed a rotational sensation, whereas as high as 90% or more of patients with peripheral vestibular problems will have vertigo.

2. Dizziness accompanied by only eighth-nerve manifestations (deafness, tinnitus) is usually not vascular in origin. When dizziness accompanied by eighth-nerve symptoms is due to a vascular cause, other brainstem manifestations (diplopia, dysarthria, weakness, headache, numbness, ataxia, and visual impairment) are usually present.

3. Dizzy spells that have recurred for more than six weeks without other manifestations are usually (but not always) not vascular.

4. Positional vertigo is not due to cerebrovascular disease.

Epilepsy can on occasion present as dizziness. Hughes and Drachman studied seizure patients with reference to their complaints of dizziness. They concluded that dizziness associated with "syncopal-like" symptoms (dim vision, pallor, limpness, roaring in ears) could be the manifestation of seizure activity, and when this association is suspected, an EEG and other appropriate investigations should be performed.

Meniere's disease has hearing loss and tinnitus, in addition to vertigo. Cerebellopontine tumors can also produce dizziness and vertigo and, thus, must be included in the differential diagnosis.

Positional dizziness is a relatively frequent complaint of hypertensive patients receiving pharmacologic therapy. Most patients with essential hypertension have a lower than normal plasma volume. Further reduction of plasma volume by diuretic therapy may lead to either symptomatic or asymptomatic orthostatic hypotension. Sympatholytic therapy in the form of beta-blockade, alpha methyl dopa, reserpine, guanethidine, or clonidine may also impair the normal sympathetic response to standing. Basline and follow-up standing (one to three minutes) blood pressure measurements should thus be obtained in all hypertensive patients. Patients are not infrequently seen with a complaint of dizziness (especially matutinal dizziness) without a documented fall in the standing blood pressure. In such situations, it is wise to measure the standing blood pressure again after mild exercise or walking.

Selected References

1. Drachman DA, Hart CW: An approach to the dizzy patient. *Neurology* 22:323–334, 1972.
2. Hughes JR, Drachman DA: Dizziness, epilepsy and the EEG. *Diseases of the Nervous System* 38(6):431–435, 1977.
3. Fisher CM: Vertigo in cerebrovascular disease. *Arch Otolaryng* 85: 529–534, 1967.
4. Frederickson JM, Figge U, Scheid P, Kornhuber HH: Vestibular nerve projection to the cerebral cortex of the rhesus monkey. *Exp Brain Res* 2:318–327, 1966.
5. Brodal A: *Neurological Anatomy.* New York, Oxford University Press, 1969.
6. Carpenter MB: *Human Neuroanatomy.* Baltimore, Williams and Wilkins, 1976.
7. Adams RD, Victor M: *Principles of Neurology.* New York, McGraw-Hill, 1977, pp 178–192.
8. Currens JH: A comparison of the blood pressure in the lying and standing positions: A study of five hundred men and five hundred women. *Am Heart J* 35:646 654, 1948.
9. Hickler RB, Hoskins RG, Hamlin JT III: The clinical evaluation of faulty orthostatic mechanisms. *Med Clin N Am* 44(5):1237–1250, 1960.
10. Talbot S, Smith AJ: Factors predisposing to postural hypotensive symptoms in the treatment of high blood pressure. *Br. Heart J* 37: 1059–1063, 1951.

6. Heat or Cold Intolerance

JOHN A. WARD, MD

Definition

Changes in the metabolism of an organism will affect the way in which the organism will perceive its environment. The patient whose metabolic rate is stimulated by excess thyroid hormones will feel uncomfortable in warm temperatures (heat intolerant). The patient whose metabolic rate is low from lack of normal amounts of thyroid hormones will be abnormally sensitive to cold (cold intolerant).

Technique

Perhaps the simplest direct question is: Do you prefer hot weather or cold weather? Many patients respond by saying, "neither." If the patient does indicate a positive response, the examiner must then determine why. Some patients prefer cold weather because they like winter sports. One patient preferred cold weather because there were no flies in the winter.

If the patient has given a positive response, the second question that is sometimes helpful is: Do you use more or less bedcovers than other members of your household? The answer to this question gives the examiner an indication of how the patient tolerates temperatures in relation to other members of the household.

Determine if there has been a change in heat or cold tolerance. If a change in thyroid function is recent, the patient may not have experienced a summer since becoming hyperthyroid or a winter since becoming hypothyroid. In such a situation a positive response can easily be missed.

Background Information

The immediate control of body temperature is regulated by centers in the hypothalamus that exert autonomic control of both sweating and blood flow to the skin. Thyroid hormones also play a role in body temperature regulation by stimulating the production of calories. The thyroid is normally under the control of the hypothalamus, which secretes thyrotropin-releasing factor (TRF). TRF stimulates the pituitary to release thyroid-stimulating hormone (TSH) which then stimulates the thyroid gland to release thyroxine (T4) and triiodothyronine (T3). The thyroid hormones exert feedback effects on both the hypothalamus and the pituitary.

If the thyroid becomes overactive, it tends to lose normal autoregulatory mechanisms and induces production of too many calories. To remove these excess calories, the body increases blood flow through the skin. Heat loss occurs by radiation, convection, and conduction from the skin surface. If the external temperature is high, the dissipation of heat proceeds slowly and the body produces sweat to utilize the heat of vaporization to divest itself of the unwanted calories. Therefore, hot weather makes the hyperthyroid patient sweaty and uncomfortable. Cold weather provides a greater temperature gradient between the ambient air and the body, making heat transfer from the body to the air more easily accomplished. Thus, the hyperthyroid patient is comfortable in cooler weather. Conversely, the hypothyroid patient has less heat production than normal and tries to conserve heat by using more clothing for insulation.

Clinical Significance

One may make certain objective observations, eg, by shaking hands with the patient. A warm, moist hand suggests hyperthyroidism. A cool dry hand suggests hypothyroidism.

If the patient is dressed in street clothes, it is sometimes helpful to note whether the patient is dressed appropriately for the weather. The hypothyroid patient may wear a sweater on a hot day in July, whereas the hyperthyroid patient may wear a short-sleeved shirt and go without a coat on a cold blustery winter day.

Hypothermia in a comatose patient should suggest myxedema (hypothyroid) coma as well as hypoglycemia.

Changes in heat or cold tolerance are not specific for thyroid disease. Obese patients may complain of heat intolerance; anemic patients often complain of cold intolerance.

Selected References

1. Scott JW: The body temperature, in Best EH, Taylor NB (eds): *The Physiological Basis of Medical Practice,* ed 8. Baltimore, Williams and Wilkins, 1966, chap 70, pp 1413–1427.
2. Ingbar SH, Woeber KA: The thyroid gland: Effects on calorigenesis, in Williams RH (ed): *Textbook of Endocrinology,* ed 5. Philadelphia, WB Saunders, 1974, chap 4, pp 152–153.

3.   Brown J, Chopra IJ, Cornell JS, et al: Thyroid physiology in health and disease. *Ann Intern Med* 81:68–81, 1974.
4.   Hardy JD, Gagge AP, Stolwijk JAJ: *Physiological and Behavioral Temperature Regulation.* Springfield, Ill, Charles C Thomas, 1970.
5.   Hadland DG, Stock JF, Hewitt MI: Heat and cold tolerance: Relation to body weight. *Postgrad Med* 55(4):75–80, 1974.

7.   Thyroid Problems

JOHN A. WARD, MD

Definition

Two major aspects of thyroid problems interest the clinician. The first is the past history of thyroid disease including conditions that could logically affect the function of the thyroid gland. The second is the family history of thyroid disease, since thyroid disorders frequently have a familial incidence.

Technique

Ask: Have you or any member of your family been treated for a goiter or thyroid condition? Since thyroidal enlargement or thyromegaly may be referred to as a goiter, it is best to use the terms "goiter" and "thyroid condition." Positive responses should be recorded on the data base, including the family member's relationship to the patient.

Obtain a history of any surgical operation on the thyroid, the use of thyroid hormones, the use of antithyroid drugs, the use iodine or iodines, and the treatment with radioactive iodine.

If a positive history of thyroid disorder is found in the patient or family member, determine if possible, whether the condition involved a hyperfunctioning gland (hyperthyroidism), a normal functioning gland (euthyroidism), or a hypofunctioning gland (hypothyroidism). A partial list of symptoms of hyperthyroidism would include weight loss, nervousness, irritability, increased sweating, heat intolerance, palpitations, and easy fatigability. Some symptoms of hypothyroidism would include lethargy, cold intolerance, constipation, coarseness of the skin and hair, and swelling of the eyelids.

Inquire about deafness associated with a goiter (Pendred's syndrome). If there is a history of medullary carcinoma of the thyroid, inquire about associated dysfunction of the parathyroid glands (hyperparathyroidism), adrenal medulla (pheochromocytoma), and adrenal cortex (Cushing's disease).

Background Information

The hormones secreted by the thyroid gland are thyroxine (T4) and 3,5,3′ triiodothyronine (T3) (Fig 4). There is now evidence that most of the T3 in the peripheral circulation is derived from T4 by deiodination by cells outside of the thyroid gland. T3 is physiologically more active than T4. A third chemical variety of thyroid hormone, reverse T3, has been recently noted. If the 5-position iodine is deiodinated rather than the 5′ position, the compound 3,3′5′ triiodothyronine (reverse T3) is formed. In certain conditions the blood levels of free T3 are low while the reverse T3 levels are increased. In these conditions the patients may be euthyroid.

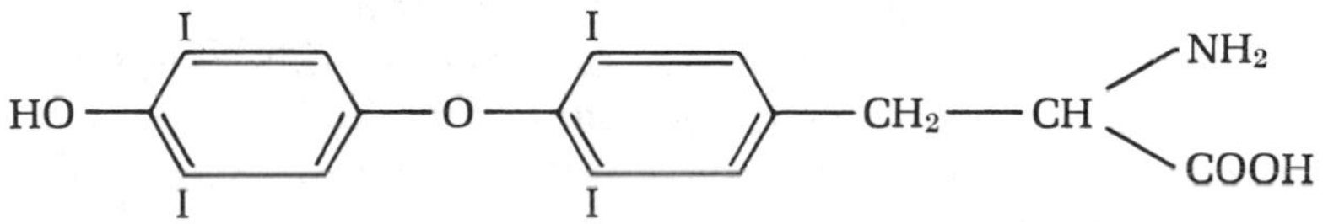

3,5,3′,5′ TETRAIODOTHYRONINE (THYROXINE, T4)

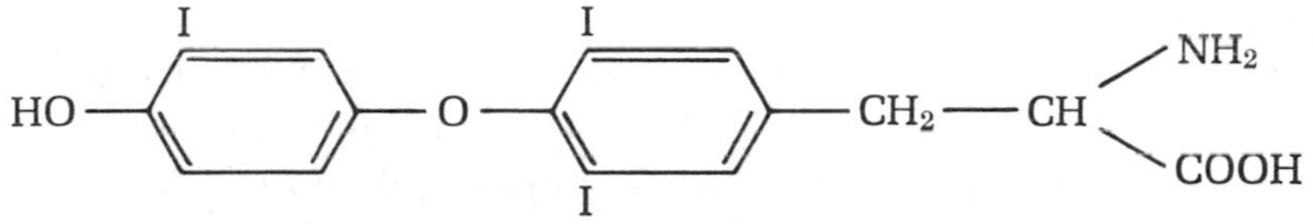

3,5,3′ TRIIODOTHYRONINE (T3)

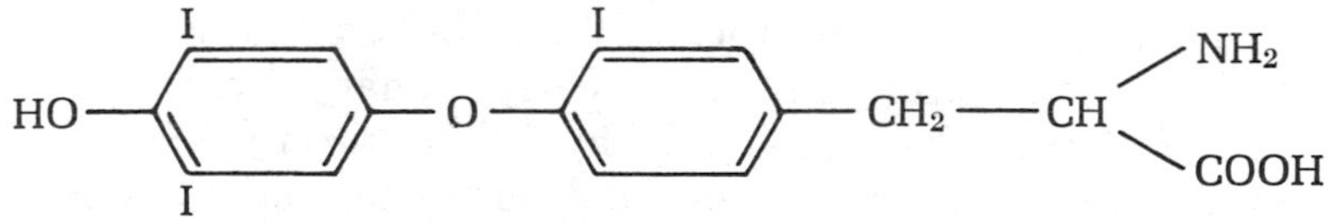

3,3′,′5 TRIIODOTHYRONINE (REVERSE T3)

Figure 4. Hormones secreted by the thyroid gland.

Reverse T3 determinations await further evaluation as to clinical usefulness.

The serum T4, or serum thyroxine, or total T4, is a measurement of the total serum thyroxine. This test is therefore affected by the patient's thyroxine-binding proteins in the serum. The three major plasma proteins that bind thyroxine are albumin, thyroxine-binding globulin (TBG), and thyroxine-binding prealbumin (TBPA). The results of the total serum thyroxine test may be misleading as to the activity of the thyroid since many drugs alter thyroxine binding and many disease states decrease or increase the various thyroxine-binding proteins.

The T3 uptake, or resin triiodothyronine uptake (RT3U), is a measurement of the ability of a patient's serum protein to bind radioactive T3 added to the serum. A secondary binder such as an ion exchange resin binds the radioactive tagged T3 not bound to the patient's thyroxine-binding proteins. Thus, an elevated T4 and T3 uptake is usually seen with hyperthyroidism; a low T4 and T3 uptake, with hypothyroidism. If the T3 uptake is high and the T4 is low, or if the T3 uptake is low and the T4 is high, there is usually an abnormality of the serum thyroxine-binding proteins.

The free thyroxine index is a calculation utilizing the values of the serum T4 and T3 uptake to compensate for abnormalities in the thyroxine-binding proteins. It provides an indirect estimate of the free thyroxine level.

The FT4, or "free" thyroxine, or "free" T4, directly estimates the circulating plasma thyroxine not bound to proteins. This determination bypasses the problems with thyroxine-binding protein. The test may not be available locally but is offered through several commercial laboratories. It may be very helpful in assessing thyroid state in patients with conditions known to alter thyroxine-binding proteins such as pregnancy, low protein states, or the taking of drugs known to alter thyroxine protein binding in the serum.

The T3 RIA, or triiodothyronine by radioimmunoassay, is a measure of the total T3. This test is particularly helpful in hyperthyroidism when the T4 is not elevated and the patient is clinically toxic (T3 toxicosis or T3 hyperthyroidism), although low levels are poor indicators of hypothyroidism.

TSH (thyroid-stimulating hormone) is not a thyroid hormone but a pituitary hormone. The test is performed by radioimmunoassay. An elevated level of TSH is a sensitive index of early primary thyroidal failure. The elevation of TSH in the presence of hypothyroidism helps eliminate the pituitary and the hypothalamus as the cause of thyroidal failure.

The radioiodine uptake by the thyroid measures thyroid trapping of radioactive iodine, usually administered 24 hours earlier. The test is occasionally helpful in factitious hyperthyroidism. In this case the patient is secretly taking thyroid hormone which suppresses the radioiodine uptake in the presence of laboratory and clinical hyperthyroidism. In such cases it would be wise to check iodine uptake over the ovary and base of the tongue to rule out ectopic thyroid tissue.

LATS refers to long-acting thyroid stimulator. The assay is available and is often but not always positive in Graves' disease. A new assay for TSI (thyroid stimulator immunoglobulin) may become available to aid in the evaluation of Graves' disease.

Other tests helpful in thyroid diagnosis are thyroid autoantibodies, particularly in the diagnosis of autoimmune thyroiditis. Thyroid antibodies include antithyroglobulin and antimicrosomal types of antibodies.

Clinical Significance

Hyperthyroidism may have been treated in the past with the antithyroid drugs methimazole or propylthiouracil; surgery; or radioactive iodine, sometimes referred to as the "atomic cocktail." Other drugs such as propranolol, reserpine, or guanethidine have been used as adjunctive therapy with the antithyroid drugs.

Hypothyroidism occurs if the thyroid gland is not producing enough hormone. The patient may be treated with the thyroid hormones L-thyroxine (T4) or triiodothyronine (T3) or with combinations such as desiccated thyroid or thyroid extract. Hypothyroidism may result from primary thyroidal disease such as chronic thyroiditis, pituitary disease with a failure of thyrotropin or thyroid-stimulating hormone (TSH), or hypothalamic disease with a failure of thyrotropin-releasing hormone (TRH). In some instances in which the production of thyroid hormone is suboptimal, such as occurs in the biosynthetic defects of thyroid hormones, TSH from the pituitary induces thyroid hypertrophy, which regresses when thyrotropin is suppressed by the administration of thyroid hormones. These defects in thyroid hormone synthesis are often inherited in several family members. A history of goiters in small children, particularly if the children are cretins, should strongly suggest a defect in thyroid hormone synthesis.

Other thyroid conditions are also important in the patient history. Surgery may have been performed on the thyroid for removal of cosmetically undesirable goiter, removal of a goiter causing obstructive symptoms in the thoracic inlet, or to exclude or remove a thyroid neoplasm. The last is so important that it is good practice to verify the diagnosis by contacting the institution where the surgery was performed. If a tumor was present, try to ascertain the histologic type. A history of thyroid surgery should alert the examiner to evaluate the patient's current thyroid function. Also make certain the parathyroid function is normal, evidenced by a normal serum calcium concentration.

Thyroid hormones may have been utilized in the past both for the treatment of hypothyroidism or to suppress thyroid-stimulating hormone in patients with neoplasms of the thyroid. It is most important to remember that hypothyroidism may be secondary to pituitary or hypothalamic disease and that other endocrine glands may not have normal function. Occasionally, patients without thyroid disease may be taking thyroid hormones for conditions in which they are not indicated.

Iodides are often used in thyroid disease in preparation for surgery. They have also been used for the treatment of iodine-deficient goiters. A history of medications containing iodides or the use of radiographic contrast material containing iodides should be noted because these materials interfere with the radioiodine uptake and scan of the thyroid.

A past history of radioactive iodine treatment is very important because of the increased incidence of hypothyroidism following such therapy. These patients need periodic evaluation for developing hypothyroidism.

Subacute thyroiditis may have been manifested primarily as a pain in the region of the thyroid. Hashimoto's thyroiditis may have been painless but nevertheless resulted in a state of hypothyroidism. A history of an autoimmune thyroiditis (such as Hashimoto's thyroiditis) should alert the examiner not to overlook other autoimmune disorders in the patient.

The long-acting thyroid stimulator (LATS) is an immunoglobulin related to the thyrotoxicosis of Graves' disease. LATS is sometimes detectable in the serum of euthyroid relatives of thyrotoxic patients.

Medullary carcinoma of the thyroid may be a part of a syndrome of multiple endocrine adenomatosis. One should be alert for associated parathyroid adenomas and pheochromocytomas. Parathyroid adenomas may be manifested by renal stones, peptic ulcer disease, pancreatitis, or the bone disease known as osteitis fibrosa cystica. Pheochromocytomas are usually manifested by the complex of hypertension, headaches, palpitations, and sweating.

Selected References

1. Stanbury JB: Familial goiter, in Stanbury JB, Wyngaarden JB, Fredrickson DS: *The Metabolic Basis of Inherited Disease,* ed 2. New York, McGraw-Hill, 1966, chap 10, pp 215–257.

2. McGirr EM: Inherited defects in thyroid hormone synthesis. *Ann Clin Res* 4:200–203, 1972.

3. Fraser GR: The genetics of thyroid disease, in Steinberg AG, Bearn AG (eds): *Progress in Medical Genetics.* New York, Grune and Stratton, 1969, vol 6, chap 3, pp 89–115.

4. Wall JR, Good BF, Hetzel BS: Long-acting thyroid stimulator in euthyroid relatives of thyrotoxic patients. *Lancet* 2:1024–1026, 1969.

5. Steiner AL, Goodman AD, Powers SR: Study of a kindred with pheo-

chromocytoma, medullary thyroid carcinoma, hyperparathyroidism and Cushing's disease: Multiple neoplasia type 2. *Medicine* 47:371–409, 1968.

6. Ingbar SH, Woeber KA: The thyroid gland, in Williams RH (ed): *Textbook of Endocrinology,* ed 5. Philadelphia, WB Saunders, 1974, pp 175–184, 208–210.

7. Soloman DH, Thomas CG Jr, Werner SC: Treatment: Antithyroid drugs; surgery; radioactive iodine, in Werner SC, Ingbar SH (eds): *The Thyroid,* ed 3. New York, Harper and Row, 1971, chap 44, pp 682–711.

8. Robbins J, Rall JE, Gorden P: The thyroid and iodine metabolism in thyroid diseases, nontoxic goiter and thyroid neoplasia: Treatment, in Bondy PK, Rosenberg LE (eds): *(Duncan's Disease of Metabolism: Endocrinology,* ed 7. Philadelphia, WB Saunders, 1974, vol 2, pp 1057–1060.

9. Glennon JA, Gordon ES, Sawin CT: Hypothyroidism after low-dose ^{131}I treatment of hyperthyroidism. *Ann Intern Med* 76(5):721–723, 1972.

10. Dunn JT, Chapman EM: Rising incidence of hypothyroidism after radioactive-iodine therapy in thyrotoxicosis. *N Engl J Med* 271:1037–1042, 1964.

11. Schimmel M, Utiger RD: Thyroidal and peripheral production of thyroid hormones. *Ann Intern Med* 87(6):760–767, 1977.

12. Brown J, Solomon DH, Beall GN, et al: Autoimmune thyroid diseases: Graves' and Hashimoto's. *Ann Intern Med* 83(3):379–391, 1978.

8.   Neck Surgery or Irradiation to the Neck

JOHN A. WARD, MD

Definition

Recent studies show that irradiation to the head or neck increases the risk of thyroid cancer. Past history of surgery to the neck usually indicates previous thyroid or parathyroid disease and may offer the first clue to insufficiency of these glands.

Technique

Begin by asking: Have you had any neck surgery or x-ray treatment to your head and neck? There are many surgical procedures performed on the neck, but the ones pertinent to the endocrine system are those involving the thyroid gland or the parathyroid glands. Any surgery on the thyroid gland should bring forth very specific inquiries about the procedure: Was it total thyroidectomy? subtotal thyroidectomy? hemithyroidectomy? When was the procedure done? And most important, why was it done? Inquire also whether or not the patient is taking or ever received thyroid hormones, calcium, or vitamin D. Further information may be obtained from the hospital or surgeon involved with the procedure.

In patients with positive responses, inquire about symptoms of hypothyroidism such as lethargy, cold intolerance, constipation, or a change in voice. Also inquire about hypoparathyroid symptoms such as numbness and tingling of the extremities, or tetany.

Background Information

Total thyroidectomy may have been performed for carcinoma of the thyroid. Thyroid hormones may be given to suppress thyroid-stimulating hormone (TSH) or they may have been given as replacement therapy if thyroid function was inadequate after surgery.

Radiation therapy to the head and neck in childhood may be associated with carcinoma of the thyroid in later life. Formerly, x-ray therapy was given to infants for presumed enlargement of the thymus. It has also been used for dermatologic conditions of the scalp, as well as for treatment of diseased tonsils and adenoids. The history of irradiation in childhood may not be remembered by the patient, and may be available only from family members.

Clinical Significance

The individual who has had thyroid surgery may now have no thyroid tissue. If the patient had a total thyroidectomy for thyroid cancer, the examiner should be alert for recurrence of the disease, as well as for evidence of metastatic disease. Thyroid cancer is somewhat unusual in that metastatic disease may be first detected many years after the original cancer was removed.

One should also be aware that thyroid surgery may have been performed for a thyroid disease which could eventuate in destruction of the remaining thyroid gland. Thyroiditis (such as Hashimoto's thyroiditis) may have presented as a mass in the thyroid with resultant surgery. The disease may have progressed to destroy the remaining thyroid tissue, leaving the patient in a hypothyroid state. Thus the history of thyroid surgery should alert the examiner to the possibility of abnormal thyroid function.

Since the parathyroid glands are usually associated with the thyroid, one should bear in mind that surgery of the thyroid may have damaged parathyroid function. The examiner should always be sure that the serum calcium is normal.

Ionizing radiation given to the head and neck in childhood should particularly alert the examiner to pay close attention to palpation for thyroid nodules, and to observe the patient carefully for parotid tumors. Recent observations in patients with parathyroid adenomas also reveal an unexpectedly high prevalence of past neck radiation.

Selected References

1. Ingbar SH, Woeber KA: The thyroid gland, in Williams RH (ed): *Textbook of Endocrinology,* ed 5. Philadelphia, WB Saunders, 1974, pp 221–222.
2. Refetoff S, Harrison J, Karanfilski BT, et al: Thyroid carcinoma after irradiation to the neck in infancy and childhood. *N Engl J Med* 292:171–175, 1975.
3. Becker FO, Economou SG: Parotid tumor and thyroid cancer: Simultaneous occurrence after irradiation of the neck in childhood. *JAMA* 232:512–514, 1975.
4. Modan B, Baidatz D, Mart H, et al: Radiation-induced head and neck tumors. *Lancet* 1:277–279, 1974.
5. Information for Physicians: *Irradiation Related Thyroid Cancer.* DHEW Publication No. (NIH) 77–1120.
6. Christensson T, Hyperparathyroidism and radiation therapy. *Ann Intern Med* 89(2):216–217, 1978.

9.　Diabetes and Diabetic Indicators

JOHN K. DAVIDSON, MD, PhD
HARRY DELCHER, MD

Definition

A data base item intended to ascertain if there are historical indicators suggesting the possibility of diabetes. An example of such an indicator would be a positive family history for diabetes.

Technique

Diabetes mellitus may be an unfamiliar term, but the patient may remember a relative who had high blood sugar or who was tested for urine sugar. Ask: Do you know of anyone in your family who has or had diabetes mellitus, high blood sugar, or sugar in the urine? Did anyone ever have to take shots (insulin) every day?

Background Information

The exact genetics of diabetes has been a subject of controversy. Many authorities think that the data best fit the hypothesis of multifactorial inheritance. References 2 through 5 provide statistical guides for the risk of an individual's developing diabetes if certain members or combinations of members of the family have diabetes.

Clinical Significance

The main significance of a positive family history of diabetes is to identify the individual whom one may wish to screen more carefully for diabetes mellitus.

The following 15 additional items obtained from the patient history may be indicators of the presence of diabetes mellitus: unexplained weight loss, polyuria, polydipsia, polyphagia, blurred vision, weakness, pruritis, dry mouth, leg cramps or pains, burning feet; large babies (more than 9 lbs), complications of pregnancy (abortions, toxemia, hydramnios, stillborns who have congenital defects or large islets on autopsy), reactive hypoglycemia, vascular disease, and impotence.

Certain items of information obtained from the physical examination may also indicate the presence of diabetes mellitus. These include obesity; cataracts; glaucoma; retinal hemorrhages; exudates or microaneurysms; vascular bruits; signs of cerebral, coronary, or peripheral vascular disease; hypertension; neuropathy (peripheral, spinal cord and roots, autonomic nervous system or cranial nerves); amytrophic lateral sclerosis; genitourinary abnormalities (Candida vulvovaginitis, Candida balanitis, bacterial bladder and kidney infections, renal failure, nephrotic syndrome); Dupuytren's contracture; xanthomatosis; skin abnormalities (necrobiosis lipoidica diabeticorum, granuloma annulare, alopecia, pyogenic or fungal infections); foot abnormalities (dermatophytosis, onychomycosis, trophic ulcers, arterial insufficiency, gangrene); peridontal disease; and other infections including tuberculosis and mucormycosis.

The patient with a positive family history of diabetes mellitus should be familiar with classic symptoms of diabetes mellitus such as polydipsia, polyuria, polyphagia, and weight loss. The patient should be encouraged to seek medical attention if these symptoms occur.

Selected References

1. Simpson NE: Genetic considerations, in *Diabetes Mellitus: Diagnosis and Treatment* New York, American Diabetes Assoc, 1971, vol 3, pp 71–75.
2. Rimoin DL: Inheritance in diabetes mellitus. *Med Clin N Am* 55(4): 807–819, 1971.
3. Smith C, Falconer DS, Duncan LJP: A statistical and genetical study of diabetes: II. Heritability of liability. *Ann Hum Genet* 35(3):281–299, 1972.
4. Darlow JM, Smith C, Duncan LJP: A statistical and genetical study of diabetes: III. Empiric risks to relatives. *Ann Hum Genet* 37(2):157–174, 1973.
5. Thompson GS: Genetics of diabetes mellitus in man. *Horm Metab Res* 4(suppl):123–128, 1974.
6. Baumslag N, Yodaiken RE: Should diabetics marry? *Lancet* 2:59, 1969.

10. Visual Dysfunction

FRANK C. BELL, MD

Definition

Visual dysfunction is a subjective decrease in visual acuity described by the patient as blurred vision, or an objective decrease in vision to less than 20/20 acuity. Other visual complaints may include ocular discomfort or a changed appearance of the eyes.

Technique

The first question to ask the patient is whether he has any eye difficulty. If the answer is yes, describe and record the nature of the complaint in the patient's own words. State whether or not the patient wears glasses.

A series of leading questions should be asked regarding the symptoms of eye diseases, since many patients cannot easily describe their ocular difficulties. Inquire whether there is any visual disturbance, pain, or discomfort in the eyes, and whether there has been any change in appearance of the eyes of surrounding structures. Ask about any previous eye injury or operation and any eye medications currently being used. Finally, ask if there is a family history of eye disease such as glaucoma, cataract, retinal detachment, crossed or deviating eyes (strabismus), or eye tumors.

Background Information

There are many causes of eye difficulties, some easily understood and others obscure even to the ophthalmologist. Visual disturbances can result from anatomical or physiological abnormalities of the eyes, optic nerves, or brain. Pain or discomfort in the eyes is a cardinal symptom of ocular diseases, but not all serious ocular diseases cause pain. A changed appearance of the eyes occurs in a wide variety of pathologic conditions.

These changes may indicate ocular pathology or eye involvement by systemic disease.

Clinical Significance

Disturbance of vision must always be explained. The most common cause is refractive error, and this is corrected with glasses. There are many other visual symptoms that have commonly associated causes. Some of these are listed below.

Visual Symptoms	Common Causes
Loss of central (reading) vision	Cataract, retinal detachment, vitreous hemorrhage
Loss of peripheral (side) vision	Glaucoma, retinitis pigmentosa, hemianopsia
Distorted vision	Retinal degeneration, temporal lobe disease
Flashes of light; floating spots	Retinal detachment, migraine, occipital lobe disease
Double vision (diplopia)	Third, fourth, sixth cranial nerve paresis, trauma, anticholinergic drugs
Halos around lights	Glaucoma, corneal disease
Transient loss or obscuration of vision (amaurosis fugax)	Arterial disease or emboli, papilledema, multiple sclerosis
Colored vision	Digitalis toxicity

Pain in the eye is most frequently of ocular origin, but is sometimes referred to the eye from the sinuses and extracranial structures. In acute glaucoma, pain may be referred to the abdominal area and be associated with nausea and vomiting. Listed below are painful complaints regarding the eyes and some likely causes.

Pain Symptoms	Common Causes
Sharp acute pain in eye	Corneal foreign body, acute glaucoma, other causes
Dull aching pain in eye	Intraocular inflammation, glaucoma, other causes
Sensitivity to light	Corneal disease or intraocular inflammation
Headaches above eyes	Rarely due to refractive error or muscle imbalance
Pain behind eye	Retrobulbar neuritis
Burning, stinging, gritty sensation	Conjunctival inflammation or tear deficiency

A change in the appearance of the eyes suggests either a specific disease of the eye or a sign of a systemic disease affecting the eye. Listed next are some observed changes in the eye and possible causes.

Observed Change	*Common Causes*
Red eye	Conjunctivitis, corneal foreign body, acute glaucoma, intraocular inflammation
Yellow discoloration of conjunctiva	Jaundice
Mucopurulent discharge	Conjunctivitis, allergy
Excessive tearing	Blocked tear ducts, ocular inflammation
Involuntary rhythmic movements of eyes (nystagmus)	Neurological defects, blindness in infancy
Elevated yellow deposits medial to upper lids (xanthelasma)	Hyperlipidemia
Subconjunctival hemorrhage	Usually idiopathic
Crossed or deviating eye (strabismus)	Nerve paralysis, idiopathic
Bulging eye (exophthalmos)	Thyroid disease, orbital tumor
Blue sclera	Osteogenesis imperfecta

Selected References

1. Scheie HG, Albert DM: Symptomatology of eye diseases, in *Textbook of Ophthalmology,* ed 7. Philadelphia, WB Saunders, 1977, pp 159–168.
2. Vaughn D, Asbury T: *General Ophthalmology,* ed 8. Los Altos, Calif, Lange Medical Publications, 1977, pp 14–16.
3. Roy FH: *Ocular Differential Diagnosis,* ed 2. Philadelphia, Lea and Febiger, 1975.

11. Difficulty Hearing or Deaf

JOHN H. PER-LEE, MD

Definition

Decreased perception of loudness and/or diminished speech intelligibility. The quantitative unit of loudness is the decibel. Normal hearing threshold is 0–10 decibels. When one says a person has lost 40 decibels of hearing, it is the same as saying that person has a threshold of 40 decibels. This unit can apply to a discrete frequency (pitch) or to human speech, a complex of many frequencies. Decrease in speech intelligibility implies an inability to understand speech. While an abnormal threshold accompanies diminished understanding, it does not determine the degree of impaired discrimination.

Technique

With questioning to determine whether the hearing loss seems unilateral or bilateral, try to have the patient distinguish between loss of loudness acuity and loss of speech intelligibility. In the former category it is difficult to hear; in the latter, difficult to understand. Of additional importance is whether the hearing loss is stable, progressive, or fluctuating and when the patient thinks the symptom began.

A patient's subjective sense of loss is not a linear function of the actual loss. An initial 10–15-decibel threshold drop may not be noticed. Furthermore, awareness of sound is a function of how critical one's hearing requirements may be and how carefully the listener concentrates. By the time a loss for speech averages 20–25 decibels, an alert patient will perceive the problem. A loss exceeding 30–40 decibels for the speech frequencies (300–3,000 cycles) is unacceptable for conversational communication. Yet, a patient has to lose hearing through a range of 110 decibels before his hearing could be considered totally gone. These generalizations apply if a loss is present in both ears. On the other hand, unilateral hearing loss, even when total, does not interfere with normal face-to-face communication even though competing noise and sound localization are more of a problem.

One can elicit historical clues that suggest a patient's hearing problem to be one of two types. These are defined as conductive and sensorineural hearing losses. The next section will define each of these. Discrimination is generally unimpaired with a conductive hearing loss. A patient with such a loss will note sound to be dimmed. Yet, when it is sufficiently amplified, it is clear and intelligible. Such impairment causes the patient to seem to hear better than a person who hears normally in a noisy environment. This is because the patient's loss attenuates the background noise that would otherwise interfere or mask the speech he or she wishes to hear. The opposite is true of the neurally impaired patient. In this instance environmental noise interferes even more than normal with speech perception. Under ideal listening conditions, ie, in a quiet environment, the functional disability of a sensorineural hearing loss relates to the frequencies involved and the quantity for each frequency.

Background Information

Hearing function is conveniently considered as occurring in two phases. Phase one is the conductive phase and involves the collection and passage of mechanical vibratory sound energy from the gaseous medium of the environment to the fluid medium of the inner ear. Since energy is largely reflected at the interface of air and water, an efficient impedance-matching system with a mechanical advantage of 23:1 serves to prevent this energy loss. This system comprises the eardrum and its attached ossicles. Diseases of this anatomy attenuate loudness, but distort sound's other physical qualities very little.

The second phase is the sensorineural phase. It begins in the cochlea where the hair cells of the Corti organ transduce vibratory energy into electric potentials. The coding of loudness and pitch occur here. This information is transmitted via the auditory nerve and brainstem through several intervening nuclear synapses to the auditory cortex for decoding and understanding. Disease or damage in this sensorineural system reduces loudness and distorts sound quality. Thus, in summary, hearing loss is labeled conductive when disease affects phase-one structures and sensorineural when it affects phase-two structures.

Sensorineural loss is further divided into cochlear and retrocochlear categories. Special tests enable one to differentiate cochlear and retrocochlear lesions. Such differentiation is sophisticated and requires especially skilled personnel to accomplish it. However, accurate diagnosis requires it to be done when the locus and etiology of a loss is not otherwise clear. For one thing, the etiology and complications of retrocochlear disease tend to be more threatening to the patient's welfare. In the adult, sensorineural loss is statistically much more common than conductive loss. The reverse is true for children and adults to age 40. For the neurally impaired, cochlear loss is several times more common than retrocochlear loss.

The audible sound spectrum ranges 16–16,000 cycles per second (cps). The majority of human speech sounds are bracketed by the frequencies 300–3,000 cps. The highest frequency phonemes and the overtones which refine speech quality, however, exceed 3,000 cps. Thus, loss of acuity above this frequency, often the only deficit seen in early sensorineural lesions, will generally affect discrimination of clarity of sound. Such adversity is noted more in a noisy environment.

Loudness is measured in decibels. One decibel equals 2×10^{-4} dynes per square centimeter. A loudness scale is logarithmic. For example, a 20-decibel tone has 100 times more energy than a 1-decibel tone. A 30-decibel tone contains 1,000 times more energy than a 1-decibel tone. The examiner seeks to know how many decibels of loudness it takes for a patient to hear a discrete frequency or human speech. Loudness threshold is the least intense sound perceived by the individual, or stated differently, the weakest sound audible to the patient. Standard normal threshold was derived by testing thousands of people. This normal is arbitrarily considered zero decibels. Techniques using tuning forks can differentiate conductive from sensorineural loss. The audiometer, designed to produce variably loud discrete frequency tones and variably loud speech signals, measures the exact loss and also differentiates the two types of loss.

The labyrinth or peripheral balance receptor is located within the otic capsule of each temporal bone. Information from each side is integrated in the central nervous system. Disturbance of this function produces a special disorientation called vertigo. While not discussed here, it is mentioned to remind the reader that disease in the otic capsule affecting the cochlea often involves the labyrinth too. By the same token since the VIIIth cranial nerve carries impulses subserving both functions, cerebral pontine angle lesions affecting one function often affect both.

Clinical Significance

Etiology of Hearing Loss

I. Conductive
   A. External canal obstruction: cerumen, foreign body, discharge, tumor, polyp, atresia
   B. Perforated eardrum: infection, trauma
   C. Intact but limited eardrum motion: middle ear fluid, exudate, fibrosis, and adhesions

D. Fixation or disruption of ossicles
   1. Fibrosis: tympanosclerosis, adhesions
   2. Atrophy and necrosis
   3. Bone proliferation: otosclerosis, postinflammatory osteoplasia
   4. Congenital
   5. Neoplasm
E. Other

II. Sensorineural
   A. Congenital: lesions and hearing loss bilateral and symmetrical
      1. Endogenous: inherited defect, positive family history
      2. Exogenous: damage during intrauterine life or during birth process: anoxia, rubella, RH incompatibility
   B. Toxic
      1. Febrile: eg, measles, flu, pneumonia
      2. Drugs: dihydrostreptomycin, neomycin, kanamycin, gentamycin
   C. Degeneration: hair cells, supporting cells, ganglion cells
      1. Vascular insufficiency: loss either symmetrical or asymmetrical, either progressive or more stable
      2. Aging: loss symmetrical, usually progressive
      3. Deteriorating biochemistry: loss either asymmetrical or symmetrical, either progressive or stable
      4. Hereditary: loss symmetrical and progressive, early, late
   D. Insults: generally unilateral but can be bilateral: loss asymmetrical and if pathology controlled, stable
      1. Infection
         a. Cochlear: viral (most common cause of sudden hearing loss), bacteria, syphilis (congenital and acquired)
         b. Retrocochlear: meningitis
      2. Trauma: Fractures, concussive
      3. Acute vascular insufficiency
   E. Tumor temporal bone and cerebral pontine angle: loss generally unilateral and progressive—acoustic neuroma, metastatic tumor
   F. Endolymphatic hydrops: loss unilateral in 80% and bilateral in 20%, usually asymmetrical and fluctuating—Meniere's disease, fluctuating hearing loss
   G. Other inflammatory disorders: loss both unilateral and bilateral—collagen disease, vasculitis

H. Noise-induced: loss bilateral, asymmetrical, progressive—acoustic trauma, concussive

I. Functional hearing loss: loss unilateral, bilateral, asymmetrical: psychogenic, malingering

J. Central nervous system: loss fluctuating and/or progressive —multiple sclerosis, other neuropathies, tumor, vascular insufficiency

Selected References

1. Paparella M, Shumrick D (eds): *Otolaryngology: Basic Sciences and Related Disciplines*. Philadelphia, WB Saunders, 1973, vol 1, pp 241–317, 943–985.

2. Paparella M, Shumrick D (eds): *Otolaryngology: Ear*. Philadelphia, WB Saunders, 1973, vol 2, pp 55–262, 309–425, 439–468.

3. Shambaugh GE Jr (ed): *Surgery of the Ear*, ed 2. Philadelphia, WB Saunders, 1967, pp 71–98, 369–400.

12. Tinnitus

MICHAEL F. LUBIN, MD

Definition

Any sound perceived for which there is no external source. It may be unilateral or bilateral. Tinnitus can be classified into cranial, aural, and neural origins (see Table 3). It can also be divided into subjective tinnitus, which is evident only to the patient; and objective tinnitus, which can be perceived by another person. Subjective tinnitus constitutes the vast majority, about 99% of patients.

Technique

The symptom of tinnitus is easily established by asking about any ringing or noise in the ears. Ask the patient if the sound is unilateral or bilateral and if vertigo or hearing loss are associated symptoms. Other

Table 3. Etiologies of tinnitus.*

Cranial	Aural	Neural
Cervical venous hums	*External ear*	*Cochlear*
Carotid bruits	Cerumen	Otosclerosis
Cardiac murmurs	Otitis externa	Meniere's disease
Arteriovenous	Tympanic membrane	Labyrinthitis
malformations	perforation	Cochlear contusion
Hyperdynamic circula-	Myringitis	Presbycusis
tion, eg, anemia	Foreign body	Noise exposure
Essential objective		
tinnitus		
Temporomandibular	*Middle ear*	*Central pathways*
joint sounds	Otitis media	Acoustic neuroma
	Otosclerosis	Cerebellar pontine
	Traumatic ossicular	angle tumors
	disruption	Concussion
	Barotrauma (skin	Cortical tumors
	diving, flying)	Seizure disorders
	Middle-ear tumors	*Drugs*
	Neuromuscular tics	Excessive alcohol,
		tea, coffee
		Aspirin
		Aminoglycoside
		antibiotics
		Quinine
		Furosemide

* Idiopathic: the most frequent cause.

important features include the duration of the sound, ie, continuous or intermittent; the duration of the symptom, ie, days, weeks, or months.

Additional history that may give clues to etiology includes age; occupational history, especially noise exposure; emotional problems; ear infections; ear or head trauma; drug history (particularly salicylates); and neurologic disease or symptoms, especially dizziness or vertigo.

Physical examination should include the external canal, tympanic membrane, and hearing, including Weber and Rinne tests. On the general examination listen carefully for orbital, cranial, or carotid bruits as well as cardiac murmurs and venous hums. A careful cranial nerve examination should be performed.

Figure 5 demonstrates a technique of occasional value if the sound is suspected to be of vascular or muscular origin, ie, objective tinnitus. Take the ear pieces and tubing from one stethoscope and connect them with

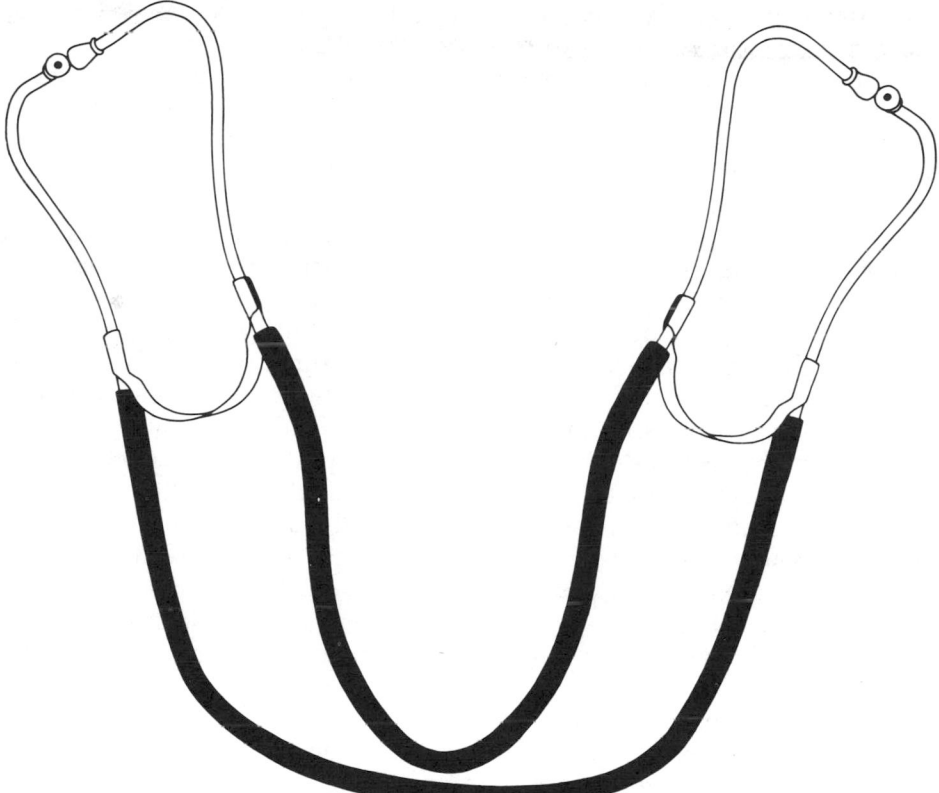

Figure 5. A method of connecting stethoscopes that will enable physician and patient to listen together for tinnitus.

the ear pieces of another. Then the patient and physician each have a pair of ear pieces, and the sound may be audible to the physician as well.

Background Information

The origins of objective tinnitus require little explanation. Clearly cranial sources of vibration beyond those to which the auditory system is accustomed to receiving, eg, vascular bruit, cardiac murmur, or ear muscle contraction, may force an unbidden intrusion of sound upon the consciousness of the individual.

The physiologic basis of aural tinnitus is akin to that of cranial origin. It has been postulated that forces which decrease the ability of the outside sounds to stimulate the auditory apparatus, such as cerumen, middle-ear infections, may allow certain internal vibrations or sounds which are usually masked by ambient noise to become audible.

The understanding of neural disorders producing tinnitus is more complex. Sensory nerve fibers carry only their own sensory stimulus; thus, when the auditory nerve is stimulated the only sensation perceived is hearing. Hearing will not result unless the areas of the auditory cortex are stimulated by the mechanical and neural mechanisms of the auditory apparatus. It seems reasonable to conclude that in some way all the various causes of neural tinnitus have a final common pathway of stimulating the auditory system somewhere along its path to the auditory cortex.

The centerpiece of a discussion of neural tinnitus is the cochlear division of the membranous labyrinth. This formation, with its precision of structure and function, is akin to a microcomputer. The cochlear hair cells mounted upon the basilar membrane and surrounded by endolymph are resonant with a surprisingly broad vibratory spectrum (20–20,000 Hz). It is subject to damage by a large number of offending conditions, and tinnitus may result when the auditory epithelium, basilar membrane, or endolymph is subjected to various disease processes. However, total ablation of the cochlea with a labyrinthectomy or section of the cochlear division of the eighth nerve may still leave the patient with subjective tinnitus. This is centrally mediated although the end-organ disorder may have been the inciting event.

Any insult to the cochlear or auditory apparatus will produce, to an independently variable degree, both deafness and tinnitus. A few examples will follow with comments upon possible physiologic mechanisms:

1. Noise exposure. If the basilar membrane is forced to vibrate beyond its accustomed amplitude for too long, the auditory epithelium will be damaged. In some unknown way, this receptive surface will then spontaneously discharge impulses to the auditory axons, thus producing an extraneous buzzing or hissing high-pitched sound since the segment of basilar membrane housing the higher frequencies is more sensitive to noise effect.

2. Meniere's disease. This fairly common disorder of unknown etiology besets the entire membranous labyrinth with symptoms characteristically intermittent of severe vertigo and tinnitus. Its pathology involves the endolymph, the fluid which bathes the auditory epithelium in the cochlea.

3. Auditory nerve lesions. Lesions affecting the auditory nerve will produce a decrement in hearing and may also cause tinnitus. The mechanism may well be secondary to nerve damage which, akin to peripheral nerve damage, may lead to abnormal sensation as well as loss of sensation; that is, tinnitus and hearing loss. Loss of myelin may perhaps be the common pathogenetic factor. An example of this type of lesion is acoustic neuroma.

4. Central lesions. Central lesions that directly involve the audi-
    tory cortex may be caused by an epileptiform discharge and
    cause several auditory experiences, including tinnitus or more
    complex auditory hallucinations.

Clinical Significance

Extraneural tinnitus of the vascular type may be described as pul-
sating or rusing and is often found to be associated with cardiac murmurs
or carotid bruits. This type of sound may also be associated with arteriovenous malformations. If the tinnitus is described as humming and is affected by light pressure on the neck or head position (occluding cervical
veins), it may be a cervical venous hum (see section 142).

Tinnitus of the aural type may be related to neuromuscular tics of
the stapedius, tensor tympani, or tensor palati muscles, or the opening and
closing of the eustachian tube, as in pharyngeal disorders. These sounds
are usually described as clicking or fluttering and are always low in pitch.

Neural tinnitus is a broader and more difficult topic. However, there
are a number of causes that are easily discovered during the history or
physical examination. Particularly in younger patients, there are a multitude of ear inflammations, usually of the middle ear, that extend to involve
the labyrinth. The importance of noise exposure in this group of young
patients cannot be overemphasized since it is a preventable cause of tinnitus and hearing loss.

More obscure causes of tinnitus include Meniere's disease and acute
idiopathic labyrinthitis. These conditions are usually accompanied by severe vertigo with nausea and vomiting as well as variable hearing loss.
Labyrinthitis is self-limited, and Meniere's disease is usually recurrent.

The most difficult group to sort out are those disorders without obvious cause. These patients constitute the vast majority of tinnitus. A part
of this large group should perhaps include presbycusis, the tinnitus of old
age. The only historical and physical examination information of note is
that the sound is usually bilateral, continuous, of long duration, and associated with subjective and objective evidence of hearing loss. Unfortunately, in this large group of patients, virtually nothing can be done to
alleviate the symptom. There is no known medical or surgical therapy that
has proved efficacious.

A more imperative example of subjective tinnitus is that which is
unilateral; cerebellopontine angle tumor, most often acoustic neuroma,
must then be considered. In this condition the tinnitus is usually continuous, most often of long duration, and associated with progressive unilateral hearing loss. Acoustic neuromas occur most frequently in young and
middle-aged adults. The diagnosis is made with sophisticated audiometric
and radiologic examination.

Selected References

1.   Simonson KM: Tinnitus. *Postgrad Med* 34:445–448, 1963.
2.   Parkin JL: Tinnitus evaluation. *Am Famil Physician* 8:151–155, 1973.
3.   Kiang NYS, Moxon EC, Levine RA: Auditory nerve activity in cats with normal and abnormal cochleas, in Wolstenholme GEW, Knight J (eds): *Sensorineural Hearing Loss*. London, Churchill, 1970, pp 268–273.
4.   Donaldson I: Tinnitus: A theoretical view and a therapeutic study using amylobarbitone. *J Laryng Otol* 92:123–130, 1978.

---

13.   Epistaxis

JOHN H. PER-LEE, MD

Definition

Epistaxis implies bleeding from the nose; however, the anatomical origin can be a contiguous structure such as the paranasal sinus or the nasopharynx. In those instances in which the origin is other than the nose proper, the nose is simply a conduit to the outside.

Technique

There is little difficulty eliciting this symptom. The distinctive visual qualities of blood are not mimicked by other potential nasal secretions. Bleeding varies in amount, frequency, and side of nose from which it comes. If a patient is seen during an episode, one can see the nose and throat to confirm bleeding. On the other hand, if bleeding has ceased and especially if the patient complains of blood expectoration rather than nosebleed, one has to consider not only a nasal source but one from the mouth, pharynx, larynx, endobronchial tree, and esophagus.

Nasal bleeding is conveniently subdivided into anterior and posterior sites. In the upright patient an anterior origin will expel blood primarily through the nares. A posterior site causes a flow primarily into the pharynx. The supine patient, of course, will drain all bleeding into the pharynx. Ultimate localization requires a careful examination.

In addition to localizing the bleeding point, the historian should seek clues as to the underlying etiology. Etiology is always local and can be systemic. One seeks clues of local inflammation, trauma, tumor, and environmental irritation. The clinician looks for evidence of blood dyscrasia, vascular disease, chronic illness, hypertension, and liver disease.

Background Information

The internal nose is well supplied with blood vessels. They originate in both the external and internal carotid circulation. Nasal palatine and sphenopalatine branches of the internal maxillary artery supply two-thirds of the nose, chiefly the posterior and inferior tissues. This contrasts with the internal carotid supply that nourishes the anterior superior one-third of the nose via the anterior and posterior ethmoidal arteries. This anatomy can vary from patient to patient. These two systems converge and anastomose at the caudal end of the nasal septum in what is called Kiesselbach's triangle. This is located just behind the nares. This area is the site of most anterior bleeding. For example, 95% of pediatric nosebleeds come from here. Subject as it is to trauma (nose blowing, wiping, picking), drying, and irritation, it is easy to see why bleeding frequently occurs at this site. The inferior meatus and the sphenoethmoid recess are the most common posterior bleeding sites. Adults are more likely to bleed from these places.

Epistaxis requires you to look for local and systemic causes. There is always a local reason; there may be a systemic contributor.

Clinical Significance

Local	*Systemic*
1. Inflammation	1. Hypertension
a. Acute infection	2. Arteriosclerotic disease
b. Allergic reaction	3. Blood dyscrasia
c. Parasympathetic reaction	a. Malignant disease, eg, leukemia
d. Granulomatous disease	b. Clotting defect
e. Vasculitis and unusual autoimmune states	4. Liver disease
2. Trauma	5. Chronic renal disease and chronic illness in general

Local	*Systemic*

3. Drying
   a. Atrophic mucosa
   b. Anatomical irregulari-
      ties
4. Tumor
5. Foreign body
6. Telangiectasia and vascular
   incompetency

6. Osler-Weber-Rendu disease
   (familial hemorrhagic
   telangiectasia)

Selected References

1. Paparella M, Shumrick D (eds): *Otolaryngology: Head and Neck.* Philadelphia, WB Saunders, 1973, vol 3, pp 48–62.
2. Paparella M, Shumrick D (eds): *Otolaryngology: Basic Sciences and Related Disciplines.* Philadelphia, WB Saunders, 1973, vol 1, pp 704–710.

14. Hoarseness

JOHN S. TURNER, MD

Definition

Any change in the quality of the normal voice may be called hoarseness or laryngitis by the patient.

Technique

The complaint of hoarseness can be evaluated only by viewing the hypopharynx and larynx with a laryngeal mirror and headlight. The proper technique can be mastered only by practice on a laryngeal manikin and on fellow students in the clinic.

Background Information

Vocal quality depends on the smooth flow of a column of air past the vibrating edge of a true vocal cord. Cord tension is maintained by the function of the adductor and abductor muscles of the larynx, which are innervated by the vagus nerve, superior and recurrent laryngeal branches (see reference 2).

Hoarseness may be created by abnormal function of these nerves or by lesions which inhibit airflow or restrict movement of the larynx and adjacent tissues.

Clinical Significance

Hoarseness may be a harmless sign of very minor vocal abuse (football cheerleading) or an extremely serious major cancer in the hypopharynx, larynx, thyroid, or lung.

Hoarseness that has been present for longer than three weeks must be evaluated by mirror examination, neck palpation, chest x-ray, and perhaps barium swallow or laryngeal tomograms and a complete blood count.

Cigarette smoking is very common; therefore hoarseness as a symptom of a minor or major illness is very common.

Selected References

1. Bryce DP (ed): *Differential Diagnosis and Treatment of Hoarseness.* Springfield, Ill, Charles C Thomas, 1974.
2. Saunders WH: The larynx. *Ciba Clin Symp* 16(3):67–99, 1964.
3. Becker W (ed): *Atlas of Otorhinolaryngology and Bronchoesophagology.* Philadelphia, WB Saunders, 1969.

15. Sinusitis

JOHN H. PER-LEE, MD

Definition

Sinusitis is an expression used by patients when the symptom is facial pain, headache, nasal congestion, or occasionally nasal airway obstruction.

Technique

The word "sinus" is a misnomer that the patient substitutes for the aforementioned symptoms. It may also be a substitute for tightness, drawing, and dryness. The examiner needs to translate the patient's complaint of sinus into a more accurate description. It is easy, for example, to ask about obstruction, discharge, and pain.

Sinus pathology produces pain in the area of the involved sinus: maxillary sinus (cheek), ethmoid sinus (nasal root and eye), frontal sinus (midfrontal region), sphenoid sinus (deep head or vortex). However, sinus pain can radiate to a higher or more distal site. Such pain is generally aching in quality. Body position influences its severity. For example, maxillary sinus pain is likely to increase in the upright position and decrease after the patient reclines. The maxillary ostia open high on the media sinus wall, a position from which retained secretion is less likely to drain when the patient is in an upright position. Conversely, frontal and/or ethmoid pathology will cause greater discomfort in the recumbent position. While sinus disease can produce headache, 85% of all headaches are not a reflection of sinus, eye, or intracranial pathology. They are categorized as either vascular or tension headache.

Obstruction implies, of course, an inability to breathe air through the nose. Is it unilateral, bilateral, or fluctuating? Is it related to environment, season, or accompanied by any of the aforementioned symptoms?

Relative to drainage, one desires to know the amount, color, and viscosity. The normal nose secretes a pint of low-viscosity seromucus per 24 hours. Decreases are associated with increased viscosity. So-called postnasal drip is a reflection of this increased viscosity. Increases are usually of lower-viscosity material and associated with abnormal stimulation, as with an acute insult (viral, allergenic, trauma). The abundant thick mucus produced in cystic fibrosis is an exception to this tendency.

Tightness, drawing, and dryness are associated with reduced function and atrophy. The patient mistakes these symptoms for "congestion." True congestion implies increased nasal activity. The notion that the patient with such congestion has exaggerated nasal activity leads to an inappropriate prescription of nasal drying agents. A simple nasal examination will prevent this error.

Background Information

The paranasal sinuses consist of four paired pneumatic cavities in immediate relation to the nose. They develop as contiguous extensions of the nasal chambers and are subject to many of the same insults.

Clinically, the sinuses are more usefully divided into two groups: the anterior and posterior groups. The anterior group consists of the frontal, maxillary, and anterior ethmoidal sinuses. The ethmoidal sinus is a labyrinth of 3–15 cells, and is divided by the root of the middle turbinate into an anterior and posterior half. The anterior sinuses have in common the fact that they ventilate and drain through the middle meatus. The posterior sinuses include the posterior ethmoid and sphenoid sinuses and communicate with the nose through the superior meatus. Protruding from the lateral nasal wall are three hanging ledges, the turbinates, whose function is to offer a large surface area over which air can flow in streamlined fashion.

The nasal mucosa is covered by respiratory pseudostratified columnar epithelium topped with cilia which beat posteriorly and exchange the surface mucous blanket every 10 minutes. The submucosal stroma, especially of the middle and inferior turbinates, is richly endowed with mixed scromucinous glands and blood sinusoidal spaces. The former dominate the middle turbinate; the latter, the inferior turbinate.

The nose is under autonomic control and has a marked capacity for moisture production and tissue swelling. A partial capacity for bacterial and viral neutralization exists, but the chief purpose served by the nose other than olfaction is the warming, moistening, and cleaning of air on its way to the lungs. Noxious stimuli, sensitizing foreign proteins (allergens), infectious agents, and emotional conflict, to mention the more common offenders, all induce an exaggeration of what is otherwise normal physiologic activity. Increased secretion and swelling are translated into symptoms of runny nose (rhinorrhea), airway obstruction, fullness, or maybe even aching pain.

Pain receptors are abundant around the sinus ostia. Sufficient swelling and pressure there can produce an ache felt anywhere around the nose, eyes, nasal root, or frontal region, even over the vortex if the posterior sinuses are obstructed.

Obstruction to the ventilation of a sinus produces discomfort if there is a sufficient drop in intrasinus pressure. Gas (oxygen, then nitrogen) is absorbed by the mucosa and is not replaced until ventilation is restored. Obstruction also produces secretion stasis and, in time, infection since pathogens are in the environment. Obstruction, stasis, infection—this is the pathogenesis of infectious sinusitis.

For various reasons the nose may become hypofunctional, even atrophic. Given sufficient dryness, the nasal mucous blanket ceases to clear unwanted matter and invading microorganisms. As previously pointed out, such a state produces many of the same symptoms common to a hyperfunctioning nose. To review, these include a congestive feeling, fullness, and at times an ache. The atrophic nose may burn and feel drawn or tight.

Clinical Significance

Again, the word "sinus" suggests any of the following: ache, pain, discharge, obstruction, congestion, tightness, burning, and dryness.

It is useful first to organize one's thinking around deviations from normal nasal function.

I.   Obstruction, discharge, maybe ache or pain, and congestion
    A.   Inflammatory disease (rhinitis and sinusitis)
        1.   Acute and chronic infection: viral, bacterial, fungal (rare)
        2.   Common hypersensitivity states: acute hay fever, chronic allergic rhinitis, nasal polyposis
        3.   Rare hypersensitivity states: vasculitis, granulomatosis (autoimmune mechanism), sarcoidosis
        4.   Nonspecific rhinitis
            a.   Air irritants (eg, smoke)
            b.   Excessive nosedrop usage
        5.   Cystic fibrosis
    B.   Parasympathetic dominance (vasomotor rhinitis in contrast to specific allergic rhinitis)
        1.   Psychogenic
        2.   Hypothyroidism
        3.   Pregnancy

II.   Burning, dryness, tightness, "congestion": tissues inflamed by virtue of lost moisture and organism defense; mucous blanket

diminished or gone; cilia nonfunctional; bacteria can be cultured; crusts form if membranes are dry enough
A.   Longstanding inflammation of any etiology
B.   Iatrogenic: surgery, medication
C.   Premature degeneration of functional nasal elements, etiology unknown
D.   Segmental, one chamber or the other becomes atrophic as a result of anatomical distortions and altered air current flow

The commonest problems in the aforementioned outline are the hyperfunctional inflammatory states such as an acute rhinitis (an element of an acute upper respiratory infection) and allergic rhinitis. The presence of an obstructed infected sinus as distinguished from simple nasal pathology depends upon physical examination. However, local facial pain in the setting of acute infection suggests the possibility.

Other disease processes associated with nasal symptomatology are as follows:

I. Obstruction
    A. Anatomical distortions
        1. Congenital and traumatic: deviated nasal septum, stenotic nares
        2. Hypertrophic turbinates
    B. Tumor
        1. Benign: papilloma, neuroesthesioma, nasopharyngeal angiofibroma, cordoma (commonly, the inflammatory polyp)
        2. Malignant: squamous cell carcinoma, sarcoma, others (rare)
    C. Foreign body
    D. Congenital anomalies: choanal atresia, stenosis

II. Discharge
    A. Total obstruction, choanal atresia
    B. Foreign body (secretion is purulent)
    C. Cerebral spinal fluid fistula
        1. Erosion
        2. Fracture

III. Ache or pain
    A. Neoplasms and occasionally cysts
    B. Complications of sinus infection (would expect a history of nasal sinus infection): orbital cellulitis, osteomyelitis, epidural and subdural abscess, meningitis

C. Neurologic states, variations of trigeminal neuralgia: thorough physical examination, x-ray studies of the nerve's anatomical course required

Selected References

1. Paparella M, Shumrick D (eds): *Otolaryngology: Basic Sciences and Related Disciplines*. Philadelphia, WB Saunders, 1973, vol 1, pp 329–346, 551–562.
2. Paparella M, Shumrick D (eds): *Otolaryngology: Head and Neck*. Philadelphia, WB Saunders, 1973, vol 3, pp 3–158.

16. Vertigo

STUART G. YEOMAN, MD

Definition

The subjective feeling of disorientation in space combined with a sensation of motion. Disorientation in space without the sensation of motion is not vertigo. The sensation of motion is almost universally rotary in nature: (1) The patient feels stationary with the environment in motion; (2) The patient feels that the environment is stationary and that the movement is internal. Both are characteristic of vertigo. Symptoms such as pallor, sweating, and the feeling of nausea are very common with vertigo but are not necessary in its definition.

Technique

There are many patients with various initial complaints that upon further investigation may represent vertigo. These complaints include: dizziness, faintness, light-headedness, swimming head, giddiness, blurred vision, near-syncope, syncope, weakness, clumsiness, and others. The examiner must ascertain which of these complaints is vertigo with a feeling of disorientation in space and motion. The history is of prime importance, for often vertigo is episodic and the patient may be totally asymptomatic at the time of questioning. Questions should be structured so as to elicit the symptoms of vertigo and to help differentiate them from other symptoms. A questionnaire (Table 4) is often useful. Remember that many drugs can give rise to sensations of dysequilibrium of various types. Psychogenic disorders such as anxiety and hyperventilation syndrome are important causes of subjective dizziness. The examiner cannot ascribe symptoms to vertigo if the patient complains of loss of consciousness as part of the history.

Once the physician is convinced that the patient is suffering from vertigo, he still faces the problem of diagnosing the pathological process responsible. The causes of vertigo are multiple, and a scheme for classification is difficult. In fact, the only common thread among the various etiologies is the existence of vertigo.

The vestibular system consists of the vestibular structures of the inner ear, the eighth cranial nerve, and the vestibular nuclei in the brain-stem with their various interconnections in the central nervous system. Any disease that alters the function of some part of the vestibular system can potentially give rise to vertigo. Here again, a skilled history is essential.

Table 4. Questionnaire for the dizzy patient.

---

1. Can you describe your symptoms without using the word dizzy?
2. Syncopal episodes? (blackout)
3. Any tendency to fall?
4. Loss of balance with walking?
5. Does position affect your symptoms?
   a. Does getting up from bed worsen your symptoms?
   b. Does rolling over in bed worsen your symptoms?
6. Any headache?
7. Any nausea or vomiting?
8. Is dizziness constant or episodic?
   a. What makes it start?
   b. Can you stop dizziness or make it worse?
9. Allergies?
10. Use tobacco or alcohol?
11. On any medications?
*12. Any sensation of movement?
   a. You?
   b. The things around?

---

* If not present, not vertigo.

Table 5.   Causes of vertigo.

I. Peripheral
  1. Vestibular apparatus of ear
     a. Meniere's
     b. Benign positional vertigo.
  2. Peripheral nerve
     a. Acoustic neuroma
     b. Vestibular neuronitis
     c. Diabetic neuropathy
  3. Trauma: temporal bone fracture
  4. Vascular: acoustic artery occlusion
  5. Eye disorders

II. Central
  1. Vascular
     a. Vertebrobasilar insufficiency → infarcts
     b. Postural hypotension with preexistent vascular disease
  2. Tumors: cerebellopontine angle tumors
  3. Seizures: temporal lobe
  4. Multiple sclerosis
  5. Trauma: whiplash
  6. Meningitis

III. Drugs: alcohol, barbiturates

IV. Metabolic: thyroid disease (hypothyroidism)

Classification of vertigo in arbitrary groups of peripheral (inner ear or peripheral nerve) and central (in central nervous system) can help direct the examiner in the quest for an etiologic agent (see Table 5). The examiner must first find the anatomic site of the lesion and then determine the pathologic process involved. By dividing causes into peripheral and central, the physician can conduct the history by searching for evidence of disturbed function in systems other than the vestibular system. Thus, associated inner ear disease indicates probable peripheral cause of vertigo, whereas existence of other neurological deficits (that is, ataxia and Horner's syndrome unilaterally) would point to a CNS lesion as the responsible agent. Except for the vestibular apparatus in the ear and the eighth nerve, the vestibular system is in close proximity with neural pathways subserving other systems. Is is with this in mind that the physician structures the history and physical, primarily searching for associated disease in systems in close anatomical proximity with the various parts of the vestibular system (Table 6).

Table 6.   Questionnaire for vertigo.

I. Hearing
   1. Any hearing difficulty?
   2. Any tinnitus?
   3. Sensation of fullness in ears?

II. Neurological review
   1. Double vision?
   2. Any numbness on face or extremities?
   3. Blurred vision or blindness?
   4. Weakness in extremities?
   5. Coordination difficulties?
   6. Any speech disturbances?
   7. Any difficulty swallowing?

Background Information

Vertigo is caused by dysfunction of the vestibular system. The vestibular system can be arbitrarily divided into two parts: the peripheral and the central. The peripheral consists of the vestibular apparatus of the ear (the semicircular canals, macula utricle, saccule) and the eighth cranial nerve. The central consists of the four vestibular nuclei and their various connections in the CNS. The vestibular nuclei (lateral, medial, inferior, and superior) lie below the floor of the fourth ventricle in the pons near the pontine medullary junction. They are supplied by perforating arteries of the vertebrobasilar system. Their intraneural connections are myriad and complex. They monitor our spatial orientation with our environment through afferent and efferent connections with the temporal lobe cortex via the thalamus, the cerebellum, the midbrain, and reticular formation of the brainstem. Vestibular nuclei receive fibers from the posterior spinocerebellar tract, and they contribute to the medial longitudinal fasciculus which runs near the midline in the floor of the fourth ventricle. The medial longitudinal fasciculus provides connections between the vestibular nuclei and the eighth, fourth, and sixth cranial nuclei.

The student can readily see how a lesion anywhere in the labyrinth system of the ear, the peripheral eighth nerve, the vestibular nuclei, in the brainstem interrupting vestibular connections, in the cerebellum, or in the temporal lobe has the potential of creating the symptom of vertigo. A sound knowledge of neuroanatomy helps to localize the lesion to one of these sites in the vestibular system.

Clinical Significance

The significance of vertigo lies in determining the cause. The etiologies range from benign to life-threatening. Various causes of vertigo (see Table 5) will be discussed briefly here. For a more detailed discussion, the student is referred to the selected references.

In the majority of patients vertigo represents a benign and self-limited condition. Due to the lack of pathological correlation, classification in this situation is primarily on a clinical basis. Patients are accordingly separated into two major groups: (1) benign positional vertigo, and (2) vestibular neuronitis. Both groups represent disease in the peripheral vestibular system and generally clear spontaneously with time.

In a large number of patients vertigo represents significant diseases that require therapeutic intervention.

1. Meniere's disease has associated hearing loss and tinnitus. It is associated with peripheral vestibular disease.
2. CNS tumors producing vertigo are usually located in the cerebellopontine angle. Acoustic neuroma is the most common example.
3. Multiple sclerosis can have vertigo as a presenting symptom or during the course of the disease.
4. Temporal lobe mass lesions or seizures can present as vertigo with some associated findings.
5. Vertigo can occur with vascular insufficiency either of the peripheral acoustic artery or secondary to vertebrobasilar disease. This is more common in the elderly patient.
6. Drugs, with alcohol and barbiturates the leading offenders, may give subjective symptoms of vertigo. A good practice would be to stop all medications if possible in evaluation of the patient with vertigo.
7. Other miscellaneous causes of vertigo include traumatic skull fracture and diabetic neuropathy involving the eighth cranial nerve.

The history and review of systems must be thorough. Careful physical examination is indicated with particular attention to the neurological examination. The physical examination should include evaluating the patient for nystagmus, hearing and audiometry testing, and assessing the function of the inner ear vestibular apparatus with caloric stimulation.

Selected References

1.   Symposium on Vertigo. *Otolaryngol Clin N Amer,* vol 6, Feb 1973.
2.   Romanes GV (ed): *Cunningham's Textbook of Anatomy,* ed 11. New York, Oxford University Press, 1972, pp 824–830.

GASTROINTESTINAL SYSTEM

17. Nausea and Retching

HORACIO JINICH, MD
THEODORE HERSH, MD

Definition

Nausea is a psychic experience that is difficult to define but may be best described by the circumstances that surround it, such as "a feeling of imminent desire to vomit," "the disagreeable feeling which usually precedes vomiting."

Retching is defined as a series of spasmodic and abortive respiratory movements, with closed glottis and mouth and with simultaneous but antagonistic contractions of the abdominal muscles, accompanied by nausea and by a set of autonomic symptoms (salivation, pallor, tachycardia, faintness, weakness, and dizziness) that immediately precede vomiting. Also called "dry heaves" because the sensation simulates motions of vomiting but no gastric contents are expelled.

Technique

The patient refers to nausea by the same name, or with terms such as a "sick feeling," a "tightness in the throat," a "sinking sensation," or a "feeling of vomiting." It is usually accompanied by salivation, pallor, weakness, dizziness, faintness, and tachycardia. Nausea may be followed by attempts to vomit (retching). Nausea is frequently relieved by vomiting.

Background Information

The spasmodic and abortive respiratory movements are such that during inspiratory movements of the chest wall and diaphragm there is opposing expiratory contraction of the abdominal musculature. The diaphragm moves violently downward, but its range of motion is slight and it remains in a high position throughout this stage. At the same time, the antral portion of the stomach is contracted and the upper stomach is relaxed.

During nausea, gastric tone and peristalsis have been found to be reduced; the tone of the duodenum and proximal jejunum is increased so that their contents may readily reflux through the pylorus into the stomach. The symptom is produced by a wide variety of stimuli, including psychic experiences, intracranial vasomotor changes, olfactory, visual, vestibular, taste, laryngeal, pharyngeal, esophageal, and gastrointestinal stimuli, and exogenous or endogenous toxins. All these stimuli, in fact, also serve to initiate the act of vomiting.

Clinical Significance

Nausea is so closely associated with vomiting that a full discussion of its clinical significance will be presented with vomiting. However, it is worth stressing that there are conditions where nausea is present but vomiting is absent or, at least, infrequent and ineffective in relieving the nausea. These conditions include:

1. Drug side effects. A growing number of drugs are responsible for causing nausea, especially if their dosage is excessive. The most common are: digitalis products, emethine, l-dopa, metronidazol, codeine, morphine, Talwin, antibiotics, antimetabolite and cytotoxic agents, and oral contraceptives.
2. Irradiation
3. Uremia
4. Hypercalcemia
5. Liver disease
6. Prodromal stage of infectious diseases
7. Motion sickness (air or sea sickness)
8. Pregnancy
9. Alcoholism

Selected References

1. Wolf S: Studies on nausea: Effect of ipecac and other emetics on the human stomach and duodenum. *Gastroenterology* 12:212–218, 1949.

2. Borison HL, Wang SC: Physiology and pharmacology of vomiting. *Pharm Rev* 5:193–230, 1953.

3. Lumsden K, Holden WS: The act of vomiting in man. *Gut* 10:173–179, 1969.

4. Fordtran JS: Vomiting, in Sleisenger MH, Fordtran JS (eds): *Gastrointestinal Disease*. Philadelphia, WB Saunders, 1973, pp 127–143.

---

18. Vomiting

THEODORE HERSH, MD
HORACIO JINICH, MD

Definition

The forceful expulsion of gastric contents.

Technique

Vomiting, most often associated with the sensations of nausea and retching, can be readily recognized by all patients. Inquire whether the patient has ever had episodes of vomiting or has vomited recently. If the patient notes that he has expelled gastrointestinal secretions or food previously ingested, then the first distinction should be whether this is actual vomiting or regurgitation. Vomiting is usually associated with forceful expulsion of gastric contents. Regurgitation is an indication of an incompetent lower esophageal sphincter, allowing the gastric contents to pass into the esophagus; nausea and retching do not occur and the events are not forceful. If the patient describes episodes of vomiting, he will also have experienced symptoms of nausea and retching immediately antedating the vomitus. Questions are then directed to a description of the vomitus: frequency; relation to meals, drugs, or alcohol; association with other gastrointestinal symptoms such as abdominal pain, fever, chills, jaundice, diarrhea. History of previous gastric resection, diagnosis for which surgery was performed, and type of operation done may be helpful in explaining the cause of vomiting. An estimate of the quantity of vomitis needs to be established. In addition, a description of its color, contents, odor, and taste may yield clues to the etiology of the vomiting.

Vomitus which contains blood or coffee-ground-like material indicates bleeding from the upper gastrointestinal tract, most likely proximal to the ligament of Treitz. Coffee ground material implies that the blood has undergone changes in time by gastric contents, including acid, digestive enzymes, and perhaps bacteria. The vomitus may be yellow or green indicating presence of bile, or it may be clear and acid indicating mainly gastric juice. The vomitus may in addition contain food particles ingested hours earlier suggesting upper gastric outlet obstruction or impaired gastric emptying.

Background Information

Vomiting in humans is characterized by prior nausea and retching before the expulsion of food. Complex central nervous system and local regulating mechanisms are at work during the course of vomiting. Nausea and hypersalivation often precede the act of vomiting. The latter may be related to the proximity of the salivary center to the vomiting center in the medulla oblongata. The vomiting center in the medulla receives afferent impulses from two types of receptors: those in the viscera that respond to food or ingested drugs (ie, ipecac or copper salts) and those receptors in the brainstem that respond to blood-borne compounds.

Retching and vomiting follow changes in respiration and motility of the stomach and esophagus. The antrum of the stomach first contracts. There is concomitant abortive respiratory movements with the glottis closed: forceful sustained contractions of the abdominal muscles are associated by descent of the diaphragm at a time when the cardia of the stomach is raised and the gastroesophageal sphincter is relaxed. Duodenal tone has increased during the act of nausea with expulsion of duodenal contents into the stomach. The gastric contents are then forcefully brought up into the mouth.

Clinical Significance

There are many medical conditions that are associated with vomiting. Vomiting may be an expression of an organic obstruction of the upper gastrointestinal tract, such as cancer of the stomach or duodenum, pyloric stenosis, or chronic ulcer disease. Vomiting may be an expression of impaired gastric emptying with retention of gastric juice and food, such as occurs in the neuropathy of diabetes mellitus or after vagotomy. Many extra gastrointestinal conditions listed below have vomiting as a prominent symptom; the etiology is varied.

1. Vomiting caused by disturbances of the digestive system
   a. Esophageal: because of the absence of nausea and retching, more properly termed regurgitation
   b. Gastroduodenal: gastric outlet obstruction, gastric ulcer, duodenal ulcer, gastric atony, postvagotomy impaired gastric emptying, gastroparesis diabeticorum, tumors of the stomach and duodenum
   c. Intestinal: intestinal obstruction, appendicitis
   d. Colonic: obstruction, fistula
   e. Hepatic: acute hepatitis, cirrhosis
   f. Biliary: biliary colic, acute cholecystitis
   g. Pancreatic: acute pancreatitis; carcinoma of the pancreas
   h. Peritoneal: peritonitis
2. Vomiting caused by renal disease
   a. Acute or chronic renal failure
   b. Renal colic
3. Vomiting of gynecologic origin
   a. Pelvic tumors or inflammatory processes
   b. Pregnancy
4. Vomiting of neurologic origin
   a. Increased intracranial pressure
   b. Meningitis
   c. Epilepsy
   d. Migraine
   e. Vertigo
   f. Motion sickness
   g. Malignant hypertension
5. Vomiting of psychic origin
6. Vomiting of toxic origin
   a. Drugs
   b. Chemicals
   c. Food poisoning
   d. Toxins
7. Vomiting of metabolic origin (endogenous toxins)
   a. Uremia
   b. Ketosis
   c. Hypercalcemia
8. Vomiting of infectious origin
9. Vomiting of cardiovascular origin
   a. Myocardial infarction
10. Vomiting of respiratory origin
    a. Any condition with violent coughing

When vomiting is accompanied by blood or coffee-ground-like material, it indicates a bleeding lesion in the upper gastrointestinal tract. When blood follows prolonged periods of retching of nonbloody vomitus, it may signify a mucosal tear in the esophagus (Mallory-Weiss syndrome). When vomiting contains mainly clear gastric contents and is associated with other gastrointestinal symptoms, particularly pain, it may be a result of an associated acute gastrointestinal condition, such as cholecystitis, pancreatitis, or peritonitis. When the vomitus contains food ingested hours earlier but no bile, gastric outlet obstruction is present. When the vomitus contains bile it suggests patency of the pylorus, allowing expulsion of duodenal contents. It may occur in acute gastrointestinal conditions, such as pancreatitis and cholecystitis, high-intestine obstructions, or may follow gastric surgery for ulcer disease, as in bile reflux gastritis. Feculent vomitus occurs with low-intestine obstructive lesions as a result of gastrocolic fistulas.

Selected References

1. Borison HL, Wang SC: Physiology and pharmacology of vomiting. *Pharm Rev* 5:193–230, 1953.
2. Rimer DG: Gastric retention without mechanical obstruction. *Arch Intern Med* 117:287–299, 1966.
3. Hill OW: Psychogenic vomiting. *Gut* 9:348–352, 1968.
4. Fordtran JS: Vomiting, in Sleisenger MH, Fordtran JS (eds): *Gastrointestinal Diseases*. Philadelphia, WB Saunders, 1973, pp 127–143.

19. Hematemesis

HORACIO JINICH, MD
THEODORE HERSH, MD

Definition

The vomiting of gross blood.

Technique

No other symptom in medicine is easier to identify. Vomited blood may be fresh and bright red in color; often it contains clots. The bloody vomitus may be dark brown or appear like coffee ground material when, having remained in the stomach for some time, the blood has been altered by the action of gastric acid and pepsin. The examiner should then ask the patient if he has vomited blood, or if the vomitus was dark brown in color or appeared as coffee-ground-like material. An attempt to determine the amount of blood actually vomited should be made by talking in terms of teaspoonfuls or cupfuls of blood vomited. The duration of bloody vomitus and the frequency are important, as is the relation to retching or vomiting of gastric contents, the relation to ingestion of meals, alcohol, or drugs, especially aspirin products.

The concomitant appearance of symptoms of anemia and shock (such as fatigue, weakness, perspiration, and pallor) should always be investigated to determine the magnitude of the hemorrhage. Also, a history of previous episodes of hematemesis and the diagnosis of their cause should be investigated. Family history for bleeding disorder should be checked. History of cardiovascular disease may hint at use of an anticoagulant.

Occasionally there may be a source of confusion between hemoptysis and hematemesis. In the first case, the blood from the air passages is bright red in color, foamy, and its expulsion follows coughing, not vomiting. Rarely a patient with profuse nosebleeds (epistaxis) will swallow blood and subsequently vomit it. Even though technically this can be called hematemesis, an adequate history will establish that the primary source of bleeding is from the nose and not from the upper gastrointestinal tract.

Background Information

Hematemesis is the result of a hemorrhage in the upper gastrointestinal tract usually proximal to the area at the ligament of Treitz. The mechanism results from either rupture of arterial or venous vessels, capillary injury, or a coagulation disorder. The rupture of an arterial or venous vessel results from the digestive action of gastric acid and pepsin secretion on gastric or duodenal mucosa. The gastric acid may reflux into the esophagus and cause bleeding from esophageal ulcer or severe esophagitis. Ulcer disease is a very common cause of hematemesis. Necrosis in a gastric carcinoma with ulceration less often presents with hematemesis. Leakage of blood cells across the submucosal capillaries occurs when the gastric mucosal barrier is ruptured allowing back diffusion of hydrochloric acid; this may occur after ingestion of substances such as aspirin, indomethacin, and ethanol. Bile salts refluxing into the stomach may cause similar mucosal damage and bleeding. Increased pressure in esophageal varices with rupture presents as an acute bout of hematemesis. Less frequently, the cause of hematemesis is hemorrhagic diathesis with concomitant bleeding in other sites.

Clinical Significance

The sources of upper gastrointestinal hemorrhage and hematemesis are as follows:

I. Esophageal
    A.   Reflux esophagitis
    B.   Varices
    C.   Laceration of the gastroesophageal junction (Mallory-Weiss syndrome)
    D.   Esophageal cancer
    E.   Ruptured aortic aneurysm

II. Gastric and duodenal
    A.   Peptic ulcer
    B.   Acute (stress) ulcers
    C.   Gastric varices
    D.   Gastritis (aspirin, alcohol)
    E.   Hereditary hemorrhagic telangiectasia
    F.   Tumors
        1.   Carcinoma
        2.   Sarcoma
        3.   Benign tumors

III. Other
    A.   Aortointestinal fistula
    B.   Pancreatitis
    C.   Hematobilia
    D.   Blood dyscrasias
    E.   Anticoagulation therapy
    F.   Collagen disease
    G.   Uremia

However, in clinical practice the most frequent causes are duodenal ulcer, gastric ulcer, erosive gastritis (alcohol or aspirin induced), esophageal varices, and reflux esophagitis.

Selected References

1.   Law DH, Gregory DH: Gastro-intestinal bleeding, in Sleisenger MH, Fordtran JS (eds): *Gastrointestinal Disease.* Philadelphia, WB Saunders, 1973, pp 195–215.
2.   Baum S, Nusbaum M, Clearfield HF, et al: Angiography in the diagnosis of gastro-intestinal bleeding. *Arch Intern Med* 119:16–24, 1967.

3. Wilson DE, Chalmers TC: Acute hemorrhage from the upper gastro-intestinal tract. *N Eng J Med* 274:1368–1371, 1966.
4. Palmer ED: *Diagnosis of Upper Gastro-intestinal Bleeding*. Springfield, Ill, Charles C Thomas, 1961.
5. Belber JP: Gastroscopy and duodenoscopy, in Sleisenger MH, Fordtran JS (eds): *Gastrointestinal Disease*. Philadelphia, WB Saunders, 1973, pp 521–535.

20. Melena

H. KENNETH WALKER, MD

Definition

The passage of black, tarry stools.

Technique

Begin by asking the patient open-ended questions: Tell me about your bowel movements. Have you noticed any change in your bowel movements? Do you have any trouble with your bowel movements?

Note that each question is slightly more specific or directive than the preceding one. The goal is to get the patient to say spontaneously, "My stool has turned black recently." A useful aid is to take a coal-black pen and in a casual fashion hold it in such a way that the patient's eyes are drawn to it, giving him the opportunity to say the stools have become the color of the pen.

If these questions don't elicit a history of coal-black stools, then become more specific: Has there been a change in the color of your stools and if so, what change? Are your stools black?

An associated complaint that patients sometimes note is that melena is often difficult to remove satisfactorily from the skin. So you can ask: Is it hard to clean yourself after a bowel movement? Is the stool sticky? The stool does frequently have a characteristic odor, but this is helpful only when the patient has had a recognized experience with melena previously. If the answer to the question is no, then move on. If the answer is yes, then you must rule out causes of melena other than blood. Iron and bismuth (peptobismol) compounds commonly cause melena.

Background Information

There is some controversy over the origin of melena. The classical view is that melena is caused by the exposure of blood to gastric acid. Thus, the source of bleeding must be proximal to the jejunum in order for this to occur. A more recent view, brought about by the observation that blood instilled experimentally into the colon during appendectomy can cause melena, is that melena is due to the action of intestinal bacteria on blood as the blood passes through the gastrointestinal tract. In the latter case the clinical observation that melena indicates upper gastrointestinal bleeding is explained by the longer transit time of the blood. That is, the bacteria have enough time to cause melena only when the bleeding is high enough to allow prolonged transit time.

As little as 60 ml of blood can cause melena. After a single gastrointestinal hemorrhage tarry stools can persist for 7 to 10 days, depending upon transit time in the gastrointestinal tract. The time the blood remains in the gastrointestinal tract probably influences the color.

Clinical Significance

Melena usually indicates gastrointestinal bleeding in the esophagus, stomach, or duodenum, since blood distal to the duodenum usually does not have an opportunity to react with stomach acid or enough time for bacteria to act on it. Peptic ulcer, gastritis, and esophageal varices are the commonest causes of melena. Other important causes are carcinoma of the stomach, hiatal hernia with esophagitis, polyps, and other tumors. Blood from epistaxis, hemoptysis, or tooth extraction can be swallowed and cause melena. The history of melena may be confirmed by testing the stool for occult blood if the patient still has melena. But a positive history of melena must be approached in the same fashion regardless of the results of the occult blood test. This is because many of the causes of melena do produce intermittent bleeding, and at the same time are problems one cannot afford to overlook, eg, carcinoma of the stomach. An associated finding highly suggestive of gastrointestinal bleeding is iron deficiency anemia. If the blood loss has occurred rapidly, orthostatic hypotension and even syncope upon standing may be present. Other symptoms and signs if present will, of course, be associated with the cause for the bleeding, eg, abdominal pain with peptic ulcer. The work-up is aimed at identifying the site of bleeding and usually includes nasogastric aspiration, gastroscopy, panendoscopy, and radiography of the gastrointestinal tract.

Selected References

1. Daniel WA, Jr, Egan S: Quantity of blood required to produce tarry stool. *JAMA* 113:2232, 1939.
2. Luke RG, et al: Appearances of the stools after the introduction of blood into the caecum. *Gut* 5:77–79, 1964.
3. Walls WD, et al: Early investigation of hematemesis and melena. *Lancet* 2:387–390, 1971.
4. Hardy KJ: Hemaetemesis and melaena. *Med J Australia* 1:785–790, 1971.
5. Barany F, Nilsson L: Diagnostic procedure in bleeding of obscure origin from the alimentary canal. *Gut* 11:307–313, 1970.

---

21. Dysphagia

THEODORE HERSH, MD
HORACIO JINICH, MD

Definition

Difficulty in swallowing or in the passage of food through the esophagus.

Technique

Ask the patient: Do you have any trouble swallowing? Does food stick? If the patient answers affirmatively, then proceed to find out more specifically about this difficulty in swallowing. The problem may be in initiating a swallow as in neuromuscular disorders or central nervous system disease, so the question would be: Do you have trouble starting a swallow? If the patient can initiate the swallow but there is stoppage of the bolus, the patient can be asked to point to the area where he feels the food sticks. Dysphagia caused by neuromuscular disorder is usually associated with choking, a symptom that should be investigated at this point. One may proceed with questions about difficulty in swallowing by inquiring about whether it occurs with solid food or with liquids. Does the difficulty occur at the beginning of the meal? that is, with the first swallows, or at the end of the meal? One needs to inquire whether the difficulty occurs only with liquids and whether this is aggravated by the extremes of temperature such as the dysphagia of spasm, particularly with cold liquids. Further questions relate to whether this occurs with every meal or only episodically; whether the difficulty is progressive or if it has remained unchanged. The patient with progressive dysphagia will very frequently reply affirmatively to the problem of dysphagia initially with solids, progressing to difficulty with soft foods, and finally with liquids. Associated questions relate to the problem of whether food is brought back into the throat or regurgitated in relation to the previous meal in which this occurs or to food ingested in previous meals. The other question which relates to difficulty in swallowing is whether it is associated with pain; that is, odynophagia. The latter occurs most often when the esophageal muscle goes into spasm during the act of swallowing.

Background Information

The act of deglutition is traditionally divided into three stages: (1) oral, (2) pharyngeal, and (3) esophageal. The oral phase follows mastication: the bolus is thrown backward by the tongue while the soft palate, fauces, and posterior wall of the oropharynx are approximated to close the opening into the nasopharynx. Then the bolus is displaced into the oropharynx by contraction of the soft palate and a posterior movement of the tongue. During the pharyngeal phase a stripping peristaltic wave is created which propels the bolus distally. With the entrance of material into the oropharynx, the hyoid bone and the larynx are abruptly elevated and the larynx simultaneously moves forward and tilts posteriorly creating a pulling force and increasing the A-P diameter of the laryngopharynx and producing a zone of negative pressure which "sucks" the bolus into the laryngopharynx. The air conduit is closed by contraction of the intrinsic laryngeal muscles and by shortening and widening of the aryepiglottic folds as well as the true and false bands. The epiglottis is tipped downward. The cricopharyngeal muscles relax prior to the entrance of the bolus into the hypopharynx and, once the peristaltic wave has traversed it, the muscle contracts, closing the esophagus superiorly and marking the end of the pharyngeal phase of swallowing.

There are two kinds of dysphagia: dysphagia of the first stage of swallowing, or difficulty in swallowing (pharyngeal dysphagia); and dysphagia of the second stage of swallowing, or difficulty in the passage of food through the esophagus (esophageal dysphagia).

The first stage of swallowing is a voluntary act and, accordingly, more prone to be influenced by nervous factors. The second stage is an involuntary act of which we are usually unconscious unless we swallow a piece of food which is too large, hard, sticky, hot, or cold.

Clinical Significance

Dysphagia is one of the symptoms where a well-taken history may establish the diagnosis. Patients who have difficulty in initiating a swallow usually have neuromuscular disease. As mentioned before, there is usually associated choking from aspiration into the airway. Dysphagia may also occur when there are motor disorders in the esophagus whereby the waves of contraction are no longer peristaltic but occur simultaneously and repetitively. Occasionally there is no peristalsis recorded by esophageal manometric study. These entities include scleroderma and diabetes mellitus when there is an autonomic neuropathy as a complication. Dysphagia also occurs when the disordered motility includes repetitive high pressure contractions. In this case a segment of the esophagus remains contracted following a swallow, thereby acting as an obstruction. This is represented by the entity called diffuse esophageal spasm, frequently causing painful swallowing (odynophagia). Patients with diffuse spasm have intermittent dysphagia related to ingestion of liquids, particularly cold liquids. Patients with a vigorous type of achalasia may also have dysphagia and pain on swallowing. Another motor disorder of the esophagus that presents with dysphagia is achalasia. These cases often start with dysphagia to liquids. In this disorder there is a combination of ineffective peristalsis in the body of the esophagus and a failure of relaxation of the lower esophageal sphincter. In time, the esophagus dilates and the patient has difficulty with both liquids and solids and has frequent regurgitation of food that has remained in the esophagus. Dysphagia to solids occurs episodically, particularly when there is ingestion of a large bolus of meat in a condition where there is a mucosal ring in the lower esophagus. This is called a Schatzki ring and is usually associated with a hiatus hernia. This episodic dysphagia, or the steakhouse syndrome, occurs when the diameter of the ring is less than 12 mm. Progressive dysphagia, particularly to solids, occurs with areas of narrowing of the lumen of the esophagus as in patients with a tumor of the esophagus or of the cardia of the stomach invading the esophagus submucosally. Extrinsic compressions from other malignancies or vascular lesions may also cause progressive dysphagia. Dysphagia due to cicatricial stenosis occurs in the background of a history of lye ingestion, chronic reflux esophagitis, or following prolonged periods of vomiting or nasogastric intubation. The following is a classification of dysphagia.

1. Dysphagia caused by oral lesions: stomatitis, cancer
2. Dysphagia caused by salivary gland lesions

3. Dysphagia caused by laryngeal and pharyngeal lesions
4. Dysphagia caused by paralysis of the pharyngeal muscles: diphtheria, botulism, bulbar lesions, myasthenia gravis
5. Dysphagia caused by spasm of the pharyngeal muscles: hydrophobia, tetanus, strychnine intoxication, hysteria
6. Dysphagia caused by esophageal lesions: foreign bodies, cicatricial stenosis, cancer of the esophagus, cancer of the stomach and cardies, ulcers, esophagitis, rings, diverticuli, achalasia, scleroderma
7. Dysphagia caused by compression by neighboring organs: goiter, tumors, aneurysms

Selected References

1. Code CF, Creamer B, Schlegel JF, et al: *An Atlas of Esophageal Motility in Health and Disease.* Springfield, Ill, Charles C Thomas, 1958.
2. Ellis FH, Olsen AM: *Achalasia of the Esophagus.* Philadelphia, WB Saunders, 1969.
3. Bennett JR, Hendrix TR: Diffuse esophageal spasm: A disorder with more than one cause. *Gastroenterology* 59:273–279, 1970.
4. Bayless TM (ed): *Management of Esophageal Disease: Modern Treatment.* New York, Harper and Row, 1970, vol 7, no 6.
5. Netter FH: *Digestive System, Part I: Upper Digestive Tract.* The Ciba Collection of Medical Illustrations, Summit, NJ, Ciba Pharm. Co. 1959, pp 74–77.

22. Indigestion

THEODORE HERSH, MD
HORACIO JINICH, MD

Definition

Indigestion is a term that is vague and hard to define. Patients complaining of indigestion describe different conditions, which the physician should try to clarify. Frequently the patient equates indigestion with heartburn, but the term may be employed to mean: a feeling of fullness in the upper abdomen; a discomfort in the same area which is "not yet painful"; excessive belching, nausea, gaseousness, or flatulence; a bad taste in the mouth or a coated tongue; and, less often, fatigue, somnolence, or headaches. When any or several of these symptoms tend to occur postprandially, they are attributed by the patient to faulty function of the digestive system; in other words, indigestion. Physicians sometimes use the word "dyspepsia" for these vague symptoms.

Technique

First clarify what the patient means by "indigestion." The patient may express his own definition of this complaint or may need to be meticulously quizzed: Is it nausea, heartburn, belching, fatigue, somnolence, headache? Is it a bad taste in the mouth or a coated tongue? Is there a feeling of fullness and discomfort in the upper abdomen, excessive belching, gaseousness, or flatulence after meals? Do the symptoms occur after each meal or only after some meals? Are they related to the quantity or to the quality of food ingested, such as spices, fats, milk, or beans? In relation to indigestion, what are the patient's eating habits? Does he eat too fast? Does he chew the food properly? Is he subject to nervous tensions during meals? Does the indigestion disappear when he is relaxed? Are there evidences of psychic tensions or emotional conflicts?

Indigestion may be the result of gastric disorders, such as a delay in emptying the stomach or excessive amounts of gas in the gastrointestinal tract. It may also be due to extragastric disorders; therefore, the clinical history must include a careful search for other signs and symptoms of gastrointestinal, hepatic, biliary, pancreatic, psychological, genitourinary, cardiovascular, and metabolic diseases.

Background Information

The feeling of fullness in the upper abdomen, occurring postprandially and lasting an excessive amount of time, if not the result of the intake of an inordinate amount of food, is usually caused by aerophagia with gastric distention or by delay in emptying of the stomach (gastric atony). Retention of food in the esophagus by obstruction as in achalasia or stricture may cause this feeling and be related as indigestion.

Functionally, the stomach may be divided into two areas: the proximal stomach, or reservoir, and the distal stomach, or antrum, where food is mixed and triturated and where the process of emptying takes place. This process is governed by a clock; the electrical slow wave is modified by a set of complex nervous and humoral influences which determine whether or not the antral pump responds to the slow wave, as well as to the force and depth of the contractions.

The volume and fluidity of the meal influences the rate of gastric emptying; liquids leave the stomach faster than solids. Gastric emptying is inhibited through the stimulation of specific receptors that are probably located in the duodenum. Gastric emptying may be inhibited by meals with high osmotic pressure, high acidity, or high fat content. (Electrolytes, carbohydrates and amino acids create high osmotic pressure.) The inhibitory activity is mediated by nervous and humoral mechanisms. The sympathetic motor innervation of the stomach, enterogastric reflexes involving the vagus nerve, and the newly described noradrenergic nerves are probably involved. Also, several gastrointestinal hormones such as gastrin, secretin, and cholecystokinin are known to exert an inhibitory action on gastric emptying. Enterogastrone, a hormone not yet isolated in pure form, is liberated from the duodenum by micellar fat and also inhibits gastric emptying and gastric acid secretion. More recently another hormone, motilin, has been found to be released from the upper small bowel and to be capable of influencing the motor activity of the antral pump.

The emptying of the stomach may be influenced by many other factors. Stressful stimuli, such as pain, inhibit gastric emptying by way of the sympathetic innervation of the stomach. Distention of the intestine has the same effect. Classical experiments in animals and humans have shown the inhibitory effect of a wide variety of emotional experiences on gastric motility and acid secretion. Conflicts arousing feelings of anxiety, fear, or guilt are particularly likely to inhibit gastric emptying. The mechanisms by which metabolic disorders such as uremia and diabetic ketoacidosis interfere with gastric emptying are unknown. An autonomic neuropathy may be the reason why gastric disturbance exists as a complication of diabetes mellitus. Gastric emptying is delayed in patients with gastric ulcer and atrophic gastritis. The mechanism is unclear, but all three conditions are associated with an elevation of serum gastrin. Delayed emptying is also present after vagotomy for ulcer disease. Finally, many drugs with anticholinergic action are known to delay the emptying processes of the stomach.

Gastrointestinal gas has two main sources: swallowed air and intraluminal production from bacterial activity. The relative importance of the two mechanisms has not been entirely clarified and probably varies from one subject to another. Epigastric discomfort and excessive belching and gaseousness after meals is very likely due to excessive swallowing of air, aerophagia. This phenomenon is quite common in anxious individuals as well as in all those who make frequent swallowing movements while the mouth is empty, such as patients who have hypersalivation or a dry mouth that they attempt to moisten, or who have postnasal drip or chew tobacco or gum. Attempts to eructate in order to get rid of the abdominal discomfort often result in more atmospheric air entering the stomach, thus aggravating this disturbance.

Clinical Significance

A feeling of upper abdominal distention and discomfort after meals suggests aerophagia or delayed emptying of the stomach, which, in turn, can be caused by at least three distinct mechanisms: (1) organic obstruction at or near the pylorus; (2) atony and hypomobility of the stomach caused by nervous (reflex) or humoral factors; (3) emotional influences.

The most important causes of organic obstruction of the stomach outlet are: tumors of the distal stomach (carcinoma, polyps); pyloric stenosis secondary to inflammation and edema in peptic ulcer disease of the duodenum, antrum, or pyloric channel; scarring secondary to peptic ulcer disease; idiopathic hypertrophy of the pyloric muscle. Other organic conditions that may interfere with the emptying mechanism of the stomach are any neoplastic or chronic inflammatory processes of the stomach and extragastric diseases, such as tumors and inflammatory masses originating in the pancreas, gallbladder, or other neighboring organs, causing extrinsic compression on the gastric outlet.

Reflex atony of the stomach and, perhaps, pylorospasm appear frequently in many digestive and extradigestive conditions. Such is the case in cholecystitis, acute and chronic liver disease, pancreatic disease, pregnancy, pelvic inflammatory disease and tumors, coronary heart disease, and migraine. The mechanisms involved are not known. Delayed gastric emptying follows vagotomy and is one of the complications of diabetes mellitus and of psychotropic drugs with anticholinergic features.

Finally, in the vast majority of patients complaining of indigestion, exhaustive clinical studies fail to show any organic explanation. The personal history of such patients often reveals that they are suffering from anxiety, nervous fatigue, depression, fear, or guilt. Thus, a personal history of the patient, including the search for evidence of nervous tension and emotional conflict should be an essential part of the study of any patient complaining of indigestion.

Selected References

1.   Thomas JE, Baldwin MV: Pathways and mechanisms of regulation of gastric motility, in Code CF (ed): *Handbook of Physiology*. Washington, DC, American Physiological Society, 1968, sect 6, vol IV, pp 1937–1968.
2.   Cooke AR, Christensen J: Motor functions of the stomach, in Sleisenger MH, Fordtran JS (eds): *Gastrointestinal Disease*. Philadelphia, WB Saunders, 1973, pp 115–126.
3.   Wolf S, Wolff HG: *Human Gastric Function*. New York, Oxford University Press, 1943.
4.   Alvarez WC: *Nervousness, Indigestion and Pain*. New York, PB Hoeber, 1943.

24. Heartburn

THEODORE HERSH, MD
HORACIO JINICH, MD

Definition

Substernal burning pain.

Technique

Heartburn is a symptom that most people have experienced, albeit infrequently. The question may thus be posed: Do you have or have you ever suffered from heartburn? If the answer is affirmative, it is important for the patient to define his symptom of heartburn and to point to where it occurs. The patient will usually describe heartburn as a substernal burning pain and may frequently relate it to meals or specific types of foods or liquids. One should also determine if the symptom is brought on by lying down or bending and whether it occurs at night. Often the patient may feel that some food previously ingested comes up to the throat and causes a burning sensation. Acid reflux into the esophagus may induce spasm, and patients complain of concomitant chest pain with the heartburn.

Background Information

Heartburn represents a symptom reflecting a pH-sensitive esophagus. Most often this is due to an inflammation of the mucosa of the distal esophagus which is periodically being bathed by refluxing gastric acid contents. Multiple factors contribute to the production of reflux esophagitis (Table 7). This most often results from an incompetent lower esophageal sphincter (LES). Ordinarily this is an area of a few centimeters separating the stomach and the esophagus that maintains a high-pressure zone which persists through the interdigestive phase. This prevents gastric acid contents and ingested food from refluxing back into the esophagus. When the lower esophageal sphincter is incompetent, gastric contents may reflux

Table 7. Determinants of reflux esophagitis

Competency of Antireflux Mechanism	Potency and Volume of refluxed Material	Esophageal Emptying	Tissue Resistance

I. Intrinsic LES
  A. Resting tone
  B. Response to abdominal pressure changes
  C. Endogenous enteric hormones
  D. Other factors: smoking, fatty foods, alcohol, drugs
II. Mechanical factors
  A. Valve mechanism
  B. Extrinsic compression
  C. Intraabdominal esophageal segment
  D. Mucosal choke
III. Postoperative alterations
  A. Vagotomy
  B. LES resection
	I. Potency
	  A. Peptic esophagitis
	    1. Acid
	    2. Pepsin
	  B. Alkaline esophagitis
	    1. Bile acids
	    2. Pancreatic enzymes
	II. Volume of material available for reflux
	  A. Gastric secretory rate
	  B. Gastric emptying rate
	    1. Obstruction
	    2. Abnormal motility
	    3. Vagotomy
	    4. Drugs
	    5. Disease, ie, diabetes
		I. Contact time
		II. Primary peristalsis
		III. Secondary peristalsis
		IV. Salivation
			I. Type epithelium
			II. Patient age
			III. Blood supply
			IV. Insult frequency
			V. Healing rate

From Dodds WJ, Hogan WJ, Miller WN: Reflux esophagitis. Am J Dig Dis 21:49–67, 1976. Used with permission.

into the esophagus. On a chronic basis and with increased contact time between the low pH juice and the mucosa, the reflux causes an inflammation in the esophagus which is reflected by the symptom of heartburn (reflux esophagitis). Patients may note aggravation of this symptom with the ingestion of citrus products, spicy foods, coffee, and alcohol.

After gastric resections and reconstruction of gastroenterostomies, alkaline duodenal contents containing bile and pancreatic secretions may reflux into the stomach and the esophagus. An alkali (bile) reflux gastritis and esophagitis may ensue and present with the symptom complex of heartburn, regurgitation, epigastric and chest pain, and nausea and bilious vomiting.

Clinical Significance

Heartburn usually reflects reflux esophagitis. One can demonstrate reflux of gastric contents by barium swallow studies. The barium meal refluxes into the esophagus. Ingested radioisotopes may also appear on scans in the esophagus due to reflux of gastric contents. An acid perfusion (Bernstein test) of the esophagus may elicit heartburn with the infused acid, but not when the esophagus is perfused with saline during the test. Another method of study with pH probes records low pH in the lower esophagus, reflecting reflux of acid gastric juice. Esophageal motility studies usually show a low or absent high pressure zone in the gastroesophageal area in patients with heartburn. The usual high-pressure zone of the lower esophageal sphincter is not detected in patients with reflux esophagitis.

Selected References

1. Dodds WJ, Hogan WJ, Miller WN: Reflux esophagitis. *Am J Dig Dis* 21:49–67, 1976.
2. Pope CE: Pathophysiology and diagnosis of reflux esophagitis. *Gastroenterology* 70:445–454, 1976.
3. Cohen S, Harris LD: The lower esophageal sphincter. *Gastroenterology* 63:1066–1073, 1972.
4. Wickbom G, Bushkin FL, Woodward ER: Alkaline reflux esophagitis, *Surg Gyn Obstet* 139:267–271, 1974.

24. Abdominal Pain

HORACIO JINICH, MD
THEODORE HERSH, MD

Definition

Pain in the abdomen.

Technique

A patient complaining of abdominal pain should be asked the following questions:

1. Where is the pain located? Because patients usually either do not know anatomical terms or employ them erroneously, ask them to point with a finger to the exact location of the pain. However, this method can also be misleading if the patient is sitting in front of the physician. If possible, ask the patient to stand up, to uncover the abdominal wall, and to point out the exact area; recheck when the patient is lying down during the physical examination.

2. Where does the pain radiate to, or does it originate elsewhere and move to the abdomen? The same technique should be followed regarding this question.

3. What kind of pain is it? Being a subjective experience, the patient may find it very difficult to answer. Help the patient to describe the pain by suggesting a series of comparisons or similarities. Is it like a hunger pain? a gnawing sensation? a cramp? Is it burning in character? Is it like acidity, heat, pressure? Is it a sticking pain?

4. How severe is it? Does it allow you to go ahead with your activities or does it force you to stop? to lie down? Does it require pain medicine? Has the pain been severe enough to require a visit to the emergency room of the hospital?

5. What other symptoms accompany the pain? Is it accompanied by nausea, vomiting, abdominal distention, diarrhea, constipation, heartburn, chills and fever, urinary frequency, changes in the color of the urine? Is jaundice present with attacks of pain?

6. What factors bring it about? Does it occur immediately after eating or several hours after a meal? Does the pain occur after eating any particular kind of food? drinking alcohol? taking any medication or drug? Is it brought on by nervous tension? moving your bowels? movements of the body? the position of the body?

7. What factors cause relief of pain? eating? taking antacids, antispasmodics, analgesics? expelling gas, having a bowel movement? vomiting, belching? emptying the bladder? acquiring any particular posture?

8. In chronic abdominal pain inquire about the patients' day. A description of routine activities and meals in reference to occurrence and disappearance of pain is important. Do they have the pain during the night? Are they awakened by it? Do they have pain when waking up in the morning? Is the pain present when they have breakfast? after breakfast? Before they move the bowels, after moving the bowels? Do they have pain during the morning? at what time? Is there any pain before lunch? after lunch? in the afternoon? before dinner? after dinner? before going to bed? Does it awaken them from sleep? This rhythmicity of pain is particularly useful in the diagnosis of pain caused by peptic ulcer disease.

9. Again in chronic pain it is useful to inquire about the periodicity of the pain. Does it tend to appear during some periods of the year? Is it related to seasons or to times when patients are under particular periods of stress? Is it related to the menstrual cycle?

Background Information

It is convenient to classify the nervous pathways conveying painful stimuli from the abdomen into two groups: fibers which transmit painful stimuli arising from the viscera (visceral pain) and those which transmit painful stimuli from nonvisceral structures of the abdomen (somatic pain). With few exceptions, visceral pain is transmitted by fibers which accompany the sympathetic nerves. The receptors consist of the corpuscles of Pacini and free nerve endings, and they are located in the walls of each of the abdominal viscera. These receptors are sensitive to stretch and to spasm, whereas they are insensitive to nerve section or temperature. The axons follow the blood vessels reaching the abdominal aorta; they traverse without synapse to the sympathetic ganglia entering the splanchnic nerves, and there follow pathways of other afferent pain fibers and course with the neurons of the spinothalamic tract. Thus, they reach the ventral posterior nucleus of the thalamus where there is a synapse with a third neuron, which carries the impulses to the posterocentral area of the cerebral cortex. In the cortex there are connections with the highest levels of integration where interpretation of the painful stimuli takes place.

Somatic pain is transmitted by the somatic fibers which innervate the walls of the abdominal cavity. Their receptors arc located in the parietal peritoneum, mesentery, and the peripheral part of the diaphragm. The receptors are sensitive to pressure, friction, torsion, traction, chemical agents, toxins, enzymes, infiltrative processes, and edema. The axons are incorporated in the dorsal and superior lumbar spinal nerves. Other receptors located in the central parts of the diaphragm and in the biliary tract have axons which join the phrenic nerve.

Abdominal Structures Capable of Causing Pain

ABDOMINAL CAVITY

Only 75 years ago it was commonly held that the viscera were insensitive to pain. This erroneous belief arose from the fact that human beings did not experience pain when they received various stimuli on the thoracic or abdominal viscera, which would have given rise to comparatively severe pain when applied to the skin. At that time it was also erroneously felt that the autonomic nervous system was exclusively efferent and that it did not include afferent fibers. Now we know that the viscera are innervated by fibers which are similar to those of the skin, although their number is relatively smaller and they are of lesser caliber. These fibers are insensitive to the stimuli which usually are effective in skin receptors such as pressure, traction, pinching, cutting, and temperature extremes. On the other hand, they are sensitive to a specific stimulation, that is, to an increase in intravisceral pressure provoked by distention or contraction. Thus, the introduction of rubber balloons distended with air in the digestive tract causes pain.

Jones, who performed the classic experiments, introduced a rubber balloon connected to a catheter and placed it at various levels of the gut. The distention of the balloon caused pain which the volunteer was asked to describe with precision. The distention of the superior esophagus immediately above the aortic arch caused pain at a level of the sternal notch or behind the head of the sternum. It was felt in a circumscribed area, although occasionally it was rather diffuse and some subjects referred it to an added discomfort in the posterior part of the throat or in the cervical region. The distention of the middle esophagus caused pain at the same level in the midsternum area, although some subjects referred it to the sternal notch or to the xyphoid. Further distention of the balloon caused the pain to radiate to both sides of the chest or to the dorsal area. The distention of the lower esophagus immediately above the cardia caused pain which was usually felt at a level of the xyphoid, although in some subjects it was felt in the midsternal and even in the upper sternal area. The pain in all these experiments was usually described as a pressure or fullness when the distention took place in the upper third of the esophagus. It was described as distention or fullness, as burning and like angina pain when the distention took place in the middle esophagus. Distention of the lower third of the esophagus was frequently described as heartburn.

Gastric distention caused pain which was referred to the midepigastric area. When stimulation was applied closer to the cardia, the pain was referred to an area closer to the xyphoid, whereas distention near the pylorus elicited pain in the midepigastric area. The distention of the duodenal bulb caused midepigastric pain and sometimes pain in the interscapular region. The location of the pain had a tendency to descend further down when the stimulation took place at more distant levels of the duodenum.

The distention of the small bowel at any level caused pain which was usually felt in the periumbilical region. The only exception was the distention of the distal ileum which caused the pain to radiate to the right iliac fossa or to the hypogastric area. The distention of the cecum also caused pain in the right iliac fossa, but in some subjects it radiated to the midline or to the umbilicus. The distention of the ascending colon caused infraumbilical pain, whereas distention in the hepatic flexure caused pain in the right flank. The distention of the transverse colon caused infraumbilical pain in the majority of the subjects, while distention of the splenic flexure caused pain in the left flank. Distention of the descending colon and sigmoid caused left-lower-quadrant or infraumbilical pain, and distention of the rectum and sigmoid caused pain in the suprapubic area.

Even though the viscera do not give rise to pain except when subjected to excessive distention or spasm, it is a fact that visceral mucosa may become sensitive to other kinds of stimuli when the viscera are inflamed. This is a possible explanation of the pain present in peptic ulcer disease. The painful stimulation of the pancreas (experimentally induced) gives rise to pain which is referred to the epigastrium. The pain is more apt to be to the right of the midline when the stimulation originates in the head of the pancreas, or in the left side of the epigastrium if the tail of the pancreas is stimulated. If the whole length of the organ is stimulated with wire electrodes, the pain is felt in the whole epigastric area and the upper quadrants and it radiates to the dorsal area.

ABDOMINAL WALL

Skin. Several dermatologic conditions may cause abdominal pain, such as keloid scars, acute porphyria, and herpes zoster. The pain preceding the skin eruption in herpes may cause the physician to suspect an acute abdominal condition.

Parietal peritoneum. This structure has a rich innervation of somatic receptors. It is sensitive to traction, pressure, and inflammation, as are also the mesentery and the lesser omentum. On the other hand, the visceral peritoneum is virtually insensitive. When the parietal peritoneum is stimulated adequately, the pain is referred to the adjacent cutaneous area. The symptom is usually exacerbated by local pressure, movements, changing position, jarring deep respiration, and cough. It is severe, sharply localized, and circumscribed. This is the kind of pain which is felt in cases of acute appendicitis, diverticulitis, or cholecystitis when the inflamed organs are in close contact with the peritoneum. When the diaphragmatic peritoneum is stimulated, the pain is referred to the anterior part of the abdomen which corresponds to the last six thoracic segments. Diaphragmatic pain may also be felt in the shoulder and neck, in the dermatomes which correspond to C3 and C4, the roots of which constitute the afferent fibers of the phrenic nerve.

Capsules of solid viscera. The capsules of the liver, spleen, and kidneys have sensitive receptors which are responsive to distention; they are stimulated when there is a rapid increase in the size of these organs.

RETROPERITONEAL AREA

The structures located in the retroperitoneal area, such as the urinary organs, have rich innervation and give rise to abdominal pain which is transmitted through the tenth and twelfth thoracic roots and the lumbar roots; the pain is then referred to the corresponding dermatome. This is the reason why many kidney and urethral lesions give rise to abdominal pain. Similar pain emanates from other retroperitoneal lesions such as infections, collections of fluid, and neoplastic processes in the retroperitoneum.

Extraabdominal Structures Capable of Causing Abdominal Pain

The heart, lungs, and pleura can cause abdominal pain. Pericarditis, myocardial infarction, pulmonary infarction, and basal lobe pneumonia may cause inflammatory reactions in the diaphragmatic pleura and cause pain which is usually felt in the right or left subcostal areas, or in the epigastrium.

Clinical Significance

Many pathologic processes taking place in any of the abdominal and various extraabdominal structures may cause abdominal pain. A meticulous analysis of this symptom is essential and may be highly rewarding in the diagnostic evaluation of patients complaining of abdominal pain. Epigastric pain is most frequently caused by gastric, duodenal, biliary, or pancreatic lesions. The epigastric pain of gastric origin may be caused by stimulation of visceral afferent fibers. It is felt in the midline, and is poorly localized, vague, and often related to the intake of food. When the lesion is either benign ulcer disease or an ulcerated carcinoma, abdominal pain is usually present when the lesion is bathed by the gastric acid, whereas the ingestion of food or antacids neutralizes the acid and affords prompt relief. On the other hand, when the pain of gastric origin is caused by distention of the organ, as may occur secondary to an obstruction at its outlet, the pain follows the intake of food and is relieved by vomiting. In these cases vomiting occurs spontaneously or may be provoked by the patient to alleviate the pain. The vomitus does not usually contain bile, and food particles are readily identified.

The pain originating from duodenal ulcer is not unlike the pain of gastric ulcer, although it may be located at a slightly lower level of the epigastric area and to the right side. It tends to appear before lunch, before dinner, and at midnight, when greater amounts of gastric acid are being secreted by the stomach and are not buffered. This type of pain is relieved by the intake of food or antacids. When the pathologic process in the stomach or duodenum penetrates beyond the wall of the organ and reaches the retroperitoneal space, the lesser omentum, or the diaphragmatic peritoneum, somatic afferent nerve fibers are stimulated. The pain becomes sharp and severe and is less dependent on the effects of fasting or the ingestion of food or antacids. This pain may be influenced by local pressure, jarring movements, or changes in position, and it is located in the dermatome corresponding to the somatic roots being stimulated.

The pain of gallbladder origin is located in the epigastrium or right upper quadrant. When it is caused by a spasm of the biliary ducts, it is paroxysmal and severe, and radiates to the upper right quadrant and right subscapular area. On the other hand, when it is caused by inflammation of the walls of the gallbladder and if the inflammatory process is in contact with or involves the parietal peritoneum, the pain becomes localized in the subcostal area precisely at the location of the gallbladder and acquires the characteristics of somatic pain.

Pain of pancreatic origin is also epigastric. Since the pancreas is a retroperitoneal organ, its pathologic processes such as pancreatitis or pancreatic cancer stimulate somatic nerve endings. Thus, the pain is somatic in character and severe, and it radiates to the right or left upper quadrants or the back and the left shoulder, depending on the extent and location of the pathologic process. The patient describes the pain as epigastric going through to the back, worse on lying down, and improved on sitting up or bending forward. Even though it may be more intense after pancreatic stimulation following a meal, the pain is more constant and lasts many hours or even days following an attack of recurrent pancreatitis. In cancer of the pancreas this pain persists for months.

Pain in the right upper quadrant of the abdomen may be caused by distention of the capsule of Glisson when there is rapid enlargement of the liver by inflammatory or neoplastic processes. This pain may also follow other lesions involving contiguous inflammatory or neoplastic processes of the gallbladder and the head of the pancreas, and penetrating duodenal ulcers. In these conditions, the pain is caused by stimulation of somatic afferent fibers and thus has the characteristics of somatic pain. It is important to remember that disease of the right kidney and thoracic processes involving diaphragmatic pleura can also cause right upper quadrant pain. Pain in this area is also caused by stimuli from the hepatic flexure of the colon. Similarly, left-upper-quadrant pain may be caused by enlargement of the spleen or infarcts of the spleen, whereby the splenic capsule is affected. Contiguous organs cause similar pain by inflammatory or neoplastic processes of the tail of the pancreas, by perforated ulcers of the greater curvature of the stomach, by diseases of the left kidney or the left thoracic cavity involving the diaphragmatic pleura, as well as by pathologic processes involving the splenic flexure of the colon.

Periumbilical pain suggests disease of the small bowel, with the exception of the terminal ileum which more commonly causes pain in the right lower quadrant of the abdomen. In acute appendicitis, the pain characteristically starts in the epigastrium, but a few hours later it moves toward the right lower abdomen, acquiring the characteristics of somatic pain as the process involves the visceral and the neighboring parietal peritoneum. Pain of colonic origin is usually central and infraumbilical, except when it arises from the hepatic flexure, splenic flexure, or sigmoid, when it might be located in the right upper quadrant, left upper quadrant, and left lower quadrant, respectively. Pain of rectal origin is felt very low in the abdomen and in the suprapubic area. The pain of renal origin is felt in the lumbar area, but radiates to the upper and lower quadrants, to the groin, and to the testicles or labia. The pain of pelvic origin is felt in the suprapubic area, lower abdominal quadrants, and deep in the pelvis.

Selected References

1. Cope Z: *The Early Diagnosis of the Acute Abdomen,* ed 13. New York, Oxford University Press, 1968.
2. Sweet WH: Pain, in Code CF (ed): *Handbook of Physiology.* Washington, DC, American Physiological Society, 1959, vol 1, sect 1, pp 459–506.
3. Way LW: Abdominal pain, in Sleisenger MH, Fordtran JS (eds): *Gastrointestinal Disease.* Philadelphia, WB Saunders, 1973, pp 326–337.
4. Smith L: Sites and behaviors of pain in certain common diseases of the upper abdomen, in *Atlas of Pain Patterns.* Springfield, Ill, Charles C Thomas, 1961, p 54.
5. Jones CM: *Digestive Tract Pain: Diagnosis and Treatment: Experimental Observations.* New York, Macmillan, 1938.

6. Smith LA, Christensen NA, Hansen NO, et al: *An Atlas of Pain Patterns: Sites and Behavior of Pain in Certain Common Diseases of the Upper Abdomen.* Springfield, Ill, Charles C Thomas, 1961.

25. Abdominal Swelling

THEODORE HERSH, MD
HORACIO JINICH, MD

Definition

Enlargement of abdominal girth and/or distention of the abdomen.

Technique

To discover whether there has been any "swelling" of the abdomen, ask about distention or ask whether there has been any change in the size of the garments worn. Use the terms "swelling," "distention," or "enlargement of the abdomen." Some patients may refer to this phenomenon as swelling of the "stomach." The patient may indicate an increase in abdominal girth by having to wear looser garments, letting the belt out, or unbuttoning the pants.

Once the presence of abdominal "swelling" has been ascertained, find out if it is intermittent or constant, recent or progressive, chronic or static. In the first case, find out if swelling appears after meals and if it is proportional to the amount of food ingested; also find out if it is relieved by the expulsion of gas or feces per rectum, or by belching or vomiting. Some patients induce vomiting as a means of relieving the feeling of distention. The nature of the material being vomited should be determined because it can locate the possible site of an obstructive process in the digestive tract (presence or absence of bile, presence or absence of food particles and when these were first ingested).

If the abdominal swelling is constant, one needs to inquire whether or not it has been associated with weight gain, with the development of obesity, with the appearance of edema in the lower extremities, with less frequent urination; and whether the swelling has occurred abruptly or over a period of time, whether it has remained stable or has been progressive and whether it involves the whole abdomen or only part of it.

Because of the possibility of the abdominal swelling being caused by pregnancy or by tumors of the pelvic organs in the female, a careful gynecologic history should be taken, including the date of the last menstrual period.

Background Information

Depending on the etiology, abdominal swelling may be either acute or chronic in nature. The increase in abdominal girth may be due to distention from gas, liquid, or solid. Depending on the pathology present, the swelling may result from a localized lesion in the abdomen, or it may indeed be a generalized swelling of the abdominal cavity. The physical examination provides information regarding the type of distention present and thereby gives a clue to the etiology.

Clinical Significance

The clinical significance of abdominal swelling can be best ascertained by studying the classification that follows:

I. Swelling due to gas
    A. Paralytic ileus
    B. Intestinal obstruction
    C. Gastric dilatation
        1. Acute (postoperative, infectious diseases)
        2. Chronic, caused by pyloric stenosis
        3. Chronic, caused by gastric atony
    D. Aerophagia
    E. Malabsorption syndrome
    F. Lactase deficiency with lactose intolerance
    G. Megacolon
    H. Reflex ileus (kidney colic, biliary colic)

II. Swelling due to fluid (see Ascites)

III. Swelling due to solid
    A. Organ enlargement
        1. Hepatomegaly
        2. Splenomegaly
        3. Pregnancy
        4. Enlarged urinary bladder secondary to prostatic enlargement

B.   Tumor
   1.   Of the abdominal wall (lipoma, hernia, abscess)
   2.   Intra-abdominal (liver, gallbladder, spleen, stomach, small and large bowel, peritoneum, bladder, uterus, ovary)
   3.   Retroperitoneal (pancreas, lymph nodes, aneurysm, kidney, adrenals)

An acute distention of the abdomen may result from an obstructive lesion in the gastrointestinal tract, from a paralytic obstruction (ileus), or from the rapid accumulation of fluid. Transient distention may be due to conditions of colonic or small intestinal pseudoobstruction syndromes where the bowel distends without an obstructive lesion. Chronic partial intermittent obstruction may present as distention; contracting loops of bowel may be visible on inspection of the abdomen. Occasionally patients with significant lactase deficiency and lactose intolerance will have abdominal distention following ingestion of large quantities of dairy products. The osmotic effect of the undigested lactose causes fluid to enter the lumen of the gut, and colonic bacteria will then ferment the lactose with production of gas. Gaseous distention may follow surgery or trauma to the abdomen.

Chronic persistent swelling due to accumulation of fluid, ascites, has various etiologies. (The physical examination will confirm the presence of fluid in abdomen.) Ascites may be due to conditions with a decrease in serum albumin and an increase in pressure in the portal venous system, such as in the various types of cirrhosis of the liver, hepatic vein thrombosis, constrictive pericarditis, and chronic right-sided congestive heart failure. Ascites is also present in other hypoalbuminemic states such as renal failure and protein-losing gastroenteropathy syndromes. Obstructed lymphatic syndromes may present as chylous ascites. Ascites with high protein content is the result of inflammatory processes such as tuberculous peritonitis or carcinomatous involvement of the peritoneum. In addition, ruptured pseudocysts of the pancreas or pancreatic ducts will ooze out high protein fluid high in amylase content; this entity is known as pancreatic ascites.

Abdominal swelling with increase in body weight occurs in obesity. Colonic obstruction with obstipation may present as abdominal swelling as a result of congenital megacolon in children or tumors or strictures in adults. Large ovarian tumors or cysts can present as localized abdominal swelling. Localized swelling in the female may represent pregnancy. Abdominal swelling is often a phenomenon of a large urinary bladder resulting from obstruction of the prostate. Apparent increase of the abdominal girth occurs with exaggeration of the lordotic curve of the spine as in the entity of pseudocyesis.

Selected References

1. Miller LD, Mackie JA, Rhoades JE: The pathophysiology and management of intestinal obstruction. *Surg Clin N Am* 42:1285–1309, 1962.
2. Witte MH, Witte CL, Dumont AE: Physiologic factors involved in causation of cirrhotic ascites. *Gastroenterology* 61:742–750, 1971.
3. Keeffe EJ, Gagliardi RA, Pfister RC: The roentgenologic evaluation of ascites. *Am J Roent* 101:388–396, 1967.

26. Jaundice

HORACIO JINICH, MD
THEODORE HERSH, MD

Definition

The yellow discoloration (pigmentation) of the skin and mucosas caused by the accumulation of bile pigments (bilirubin).

Technique

The first step in the diagnosis of the patient with jaundice is to ascertain that he actually has jaundice and not one of the following conditions with which it may be confused:

1. Pallor
2. Subconjunctival fat
3. Concentrated urine
4. Pigmentation from carotene and other carotenoid pigments.
5. Pigmentation from atabrine, picric acid, acriflavin or fluorescein.

Patients with pallor are sometimes erroneously considered to have a yellow appearance, mistaken for icterus. A careful examination of the sclerae will usually suffice to rectify the mistake. Adequate lighting is essential for this purpose and, in general, for the identification of jaundice, which can readily be overlooked in artificial light. During the recollection of the past medical history, it is not unusual for patients to mention "jaundice," a sign confused with pallor. A previous history of jaundice should be confirmed. The patient with pernicious anemia may indeed have pallor and icterus resulting from the macrocytic anemia and hemolysis found in these patients. Other patients with hemolytic anemias may similarly have pallor from the anemia and icterus from the resulting high serum bilirubin levels.

Subconjunctival fat must not be confused with jaundice. It frequently appears in spots or patches and is not evenly distributed. The careful examination of the floor of the mouth, skin, and urine will suffice to establish presence of jaundice, but occasionally it may be necessary to resort to chemical tests of the blood or urine in order to ascertain the presence of bile pigments.

Concentrated urine may be mistakenly diagnosed as bile pigments in urine (choluria). It is easy to avoid the mistake: urine collected in a transparent container is shaken until foam is formed. If the foam is white, then the urine is concentrated. Yellow foam denotes the presence of bile pigments. This useful procedure has the further advantage of allowing an early diagnosis of jaundice, particularly since bile pigments usually appear in the urine before color appears in the skin or on mucous membranes in conditions such as acute viral hepatitis or obstructive lesions leading to jaundice.

Prolonged ingestion of foods rich in carotene and other carotenoid pigments (carrots, tomatoes, papaya) causes an orange-yellow pigmentation of the skin which not infrequently causes the patient to consult the physician with the mistaken notion that he is jaundiced. Diagnosis should be easy since this pigmentation affects the palms and soles, while the sclerae and the urine maintain their normal color. Furthermore, the dietary history of ingestion of these foods supports the impression of carotenemia. A high serum carotene level is confirmatory.

Drugs may cause a yellow hue, but not jaundice (hyperbilirubinemia). When atabrine was widely employed for the treatment of malaria, it was not unusual to find patients with a generalized yellow pigmentation, especially marked in the dorsum of the arms, hands and feet. However, the sclerae are usually not affected, and it is easy to determine the true cause of this pigmentation by questioning the patient about use of this medication. In addition, the intake of picric acid, fluorescein, and acriflavin can give rise to a pseudoicteric pigmentation of the skin. If the patient is psychotic or a malingerer, it may be necessary to resort to chemical tests of the blood and urine to rule out the presence of increased amounts of bile pigments in blood.

Background Information

Normal metabolism of bile pigments can be conveniently divided into the following stages: formation of bilirubin, transport of bilirubin into the hepatocytes, conjugation within the hepatocyte with glucuronic acid, transport into the bile canaliculi, and excretion into bile ducts and duodenum.

Formation of bilirubin. The average life span of erythrocytes is 120 days. After this time, they are destroyed in the reticuloendothelial system. The components of the hemoglobin molecule are metabolized differently: iron is kept in the organism and reutilized in the synthesis of new hemoglobin molecule and other iron-containing compounds. Globin is subsequently metabolized. The enzyme heme-oxygenase converts heme into biliverdin which is then rapidly converted into bilirubin by another enzyme, biliverdin reductase. Bilirubin, which is lipid soluble, diffuses freely across cell membranes into the cells where it could interfere with the normal process of oxidative phosphorylation in the mitochondria. The organism, however, prevents this diffusion of the pigment into the cells by linking bilirubin with circulating albumin. The subsequent excretion of the pigment is made possible by its conjugation with glucuronic acid, thus becoming more polar, water soluble, and amenable to excretion via biliary system and intestine. Bilirubin is also formed through another metabolic pathway: intravascular lysis of red blood cells whereby hemoglobin is set free, bound by haptoglobin, and subsequently taken up by the hepatocytes.

Transport of bilirubin into the liver cells. The liver cell membrane is extremely permeable to bilirubin. Two cytoplasmic proteins, protein Y, or ligandin, and protein Z, bind the pigment and apparently transport it in the hepatocyte to the site of conjugation.

Conjugation of bilirubin. Conjugation with glucuronic acid and, possibly to a lesser extent, with other radicals such as sulfates, converts free bilirubin into conjugated bilirubin. The conjugation takes place in the smooth endoplasmic reticulum, mediated by the enzyme glucuronyl transferase.

Transport of conjugated bilirubin into the bile canaliculi. The process of secreting bilirubin out of the hepatocyte is an active process involving the participation of the endoplasmic reticulum, the Golgi apparatus, the lysosomes, and the microvilli lining the bile canaliculi.

Excretion of conjugated bilirubin. Conjugated bilirubin reaches the small intestine through the various branches of the biliary system. Since it is a polar compound, it cannot be absorbed. In the colon, bilirubin is reduced by the activity of the colonic flora into a set of compounds known by the genetic name of urobilinogens. Most urobilinogen is excreted with the feces; only a small amount is absorbed and then reaches the liver where it is reexcreted into the bile. A very small amount of urobilinogen escapes into the systemic circulation and is excreted by the kidney (less than 2.5 mg per 24 lb).

Bile pigments accumulate in the body giving rise to jaundice under the following circumstances:

1. Excessive formation of bilirubin. This is usually the result of accelerated hemolysis (hemolytic anemia).
2. Defective conjugation of bilirubin, secondary to a deficiency of the enzyme glucuronyl transferase or the defective uptake into the liver cells.
3. Cholestasis, secondary to defects in the active transport of conjugated bilirubin into the biliary tract, to structural damage of the liver cells and to actual intra or extrahepatic obstruction of the biliary tract caused by calculi, tumor, or strictures.

In any of these conditions, the concentration of bilirubin in the blood and then in tissues rises, and jaundice becomes apparent. However, in the groups of conditions listed in (1) and (2), free (unconjugated) bilirubin is the fraction which is present in high concentration; in condition (3) it is both unconjugated and conjugated bilirubin.

Clinical Significance

Jaundice is the result of many varied pathophysiologic processes. It is the function of the clinician to utilize all the clinical evidence, and to gather all the available information derived from the laboratory tests, radiologic studies, and special procedures in order to clearly define the etiology and mechanism in every case of jaundice. If there is no other history suggestive of liver disease, usually the first step is to determine whether the elevation of bilirubin is caused by the free or the conjugated form of the pigment. If it is free bilirubin, the clinician will next have to know whether there is hemolysis by determination of hemoglobin level, reticulocyte count and special studies of hemoglobin electrophoresis and red cell survival if necessary. Unconjugated hyperbilirubinemia is often due to slow uptake by the hepatocyte (Gilbert's disease). More often, jaundice is caused by an elevation of conjugated bilirubin, and the differential diagnosis becomes one of determining whether the hepatic cause of the jaundice is parenchymal damage (hepatocellular jaundice) or stasis of bile in the biliary tract (cholestatic jaundice). If the diagnosis of cholestasis is established, then it must be decided if it is intrahepatic such as that resulting from drugs, alcohol, or viral hepatitis or extrahepatic as in common duct calculi or carcinoma of the head of the pancreas.

Selected References

1. Fleischner G, Arias IM: Recent advances in bilirubin formation, transport, metabolism, and excretion. *Am J Med* 49:576–589, 1970.
2. Bissell DH. Formation and elimination of bilirubin. *Gastroenterology* 69:519–538, 1975.
3. Berk PD: Unconjugated hyperbilirubinemia: Physiologic evaluation and experimental approaches to therapy. *Ann Intern Med* 82:552–570, 1975.
4. Ostrow JD: Jaundice in older children and adults: Algorithms for diagnosis. *JAMA* 234:522–526, 1975.

27. Hematochezia

THEODORE HERSH, MD
HORACIO JINICH, MD

Definition

The passage of fresh blood per rectum.

Technique

The examiner first inquires about a patient's bowel habits. It is important to note if there has been any change in the frequency of defecation or in the quality or size of the stool. The presence or absence of blood in the evacuation needs to be established. A direct question is the best approach: Did you ever notice any blood in your stools? If the patient has noted blood in the stool, ascertain whether the blood is on the outside of the stool, on the toilet paper, or mixed in with the stool. Is the blood only on the garments? The blood may be passed independent of a bowel movement. An estimate should be made about the amount, frequency, and duration of rectal bleeding. Is the blood present with diarrheal stools? Is this an acute or chronic situation? Are there other symptoms such as chills, fever, abdominal pain, weight loss? Is there any history of a bleeding disorder? Has there been a change in bowel habits?

Background Information

Blood per rectum signifies a bleeding lesion of the lower gastrointestinal tract. Occasionally in the acutely bleeding patient, bright red blood may be coming from the upper gastrointestinal tract, such as from a massively bleeding duodenal ulcer or a ruptured aortic aneurysm; however, bleeding proximal to the ligament of Treitz usually presents as melena. In patients where rectal bleeding is associated with other symptoms, such as diarrhea and fever, the presence of blood with the stools may indicate an inflammatory lesion of the gastrointestinal tract. Ulcerative lesions present with blood mixed with diarrheal stools and mucus. Blood is mixed in with a formed stool when there is a circumscribed lesion in the colon, since the remaining distal bowel can continue to fulfill its function of absorbing fluid. An example of this lesion is a carcinoma of the left colon. Rupture of blood vessels and vascular insufficiency to the colon may cause rectal bleeding. Blood covering the stool is likely to be from the lower portion of the rectum or the anus.

Clinical Significance

Acute loss of blood per rectum indicates an actively bleeding lesion in the lower gastrointestinal tract. In children this may represent a bleeding Meckel's diverticulum; in the adult, bleeding from diverticula, particularly in the right colon, may present with hematochezia. Ruptured vessels such as the low perfusion syndrome of ischemic proctitis manifest as rectal bleeding. Acute blood loss via bright red blood per rectum plus shock may even indicate lesions in the upper intestinal tract, such as duodenal ulcer or ruptured aortic aneurysm. Bloody diarrhea may represent ulcerative lesions such as amebiasis, bacillary dysentery, chronic ulcerative colitis, or ulcerative proctitis. Blood mixed in with the stool most often signifies a lower colonic carcinoma. Blood covering the stool usually represents hemorrhoids or fissure. Coagulation disorders need to be ruled out in cases where no etiology for hematochezia is apparent. The following is a classification of hematochezia:

1. Internal hemorrhoids
2. Nonspecific chronic ulcerative colitis; granulomatous colitis
3. Amebiasis or bacillary dysentery
4. Gonococcal proctitis
5. Radiation enteritis

6. Cancer of the recum and colon
7. Polyps and other benign tumors of the rectum and colon
8. Fissures (anal)

Selected References

1. Noer RJ, Hamilton JE, Williams DJ, Broughton, DS: Rectal hemorrhage: Moderate and severe. *Ann Surg* 155:794–805, 1962.
2. Baum S, Nusbaum N: The control of gastrointestinal hemorrhage by selective mesenteric arterial infusion of vasopressin. *Radiology* 98:497–505, 1971.
3. Byrne JJ, Wittenberg J, Grimes ET, et al: Ischemic diseases of the bowel: II. Ischemic colitis. *Dis Col Rect* 13:283–289, 1970.

28. Diarrhea

THEODORE HERSH, MD
HORACIO JINICH, MD

Definition

The frequent passage of watery stool.

Technique

Take a general approach: How are your bowel movements? What is your regular (usual) pattern? Have you had a recent change in bowel movement habits? Answers to these questions may not reveal a chronic gastrointestinal condition; therefore, ask the patient to describe the frequency of his bowel movements in terms of number of times per day or per week. Follow with questions relevant to a description of the consistency of the stool, using words like "formed," "soft," "liquid." Consider whether the described frequency represents a change in the pattern of defecation. Questions can then be directed to the color and contents of the stool, which may be described as various shades of brown, green, black, yellow, or colorless, bloody, or watery. Comparison to standard objects or to colors in the examining room is helpful. Once the color is established, inquire whether this represents a change. Inquire whether food particles have been recognized, and ask the patient to list these foodstuffs. Associated symptoms collected from the remainder of the gastrointestinal questions are vital, including the presence or absence of abdominal pain, abdominal distention, urgency to defecate, passage of flatus, the passage of mucus with stools, watery discharge independent of stools, rectal seepage of oil independent of stools. The latter two may be actually described by the patient as diarrhea, because of the liquid nature of both secretions.

Background Information

Diarrhea represents an increase in the frequency, fluidity, or volume of bowel movements that may result from a variety of alterations in the absorption and secretion of fluids in the gastrointestinal tract. Mean daily fecal weight is usually less than 200 gm with water content constituting about 70%; however, in liquid stools the water content may increase up to 90%. Although the content of water in the stool may be the best indicator of diarrhea, there are many situations in which there is more volume of stool, particularly when the alteration is in the distal colon. Stools are normally formed because the bowel has remarkable efficiency for reabsorbing fluid and returning it to the extracellular space. The jejunum and ileum absorb significant quantities of exogenous and endogenous fluids from gastric, biliary and pancreatic secretions, but the luminal contents in the distal ileum and ascending colon are still liquid. The great efficiency of absorption of fluids by the colon accounts for solid stools.

Diarrhea can be caused by a number of mechanisms.

1. *Osmotic diarrhea.* In this case, large amounts of poorly absorbable, osmotically active substances are present in the lumen of the gut. Water and electrolyte absorption is retarded; the osmotic effect tends to cause net water movement from plasma to the lumen of the gut since the osmotic pressure of the nonabsorbable luminal contents is higher than that of plasma. Subtypes of osmotic diarrhea can be recognized; namely, ingestion of poorly absorbed compounds such as laxatives and poor digestion of certain foods.

2. *Disorders of intestinal secretion.* In the normal bowel, there is both absorption and secretion of fluid and electrolytes. Diarrhea may ensue when there is an increased secretion of fluid into the lumen of the gut. This may come from toxins that occur in gastrointestinal infections such as cholera, or infections by *Staphylococci* and *Escherichia coli*. Diarrhea may also be produced by the action of various hormones, in-

cluding excess quantities of gastrin, which stimulates copious amounts of gastric acid; vasoactive intestinal polypeptide released from various tumors, which causes secretion from the small bowel, or calcitonin released from medullary thyroid cancer.

3. *Exudative diarrheas.* In many conditions, diarrhea is caused by exudation of serum proteins, blood mucus, or pus from sites of inflammation, ulceration, or diseases which infiltrate the gastrointestinal mucosa. The exudation increases the fluid in the lumen of the gut; alterations in the mucosa of the bowel result in a decrease of fluid absorption. There is an increase in water excretion and thus diarrheal stools.

4. *Disorder of absorptive surface.* Diarrhea may also ensue if the absorptive surface of the gastrointestinal tract is altered by disease or if its absence is due to bypass or previous resection. Rapid intestinal transit such as occurs in hyperthyroidism may cause diarrhea. Altered absorption occurs in diseases with small bowel villous atrophy. Decrease in the absorptive surface area follows massive intestinal resections or the jejunoileal bypass for morbid obesity. Absorptive areas of bowel are also bypassed when enteroenteric fistulas have formed.

5. *Altered motility.* Diarrhea may result from alterations in intestinal motility, particularly delayed intestinal transit, which promotes stasis of fluid and food contents in the lumen of the gastrointestinal tract. This is followed by an overgrowth of intestinal bacteria which deconjugate the bile salts that are normally needed to form micelles for absorption of dietary fat. In addition, unconjugated (free) bile acids may have "inhibitory" effects on the intestinal mucosal absorptive processes.

6. *Steatorrhea.* Another type of "diarrhea" needs to be recognized when the patient describes his stools as being soft or liquid, bulky, yellow, frothy, and malodorous. This stool may contain recognizable food particles. The cause is increased fat content in the stool (steatorrhea) and represents a maldigestion or malabsorption syndrome.

Clinical Significance

The history is most important in providing information regarding the etiology of diarrhea. Even the quality and quantity of the stools may point to the area of involvement of the gastrointestinal tract. A distinction by history may be made between "large" stool or "small" stool diarrhea. The former would likely indicate a disorder of the upper gastrointestinal tract or, less frequently, of the proximal colon. These stools are likely to be lighter in color and contain excess water; they may be frothy or soupy. When diseases of the pancreas or small intestinal mucosa are present, the stool may contain excess fat, and thereby be greasy, foul smelling, and yellow. Dietary long-chain triglycerides in stool reflect undigested dietary fat due to exocrine pancreatic insufficiency (decrease in lipase), while fatty acids in stool tend to signify malabsorption. Bacterial enzymes, however, can digest fat. Undigested food particles may be present. These patients may experience periumbilical cramping, abdominal pain, gas, and distension. In contrast, small-volume diarrhea, particularly when there is a significant urgency to defecate, suggests that the disease is likely to be in the distal colon. These patients will frequently pass only flatus or small quantities of mucus. Stools may be mushy and contain blood when the mucosa is inflamed.

Diarrhea of recent onset, particularly when accompanied by systemic symptoms, such as chills and fever, nausea, or vomiting suggests an infectious origin, such as *Salmonella, Shigella, Escherichia coli* diarrheas, and viral gastroenteritis. Travel to a recent country may uncover an *E. coli* diarrhea (traveler's diarrhea), giardiasis, or amebiasis. Staphylococcus food poisoning, which may affect more than one family member, causes an acute gastrointestinal attack with diarrhea. Diarrhea associated with ingestion of various foodstuffs, particularly carbohydrates such as lactose in dairy products and sucrose, suggests deficiencies of disaccharidases in the small intestinal mucosa, with inability to digest the disaccharide into its component monosaccharides. The undigested sugar in the lumen of the bowel causes an osmotic diarrhea. In the newborn, diarrhea following ingestion of sugar solutions suggests the entity of glucose-galactose malabsorption.

Many medications are associated with diarrhea. Frequently, one just has to inquire whether the patient has been taking laxatives for the treatment of "constipation." Laxatives that include the saline cathartics increase fecal water as a result of the slow and incomplete absorption of these ions, such as occurs following preparations with magnesium sulfate and phosphate. Some antacids for the treatment of peptic ulcer cause diarrhea because of their excess content of saline cathartics. Other laxatives, such as castor oil, senna, bisacodyl, cascara, and phenolphthalein may cause diarrhea by increasing intestinal secretion or enhancing intestinal motility. Antibiotics have also been noted to cause diarrhea by various mechanisms, perhaps altering the bacterial flora; the most common offenders include lincomycin, clindamycin, and neomycin. In some of these patients a fulminant diarrheal disorder named pseudomembranous enterocolitis has been described. Alcohol causes diarrhea by mechanisms that have not yet been elucidated. Prostaglandins may cause diarrhea by increasing intestinal secretion; antimetabolites and radiation therapy, by their effect on small intestinal mucosa. Radiation and previous ischemia can form strictures in the bowel with consequent alterations in bacterial populations.

Small-intestinal diarrhea may, in addition to infectious agents, be due to hormones produced by the gastrointestinal tract or other organs. When there is an excess circulating gastrin synthesized by pancreatic islet cell tumors (Zollinger-Ellison syndrome), there is an increase in secretion of gastric acid. The diarrhea resulting from this hypergastrinemia depends on an increased load provided to the bowel; in addition, the high volume and low pH fluid damage the intestinal mucosa, render pancreatic lipase inactive, and result in an inadequate pH for proper micelle formation. Other pancreatic tumors produce hormones that may cause diarrhea, including vasoactive intestinal polypeptide, the likely culprit in the entity of pancreatic cholera. In this syndrome there is an inhibition of gastric acid and a loss of potassium from the bowel. These patients present with profound diarrhea and hypokalemia. Calcitonin causes a secretory diarrhea in patients with medullary thyroid cancer. Bile acids may also be included as mucosal secretagogues. When there is an increase of bile acids entering the colon with involvement of the terminal ileum, as occurs in Crohn's disease, or when the ileum has been resected or bypassed, large quantities of bile acids enter the colon and produce diarrhea. The loss of bile acids due to ileal disease decreases the pool size, and there is concomitant decrease in their concentration in the duodenum. Impaired micelle formation occurs and, there is steatorrhea. The long-chained fatty acids that are present in the colon in the various steatorrheal syndromes may increase fecal water as a result of their action on the colonic mucosa.

Inflammatory bowel diseases, including ulcerative colitis and granulomatous colitis, are exudative states with consequent bloody diarrhea. Ischemia and radiation also damage the colonic mucosa and present as bloody diarrhea.

Intestinal neoplasms may cause diarrhea, particularly the villous adenomas of the rectum where there is a large surface area with secretion of water and potassium. The loss is often significant enough to cause severe hypokalemia. When the adenoma is located close to the rectum, the passage of water may be independent of stools. Other tumors may cause diarrhea by causing intestinal obstruction. Lymphoma may involve the small bowel and cause diarrhea and malabsorption by alterations in absorptive processes and lymphatic blockage. Often, intestinal lymphatic obstruction results in a syndrome of protein-losing enteropathy, which includes diarrhea, steatorrhea, and edema resulting from hypoalbuminemia.

Metabolic diseases, such as hyperthyroidism by rapid transit time, Addison's disease, the carcinoid syndrome, and mastocytosis may also cause diarrhea. Nocturnal diarrhea of diabetes mellitus is well known, and probably results from the alterations in gastrointestinal motor function.

Steatorrheal disorders, the passage of excess fat in the stools, may result from diseases of the pancreas, biliary tract, or small bowel. Exocrine pancreatic insufficiency results in maldigestion of fats and consequent steatorrhea. Often these patients will have a history of chronic recurrent abdominal pain of pancreatitis and diabetes mellitus. Undigested food particles are more commonly seen in the steatorrheal stools of pancreatic insufficiency. Occasionally, these patients report rectal seepage of oil independent of bowel movement. Steatorrhea due to small-bowel disease has diverse etiologies. In nontropical areas of the world, celiac disease (gluten enteropathy) is probably the most common cause of malabsorption. Its onset may be in childhood. In the tropics the entity of tropical sprue occurs with varying degrees of intestinal mucosal atrophy and is associated with steatorrhea. Absence of conjugated bile salts in the intestinal lumen, such as in patients with obstruction to the common bile duct by a tumor or calculus or presence of a stricture, may result in steatorrhea due to an inadequate concentration of the bile acids for micelle formation.

Selected References

1. Fordtran JS: Speculations on pathogenesis of diarrhea. *Fed Proc* 26:1405–1414, 1967.
2. Fordtran JS, Dietschy JM: Water and electrolyte movement in the intestine. *Gastroenterology* 50:263–285, 1966.
3. Wilson FA, Dietschy JM: Differential diagnostic approach to clinical problems of malabsorption. *Gastroenterology* 61:911–931, 1971.
4. Gray GM: Intestinal digestion and maldigestion of dietary carbohydrates. *Ann Rev Med* 22:391–404, 1971.
5. Phillips SF: Diarrhea: A current view of the pathophysiology. *Gastroenterology* 63:495–518, 1972.
6. Grady FG, Keusch GT: Pathogenesis of bacterial diarrheas. *New Eng J Med* 285:831–841, 1971.
7. Brooks FP (ed): *Gastrointestinal Pathophysiology,* ed 2. New York, Oxford University Press, 1978.

29. Constipation

THEODORE HERSH, MD
HORACIO JINICH, MD

Definition

The passage of stools with decreased frequency or stools of insufficient size or of excessive dryness. This definition is necessarily relative because there is no absolute standard for comparison. Healthy people move their bowels from three or more times a day to once every seven or more days. The basis for comparison, then, must be the average for the population in a given culture and, mainly, the previous or usual bowel habits of that particular individual. Thus, in our urban American culture we tend to employ the term constipation if the stools are less often than every other day, weigh less than 50 gm per day, or, because of their dryness, demand strenuous efforts on the part of the patient during defecation. On the other hand, the individual who is used to having one average bowel movement a day would be concerned if the frequency of bowel movements decreased to once every other day or longer. There is also concern when stools are smaller with straining which had not previously been present during defecation.

Technique

The patient who suffers from constipation will usually consult the physician for different reasons: (1) he has noticed a change in his bowel habits; (2) he requests a new laxative complaining that the one he has been using does not work any more; (3) even though he has no complaints except for habitual infrequent bowel movements, he has been informed and even warned and frightened by other people or newspaper ads about his "abnormal and potentially dangerous habit," (4) he complains of a set of symptoms attributed to constipation such as: a subjective sensation of incomplete emptying of the rectum; lower abdominal discomfort, malaise, anorexia, halitosis, coated tongue, abdominal distension, and flatulence.

The physician should first of all clarify what the patient means by the term "constipation." Ask the patient: Do you mean you don't move your bowels as often as before? How did you move your bowels before when you were all right? How often do you move your bowels now? Do you mean your stools have become smaller? thinner? harder? dryer? more difficult to expel? Do you feel that there is stool remaining in your rectum?

If the patient does not complain of constipation spontaneously, the physician should ask simple questions such as: How often do you move your bowels? Have you noticed any change in your bowel habits? Have you noticed any change in the bulk of your stools? Do you feel that you have emptied your bowels entirely after you go to the toilet?

Background Information

Conditions that may lead to constipation may be divided into those affecting the filling and those affecting the emptying of the rectum. The filling of the rectum occurs as the logical end result of the normal function of the large bowel which includes: storage of intestinal contents prior to discharge, absorption of water, electrolytes, and bile salts. While the absorptive processes take place, the colonic contents move in a caudad direction, finally reaching the rectum because of effective propulsive mechanisms that occur mainly by way of mass movements. Usually the entry of food into the upper small bowel initiates a reflex response leading to passage of material from the distal small intestine into the cecum (gastroileal reflex). After a time lag necessary for adequate distention of the cecum and right colon, the mass movement takes place. The participation of several hormones such as gastrin, secretin, and particularly cholecystokinin-pancrozymin remains to be determined. The response does not depend upon the vagus nerve because it is present after vagotomy.

The emptying of the rectum is a result of the defecation reflex: the pressure on the wall of the rectum caused by the arrival of feces stimulates receptors and gives rise to a feeling of dull discomfort and to afferent impulses that reach a center in the sacral portion of the spinal cord. The efferent limb of the reflex causes relaxation of the internal anal sphincter, descent of the diaphragm, contraction of the abdominal wall musculature, and a Valsalva maneuver that increases intraabdominal pressure. This set of integrated events leads to the expulsion of the rectal contents, which is facilitated by the elevation of the muscles of the pelvic floor. It has been pointed out that the squatting posture assumed by our ancestors during the act of defecation favors the emptying of the rectum by increasing intra-abdominal pressure and aligning rectum and lower sigmoid more nearly in the vertical axis of the body.

Constipation due to inadequate filling of the rectum will result from the following causes:

1. Ineffective propulsive motility. In most instances there is exaggeration and persistence of segmental nonpropulsive motility, particularly in the distal colon. This is one of the most frequent causes of constipation and is usually called "spastic constipation" or "irritable bowel syndrome with constipation." It is generally acknowledged that this disorder is caused by emotional factors, although occasionally it may be the result of toxic products, as in lead poisoning. In some instances the ineffective propulsive motility of the colon is due to diminished irritability of the smooth muscle, as in pregnancy, hypothyroidism, hypercalcemic states, and depression.
2. Organic obstruction of the colon.
3. Congenital aganglionic megacolon (Hirschsprung's disease).
4. Iatrogenic pharmacologic factors (opiates, anticholinergic drugs, antidepressants, ganglionic blockers, antacids).

The defecation reflex and, therefore, the emptying of the rectum can be interfered with, leading to constipation, at several points:

1. Neurologic damage of the afferent or efferent fibers or the sacral spinal cord center. This cause is fortunately rare.
2. Rise in threshold of pressure for the perception of rectal distention and the initiation of defecation reflex. This phenomenon is an important cause of constipation in old people and in individuals with faulty habits who tend to disregard the urge to defecate.
3. Local disease of the anus preventing the adequate relaxation of the anal sphincter, as in cases with thrombosed hemorrhoids.
4. Malignant or benign strictures of the anus and rectum.
5. Weakness of the effector muscles of the abdominal wall, as in pregnancy, obesity, debilitating disease, old age.
6. Departure from the squatting posture.
7. Psychogenic factors. Through the process of toilet training the child learns to inhibit the reflex until such time as defecation is socially acceptable. Eventually the defecation reflex becomes dependent on a complex set of conditioning factors such as time and place, rituals, kind of food, state of mind, etc.

Clinical Significance

Constipation may be an irrelevant symptom or the expression of a serious illness. It may be the consequence of faulty habits or psychological disturbances; the result of toxic, pharmacologic, or metabolic influences; the consequence of decreased irritability of the smooth muscle or of weakness of the abdominal wall. It occurs because of local disease of the rectum or anus, including both benign and malignant conditions. A change of bowel habit in individuals over 40 with less frequent motions or thinner (pencillike) stools makes it mandatory to rule out a rectal carcinoma. Finally, it can be caused by neurological diseases affecting the spinal cord, the afferent or efferent pathways or the intrinsic innervation of the colon. Thus, any patient with constipation should be subjected to a careful evaluation. A systematic consideration of all the causes and mechanisms discussed under Background Information will be most useful.

Selected References

1.   Connell AM: Motor action of the large bowel, in Code CF, Heidel W (eds): *Handbook of Physiology*. Washington, DC, American Physiological Society, 1968, vol 4, sect 6, pp 2075–2093.
2.   Almy TP: Constipation, in Sleisenger MH, Fortram JS (eds): *Gastrointestinal Disease*. Philadelphia, WB Saunders, 1973, pp 320–325.

30. Hernia

THEODORE HERSH, MD
HORACIO JINICH, MD

Definition

The protrusion of a loop of bowel or part of an organ through an opening is termed hernia.

Technique

There are many types of hernias in the body, but most patients use this word to refer to hernias in the inguinal region. Probably the second most common use of the word "hernia" relates to a hiatus hernia. The patient has been told that his symptoms of heartburn and indigestion are due to the esophagitis resulting from the hiatus hernia. Thus, the frequent and common use of this term allows the examiner to ask the patient: Have you ever had a hernia? If the answer is affirmative, then the next question is: Where is your hernia? The next set of questions relates to known duration of the hernia, how it was uncovered, and what kind of symptoms it produced, if any. When hernias are symptomatic, what does the patient do to prevent symptoms or to alleviate these when they become manifest? Has the patient had any complications of hernia, or has there been surgical repair of the hernia? Occasionally, hernias appear after abdominal operations, and the patient would probably describe this as a hernia appearing at the site of the incision. Inguinal and umbilical hernias are not uncommon in children, and the patient may recall that his was repaired.

Background Information

There are many types of hernias, particularly in relation to an abdominal cavity. The most common include the direct and indirect inguinal hernias. These may appear soon after birth or later in life. The direct inguinal hernia is due to a weakness in the abdominal musculature with protrusions through the region of Hesselbach's triangle. The indirect hernia goes through the internal inguinal ring, and a hernial sac descends beside the spermatic cord or into the scrotum. Occasionally, the hernia is large enough for the contents to enter the scrotum with the contents of the spermatic cord. Femoral hernia occurs when there is a defect in the abdominal wall along the femoral canal. Then the hernia sac enters deeply into the inguinal ligament. An umbilical hernia protrudes through the umbilical ring, and an epigastric hernia occurs through weakness in the linea alba between the xyphoid and the umbilicus.

The patient may use the word "hernia" to refer to a hiatus hernia that caused symptoms of indigestion and was uncovered by an upper gastrointestinal radiologic study. Other usage of the word "hernia" pertains to incisional hernias, where, as the name implies, there is a defect secondary to an incision. The defect may have occurred because of poor wound healing or closure, postoperative vomiting, partial wound disruption, or obesity. Diaphragmatic hernias occur through defects in the diaphragm that allow the protrusion of abdominal viscera into the thoracic cavity. These may be congenital, where frequently some portion of the diaphragm is absent, or they may follow trauma. Of the acquired diaphragmatic variety, the most common is the hiatus hernia, usually referred to as a sliding hernia, and the para-esophageal hernia.

Clinical Significance

Hernias may cause symptoms because of complications, particularly if there is impairment of the blood supply to the contents of the hernial sac. Particularly, in the inguinal area, incarcerated hernias occur when the contents cannot be returned to the abdominal cavity although there is no interference with blood supply. These patients may have abrupt symptoms of pain. In contrast, the strangulated hernia is one in which the blood supply to the viscera within the hernial sac has become obstructed, and there is concomitant necrosis of tissue. Umbilical hernias may also become strangulated and require emergency repair. Hiatus hernia by disruption of the high pressure zone in the lower esophageal sphincter allows reflux of gastric acid into the esophagus with consequent esophagitis. Not infrequently, the area of the esophagitis may narrow and the ensuing stricture may require dilatation or colon bypass because of symptoms of dysphagia. Symptomatic hernias may be successfully repaired when symptoms are intractable before complications ensue.

Selected References

1. Morton JH: Abdominal wall hernias, in Schwartz SI (ed): *Principles of Surgery.* New York, McGraw-Hill, 1969, pp 1201–1216.
2. Maingot R: Hernia, in *Abdominal Operations,* ed 5. New York, Appleton-Century-Crofts, 1969, pp 1219–1306.

31. Hemorrhoids

THEODORE HERSH, MD
HORACIO JINICH, MD

Definition

Hemorrhoids are varicosities of the venous system comprising the hemorrhoidal venous plexus. They are commonly known as piles.

Technique

Most patients are aware of the presence of hemorrhoids or piles. The question can be posed directly: Have you ever been troubled by hemorrhoids? Questions about the presence and symptoms emanating from hemorrhoids relate to prolapse of internal hemorrhoids forming an anal mass and causing bleeding. The examiner would have already inquired about rectal bleeding. Internal hemorrhoids protrude during defecation but can retract early in the course of the disease. In addition, hemorrhoids can cause discharge of mucus from the anus, and this, of course, worsens as the hemorrhoids get larger and prolapse increases. The development of pruritis causes further destruction of the thin tissue overlying the hemorrhoids.

The main symptom resulting from hemorrhoids is bleeding. It is often intermittent and occurs mainly with defecation, particularly if there is a hard stool or there is excessive straining during the act of defecation. The patient will describe this as bright red streaks on the outside of the stool or on the toilet paper. Less frequently the patient will note gross bleeding during the act of defecation, coloring the water in the toilet bowl.

External hemorrhoids are found outside the anal orifice and frequently develop after straining during defecation. They are covered by skin rather than rectal mucosa. Although external piles can bleed, frequent symptom is pain from venous thrombosis or from rupture of the venules, forming a hematoma below the skin. The patient will have noted a painful lump in the anus. These symptoms are worsened by defecation.

Background Information

Hemorrhoids appear to be related to the erect position. An increase in pressure in the hemorrhoidal veins has been noted when the subject assumes an erect position. Straining during the act of defecation increases the hydrostatic pressure in the superior hemorrhoidal veins following the increase in intra-abdominal pressure. Over the years, there may then ensue greater distensibility of these veins, resulting in the large internal hemorrhoids. Weakness in the supporting anal tissues probably contributes to higher incidence of hemorrhoids as persons become older. Hemorrhoids are also common in conditions that increase pressure in the portal venous system, including the portal hypertension found in cirrhosis, thrombosis of the portal vein, and chronic heart failure. Hemorrhoids are also common in diseases associated with excessive straining during the act of defecation, including chronic constipation or chronic diarrhea. They are also common during pregnancy.

Clinical Significance

Hemorrhoids cause significant anal symptoms in many patients, requiring local therapy. When they occur as complications of diseases such as cirrhosis and heart failure, other disease manifestations predominate. Thus, hemorrhoids do not provide significant diagnostic clues to other diseases. Local therapy, as well as improvement of the causative mechanism, are important to relieve symptoms. Not infrequently, surgical therapy for hemorrhoids is indicated when there is bleeding, protrusion of the hemorrhoids, thrombosis, ulceration, or infection.

Selected References

1.   Turrell R: Present status and modern treatment of hemorrhoids. *NY State J Med* 56:2245–2250, 1956.
2.   Lockwood RA: *Atlas of Anorectal Surgery.* New York, McGraw-Hill, 1964.
3.   Spiro HM: *Clinical Gastroenterology.* New York, Macmillan, 1970, pp 707–714.

32. History of Peptic Ulcer Disease

THEODORE HERSH, MD
HORACIO JINICH, MD

Definition

With a past clinical history of peptic ulcer, patients may recognize the specific site of the ulcer as the stomach (gastric) or the duodenum.

Technique

The examiner will have already inquired whether abdominal pain is a component of the patient's main complaint or a separate problem. Most patients are familiar with the word "ulcer" or "peptic ulcer"; those who indeed have had ulcer disease may actually know the site of the ulceration, namely the duodenum or the stomach, or less commonly the esophagus. If the patient has a positive history of ulcer disease, one needs to establish the location of the ulcer, the character of the pain, the way the diagnosis was established, and whether there have been any complications of ulcer disease, including bleeding, perforation, or obstruction. If radiologic studies were performed, an attempt should be made to obtain the films, or at least a copy of the radiologic report. If the ulcer was located in the stomach, the examiner must ascertain whether the patient was followed through complete healing of the ulcer, since gastric malignancies may present as nonhealing or poorly healing gastric ulcers. In addition, if there is a history of recurrence, the investigator should ascertain whether this was gastric or duodenal.

The pain of peptic ulcer, when not complicated by penetration into the pancreas or a free perforation, may be poorly localized but is usually located in the midline. Referred pain is unusual unless there is a complication such as a penetration or perforation. The patient may describe the pain as burning, boring, aching, or gnawing. Often he can compare it to severe hungerlike pain sensations. Most commonly, this pain occurs in relation to meals, usually appearing from one to three hours postprandially. Another very common feature of this pain is that it responds promptly either to ingestion of food (especially milk or protein-rich foods) or to one of many commercial antacid preparations. Duodenal ulcer pain is more likely to be in the middle of the epigastrium or just to the right of the midline; that of the gastric ulcer is in the epigastrium but more likely to the left of the midline. The pain of peptic ulcer disease may awaken the patient after a few hours of sleep but is rarely present upon awakening. The nocturnal pain that occurs in about 50% of patients with ulcer disease is also characteristically relieved by food or antacid therapy. Not infrequently, vomiting relieves the pain of ulcer disease.

Since duodenal ulcer disease is chronic and recurrent, there is a tendency to complete healing of the ulcer and then recurrence. This pattern is referred to as "periodicity." Pain of duodenal ulcer disease lasts for days or weeks, depending on treatment: a diagnosis of ulcer often cannot be made in a patient who experiences pain for one or two days throughout the year, although the description may fit ulcer disease. The periods of remission are usually longer than the episodes of pain. It has been said that ulcer disease most commonly recurs in the spring and fall.

If the pain pattern is suggestive of ulcer disease, then the examiner must ascertain whether the patient has experienced any of the complications of this disease. Complications may occur in both duodenal and gastric ulcers. It is particularly important to know whether a gastric ulcer has been followed to complete healing, verified by a review of radiologic studies or endoscopic reports. A gastric malignancy may then be ruled out. Ulcer disease may present as an acute abdomen when there is free perforation. These patients will likely have required surgery for closure of the perforation. Ulcers may penetrate through the serosa or into adjacent organs, such as the pancreas. Then the pain pattern, in addition to the visceral component described above, elicits somatic pain. This pain is reported as localized and steady, with appropriately referred pain. There is historically a less clear-cut association with ingestion of food and relief with food or antacids, but amelioration of symptoms may also occur.

Ulcers may present with gastrointestinal bleeding, either hematemesis or melena. The frequency and severity of the bleeding episodes associated with ulcer disease must be established. Inquire whether surgery has been performed for bleeding ulcer disease. During the course of recurrent ulcer disease, a patient may present with nausea and vomiting secondary to gastric retention of acid and food contents when there is gastric outlet obstruction. This may occur as a consequence of chronic ulcer disease with scarring or as a result of acute inflammatory reaction from an active ulcer.

Finally, the patient with ulcer disease may have had surgery not only for one of the above-mentioned complications but also for chronicity or intractability of the ulcer. The type of surgery performed must be ascertained either from the patient or the referring physician or, more precisely, from a copy of the operative report. Patients with recurrent ulcers after surgery, ie, marginal ulcers, may have undergone a preoperative gastric analysis or a serum gastrin level test. These tests must be obtained or repeated to rule out a gastrin-secreting tumor, the Zollinger-Ellison syndrome. Inadequate surgery (vagotomy) may also lead to marginal ulcer.

Selected References

1.   Blumenthal IS: Digestive disease as a national problem: III. Social cost of peptic ulcer. *Gastroenterology* 54:86–92, 1968.
2.   Fordtran JS, Collyns JA: Antacid pharmacology in duodenal ulcer. *N Eng J Med* 274:921–927, 1966.
3.   Spiro HM: *Clinical Gastroenterology.* New York, Macmillan, 1970, pp 214–305.
4.   Walker CO: Chronic duodenal ulcer, in Sleisenger MH, Fordtran JS (eds): *Gastrointestinal Disease.* Philadelphia, WB Saunders, 1973, pp 665–691.

33. History of Gallbladder Disease

THEODORE HERSH, MD
HORACIO JINICH, MD

Definition

The most common diseases of the gallbladder involve the presence of gallstones and inflammation of the organ. Carcinoma of the gallbladder is rare, and most of these cases have associated gallstone disease.

Technique

A patient may first be asked: Do you have any trouble with your gallbladder? Have you ever had an attack of gallbladder pain? Have you ever been told that you have gallstones? Have you ever had an x-ray of your gallbladder? If any of these general questions are answered affirmatively, then inquire about the symptoms that may have led to a diagnosis of gallbladder disease, such as a history of pain in the epigastrium or right upper abdominal quadrant beginning abruptly and associated with nausea or vomiting, chills, and fever. Was the patient jaundiced or was there a change in the color of the urine or stool? Gallbladder pain may radiate to the right shoulder or to the back. The patient may have required narcotics for pain. If a physician was consulted, was there any tenderness in the area of the gallbladder fossa and were x-ray studies of the gallbladder done then or later? If these tests were done, what were the results, that is, did the gallbladder visualize with the contrast media given? Was the study done by administration of oral dye (many tablets taken the night before the x-ray study) or by intravenous route? Was the diagnosis of gallstones established by an ultrasound study? Where and when were the radiologic studies done? These can be requested for review or the report obtained. If the gallbladder visualized, were there any calculi in it? Did the patient require a second study with more tablets? What was the result?

Since gallstones are often asymptomatic, the history of gallbladder disease may have been elicited because of nonspecific gastrointestinal symptoms such as dyspepsia, fatty food intolerance, or gaseousness. If a gallbladder x-ray was done to evaluate these nonspecific symptoms, the presence of calculi may have been noted. In the case of an acute attack of pain and jaundice, was the common duct evaluated by x-ray study? Was surgery necessary?

Background Information

Inflammation of the gallbladder, cholecystitis, is most often associated with gallstone disease; however, acalculus cholecystitis presenting as an acute abdomen may also occur. Gallstones may be composed of bilirubin pigment, as a result of a chronic hemolytic process with an increased excretion of bilirubin by the liver. Bilirubin stones often appear as calcified stones on x-ray studies. The most common type of gallstone, however, is composed of cholesterol. The etiology of cholesterol gallstones is related to an increase in the rate of hepatic synthesis and secretion of cholesterol in bile with a relative decrease in the biliary concentration of bile acids. That is, cholesterol now exists in a saturated or supersaturated solution ("lithogenic bile"); cholesterol may then precipitate out of solution forming cholesterol crystals and stones in the gallbladder. Since bile is stored in the gallbladder during the interdigestive phases, cholesterol may readily precipitate and form the characteristic radiolucent gallstones. The exact mechanism by which an acute inflammatory process occurs in the gallbladder with calculi is not apparent but may be related to an infection occurring behind the stones, particularly when these obstruct the cystic duct. Often gallstones may leave the gallbladder and block the common duct causing biliary colic and jaundice. The obstruction from gallstone disease in the common duct must be relieved surgically when the stone does not pass spontaneously into the intestinal lumen.

Clinical Significance

An inflamed gallbladder with or without stones requires medical or surgical therapy. With the advent of antibiotics, cholecystitis can be controlled medically. In many patients an emergency cholecystectomy is performed. If the gallbladder contains gallstones, particularly if these are multiple and small with opportunity to pass into the common duct, cholecystectomy is advised. In many asymptomatic persons, cholecystectomy is performed for prophylactic measures. A new method of therapy for cholesterol gallstones currently being evaluated is the administration of chenodeoxycholic acid over prolonged periods to dissolve the gallstones.

Selected References

1. Friedman GD, Kannel WB, Dawber TR: The epidemiology of gall-bladder disease: Observations in the Framingham study. *J Chron Dis* 19:273–292, 1966.
2. Thistle JL, Hoffman AF: Efficacy and specificity of chenodeoxycholic acid therapy for dissolving gallstones, *N Eng J Med* 289:655–659, 1973.
3. Linden W van der, Sunzel H: Early versus delayed operation for acute cholecystitis: A controlled clinical trial, *Am J Surg* 120:7–13, 1970.
4. Way LW, Admisrand WH, Dunphy JE: Management of choledocho-lithiasis. *Ann Surg* 176:347–359, 1972.

34. History of Pancreatitis

THEODORE HERSH, MD

HORACIO JINICH, MD

Definition

Pancreatitis is an inflammatory disease of the pancreas and causes a symptom complex of abdominal pain, fever, nausea, and vomiting. Pancreatitis may occur as an acute attack or as a series of recurrent attacks of abdominal pain. It is classified as acute pancreatitis, acute recurrent pancreatitis, chronic relapsing pancreatitis, and chronic pancreatitis (exocrine insufficiency).

Technique

The patient who has had an attack of abdominal pain caused by pancreatitis will readily remember the episode. Ask the patient: Have you ever had a problem with your pancreas or an attack of pancreatitis? Some individuals may not recall their physician using this word as a diagnosis for their acute abdomen. One might elicit a history suggestive of an attack of pancreatitis: abrupt onset of epigastric pain, mainly in midepigastrium, often radiating through to the back and accompanied by nausea, vomiting, chills, and fever. In this instance one might ask whether the physician reported that one or more of the serum pancreatic enzyme levels, particularly amylase and lipase, were elevated during the attack. Did the attack follow ingestion of alcohol or large meals? Was the patient jaundiced? Furthermore, one needs to inquire whether hospitalization occurred for this or for repeated attacks of pain. What is the frequency of the attacks? Was there use of nasogastric suction and intravenous fluid replacement? Was the patient examined during one of these attacks of pain to confirm the diagnosis of pancreatitis or was there surgery for one of the complications of this disease? Of course, if the patient who is suspected of having experienced one bout of pancreatitis or recurrent attacks of pancreatitis cannot provide more information, then a call or a letter to the physician or the hospital will help establish the background on which the diagnosis of pancreatitis was made. Other information needed includes history of alcoholism, gallbladder disease, trauma, family history of pancreatitis, and disorders of calcium and lipid metabolism.

Background Information

Acute pancreatitis is an inflammation of the pancreas with various etiologies. Regardless of etiology, the most popular theory regarding the pathogenesis of the disease suggests that there is a release of proteolytic enzymes in the parenchyma of the gland; the liberated enzymes then set up an inflammatory reaction in the pancreas. The activation of the pancreatic enzyme elastase from its proenzyme by trypsin digests the elastic tissue of local blood vessels and causes hemorrhage into the pancreas. This results in a severe attack, hemorrhagic pancreatitis. The enzyme lipase causes lipolysis in the pancreas and in the mesentery with release of fatty acids and deposition of calcium soaps. This may be one mechanism contributing to the hypocalcemia of pancreatitis.

In many institutions the most common cause of pancreatitis is related to chronic alcoholism. The mechanism by which alcohol induces pancreatitis has not been established but one theory notes that there is chronic, partial ductal obstruction; pancreatic hypersecretion results from stimulation by the alcohol-induced gastric acid secretion which in turn releases the hormone secretin from the proximal small intestine. Pancreatitis results from hypersecretion against the background of ductal obstruction with the consequent release of activated proteolytic enzymes into the pancreatic parenchyma. An inflammatory process then sets in. If the inciting cause is not eliminated, these patients will go on to develop recurrent attacks of pancreatitis with further destruction of the gland and alterations of the ductal system. Chronic relapsing pancreatitis ensues with its complications of pancreatic parenchymal calcification and ductal calculi, diabetes mellitus, exocrine pancreatic insufficiency, and the formation of pseudocysts. The recurrent attacks of abdominal pain requiring narcotics may be complicated by addiction.

Pancreatitis may also be associated with calculi in the gallbladder. The mechanism by which pancreatitis is associated with gallstone disease and cholecystitis is not known, but "infected" bile and an increase of pressure in the biliary tract reportedly may initiate an attack of pancreatitis. In these cases, elimination of gallstone disease early in the course of the pancreatic disease will prevent further attacks of pancreatitis. Less frequent conditions associated with pancreatitis include a history of abdominal trauma which has caused previous damage to the pancreatic ducts. Pancreatitis may also be present as attacks of abdominal pain in some patients with hypercalcemic syndromes and in cases with hyperlipidemia. Attacks of pain simulating pancreatitis may be caused by pancreatic infarction, which may be present in patients with vasculitis from collagen diseases or malignant hypertension. Recurrent attacks of pancreatitis have also been described in families; some of these cases have had an associated aminoaciduria, particularly increased urinary levels of lysine, arginine, and cystine.

Clinical Significance

Pancreatitis is an inflammatory disease of the pancreas occurring de novo or as a result of other underlying disorders. As stated, pancreatitis may be a complication of other diseases, and the inciting factor must be uncovered and, if possible, eliminated to reduce or eliminate recurrent attacks of pancreatitis. The ingestion of alcohol should be discontinued in patients with recurrent attacks of pancreatitis. If gallbladder disease has been complicated by an attack of pancreatitis, cholecystectomy is definitely indicated. Diagnosis and therapy of the cause of hypercalcemia should be established and when corrected, attacks of pancreatitis should no longer occur or at least become less frequent. Hyperparathyroidism is often uncovered after an attack of unexplained pancreatitis. Dietary or drug therapy for an existing hyperlipidemia should be instituted and again attacks of pancreatitis may become less frequent.

When the patient has had various attacks of pancreatitis and one or more of the complications of pancreatitis has become manifest, correction of pancreatic ductal pathology should be attempted. Pancreatography will outline the obstruction or presence of pseudocysts, and surgical approach follows. Pseudocysts that persist and that are associated with recurrent episodes of abdominal pain should be surgically drained.

Selected References

1.   Howat HT (ed): *The Exocrine Pancreas: Clinics in Gastroenterology.* Philadelphia, WB Saunders, 1972.
2.   Sarles H, Sarles JC, Camatte R, et al: Observations on 205 confirmed cases of acute pancreatitis, recurring pancreatitis, and chronic pancreatitis. *Gut* 6:545–555, 1965.
3.   Dreiling DA, Janowitz HD, Pernier CV: *Pancreatic Inflammatory Disease: A Physiologic Approach.* New York, Paul B Hoeber, 1964.
4.   Strum WB, Spiro HM: Chronic pancreatitis. *Ann Intern Med* 74:264–277, 1971.

35. History of Gastrointestinal Surgery

THEODORE HERSH, MD
HORACIO JINICH, MD

Definition

This refers to a history of a surgical procedure on the gastrointestinal tract, pancreas, biliary tract, or liver.

Technique

The examiner should inquire whether the patient has ever had an operation. If the patient responds affirmatively, the diagnosis for which the operation was performed and the type of surgery should be elucidated. The names of the attending physician and surgeon should be obtained, as well as the date of the operation and the name and location of the hospital. These will serve as important reference points in case the information is scant or missing. The symptoms, tests, and other details leading to surgery should be recorded. Ask why the doctors recommended surgery. The results of the operation should then be sought: What was found at the time of surgery and what did they do? In many instances, the removal of tumors or biopsies at the time of surgery are required to determine the existence of a benign or malignant lesion. If the patient cannot give adequate confirmation of the operative findings, the examiner may request loan of the microscopic slides for review by his own pathologist, in addition to the operative record and pathology report.

Background Information

List all operative procedures and diagnosis on the patient's data base. If the current symptoms and problem are related to the past operation, further clarification of the operative findings may be necessary. The patient's statements can be verified or clarified if necessary by obtaining a verbal or a written report from the physician or hospital record room where the surgery was performed; furthermore, in cases where there is a question of a malignant lesion, one can request the microscopic slides of tissue sections.

Clinical Significance

Depending on the symptom currently being evaluated, past abdominal operations may be important. For instance, intestinal obstructions may result from adhesive bands from previous abdominal surgery or from recurrent malignant disease causing intrinsic or extrinsic compression of the loops of bowel. The latter would more correctly establish a diagnosis if one knew that malignancy had been resected. The amount of bowel resected, the area of involvement, and the anastomosis created may be important in management of the short-gut syndrome.

Operations for peptic ulcer disease may cause new gastrointestinal syndromes; definition of the exact nature of the procedure is necessary, for example, the type of anastomosis performed after gastrectomies such as gastroduodenostomy or gastrojejunostomy procedures. Whether a vagotomy was performed in the treatment of ulcer disease is of particular note since recurrent ulceration or marginal ulcers may be related to persistently high quantities of gastric acid secretion, and a subsequent operative procedure might require either further resection of the secreting gastric pouch or a vagotomy to reduce the secretion of gastric acid. Roux-en-Y procedures are often second operations in the treatment of peptic ulcer disease to alleviate one of the complications of ulcer surgery, namely, bile reflux gastritis.

Cholecystectomies may be performed for aculculus cholecystitis or for gallstone disease. The presence or absence of jaundice indicates whether the common duct may have been obstructed preoperatively by a calculus. An inquiry into the patient's history regarding tube drainage of bile would suggest that the common duct was explored. Consequently, appearance of symptoms suggesting cholangitis or appearance of jaundice after gallbladder surgery would tend to suggest either a stricture complicating previous common duct exploration or common duct obstruction from recurrent biliary tract calculi.

Knowledge of amount and site of resections of segments of small or large intestine in patients with inflammatory disease of the bowel helps in the management of recurrent gastrointestinal symptoms, particularly chronic diarrhea. Distal ileal resections more commonly cause diarrhea and steatorrhea. Occasionally, in Crohn's disease, a diseased segment is merely bypassed rather than resected, and there are persistent systemic symptoms. In exploratory laparotomies or gynecologic operations, it is important to know whether an incidental appendectomy has been performed.

Selected References

1. McLelland RN: Indications for surgery and selection of operation in peptic ulcer disease, in Sleisenger MH, Fordtran JS (eds): *Gastrointestinal Disease*. Philadelphia, WB Saunders, 1973, pp 772–790.
2. Johnston D, Tickford IR, Walker BE, et al: Highly selective vagotomy for duodenal ulcer. *Br Med J* 1:716–718, 1975.
3. Smith R: Operative management of exocrine pancreatic disease, in *Clinics in Gastroenterology*. Philadelphia, WB Saunders, 1972, vol 1, pp 239–256.
4. Haff RC, Butcher HR Jr, Ballinger, WS: Biliary tract operations: A review of 1,000 patients. *Arch Surg* 98:428–434, 1969.
5. Welch CE: Abdominal surgery. *N Eng J Med* 293:957, 1975.

36. History of Alcoholic Intake

HORACIO JINICH, MD
THEODORE HERSH, MD

Definition

The account of the alcoholic content of beverages consumed and the amount, frequency, and duration of alcoholic intake.

Technique

Patients are unreliable when it comes to answering such questions as: How much do you drink? What do you drink? When and where do you drink? The more severe their problem, the less accurate their reporting. More accurate information will usually be obtained from the patient's closest relatives. The severity and duration of alcoholic intake has important diagnostic and prognostic implications. It is also important to try to learn what effect the patient's drinking has on his life.

Several key questions help determine whether the patient's drinking pattern shows a psychological or physical dependence on alcohol. Does he use alcohol as a tranquilizer or antidepressant? for relief or escape? Is there conflict, internal or external, over the use of alcohol? Are there quarrels with spouse or friends, ultimatums, hiding liquor? Are there signs of internal conflict, such as guilt, shame, remorse, denial? Has drinking been associated with some definite harmful effects such as losing a job, having familial or financial difficulties, or suffering impairment of health? Other questions helpful in evaluating the pharmacological status of the patient are: Has he had blackout spells? Has his capacity for alcohol increased? Is the patient physically dependent on alcohol?

Information of this sort will help the physician evaluate not only the importance of alcohol as an etiologic factor in many organic diseases but also the disease alcoholism itself, the most common form of drug abuse in the United States and a great scourge of our society.

Background Information

Ethyl alcohol, or ethanol, is the chief ingredient in beer, wine, whiskey, gin, brandy, vodka, and other alcoholic beverages. The ethanol content of alcoholic drinks in grams is shown in Table 8.

Alcohol is absorbed unaltered from the stomach (20%) and intestine (80%). It is carried in the plasma and enters the various organs of the body as well as the spinal fluid, the urine, and the expired air. It is oxidized, liberating 7 Kcal/gm. The metabolism of alcohol takes place mainly in the liver, where it is first oxidized to acetaldehyde through the intervention of the enzyme alcoholic dehydrogenase, and then acetaldehyde is converted to acetate, most of which is released into the bloodstream. As a net result, hydrogen is transferred from ethanol and acetaldehyde to the cofactor nicotinamide adenine dinucleotide (NAD) which is converted to its reduced form (NADH). The resulting enhanced NADH/NAD ratio, in turn, disturbs the redox system and produces a change in the rates of those metabolites that are dependent for reduction on the NADH/NAD couple; the concentration of alpha-glycerophosphate rises, fatty acids are trapped, and hepatic glyceride accumulation is favored; fatty acid syn-

Table 8. Ethanol content of alcoholic drinks in grams.

Whiskey			Wine			Beer		
Size	% V/V	Gm	Size	% V/V	Gm	Size	% V/V	Gm
1 oz	43	10	liter	10	79	12 oz	6	17
100 ml	43	34.1	fifth	10	75	14 oz	6	20
100 ml	50	39.7	fifth	12	90	16 oz	6	23
pint	43	163	fifth	14	106			
fifth	43	258						
fifth	50	300						
quart	43	322						
quart	50	375						

50% V/V = 100 proof; 43% V/V = 86 proof

thesis is promoted, fatty acid oxidation is decreased, and as a result, dietary fat and endogenous fatty acids are deposited in the liver, causing steatosis. Other metabolic consequences occur such as increased ketogenesis, enhanced secretion of lipoproteins, an increased lactate-pyruvate ratio resulting in hyperlactacidemia, which contributes to acidosis and also reduces the capacity of the kidney to excrete uric acid, leading to secondary hyperuricemia. It is possible that the increased availability of lactate may stimulate the production of collagen. Finally, severe hypoglycemia may occur as a result of acute alcohol abuse, through the block of hepatic gluconeogenesis in subjects with depleted glycogen stores.

Ethanol damages the mitochondria and other organelles of the liver cell and leads to the development of central hyaline necrosis. The proliferation of the smooth endoplastic reticulum is also stimulated.

Clinical Significance

Alcoholism is a chronic disease and a disorder of behavior characterized by the repeated drinking of alcoholic beverages to an extent that exceeds customary dietary use or surpasses the social drinking customs of the community and that interferes with the drinker's health, interpersonal relations and economic functioning. In other words, it creates medical, psychologic, and sociologic problems.

Alcoholic intake is responsible for many symptoms and diseases of the digestive system. It causes morning nausea and vomiting, gastritis, and an increased incidence of peptic ulcer. The most important pathologic consequence of alcoholism is liver disease. If alcohol is taken in sufficient amounts, it causes progressive liver injury ranging from fatty infiltration to alcoholic hepatitis and cirrhosis. Alcoholic hepatitis usually develops after years of excessive drinking; the probability of developing the disease is small in those who drink less than 80 gm per day of ethanol (approximately 8 ounces of 86 proof whiskey or 1 liter of wine), or if ethanol provides less than 20% of their calories. As the daily alcohol consumption increases from 80 to 160 gm per day and the duration of drinking becomes longer, the risk of developing alcoholic liver disease increases. Excessive use of alcohol is also a significant factor in causing pancreatitis, probably by increasing pancreatic secretion of proteins which precipitate in the ducts, thus forming protein plugs and stones which, in the face of hypersecretion (also determined by the intake of alcohol), will cause the disease.

Alcohol is a depressant of the nervous system and is associated with a large number of neurologic disorders such as alcoholic intoxication (drunkenness, coma, excitement), the abstinence or withdrawal syndrome (tremulousness, hallucinosis, "rum fits," delirium tremens, auditory hallucinosis); nutritional diseases of the nervous system secondary to alcoholism (Wernicke-Korsakoff syndrome, polyneuropathy, retrobulbar neuropathy, pellagra), and diseases of uncertain pathogenesis, associated with alcoholism (cerebellar degeneration, Marchiafava-Bignami disease, central pontine myelinolysis, cerebral atrophy).

The cardiovascular system is also involved by the toxicity of alcohol; it produces a cardiomyopathy manifested by congestive heart failure after ingestion of large quantities of the toxin. Repeated insults may lead to irreparable damage.

Selected References

1. Lieber C: Liver adaptation and injury in alcoholism. *New Eng J Med* 288:356–362, 1973.
2. Victor M, Adams RC: Alcohol, in Wintrobe MW, et al (eds): *Harrison's Principles of Internal Medicine*, ed 8: New York, McGraw-Hill, 1977, pp 707–716.
3. Galambos JT: Alcoholic hepatitis, in Schaffner F, et al (eds): *The Liver and Its Diseases*. New York. Stratton Intercontinental Medical Book Corp, 1974, pp 255–267.
4. Sarles H, Gerolami A: Chronic pancreatitis. *Clin Gastroent* 1:1, 1972.

37. Dyspnea, Breathlessness, and Shortness of Breath

P. BAILEY FRANCIS, MD

Definition

An uncomfortable awareness of the necessity for increased respiratory effort is normal after heavy exertion or at high altitude, abnormal at rest or when inappropriate to the level of exertion.

Technique

Begin with open-ended, nonleading questions: Do you have any problems with your breathing? If so, can you describe this for me? If the description suggests dyspnea, first determine whether it is continuous or intermittent. More specific questions should then include when the patient first became aware of it; whether it is worse, better, or unchanged since its onset; if there are circumstances in which it is made worse or better, specifically exertion, emotional upset, lying supine or on either side, during certain seasons of the year, or while in specific environments; and the effects of any medications taken. If dyspnea is intermittent, additional information should include the frequency and duration of episodes and any apparent precipitating or ameliorating factors.

If dyspnea occurs with or is worsened by exertion, quantitation is necessary to estimate the severity of the underlying illness, if any. The milder the clinical problem, the greater the exertion necessary to cause dyspnea. Walking and climbing stairs are forms of exertion experienced by most people. Dyspnea on climbing stairs can be quantitated in terms of the number of flights that must be climbed without rest to produce dyspnea, that is, the patient has two-flight dyspnea. If the patient does not have occasion to climb stairs, a similar exertion would be walking up a steep grade. Likewise, a lesser exertion, walking on level ground, may be

152

expressed in terms of city-block lengths, that is, three-block dyspnea. It is important to ask how fast the patient walks this distance, since many patients slow their pace considerably to avoid dyspnea. In housewives, a good question to ask is if dyspnea occurs with mopping the floor, since this requires considerable energy expenditure. Decreased exercise tolerance as a result of advancing age or poor physical conditioning should not be confused with true exertional dyspnea.

Background Information

Although quiet breathing occurs at a subconscious level, many factors may cause an individual to become aware of his breathing, dyspnea being an extreme example. Of several neural receptors present in the chest wall and lungs, two are postulated to play a role in the pathogenesis of dyspnea. Dyspnea may relate to the muscle spindles within the intercostal muscles. It is thought to be sensed as a result of alterations in length-tension relationships between the intrafusal muscle fibers of the muscle spindle and the extrafusal fibers of the intercostal muscles. Impulses from these muscle spindles travel along the intercostal nerves to the spinal cord. Dyspnea may also relate to small sensory end-organs called j-receptors, which are found in the interstitial spaces surrounding the alveoli of the lung. These receptors are thought to be stimulated by stretching and distortion, as might occur with interstitial pulmonary edema or fibrosis. Afferent impulses from j-receptors are carried by vagal c fibers.

Dyspnea may occur with cardiopulmonary diseases that increase the frictional resistance (asthma, emphysema, chronic bronchitis) and the elastic resistance (fibrosing alveolitis, pulmonary edema) to breathing. It may also occur in the setting of diminished ventilatory capacity (weak respiratory muscles, chest wall abnormalities, pleural effusion and fibrosis, postpneumonectomy). It may be associated with or aggravated by increased ventilatory requirements (exercise, arterial hypoxemia and hypercapnia, severe anemia, fever, or metabolic acidosis), although these factors alone do not produce true dyspnea. Multiple factors are almost always present.

Thus, dyspnea tends to correlate with the work performed by the respiratory muscles to maintain a certain level of ventilation and tends to be worse with an increasing work of breathing. The degree of dyspnea is also a function of the rapidity of onset of an increased work of breathing. Patients who have gradual increases in work of breathing over several years, as occurs with emphysema, may not experience resting dyspnea; whereas patients with acute increases in work of breathing, as with an asthma attack or a pulmonary embolus, may experience extreme dyspnea.

Clinical Significance

A sudden onset of dyspnea suggests pulmonary embolism, acute myocardial infarction with pulmonary edema, acute bronchoconstriction including anaphylaxis, a paroxysmal cardiac arrhythmia, aspiration, spontaneous pneumothorax, or anxiety with hyperventilation. Diagnostic difficulty may arise in differentiating the dyspnea of pulmonary embolism from the breathlessness of anxiety with hyperventilation. The latter tends to occur in the setting of emotional stress, tends to be recurrent over a number of years without significantly worsening, and complaints often take the form of not being able to "get enough air in." Dyspnea from chronic left ventricular failure tends to be more gradual in onset but without treatment relentlessly worsens over a period of months to a few years. It is usually associated with orthopnea and paroxysmal nocturnal dyspnea. The dyspnea of chronic obstructive lung disease is likely to be even more gradual in onset and to have been present for several years. It is often worsened in cold, damp weather and during upper respiratory tract infections. The coexistence of chronic lung disease and left heart failure provides a difficult diagnostic challenge, since some patients with severe chronic obstructive lung disease experience a supine dyspnea that mimics orthopnea. Dyspnea in the absence of mechanical pulmonary or cardiac dysfunction may result from primary pulmonary vascular diseases such as multiple pulmonary emboli or primary pulmonary hypertension. Patients with unilateral pulmonary disease, such as pneumonia, may be more dyspneic when they lie on the affected side.

Selected References

1.   Means JH: Dyspnoea. *Medicine* 3:309–416, 1924.
2.   Woolf CR: The relationships between dyspnea, pulmonary function, and intracardiac pressures in adults with left heart valve lesions. *Dis Chest* 49:225–240, 1966.
3.   Howell JBL, Campbell EJM: Breathlessness in pulmonary disease. *Scand J Resp Dis* 48:321–329, 1967.
4.   Rappaport E: Dyspnea: Pathophysiology and differential diagnosis. *Prog Cardiovasc Dis* 13:532–545, 1971.

38. Cough and Sputum Production

P. BAILEY FRANCIS, MD

Definition

A cough is a sudden audible expulsion of air from the lungs. It is normal when transient in response to inhaled irritants and abnormal when persistent or recurrent. Sputum production is the expectoration of semi-solid material originating in the upper or lower airway and is almost always abnormal.

Technique

An accurate history of cough and sputum production is difficult to obtain because: (1) many cigarette smokers deny or minimize symptoms related to their smoking; (2) patients commonly underestimate their true cough frequency; (3) some patients swallow their sputum rather than expectorate it; and (4) some patients may exaggerate their symptoms in an attempt to gain compensation resulting from a "dusty" work environment. For patients whose initial complaints do not include a cough, a good beginning is to ask: Do you cough or clear your throat when you get up in the morning? For known smokers, a good question is: Do you have a smoker's cough? If so: Do you bring up phlegm when you cough?

It should be determined whether the patient coughs and produces sputum throughout the day, whether this occurs most days of the week, whether it is seasonal or year-round, and when the patient first became aware of it. If the initial complaint includes a cough, the duration, production of sputum, and course should be noted. For intermittent chronic coughs, it is also helpful to ask about precipitating factors (environment, body positions, eating).

If the patient produces sputum, he may be able to relate whether it seems to come from the throat or chest. Further characterization of the sputum should include the average daily amount, the color (clear, white, gray, yellow, green), the consistency (thin and watery, thick and tenacious), and whether the patient is aware of a bad taste or odor related to it.

Background Information

Coughing may be initiated by any physical or chemical irritation of the pharyngeal, laryngeal, or tracheobronchial epithelium. Subepithelial irritant or cough receptors are the afferent sensory end-organs. They are most numerous in the trachea and larger airways of the lungs and are absent beyond the level of the respiratory bronchiole. Afferent impulses travel primarily along the vagus and glossopharyngeal nerves to the "cough center" in the medulla from which efferents to the involved muscles complete the complex reflex arc. Mechanically, a cough is preceded by a deep inspiration, glottic closure, and compression of the gas within the thorax by the expiratory musculature. A sudden opening of the glottis and a rapid expulsion of the compressed thoracic gas ensues. Intrapulmonary pressures may approach 300 mm Hg above atmospheric pressure. The resultant dynamic airway compression aids maximal flow, which commonly exceeds 500 liters/min. A sheering stress is thus produced along the tracheobronchial epithelium that dislodges material in the airways. Coughing at high lung volumes tends to empty larger airways; coughing at lower lung volumes, the smaller airways.

A second mechanism for airway clearance is mucociliary flow. The volume of secretions cleared daily from the lungs in an adult may approach 100 ml; however, this is swallowed and rarely expectorated. Normal tracheobronchial fluid is made up of secretions from the bronchial glands and goblet cells and from transudation of serum. Normal constituents include exfoliated epithelial cells, glycoproteins, bacteriostatic agents including lysozyme, lactoferrin, and secretory IgA, and serum proteins, primarily albumin. This material makes up the mucous blanket overlying the cilia that serves as a medium to remove foreign particles, kill bacteria, and protect the respiratory epithelium from water loss. During acute or chronic inflammation, irritation, or certain pathological states, the volume of material may increase so that some of it is expectorated. The excessive production of mucous and serous secretions by the bronchial glands and goblet cells and the increased exudation of serum result in mucoid sputum. With large numbers of polymorphonuclear leukocytes, the sputum becomes mucopurulent or purulent. Sputum which is purulent (yellow-green, opaque to light) is more viscous and less elastic rheologically than that which is mucoid (colorless, translucent to light), and clinically, purulent sputum is more difficult to raise by coughing. A purulent appearance may be misleading since a greenish color can result from the presence of verdoperoxidase (myeloperoxidase), a leukocyte enzyme, without active bacterial infection.

Clinical Significance

A laryngeal cough is one in which the expectoration of sputum results from clearing the throat, or "hawking." In this instance the sputum originates from above the larynx, the most common etiologies being allergic rhinitis or chronic sinusitis with postnasal drainage. These are the most common causes of chronic sputum production in nonsmokers. However, a persistent feeling of an inability to clear the throat may be an indication of a pharyngeal or laryngeal tumor. More important are bronchial coughs which originate below the larynx. These may be classified as productive (of sputum) or nonproductive, and as acute or chronic. An acute nonproductive bronchial cough is commonly associated with viral tracheobronchitis and/or pneumonia, Mycoplasma pneumonia, acute fungal infections of the lung, an aspirated foreign body, or recent exposure to inhaled irritants. A nonproductive postinfluenza cough may persist for several weeks. A nonproductive cough occurring in the supine position that often awakes the patient from sleep is sometimes seen in left ventricular failure. A supine cough caused by aspiration may be seen in patients with a pharyngeal diverticulum, achalasia of the esophagus, or gastroesophageal reflux from an incompetent lower esophageal sphincter. Paroxysms of coughing following liquid ingestion suggest incompetence of laryngeal function or an esophagopulmonary fistula. Chronic nonproductive coughs may be related to smoking or other inhaled irritants, but can also be caused by lesions such as a substernal thyroid or aortic aneurysm pressing against the trachea. The earliest symptom of carcinoma of the lung is often the onset of or increase in a cough.

An acute onset of a bronchial cough productive of purulent sputum often indicates bacterial infection of the lung or bronchial tree. Abrupt onset of chills, fever, and rusty-hued purulent sputum suggests pneumococcal pneumonia. A similar clinical history with extremely thick, tenacious, purulent sputum in an alcoholic is characteristic of Klebsiella pneumonia. Low-grade fever and copious purulent sputum production, which may be extremely foul smelling, for several weeks suggests a suppurative lung abscess. A persistent cough, productive or nonproductive, associated with weight loss and night sweats, should raise the possibility of tuberculosis.

Chronic productive coughs from chronic bronchitis or asthma usually raise mucoid sputum that tends to become purulent during bouts of acute respiratory infection. Patients with bronchiectasis expectorate large amounts of usually purulent sputum, often causing an unpleasant odor to their breath. Extremely thick sputum may be seen in mucoviscidosis, asthma, and dehydration.

Bile ptyalism, or yellow sputum, may be seen in jaundiced patients. A red or reddish brown color suggests the presence of blood, but a reddish tint may also result from certain aerosol bronchodilators and, in glass sanders, iron oxide. A gray or black discoloration occurs in coal miners, a blue discoloration in copper miners. Additional discoloration may result from contamination with pigmented foods or liquids ingested by the patient.

Selected References

1. Phillips AM, Phillips RW, Thompson JL: Chronic cough: Analysis of etiologic factors in a survey of 1,274 men. *Ann Intern Med* 45:216–231, 1956.
2. Wynder EL, Lemon FR, Mantel N: Epidemiology of persistent cough. *Am Rev Resp Dis* 91:679–700, 1965.
3. Spicer SS, Chakrin LW, Wardell JR Jr: Respiratory mucous secretion, in Dulfano MJ: *Sputum*. Springfield, Ill., Charles C Thomas, 1973, pp 22–68.
4. Dulfano MJ, Philippoff W: Physical properties, in Dulfano MJ: *Sputum*. Springfield, Ill. Charles C Thomas, 1973, pp 201–242.
5. Irwin RS, Rosen MJ, Braman SS: Cough: A comprehensive review. *Arch Intern Med* 137:1186–1191, 1977.

39. Hemoptysis

P. BAILEY FRANCIS, MD

Definition

The expectoration of blood or blood-tinged material arising from the lungs or tracheobronchial tree is called hemoptysis.

Technique

Hemoptysis is a frightening symptom to most patients and is often the presenting complaint. This complaint frequently takes the form of "spitting up blood," and the physician as well as the patient may be in doubt as to its origin. True hemoptysis is usually produced as a result of coughing. Bleeding from the oral cavity, nasopharynx, or oropharynx tends to appear in the mouth or upper airway in the absence of coughing. Likewise, the regurgitation of blood from the upper gastrointestinal tract is not usually associated with coughing unless it is aspirated onto the vocal cords or into the trachea.

If hemoptysis is not a presenting complaint, then as part of a complete history, the clinician should ask: Have you ever coughed up any blood or blood-streaked phlegm? Next, the amount, color, character, and duration should be noted. If the patient has difficulty spontaneously quantitating the hemoptysis, suggest some examples with which he is likely to be familiar; eg, a teaspoonful, cupful, or quartful. The color will usually be pink, rust, bright red, or dark red. It may be blood mixed with mucus or frank blood and may contain clots. The duration should be recorded as hours, days, or weeks, and the clinician should determine if this is a single episode or a problem of recurrent hemoptysis with periods of clear sputum in between.

It is also important to determine any associated or precipitating factors such as exertion, anticoagulant therapy, or chest trauma. Occasionally, a patient may note a bubbly sensation in the chest localized to the side from which the blood is coming. Obviously, a history of hemoptysis should lead the examiner to ask about other related symptoms, especially cough, dyspnea, sputum production, weight loss, and cigarette smoking.

Background Information

The lungs contain branches of the bronchial arteries and veins as well as those of the pulmonary vascular system. Hemoptysis may occur from necrosis, erosion, invasion, engorgement, or traumatic disruption of these vessels into a conducting airway. Specifically, active tuberculosis may produce hemoptysis from caseous necrosis of the lung parenchyma or from endobronchial infection. Arrested tuberculosis may produce hemoptysis by the rupture of a blood vessel in the wall of a healed cavity, from the erosion of a bronchus by a calcified tuberculous lymph node, from posttuberculous bronchiectasis, or from the presence of an aspergilloma (fungus ball) in an old healed cavity. Other inflammatory airway diseases such as bronchitis or bronchiectasis produce hemoptysis as a result of the increased vascularity of the inflamed, friable mucosa, coupled with traumatic disruption from the sheering stress of coughing. Pulmonary neoplasms may bleed either from necrosis of the tumor itself or invasion into a blood vessel. The hemoptysis of mitral stenosis is thought to occur from the rupture of dilated anastomoses between the bronchial and pulmonary veins in the bronchial walls. Bleeding from parenchymal vascular necrosis may occur with lung abscess, pulmonary infarction, necrotizing pneumonia, and vasculitis.

Clinical Significance

Although no definite etiology may ultimately be found in up to 40% of cases, hemoptysis of any amount, especially in a patient over 40 years of age, should be considered to result from a potentially serious underlying process. The volume of blood is not very helpful in differential diagnosis, but if massive (600 ml or more within a 48-hour period), it should alert the clinician that prompt surgical intervention may be necessary. Massive hemoptysis is more likely to be associated with a malignancy, tuberculosis, or acute pulmonary suppuration.

The clinical setting and associated symptoms will often suggest the diagnosis. Chronic sputum production in a relatively young patient with a history of recurrent pulmonary infection suggests bronchiectasis. Putrid sputum suggests lung abscess. Dyspnea, pleuritic chest pain, and small amounts of dark red hemoptysis often indicate pulmonary infarction. Recurrent, scant, bright red hemoptysis in a cigarette smoker over 40 years of age is often due to primary lung cancer. Intermittent mild hemoptysis over an interval of time up to two years in an otherwise healthy young woman suggests a bronchial adenoma. Although spontaneous bleeding from the chest may occur in patients on anticoagulants, the clinician should be alert to the possibility of an underlying lung lesion such as a carcinoma as the source. Cutaneous telangiectasias may be a clue to bleeding from corresponding intrapulmonary lesions in hereditary hemorrhagic telangiectasia. The presence of renal disease in association with hemoptysis suggests Goodpasture's syndrome, Wegener's granulomatosis, or polyarteritis nodosa.

Some patients with psychiatric problems may feign hemoptysis by mixing blood from some other site with their sputum. Other causes of reddish sputum which must be differentiated from hemoptysis include the iron oxide discoloration seen in glass sanders, the reddish purulent sputum seen in pneumonias caused by pigmented *Serratia marcescens,* and the "anchovy paste" sputum that results from the rupture of an amoebic abscess into a bronchus.

Selected References

1. Jackson CL, Diamond S: Haemorrhage from the trachea, bronchi, and lungs of nontuberculous origin. *Am Rev Tuberc* 46:126–138, 1942.
2. Abbott OA: The clinical significance of pulmonary hemorrhage: A study of 1316 patients with chest disease. *Dis Chest* 14:824–839, 1948.
3. Statement by the Committee on Therapy: Managment of hemoptysis. *Am Rev Resp Dis* 93:471–474, 1966.
4. Wolfe JD, Simmons DH: Hemoptysis: Diagnosis and management. *West J Med* 127:383–390, 1977.

40. Wheezing and Asthma

P. BAILEY FRANCIS, MD

Definition

Wheeze (rhonchus): a high-pitched, musical, adventitious sound or vibration in the lungs during respiration.

Asthma: an increased responsiveness of the airways to various stimuli and characterized by recurrent attacks of wheezing, cough, dyspnea, and chest tightness as a result of widespread narrowing of the airways, which is almost always reversible.

Technique

Wheezing is rarely a chief complaint even when severe, and the patient usually either complains of difficult breathing or presents with a diagnosis; that is, "I'm having an asthma attack," or "I have emphysema."

Generally, for wheezing, the examiner might ask: Do you or have you ever had problems with wheezing when you breathe? Specifically, for asthma, the examiner might ask: Do you have asthma or have you ever been told that you had asthma? Because of the tendency for patients (and many physicians) to ascribe all wheezing to asthma, the wary clinician should regard a history of asthma as probable wheezing, etiology to be determined.

If wheezing (or asthma) is or has been present, determine when this first began, whether it is continuous or intermittent, and what the course has been since the onset. If episodic, the frequency and duration of attacks should be recorded. Relationships such as specific seasons of the year and specific environments should be sought. Precipitating factors such as weather, respiratory tract infections, drugs (especially aspirin), body position, exercise, dusts, pollens, noxious fumes and odors, and emotional upset should also be sought. If the patient has taken any drugs for wheezing, the name of the drug and any apparent benefit should be noted. The patient should also be asked about a history of atopy (allergic rhinitis, infantile eczema) and about a family history of both asthma and atopy.

Background Information

Wheezing may result from localized or diffuse airway narrowing from the hypopharynx down to the level of small bronchi and perhaps bronchioles. According to Poiseuille's law for flow through smooth-bore conduits, the resistance to flow varies inversely with the fourth power of the internal radius. It is this markedly increased resistance to the flow of air through the narrowed airways, the energy expenditure of the respiratory apparatus to attempt to compensate, and the subsequent effects on respiratory gas exchange that account for most of the acute symptoms.

Although many cases of asthma are difficult to categorize, there are several classical subtypes. Allergic (extrinsic) asthma is a type I, IgE-mediated immunologic reaction from various allergens, including pollens, dusts, feathers, and animal hair. Infective (intrinsic) asthma is probably not allergic in etiology, but a reaction to nonspecific stimuli such as respiratory tract infections, dusts, and fumes. The best current theory to explain these two major types as well as other variations is that patients with asthma have a defect in beta-adrenergic responsiveness, specifically the beta$_2$ receptor. Response of the beta$_2$ system is thought to be mediated by the production of cyclic 3',5'-adenosine monophosphate (cAMP) at the cellular level, and this results in bronchodilation. Thus, a stimulus to bronchoconstriction (allergic or nonspecific) in the asthmatic cannot be counterbalanced by the defective beta$_2$ system. In allergic asthma, the stimulus comes from the release of bronchoconstrictor amines from mast cells in the lung when the antigen combines with specific IgE on the cell surface.

Other forms of asthma include mixed allergic-infective types, allergic bronchopulmonary aspergillosis due to a type III (arthus) immunologic reaction to *Aspergillus fumigatus,* aspirin-sensitive types, and occupational asthma syndromes.

Clinical Significance

Acute wheezing in a small child with no history of previous difficulty suggests bronchiolitis, but could be the onset of asthma. Wheezing that is worse during inspiration in a child suggests laryngotracheobronchitis (croup) or acute epiglottitis. Chronic wheezing and respiratory infections in a child should raise the possibility of mucoviscidosis.

Asthma, beginning in childhood or adolescence, which is seasonal and associated with multiple allergies and a family history of atopy is characteristic of allergic asthma. Adult-onset asthma, which is not seasonal and not associated with allergies (but may have a family history of asthma alone) suggests infective asthma. A picture of infective asthma, wheezing with aspirin ingestion, and hyperplastic rhinitis (especially with polyps) make up the triad of aspirin sensitivity. An asthmalike syndrome may be related to occupation (see section on Environmental Inhalation).

Adult-onset wheezing (which may be called "asthma") of only a few months duration should bring to mind the possibility of a mechanical obstruction of the larynx, trachea, or a mainstem bronchus, especially by a neoplasm.

A long history of wheezing, progressive dyspnea on exertion, and chronic sputum production in an older cigarette smoker suggests chronic bronchitis and emphysema. Wheezing in the supine position in a patient with heart disease suggests left ventricular failure.

Episodic wheezing may be seen in the metastatic carcinoid syndrome. Transient wheezing may occur following a pulmonary embolus. Almost any acute or chronic pulmonary disease may, on occasion, produce wheezing of which the patient may be aware. The astute clinician must always bear in mind that "all that wheezes is not asthma."

Selected References

1.   Statement by the Committee on Diagnostic Standards for Nontuberculous Respiratory Disease: Chronic bronchitis, asthma, and pulmonary emphysema. *Am Rev Resp Dis* 85:762–768, 1962.

2.   Dines DE, Henderson LL: All that wheezes is not asthma. *Postgrad Med* 44:64–71, 1968.

3.   Radermecker M, Rose B: Bronchial asthma: Clinical course and treatment, in Samter M: *Immunological Diseases.* Boston, Little, Brown, 1971, pp 878 892.

4.   Terr AI: Bronchial asthma, in Baum GL: *Textbook of Pulmonary Diseases.* Boston, Little, Brown, 1974, pp 421–443.

41. Tuberculosis or Exposure to Tuberculosis

JOHN E. MCGOWAN, JR., MD

Definition

Personal experience with or contact with another person who has had a clinical infection due to *Mycobacterium tuberculosis.*

Technique

Currently tuberculosis is a disease that is reasonably well known to the nonmedical population of the United States. Thus, one may begin by inquiring whether the patient has had tuberculosis, or whether members of the patient's family have had tuberculosis. In the past, a large number of the patients said to be suffering from "consumption," "phthisis," or a "spot on the lung" were victims of tuberculosis. Inquiring whether the patient, members of the patient's family, or other close contacts have been in a sanatorium is sometimes helpful, although the trend in recent years to treat this disease in the general hospital or outpatient setting means that a negative answer to this question does not exclude the possibility of tuberculosis.

If the patient does not recall previous experience with the disease by name, a prior history of tuberculosis may be difficult to document. Unfortunately, the clinical manifestations of tuberculosis can be so varied that there are no pathognomonic symptoms whose presence would indicate a prior exposure to the tubercle bacillus.

Background Information

Few diseases that are encountered as frequently as tuberculosis can present in as many different fashions, or can resemble so many other diseases. In part, this is because the natural history of tuberculosis is progression through a number of different phases with involvement of different organs or involvement of the same organ in a different fashion in each phase. For example, uncomplicated primary tuberculosis usually is either asymptomatic or produces only symptoms simulating a mild respiratory infection. On occasion, however, the infection progresses to dissemination via the bloodstream or through the lung. Postprimary pulmonary tuberculosis is usually insidious in onset; many cases are discovered only on x-rays taken for another purpose. When present, the earliest symptoms are often fever and tiredness or night sweats, or both. Weight loss may occur before other symptoms or may not be seen until the disease is fairly advanced. Likewise, cough and sputum production may be present either early or late in the course of the disease. Because these two phases of tuberculosis are often clinically inapparent, patients may present initially with complications of postprimary pulmonary tuberculosis. Since *M. tuberculosis* can invade virtually any organ or tissue, presenting signs and symptoms may be extremely variable. Generally, patients present with two different syndromes (see reference 4):

1. Localized tuberculosis with manifestations originating from specific organs or tissues, for example, lungs, nervous system, kidneys and skin. One common presentation is unilateral pleural effusion.
2. A type characterized by fever and other constitutional manifestations but without definite localizing signs, for example, miliary and disseminated.

Clinical Significance

Because of the protean manifestations with which tuberculosis can present, a past history of the disease will be useful in distinguishing this disease from others that it closely resembles. Tuberculosis today is a disease that can be completely cured with therapy, but may be fatal if undetected. Because of the drastic consequences of missing the diagnosis, the physician must have an extremely high index of suspicion for the occurrence of this disease. Tuberculosis is spread from person to person, and the majority of new cases originate from contact with an unsuspected carrier. Thus, routine attempts in all patients to determine previous history of tuberculosis not only may lead to therapy for those who are afflicted but also may decrease the number of unsuspected cases likely to infect others.

Selected References

1. Stead WW: *Fundamentals of Tuberculosis Today for Students in the Health Profession*, ed 2. Milwaukee, Central Press, 1973.

2.   Maycock RL, Macgregor RR: Diagnosis, prevention, and early ther-apy of tuberculosis. *Disease-a-Month.* May 1976, pp 1–60.
3.   Diagnosis, in *Diagnostic Standards and Classification of Tuberculo-sis and Other Mycobacterial Diseases.* New York, American Lung Association, 1974, chap 3.
4.   Harvey AM, Bordley J: Special diagnostic problems, in *Differential Diagnosis: The Interpretation of Clinical Evidence,* ed 2. Philadel-phia, WB Saunders, 1972, chapter 16, pp 619–620.
5.   Furey WW, Stefanic MF: Tuberculosis in a community hospital. A five-year review. *JAMA* 235:168–171, 1976.

42. PPD Test

JOHN E. MCGOWAN, JR., MD

Definition

To determine whether the patient has had an intradermal skin test for detection of infection with tuberculosis. If the patient has had such a test, to determine and record the result.

Technique

Begin by asking whether the patient has ever had a skin test for tuberculosis. Some patients may recognize the term "PPD Skin Test." If the patient recalls such a test, ask whether it was positive or negative.

If the patient does not know or cannot recall, ask whether a bump appeared after the test was done. Interpretation of this test depends on a quantitative measurement, since a patient can have some reaction at the site but still have a test that is reported as negative (see laboratory section on PPD Tuberculin Skin Test). Thus, history from the patient who indicates a reaction at the site of intradermal injection often will not be interpretable as a positive or negative reaction. A history of no reaction at the site is more frequently useful as an indication of a negative PPD test, although there are factors that may lead to false negative tests. Thus, interpreting the data provided by the patient is problematic. An effort to recover objective information about the actual interpretation of previous PPD skin tests may include inquiry into other physicians' records or records of schools, employers, or local health departments.

Background Information

Information underlying the immunobiology of the PPD test is given in the laboratory section on PPD Tuberculin Skin Test. The clinical utility of the PPD skin test has been shown by epidemiologic studies demonstrating increased frequency of positive skin tests in patients with culture-proved *M. tuberculosis* infections, when compared with the frequency in "control" subjects without such infections. Similar studies have shown that individuals with positive PPD response have a greater likelihood to subsequently develop clinical tuberculosis than those with a negative PPD response.

In most individuals the reaction to the tuberculin skin test tends to persist throughout life. However, cell-mediated responses such as the tuberculin reaction may decrease with age or disappear temporarily during any severe or febrile illness, certain viral infections or immunization with live virus vaccine, Hodgkin's disease, overwhelming miliary or pulmonary tuberculosis, and after the administration of adrenal corticosteroids or other immunosuppressive drugs. In addition, factors such as variability in antigens and techniques used for testing and faulty recollection of the subject may also lead to incorrect history of a negative tuberculin skin test (see references 2 and 3).

Clinical Significance

A positive PPD skin test indicates that at some time in the past the patient has been infected with the tubercle bacillus, but does not indicate when the infection with *M. tuberculosis* occurred or how severe it was. Therefore, a reliable history of positive or negative PPD skin test in the past can be of use in determining when infection with *M. tuberculosis* might have occurred. In addition, when any of the factors that interfere with skin testing are present, results from a previous PPD skin test may be of great utility if the test was done at a time when the interfering factor was not present.

Selected References

1. *Diagnostic standards and classification of tuberculosis and other mycobacterial diseases.* New York, American Lung Association, 1974, pp 17–21.

2.   Reichman LB, O'Day R: The influence of a history of previous test on the prevalence and size of reactions to tuberculin. *Am Rev Resp Dis* 115:737–741, 1977.

3.   Comstock GW: False tuberculin test results. *Chest* 68(suppl):465–469, 1975.

43. Previous Chest Radiograph

P. BAILEY FRANCIS, MD

Definition

To identify sources of previous chest radiographs for comparison to the patient's present one.

Technique

In the average patient, it is sufficient to ask: When did you last have a chest x-ray? If there is a recent past radiograph, the date, place of the examination, physician, and hospital should be noted. In a patient whose present chest radiograph exhibits an abnormality, further diagnostic work-up and treatment may be altered (perhaps saving the patient time, misery, and money) if a previous chest radiograph, especially a recent one, can be located and obtained. In such an instance, a more careful history is required. In addition to physicians and hospitals, potential sources (which the patient may temporarily have forgotten) include military induction or discharge physical examinations and city or county health department radiographs, which are often taken in cases of food handlers, beauticians, dental hygienists, nursery attendants, and those investigated as tuberculosis contacts. Unfortunately, such x-rays are often destroyed five years after the file becomes inactive. Large-scale employers often require periodic radiographs of employees and may keep them on file for a longer period of time. In requesting past radiographs, much time may be saved by including a form signed by the patient authorizing release of medical information.

Background Information

In the case of noncalcified pulmonary nodules (coin lesions) in patients over 35 years of age, a fairly accurate (but not infallible) estimate of whether the lesion is benign or malignant can be made from its growth rate. Malignant lesions of the lung up to a diameter of 2–3 cm appear to grow logarithmically, resulting in periodic doublings by cell division. The doubling time, based on a twofold increase in the volume of the lesion, can be estimated by comparing previous chest radiographs to the present one and calculating volume (if fairly spherical) by the formula $4/3\pi r^3$. The doubling time of malignant nodules in the lungs is rarely less than 1 month or more than 18 months. Notable exceptions include metastases from choriocarcinomas, testicular tumors, and osteosarcomas which may double within 2 weeks, and rare primary lung tumors which may appear stable in size for 1–2 years. Interestingly, by average tumor growth rates, it may be calculated that a squamous cell carcinoma of the lung beginning from a single malignant cell requires 8 years to become a nodule 2 cm in diameter.

Clinical Significance

A previous chest radiograph in an older patient with a solitary pulmonary nodule may save the patient a major operation if it can be shown that the growth rate is too fast or slow to be a malignancy (keeping in mind the rare exceptions). On the other hand, if the lesion was not visible on a recent past radiograph, more serious thought may be given to removing it. A paralyzed hemidiaphragm suggests malignancy, and an exhaustive work-up for a primary tumor may ensue. A chest radiograph five years earlier showing the same elevated hemidiaphragm would point to a more benign etiology.

Other uses of previous radiographs include assessment of the rapidity of development or progression of numerous diffuse and localized pulmonary diseases. In regard to the cardiac silhouette, a rapid increase in size might suggest a pericardial effusion; a more gradual increase would point toward cardiac enlargement from dilatation or hypertrophy.

Selected References

1. Nathan MH, Collins VP, Adams RA: Differentiation of benign and malignant pulmonary nodules by growth rate. *Radiology* 79:221–232, 1962.
2. Lillington GA: The solitary pulmonary nodule. *Am Rev Resp Dis* 110:699–707, 1974.

44. Respiratory Infections and Pneumonia

P. BAILEY FRANCIS, MD

Definition

Upper respiratory infection (URI): inflammation of the nasal, pharyn-geal, or laryngeal mucosa produced by an infectious agent.

Lower respiratory infection (LRI): inflammation of the tracheobron-chial tree or lung parenchyma by an infectious agent.

Pneumonia: inflammation of the lungs manifested by a radiographic density and/or physical signs of consolidation of lung parenchyma or pathologic evidence of an inflammatory exudate in the alveoli.

Recurrent URI: more than three separate episodes in a year in an adult.

Recurrent pneumonia: two or more separate documented episodes of pneumonia with complete interim clearing, especially if the interval is less than two years.

Technique

If the patient's presenting complaints suggest a current respiratory tract infection, a complete chronologic list of the symptoms should be recorded from the beginning of the illness. Symptoms suggestive of upper respiratory involvement include rhinorrhea, stuffy nose, sore throat, post-nasal drainage, hoarseness, and occasionally neck tenderness from in-flamed cervical lymph nodes. Symptoms suggesting lower respiratory involvement include cough with or without sputum production and chest discomfort. Accompanying these specific symptoms may be headache, myalgias, malaise, fever, and chills or chilly sensations. The history should also include exposure to other persons with a similar illness and any ap-parent precipitating conditions of which the patient may be aware.

In all patients, regardless of presenting complaints, the clinician should inquire about past respiratory infections. Possible questions in-clude: Do you have colds or sore throats very often? If so: How often? When did you first become aware of this? Have you ever had pneumonia? How many times? When did this (these) occur?

In a patient who says he has had pneumonia, it should be determined if this was a physician's diagnosis based on examination or x-ray, or if this was the patient's self-diagnosis. If seen by a physician or hospitalized for this, names and locations of the physicians and hospitals should be recorded so that the records may be requested. If there have been two or more episodes of pneumonia, some patients may have been told whether the pneumonias occurred in the same or different areas of the lung.

Background Information

Since the majority of URIs of viral etiology are merely nuisances to the patient and afflict most of us periodically, their pathogenesis will not be considered here. However, LRIs (excluding viral etiology), especially bacterial pneumonias, are rather uncommon unless there has been a major breakdown of the host's normal defense mechanisms.

The mucosa of the lower respiratory tract is exposed to the inhalation of dust and droplet particles that may contain any type of infectious agent. In addition to the mechanical removal by cough and mucociliary flow, several mechanisms are present to inactivate and kill inhaled or aspirated organisms, especially bacteria. Cellular mechanisms include phagocytosis by alveolar macrophages and polymorphonuclear leukocytes. Humoral mechanisms include specific IgG or IgM, secretory IgA, and nonspecific proteins such as lysozyme, interferon, lactoferrin, complement, and granulocyte proteases.

A single episode of bacterial pneumonia may occur during a time of temporary loss of host resistance, as occurs with acute influenza, a drunken stupor, or exposure. Bacterial pneumonia may occur repetitively if host resistance is impaired for an extended period of time or permanently. The latter category includes general debilitating diseases such as alcoholism, diabetes mellitus, congestive heart failure, and carcinomatosis; diseases affecting humoral or cellular immunity such as lymphoma, leukemia, multiple myeloma, and congenital or acquired immunoglobulin deficiencies; diffuse lung diseases including chronic bronchitis, emphysema, bronchiectasis, and mucoviscidosis; focal mechanical obstructions including aspiration of a foreign body, broncholithiasis, and endobronchial tumors; recurrent aspiration as may occur with achalasia or certain neurological diseases; and ineffective ventilation and cough as may occur in myasthenia gravis or muscular dystrophy.

Clinical Significance

Little clinical significance can be made of acute viral URIs. Frequent viral URIs in both children and adults have been associated with high urban air pollution, cigarette smoking in the home, and overcrowding;

however, patients who appear to have frequent URIs may actually have allergic rhinitis, chronic sinusitis or both. Recurrent streptococcal pharyngitis is the most significant common URI because of the potential of post-streptococcal glomerulonephritis and rheumatic fever.

Acute bacterial pneumonia, especially pneumococcal, presents with the abrupt onset of shaking, teeth-chattering chills, fever, cough with purulent sputum, and chest pain. Symptoms suggestive of a viral URI often precede this onset by several days. Viral and *Mycoplasma* pneumonias tend to present with a somewhat longer, more gradual onset, a nonproductive cough, and fever with chilly sensations, but not true shaking chills. (For in-depth reading of the clinical presentation of various pneumonias, consult a textbook of medicine or pulmonary diseases.)

Recurrent acute LRIs without pneumonia in adults often involve primary or secondary bacterial infection, and tend to occur in patients with diffuse chronic lung diseases, especially those related to cigarette smoking.

If a history of recurrent pneumonia has been elicited, a careful search for one or more of the predisposing conditions listed in the previous section is mandatory. Recurrent pneumonia in the same lobe or lobes of a lung suggests one of the focal mechanical problems including bronchiectasis. Recurrent pneumonia occurring in different areas suggests one or more of the aforementioned systemic disorders. Although most of these diseases predispose primarily to the more common bacterial pathogens, the disorders of immunity also predispose to unusual bacterial infections, tuberculosis, and various fungal infections of the lung.

A history of pneumonia does not have to imply infection since recurrent and chronic infiltrates may result from the inhalation of toxic substances including hydrocarbons and lipids. Recurrent pneumonia must be differentiated from the chronic pneumonic processes in which there is little or no interim clearing.

Selected References

1.   Cecil RL, Baldwin HS, Larsen NP: Lobar pneumonia: A clinical and bacteriologic study of 2,000 typed cases. *Arch Intern Med* 40:253–280, 1927.
2.   Green GM: Pulmonary clearance of infectious agents. *Ann Rev Med* 19:315–336, 1968.
3.   Winterbauer RH, Bedon GA, Ball WC Jr: Recurrent pneumonia: Predisposing illness and clinical patterns in 158 patients. *Ann Intern Med* 70:689–700, 1969.
4.   Sullivan RJ, Dowdle WR, Marine WM, et al: Adult pneumonia in a general hospital. *Arch Intern Med* 129:935–942, 1972.
5.   Bode FR, Paré JAP, Fraser RG: Pulmonary disease in the compromised host. *Medicine* 53:255–293, 1974.

45. Smoking History

P. BAILEY FRANCIS, MD

Definition

The habitual purposeful inhalation of the smoke produced from smoldering dried plant material (usually tobacco leaves) into the upper and lower airways.

Technique

Although certain patients have always falsely stated that they do not smoke, or that they smoke less heavily than they actually do, the likelihood of the patient's understating the amount of smoking has risen in recent years due to increasing public awareness of the health consequences of smoking and the increasing militancy of nonsmokers toward smokers. Accusatively asking the patient, "Do you smoke?" may get a negative reply because the patient fears the wrath of the physician. A more reliable answer may be obtained if it is assumed that the patient does smoke and is asked casually, "How much do you smoke?" This question is also more appropriate for the individual with a telltale pack of cigarettes. If the answer is no, the next question should be, "Have you ever smoked?" since some patients may have ceased smoking prior to seeking medical attention. Since smoking and tobacco are nearly synonymous, patients should also be queried specifically about other substances such as marijuana.

Cigarette smoking is usually quantitated in pack-years. The number of pack-years equals the average number of packs (20 cigarettes each) smoked during each 24-hour period multiplied by the total number of years of smoking. Hence, a 40-pack-year smoker may have smoked 1 pack daily for 40 years or 2 packs daily for 20 years. Additionally, it should be noted whether the patient smokes filtered or unfiltered cigarettes, and whether he usually inhales the smoke into the lungs. Cigar smoking is obviously recorded as the number of cigars smoked per day, and pipe smoking as the number of pipefuls per day.

173

Background Information

Although the statistical association between smoking and various diseases is unquestionable, the exact mechanisms are not fully understood. Nicotine, in the amounts obtained from cigarette smoking, causes stimulation of sympathetic ganglia resulting in arterial vasoconstriction. Cigarette smoking has been shown to reduce blood flow in the extremities and to elevate blood pressure and heart rate in certain individuals. Numerous carcinogenic materials have been isolated from tobacco tars, including polynuclear and n-heterocyclic aromatic hydrocarbons. Other agents which have been implicated as carcinogens include the n-nitrosamines and radioactive materials concentrated in tobacco leaves. Carbon monoxide is absorbed through the lungs from cigarette smoke and is present in the blood as carboxyhemoglobin in levels up to 15% saturation in some smokers. Recent studies suggest it may play a role in atherogenesis as well as its effect on tissue oxygenation by shifting the oxyhemoglobin dissociation curve to the left. Gases such as the oxides of nitrogen liberated from burning tobacco have been shown to induce changes in the bronchioles of experimental animals similar to lesions found in the lungs of young cigarette smokers, and they may play a causative role in chronic bronchitis and emphysema. The inhalation of cigarette smoke has been shown to temporarily paralyze ciliary motion in the tracheobronchial tree. Evidence also suggests that urban air pollution potentiates the inflammatory and structural damage in the lung resulting from chronic cigarette smoking.

Clinical Significance

Cigarette smoking, and to a much lesser extent cigar and pipe smoking, are associated with an increased morbidity and mortality from a variety of diseases including carcinomas of the oral and pharyngeal cavities, larynx, lung, esophagus, and bladder; chronic bronchitis and emphysema; coronary artery disease and atherosclerosis, Buerger's disease, and cerebrovascular disease, especially in women. It is also associated with respiratory tract infections, peptic ulcer disease, and premature facial wrinkling. The increased morbidity and mortality correlate directly with the amount and duration of smoking, the smoking of unfiltered cigarettes, and inhalation of the smoke. The cessation of smoking is associated with a gradual fall of morbidity and mortality rates toward those of nonsmokers; therefore, it is imperative to inform patients of the dangers of smoking and urge them to stop.

Selected References

1. Auerbach O, Stout AP, Hammond EC, et al: Smoking habits and age in relation to pulmonary changes. *N Eng J Med* 269:1045–1054, 1963.
2. Doll R, Hill AB: Mortality in relation to smoking: Ten years' observations in British doctors. *Br Med J* 1:1399–1410, 1964.
3. Root E: Smoking and mortality among US veterans. *J Chron Dis* 27:189–203, 1974.
4. Ochsner A: Smoke at your own risk, in *Smoking: Your Choice between Life and Death.* New York, Simon and Schuster, 1970, pp 9–44.

46. Environmental Inhalation

P. BAILEY FRANCIS, MD

Definition

A history of inhalational exposure to dusts, gases, fumes, or infectious agents as a result of an occupation or some other aspect of daily living.

Technique

Detailed information regarding the patient's environment and occupation is an essential part of every medical history, especially if respiratory symptoms are present. The sophistication of modern industry has created potential exposure to numerous fumes and dusts, the nature and toxicity of which may not be fully known. The clinician should use caution in obtaining and interpreting such a history. Patients seeking compensation may exaggerate symptoms, and patients who fear retaliation from their supervisors may hesitate to incriminate their work environment and thereby minimize their symptoms.

First, a detailed lifetime chronologic work history should be listed including length of time spent at each job. For each job, the patient should be asked about the type of work performed by him and others in the immediate area, the nature of any materials handled, and if safety devices and masks were used.

Second, a detailed residential history should be noted, including inhalational exposure from proximity to industries near the home or from materials used around the home. Patients should also be asked about exposure to animals or fowl in or around the home.

Third, a detailed respiratory history should note the presence and duration of dyspnea, cough, sputum production, and wheezing. If the symptoms are intermittent and recurrent, the timing of onset and relation to work should be obtained. It is equally important to ask about similar symptoms in other employees working nearby.

Last, in patients with respiratory symptoms, detailed allergy and smoking histories are necessary, since these factors may add to the effects of environmental inhalation exposure.

Background Information

Particles small enough to be inhaled and deposited into the lower respiratory tract may affect the patient by: (1) absorption and systemic toxicity; (2) directly producing an acute or chronic inflammatory reaction in the lung; (3) indirectly producing an acute or chronic inflammatory reaction by a hypersensitivity mechanism; or (4) acting as carcinogen.

Systemic toxicity with little or no primary respiratory reaction may be seen acutely with carbon monoxide and chronically with exposure to lead, mercury, or cadmium. Acute direct alveolar injury may result from accidental inhalation of irritant gases such as chlorine or nitrogen dioxide. A more chronic direct lung injury, usually resulting in varying degrees of fibrosis, may occur with exposure to inorganic dusts including the pneumoconioses from silica, asbestos, and coal dusts, or from various metallic vapors and fumes. The degree of lung damage is dependent primarily on the fibrogenicity of the specific materials involved but may be potentiated by cigarette smoking.

Acute alveolitis and small airway obstruction may occur as a result of hypersensitivity to various vegetable, animal, or fungal spore dusts. This produces a multitude of specific syndromes, called the hypersensitivity pneumonitides, which include farmer's lung, bagassosis, suberosis, sequoiosis, malt worker's lung, parakeet fancier's lung, pigeon breeder's lung, maple-bark stripper's lung, mushroom picker's lung, and many others. Repeated exposures may result in chronic lung damage and fibrosis. An asthmalike illness may result from exposure and hypersensitivity to western-red cedar, proteolytic enzymes used in the detergent industry, several heavy metals, and isocyanates. Byssinosis, from exposure to cotton dust, does not appear to have a hypersensitivity mechanism.

Infectious respiratory diseases with environmental associations are tuberculosis (doctors, nurses), anthrax (exposure to wool, mohair, alpaca), psittacosis (exposure to infected birds), coccidioidomycosis (ditch and canal diggers), histoplasmosis and cryptococcosis (exposure to chicken and pigeon droppings).

Although ozone and nitrogen dioxide, major components of urban air pollution, cause acute irritative symptoms in humans and chronic lung damage in experimental animals, their role in human chronic lung disease remains unclear.

Clinical Significance

Although individual reactions to a specific inhalant may vary, some basic patterns of symptoms may be found. However, it may be difficult to distinguish between symptoms from environmental inhalation and those from cigarette smoking.

The inorganic dust pneumoconioses usually present as a slowly progressive dyspnea on exertion, although silicosis, especially from sandblasting, may be quite rapidly progressive. Symptoms related to silica and asbestos exposure often progress even after exposure has ceased.

The hypersensitivity pneumonitides usually present as acute episodes of dyspnea, malaise, fever, and chills which begin 4–6 hours after exposure and resolve within 24–48 hours. They may also present as a more chronic progressive dyspnea. The dyspnea of byssinosis tends to be worse early in the work week (Monday asthma), and headache may be quite prominent in enzyme workers. Evaluation of any patient presenting with adult-onset, intrinsic asthma should include a careful attempt to relate the symptoms to environmental inhalation exposure.

Mesotheliomas have been associated with asbestos exposure. An increased incidence of carcinoma of the lung has been reported with asbestos exposure in cigarette smokers, in radioactive-ore miners, and with chronic exposure to arsenic, beryllium, coal tars from oven fumes, and other industrial materials.

A carefully taken history that leads the clinician to diagnose an occupational respiratory syndrome may not only save the patient from subsequent exposures that could lead to irreversible pulmonary disability, but may also lead to the prevention of similar problems in other workers exposed to the same environment.

Selected References

1.   Perry KMA: Diseases of the lung resulting from occupational dusts other than silica. *Thorax* 2:91–120, 1947.

2. Second Skytop Conference: Respiratory disease in industry. *J Occup Med* 15:165–307, 1973.
3. Fitzgerald MX, Carrington CB, Gaensler EA: Environmental lung disease. *Med Clin N Am* 57:593–622, 1973.
4. Kilburn KH (ed): Pulmonary reactions to organic materials. *Ann NY Acad Sci,* 221:5–390, 1974.

CARDIOVASCULAR SYSTEM

47. Exercise Level

CHARLES A. GILBERT, MD

Definition

The amount of physical activity that the patient ordinarily engages in. The exercise level should include occupational physical exertion, avocational or sport activities, and daily living activities.

Technique

Usual activities. Ask the patient to tell you what he did yesterday (or the day before admission), hour by hour. Then ask if the day in question was a workday (or regular day, if unemployed), a day-off, or a holiday. Finally, ask if the day in question was typical or unusual with regard to physical activity. It may be necessary to go through more than one day if the original day was unusual or not typical for the patient. After the interview and listing of the usual day's activities, some qualitative classification might be attempted based on walking or climbing stairs, as below.

	Walking	*Climbing stairs*
Sedentary	Less than 6 blocks	Less than 3 flights
Light active	6–10 blocks	3–5 flights
Active	11–20 blocks	6–10 flights
Vigorous	21 or more blocks	11 or more flights

Special activity. For each day of the week ending yesterday (or the day before admission), ask the patient to tell you about special or unusual activities. Special activities are those in which he does not usually engage.

Background Information

The ability to do physical work depends on many factors such as body build; neuromuscular, cardiac, and pulmonary function; aerobic and anaerobic energy supply; motivation; and skill. The environment in which the physical work is carried out is an important determinant of total physical work. Less work is possible under the conditions of a hot, humid climate, at high altitudes, or in the presence of certain polluting air contaminants.

In a controlled environment physical working capacity varies, depending on sex, age, and the level of usual physical activity or training. Diseases affecting the neuromuscular systems, or any part of the oxygen delivery system, can also limit physical working capacity.

Maximal oxygen consumption ($VO_{2\ max}$) is a frequently employed measurement to determine the body's ability to exercise at a peak level. $VO_{2\ max}$ requires special laboratory and testing equipment but is sometimes useful in correlating with history-obtained information on exercise level. $VO_{2\ max}$ is expressed as milliliter per minute, or milliliter per kilogram body weight per minute. In a patient with cardiac or pulmonary disease, a true maximal test may not be possible, and the oxygen consumption at a work level which produces symptoms is called the peak, or symptom-limited oxygen consumption. Another commonly used term to express energy expenditure is the MET. One MET is the amount of energy expended while resting and is roughly equivalent to an oxygen consumption of 250 ml/min or 3.5 ml/kg body weight/min for a 70-kg person. One MET may be considered equivalent to 1 calorie. A table of energy expenditure for common vocational and recreational activities is given in Table 9.

Clinical Significance

It is important to determine as precisely as possible what physical work a patient does and whether it causes any symptoms such as dyspnea, fatigue, chest pain, or leg cramps. A patient may complain of shortness of breath with physical exertion, but the amount of exertion should be quantitated. Shortness of breath would be interpreted differently if it were provoked by walking slowly from room to room than it would be if it were brought on only when climbing three flights of stairs in a brisk manner. Also, it is important to know what a patient's usual exercise level is to aid in advising about disease prevention or treatment. One of the

Table 9. Approximate energy requirements of activities.*

Descriptor	Energy requirement (includes resting energy needs)	Occupational activities	Recreational activities
Light	1½–3 METS 4–11 ml O_2/kg/min 2–4 kcal/min (70-kg person)	Desk calculator operation Bench work: radio, TV repair Light auto repair Driving auto Desk work Typing	Walking 1–2 mi/hr Playing cards Sewing Riding lawn mower Piano playing Golf (ride cart)
Light-moderate	3–5 METS 11–18 ml O_2/kg/min 4–6 kcal/min	Most construction/building trades (brick laying, plastering, painting, light carpentry) Welding Cleaning windows Trailer truck in traffic	Walking 3 mi/hr Golf (pull cart or carry clubs) Sailing (handle small boat) Pitching horse shoes Noncompetitive volleyball Pushing light power mower
Moderate-heavy	5–7 METS 18–25 ml O_2/kg/min 6–8 kcal/min	Digging garden Shoveling light earth (10/min; 4.5 kg/shovel) Splitting wood	Tennis (singles) Ice or roller skating Cycling (10–11 mi/hr) Canoeing (4 mi/hr) Square dancing Cross-country skiing (2.5 mi/hr)
Heavy	7–9 METS 25–32 ml O_2/kg/min 8–11 kcal/min	Digging ditches Shoveling (10/min; 5–5.5 kg) Carrying 36 kg Sawing hardwood	Jogging 5 mi/hr Basketball Mountain climbing Ice hockey Paddleball Squash/handball (social)

"minor" coronary risk factors is physical inactivity. For the sedentary, obese, middle-aged male, a regular program of physical activity may be important in delaying or preventing heart disease. Conversely, in certain disease processes (acute arthritis, heart failure) a vigorous, active person needs to be cautioned to curtail activity, and bed rest may be indicated.

When an interview technique to assess a patient's level or work capacity is not sufficiently accurate or is contradictory to other history or physical examination data, then an exercise stress test is indicated. Stress testing for functional capacity may be done by a variety of methods, which may include the use of a bicycle ergometer, treadmill, or other standardized work load. Measurements commonly taken during an exercise test are heart rate, blood pressure, oxygen consumption, ECG wave form, and, occasionally, peripheral blood lactates. The results of serial exercise tests are used in judging the results of pharmacologic, surgical, or physical therapy of various types.

Selected References

1.   Astrand P-O, Rodahl K: *Textbook of Work Physiology,* ed 2. New York, McGraw-Hill, 1977.
2.   *Exercise Testing and Training of Apparently Healthy Individuals: A Handbook for Physicians.* New York, American Heart Association, 1972.
3.   Fox SM: Relationship of activity habits to coronary heart disease, in Naughton JP, Hellerstein HK: *Exercise Testing and Exercise Training in Coronary Heart Disease.* New York, Academic Press, 1973, pp 3–22.
4.   Fox SM, Naughton JP, Gorman PA: Physical activity and cardiovascular health: III. The exercise prescription: Frequency and type of activity. *Mod Concepts CV Dis* 41:6, 1972.

48. Orthopnea and Paroxysmal Nocturnal Dyspnea

DOUGLAS C. MORRIS, MD

Definition

Orthopnea: the sensation of shortness of breath or distress in breathing experienced in the recumbent position and eased or relieved by elevating the upper torso.

Paroxysmal nocturnal dyspnea (PND): paroxysmal breathlessness or respiratory distress that awakens the patient after an hour or two of sleep.

Technique

Begin by asking whether the patient is ever short of breath or has difficulty catching his breath. An affirmative response is often followed by a spontaneous description of the occasions when shortness of breath is experienced. Direct inquiry is necessary if the patient does not spontaneously describe the nature and time of occurrence of the shortness of breath. A failure to evoke a history of dyspnea upon or during recumbency should lead to further inquiry. One line of questioning would include the following: How many pillows do you use under your head at night? Do you ever have to sleep sitting up? Do you ever develop a wheeze or cough upon lying down? Do you ever awaken at night short of breath? Do you ever have to sit up to catch your breath? If the answers to any or all of these questions suggest respiratory distress during recumbency, the clinician should next inquire about efforts made to relieve the distress. Characteristically, the patient with left heart failure will sit up in bed or next to the bed and will otherwise remain immobile. There seems to be an innate awareness that greater amounts of ambulation will accentuate the distress. One should be reluctant to ascribe the respiratory distress to heart failure in those patients who gain relief by getting up and walking around.

The duration and severity of symptoms must be ascertained. A reasonably accurate timing of the onset of orthopnea or PND may provide a clue to the precipitating event. The severity of orthopnea is usually assessed in terms of the number of pillows necessary to prevent its occurrence, while the severity of PND is usually measured in terms of the frequency of its occurrence. Ask whether or not any medical intervention has reduced the severity of the symptoms.

Background Information

Despite extensive research, there is no consensus concerning the origin of the sensation accompanying labored breathing. However, the associated physiologic disturbances are reasonably well documented.

The precipitating factor in orthopnea is augmentation of intrathoracic blood volume during recumbency. Upon reclining, an alteration in gravitational forces acts on the vascular beds causing redistribution of a portion of the blood volume from the lower extremities and splanchnic beds to the lungs. Pulmonary blood volume in the horizontal position may exceed that in the erect position by as much as 500 cc. This augmentation of intrathoracic blood volume contributes to a reduction of the vital capacity of the lungs. In normal subjects this reduction is slight, but in patients with orthopnea, decreases of 25–35% have been reported. The earlier impression was that the reduced vital capacity was related to cardiac enlargement, pulmonary vessel engorgement, and an elevated diaphragm. However, recent evidence suggests that reduced pulmonary compliance may be a more important factor. A greater intrathoracic pressure is required to produce a given volume change in the congested lung. This reduced pulmonary compliance dictates that an increase in muscular effort is required to achieve any given level of ventilation. Perhaps the awareness of this discrepancy between muscular effort and the volume of ventilation accounts for the sensation of dyspnea.

On assuming a more erect posture, the patient once again has a redistribution of blood volume. The right atrium is returned to a level above the splanchnic and lower extremity beds, and there is decreased venous return from these areas. Consequently, pulmonary engorgement is decreased and pulmonary compliance and vital capacity are increased. With these physiologic alterations, the sensation of orthopnea clears.

Paroxysmal nocturnal dyspnea is also associated with pulmonary congestion. The pulmonary congestion is directly dependent upon a sudden disproportion in the output from a failing left ventricle and a more normally functioning right ventricle. The disproportionate cardiac output between the two ventricles probably arises from an increased venous return to the right ventricle. In some patients, the mechanism is identical to that of orthopnea. The patient would begin sleeping comfortably with the head elevated and develop dyspnea only after slipping to a more hori-

zontal position. Additional mechanisms must be operative in those patients who can comfortably assume the recumbent position while awake
but develop paroxysmal nocturnal dyspnea after an hour or two of sleep.
An augmented recumbent venous return can result from an increased
intravascular volume caused by reabsorption of edema fluid from previously dependent portions of the body. Augmented venous return can also
result in an increase in influx of blood to the right ventricle. This might
occur during sudden muscular movement of the extremities during a
dream or during increased respiratory effort associated with coughing.
Other factors which may be operative during sleep include decreased excitability of the nervous system, which allows pulmonary congestion to
reach an intensity beyond that which the awake patient would permit;
and a further impairment of ventricular function because of reduced adrenergic stimulation of the myocardium.

An additional factor important in cardiac asthma is bronchospasm,
which increases the resistance to airflow and further increases the effort
of breathing. The exact mechanism of recumbent bronchospasm is as yet
undefined, but edema fluid in the bronchial walls likely plays a role.

Clinical Significance

Orthopnea and PND are most characteristic of those forms of heart
failure associated with elevations of pulmonary venous and pulmonary
capillary pressure, namely, left ventricular failure and severe mitral stenosis. However, neither symptom is pathognomonic for these conditions.
Orthopnea is often found in bronchial asthma, pulmonary emphysema,
severe pneumonia, pneumothorax, and large pleural effusions. Any patient
with pulmonary disease sufficient to require the use of accessory respiratory muscles may experience orthopnea because a supine position impairs
use of these muscles. Massive ascites may also be associated with orthopnea, probably because of accentuated elevation of the diaphragm during recumbency.

Orthopnea and PND are usually more advanced symptoms of left
ventricular dysfunction than is exertional dyspnea. However, either may
be the earliest symptom of cardiac failure in patients with a sedentary
life-style.

The severity of orthopnea is a reasonable reflection of the severity
of cardiac failure. However, if right ventricular dysfunction develops, the
degree of pulmonary congestion may decrease and the symptoms of orthopnea can occasionally improve despite continued deterioration of cardiac function.

Patients with PND must be distinguished from those with bronchitis
or bronchiectasis who awaken with a paroxysm of coughing or even
wheezing. The latter group's symptoms are usually improved with expec-

toration of accumulated bronchial secretions, unlike the case with PND.

In cases of paroxysmal nocturnal dyspnea, the feeling of suffocation is often associated with coughing and wheezing (cardiac asthma). The patient may complain of palpitations, faintness, substernal tightness, or profuse sweating. The struggle to breathe usually lasts 10–20 minutes, then subsides spontaneously with assumption of the upright posture. On occasion, the attack is not aborted and overt pulmonary edema develops. Immediate medical therapy is obviously indicated in this setting.

Selected References

1.   Harrison TR: The mechanism of orthopnea, in Harrison TR: *Failure of the Circulation*. Baltimore, Williams and Wilkins, 1935, pp 166–192.
2.   Christie RV: Dysponea: A review. *Quart J Med* 31:421–454, 1938.
3.   Wood P: Heart failure, in Wood P: *Diseases of the Heart and Circulation*. Philadelphia, JB Lippincott, 1956, pp 272–276.
4.   Ebert RV: The lung in congestive heart failure. *Arch Intern Med* 107:450–459, 1961.
5.   Kettel LJ, Moran F, Cugell DW: Pulmonary function in patients with heart disease. *Med Clin N Am* 50:141–157, 1966.

49. Chest Discomfort or Pain

MARK E. SILVERMAN, MD

Definition

Any painful or uncomfortable sensation originating in or extending to the chest.

Technique

Chest pain or discomfort is a very common and often perplexing symptom confronting the clinician. The task of the clinician is to clarify the symptoms as fully as possible so that all important etiologies are considered. The essential information is obtained by developing the following lines of questions:

1.   Bodily location. Define the area of origin and radiation of the symptom as precisely as possible.
2.   Quality. The quality is the flavor imparted by the symptom, such as sharp, heavy, crampy, crushing, or tingling. An inability to describe the quality may also be informative.
3.   Quantity. This includes the severity, the number of times experienced, and the duration of the symptom.
4.   Chronology. The chronology of a symptom implies the onset of the symptom, as exactly as possible, and its sequential development until the present.
5.   Setting. The symptoms should be related to the time of day or night, whether the patient was active or resting, eating or fasting, emotionally upset or relaxed, at home or at work.
6.   Aggravating or alleviating factors. Clarify the symptom further by asking what was done to gain relief, what position was sought, and the effect of movement, respiration, and medication.
7.   Associated symptoms. Many diseases are manifest as a constellation of associated symptoms that support a diagnosis when linked together. The patient should be asked to describe other sensations occurring before, during, or after the major symptom.

The question, "Do you have chest pain?" may be firmly denied by the patient who does not interpret burning, tightness, aching, heaviness, or indigestion as pain. For this reason, a more productive question is: Do you have any discomfort or disagreeable sensation in your chest? Trace the symptom from its inception to the present. Some patients can relate their symptoms with accuracy and detail; others become confused or frustrated if pressed for exact chronologic information. In the latter situation, the physician should sacrifice chronology for a better comprehension of the nature of the symptom. For example, the physician might ask: Can you describe a typical attack? What time of day or night do the attacks occur? How long is the shortest attack? the longest? the usual? Approximately how many attacks of chest discomfort do you have each week? Have these recently increased in frequency, duration, or severity?

Eventually enough information should be available to suggest a differential diagnosis. Specific questions are then directed for exploration of the possible etiologies. For example, if the nature of the chest discomfort suggests a hiatal hernia, ask specifically about precipitation of the pain by leaning forward or lying flat. The patient may or may not volunteer important information such as a close friend or relative who has recently died of a heart attack, a previous evaluation that demonstrated an abnormal electrocardiogram or duodenal ulcer, trauma to the chest from sports or a car accident, or reproducibility of the pain by prodding the chest wall.

Experienced clinicians realize that it is virtually impossible to evaluate chest discomfort as sifted through another physician's ears, vision, or descriptive talents. The emphasis placed by the patient on the severity of the pain and the facial expressions and mannerisms directly perceived by the clinician are almost as important as the content.

Background Information

Since William Heberden's original description of angina pectoris in 1768, physicians have struggled to correlate the symptom of chest pain with more objective evidence for or against coronary disease. The development of selective coronary arteriography has recently been utilized to correlate coronary anatomy with the clinical history. This method provides detailed objective information about the anatomy of the coronary vessels and, at first glance, provides the definitive answer to the question of whether the patient has angina pectoris due to coronary disease. Unfortunately, the association is not precise because of the following findings:

1. The patient may have grossly obstructed coronary arteries and have no chest pain.
2. There is no guarantee that the chest pain is due to any coronary abnormalities noted.
3. A significant number of patients (10–15%) experience "angina pectoris" and yet have normal coronary arteriograms.
4. Patients with normal coronary arteriograms have had documented myocardial infarctions.

Despite these flaws in the diagnosis of angina pectoris based on the arteriographic findings, two comprehensive studies by Friesinger et al and Proudfit et al have shown the following:

1. Approximately 90% of patients with typical angina pectoris (defined as chest pain or discomfort precipitated by exertion and relieved by rest) have 30% or greater narrowing of one or more major vessels. About 75% of patients with typical angina have at least 90% occlusion of one vessel or more.
2. Approximately 65% of patients with atypical angina (defined as pain probably due to myocardial ischemia but not fulfilling one criterion or more for typical angina pectoris) have moderate or severe coronary artery obstruction.
3. Approximately 80% of patients with uncertain chest pain (de-

fined as probably not angina pectoris but with some suggestive features) have normal coronary arteriograms.

4. Greater than 90% of patients with chest pain thought not to be coronary disease have normal coronary arteriograms.

These two studies substantiate that chest pain brought on by exertion and relieved by rest is the best clinical diagnostic feature of angina pectoris. Patients with chest discomfort highly suggestive of myocardial ischemia but occurring at rest or lasting for a prolonged period remain a diagnostic problem since 20% of these patients have no significant obstruction. Chest pain due to coronary artery disease is particularly difficult to diagnose in women. Fifty percent of women thought to have angina pectoris are found to have normal coronary arteriograms.

The response to nitroglycerin has also been correlated with the coronary anatomy by Horwitz et al. In this study 90% of patients with prompt relief had coronary artery disease (total occlusion or stenosis greater than 75%). Three-fourths of patients had relief of chest pain within three minutes while about one of six patients required a longer period. Patients with coronary artery disease who exhibited a delayed or absent response tended to have more severe obstructive disease and wall motion abnormalities than the group experiencing prompt relief. In contrast, 19% of a group of patients without coronary disease had consistent relief of chest pain in three minutes or less.

Clinical Significance

There are numerous causes of chest pain. Cardiovascular diseases that can produce chest pain include myocardial ischemia or infarction, pericarditis, pulmonary embolus, aortic aneurysm or dissection, cardiomyopathy, pulmonary hypertension, arrhythmia, and mitral valve prolapse. Noncardiac causes that can produce chest pain and must often be considered in the differential diagnosis include anxiety, chest wall pain, hyperventilation, hiatal hernia, esophageal spasm, esophagitis, gastritis, duodenal or gastric ulcer, cholecystitis, pancreatitis, cervical or thoracic spine disease, rib fracture, pleurisy, pneumonia, herpes zoster, and pneumothorax.

Although many of the above diseases have characteristic "textbook" profiles that suggest an immediate diagnosis, there is often considerable overlap. Indeed, an "atypical" pattern seems to be quite common. The following brief discussion points out certain characteristic features of important cardiovascular causes of chest pain.

Angina pectoris. The pain may be located anywhere in the chest but is more commonly substernal or across the anterior chest. Location or radiation to the neck, jaw, upper arms, or elbows is highly suggestive, though not diagnostic. An aching, heaviness, or lifeless sensation in the arms is particularly noteworthy and bilateral pain in the wrists or elbows carries additional specificity. The pain is seldom localized with one finger but rather encompasses an area indicated by a sweep of the hand. It is unusual for the pain to be localized to the apex, left lateral chest, or right chest, or to be located above the jaw or below the epigastrium.

The most characteristic types of pain due to myocardial ischemia are tightness, squeezing, heaviness, pressure, constriction, and indescribable pain. Indigestion, aching, burning, throbbing, tingling, "like gas," and sharp pain are less frequent descriptions offered by the patient. The discomfort is seldom referred to as catching, stabbing, or "like a needle."

Angina pectoris is often precipitated by stress and alleviated by reducing or eliminating the stress. Cardiac stress includes emotional as well as physical stress and therefore may occur when the patient is inactive or sleeping. Precipitation of the pain by a cold wind, walking up an incline, eating a heavy meal, or performing isometric exercises are helpful clues.

Angina pectoris is usually brief, varying from several minutes to about half an hour. Relief of the pain within three minutes by nitroglycerin is a common feature. Nitroglycerin can also abate the pain of other diseases, particularly esophageal spasm; therefore, this response does not necessarily clinch the diagnosis. Conversely, some patients with coronary disease do not gain relief from nitroglycerin or other nitrates.

Myocardial infarction. This pain is usually, although not always, more intense than angina pectoris, and may last from minutes to several hours. Nitrates are not usually effective. The type of pain may be described as crushing, choking, "like a heavy weight," intolerable, and indescribable, with wide radiation across the chest or to the neck and arms. Associated symptoms, including diaphoresis, nausea, vomiting, dizziness, weakness, and dyspnea are common. Occasionally the associated symptoms are more prominent than the chest pain. Sometimes the pain is insignificant or absent and the occurrence of a myocardial infarction is suspected only because of heart failure, unexplained severe weakness, sweating, syncope, arrhythmias, or peripheral embolism. Finally, some patients (estimated to be up to one-third of patients with myocardial infarction) have recognized no symptoms, yet are found to have evidence of a myocardial infarction by routine electrocardiogram.

Pericarditis. This is suspected when the patient describes the pain as sharp and accentuated by breathing, lying down, or other thoracic movement. It is typically improved by sitting up. Radiation of the pain to the left scapula, shoulder and trapezius area, and an awareness that the pain is related to each heart beat are characteristic. The retrosternal location and radiation to the shoulder and arm are similar to myocardial ischemia. Some patients have positional neck or shoulder discomfort with minimal chest pain. On occasion, the pain of pericarditis is indistinguishable from myocardial infarction.

Pulmonary embolus. Pulmonary emboli are often suspected when the patient complains of chest pain accentuated by inspiration, particularly if dyspnea and hemoptysis also occur. More commonly, however, a pulmonary embolus does not announce itself so blatantly. Pain is often absent or insignificant; hemoptysis is uncommon. The diagnosis of pulmonary embolus should be considered with any unexplained dyspnea, particularly if the dyspnea is acute and episodic. Additional clues include atrial arrhythmias, cyanosis, sinus tachycardia, fever, unexplained congestive heart failure, recent bed rest, recent leg trauma, use of estrogen-containing oral contraceptives, and the postpartum state.

Aortic aneurysm. Localized thoracic aneurysms are usually asymptomatic until they rupture or impinge upon a neighboring structure. Erosion into the anterior chest wall or posterior spine may produce significant pain in and around the area. A dissection of the aorta is usually associated with sudden, severe midline pain often described as tearing or ripping. The pain may radiate from front to back or extend down into the abdomen. The peak severity of the pain is classically at the onset, followed by symptoms representing vascular involvement of other areas. A clinical presentation, such as pericardial tamponade, cerebrovascular accident, or anuria, may mask the earlier chest pain.

Mitral valve prolapse. Patients with systolic click(s) and mid-late systolic murmurs due to mitral valve prolapse often present because of chest pain. The chest pain tends to be sharp, fleeting, nonexertional, and located near the cardiac apex on the left lateral chest. On occasion the pain is substernal and simulates the pain of angina pectoris or myocardial infarction.

Cardiomyopathy. Various types of cardiomyopathy may be associated with chest discomfort. This often resembles angina pectoris or myocardial infarction and leads to a false positive diagnosis of coronary artery disease, particularly when there are associated abnormalities in the electrocardiogram.

Pulmonary hypertension. The chest discomfort related to pulmonary hypertension has been attributed to right ventricular ischemia and is often associated with marked dyspnea. Relief is sometimes, but not always, obtained with nitroglycerin.

Arrhythmia. The patient is often aware of extrasystoles, particularly the enhanced contraction following a premature beat, as a fluttering, bumping, choking, or jerking inside the chest. A tachyarrhythmia, such as paroxysmal atrial tachycardia, may elicit an alarming tightness or fullness in the chest or neck.

Selected References

1. Morgan WL Jr, Engel GL: *The Clinical Approach to the Patient.* Philadelphia, WB Saunders, 1969, pp 1–79.
2. Friesinger GC, Page EE, Ross RS: Prognostic significance of coronary arteriography. *Trans Assoc Am Physicians* 83:78–92, 1970.
3. Proudfit WL, Shirey EK, Sones FM: Selective cine coronary arteriography: Correlation with clinical findings in 1000 patients. *Circulation* 33:901–910, 1966.
4. Horwitz LD, Herman MV, Gorlin R: Clinical response to nitroglycerin as a diagnostic test for coronary artery disease. *Am J Cardiol* 29:149–153, 1972.
5. Sampson JJ, Cheitlin MD: Pathophysiology and differential diagnosis of cardiac pain. *Prog Cardiovasc Dis* 13:507–531, 1971.
6. Short D, Stowers M: Earliest symptoms of heart disease and their recognition. *Br Med J* 2:387–391, 1972.
7. Levene DL, Billings RF, Davies GM, et al: *Chest Pain: An Integrated Diagnostic Approach.* Philadelphia, Lea and Febiger, 1977.
8. Waters DD, Halphen C, Theroux P, et al: Coronary artery disease in young women: Clinical and angiographic features and correlation with risk factors. *Am J Cardiol* 42:41–47, 1978.
9. Malcolm AD, Boughner DR, Kostuk WJ, et al: Clinical features and investigative findings in presence of mitral leaflet prolapse: Study of 85 consecutive patients. *Br Heart J* 38:244–256, 1976.

50. Palpitation

BARRY SILVERMAN, MD

Definition

Palpitation refers to a disagreeable awareness of the heart beat, described as a thumping, pounding, skipping, flopping, stopping, jumping, racing, or expanding sensation in the chest.

Technique

First, ask the patient to describe the frequency and duration of each episode, since it is important to determine if the episode lasts a few seconds or a few minutes. Question the patient whether palpitations are associated with excitement, anxiety, unusual work hours, smoking, coffee, alcohol, diet pills, or other drugs such as nasal decongestants.

Second, ask the patient to tap out the rhythm or cadence of the sensation he feels. If the patient is unable to do this, tap out the cadence of various arrhythmias and ask the patient to identify the one that best fits his situation.

Background Information

Precise pathophysiology of palpitations is not clearly understood. Some patients are very sensitive to variations in heart rate and force of contraction and can appreciate an atrial premature beat or the more forceful contraction of a postextrasystolic beat. Other patients with serious life-threatening arrhythmias, such as ventricular tachycardia, have no sensation of the event. There are a number of efferent neural pathways leading from the atria, ventricles, and great vessels which follow the cervical sympathetic chain to the hypothalamus and detect changes in the rate and force of contraction. The shape and size of the chest cavity and the position of the heart within the chest cavity may also be related to recognition of these sensations.

Clinical Significance

The sensation of palpitations may have no clinical significance. Many patients detect changes in rhythm and strength of contraction from atrial or ventricular ectopic beats without underlying organic heart disease. This sensation is frequently appreciated at times of excitement, exertion, or intake of coffee, alcohol, nicotine, diet pills, or other stimulatory drugs. Like tinnitus, palpitations are often more noticeable at night when extraneous noises are removed from the environment. Emotions and anxiety, however, do not produce serious cardiac arrhythmias without underlying heart disease. Patients who are begun on digitalis may notice a change in the forcefulness of contraction. This sensation is often a complaint of patients with thyrotoxicosis, anemia, or pheochromocytoma.

Patients with a large stroke volume, as in aortic regurgitation, may be troubled with an abnormal sensation of the heart beat. A complaint of frequent palpitations may also be noted in patients with atrial fibrillation, such as those with undetected mitral stenosis or thyrotoxicosis. A racing heart sensation which begins and ends abruptly (within minutes) may represent paroxysmal atrial tachycardia. Patients with paroxysmal atrial tachycardia sometimes give a history of learning how to abort the palpitations by straining, pressing on their necks, or gagging themselves. Their electrocardiograms should be carefully analyzed for the presence of a short P-Q interval, delta waves, and a widened QRS complex characteristic of the Wolff-Parkinson-White syndrome.

Selected References

1. Hurst JW (ed-in-chief), Logue RB, Schlant RC, Wenger NK (eds): *The Heart*, ed 4. McGraw-Hill, 1978.
2. Katz LN, Winston SS, Megibow RS: Psychosomatic aspects of cardiac arrhythmias: A physiologic dynamic approach. *Ann Intern Med* 27:261-274, 1947.
3. Wintrobe MM, Thorn GW, Adams RD, et al (eds): *Harrison's Principles of Internal Medicine*, ed 7. New York, McGraw-Hill, 1974, pp 182-183.
4. Pickering TG, Johnston J, Honour AJ: Comparison of the effects of sleep, exercise and autonomic drugs on ventricular extrasystoles, using ambulatory monitoring of electrocardiogram and electroencephalogram. *Am J Med* 65:575-583, 1978.

51. Syncope

NANETTE K. WENGER, MD

Definition

Syncope is a sudden, temporary loss of consciousness, associated with inability to maintain postural tone. Syncopal episodes are generally abrupt in onset, of brief duration, and characterized by complete recovery within a few minutes. Symptoms such as faintness, light-headedness, and giddiness also imply an impairment, although not an actual loss, of consciousness; when these occur in the sitting or recumbent position, they must be considered as syncope equivalents because true syncope might have occurred with the patient upright.

Technique

The physician is usually unable to observe most patients during their syncopal episode, but rather sees them after the fact. Thus, a detailed history is of great importance in determining the etiology of the alteration of consciousness (see also section 87, Episodic Neurological Symptoms).

Syncope is an unfamiliar term to most patients and the questioning should concern loss of consciousness or, more simply, fainting, falling out spells, or blackouts.

In addition to identifying the patient's age at onset of syncope and the frequency and duration of attacks, establish the relationship to activity or exercise; postural or positional change (with emphasis on head turning or neck pressure); anxiety, fear, or emotional stress (eg, the sight of blood, a hypodermic injection); hunger; urination; or a coughing paroxysm. Was there a warning of the attack?

Inquire about premonitory or associated palpitations; chest discomfort; headaches; loss of vision, speech, or motor function; loss of bladder or bowel control; or autonomic manifestations: pallor, nausea, yawning, sweating.

Ascertain the presence of known cardiovascular disease or a disturbance of cardiac rhythm; central nervous system disease, eg, stroke or seizure disorder; recent prolonged immobilization or blood loss; the use of antihypertensive agents; other states or diseases altering autonomic activity: the postsympathectomy state, diabetic neuropathy, or syringomyelia; or use of diuretic or vasodilator drugs. Determine if there is a family history of syncope.

Obtain an observer's description of the patient during an attack regarding appearance, vital signs, the presence of tonic or clonic movements, postsyncopal weakness, or confusion.

Background Information

The loss of consciousness in the varied types of syncope is thought to be due to an abnormality in cerebral cellular metabolism in those parts of the brain which subserve consciousness. This abnormality in cerebral metabolism is most frequently due to a reduction in cerebral blood flow, and this reduction in cerebral blood flow in turn results from a sudden decrease either in peripheral resistance or in cardiac output. Cerebral blood flow normally represents about 15% of the total cardiac output. Qualitative changes in the blood, such as a decrease in the PCO_2 or in the blood glucose level, may also impair consciousness by altering cerebral cellular metabolism.

Syncope can be discussed in three major categories: (1) peripheral circulatory failure, (2) cardiac disorders, and (3) miscellaneous diseases responsible for alterations of consciousness.

Peripheral circulatory failure. In this category, "vasodepressor syncope" (the common faint) is the most frequent cause of a transient loss of consciousness. It represents a response to an emotional or physical stimulus which would ordinarily call for immediate physical activity, the fight or flight reaction. When this physical activity does not occur, there is sudden peripheral vasodilation, particularly of the skeletal muscles, without a compensatory increase in cardiac output. This results in a fall of the systemic blood pressure and decreased cerebral perfusion with loss of consciousness.

A number of pharmacologic agents, particularly antihypertensive drugs which suppress sympathetic nerve activity, and the injudicious or excessive use of potent diuretic agents are frequent causes of "orthostatic hypotension." Potent diuretic agents rapidly deplete the circulating blood volume and cause the blood pressure to fall when the patient is in an upright position. Various nitrite preparations may also cause orthostatic hypotension with syncope. Orthostatic hypotension is also seen in the patient who has had a sympathectomy and in a number of diseases involving the autonomic nervous system, particularly tabes dorsalis, diabetic neuropathy, and syringomyelia; the patient with severe varicose veins is also subject to orthostatic hypotension, presumably because large amounts of blood pool in the dilated venous beds of the leg.

"Tussive syncope," another cause of peripheral circulatory failure, follows a paroxysm of vigorous coughing; it is most common in men with chronic bronchitis or in children. The loss of consciousness seems due to an increase in intrathoracic pressure during the coughing episode, which interferes with venous return to the heart and thus impairs cardiac output and cerebral perfusion; alternatively, the paroxysm of vigorous coughing may increase intracerebral pressure and limit cerebral perfusion.

"Micturition syncope" is most often seen in older men with nocturia, who leave a warm bed and stand to void. There is a sudden loss of consciousness during or immediately after voiding, generally without premonitory symptoms. The mechanism appears to be a combination of peripheral vasodilatation and increased intrathoracic pressure from straining.

"Prank" fainting is common in teenagers who induce syncope by suddenly increasing intrathoracic pressure, thus decreasing venous return, cardiac output, and cerebral blood flow. The person hyperventilates, decreasing PCO_2 and thereby cerebral blood flow; sudden manual chest compression induces the above hemodynamic alterations and results in syncope.

Cardiac disorders. Fainting of cardiac origin is due to a sudden, marked decrease in cardiac output with decreased cerebral perfusion. This may be due to a disturbance of the heart rate or rhythm, or to any disorder characterized by an inability to increase cardiac output in response to a fall in peripheral resistance.

Patients who are elderly or who have organic heart disease or arrhythmias with very rapid ventricular rates are most prone to develop symptoms from the arrhythmias. Tachycardia, even in a patient with a normal heart, is associated with a significant reduction in peripheral perfusion when the heart rate is greater than 140 or 160 beats per minute. This decrease in peripheral and, of course, cerebral perfusion occurs at a slower heart rate in the patient with heart disease.

"Effort syncope," with a fall in peripheral resistance most commonly induced by exercise, is seen in patients with aortic outflow obstruction, primary pulmonary hypertension, tetralogy of Fallot, and congenital cardiac lesions with the Eisenmenger physiology. These patients cannot increase their cardiac output to compensate for the decreased peripheral resistance. Syncope related to a change in position should suggest mechanical obstruction either of the tricuspid or mitral valve orifice, as seen with a ball valve thrombus or atrial myxoma.

In patients with carotid sinus hypersensitivity, stimulation of the carotid sinus is followed by a marked slowing of the heart rate: sinus bradycardia or sinoatrial or atrioventricular block. Carotid sinus stimulation may also be associated with a profound decrease in peripheral resistance, or indeed, with a combination of slowing of the heart rate and decreased peripheral resistance and resultant hypotension.

Swallowing, as an unusual cause of syncope, is encountered in patients with esophageal spasm, strictures, diverticulae, and neoplasms. A reflex vasovagal mechanism is thought to precipitate atrioventricular conduction disturbances, which may be abolished by atropine.

Miscellaneous diseases.   Akinetic epilepsy and bona fide cerebral vascular disease must be included in the differential diagnosis of syncope, as must hysterical fainting

Fainting in the hyperventilation syndrome results from a decreased PCO_2 secondary to overbreathing, with consequent cerebral vasoconstriction and peripheral vasodilatation.

Clinical Significance

Vasodepressor syncope, the common faint, may occur in normal individuals or in patients with varying types and severities of illness. Useful in the clinical history are the presyncopal autonomic manifestations, particularly pallor, nausea, and sweating. Following this, there may be yawning, dilation of the pupils, hyperventilation, and bradycardia. Often headache, weakness, and slight mental confusion occur after the faint has been terminated. Vasodepressor syncope generally occurs in the upright posture, and there is a prompt return of consciousness once the patient is recumbent. Common precipitating events for vasodepressor syncope include hypodermic injections, minor surgery, trauma, prolonged standing in one position, a sudden emotional shock, or even the sight of blood. Syncope may recur if the patient too rapidly resumes the upright posture.

Syncope that occurs when a patient suddenly arises from the recumbent position should suggest orthostatic hypotension. It is common after prolonged immobilization or bed rest, especially when the patient is elderly; it may be seen with prolonged standing and in patients receiving antihypertensive drugs, excessive diuretic therapy, or nitrite or other vasodilator drugs. This phenomenon is readily documented by abruptly placing the patient in the upright position and observing the symptoms and the heart rate and blood pressure response.

An interesting rare condition is "chronic idiopathic orthostatic hypotension." Syncope is due to failure of the normal compensatory autonomic and humoral factors and occurs when the patient assumes the upright posture. The fall in blood pressure is prompt and the usual prodromal symptoms of vasodepressor syncope are absent. These patients may have other manifestations of autonomic dysfunction, eg, impotence, loss of sweating, and bladder disturbances, which may provide a clue to the diagnosis.

Syncope may be related to tachycardia, to bradycardia, to ectopic ventricular beats, or to complete atrioventricular block, all of which may interfere with cardiac output and cerebral perfusion. Syncope caused by complete heart block, in contrast to syncope of most other causes, is unlikely to be related to posture, an important diagnostic consideration. The loss of consciousness is sudden and is not preceded by premonitory symptoms. Patients with this Stokes-Adams syncope may even deny their brief episodes of unconsciousness. If cardiac standstill is prolonged, a convulsion may occur. Syncope due to paroxysmal tachycardia occurs most commonly when the patient is upright. Frequently the patient is aware of rapid heart action or reports palpitations before there is an alteration of consciousness, but not invariably so. Absence of reported rapid heart action should not exclude suspicion of tachycardia, as some patients may be completely unaware of heart rates of 175–200 beats per minute or of multiple ectopic beats.

Syncope associated with chest pain may reflect an inadequate cardiac output due to left ventricular ischemic paralysis both in patients with classical Heberden's angina and patients with Prinzmetal or variant angina. More typically, though, arrhythmia is the cause of syncope in patients with severe coronary disease.

Carotid sinus hypersensitivity is most common in elderly men. Syncope may be initiated by motion of the head, by shaving over the carotid sinus areas, or even by a tight collar. Many older patients may have reflex slowing of the heart rate or a fall in blood pressure when the physician massages the carotid sinus, but only a few who exhibit this response will actually lose consciousness. The most important observation to document carotid sinus hypersensitivity is not whether hemodynamic changes are produced by carotid sinus massage, but whether the symptoms produced are those which occur with the spontaneous attacks; this observation makes the diagnosis. A concomitant electrocardiographic recording is mandatory for safety during carotid sinus stimulation. Also, listening for bruits over both carotid vessels and palpation for patency of the contralateral carotid artery is requisite prior to carotid sinus massage; carotid sinus stimulation may precipitate syncope when there is atheromatous narrowing of the contralateral carotid or basilar artery.

Patients with cerebral atherosclerosis who have repeated episodes of impairment of consciousness often have these attacks accompanied by a focal neurologic deficit.

Hysterical fainting is seen almost exclusively in young women with emotional illnesses. The diagnosis can usually be easily made based on the clinical setting and the virtual absence of abnormalities of heart rate, blood pressure, and skin color.

Fainting can occur with the hyperventilation syndrome, a symptom complex which includes dizziness, perioral and digital paresthesias, palpitations, and a sensation of tightness in the chest. It is a common cause of recurrent faintness without actual loss of consciousness. Clues to differentiate hyperventilation attacks from other forms of light-headedness include the occurrence of attacks with any body position, the absence of a marked drop in blood pressure, and particularly the failure to relieve the symptoms when the patient assumes the recumbent position. Symptoms can often be reproduced by having the patient voluntarily hyperventilate for several minutes.

Hypoglycemia is another common cause of episodic weakness, sweating, and mental confusion; it is often accompanied by a sensation of hunger. An awareness of the conditions which may produce hypoglycemia alert the physician to this diagnosis. Temporal relationship to meals is important, as is relief by glucose administration.

Selected References

1. Friedberg CK: Syncope: Pathological physiology: Differential diagnosis and treatment. *Mod Conc Cardiovasc Dis* 40:55–63, 1971.
2. Noble RJ: The patient with syncope. *JAMA* 237:1372–1376, 1977.
3. Vaisrub S: Bizarre blackouts. *JAMA* 233:452, 1975.
4. Van Durme JP: Tachyarrhythmias and transient cerebral ischemic attacks. *Am Heart J* 89:538–540, 1975.
5. Walter PF, Reid SD Jr, Wenger NK: Transient cerebral ischemia due to arrhythmia. *Ann Intern Med* 72:471–474, 1970.
6. Wright KE, McIntosh HD: Syncope: A review of pathophysiological mechanisms. *Prog Cardiovasc Dis* 13:580–594, 1971.

52. Edema

See section 164.

53. Phlebitis

See section 165.

54. Claudication

ROBERT B. SMITH III, MD

Definition

Pain or weakness in the muscles of the lower extremities related to exercise.

Technique

A general question related to function of the lower extremities usually results in a characteristic description of symptoms by patients with intermittent claudication. One may ask simply, "Do you have any difficulty walking?" or, "How far can you walk without stopping to rest?" If the patient gives an indication in the reply that his ability to walk is limited by discomfort in the legs or that he is unable to walk 8–10 city blocks without stopping to rest, the examiner should encourage him to describe what happens when he tries to walk. The patient may then relate the typical sequence of walk, pain, rest, relief. But leading questions are useful in getting the full story: Does he have pain with exercise? If so, in what part of the leg? How long does it last? What can he do to relieve it? If it disappears with rest, as is typical of claudication, can he walk again for the same distance? What is the effect of more strenuous muscular exertion, such as climbing hills or steps or jogging? Many patients do not recognize the disability as a pain, but instead talk of aching, cramping, burning, tiredness, numbness, or weakness in the calf, thigh, or buttock muscles related to activity. Some individuals mention that the discomfort always begins in one leg before the other, or that it begins in the calf and then spreads to the thigh or buttock. Others will say that the first sensation is fatigue or weakness and that real pain develops only if they persist in exercising without pausing to rest when the first symptoms appear.

It is important in the questioning to establish that the pain does not occur simply upon standing up, and that it does not persist for more than a few minutes after stopping to rest. The latter symptoms would be more suggestive of pain due to musculoskeletal or neurologic disorders. Night cramps, which occur while in bed, and pain on prolonged standing due to venous insufficiency likewise should be differentiated by history. If the patient is uncertain about these points, or gives a history that is suggestive of claudication, but not typical, the examiner may ask the individual to reproduce his symptoms by having the patient walk briskly or perform treadmill exercise under observation. When the claudicatory pain appears, its nature, duration, and response to rest can be recorded and the affected extremity examined.

Background Information

Intermittent claudication is not a diagnosis but a symptom. It refers to a condition of lameness and pain in the lower extremity, precipitated by exercise and relieved by rest. When present, it is a rather specific and reliable indicator of arterial insufficiency of the leg. The blood flow may be adequate to maintain a comfortable limb at rest or with limited activity, but upon more vigorous exercise the major muscle groups distal to a level of arterial obstruction receive inadequate circulation to meet metabolic demands. The resulting pain is thought to be due to accumulation of irritating metabolic products in the ischemic muscle, causing stimulation of sensory nerves. Similar pain can be produced by having experimental subjects exercise with a proximally applied arterial tourniquet on the limb. When patients with claudication stop to rest, they achieve relief of pain by allowing the blood supply to catch up with the previous metabolic activity. The subjects may then walk for the same distance, with the same sequence of events. Although rest generally affords prompt relief of claudicatory pain, patients may have persistent tenderness, soreness, or fatigue of the affected muscles for some time. While the pain of claudication is usually of a dull, aching type, on occasion it may be excruciating or totally disabling, especially if the individual persists in walking despite ischemic symptoms.

Intermittent claudication is the most common presenting complaint in patients with arterial insufficiency of the lower extremity and may be the only symptom that patients experience for many years. The severity of the underlying arterial occlusive disease can be estimated by the distance at which claudication appears, the relationship to how rapidly the patients were walking at the time, and the duration of rest necessary to allow subsidence of pain. Symptoms may vary from day to day in the same person, depending upon the incline and condition of terrain traveled, or the environmental temperature and wind resistance encountered.

Similar claudication pain may occur in the forearm or hand in a patient with upper extremity vascular compromise, but it is uncommon in that setting because of more adequate collateral systems in the arm and less vigorous muscular activity of that extremity, as compared to the leg. Persons who perform heavy physical labor or athletes involved in sports that require repetitive arm motion are more likely to complain of arm claudication than other, more sedentary individuals, with the same degree of vascular obstruction.

Clinical Significance

Intermittent claudication most commonly occurs in atherosclerotic occlusive disease. Although atherosclerosis is a diffuse process, the more severe arterial obstructions are segmental in location. As the lesions progress, collateral circulation develops and may be sufficient to preserve viability and to prevent symptoms at rest. Claudication occurs when the collateral circulation is not adequate to supply the increased demand of exercising muscles distal to a major obstruction. The severity of the patient's symptoms depends upon the pattern of occlusion, the degree of narrowing, the rate of progression, and the adequacy of collateral flow. Claudication may worsen as the underlying disease progresses, or it may remain stable for many years. If the collateral bed gradually enlarges with time, claudication symptoms may actually improve. If, on the other hand, the collateral itself becomes occluded or another major arterial block develops, claudication may suddenly worsen and progress to pain at rest, ulceration of the skin, or ischemic gangrene of the limb. It is estimated, however, that only 10% of patients who present with intermittent claudication on the basis of atherosclerosis eventually go on to gangrenous changes.

The location of claudication pain can be used to predict the site of major arterial obstruction, since the affected muscle group is always distal to the level of vascular occlusion. If the pain is confined to the foot, tibial segment obstruction is indicated; if the pain is also in the calf, the superficial femoral segment; if in the thigh, the iliofemoral segment; and if in the hip and buttock, the aortoiliac segment. Usually, the physical findings corroborate these principles, but arteriography is necessary to define the extent of disease with precision. Claudication pain is also seen in other forms of vascular insufficiency, including embolic occlusion, Buerger's disease, extrinsic vascular compression, and arteriospastic disorders such as ergotism.

The assessment of vascular insufficiency symptoms must be individualized according to the patients' life-style and general health status. Certainly, a 60-year-old person who cannot walk 2–3 blocks at a moderate pace has a significant disability. This disability might be only an annoyance if he is retired and troubled by cardiac disease, but it could constitute a real threat if the individual is otherwise in good health and has to walk to keep his job. A thorough knowledge of all these factors is required before any decision can be made regarding further diagnostic studies or possible surgical treatment.

Selected References

1. Fairburn JF II, Juergens JL, Spittell JA Jr: *Peripheral Vascular Disease*, ed 4. Philadelphia, WB Saunders, 1972.
2. Eastcott HHG: *Arterial Surgery*, id 2. Philadelphia, JP Lippincott, 1973.
3. Hershey FB, Calman CH: *Atlas of Vascular Surgery*, ed 2. St. Louis, CV Mosby, 1967.

55. Hypertension

ELBERT P. TUTTLE, JR., MD

Definition

Elevated blood pressure. When used unmodified, hypertension usually means high systemic arterial blood pressure. Since blood pressure is a continuous variable that is unimodally distributed in the population, the definition of what is "high" is arbitrary and varies considerably in different areas. The World Health Organization has defined hypertension in adults as blood pressure over 160 mm Hg systolic or 95 mm Hg diastolic, or both. Many studies in the United States have considered the upper limit of normal blood pressure to be 140/90 mm Hg. Others would define hypertension as a diastolic blood pressure above 90 mm Hg, or a mean arterial blood pressure greater than 107 mm Hg. Mean arterial blood pressure is approximately equal to:

$$\frac{\text{systolic BP} + 2\,(\text{diastolic BP})}{3}$$

Labile or borderline hypertension is usually defined as blood pressure intermittently elevated (one or two out of three measurements) and near the above dividing values.

Technique

The technique of eliciting a history of hypertension consists first of asking the simple direct question: Have you ever had high blood pressure? There are some communities in which the common term is "high blood." In others the disturbance might be termed "hypertension." If there is doubt about recall, ask explicitly: What about at times of athletic examinations, military induction or discharge, insurance examinations, or pregnancy? A third relevant question is whether the patient has ever taken high blood pressure medication such as diuretics (water pills). The latter may become so routine as not to be remembered by the patient.

Background Information

The analysis of the determinants of hypertension is well set forth in the writings of Dr. Arthur Guyton. The blood pressure is the force generated by the cardiac output, the elastic character of the great vessels, and peripheral vascular resistance of the arterioles. The relative contribution of cardiac output and peripheral resistance varies in different disease states and at different times in the course of a disease. Often hypertension of recent onset and labile character is associated with high cardiac output, while longer standing hypertension is usually associated with high peripheral resistance. The first may become converted to the second with the passage of time.

Hypertension is more than twice as prevalent in black as in white populations in the United States. An excess of hypertension occurs in first-order relatives of patients with hypertension. It is therefore of value to inquire about a family history of hypertension. Do members of your immediate family have high blood pressure? In a more circuitous form the question may be asked: Are your mother and father alive? If not, did your deceased parent die of a stroke, uremic poisoning or heart failure? An affirmative answer increases the probability of familial hypertension. On the other hand, the answer no to any of the above may simply mean that the patient does not know.

Clinical Significance

The date of onset of transient or persistent hypertension is of clinical significance in the differential diagnosis of its cause, the extent of target organ damage, the relationship to coexistent disease of specific organs, and the probable response to therapy. For example, long-standing hypertension will more frequently be associated with hypertensive retinopathy, left ventricular hypertrophy, and elevated serum creatinine. In cases of renal artery stenosis, duration of hypertension of more than three years is associated with a decreased chance of response to operation.

The highest incidence of essential hypertension is in middle age. Thus, when hypertension appears in the young or the old, a somewhat higher probability exists that it is due to a specific and diagnosable cause. The search for correctable causes such as renal parenchymal disease, renal artery stenosis, aortic coarctation, aldosterone-secreting tumor, pheochromocytoma, or hyperparathyroidism is indicated by an onset of hypertension in the young, in the old, in the recent past, or at intermittent times.

On the other hand, a history of confirmed hypertension in the past, but now no longer present, suggests either good pharmacologic management or some counteracting occurrence. Examples of events which may counteract hypertension include termination of a toxemic pregnancy, remission of a renal disease, occurrence of a myocardial infarct, development of intravascular volume contraction, or the presence of pericarditis with tamponade.

Renal disease causing hypertension may be either renovascular or renal parenchymal hypertension. Hypertension may also lead to renal disease, known as nephrosclerosis. The differentiation of these two conditions often depends on an accurate history of which occurred first.

With long duration of uncontrolled hypertension, target organ damage can be anticipated. Such target organ damage includes retinopathy, increased atherosclerosis, myocardial hypertrophy, cerebrovascular disease, and nephrosclerosis. The reversibility of hypertension is related to its duration. Long-standing hypertension is more likely to persist after removal of a putative cause. It is thus preferable to identify correctable causes as soon as possible after initial confirmation of hypertension.

Selected References

1. Guyton AC, Coleman TG, Cowley AW Jr, et al: A systems analysis approach to understanding long-range arterial blood pressure control and hypertension. *Circ Res* 35:159–176, 1974.
2. Report of the Joint National Committee on detection, evaluation and treatment of high blood pressure: A cooperative study. *JAMA* 237: 255–261, 1977.
3. Pickering G: Hypertension: Definitions, natural histories, and consequences, in Laragh JH (ed): *Hypertension Manual.* New York, Dun-Donnelly Publishing Corp., 1973, pp 3–30.
4. Foster JH, Maxwell MH, Franklin SS, et al: Renovascular occlusive disease. Results of operative treatment. *JAMA* 231:1043–1048, 1975.

56. Rheumatic Fever

DONNA GIBBAS, MD

Definition

A systemic disease precipitated by an immune reaction to group A streptococcal throat infections characterized by recurring episodes of fever, arthritis, and carditis.

Technique

A good history of rheumatic fever is often difficult to obtain. Make every effort to characterize the clinical manifestations of each attack. Careful patient interviews and thorough review of previous chart data will often yield a suggestive history. Not infrequently, however, a patient presents with rheumatic heart disease, yet gives no history of an acute illness resembling rheumatic fever. A logical approach is to seek information contained in the Jones criteria for the diagnosis of rheumatic fever. These criteria were first proposed by T. D. Jones in 1944. They were revised in 1965 and are reevaluated annually by the American Heart Association. The Jones criteria have proved helpful in reducing overdiagnosis. They also assist in distinguishing rheumatic fever from collagen and infectious diseases.

Using these standards, either two major or one major and two minor criteria indicate a high probability of rheumatic fever, provided there is evidence for a preceding streptococcal infection. The latter is required except in cases in which the acute illness occurred several months earlier, such as chorea.

Jones Criteria (revised 1965)

Major
Carditis
Polyarthritis
Chorea
Erythema marginatum
Subcutaneous nodules

Minor
Fever
Arthralgia
History of previous rheumatic fever or rheumatic heart disease
Abnormal acute phase reactions (elevated sedimentation rate, positive C-reactive protein, leukocytosis)
Prolonged P-R interval

Supporting evidence of streptococcal infection
Increased titer of streptococcal antibodies (antistreptolysin O or others)
Positive throat culture for group A streptococcus
Recent scarlet fever

Ask details about any long-term childhood illness or hospitalization: What was the extent and nature of the child's confinement? Were physical activities limited? To what degree and for what length of time? Did the patient ever receive long-term injections or oral antibiotics? Were frequent sore throats or diagnosed streptococcal infections a problem? How much school was missed for this reason? When was the last episode of pharyngitis? How was it treated? What was the risk of exposure to streptococcus? Specific questions should then be asked using the major Jones criteria as guides:

1. *Carditis.* Was the patient ever told of a heart murmur? At which age was it first detected? Is it still present? Was it considered a significant murmur? If the patient describes previous carditis, was cardiomegaly or congestive heart failure present? Has the patient ever received medication for a heart condition?
2. *Polyarthritis.* Has the patient ever experienced arthritis or arthralgias? Which joints were involved? How long did each joint symptom persist? Was the arthritis migratory or did all joint symptoms occur together? Was there much swelling, erythema, pain, or limitation of joint motion? Did the patient receive aspirin? What was the response? Did the patient ever have growing pains or shin splints as a child? If so, what were the symptoms?
3. *Chorea.* Has the patient ever noted a movement disorder? What description can be given? Were the movements repetitive? Could the movements be controlled? How long did the disorder persist? Did anyone ever mention St. Vitus' dance? Did teachers or parents ever complain of decreased school performance, marked deterioration of handwriting, clumsiness or onset of labile temper in a previously good student?
4. *Erythema marginatum.* Was a rash ever associated with an un-

diagnosed acute illness? What was the description of the rash, including color, texture, and distribution? How long did the rash persist? What if anything would make the rash more prominent? Was it pruritic? What were the associated symptoms?

5. *Subcutaneous nodules.* Were nodules ever noted either by the patient or physician? What was their size and distribution? Were they movable or painful? Was there a preceding or associated illness? Was a heart murmur noted? If arthritis was present, how did it manifest?

Background Information

The greatest occurrence of initial rheumatic fever cases is between the ages of 6 and 15 years. Initial attacks decline markedly after puberty, but one-third of recurrences are between the ages of 20 and 40. For patients with rheumatic heart disease, the risk of recurrence persists for life.

Rheumatic fever is considered an autoimmune disease. Cross-reaction between streptococcal components and myocardial fibers has been noted, as has cross-reaction between the group A streptococcal polysaccharide and heart valve glycoproteins. Antiheart antibodies are found in more than half of patients with carditis. These antibodies may also occur in rheumatic fever without carditis, as well as in nonrheumatic causes of myocardial damage. In contrast to poststreptococcal glomerulonephritis, rheumatic fever does not tend to be associated with either skin infections or specific strains of group A streptococci.

The histological lesions of rheumatic fever are proliferative and exudative inflammatory reactions. They are found in the mesenchymal supporting tissue of the heart, joints, blood vessels, and subcutaneous tissues. The most distinctive lesion is the Aschoff body, described in 1904. It is an oval perivascular aggregation of large cells with polymorphous nuclei and basophilic cytoplasm arranged as a rosette around an avascular core of fibrinoid or necrotic protoplasm. Aschoff cells resemble histiocytes and macrophages, and are probably derived from connective tissue cells. Aschoff bodies can be classified as active or senescent. Active bodies are seen in active carditis and in those patients with clinically inactive disease but persistently elevated sedimentation rates. Senescent or more scarred Aschoff bodies probably represent healing or inactive disease.

The cardiac lesions of acute rheumatic fever can be divided into myocarditis, endocarditis, or pericarditis. During the acute stages of myocarditis, sparse inflammatory infiltration is present. As the disease progresses, Aschoff bodies appear in all areas of the myocardium, particularly the subendocardial regions of the left ventricle and the interventricular septum. Residual fibrosis occurs with varying severity. Nonbacterial endocarditis affects the mural endocardium and the valves. The most characteristic mural lesion is a thickened, opaque area at the base of the posterior mitral leaflet. The valvular lesion consists of edema and inflammatory cellular reaction involving the leaflets and chordae tendinae. Verrucae appear as hyaline masses on the lines of valve closure. These heal, leaving the valves thickened, deformed, fused, or calcified. The valve most often involved is the mitral, manifesting regurgitation initially and stenosis a variable number of years later. The apical middiastolic murmur (Carey-Coombs) heard in active disease is due to relative rigidity of the mitral valve in relation to a dilated ventricle. The second most commonly involved valve is the aortic, manifesting significant regurgitation initially and stenosis or insufficency many years later. The tricuspid valve is seldom affected and involvement of the pulmonary valve is rare. The pericarditis is predominantly exudative, with fibrinous involvement of both the visceral and parietal pericardium. Cardiac tamponade is rare, as is the development of subsequent constrictive pericarditis.

The joint inflammation of acute rheumatic fever is chiefly exudative, with edema and fibrinoid degeneration of the synovium. The cartilage is characteristically spared. The periarticular tissues are edematous, and lesions similar to Aschoff bodies may be found.

Subcutaneous nodules consist of a central area of fibrinoid necrosis surrounded by connective tissue cells and lymphocytes.

Perivascular round cell hemorrhages, petechiae, and hyalinization of small vessels have been seen scattered throughout the cortex, cerebellum, and basal ganglia of the central nervous system. No site is consistently involved, and Aschoff bodies have never been found.

Clinical Significance

Crowded living conditions of lower socioeconomic groups render members of these groups more susceptible to rheumatic fever. Also at risk are students, military populations, mothers of young children, and persons in occupations involving contact with children.

The appearance of a murmur in a patient with a previously normal examination is of particular importance. Most typical of acute rheumatic fever is a systolic or middiastolic murmur at the apex, or a diastolic murmur at the base. Report of a changing or new murmur in a patient with previous rheumatic heart disease may be suggestive of previous valvular damage, recurrent acute rheumatic fever, or bacterial endocarditis.

The severity of previous carditis is important since subsequent rheumatic heart disease and the frequency of recurrent rheumatic fever increase in direct proportion to the severity of the previous carditis.

Polyarthritis is the most common major criterion for rheumatic fever. It is usually migratory and evinced by intense pain and limitation of motion disproportionate to the clinical signs of inflammation. The polyarthritis is of short duration, is extremely sensitive to aspirin, and resolves without joint destruction. Although a genuine rheumatic sign, arthralgias should be given careful but not excessive consideration in forming the diagnosis. Occasionally a patient notes that he had growing pains or shin splints as a child. These typically occur in the muscles of the thighs and legs at the end of the day. The pains are only vaguely localized and are usually relieved by heat or massage. True growing pains or shin splints are not associated with rheumatic fever.

Sydenham's chorea, also called St. Vitus' dance, is an important criterion but often exceedingly difficult to uncover. Chorea consists of involuntary, purposeless, rapid movements often associated with muscle weakness and emotional lability. It is easy to note in retrospect, but the onset can be insidious, with changes in behavior in school, deteriorating handwriting, clumsiness, or temper tantrums. The history must be carefully distinguished from normal childhood hyperactivity and tics (stereotyped, repetitive movements).

Erythema marginatum is characterized by evanescent, serpiginous, slightly raised lesions with pale centers found mainly on the trunk and proximal extremities. Erythema marginatum is never seen on the face, is nonpruritic, and can be brought out by a warm bath. Like chorea, the appearance of the rash is often late. It responds poorly to systemic anti-inflammatory drugs. Erythema marginatum is almost always associated with carditis, but has no other relationship to severity. Urticaria is more commonly seen than the classic rash of erythema marginatum.

Like erythema marginatum, subcutaneous nodules are associated with prolonged active carditis and usually do not occur until several weeks after the onset of the attack. The nodules are firm, painless, freely movable, and vary in size from pinpoint to 1 cm. They are seen, or more often felt, over the extensor surfaces of the large joints. Rheumatic nodules are more frequently noted in children, while rheumatoid arthritis nodules occur more often in adults.

Certain combinations of Jones criteria are relatively weak in validating a rheumatic fever diagnosis. Such combinations would include polyarthritis plus two minor criteria. Rheumatic fever is a major consideration, but an element of doubt should remain. A history of previous rheumatic fever or rheumatic heart disease is a minor Jones criterion. Such a history strongly suggests the possibility of a recurrence in a patient presenting with compatible symptomatology, that is, any of the five major criteria. It also requires a careful search for residual and often occult valvular heart disease such as mitral stenosis, mitral regurgitation, or aortic insufficiency.

Antibiotic prophylaxis against streptococcal infection must be restarted or continued in any patient with previous rheumatic carditis. A history of isolated Sydenham's chorea (perhaps also subcutaneous nodules) also requires prophylaxis since 20% of patients presenting with only chorea will later develop cardiac sequelae. A debate centers around those cases without initial carditis. Certainly, patients in high-exposure ages and environments require prophylaxis. Some physicians recommend that prophylaxis be continued for life despite the lower risk of recurrence and subsequent carditis.

Antibiotic prophylaxis against bacterial endocarditis is required for patients with rheumatic heart disease. This should be instituted for any of the following procedures: dental extractions or cleaning; major or minor surgery; instrumentation such as bronchoscopy, cystoscopy, or endoscopy of the gastrointestinal tract; labor and delivery.

Selected References

1. Jones Criteria (Revised) for Guidance in the Diagnosis of Rheumatic Fever, Council on Rheumatic Fever and Congenital Heart Disease of the American Heart Association, in Schaffer A (ed): *Major Problems of Clinical Pediatrics,* ed 2. Philadelphia, WB Saunders, 1972, vol 2, pp 247–255.
2. Markowitz M, Gordis L: Rheumatic Fever, ed 2. Philadelphia, WB Saunders, 1972, vol 2.
3. Hollander JL, McCarty DJ: *Arthritis and Allied Conditions.* Philadelphia, Lea and Febiger, 1972, pp 736–820.

57. Past Heart Disease

MARK E. SILVERMAN, MD

Definition

The presence or absence of symptoms or other historical evidence of heart disease.

Technique

A thorough search for current or previous heart disease is accomplished by directing questions that explore the following four general areas:

1. Historical evidence of cardiovascular disease: Have you had an illness or problem of any sort related to your heart or blood vessels? Have you ever been told that you have an enlarged heart? a rheumatic heart? a heart murmur or leaky valve? a heart attack or coronary? heart failure or congestion? a blood clot in your lung? poor circulation? stroke? pericarditis? Have you ever been rejected from the armed services? failed an examination for insurance or athletics? had a high rating on an insurance examination? had an abnormal electrocardiogram, Master's exercise stress test, or coronary arteriograms? Have you ever taken digitalis, heart pills, water pills, pills to lower your blood pressure or cholesterol, pills you put under your tongue, blood thinners, or paste on your arms?

2. Symptoms that may suggest the presence of heart disease: Have you experienced chest discomfort or pain? shortness of breath on exertion? shortness of breath when recumbent? swelling of your ankles? dizziness or passing out spells? palpitations, skipped beats, or rapid heart beat? significant unexplained fatigue? coughing at night? coughing up blood? cramps in your calves, thighs, or hips that occur while walking and are relieved by rest? Do you have to sleep on more than one pillow to breathe comfortably at night? Do you arise several times during the night to urinate? Do you have tender or swollen calves? varicose veins?

3. Information that suggests a disease known to involve the cardiovascular system: Complexes of disease-specific questions are asked to probe for diseases that are known to cause cardiovascular disease (these subjects are treated in their respective sections). The following diseases are listed as etiologies for cardiovascular disease by the New York Heart Association Committee on Nomenclature and Criteria for Diagnosis of Diseases of the Heart and Great Vessels:

Acromegaly	Hypertension	Pulmonary disease
Alcoholism	Hyperthyroidism	(cor pulmonale)
Amyloidosis	Hypothyroidism	Reiter's syndrome
Anemia	Infection	Rheumatic fever
Ankylosing spondy-	Marfan's syndrome	Rheumatoid ar-
litis	Mucopolysac-	thritis
Atherosclerosis	charidoses	Sarcoidosis
Carcinoid tumor	Neoplasm	Syphilis
(argentaffinoma)	Obesity	Systemic arterio-
Congenital anomaly	Polyarteritis	venous fistula
Friedreich's ataxia	nodosa	Systemic lupus
Glycogen storage	Progressive mus-	erythematosus
disease	cular dystrophy	Toxic agent
Hemochromatosis	Progressive sys-	Trauma
Hypersensitivity	temic sclerosis	Unknown
reaction	(scleroderma)	Uremia

4. Questions on the following are directed toward discovery of associated coronary risk factors: age, sex, race, smoking habits, hypertension, hypercholesterolemia, diabetes, obesity, inactivity, stress, personality, abnormal electrocardiogram, and abnormal exercise test.

Background Information

For the basic science information relative to specific cardiovascular symptoms, refer to the cardiovascular history sections (sections 47–55).

Clinical Significance

The diagnosis of heart disease is accompanied by significant emotional, economic, and prognostic consequences. The patient may be so frightened that symptoms and other important information are unconsciously submerged, made light of, or altered to suggest other faulty organs. The clinician must attempt to recognize patient denial and gently probe for the details that may lead to a correct diagnosis. Common examples of this include shortness of breath attributed to smoking, chest or epigastric discomfort interpreted as indigestion, or dizziness ascribed to rising too quickly. It is often helpful to ask what the patient thinks is the cause of the symptom. Asking directly about chest pain may elicit a misleading response. Patients will often vehemently deny chest pain, interpreting their discomfort as indigestion, an unpleasant ache, or a fullness rather than pain. On the other hand, some patients develop symptoms related to the chest because of a fear of a heart attack. In many cases this is because of a recent illness or death of a friend or relative. The patient may not mention this until the clinician specifically asks if a friend or relative has had a heart attack. Even a history of a heart attack should be subjected to careful scrutiny since this term may be used by the patient to mean heart failure, angina pectoris, an arrhythmia, or severe chest pain of some other etiology.

The history of a heart murmur can be deceiving. The wary clinician must inspect the information with great caution. A childhood innocent murmur, the noisy heart of pregnancy, anemia, tachycardia or thyrotoxicosis, and the cacophony of a normal venous hum may easily fox a naive or untutored stethoscopist. In many instances an innocent murmur or the murmur of congenital heart disease is mistakenly interpreted as rheumatic heart disease and a history of sore throat, arthralgias, or growing pains promoted to a diagnosis of acute rheumatic fever by the physician. The diagnosis of rheumatic fever is then permanently embedded in the memory of the patient or parent.

The symptoms that suggest heart disease must also be approached with caution. For example, the symptom of orthopnea suggests pulmonary congestion due to left ventricular failure. Many patients without heart disease, however, choose to sleep on several pillows. Patients with emphysema may also elevate their heads at night. The symptom of palpitation may mean an arrhythmia to the clinician but merely a forceful or rapid heart beat to the patient. Swelling of the ankles, tender calves, dizzy spells, and easy fatigability are other symptoms that must be interpreted in the context of the entire history and the physical examination.

Selected References

1.   Hurst JW: Symptoms due to diseases of the heart and blood vessels, in Hurst JW (ed in chief), Logue RB, Schlant RC, Wenger NK (eds): *The Heart*, ed 4. New York, McGraw-Hill, 1978, chap 13.
2.   Silverman ME: *Examination of the Heart, Part 1: The Clinical History*, American Heart Association Booklet, 1978.
3.   *Nomenclature and Criteria for Diagnosis of Diseases of the Heart and Great Vessels*, ed 7. The Criteria Committee of the New York Heart Association. Boston, Little, Brown, 1973.

58.   Family History of Heart Disease

MARK E. SILVERMAN, MD

Definition

The presence of cardiovascular disease or genetically determined disorders in the family that may affect the cardiovascular system of the patient or his descendants.

Technique

The clinician could superficially explore the family history with the simple question: Does anybody in your family have heart disease? This approach, although time-saving, will likely net only gross descriptions of heart disease such as, "My father had some kind of heart trouble." Important, but often subtle genetic influences will remain undetected. The following approach provides a more detailed pedigree that applies to all possible inherited illnesses. The patient (known as the proband, propositus, or index case) is asked to list all family members, living and dead, beginning with the oldest child and proceeding through each of the children, brothers, sisters, parents, uncles, aunts, and grandparents. Parental consanguinity (parents who are blood relatives) should be elicited since this will significantly increase the possibility of a rare, recessively inherited disease. The name, age, sex, location, state of health, and occurrence of congenital defects or significant illnesses should be obtained. The race, religious, and ethnic background and the occurrence of abortions, stillbirths, miscarriages, and early death are important.

The cardiovascular family history should search for three specific items: heart disease, heart murmur, or sudden death. The questions may have to be phrased in several ways utilizing slang expressions such as dropsy, congested lungs, hole in the heart, rheumatic heart, hardening of the arteries, coronary. The patient should be asked if any blood relatives had a similar problem or disease.

A family history of birth defects, mental or physical retardation, or unusual stature become particularly important if the patient has suspected congenital heart disease. The possibility of maternal rubella, drugs, or other possible teratogenic influences such as alcohol and viral infections should be considered. Genetically determined disorders vary in their expression and clinical manifestations such that examination of other family members may be required. Other family members may also provide more detailed knowledge about the family ancestors and relatives.

Background Information

An analysis by Nora and Nora (reference 5) of a large number of patients with congenital heart disease showed that about 8% of the patients had heart defects primarily related to genetic factors, 2% were environmental in origin, and 90% were multifactorial. The environmental catalysts could be drugs, viruses, maternal nutrition, maternal metabolism or fetal hemodynamics. Specific cardiovascular teratogens include drugs such as alcohol (VSD, PDA, ASD), amphetamines (VSD, PDA, ASD, TGA), the anticonvulsants hydantoin (PS, AS, PDA, coarctation of aorta) and trimethadione (TGA, tetralogy, hypoplastic left heart), lithium (Ebstein anomaly, tricuspid atresia, ASD), sex hormones (VSD, TGA, tetralogy), thalidomide (tetralogy, VSD, ASD, truncus), and disease states such as rubella (peripheral pulmonary artery stenosis, PDA, VSD, ASD), diabetes (TGA, VSD, coarctation of aorta), lupus erythematosus (heart block), and phenylketonuria (tetralogy, VSD, ASD). The multifactorial group is thought to consist of patients with a genetic predisposition to cardiovascular disease due to small, additive effects of many genes (polygenic) and an environmental trigger that produces a cardiovascular malformation. The Noras conclude that "the production of an anomaly by a teratogen requires certain conditions including: genetic predisposition to maldevelopment, genetic predisposition to react adversely to the teratogen, and exposure to the teratogen at the vulnerable period of embryonic development."

This study and others have noted that the recurrence risk for cardiovascular disease in families increases twofold to threefold where there are two affected family members, particularly when the two affected first-degree relatives are parent and child or when the index case is severely affected. The more common the prevalence of the defect in the general population, the more likely it is to recur in first-degree relatives. A history of parental consanguinity is especially important since second cousins have a 1 in 32 chance of sharing a particular gene while third cousins have a 1 in 128 likelihood.

Once the family history establishes a disorder that is inherited through Mendelian patterns, then the likelihood that the patient is similarly affected can be established. This is discussed in section 111, Family Pedigree and Heritable Disease Potential.

Clinical Significance

Inherited cardiovascular diseases may involve only the cardiovascular system or be a component of a more extensive genetic disorder such as Down's syndrome. The possibility of a genetically determined disease may be immediately apparent, as in the Ellis-Van Creveld syndrome, or be only an indirect, poorly understood influence, as in coronary atherosclerosis. Some forms of heart disease, such as mitral valve prolapse or atrial septal defect, may be genetically determined in some patients but not in others. The importance of a family history is emphasized by the number and variety of problems that can be transmitted by Mendelian inheritance, multifactorial influences, or chromosomal abnormalities. An extensive although incomplete list would include genetic diseases associated with an abnormal electrocardiogram or arrhythmia, diseases affecting the myocardium, diseases affecting the pericardium, diseases affecting the valves and septae, and diseases affecting the vascular system generally. The number following the disease refers to the listing in reference 4 where a brief description of the problem and several additional references can be located.

Genetic diseases associated with an
abnormal electrocardiogram or arrhythmia

Adrenogenital syndrome (AR-20170)
Conduction defects (AD-11390, 11508)

Friedreich's ataxia (AR-22930)
Leopard (AD-15110)
Mitral valve prolapse (AD-15770)
Muscular dystrophy (X-31020)
Myotonic dystrophy (AD-16090)
Ocular myopathy (AD-16510)
Periodic paralysis (AD-17040)
Prolonged Q-T interval (AD-22040)
Refsum's disease (AR-26650)
Wolff-Parkinson-White (AD-19420)

Genetic diseases that affect the myocardium

Amyloidosis (AD-10500)
Cardiomyopathy (AD-19260)
Friedreich's ataxia (AR-22930)
Glycogen storage disease (AR-23230)
Hemochromatosis (AD-14160)
Leopard (AD-15110)
Muscular dystrophy (X-31020)
Noonan's syndrome (AD-16395)
Refsum's disease (AR-26650)
Sickle cell (AD-14170)
Thalassemia major (AR-27350)
Tuberous sclerosis (19110)

Genetic diseases affecting the pericardium

Mulibrey nanism (AR-25325)

Genetic diseases affecting valves or septa

Alcaptonuria (AR-20350)
Aortic stenosis, supravalvular (AD-18550)
Apert (AD-10120)
Atrial septal defect (AD-108880, AR-20940)
Carpenter (AR-20100)
Chondrodysplasia punctata (AR-21510)
Chromosomal aberrations
  Trisomy 8 mosaic
  Trisomy 9 mosaic
  Trisomy 13
  Trisomy 18
  Trisomy 21
  Trisomy 22
  Trisomy 22, partial

4 p—
5 p—
13 q—
+14 q—
18 q—
Ebstein anomaly (AR-22470)
Ehlers-Danlos (AD-13000)
Ellis-Van Creveld syndrome (AR-22550)
Fanconi pancytopenia (AR-22765)
Forney (AD-not listed)
Holt-Oram syndrome (AD-14290)
Laurence-Moon-Biedl-Bardet syndrome (AR-24580)
Leopard (AD-15110)
Marfan's syndrome (AD-15470)
Mitral valve prolapse (AD-15770)
Mucopolysaccharidosis (AR-25280)
Noonan's syndrome (AD-16395)
Osteogenesis imperfecta (AD-16620)
Patent ductus arteriosus (AD-16910)
Pseudoxanthoma elasticum (AR & AD-17860)
Pulmonic stenosis (AR-26550)
Smith-Lemli-Opitz (AR-27040)
Thrombocytopenia—absent radius (AR-27400)
Treacher Collins (AD-15440)
Weill-Marchesani (AR-27760)
Zellweger (AR-21410)

Genetic diseases that affect the vascular system

Anomalous pulmonary venous return (AD-10670)
Apert (AD-10120)
Arterial tortuosity (AR-20805)
Coarctation of the aorta (AD-12000)
Coronary atherosclerosis (U)
Crouzon (AD-12350)
Cutis laxis (AD-12370 & AR-21910)
Diabetes mellitus (U)
Ehlers-Danlos (AD-13000)
Erdheim cystic medial necrosis (AD-13290)
Fabry's disease (X-30150)
Hemorrhagic telangiectasia (AD-18730)
Homocystinuria (AR-23620)
Hyperlipidemia (AD-14425)
Hypertension, essential (U-14550)
Hypotension, orthostatic (AD-14650)

Mucopolysaccharidosis (AR-25280)
Marfan's syndrome (AD-15470)
Neurofibromatosis (AD-16220)
Osteogenesis imperfecta (AD-16620)
Progeria (AR-26410)
Pseudoxanthoma elasticum (AR & AD-17785)
Pulmonary hypertension, primary (AD-17860)
Turner's syndrome (C)
Varicose veins (AD-19220)
Werner's syndrome (AR-27770)
XXXXY (C)

Abbreviations

AS = aortic stenosis
ASD = atrial septal defect
PDA = patent ductus arteriosus
PS = pulmonic stenosis
Tetralogy = tetralogy of Fallot
TGA = transposition of the great arteries
Truncus = truncus arteriosus
VSD = ventricular septal defect
AD = autosomal dominant
AR = autosomal recessive
X = sex linked
C = chromosomal
U = uncertain

Selected References

1.   Fraser FC: Taking the family history. *Am J Med* 34:585–593, 1963.
2.   Goodman RM: The family pedigree and genetic counseling, in Goodman RM (ed): *Genetic Disorders of Man.* Boston, Little, Brown, 1970, pp 87–104.
3.   Goodman RM, Gorlin RJ: *Atlas of the Face in Genetic Disorders,* ed 2. St. Louis, CV Mosby, 1977, pp 48–63.
4.   McKusick VA: *Mendelian Inheritance in Man: Catalogs of Autosomal Dominant, Autosomal Recessive and X-linked Phenotypes,* ed 4. Baltimore, Johns Hopkins Press, 1975.
5.   Nora JJ, Nora AH: The evolution of specific genetic and environmental counseling in congenital heart diseases. *Circulation* 57:205–213, 1978.
6.   Rowley PT: Genetics for the cardiologist. *Mod Concepts Cardiovas Dis* 47:63–70, 1978.

59. Urinary Frequency, Urgency, and Dysuria

KENNETH N. WALTON, MD
DAVID P. O'BRIEN, MD

Definition

Urinary frequency: abnormally frequent voiding of urine throughout the day.

Urinary urgency: the immediate desire or need to urinate.

Dysuria: usually signifies painful urination, although the derivation of the word "dysuria" implies an altered urination.

Technique

A time-voiding record of the frequency and volume of urination documents the patient's voiding pattern. An adult usually voids approximately 250–500 cc every 3–5 hours while awake. Patients voiding 500 cc every 2 hours may not complain of frequency if their bladder reservoir is larger than normal; similarly, a 2-hour period between voiding may not be impressive to the patient, yet large urine volumes may accrue over a 24-hour period. When urination persists through the night hours (nocturia), an abnormality is likely. Thus, increased urine production may cause frequency, but this frequency may be masked by a large bladder capacity. Urine volumes and voiding times together provide more meaningful information than either alone.

Ask the patient: Are you having any difficulty urinating? The patient may simply state that he has a tremendous urge to urinate immediately or that he will "lose urine" or void incontinently. The examiner should determine the frequency of urgency. Does it occur with every urination or rarely? Does the urgency occur without voiding? Is it associated with frequency, dysuria, or incontinence?

The patient generally describes painful urination as a burning feeling. In the male the painful sensation is usually most acute in the region of the glans penis even though the inflammation may be in the prostatic urethra. Prostatic urethral pain is commonly referred to the glans. Ask the patient about any associated perineal, retropubic, or suprapubic pain such as with prostatitis or cystitis.

In the female the complaint may be that the pain is in her bladder or vaginal area. Always ask about vaginal discharge or itching since vulvovaginitis may also cause dysuria, especially when the ammonia content of the urine is high. Dysuria in women may thus occur without urinary tract disease. Urine cultures obtained by catheterization or suprapubic tap may be necessary to establish or rule out true urinary infection when severe vulvovaginitis is present. A clean-catch urinalysis is otherwise a good screening test.

Background Information

Urinary frequency may be caused by a variety of factors occurring singly or in combination. Frequency may be caused by increased urine formation, diminished bladder capacity, incomplete bladder emptying or bladder irritability.

The osmotic diuresis associated with glycosuria is a classic example of increased urine formation. Nephrogenic or pituitary diabetes insipidus or the diminished concentrating ability of many renal parenchymal diseases may produce frequency. Orally administered diuretics, compulsive water drinking, or mobilization or edema fluid may also cause increased urine formation.

A diminished bladder capacity (ie, less than 200 cc) may be caused by chronic infection, operative procedures, neuropathic disorders (spastic bladder as with spinal trauma or multiple sclerosis), or a thickened inelastic bladder wall (as with chronic obstruction or radiation fibrosis).

A common cause of frequency in the absence of infection is bladder outlet obstruction. The elderly male with prostatic enlargement may have a bladder capacity of 400 cc but void 100 cc frequently while retaining the remaining 300 cc. Neuropathic disorders may produce large hypotonic bladders as well as spastic bladders. This occurs most notably in the visceral neuropathy of diabetes and in diseases of the sacral spinal cord or its roots.

An inflamed bladder or posterior urethra is sensitive to stretch and produces an urge to urinate despite small bladder volumes. Urgency and dysuria will commonly accompany this form of frequency and the bladder will often empty with each voiding.

The urge to empty the urinary bladder normally develops between the ages of 3 and 6 years. The normal urge to urinate occurs when the bladder approaches maximum capacity, that is, 250–600 cc in adults. Adults can volitionally empty a partially filled bladder, but such total control does not become manifest until adolescence. The urge to urinate is monitored in the bladder and posterior urethra by stretch receptors which are stimulated when the bladder capacity is near maximum volume. Abnormal sensitivity of these receptors can be secondary to inflammatory or neuropathic processes.

Incontinence preceded by a strong desire to urinate should be distinguished from other forms of incontinence. Incontinence without the patient's knowledge or prior to reaching the bathroom suggests a neuropathic process.

Dysuria develops in cases of inflammation of the lower urinary tract whether the etiology is bacterial, mechanical, chemical, or foreign body. Mechanical trauma may occur in conjunction with sexual intercourse. Chemical trauma may occur with various irritants such as bubble bath soaps. Foreign body trauma includes bladder stones and urethral catheters. In women the region of the trigone is the most sensitive area of the bladder. It is commonly inflamed as part of an ascending infection. Frequency, urgency, suprapubic, or retropubic pain are associated features. Cystitis is uncommon in males. Isolated urethritis in the male does not produce symptoms of bladder irritability.

Clinical Significance

The multiple causes of urinary frequency clearly indicate the importance of determining associated symptoms. Urine volumes, urine specific gravity, associated diseases, and current medications must all be documented. A residual urine in excess of 50 cc will usually be found where incomplete emptying is the cause of frequency. The residual volume is usually normal or low with bladder infections. The bladder capacity may be estimated in two ways: by catheterizing the patient or by obtaining a postvoid film during excretory urography. A cystogram will outline the shape of the bladder.

Urinary urgency is a symptom of bladder irritability and most commonly occurs in association with urinary infection. However, the other stigmata of infection should also be present. These include frequency, dysuria, pyuria, bacteriuria, and occasionally fever. In the absence of these signs and symptoms, neuropathic processes involving the bladder should be considered. Prostatic and urethral inflammations may cause urinary urgency without bacteriuria or significant pyuria. Physical examination of the urethra and prostate is thus in order. Bladder outlet obstruction and neuropathic disorders must be ruled out in the absence of an inflammatory process. Other entities that may lead to urinary urgency include foreign bodies, bladder tumors, trauma, and any inflammatory process or space-occupying lesion near the bladder.

Suprapubic, perineal, or retropubic pain may be associated with cystitis and all are likely to be associated with frequency and urgency. Cystitis is very common in women. Extreme urgency and severe dysuria are prominent symptoms. Fever is generally absent. Congestive prostatitis usually has only mild urinary symptoms and the urine culture is commonly negative. There is disagreement about the role bacteria play in this disease. Isolated urethritis in the male produces urethral pain only and produces a urethral discharge since the inflammation is distal to the external sphincter. In contrast, acute bacterial prostatitis is an uncommon condition marked by high fever, chills, dysuria, and occasionally urinary retention. Urethral instrumentation and rectal examinations may result in bacteremic episodes and should be avoided in acute febrile prostatitis.

Selected References

1. Greenfield S, Friedland G, Scifers S, et al: Protocol management of dysuria, urinary frequency, and vaginal discharge. *Ann Intern Med* 81:452–457, 1974.
2. Waters WE, Elwood PC, Asscher AW, et al: Clinical significance of dysuria in women. *Br Med J* 2:754–757, 1970.
3. Brooks D, Maudar A: Pathogenesis of the urethral syndrome in women and its diagnosis in general practice. *Lancet* 2:893–898, 1972.
4. Steensberg J, Bartels ED, Bay-Nielson H, et al: Epidemiology of urinary tract diseases in general practice. *Br Med J* 4:390–394, 1969.

60. Urinary Tract Infection

SUSAN K. FELLNER, MD

Definition

Upper urinary tract infection: infections with bacteria, yeast, or fungi above the ureteropelvic junction. Lower urinary tract infection: infections below this junction. The presence of infection must be documented with cultures.

Technique

Occasionally, bacteriuria is asymptomatic. Generally, however, patients describe dysuria, urgency, and frequency. They may have cloudy urine or hematuria. Fever, flank pain, nausea, and vomiting usually point to upper urinary tract infection. Ask the patient if the symptoms have been recurrent. A history of recent onset of sexual intercourse or of pregnancy is sought in women. Symptoms of prostatism or urethral stricture are sought in men. In both sexes look for evidence of stone disease, neurogenic bladder, and pelvic or retroperitoneal tumor or fibrosis.

Obtain carefully collected clean-catch urine for culture and urinalysis. Infection is documented by culture. The presence of casts containing white cells or organisms signifies renal parenchymal infection.

Background Information

In adults, urinary tract infection (UTI) is more common in women because of an anatomically short urethra. Fecal and perineal organisms may gain entry to the bladder, particularly during sexual intercourse. In older age, men become susceptible to UTIs when prostatic hypertrophy impairs bladder emptying. Bacterial growth in the urine is also facilitated by high osmolality, elevated pH and glucosuria. Factors which predispose to UTI include obstruction, calculi, vesicoureteral reflux, in-dwelling bladder catheters, urologic manipulation, neurologic disease of the bladder (spinal cord injury, multiple sclerosis, diabetic neuropathy) and pregnancy. The majority of upper urinary tract infections evolve from ascending coliform organism contamination of bladder urine. *Staphylococcus aureus* infections of the kidney are usually of hematogenous origin.

Clinical Significance

Asymptomatic bacteriuria, recurrent cystitis, UTI during pregnancy, and an isolated episode of acute pyelonephritis do not require extensive urologic evaluation in women. Cultures at the time of recognition and after therapy will show whether the infection has been irradicated. Subsequent bacteriuria with the same or different organisms may represent relapse or reinfection.

Any man with UTI or any woman with recurrent pyelonephritis should have a radiographic and urologic evaluation to exclude the following etiologies:

Acquired obstruction

Stones
Retroperitoneal fibrosis
Tuberculosis
Urethral stricture
Irradiation induced strictures
Neurogenic bladder

Congenital obstruction

Ureteropelvic junction narrowing
Ureteroceles
Bladder neck obstruction
Artery compressing ureter

Tumors

Prostatic cancer
Benign prostatic hypertrophy
Retroperitoneal lymphoma or metastatic cancer
Pelvic tumors

Selected Reference

1. Brenner B, Rector F (eds): *The Kidney.* Philadelphia, WB Saunders, 1973, pp 796–797, 1079–1104, 1299, 1900–1909.

61. Flank Pain

KENNETH N. WALTON, MD

Definition

Pain in the costovertebral angle. The area is bound medially by the paraspinous muscle and superiorly by the twelfth rib. The quadratus lumborum muscle is between the examiner's hand and the kidney.

Technique

The pain is often associated with tenderness and overlying muscle spasm. Examination by percussing over the rib cage, iliac crest, and contralateral angle should precede gentle percussion over the affected side.

The history should determine whether there is associated fever, or whether there are symptoms suggestive of renal colic. The latter include nausea, pain referred to the genital area, and episodes of severe flank pain.

A history of pain in the flank should be distinguished from similar pains produced by lumbosacral strain or herniated disk (usually lower and more midline) and chest conditions such as pneumonia, pulmonary embolus or rib fracture (usually higher and often pleuritic).

Background Information

In acute renal inflammation the renal capsule is distended, and there are perinephritis and regional peritonitis of the overlying posterior parietal peritoneum. These cause or contribute to the sensation of flank pain.

Acute ureteral obstruction causes capsular distention and flank pain. There is associated colic with nausea, vomiting, diaphoresis, pallor, and pain referred to the testis or labium.

Acute renal infarction may present with acute flank pain without fever or pyuria. Suspect renal infarction when flank pain occurs in patients with atrial fibrillation, recent myocardial infarction, or past renal artery bypass grafts.

Abdominal problems such as acute cholecystitis, pancreatitis, pancreatic pseudocyst, retrocecal appendicitis, or leaking abdominal aneurysm may simulate renal pain in that the pain may be referred to the back. Pulmonary infarction, pneumonia, or lower rib fractures may also masquerade as flank pain. Urinalysis and radiographic studies aid greatly in the differential diagnosis.

Clinical Significance

Acute renal infection requires immediate treatment. Such treatment is not adequate in the face of obstruction. Urography must be done where obstruction is suspected on the basis of the character of the pain, chills, septic shock, hematuria, or associated conditions such as established lower urinary tract disease.

Acute renal colic is usually dramatically painful. Nausea accompanies the waves of severe pain. There is microscopic hematuria. Treatment may be surgical or symptomatic, as when the clinician anticipates that the stone will pass spontaneously.

It is a serious error to miss the presence of an obstruction in an infected patient. The combination of renal obstruction and infection is an emergency situation since septicemia is a complication.

Selected References

1.   Waters WE: Prevalence of symptoms of urinary tract infection in women. *Br J Prev Soc Med* 23:263–266, 1969.
2.   Fairley KF, Carson NE, Gutch RC, et al: Site of infection in acute urinary tract infection in general practice. *Lancet* 2:615–618, 1971.
3.   Finlayson B: Renal lithiasis in review. *Urol Clin N Am* 1:181–212, 1974.

---

62. Nocturia

SUSAN K. FELLNER, MD

Definition

Urination, usually more than once, during usual sleeping hours.

Technique

Ask the patient if he arises from sleep to urinate or "pass water," and if so how many times and how much, ie, a few drops or a few cupfuls. Determine whether the patient then drinks a glass of water and whether it is because of thirst or from habit. Does the patient ordinarily drink tea, coffee, or other beverages in the evening? If not previously elicited, a history of stones, recurrent urinary tract infections, or pelvic surgery may be sought at this point.

Background Information

The ability to elaborate a small volume of concentrated urine during sleeping hours depends on a reduced solute and volume load to the kidneys, adequate release of vasopressin (antidiuretic hormone, ADH), and an anatomically intact countercurrent system in the renal medulla. Derangements in any of these will limit the ability to concentrate the urine and the patient may need to void during the usual 6–9 hours of sleep. Reduction in bladder capacity (from surgery or tumor) or obstruction of the bladder neck (prostatic hypertrophy) also may result in nocturia despite normal pituitary, adrenal, and renal function. Finally, patients with a variety of edema states (reduced cardiac output, hypoalbuminemia) often have a nighttime diuresis because of improved venous return to the heart in the supine posture.

Clinical Significance

Since nocturia may be a symptom of disease anywhere from the pituitary to the penis, it is important to separate disorders of urinary concentration from those structural and physiologic states associated with nighttime urination. Table 10, a chart of data from the history and physical examination, will assist in the differential diagnosis.

Table 10. Differential diagnosis of nocturia according to history and physical examination features.

| Disorder | Nocturia | Thirst | Urinary Volume | | Daytime Frequency | Edema |
			Day	Night		
Psychogenic water drinking	+	−	↑	↑	+	−
Diabetes insipidus	+	+	↑	↑	+	−
Obstructive uropathy	+	+	variable		+	−
Chronic interstitial nephritis	+	−	variable		+	−
Decreased bladder capacity	+	−	↓	↓	+	−
Congestive heart failure	+	±	↓	↑	−	+
Nephrotic syndrome	+	±	↓	↑	−	+

Selected References

1. Kleeman CR: Water metabolism, in *Clinical Disorders of Fluid and Electrolyte Metabolism*. New York, McGraw-Hill, 1972, pp 215–295.
2. Harrington JT, Cohen JJ: Clinical disorders of urine concentration and dilution. *Arch Intern Med* 131:810–825, 1973.

63. Hematuria

KENNETH N. WALTON, MD

Definition

Hematuria: blood in the urine, gross or microscopic. Total hematuria: uniformly bloody urine throughout voiding. Initial hematuria: occurs at the beginning of urination. Terminal hematuria: occurs at the end of urination.

Technique

The history of hematuria should carefully document the setting in which the hematuria occurred. Associated symptoms such as severe colicky unilateral flank and inguinal or radiating testicular pain suggest stones; urgency, dysuria, and frequency may indicate hemorrhagic cystitis; weight loss may offer a clue to hypernephroma; abuse of aspirin or phenacetin may suggest papillary necrosis due to analgesic nephropathy; repetitive flank trauma (football players, boxers) may suggest a perinephric hematoma; associated proteinuria and repetitive throat infections may signal glomerulonephritis; and episodic hematuria only during viral upper respiratory infections suggests IgA nephropathy. In addition to ascertaining these etiologic clues, always determine if the hematuria is total, initial, or terminal.

Obtain a voided urine. Observe the urine grossly and examine it under the microscope to be sure any red discoloration is due to red cells, since red urine can also result from excessive beet ingestion (beeturia), coproporphrinuria in porphyria, or drugs such as phenazopyridine (Pyridium) (deep orange). With grossly bloody urine it is not necessary to centrifuge the specimen. If the specimen is not obtained under supervision, spurious conclusions may be drawn. In female patients the blood may be menstrual. In uncircumcised males a lesion under the foreskin may be bleeding. Occasionally a patient may introduce blood into the urine specimen by pricking a finger or adding a few drops from another patient's blood sample tube. Factitious hematuria may occasionally be detected by ABO typing of the urine red cells.

Microscopic hematuria may be evaluated by the two-glass or (in men) three-glass urinalysis. The two-glass urinalysis evaluates initial and midstream samples, while the three-glass urinalysis includes a third sample collected after prostatic massage.

Background Information

As determined by Addis, normal persons excrete red cells in the urine. However, the average adult value of 600,000 red blood cells per 12 hours does not discolor the urine, is not detected by dipstick tests, and amounts to none or only occasional red blood cells per microscopic high-power field (rbc/hpf) after dilution in a large volume of urine. A history of visible hematuria is thus clearly abnormal.

Painless hematuria is more suspect for malignant disease than is painful hematuria. The latter is more typical of benign inflammations, but there is overlap. Gross and microscopic (even persistent 5–10 rbc/hpf) hematuria must be evaluated thoroughly since significant disease is generally found. One proceeds logically to discover where the bleeding is coming from and then what the pathology is at that site. If the hematuria is equal in all three glasses, it means that the urine in the reservoir (bladder) is bloody. The bleeding is commonly from somewhere above the bladder neck, although it may be prostatic with bleeding back into the bladder. Thus bleeding could be renal, ureteral, or vesical in origin.

If the hematuria is prominent in glass one and glass three in the male, the source is likely prostatic. If the hematuria is prominent only in glass one, then the source is some portion of the urethra other than the prostatic segment. Terminal hematuria (glass three) signifies a bladder or occasionally prostatic source. Painless terminal hematuria is presumed to signify a bladder tumor until proven otherwise.

Clinical Significance

Although some patients with glomerulonephritis have gross hematuria (episodic in IgA nephropathy and occasional in acute poststreptococcal glomerulonephritis), microscopic hematuria is more commonly present. Clinical indicators that the hematuria is due to glomerular disease include hypertension, heavy proteinuria, and multiple granular or any red cell casts in the urinary sediment.

One must always establish the origin of the bleeding. Cystoscopy at the time of gross bleeding will visualize bleeding points in the urethra and bladder and will demonstrate whether any efflux from one or both ureteral orifices is blood tinged. Cytology, biopsies, excretory, and retrograde pyelograms will evaluate the lining of the urinary tract for filling defects, obstruction, and deformity. If the bleeding is renal, tomography and arteriography help to evaluate the parenchyma. Occasionally renal bleeding is idiopathic. Before reaching this conclusion, serially evaluate the patient since idiopathic renal bleeding is a diagnosis of exclusion. If hematuria is renal and bilateral, it may be due to various forms of glomerulonephritis. Sickle cell trait (AS hemoglobin) is a common cause of relatively painless gross hematuria in black patients.

The evaluation of most patients with hematuria is designed to establish or rule out surgically correctable causes. Patients on anticoagulants who bleed from the urinary tract require the same evaluation.

Selected References

1. Addis T: The number of formed elements in the urinary sediment of normal individuals. *J Clin Invest* 2:409–415, 1926.
2. Northway JD: Hematuria in children. *J Ped* 78:381–396, 1971.
3. Holland JM: Cancer of the kidney: Natural history and staging. *Cancer* 32:1030–1042, 1973.
4. Zimmerman SW, Burkholder PM: Immunoglobulin A nephropathy. *Arch Intern Med* 135:1217–1223, 1975.
5. Buckalew VM, Someren A: Renal manifestations of sickle cell disease. *Arch Intern Med* 133:660–669, 1974.

64. Past Stones

JAMES O. WELLS, JR., MD

Definition

Past history of one or more calculi in the kidneys, ureters, or bladder. Some or all of the stones may have been excreted with urine, and they may or may not be present whenever the patient is examined.

Technique

The patient may already be aware of the existence of or the previous passage of stones. Ask: Have you ever passed a kidney stone? Have you ever had an x-ray of your kidneys? Ask if relatives have had stones since some types of stone disease are hereditary.

If there is no known history of stone disease, the patient may recall an episode of the acute and severe pain characteristic of a stone passing down the ureter. This pain is frequently described as an intense, sharp, knifelike flank discomfort that radiates to the inguinal area and, in males, into the scrotum. This pain is known as renal colic. The patient may also recall an episode of gross hematuria accompanying the pain. If a suggestive history is obtained, ask if the patient ever noted the passage of gravel or stones in the urine. A sudden sensation of discomfort may accompany the passage of calculi with the urinary stream. Straining the urine through gauze is helpful in obtaining specimens for analysis.

Examination of the urine in a patient suspected of having stones may be helpful. Hematuria often accompanies active stone disease but may be absent. One may see large quantities of uric acid or the characteristic flat, hexagonal crystals of cystine. An alkaline urine with many bacteria may imply that urea splitting organisms are present; urea splitting bacteria are often found in patients with magnesium-ammonium-phosphate (struvite) stones, and may predispose to their formation.

Background Information

Two to three percent of the adult population will have urinary calculi at some time. In most, the stones will recur. If a stone is found in the urine, it should be saved and submitted for chemical analysis.

Stone formation may occur whenever concentrations of mineral solutes and other constituents of urine become abnormal. For example, calcium and oxalate are much more soluble in the presence of magnesium and citrate. Uric acid and cystine are much more soluble in alkaline urine. Urine volume obviously will effect the concentrations of any solutes; thus patients with stone disease are encouraged to ingest large volumes of fluid. Foreign bodies and spaces in the urinary tract will predispose to stone formation. Crystals serve as a nidus around which other minerals may be deposited.

Uric acid and cystine stones are radiolucent, while stones containing calcium and oxalate are radiopaque. Stone disease may be active, with recurrent or enlarging calculi, or inactive, with no new stones being formed or passed.

Clinical Significance

Hypercalciuria is the most common abnormality in patients who form stones consisting primarily of calcium salts. The high calcium in the urine may be the result of excessive bone resorption (hyperparathyroidism, metastatic tumors); excessive absorption of calcium from the gut (vitamin D intoxication, milk alkali syndrome, high calcium diet); or decreased renal reabsorption of calcium. The most common of these causes of hypercalciuria is hyperparathyroidism, a disease that should be suspected whenever calcium oxalate stones are found. Calcium oxalate stones also occur with hyperoxaluria which may accompany hereditary oxalosis, inflammatory bowel disease, renal tubular acidosis, malabsorption syndromes, or chronic diarrhea. Excessive urinary oxalate excretion may also be associated with hyperglycinuria or with pyridoxine (vitamin B_6) deficiency.

Stones composed primarily of uric acid constitute approximately 5% of renal calculi. In patients with gout, uric acid stones are particularly common if the urinary excretion of uric acid exceeds 1,000 mg per 24 hours. These patients may or may not have hyperuricemia.

Cystine stones result from the rare autosomal recessive disease, cystinuria. Patients with cystinuria have excessive excretion of the dibasic amino acids, ornithine, lysine, arginine, and cystine. Of these dibasic amino acids, only cystine is insoluble and tends to precipitate.

Chronic pyelonephritis predisposes to the formation of $Mg-NH_4-PO_4$ (struvite) stones. These are usually large and wedge themselves within the pelvis of the kidney. They are often first noted on routine abdominal films. The presence of "stag horn" calculi of this type usually implies chronic infection with urea-splitting organisms.

Selected References

1.   Smith LH: Medical evaluation of urolithiasis: Etiologic aspects and diagnostic evaluation. *Urol Clin North Am* 1:241–260, 1974.

2.   Thomas WC Jr: *Renal Calculi: A Guide to Management.* Springfield, Ill, Charles C Thomas, 1976.

3.   Pak CYC: Disorders of stone formation, in Brenner BM, Rector FC Jr (eds): *The Kidney.* Philadelphia, WB Saunders, pp 1326–1354.

4.   Smith LH: Urolithiasis, in Earley LE, Gottschalk CW: *Strauss and Welt's Diseases of the Kidney,* ed 3. Boston, Little, Brown, pp 893–931, 1979.

5.   Coe FL: *Nephrolithiasis: Pathogenesis and Treatment.* Chicago, Year Book Medical Publishers, 1978.

6.   Broadus AE, Thier SO: Metabolic basis of renal-stone disease. *N Engl J Med* 300:839–845, 1979.

65. Urinary Stream Flow Abnormality: Hesitancy, Intermittency, and Incontinence

DAVID P. O'BRIEN, MD

Definition

Urinary flow is defined in terms of the size and force of the patient's stream. The caliber and force of the urinary stream vary greatly. The normal urinary stream should be continuous for at least 80% of urination.

Hesitancy is a delay in initiating urination. Intermittency describes a urinary stream which is not continuous. Incontinence is the involuntary loss of urine.

Technique

Questions regarding the size and force of the urinary stream in female patients are rarely fruitful unless extreme outlet obstruction is present. However, the importance of this question to male patients from infancy through adulthood cannot be understated, and the quality of the history reflects the tenacity and experience of the clinician. The normal caliber and force of the urinary stream varies among individuals, and the examiner should attempt to elicit the history of changes in the urinary stream rather than the specific caliber or force. Begin by asking: Have you had any decrease in the size of your stream? Then pointedly ask the patient or an infant's parent questions easily related to several reference points. For example: Can the infant urinate across the bed? Could you write your name in the snow or on a sidewalk? Are you having to stand closer to the toilet or over the toilet to prevent going on your shoes or on the floor? Is your stream as strong as it was a few years ago? Observe the patient's urinary stream. Accurate documentation of the urinary flow may be obtained by timed voided specimens or by dynamics.

Hesitancy is not usually mentioned by the patient. Ask "Do you have to wait awhile for your stream to start?" This should be distinguished from the "shy bladder" where the patient experiences difficulty voiding in the presence of a nurse, physician, or other person.

Intermittency is evaluated by asking: Once you have started urination, can you pass 80–90% in a continuous stream? This eliminates the questionably significant terminal dribbling experienced by many normal men. Two features are notable if one observes the voiding of a male patient with hesitancy and intermittency: straining is often apparent in initiating and maintaining the stream, and the stream often slows or stops when he takes a breath.

All patients should be asked if they have any difficulty controlling urination or if they have loss of urine at inappropriate times. If the response is positive, a detailed evaluation of the nature of incontinence is necessary. Determine whether incontinence occurs with or without the patient's knowledge; that is, does the patient know he is going to urinate but is unable to get to the bathroom on time, or is incontinence noted only indirectly when the clothes and bed are found to be wet. A history of stress incontinence can be elicited by asking the patient if involuntary urination occurs during coughing, sneezing, straining, or lifting heavy objects. Urgency, or urge incontinence, is suggested when the patient states that he feels a strong desire to urinate and cannot suppress the flow of urine before reaching the toilet. Ask if bedwetting occurs at night (nocturnal incontinence, or enuresis), or occurs both at night and in the daytime. Ask if urine leaks or dribbles all the time, as in total incontinence, or in intermittent small amounts, as in overflow incontinence.

Background Information

The factors controlling the caliber of the urinary stream and the force of urinary flow are primarily mechanical. However, they are secondarily influenced by volitional control. The force or pressure of the flow is initially generated by the bladder with some modification by the patient's use of accessory abdominal muscles. The caliber and force of flow are also influenced by the caliber of the bladder outlet. The bladder outlet refers to the bladder neck, posterior and anterior urethra, and the urethral meatus. Posterior urethral obstructions produce a stream with little force. Distal urethral obstructions, usually strictures, may produce a stream of markedly reduced caliber but normal force. With distal obstructions the stream may be split. Difficulty in initiating and maintaining voiding is found where there is lower urinary obstruction or ineffective bladder contractility, or both.

Stress incontinence usually results from pelvic relaxation or damage to the urinary sphincter. Urge incontinence is usually secondary to inflammatory changes in the urinary stretch receptors. Overflow incontinence occurs when there is minimal emptying of a distended bladder, leaving a high bladder volume and only a short period before the next urination. Total incontinence implies a continual discharge of urine. Enuresis is a form of involuntary nocturnal incontinence.

Clinical Significance

Alterations in the flow characteristics of the urinary stream are usually due to obstruction. This leads to a diminution in both caliber and flow. In infants and children the obstruction may be congenital with posterior urethral valves, congenital bladder neck contracture, urethral meatal stenosis, or phimosis. In adults, obstructions are commonly secondary to urethral stricture disease, prostatic hyperplasia, or carcinoma of the prostate. In females, urethral diverticula and cystoceles may lead to diminution in flow. In both males and females, the flow pattern of the urinary stream may be influenced by bladder neoplasms, urethral diverticula, or neuropathic changes of the bladder.

All forms of incontinence may be secondary to neuropathic disturbances of the bladder. Thorough investigation of each particular form should be carried out. Stress incontinence classically occurs in the multigravida or in the elderly female who has pelvic relaxation with a cystocele or urethrocele, or both. These findings are confirmed by the Valsalva maneuver during pelvic examination. Stress incontinence may also occur in patients who have had previous trauma or surgical procedures near the bladder neck and urine sphincters, thereby weakening the control of retention of urine. As previously stated, urge incontinence is usually seen in conjunction with inflammatory processes of the bladder or posterior urethra. Overflow incontinence may occur in neuropathic disturbances but is more commonly associated with bladder outlet obstruction where the patient has urinary retention and frequently voids very small amounts of urine. Total or true incontinence may occur in patients who have a neuropathic disturbance of the bladder or in whom the urinary sphincters are bypassed by the flow of urine. Examples of the latter would include patients who have vesicovaginal or urethrovaginal fistulas, and patients with ectopic ureters that empty into the vagina or urethra at a point distal to the urinary sphincters. Enuresis may be a symptom of outflow obstruction and is often difficult, in the adult, to distinguish from overflow incontinence. Classic enuresis occurs in children and is present from birth. The exact dynamics of enuresis are unknown, but rarely does investigation need to be undertaken in patients before the age of 5 or 6. Beyond the age of 6, total control of urination is present in 95% of children. Thorough neurologic examinations and urinary tract x-rays should be obtained in adult patients with enuresis because of the high prevalence of associated genitourinary pathology.

Selected References

1. Griffiths DJ: The mechanics of the urethra and of micturition. *Br J Urol* 45:497–507, 1973.
2. Zacharin RF: *Stress Incontinence of Urine.* New York, Harper and Row, 1972.
3. Issacs JH: Stress incontinence: A plan for systematic evaluation. *Postgrad Med* 54:102–105, 1973.
4. Arnold EP, Webster JR, Loose H, et al: Urodynamics of female incontinence: Factors influencing the results of surgery. *Am J Obstet Gynecol* 117:805–813, 1973.
5. Mahoney DT: Studies of enuresis: V. Classification of enuresis and the juvenile urethral incontinence syndrome. *Urology* 1:315–316, 1973.
6. Forsythe WI, Redmond A: Enuresis and spontaneous cure rate: Study of 1,129 enuretics. *Arch Dis Child* 49:259–263, 1974.

66. Urethral Discharge

NORMAN F. JACOBS, JR., MD

Definition

A urethral discharge consists of any fluid excreted through the urethral meatus except during voiding or ejaculation.

Technique

Ask the patient if stains are present on the underclothes. If so, what color are they? Male patients may notice a discharge only in the morning prior to first voiding. Female patients will usually complain of vaginal rather than urethral discharge (see section 74 on Vaginal Discharge). Ask both men and women about urinary frequency, urgency, and dysuria. If the patient gives a history of urethral discharge, try to determine if there have been any trauma, insertion of foreign bodies into the urethra, or use of chemicals (douches and deodorants). Is the patient sexually active? Is there a history of exposure to a venereal disease?

To examine men for urethral discharge, first observe for the presence of spontaneous discharge. If none is seen, have the patient gently compress the urethra at the proximal end of the penis with his fingers, and then gently strip the urethra distally. To obtain a smear for Gram stain and culture, have the patient open the meatus while you insert a swab at least 1 cm into the meatus. The swab should immediately be rolled on a glass slide for the Gram stain and then inoculated onto chocolate agar for culture. The smear and culture may show *Neisseria gonorrhoeae* even in the absence of observable discharge.

Examine women for urethral discharge and urethrocele during the pelvic examination. Gently compress the urethra against the pubic symphysis and strip it distally. Note the amount and color of any discharge. If discharge is present, a culture should be obtained. (For routine screening cultures in women, endocervical rather than urethral specimens are used.)

Background Information

The two most important causes of urethral discharge are *Neisseria gonorrhoeae*, which produces gonococcal urethritis, and *Chlamydia trachomatis*, which is reponsible for many cases of nongonococcal urethritis. Other organisms such as *Ureaplasma urealyticum* and *Trichomonas vaginalis* may occasionally cause urethritis. Noninfectious causes of urethral discharge include trauma, chemical urethritis, and tumors.

Because the gonococcus and chlamydiae are unable to penetrate healthy adult squamous epithelium, infection develops only on mucous membranes. The site of infection is initially the mucosa of the anterior urethra, but the organisms may spread into the urethral crypts and glands of Littré. The products of the organisms and the patient's cellular response are visualized as a urethral discharge. In most cases, the infection does not extend proximal to the external sphincter; thus, dysuria and discharge are the only symptoms produced. If the infection extends proximally to involve the prostate, bladder, or epididymis, systemic manifestations such as fever and malaise may. occur, as well as pain in the involved tissues. Bladder involvement leads to urinary frequency. Chronic untreated urethritis may produce a urethral stricture as the end result of the inflammatory process.

Clinical Significance

Most patients with urethral discharge will have gonorrhea or nongonococcal urethritis (NGU). A copious, thick, purulent discharge is more common in gonorrhea; a thin, clear, watery discharge is characteristic of

NGU. Smears or cultures should always be obtained to confirm the diagnosis. A bloody discharge should suggest trauma or tumor and requires further evaluation including urethroscopy.

At times, a man complaining of dysuria or urethral discharge may not have any observable discharge. Nevertheless, a urethral Gram stain should be obtained. If there are more than four polymorphonuclear leukocytes per high-power field, urethritis is present. Some men with NGU will only have an observable discharge in the morning prior to voiding. If symptoms are present but the smear shows few inflammatory cells, a repeat examination in the early morning may be useful.

Selected References

1. Jacobs NF Jr, Kraus SJ: Gonococcal and nongonococcal urethritis in men: Clinical and laboratory differentiation. *Ann Intern Med* 82:7–12, 1975.
2. Handsfield HH, Lipman TO, Harnish JP, et al: Asymptomatic gonorrhea in men: Diagnosis, natural course, prevalence, and significance. *N Engl J Med* 290:117–123, 1974.
3. US Department of Health, Education and Welfare: *Criteria and techniques for the diagnosis of gonorrhea.* Atlanta, Public Health Service, 1973.
4. Warren RM: Differential diagnosis of gonorrhea. *Practitioner* 217: 729–733, 1976.

67. Syphilis or Positive Serology

SUMNER E. THOMPSON III, MD, MPH

Definition

Untreated syphilis is a chronic, systemic disease caused by a spirochetal bacterium *Treponema pallidum.* Diverse, subtle clinical manifestations of the disease include unpredictable course, brief symptomatic episodes (primary and secondary syphilis), and a long asymptomatic interlude (latent syphilis).

Most commonly, the physician is confronted with a positive serologic test for syphilis (STS) in a patient who has not had specific anti-syphilis therapy and who has no clinical manifestations of syphilis.

Technique

Even in these days of liberated attitudes, eliciting a history of syphilis requires tact and skill. The clinician may be embarrassed and neglect to ask specific questions. Either the clinician or patient (or both) may also become uneasy and fractious during the interview; thus the chances of successfully obtaining useful information are ruined.

Helpful approaches for obtaining a positive history include a concerned, assertive attitude and language the patient can understand. Repeat the question in different ways. For example: Have you had syphilis? Have you ever had a blood test that was positive or required a course of shots? Have you ever had a sore on your penis/vagina that needed treatment? Do not begin by asking about "bad blood," a colloquialism with degrading connotations which patients almost always deny. Make sure the patient knows exactly what you are both talking about so that answers will be easier to obtain and will be more reliable. Do not let the patient's emotions engender hostility in you. Be relentless in your quest for information while remaining neutral.

Specifically seek the following information:

1. History of any venereal disease. A patient having one venereal disease is more likely to have another.
2. Specific signs and symptoms of primary or secondary syphilis such as penile or vaginal sores, rash, patchy hair loss.
3. History of syphilis in the family. Inquire about syphilis in near relatives. Ask about miscarriages and stillbirths. Inquire about siblings who have had abnormal blood test results or required a course of shots.
4. If and when blood tests for syphilis have been done. Direct questions in the following areas:
   a. Marriage. A premarital test for syphilis is required in all states except Maryland, Minnesota, Nevada, South Carolina, and Washington.
   b. Pregnancy. A serology is required on the first prenatal visit in most states. Birth certificates give the test date, but not the result.
   c. Hospitalization. A serology may be required on all newly admitted patients; check old records.
   d. Selective service. Both entrance and discharge physicals require a serology.

    e.   Employment records. Government employee and certain other jobs (beautician, barber, food handler) require pre-employment blood tests.

    f.   Blood donation. Individuals with positive serology are not accepted as blood donors.

    g.   Prisoner. Usually local control exists by prison authorities.

    h.   Insurance examination. Acceptance occasionally requires tests.

5.   Infectious disease history. Infectious processes within 3 months that might cause biological false positive (BFP) results include mononucleosis, viral pneumonia, and hepatitis.

Background Information

Despite excellent methods for diagnosing and treating syphilis, the disease is still widespread, primarily because of a silent course until the late, irreversible manifestations occur. Any organ system can be involved. These factors, coupled with a slowly progressive, capricious course, led Sir William Osler to say, "He who knows syphilis knows medicine."

The pallid spirochete that causes syphilis is one of a large group of organisms most of which are saprophytic. It is closely related to two other genera pathogenic for humans, *Leptospira* and *Borrelia*. Its characteristic corkscrew shape and rapid spiral movements allow identification of the living organism directly from lesions of primary and secondary syphilis with the darkfield microscope. Darkfield microscopy requires experience, particularly with oral lesions where naturally occurring nonpathogenic spirochetes are found. *Treponema pallidum* cannot be cultured on any known laboratory medium. Therefore, the physician must make the final diagnosis of syphilis by synthesizing evidence from the clinical picture, the site or origin of the organism, the microscopic morphology and motility, and the serological results.

Syphilis is transmitted only through direct contact with an infected lesion. Spirochetes may pass through intact mucous membranes or abraded skin to the bloodstream, and the infection becomes systemic within a few hours. The primary lesion, the chancre, develops 9–90 days after exposure. It is infective until healed (1–5 weeks). The lesions are usually painless with firm, raised edges and regional adenopathy. Pathologic examination reveals lymphocytic and plasmacytic infiltration. Treponemes can be recovered from aspirates of both chancre and lymph node.

Secondary syphilis may involve any cutaneous or mucosal surface, or any organ system. The organism may be demonstrated in all lesions but most easily in those on moist mucous membranes. All of these lesions are highly infectious. Systemic adenopathy and occasionally splenomegaly occur during this phase; serologic tests are almost always positive.

The characteristic pathologic lesion in all stages is an endarteritis and periarteritis of arterioles and capillaries. Endarteritis is a proliferation of endothelial cells causing a decrease in the luminal size of the vessel. Periarteritis is cuffing of the vessels by inflammatory cells; in this case, mononuclear cells. Like tuberculosis, syphilis is a classic example of granulomatous inflammation.

Invasion of tissue by the treponeme is associated with a complex but predictable humoral immune response. This response is first detectable in the serum 4–6 weeks after infection, that is, 1–3 weeks after the appearance of the primary chancre.

Clinical Significance

There are three reasons to diagnose syphilis as early as possible: (1) to prevent spread of infection to others; (2) to prevent irreversible, late complications; (3) to prevent congenital syphilis.

Infectiousness. There is a one-in-three chance of contracting syphilis from an infected partner. Treatment with a single adequate dose of penicillin rapidly renders lesions noninfective. Treatment instituted within a year will almost invariably revert the nontreponemal tests to negative, thus preventing stigmatization of the patient with a lifelong positive serologic test for syphilis.

Late complications. About 30% of untreated patients will eventually develop a late complication of syphilis. Central nervous system syphilis may occur in the form of either meningovascular-endarteritis and periarteritis with cerebral infarcts, or parenchymal changes with brain or spinal cord atrophy. Cardiovascular syphilis is a medial necrosis of the aorta with dilatation of the aorta or aortic valve commissures, or both. Finally, gumma formation may occur, a chronic, localized, intensely destructive lesion of any tissue, which is probably autoimmune in nature. Gumma formation is often mistaken for carcinoma.

Congenital syphilis. Most patients with untreated acquired syphilis are no longer considered to be infectious 3–4 years after acquiring the disease. They are unlikely to relapse from the latent phase to the infectious lesion secondary phase. However, an untreated woman can infect her fetus during any stage of the disease. It is now known that transplacental infection may occur at any stage of fetal development. Kassowitz's law states that the longer the duration of untreated syphilitic infection before pregnancy, the less likely the fetus is to be stillborn or infected. This rule has many exceptions. Thus, conception while the mother is in the primary or secondary stage of syphilis frequently ends in stillbirth, whereas conception during later stages of the disease may result in a clinical spectrum ranging from fulminating fatal congenital syphilis to a normal, uninfected child.

Selected References

1. Drusin LM: The diagnosis and treatment of infectious and latent syphilis. *Med Clin N Am* 56:1161–1174, 1972.
2. *Syphilis: A synopsis.* US Government Printing Office, Public Health Service Publication 1660, Jan 1968.
3. Rockwell DH, Yobo AR, Moore MB Jr: The Tuskegee study of untreated syphilis. *Arch Intern Med* 114:792–798, 1964.

68. Male Genital Lesions

SIDNEY OLANSKY, MD

Definition

A history of congenital or acquired abnormalities of the genital area including the urethra.

Technique

Most genital lesions are readily apparent on inspection and palpation of the genitalia during the physical examination. Eliciting a history of a genital lesion is rarely difficult. A comprehensive history includes the lesion's location, duration, character of onset, relation to previous intercourse, pain, trauma, size, enlargement, interference with normal function, and concomitant symptoms of urinary infection.

Background Information and Clinical Significance

Genital lesions can be found on a thorough physical examination. For the purpose of taking a history, the examiner may mentally categorize these lesions into malformations, inflammatory diseases, and scrotal swellings.

Malformations. Congenital lesions such as hypospadias and cryptorchism should be documented along with the nature of any present symptomatology or previous surgical procedures. Hypospadias is a developmental anomaly with a defect in the urethral wall such that the canal is open on the undersurface of the penis. Cryptorchism is the failure of descent of a testis.

Inflammatory diseases. Chancroid, granuloma inguinale, herpes progenitalis, and all stages of syphilis are acquired inflammatory diseases. Proper laboratory examination such as serologic tests for syphilis and bacteriology should be done for confirmation.

Of dermatologic importance, psoriasis and lichen planus frequently occur on the penis, which may be the only area involved. Fixed drug eruptions are also commonly seen on the penis. Balanitis, epididymitis, and orchitis, although more rare, produce severe symptomatology and must be recognized. Neoplasia, although uncommon, should be considered in chronic lesions, and biopsy is necessary to confirm this diagnosis.

Parasitic infections, such as scabies and pediculosis pubis, frequently occur in the genital area and are easily recognized if kept in mind. The organism of pediculosis can be easily recognized with the naked eye, and scabies can be identified under the microscope.

Scrotal swellings. The onset, duration, and character of the swelling should be documented. While a history of trauma, size, enlargement, pain, and constitutional symptoms is necessary, the physical examination is of supreme importance. Hydroceles, varicoceles, testicular tumors, and testicular torsion are examples of scrotal enlargements. The reader should refer to the following section on Testicular Mass or Pain.

Selected References

1. Campbell MF, Harrison JH: *Urology,* ed 3. Philadelphia, WB Saunders, 1970.
2. Karafin L, Kendall AR: *Urology.* Hagerstown, Md, Harper and Row, 1973.
3. King A, Nicol C: *Venereal Diseases.* Philadelphia, FA Davis Co, 1964.
4. Judge RD, Zuidema GD: *Methods of Clinical Examinations: A Physiological Approach.* Boston, Little, Brown, 1974.

69. Testicular Mass or Pain

KENNETH N. WALTON, MD

Definition

Testicular pain is what patients call the pain appreciated in one or both scrotal compartments. A ureteral stone, inguinal hernia, epididymitis, testicular disease, or psychosomatic illness may produce pain interpreted by the patient as testicular. It is important to pursue the complaint and determine the cause.

Any mass in one or both scrotal compartments is potentially testicular but may be due to other causes. It is extremely important to know whether the mass is truly testicular.

Technique

The history establishes the duration of the pain or mass and the association of fever or other symptoms. The physical examination is more important (see section 178, External Male Genitalia). The astute clinician will thus signal the history of testicular pain or swelling in seconds, preserving several minutes for careful physical examination.

Background Information

Since virtually all testicular masses are tumors and over 95% of these are malignant, all testicular masses are explored surgically. Clearly if one cannot tell clinically whether the mass is in the testes, exploration is necessary. Almost all nontesticular scrotal masses are nonmalignant. Testicular tumors are more common in cryptorchid testes even after they have been brought down surgically. Delay in the diagnosis of a testis tumor is more often due to physician than to patient delay.

The sensation of testicular pain may be diminished or absent in diabetic patients with other features of autonomic neuropathy.

Clinical Significance

Pain associated with fever and local tenderness is usually due to an inflammation in the epididymis. The testis may share in the inflammatory enlargement. Pain and swelling without fever may be due to benign conditions but are regarded as a tumor of the testis until the etiology is established. If the physical examination cannot make this distinction, surgical exploration will.

Selected References

1. Whitmore WF Jr: Germinal testis tumors in adults, in *Proceedings of the Seventh National Cancer Conference, 1973.* New York, American Cancer Society, pp 793–801.
2. Campbell IW, Ewing DJ, Clarke BF, et al: Testicular pain sensation in diabetic autonomic neuropathy. *Br Med J* 2:638–639, 1974.
3. Mostofi FK: Testicular tumors: Epidemiologic, etiologic and pathologic features. *Cancer* 32:1186–1201, 1973.

70. Impotence

W. DALLAS HALL, MD

Definition

Impotence in men may be classified into three types: loss of libido, erectile dysfunction, and ejaculatory incompetence.

Technique

Read the techniques described in the sections on Sexual History. Ask additional questions to ascertain whether the complaint of impotence is an expression of poor libido, difficulty with erection, or difficulty with ejaculation. Inquire thoroughly about libido since an intact libido may be the first clue to organic causes of impotence. Ask about life events or stresses that may have occurred near the onset of symptoms. If the complaint is erectile dysfunction, determine if this is intermittent or persistent. Ask about the presence of morning erections since both micturition and erection reflexes emanate from the same sacral segments of the spinal cord. Ask about awareness by the patient of nocturnal penile tumescence since a 10–25-mm expansion in penile circumference normally accompanies the automatic discharge associated with the rapid eye movement (REM) phase of sleep. Ask if partial or firm erection occurs in a variety of settings that may create sexual arousal. If the complaint is ejaculatory incompetence, determine if the sensation of ejaculation occurs in the absence of emission.

A thorough review of the current medication history is mandatory. Attempt to relate all new drug therapies or dosage increments to the onset of the patient's symptom. Seek a past history of depression, alcoholism, diabetes, peripheral vascular disease, or neurologic disorders such as multiple sclerosis, tabes dorsalis, and amyotrophic lateral sclerosis. Ask about any past genitourinary or abdominoperineal surgical procedures.

Background Information

Penile erection is directly associated with an increase in the volume of blood in the penis. The blood is delivered via penile branches of the internal pudental artery, a branch of the hypogastric artery. The increase in penile blood volume expands the vascular and muscular corpora cavernosa such that venous return is mechanically impaired and erection occurs. Both sympathetic and parasympathetic components of the autonomic nervous system allow vasodilatation of the internal pudental and penile arteries. Sympathetic fibers emerge from L_{2-4} and inhibit vasoconstriction; parasympathetic fibers emerge from S_{2-4} (nervi erigentes) and cause vasodilation. Afferent sensory nerve endings in the genital region are carried to the cord via the pudental nerve, from which sympathetic outflow occurs. Sympathetic outflow from the central nervous system also allows vasodilatation of penile arteries.

Ejaculation is primarily under control of the sympathetic nervous system (L_{2-4}), which controls contraction of the ejaculatory ducts and closure of the internal sphincter of the bladder. Interruption or blockade of the sympathetic nerves supplying the bladder may allow the ejaculate to enter the bladder rather than exit the urethra. This is known as retrograde ejaculation.

Lawrence and Swyer studied plasma testosterone levels in 27 normal adult men and 27 men with impotence and normal secondary sex characteristics. No significant differences were noted.

Clinical Significance

In a study by Frank et al., 40% of apparently healthy married men reported erectile or ejaculatory dysfunction. The prevalence of sexual problems uncovered by careful patient interviews illustrates both the magnitude of the problem and the considerable difficulties encountered in the design and interpretation of studies on "impotence."

Impotence has been classically considered of nonorganic etiology in more than 90% of cases. Nonorganic causes of impotence are suggested by the following features:

1. Often associated with poor libido and recent life stresses
2. Intact ability to gain erection with stimuli (full bladder, REM sleep, and so forth) other than command performances
3. Intact ability to ejaculate
4. Absence of disease processes or medications known to be associated with impotence

Organic causes of impotence have become more appreciated in the past decade. The major categories include vascular, neurologic, and drug-induced etiologies.

Vascular causes are exemplified by impotence occurring as part of the LeRiche syndrome with aortic aneurysms. Erectile dysfunction occurs because adequate blood supply does not allow engorgement of the corpora cavernosa. Stenoses of the internal pudendal artery may be particularly prominent in diabetic patients. Although they correlate poorly with the intensity of femoral artery pulsations, a strong pulsation of the dorsal penile artery weighs against a vascular etiology.

Neurologic causes of impotence are generally related to impairment of the sympathetic nerve supply from the L_{2-4} region, or of the parasympathetic nerve supply from the S_{2-4} region. Neurologic diseases that may involve multiple cord segments include multiple sclerosis, amyotrophic lateral sclerosis, tabes dorsalis, and combined system disease of pernicious anemia, as well as disorders of autonomic function associated with known (eg, diabetes mellitus) or unknown etiologies (eg, Shy-Drager syndrome). Nerve supply may also be interrupted by trauma or surgical procedures such as prostatectomy or abdominoperineal resection for rectal carcinoma.

Many pharmacologic agents may induce impotence, a particularly common occurrence in the treatment of hypertension. Antihypertensive drugs that alter central vasomotor outflow (propranolol, clonidine, and others) are occasionally associated with impotence but less often than those which directly block peripheral sympathetic ganglia (eg, guanethidine impotence typically spares erection but impairs ejaculation). Methyldopa has both a central and peripheral sympatholytic effect and, in most series, a fairly high incidence of impotence. The primary sympatholytic action of reserpine is peripheral, and impotence is an occasional side effect. Vasodilators and prazosin are relatively free of inducing impotence. Impotence is a definite side effect of spironolactone and has been reported with thiazide diuretics. Bulpitt noted that impotence was reported 2.5 times more often in patients with untreated hypertension when compared with normotensive men of similar age.

Many other therapeutic compounds have been associated with impotence as a side effect. Phenothiazines may induce decreased libido, erectile dysfunction, or inhibition of ejaculation. Impaired or retrograde ejaculation has been particularly noted with thioridazine. Varieties of impotence have also been noted with the tricyclic antidepressants and thioxanthenes. Atropine and other anticholinergics may impair parasympathetic function and cause impotence. Alcohol, cocaine, nicotine, and other drugs of abuse have been associated with impotence.

Patients who complain of any or all three varieties of impotence may have multiple etiologies. Two of the most commonly associated disease processes are diabetes mellitus and chronic alcoholism. For example, Kolodny et al. reported erectile dysfunction in 50% of adult male diabetics. A diabetic patient with impotence should have psychologic, vascular, neurologic and drug-induced etiologies thoroughly explored. Lemere and Smith surveyed 17,000 alcoholic patients and reported that 8% had total impotence. The impotence persisted in approximately 50% of those who abstained from alcohol for several months.

Selected References

1. Weiss HD: The physiology of human penile erection. *Ann Intern Med* 76:793–799, 1972.
2. Frank E, Anderson C, Rubinstein D: Frequency of sexual dysfunction in "normal" couples. *N Engl J Med* 299:111–115, 1978.
3. Mallory TR, Wein AJ: The etiology, diagnosis and surgical treatment of erectile impotence. *J Reprod Med* 20:183–194, 1978.
4. Levine SB: Marital sexual dysfunction: Erectile dysfunction. *Ann Intern Med* 85:342–350, 1976.
5. Lawrence DM, Swyer GIM: Plasma testosterone and testosterone binding affinity in men with impotence, oligospermia, azospermia and hypogonadism. *Br Med J* 1:349–351, 1974.
6. Reichgott MJ: Problems of sexual function in patients with hypertension. *Cardiovasc Med* 4(2):149–156, 1979.
7. Bulpitt CJ, Dollery CT, Carne S: Change in symptoms of hypertensive patients after referral to hospital clinic. *Br Heart J* 38:121–128, 1976.
8. Mills LC: Drug-induced impotence. *Am Fam Pract* 12:104–106, 1975.
9. Ellenberg M: Impotence in diabetes: The neurologic factor. *Ann Intern Med* 75:213–219, 1971.

10. Kolodny RC, Kahn CB, Goldstein HH, et al: Sexual dysfunction in diabetic men. *Diabetes* 23:306–309, 1974.
11. Herman A, Adar R, Rubinstein Z: Vascular lesions associated with impotence in diabetic and nondiabetic arterial occlusive disease. *Diabetes* 27:975–981, 1978.
12. Lemere F, Smith JW: Alcohol-induced sexual impotence. *Am J Psych* 130:212–213, 1973.
13. Hargreave TB, Stephenson TP: Potency and prostatectomy. *Br J Urol* 49:683–688, 1977.
14. Weinstein M, Roberts M: Sexual potency following surgery for rectal carcinoma. A followup of 44 patients. *Ann Surg* 185:295–300, 1977.

71. Family History of Renal Disease

W. DALLAS HALL, MD

Definition

The history of any type of renal disease occurring in immediate family members. Normally the family history of renal disease is negative.

Technique

Begin by asking if anyone in the family has had kidney trouble. If so, ask about special diets, kidney machines, or special treatments for kidney poisoning. Ask about nephritis or Bright's disease. Since several hereditary renal diseases are associated with deafness, inquire whether anyone in the family wears a hearing aid. Ask about family members who have had kidney stones. Some patients refer to kidney stones as "gravel."

Background Information

Hereditary renal diseases may have an autosomal dominant, autosomal recessive, or sex-linked inheritance pattern. The characteristic pedigrees of these types of Mendelian inheritance are outlined in section 111, Family Pedigree and Heritable Disease Potential.

The most frequent autosomal dominant renal disorder is the adult type of polycystic kidney disease. Another important disorder with dominant inheritance is the hereditary type of idiopathic renal tubular acidosis (RTA), also known as type I or distal RTA. Hereditary nephritis with deafness (Alport's syndrome) is frequently inherited as autosomal dominant but associated with partial X-linkage or preferential segregation and chromosomal association. It is usually detected by the onset of hematuria and deafness in young males. Females may present in the fourth or fifth decade of life and manifest only high-pitched hearing loss on audiometry. Hereditary osteo-onychodystrophy, also referred to as the nail-patella syndrome or HOOD, occurs in a dominant inheritance pattern with linkage to the ABO blood group system. This condition is usually recognized by a bitten appearance of the nails, absent or hypoplastic patellae, and pathognomonic iliac horns on plain films of the abdomen or pelvis. Relatively rare renal disorders with autosomal dominant inheritance patterns include renal glycosuria, glycinuria, and familial hyperprolinemia.

The most important autosomal recessive hereditary renal disorders are medullary cystic disease and cystinosis. Medullary cystic disease usually presents with anemia in the second or third decade of life. Characteristically there is prominent renal salt wasting with lack of edema, hypertension, or alterations in the urinary sediment. In some families the disease is inherited in an autosomal dominant pattern. Controversy among experts concerns whether medullary cystic disease can be clinically and histologically differentiated from juvenile nephronophthisis. Cystinosis is an inborn error of metabolism characterized by the presence of cystine crystals in multiple tissues. It is a common cause of end-stage renal disease in children between the ages of 6 and 12. Infrequent renal disorders with autosomal recessive inheritance patterns include the infantile type of polycystic disease, congenital nephrosis, cystinuria, Hartnup disease, and hereditary renal-retinal dysplasia with retinitis pigmentosa.

The most important X-linked renal disorder is Fabry's disease, also known as angiokeratoma corporis diffusum. This condition is characterized by intermittent fever, proteinuria, hypertension, renal failure, and angiomatous skin lesions on the trunk and genital areas. Other renal disorders with X-linked dominant or recessive inheritance patterns are relatively rare. These disorders include nephrogenic diabetes insipidus, hypophosphatemic vitamin-D-resistant rickets, and the oculocerebrorenal syndrome of Lowe.

Additional disorders which may involve the kidney and may occasionally be associated with a positive family history are systemic lupus erythematosus, diabetes mellitus, hyperparathyroidism, gout, and various developmental anomalies. Inherited renal diseases may also be linked to hereditary platelet abnormalities, either macrothrombocytosis or thrombocytopenia.

Clinical Significance

A positive family history is useful in delineating the etiology of renal disease in patients with otherwise unexplained hematuria, proteinuria, stones, or renal failure.

An autosomal dominant family history is suggestive of polycystic kidney disease in any patient over age 30 who presents with undiagnosed hematuria or renal failure. Palpable abdominal masses and a relative lack of anemia are additional clues. If the patient is female, an audiogram should be performed to exclude late onset of Alport's syndrome. The dominant inheritance form of medullary cystic disease should be particularly suspect if the patient is between age 10 and 30. If the patient is male and below age 15, Alport's syndrome should be strongly suspected.

An autosomal recessive family history is more difficult to recognize. Often, however, some type of kidney problem is known to occur intermittently in the family. Each of the seven previously mentioned recessive kidney diseases should be considered, depending on the age and setting of the patient.

X-linked renal disorders should be easily recognized by their predominant clinical expression in males within the family.

Conditions that should be considered in patients with a strong family history of renal calculi include gout, familial hyperparathyroidism, cystic diseases of the renal medulla, hypercalciuric varieties of renal tubular acidosis, glycinuria, and cystinuria.

Detection of hereditary renal disease carries more than just diagnostic implications. Depending on the age and specific disorder, parents or children should be examined and genetic counseling considered. If end-stage renal disease is present, renal transplantation may be considered to have relatively favorable results. Replacement of specific missing enzymes may be indicated.

Selected References

1. Gardner KD Jr: Evolution of clinical signs in adult-onset cystic disease of the renal medulla. *Ann Intern Med* 74:47–54, 1971.
2. Simon HB, Thompson GJ: Congenital renal polycystic disease: A clinical and therapeutic study of three hundred sixty-six cases. *JAMA* 159:657–662, 1955.
3. Perkoff GT: The hereditary renal diseases. *N Engl J Med* 277:79–85, 129–138, 1967.
4. Purriel P, Drets M, Pascale E, et al: Familial hereditary nephropathy (Alport's syndrome). *Am J Med* 49:753–772, 1970.

72. Birth Control

ROBERT A. HATCHER, MD

Definition

The fertility status of a couple (or of an individual) could be categorized in one of four ways:

1. Wish to become pregnant at the present time
2. Are ambivalent about procreation at the present time
3. Desire to avoid pregnancy at the present time (spacing)
4. Desire no further children (desire to terminate childbearing) or desire no children at all

The physician cannot know a patient's desires with regard to childbearing unless he asks the patient. The physician should determine if the patient wants to avoid pregnancy, what method of birth control is currently being used, and what medical or surgical complications might be affecting the patient's current use of a contraceptive.

Technique

Assume the patient is a woman. The following series of questions will help define current fertility goals, need for birth control, use of birth control, attitudes toward birth control, and effects of birth control on menstruation, sexual activity, and general health. These questions begin to delineate the patient's attitudes about and experience with the four basic means of fertility control: contraception, sterilization, abortion, or abstinence.

When would you like to have your next baby? What method(s) of birth control have you used? Have you ever been told not to use any specific method of birth control? Approximately how often do you have intercourse? Are you currently using any method(s) of birth control? Are you pleased with your current means of birth control? Is your partner pleased with your current means of birth control? Have you ever become

Table 11. Twelve methods of fertility control.

Method of Fertility Control	Profile of Situation Pointing to Consideration of Method	Major or Minor Contraindications	Major or Minor Complications
Abstinence	Any individual who does not wish to be sexually active; who does not enjoy intercourse; who feels guilty about intercourse; who has an active infection of the genitourinary tract; or who finds intercourse painful	Past history of sexual activity with an individual makes it relatively unlikely that this couple will avoid sexual intercourse in the future	Frustration or guilt; couple changes plans and woman is exposed to risk of unplanned pregnancy
Coitus interruptus (withdrawal)	No other method available; very infrequent intercourse; as a backup means of birth control to a second, more effective method	Tendency to premature ejaculation; inability to enjoy intercourse in this manner; lack of trust between man and woman	Frustration; inability for either partner to enjoy intercourse
Condoms (rubbers)	Teenagers; intercourse when one individual does not know the other well and where the development of a sexually transmitted infection is a concern; use as a backup to another method; temporary use while treating vaginitis or VD; postvasectomy until ejaculate is free of sperm; used to treat premature ejaculation in the male	Male impotence using condom; diminished pleasure; inability to use properly; lack of cooperation of the male	Allergy to rubber; impotence; failure to interrupt intercourse to use the method; negative associations with condoms (VD, illicit sex, one-night stands)

Method	Indications	Contraindications	Complications
Diaphragm (with cream or jelly)	Woman (or woman with partner) who is not embarrassed to insert diaphragm into vagina; patient concerned about complications of other methods	*Major:* vaginal anomaly; severe cystocele or severe retroversion or anteversion of the uterus; rectovaginal fistula; vesicovaginal fistula; complete uterine prolapse. *Minor:* inability to insert properly	Diaphragm left in place for too long (3–4 weeks); allergy to rubber (rare); cystitis and/or urethritis; inability to remove the diaphragm
Aerosol foam; vaginal spermicide (Delfen, Emko, Koromex, and Dalkon foam)	Couple wanting safe, effective contraceptive; may have experienced complication from pills or IUD	Couple unwilling to interrupt coitus or who find this method esthetically unpleasant	Vaginal or penile irritation; discharge from vagina following use; too much lubrication during act of intercourse
Foaming contraceptive suppository (Encare Oval)	Couple frustrated with all of the other contraceptive options; woman who finds the small oval more convenient than foam to carry about; couple seeking very safe approach to contraception	Couple unwilling to interrupt coitus; fear that effectiveness rates originally claimed may not be corroborated	Intercourse is interrupted; vaginal or penile irritation; vaginal discharge following use
Intrauterine devices (IUDs)	Patient desiring highly effective method not related to coitus or daily use of pills; patient with history of relatively painless menses	Pregnancy; endometritis or salpingitis; undiagnosed vaginal bleeding; very small uterus (less than 4.5 cm); bicornuate uterus; desire for a future pregnancy is a relative contraindication	Endometritis; salpingitis; sepsis; dysmenorrhea; menorrhagia, metrorrhagia, partial or complete expulsion; penile irritation; risk of miscarriage or sepsis if pregnancy occurs with IUD in place

Table 11. Twelve methods of fertility control. (Cont'd.)

Method of Fertility Control	Profile of Situation Pointing to Consideration of Method	Major or Minor Contraindications	Major or Minor Complications
Oral contraceptives with estrogen and progesterone derivatives	Patient desiring the most effective method of contraception (if she remembers to use method perfectly); patient embarrassed by or unwilling to use coitus-related methods; patient hoping to experience one of a myriad noncontraceptive side benefits of orals (dysmenorrhea improved; acne diminished; menstrual blood loss decreased; midcycle secretion and mittelschmerz eliminated; more predictable menstrual periods; breast enlargement, functional ovarian cysts less likely)	*Absolute:* thromboembolic disorders or history thereof; cerebrovascular accident or history thereof; impaired liver function; malignancy of breast or reproductive system; pregnancy *Strong relative:* migraine headaches; hypertension; gestation of 20 weeks terminated within the past 4 weeks; prediabetes or diabetes; history of cholestasis during pregnancy; undiagnosed abnormal vaginal bleeding *Other relative:* varicose veins, asthma, cardiac or renal disease; mental retardation; cholasma; family history of diabetes; uterine fibromyomata; epilepsy; depression; profile suspicious for subsequent infertility problems; late onset or very irregular menses; lactation	*Major:* gallbladder disease; thromboembolic events; myocardial infarction; stroke; hypertension; migraine headaches; depression; hepatic adenoma *Minor:* nausea; weight gain; spotting; decreased menstrual flow; chloasma; decreased libido (rare); non-migraine headaches

Method	Indications	Contraindications	Side Effects/Complications
Oral contraceptives with progestin only (mini-pills)	...lated side effects from combined pills; women over 35; women with severe headaches; sickle cell disease	Same absolute indications as estrogen-progesterone pills; other relative contraindications include undiagnosed abnormal vaginal bleeding	...creased or decreased duration and amount of menstrual flow; spotting; amenorrhea
Long-acting progesterone injections	Patient wants no more children; patient desiring to terminate menses; individual unable to use other methods of birth control; mental retardation	Pregnancy desired as soon as method discontinued; thromboembolic disorders or history thereof; malignancy of breast or reproductive system; pregnancy; undiagnosed abnormal vaginal bleeding; profile suspicious for subsequent infertility (late onset of or very irregular menses, painless menses)	Menstrual irregularities during first year; amenorrhea after first year; delayed return of fertility (6-12 months); headaches; weight gain; depression; decreased libido (rare); allergic reactions (rare); not FDA approved
Sterilization	For couple definitely wanting to terminate childbearing, sterilization is often the method of choice	Most sterilization procedures should be considered irreversible; therefore, indecision regarding future desire for pregnancy is a strong contraindication	Vasectomy: hematoma; infection; pain; sperm granuloma Tubal ligation: hemorrhage; tying off structure other than Fallopian tube; anesthesia Both vasectomy and tubal ligation may cause concern over ability to enjoy intercourse or status of normal output, ie, psychological problems
Abortion	Pregnant individual who does not wish to have a baby; women who have failed to use a contraceptive or who have had a contraceptive failure	The later the pregnancy, the less desirable for patient, medical community, and society	Hemorrhage; infection; uterine perforation; anxiety and various types of guilt reactions

pregnant when you did not plan to become pregnant? If so, what did you choose to do about your unplanned pregnancy? What are your thoughts about sterilization? How (if at all) does your current method of birth control alter your monthly periods?

Background Information

The average woman in America starts to menstruate at 12.5 years of age and ceases menses between the ages of 45 and 50. Not all cycles are ovulatory. Ovulatory cycles tend to be more regular than anovulatory cycles, are more painful than anovulatory cycles, and are associated with midcycle pain in some women. The average woman ovulates 400 times, conceives 3–4 times, and has 2–3 deliveries in a lifetime. The desired number of children per family in the United States is now about two. Close to 50% of pregnancies in the United States are unplanned. Approximately 25% of babies born are unwanted at the time of birth. In states where abortion is available, there are about 200–300 therapeutic abortions per 1,000 live births. Thus, one in four to six pregnancies may end in abortion. Abortion is not taken lightly by most American women. Most couples and clinicians consider contraception preferable to abortion. There are 11 million sexually active teenagers in the United States; of these 4.5 million are teenage girls. One million teenage girls 15–19 become pregnant each year, and one-third of these girls obtain abortions. Less than one-fourth of all sexually active teenage girls use effective contraceptives consistently. Once couples are over 30 years of age, sterilization becomes the most frequently chosen means of fertility control.

Clinical Significance

The practicing clinician must be aware of the fertility goals and practices of patients for two basic reasons: the risk of pregnancy and the risks of contraception.

Pregnancy may adversely affect the physical or psychological health of an individual, of a relationship, or of a family unit. Women at risk of having a less than ideal outcome of pregnancy for themselves or for their child include the following: those with high parity, recent delivery (less than 12 months), recurrent premature deliveries or stillbirths, a history of postpartum depression, age less than 15 or over 40 years, chronic hypertension, sickle cell disease, advanced heart disease, and perhaps the most important in this context, women who do not wish to be pregnant.

Efforts to avoid pregnancy (contraceptives) are used by great numbers of individuals. All physicians should understand the potential complications of current contraceptives. Hypertension, thrombophlebitis, pulmonary emboli, cerebral thrombosis, myocardial infarction, hyperlipidemia, glucose intolerance, migraine headaches, mesenteric vascular thrombosis, pancreatitis, gallbladder disease, small-bowel obstruction, increased menstrual blood loss or pain, pelvic inflammatory disease, sepsis, moniliasis, amenorrhea, postmethod infertility, failure of contact lens fit, chloasma, acne, alopecia, erythema nodosum, arthritis, erythema multiforme, asthma, depression, and, of course, death, have all been attributed to various contraceptives.

Table 11 summarizes the relative indications, contraindications, and complications of twelve different approaches to fertility control.

Selected References

1. Hatcher RA, Stewart GK, Guest FJ, et al: *Contraceptive Technology,* 1978–1979. New York, Irvington Publishers, 1978.
2. Population Reports. A series of articles containing references, available from the US Agency for International Aid (AID).

FEMALE GENITALIA

Introduction to the Gynecologic History

JOHN D. THOMPSON, MD

These comments are included to help the student and physician gather adequate and accurate data from the female patient with gynecologic complaints. Although many of the comments are appropriate for the general history and physical examination, they have specific significance for the gynecologic patient.

1. The gynecologic history and examination should be conducted in a completely professional and *nonjudgmental* manner. Subjects are often discussed that the patient considers private and personal. If she does not feel comfortable with her physician or if the physician does not seem to her a person that she can trust, then she will have difficulty not only in giving an adequate and accurate history but also in cooperating during the examination.

2. Women differ in how they feel about themselves as women. They

have different values and ideas about sexuality, relationships between men and women, abortion, menstruation, contraception, and childbearing which are more or less modern, liberated, traditional, or old-fashioned. The gynecologic history and examination should be conducted in such a way that the patient can feel comfortable about her individual expression of "womanhood" and "femaleness."

3. The gynecologic history cannot be taken by requiring patients to answer a series of questions in a definite written and predetermined sequence. Patients will usually answer properly a question that is properly presented by the proper person at the proper time. Judgment on the part of the physician must be exercised in order for the history to be adequate and accurate.

4. The gynecologic history must be updated continually. The date of the last menstrual period, for example, usually changes every month. Serious mistakes can be made if the patient's last menstrual period is not the same as that recorded in the chart. Other information must also be updated.

5. Gynecology patients are often unaware of what is "normal" from a gynecologic standpoint. Obtain specific data instead.

73. Pelvic Pain

JOHN D. THOMPSON, MD

Definition

A feeling of pain or discomfort in the pelvis.

Technique

A careful history is important. The intensity, onset, and relation to past events and adjacent organ systems should be carefully evaluated. Changes in the menstrual cycle, relation to the menstrual flow, relation to coitus, a history of previous pelvic surgery or of a recent gonorrheal infection, the type of contraceptive used, the sexual history, long periods of involuntary infertility—all of these and others are important in evaluating pelvic pain that may be of gynecologic origin.

Dyspareunia is pelvic pain associated with intercourse. A detailed description of the pain and its relationship to penile insertion must be obtained. Is the discomfort at the vaginal introitus and present at the moment of entry? Or, is the pain deep in the pelvis with the feeling that something tender is being hit? Or, is this a residual feeling of congestion and heaviness, particularly throughout the pelvis following intercourse without orgasm?

Background Information

A feeling of pain or discomfort in the pelvis in a female patient may be a part of a normal physiologic mechanism, may be associated with a medical crisis for which emergency therapy is needed to save the patient's life, may be associated with a chronic pelvic problem, or may remain forever and mysteriously unexplained. It should be understood, particularly by men, that some degree of pelvic discomfort and pelvic pain is a normal and natural part of human femaleness. Men rarely experience pelvic discomfort, whereas women frequently do. Pelvic pain in the female, therefore, may or may not require intervention and treatment. It will be the presenting complaint in about 20% of all gynecology patients.

Evaluation of pelvic pain is also made more difficult because the characteristics of pelvic pain are often difficult for women to describe and localize accurately. In all probability, the explanation for this lies in the fact that there are no great concentrations of sensory nerve ganglia in the pelvis, such as one encounters in the periosteum of the bone or the conjunctiva or the skin—especially perianal skin. Thus, it is difficult for the pain-perceiving centers in the brain to make a sharp differentiation as to the location, type, and severity of the pain. This is the primary reason that ovarian carcinoma has such a poor prognosis. It causes no discomfort in the early stages, even though the tumor has grown to a large size. On the other hand, great discomfort can be caused by small implants of endometriosis on the uterosacral ligaments.

Pelvic pain may be associated with a variety of acute and chronic gynecologic and nongynecologic organic diseases at the same time. It should also be stated that many of these diseases may be present without pelvic pain. Some women with chronic pelvic inflammatory disease will have pelvic pain and some will not. Some women with extensive endometriosis will have pelvic pain and some will not. The same is true of relaxations and prolapse.

Dysmenorrhea is painful menstruation. Primary dysmenorrhea is painful menstruation when the pelvic examination is normal. Secondary dysmenorrhea is diagnosed in the presence of gynecologic disease and is usually associated with such conditions as endometriosis, adenomyosis, and pelvic inflammatory disease.

Primary dysmenorrhea is not present when the menstrual cycles are anovulatory. For several cycles after the menarche, menstruation is likely to be painless because the cycles are anovulatory. When dysmenorrhea begins in young girls and the pelvic examination is normal, one can assume that ovulatory cycles are also present. It should be emphasized, however, that severe dysmenorrhea in young girls may be associated with cryptomenorrhea (hidden menstruation) because of an anomalous development (imperforate hymen, rudimentary uterine horn).

Dysmenorrhea is described as an intermittent cramping discomfort in the lower abdomen and pelvis. It may also be associated with a bearing-down sensation, backache, and epigastric discomfort and vomiting. Discomfort and cramping in the legs are not uncommon. A syndrome of "premenstrual tension" often precedes the appearance of menstrual flow. This syndrome may include headaches, constipation, fluid retention, weight gain, abdominal bloating, mild depression, and breast tenderness. Often, the constipation will be relieved with several loose stools just before the menstrual flow begins.

Clinical Significance

A complaint of pelvic pain deserves a careful evaluation at any age, but the occurrence of new pelvic pain in a premenarchial girl or a postmenopausal woman is more often found associated with significant pathology and should never be dismissed lightly.

In addition to a careful gynecologic history, a complete pelvic examination will be helpful in evaluating the complaint of pelvic pain. One should look for irritating lesions of the vulva and vagina, vaginal relations and uterine malpositions, evidence of stenosis of the cervical canal, adnexal masses, and tenderness and indurated and nodular pelvic tissue.

Unfortunately, it is not always possible to be certain about the presence or absence of disease in the pelvis, even with a properly performed examination on a completely cooperative patient. Organic pelvic disease may be present even though the pelvis is judged to be normal at the time of the examination. Also, organic pelvic disease may be absent in women who have suspicious findings on pelvic examination. Therefore, laparoscopy has a definite place in the examination of patients with pelvic pain.

Selected Reference

1.   Novak ER, Jones GS, Jones HW: *Novak's Textbook of Gynecology,* ed 9. Baltimore, Williams and Wilkins, 1975.

74. Vaginal Discharge

SUMNER E. THOMPSON III, MD, MPH
MICHAEL REIN, MD

Definition

The hallmark of vaginal infection is the complaint of discharge that is usually purulent; it must be differentiated from the mucoid, normal physiologic discharge.

Technique

The differential diagnosis of vaginal discharge centers on the demonstration of the causative agents, most of which are infectious.

Age. Patients in their sexually active years are likely to have a sexually transmitted disease such as gonorrhea or trichomoniasis; neoplasia is more common among older women. A vaginal discharge in prepubescent girls is almost never physiologic. Pediatric vaginal infections should raise the question of child abuse.

Mode of onset. Abrupt onset suggests an infectious process while gradual increase over weeks or months is more consistent with neoplasia or atrophic vaginitis. Discharge and pruritus occurring during or just after menses suggests trichomoniasis; premenstrual onset may occur with candidiasis.

Amount of discharge. This is highly variable in all conditions. Severe infection may be accompanied by only scant discharge.

Pruritus. This is most common and severe in trichomoniasis and candidiasis, and frequent in gonorrhea and *Corynebacterium vaginale* vaginitis.

Other diseases. Diabetes mellitus and hypoparathyroidism are associated with *Candida* vaginitis.

263

Medications.   A history of current and prior medication is of paramount importance. Douches, feminine hygiene products, contraceptive foams and jellies, and intravaginal medications may produce irritative or true hypersensitivity vaginitis. Patients taking broad-spectrum antibiotics, such as tetracycline, ampicillin, or metronidazole (Flagyl), are at increased risk for developing *Candida* vaginalis, as are those taking oral contraceptives or other steroids.

Sexual history.   This is important. The specific question, "Do you have a reason to suspect that you may have a venereal disease?" may give information on new sex partners, changes in contraceptive habits, or recent treatment for venereal diseases.

A physical examination should include not only a speculum and bimanual pelvic examination, but inspection and palpation of the entire perineal area and rectum to exclude extravaginal disease simulating vaginal discharge.

1. Perineal lesions
   a. Syphilitic chancre
   b. Chancroid
   c. Herpes progenitalis
   d. Intertrigo
2. Bartholinitis
3. Proctitis or inflammatory bowel disease

Once the examiner is satisfied that vaginal discharge truly exists, two simple procedures can be done rapidly to distinguish between the four most common infectious causes of vaginitis: *Trichomonas, Candida,* gonococcus, and *Corynebacterium vaginale.*

1. Direct microscopic examination of vaginal secretions—the wet mount
2. A Gram stain smear of endocervical and vaginal secretions

Technique.   At the conclusion of the speculum examination under direct vision, take a cotton-tipped swab specimen from the posterior fornical pool and make a dime-sized smear on one end of a glass microscope slide. Then place this swab in a tube containing a milliliter or so of saline and agitate well. On the other end of the slide make a similar smear from a swab rotated in the endocervix.

The wet mount should be examined within 5 minutes. Gently pass the tube through a flame or hold it near an exposed lightbulb to warm it slightly. Warming will increase trichomonal activity, making them easier to identify. Place a drop of this fluid on a slide, coverslip, and examine under high dry (100x) with the substage condenser racked down to increase contrast. Look for the motile, pear-shaped, flagellated trichomonads, which are about the size of white blood cells. If motility is lost, the organisms will be quite difficult to distinguish from white blood cells. The wet mount may also show budding yeasts with or without pseudohyphal elements suggesting *Candida* infection. One may also observe "clue cells," epithelial cells studded with bacteria giving them a coarsely granular appearance that may be dense enough to obscure the nucleus. Clue cells are said to suggest infection with *Corynebacterium vaginale.*

Prepare the Gram stain as usual on the air-dried smear. The vaginal specimen may reveal *Candida:* large blue black, oval, budding yeast forms often seen with the broad, filamentous pseudomycelia; *Corynebacterium vaginale:* sheets of large, flat, epithelial cells literally covered with small pleomorphic rods to the exclusion of all other flora and Gram variable (but often Gram negative); *Neisseria gonorrhoeae:* the typical Gram negative diplococci packed within the cytoplasm of the polymorphonuclear neutrophils. Other *Neisseria* are part of the normal flora of the female genital tract but remain extracellular. The Gram stain must not be interpreted as suggesting gonorrhea if only extracellular Gram negative diplococci are present. *Trichomonas vaginale* is not easily identified in the Gram stain preparation. One or more of these conditions may coexist within the same patient.

All women suspected of having gonorrhea should have a swab from the endocervix cultured on standard Thayer-Martin medium. All smears positive for the gonococcus should be confirmed by culture. *Trichomonas vaginalis* and *Corynebacterium vaginale* can be cultured, but these procedures are not routinely available in most hospital bacteriology laboratories. *Candida* will grow on almost any routine bacteriologic medium except Thayer-Martin, which contains nystatin.

Background Information

The most frequent causes of pathologic vaginal discharge are infectious. Four agents account for 80–90% of all cases.

Trichomonas. This protozoan parasite grows well under slightly acid conditions (pH 5.6–6.5). The normal vaginal pH of the adult vagina under hormonal influence is less than 4.0. Menstrual blood is a good buffer. Parasite loads may increase markedly and symptoms suddenly appear at the time of menses, when the pH rises. The urethra and periurethral glands are colonized in 95% of women with trichomoniasis. The endocervix is rarely infected. Systemic treatment is superior to local therapy such as douching, since organisms in extravaginal sites can result in reinfection of the vagina. *Trichomonas* is sexually transmitted. Up to 70% of the male sex partners of infected women will have trichomonads demonstrable in urine sediment or prostatic secretions. Simultaneous treatment of sex partners is necessary.

The classical clinical picture is that of reddened edematous labia with a copious, greenish white, frothy, disagreeable smelling, oozing discharge. The posterior vaginal walls and cervix are often covered with punctate hemorrhages. This so-called strawberry cervix is almost pathognomonic, but occurs within only a small percentage of infections.

Candida.   Several species of *Candida,* including *C. albicans,* normally inhabit the vagina; all may be pathogenic on certain occasions. There is no sure test which will allow one to tell when *Candida* species are actually causing vaginitis or merely part of the normal flora, but the presence of large numbers of yeast buds and mycelial elements should increase the suspicion that *Candida* is causing the disease. Certain risk factors also play a role in producing candidal vaginitis: uncontrolled diabetes mellitus, steroids, broad-spectrum antibiotic use, treatment of trichomoniasis with metronidazole (Flagyl), hypoparathyroidism, birth control pills with high estrogen content, and tight, constricting, nonventilated clothing such as pantyhose. Recurrence is frequent. In resistant cases, oral nystatin to prevent endogenous reinfection from the gastrointestinal tract, or examination of sexual partners for *C. balanitis* may help.

The discharge, usually scant, is thick and creamy white in appearance and is often likened to cottage cheese. It is usually adherent to the vaginal walls and vulva. Pruritus may be intense.

Corynebacterium vaginale.   The pathologic significance of this organism is controversial. Some feel it is a rare cause of vaginitis, others that it may cause up to 90% of vaginitis when trichomonas or candidiasis has been excluded. Up to 40% of women carrying the organism have no symptoms.

Corynebacterium vaginale, like *Candida,* can obviously be a commensal. The factors responsible for allowing pathogenic expression are not known.

The organism may be sexually transmitted, thus the infection is seen almost exclusively in sexually active women. In the majority of symptomatic cases, the organism can be recovered from the urethras of sexual partners. Some authorities advocate simultaneous treatment.

The clinical syndrome is usually mild. Vaginal discharge is scant, thin, and grayish white. Symptoms are not related to menses. There is often a mild dysuria, vaginal soreness, and a diffuse mildly red vaginal wall. The external genitalia are usually normal.

Corynebacterium vaginale is difficult to grow and identify accurately. Heavy reliance is placed on the Gram stain, where one sees sheets of the organisms on vaginal (not endocervical) material, virtually replacing the normal flora, and on the wet mount for identification of clue cells.

Gonorrhea. After puberty, circulating estrogens stimulate cornification of the vaginal epithelium. This epithelium is resistant to direct infection with *Neisseria gonorrhoeae.* Thus gonorrhea in the postpubertal woman is an infection of the endocervix, urethra, or rectum—areas lined with cuboidal, transitional, or columnar epithelium. About one-third of women with endocervical gonorrhea are seen initially because of "vaginal discharge," which actually originates in the endocervix, but is seen by the patient at the introitus.

A Gram stain of endocervical material (not vaginal) is an acceptable rapid method for making a presumptive diagnosis of gonorrhea. The method has serious limitations, however, which must be borne in mind if the technique is to be applied successfully. First, compared to the endocervical culture, the Gram stain is insensitive. In a group of women at high risk for gonorrhea, the smear will be negative in more than half who actually have gonorrhea. A negative smear can never be used to reassure a patient that she does not have gonorrhea. On the other hand, it is rarely positive if gonorrhea is not present by culture. In this situation the probability that one will correctly diagnose gonorrhea if the Gram stain is positive is greater than 80%. A drawback of the smear is that some experience in interpretation is necessary. Therefore we recommend the following: cultures should *always* be done. If the smear is positive, the patient should be treated for gonorrhea while waiting for culture results. If the smear is negative, but clinical or epidemiologic evidence makes the diagnosis of gonorrhea likely, treatment should be given pending the culture. All smears should be confirmed by culture.

The overall sensitivity of the single endocervical culture is 80–90%. Doing either a rectal culture in addition or two successive cervical cultures may increase the yield. All women should be recultured within one week after treatment.

Nonspecific vaginitis. About 10% of women with vaginitis will have negative examination for pathogenic organisms after using the tests outlined above. As the diagnostic acumen of the physician increases, the proportion of women falling into this group decreases. Since therapy of these women is unsatisfactory, a genuine search for an etiologic agent should be made. Frequently women with repeated vaginal infection are considered to have a "vaginal fixation" or are termed "vaginal cripples." If you espouse this view, so may your patient. Time and a positive, searching frame of mind are needed to solve this complex problem.

Physiologic vaginal discharge. It is important to realize that a vaginal discharge may be a normal response to high estrogen levels. Discharge may occur:

1.   At the time of ovulation: "ovulary cascade"
2.   In the immediate premenstrual period
3.   During pregnancy
4.   During oral contraceptive use

The characteristics of a normal vaginal discharge are:

1.   May leave a brownish stain on underclothing
2.   Odor is not offensive
3.   Nonpruritic, no vulvar soreness
4.   Few PMNs (Polymorphonuclear Neutrophil Leukocytes) on microscopic examination of discharge
5.   Normal vaginal flora is present (predominantly fat Gram negative rods, Döderlein's bacilli, which are probably lactobacilli)

Clinical Significance

Vaginal discharge is the complaint which most frequently brings symptomatic women to a venereal disease clinic, and accounts for over half of visits to the private gynecologist's office.

The physician should pinpoint the etiologic agent for several reasons:

1.   Correct therapy for each agent mentioned above is specific. No one drug can eradicate all forms of vaginitis. Treatment with broad-spectrum antibiotics in a blind fashion may confuse the diagnosis by allowing candidal overgrowth while suppressing the actual causative agent.
2.   Several of these agents are sexually transmitted, and in these cases examination and treatment of infected sexual partners should be considered as a part of the patient's therapy.
3.   There is morbidity associated with certain of these conditions:
   a.   Trichomoniasis: Women infected at the time of delivery are more likely to develop postpartum fever of frank endometritis than the noninfected. Consorts of infected women may be at risk for prostatitis. A heavy infestation can interfere with the diagnosis of cervical malignancy by Pap smear.
   b.   Candidiasis: Children born through an infected birth canal have a high probability of contracting neonatal thrush.
   c.   Gonorrhea: Significant local complications such as bartholinitis and pelvic inflammatory disease with irreversible sterility may occur. Systemic dissemination through the

bloodstream may occur from any infected local site with the development of septic arthritis, endocarditis, or meningitis.

Selected References

1. Trends in candidal vaginitis. *Proc R Soc Med* 70 (suppl 4), 1977.
2. Lewis JF, O'Brien SM, Ural UM, Burke T: Corynebacterium vaginale vaginitis: Review of the literature. *Am J Obstet Gyn* 112:87–90, 1972.
3. Rein MF, Chapel TA: Trichomoniasis, candidiasis and the minor venereal diseases. *Clin Obstet Gyn* 18:73–88, 1975.
4. Dykers JR: Single dose metronidazole for trichomonal vaginitis. *New Eng J Med* 293:23–24, 1975.

75. Abnormal Vaginal Bleeding

JOHN D. THOMPSON, MD
JOHN R. K. PREEDY, MD

Definition

The following information is obtained:

1. Onset of menses (menarche)
2. Cessation of menses (menopause)
3. The characteristics of the menstrual cycle
   a. The menstrual interval: time from the first day of one flow to the first day of the next flow
   b. Duration of flow: the number of days of menstrual flow
   c. Amount of flow
   d. Last monthly period
4. Postcoital bleeding (any bleeding after intercourse or in association with douching)
5. Postmenopausal bleeding (*any* bleeding occurring in the postmenopausal female)

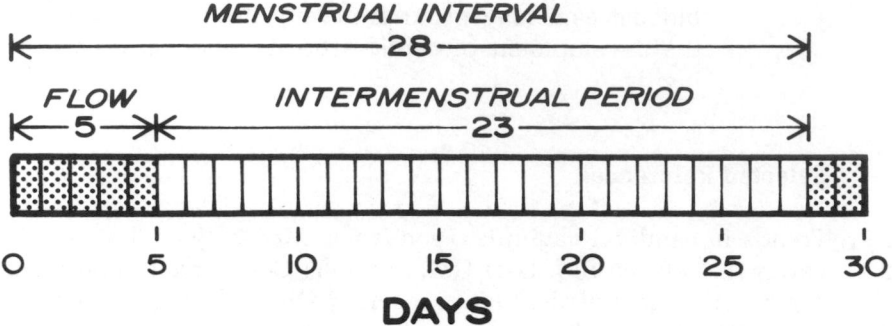

DAYS

ABNORMAL MENSTRUAL INTERVAL

1. POLYMENORRHEA(frequent menses) – Menstrual interval less than 21 days.

2. OLIGOMENORRHEA(infrequent menses) – Menstrual interval greater than 37 days and less than 90 days.

3. AMENORRHEA–Absence of menses for any period greater than 90 days.

ABNORMAL DURATION OF FLOW

1. METRORRHAGIA– Increased duration of flow beyond 7 days (continuous).

2. INTERMENSTRUAL BLEEDING–Bleeding in the inter-menstrual period(discontinuous).

Figure 6.   Terms denoting abnormal menses.

The definitions of normal and abnormal for the information listed above are given in the Background Information. Fig 6 illustrates some of the terms listed above.

Technique

Begin by asking the patient about the onset of menses, which is usually at 10–15 years of age. Then determine if the patient has ceased menstruation, which usually occurs between ages 45–50 years. Determine the menstrual interval or length of the cycle. This is counted from the first day of one flow to the first day of the next flow; ordinarily this is 26–30 days. Next ask about the duration of flow, which is usually 3–5 days. The intermenstrual period can then be determined. Count from the last day of one flow to the first day of the next flow.

The amount of flow is very important to determine. A careful history must be obtained for the flow to be properly evaluated. Simply asking a patient if her flow is normal is not sufficient. The patient may not understand whether or not her flow is normal because she has no basis for comparison. Her impression of her flow and whether it is light, normal, or heavy is important from the standpoint of knowing how she feels about herself, however. Additional helpful questions are: How many tampons or pads do you use on the heaviest day of your flow? How well soaked are these tampons or pads? A patient who is very fastidious about her menstrual flow may change pads when there is just the slightest sign of staining. She may actually use as many as 10–12 tampons or pads per day but lose less blood than another patient who uses only 4 pads per day but does not change pads until they are soaked from corner to corner. Patients who bleed very heavily may also state the necessity for using two tampons or pads at a time or sheets or towels. The passage of definite aggregates of red blood cells, or "clots," is significant and indicates heavy bleeding. Ordinarily if the menstrual flow can be controlled with the use of vaginal tampons alone, one can assume that the menstrual flow is not too heavy.

A patient may have a heavy menstrual flow with a normal hemoglobin and hematocrit value. Excess menstruation may result in iron deficiency, but iron deficiency anemia is a late manifestation of excessive menstrual flow. Therefore a history of excessive menstrual flow should not be discounted simply on the basis of a normal hematocrit value.

It is important to specifically ask the patient about her last period. Many patients will assume that the occurrence of any bleeding episode is a "period." Lack of this distinction can result in misleading information.

The date of the last menstrual period should be included in the data base of all female patients. Record the date that the menstrual flow began. Therefore simply asking a patient, "When was your last menstrual period?" is not sufficient. Ask instead, "When was the first day of your last menstrual period?" Also record the duration of flow in the number of days. The date of the previous menstrual period (PMP) should be recorded with the duration of flow. Then ask the patient if these periods were normal. Any deviation from normal should be recorded. Whenever the data base is updated, the date of the last menstrual period should also be updated.

Ask the patient if there is any evidence of bleeding after intercourse or in association with douching.

The significance of a variety of gynecologic complaints and findings changes tremendously with menopause. Any complaint of vaginal bleeding after menopause is considered abnormal. No matter how slight the bleeding, always consider this abnormal and investigate.

Background Information

Onset of menses (menarche).   Menstruation usually begins at age 10–15. Young girls who have not menstruated before age 15 or who have vaginal bleeding before age 10 should be suspected of having gynecologic disease. Menarche usually appears 1 or 2 years after thelarche, or breast development.

Cessation of menses (menopause).   The menopause with associated symptoms and cessation of menses usually occurs at age 45–50. A patient who is still menstruating regularly at age 52 should have a D and C even if she is asymptomatic. A patient who has stopped her menses for 6–12 months then begins again to have vaginal bleeding hould have a careful examination. If the examination does not reveal a gross neoplasm of the cervix, then a D and C must be done.

Characteristics of the menstrual cycle.   Three clinical characteristics of cyclic menstruation should be recorded for the adult patient:

1. The menstrual interval (length of cycle). The menstrual interval is counted from the first day of one flow to the first day of the next flow (ordinarily 26–30). The definition of a normal menstrual interval is 21–37 days. Therefore menstruation occurring more frequently than 21 days is considered abnormal (polymenorrhea), and menstruation occurring less frequently than every 37 days is considered abnormal (oligomenorrhea). If menses has been absent for 90 days, the patient is said to have amenorrhea.

2. The duration of flow. This is usually 3–5 days, but a duration of 7 days is still considered normal. If the duration of flow is greater than 7 days, the patient is said to have metrorrhagia (bleeding beyond the normal duration of flow and into the intermenstrual period). The intermenstrual period is counted from the last day of one flow to the first day of the next flow. Therefore metrorrhagia and intermenstrual bleeding are synonymous. In practical usage these terms are distinguished from each other depending on whether the bleeding is continuous into the intermenstrual period (metrorrhagia) or discontinuous into the intermenstrual period (intermenstrual bleeding). This is explained in Fig 1.

3. The amount of flow is more difficult to define. The normal amount of blood lost with each menstrual flow is 30–50 cc. However, there is no practical way to measure the amount of flow, and its evaluation is therefore rather subjective. Menorrhagia and hypermenorrhea refer to an increase in the amount of menstrual flow. Hypomenorrhea refers to a decrease in the amount of menstrual flow.

Healthy adult females usually menstruate normally. However a patient cannot be guaranteed a complete state of health simply because her menstruation is normal, even though women who menstruate normally usually feel better and think of themselves as healthy.

On the other hand, the patient is likely to consider abnormal menstruation as a sign of ill health. It may be a manifestation of either a general medical disease or a specific gynecologic problem. For example, oligomenorrhea and amenorrhea may be associated with hypothyroidism, or the same menstrual problem may be associated with tuberculosis. Thrombocytopenia may be associated with menorrhagia or metrorrhagia, or both.

ENDOCRINE CONTROL OF THE MENSES

Menarche. The inception of menses (menarche) is dependent upon the previous development of normal puberty. Menarche is the latest event in puberty. The mechanisms responsible for the start of puberty, and for the resulting menarche, are to a great extent unknown. Puberty is associated with an increased secretion of gonadotropin-releasing hormone (GnRH) from the hypothalamus, and consequent increased secretion of the gonadotropins follicle-stimulating hormone (FSH) and luteinizing hormone (LH) from the adenohypophysis. This results in increased secretion of estrogens (mostly estradiol-17β, some estrone) from the ovary. Finally cyclic secretion of GnRH, FSH, and LH is established, and in consequence cyclic secretion of estrogens and progesterone by the ovaries occurs. As a result of this, the endometrium undergoes cyclic stimulation, and menses start.

Menstrual cycle. The normal menstrual cycle depends, as mentioned above, on the cyclic secretion of GnRH by the hypothalamus, resulting in cyclic secretion of FSH and LH by the adenohypophysis, resulting in cyclic secretion of estrogens and progesterone by the ovary, resulting finally in cyclic stimulation of the endometrium.

On the first day of the menstrual flow, plasma levels of FSH, LH, estrogens, and progesterone are relatively low. Plasma estrogens rise slowly during the first 12 days and then more abruptly around the thirteenth to fifteenth day, producing a midcycle peak. The level then diminishes somewhat, to rise again about the twenty-second day to form a second (luteal) peak, and falls finally to low levels as the menstrual flow starts again. Plasma FSH and LH are also low during the menstrual flow and remain low until the thirteenth to fifteenth day, when there is a sharp and abrupt rise in concentration which rapidly subsides (midcycle peak). This peak appears to follow the midcycle estrogen peak by some hours. There is but one peak for both FSH and LH. Plasma progesterone remains low until after the midcycle. The concentration then rises to form a broad luteal peak corresponding with the luteal estrogen peak, and falls to low levels as the menstrual flow starts. The midcycle peak of gonadotropins appears to be responsible for ovulation, and the luteal estrogen and progesterone peaks correspond to the formation of and the secretion by the corpus luteum. The elevation of plasma estrogens during the first part of the midcycle estrogen peak is thought to trigger the gonadotropin peak, with subsequent ovulation.

Menopause. The menopause can be regarded as physiological ovarian failure. For reasons unknown the ovary ceases to respond to gonadotropin stimulation at around the age of 45. Plasma estradiol-17β is low, and since there is no ovulation, plasma progesterone remains low. The endometrium is therefore not stimulated and there are no menses. Plasma FSH and LH are greatly elevated and remain so for many years.

Clinical Significance

A variety of gynecologic problems is associated with abnormal menstruation. Invasive cervical cancer may cause menometrorrhagia or postcoital bleeding, or both. Tubal pregnancy may cause oligomenorrhea followed by metrorrhagia. Uterine myomata, pelvic endometriosis, pelvic inflammatory disease, adenomyosis, and dysfunctional uterine bleeding may cause menorrhagia. Adenomatous endometrial hyperplasia and endometrial adenocarcinoma may cause postmenopausal bleeding. Functioning ovarian tumors may cause a variety of menstrual abnormalities, depending upon the hormone produced by the tumor. Normal intrauterine pregnancy is the most frequent explanation for oligomenorrhea followed by amenorrhea.

Many associated findings in the history and the physical examination must be evaluated in order to determine the etiology of the abnormal bleeding. The basic general complete gynecologic history and physical examination will be extremely helpful. Ask about associated pain, discharge, bladder symptoms, nausea and vomiting, fever, infertility, and other history points. During the physical examination look for such conditions as abnormal phenotype breast development, abnormal hair distribution, thyroid enlargement, abdominal distention and tenderness, and hepatomegaly. Look for pelvic tumor, cervical lesions, polyps, and tenderness on the pelvic examination. Special diagnostic procedures such as hormonal assays, visual field, chest x-rays, laparoscopy, vaginal cytology, colposcopy, ultrasonography, culdocentesis, endometrial curretage, pelvic examination under anesthesia, and many others are helpful.

Selected Reference

1. Novak ER, Jones GS, Jones HW: *Novak's Textbook of Gynecology,* ed 9. Baltimore, Williams and Wilkins, 1975.

76. Pelvic Mass

JOHN D. THOMPSON, MD

Definition

Either a sensation of a mass in the lower abdomen or the actual discovery of one by a patient.

Technique

It is important to completely describe a mass in the data base so that subsequent examiners can determine whether or not there has been any change. This is particularly important in managing patients with an adnexal mass. Its consistency, size, shape, location, movability, and tenderness should be described in detail. The size of the mass should be described in terms of actual measurements. Use of descriptions such as "the size of a grapefruit" is not helpful, may be misleading, and should be avoided.

Background Information

A mass on the vulva may be a condyloma, a neoplasm, vulvar varicosities, or granulomatous venereal disease. Patients who have a Bartholin gland duct abscess or cyst may complain of a mass on one side of the vaginal introitus. Relaxation of the anterior vaginal wall resulting in a urethrocele and cystocele may present as a mass at the vaginal introitus.

The same is true of relaxations of the posterior vaginal wall, resulting in a rectocele and an enterocele. Uterine descensus or complete prolapse of the uterus may also be found in a patient complaining of a mass extending from the vulva.

Most of the above problems can be identified by simple inspection and palpation during the course of the complete gynecologic examination.

Clinical Significance

Gynecologic patients sometimes present with the complaint that they can feel a mass. The mass may be in the lower abdomen in the midline or on one or both sides. There also may be a mass in the groin, on the vulva, around the introitus or coming through the introitus.

A mass in the lower abdomen may or may not be associated with other complaints such as pain, pressure on the bladder and/or rectum, abdominal swelling, fever, oligomenorrhea, and amenorrhea or meno-metrorrhagia. A mass which arises from the pelvis may extend all the way to the upper abdomen. Such masses are usually either large uterine myomata or large ovarian cysts. A mass in the abdomen should always be listened to with a stethoscope for evidence of a bruit or perhaps fetal heart tones in a patient who is pregnant. Special diagnostic procedures may be helpful in determining the etiology of the mass. These would include pregnancy tests, ultrasonography, x-ray of the abdomen, barium enema, gastrointestinal series, intravenous pyelography, pelvic arteriography, and sometimes abdominal paracentesis may be necessary. The fluid should be examined cytologically.

Selected Reference

1.   Novak ER, Jones GS, Jones HW: *Novak's Textbook of Gynecology,* ed 9. Baltimore, Williams and Wilkins, 1975.

SEXUAL DIFFICULTIES

77. Introduction to the Sexual History

MALCOLM G. FREEMAN, MD

The process of taking a useful and accurate sexual history is sufficiently threatening to most clinicians to justify some special comment. It is easy for the physician to excuse the omission of a sexual history on any one of several grounds:

1.   I'm in a hurry.
2.   It isn't pertinent to this patient's illness.

3. The patient didn't mention any sexual complaint.
4. I respect the patient's privacy whenever possible.
5. If I ask sexual questions, the patient may think I'm a pervert or a nut.
6. The patient might be embarrassed.
7. I will next time.
8. Her gynecologist takes care of that.

The real reasons are more often:

1. I really don't know how to go about it.
2. I'm always in a hurry and never take a very complete history.
3. I never ask sexual questions.
4. I forgot because I was more "interested in" (comfortable with) the other problem.
5. If I asked and uncovered a problem, I wouldn't have any idea what to do about it.
6. I would be embarrassed.
7. I often forget that patients have sexual lives which are important to them.
8. You can't send everyone to a psychiatrist.
9. Hell, nobody's sex life is perfect, my own included.

Taking a sexual history serves two functions. First, it may identify problem areas which justify active treatment. Second, it serves notice to the patient that the physician sees sexual function as an important and integral part of the medical history and life-style of the patient and demonstrates that the physician is ready and willing to discuss sexual problems in the future should the patient desire.

The patient views his or her sexual life and performance as private but very important. If an illness has had or is likely to have an impact on sexual feelings and activity, the patient wants to know the facts and understand them thoroughly. The patient's sexual partner is equally involved, concerned, and anxious for information.

Partner: "Did you ask him how soon we could begin to make love?"
Postoperative (or postcoronary) patient: "He just said to take it easy for a while."
Partner: "What does that mean?"
Postoperative patient: "I don't know."

It is difficult to think of an illness that doesn't have an impact on sexual function, from tonsillitis ("How long will you be infectious?") to a broken foot ("I can't get on top with this damn cast on my leg").

Often the patient's initial complaint is intended only as an introduction, which the patient hopes will lead to a more specific discussion of sexual problems.

> *Patient:* "I'm having pains in my stomach," or, "I haven't been feeling well lately."

When a physician deals with this initial complaint summarily or dismisses it as unimportant, the patient becomes confused and angry because the hoped-for gradual disclosure has been thwarted. If, however, a sexual function history becomes a routine part of data collection, then the patient has a nonthreatening opportunity to expand on the original complaint.

Like all other parts of the data base, the type and complexity of the data collected vary according to the patient's problem. Familiarity with the various forms of human sexual inadequacy makes the physician sensitive to patient response and indicates directions for further questioning. Familiarity with normal sexual anatomy and physiology lends the physician a sense of confidence and assurance in dealing with sexually confused or dysfunctional patients.

I. SEXUAL WORDS

Words allow us to transfer complex ideas and experiences to another person rapidly. When a physician and a patient communicate, they must find some common or equally acceptable vocabulary if information, ideas, and feelings are to be exchanged effectively and comfortably. The following techniques are useful in dealing with sexual words.

1. Never accept a sexual term at face value until you are sure what the patient means by it.

> *Patient:* "I'm impotent."
> *Physician:* "Do you mean that you have trouble getting an erection, have trouble keeping the erection long enough to use it, or something else?" or "What do you mean by that? What does the term 'impotent' mean to you?"

2. Be sensitive and inquiring about the sort of terms with which the patient is comfortable. Keep a mental or written list. If it appears necessary to discuss sexual function at any length with the patient, it is permissible to ask directly about terms they use together.

> *Physician:* "When you and your husband are talking about his penis, his sexual organ, what do you call it?"

3. When your patient seems confused by terminology, it may be helpful to use several different terms in a series to convey the idea. The terms selected are usually the least "loaded" words known.

Physician: "Are you having any pain or discomfort in your vulva—your female organs—your privates?"

4. Once a patient has used a nonscientific but understandable sexual term, it is permissible for the physician to use the same term.

Patient: "I really like it when he goes down on me."
Physician: "Do you ever come—have an orgasm when he goes down on you?"

5. Rarely and cautiously a physician may introduce common or slang terms into the conversation. This is more often done with younger patients and usually only when some mutual respect and rapport have been established between the patient and physician.

Physician: "It seems to me you've been saying that there has been a lot of screwing in this marriage but not much loving."
Patient: "That's right."

Too often both physician and patient try to use the physician's vocabulary. This results in discomfort and confusion on the part of the patient who may be trying to use or understand unfamiliar or half-understood words. Communication is enhanced when the physician adapts to the patient, instead of vice versa. The effective physician must master many vocabularies and adjust his language to meet the communication needs of individual patients. This is part of the art of medicine rather than the science. It is as important a skill as surgical technique or differential diagnosis.

In American culture, sexual words are particularly difficult for patients and often for physicians as well. Instead of accepting them as simple tools for effective communication, all sorts of taboos and value judgments are made which inhibit the free use of sexual words. Words in common, everyday usage by some people are regarded as gross obscenities by others. Patients often feel that the words they know and use regularly will not be acceptable to a physician-father-authority figure. Patients, therefore, are often uncomfortable using their own words and are uncertain about the precise meaning of both scientific and other less familiar slang expressions. Many commonly used terms have multiple meanings. Some examples are:

1.   "Make out" may mean manual or oral foreplay in some contexts and sexual intercourse in others.
2.   "Go to bed" covers a range of activities from watching television to sleep to coitus.

Patients often use terms which they believe will earn approval from physicians. Many of these may be imperfectly understood or incorrectly used by the well-intentioned patient.

Patient: "I have a pain in my vagina."

No words are inherently dirty, indecent, or immoral. Physicians should use sexual words with which patients are familiar and comfortable.

II. PROBLEMS IN SEXUAL HISTORY TAKING: ASSUMPTIONS AND BIASES

In sexual history taking there is a grave risk that the examiner will assume too much about the patient from superficial clues or from the examiner's personal biases. Such assumptions put the examiner at a great disadvantage and confuse as well as embarrass the patient. The usual result of such assumptions is the loss of time, valuable information, and rapport with the patient. It is axiomatic that the examiner cannot be certain about *anything* concerning the patient's sexuality from a superficial examination of dress, manner, or style. Indeed, many patients' dress, manners, and style are deliberate or unonscious strategies to hide true sexual feelings and attitudes. It is best to approach all patients with a clean slate and allow them to express personal feelings and attitudes. Observations of dress, manners, or style coupled with history are extremely informative but must not distract the examiner from history taking.

The examiner's own biases may distract the direction of history taking. Common biases are:

Young people aren't sexual yet.
Old people aren't sexual anymore.
Dignified, mature men and women can't be very concerned about their sexuality.
Married people can't have venereal disease.
"Nice" people don't enjoy sexual variations.
Girls who dress sexy are sexy.

Effeminate men are gay.

You can always tell gay people by the way they act.

Sick people aren't sexual.

Blind, deaf, cerebral palsied, and paraplegic people aren't sexual.

Women aren't gay.

Women don't get horny.

Nobody over 35 ever heard of fellatio and cunnilingus, much less has tried them.

My mother and father never had intercourse—or at least not often—or at least not anymore.

If you are a woman, you must either want a man or already have a man.

Patients never get sexually interested in their doctors.

Doctors never get sexually interested in patients.

Fat people aren't sexual.

Ugly people aren't sexual.

Retarded people aren't sexual.

Black people are different from white people.

Oriental people are probably different from black people and white people—at least they are inscrutable and polite.

There are two kinds of women; the good kind, mothers and sisters, and the other kind.

The world is pretty much the way I see it, and normal people are pretty much like me except that I am exceptional.

Acting from these or similar biases can erase much of the effectiveness of any history taker. All people have biases of some sort, determined by their learned concept of what the world is like. Setting aside biases is a conscious act requiring practice and at best can be only partial. For that reason, each history taker should begin with a clean slate.

III. HOMOSEXUALITY

The purpose of this section is to comment on homosexuality in the context of sexual history. Questions about homosexuality are not a routine part of survey-type sexual history taking. They become appropriate when the examiner begins to feel that the patient has anxiety about his sexual role or expresses some discomfort in the area of roles.

If the patient describes himself as a homosexual, then the examiner's next concern is to determine if this represents a fact, a fear, or a self-castigating label. Homosexuals exist in two situations—covert (in the closet, secret) and overt (out, out of the closet). Traditionally in American culture to "come out" is an act of great bravery which exposes the homosexual to risk of societal and individual rejection as well as physical attacks and arrest. The person whose major erotic interest is in individuals of the same sex may reject his own feelings, may accept the feelings but be uncomfortable living with them, or may need help in adjusting to the feelings of others toward him.

Others who describe themselves as homosexual may be expressing a fear based upon one or more childhood or adolescent experiences of genital exposure, mutual masturbation, or the like. It is, of course, common for adults to have had one or more such experiences and to have found them exciting without any general preference for partners of the same sex. It is also common for individuals who have a heterosexual partner to fear rejection if their history of same-sex experience or of their occasional preference for same-sex partners became known.

Many patients who have fears that they may be homosexual can be relieved and reassured by such questions as:

> Most boys and girls can remember playing sexual games when they were very young—like playing doctor, or "I'll show you mine, if you'll show me yours." Do you remember any experiences like that when you were growing up?
>
> Many adolescents are introduced to masturbation by friends or by older children who demonstrate how to do it. How did you first learn about masturbation? Did you have any experience with other people or was it always by yourself?
>
> Can you ever remember a time when you were approached by a homosexual? Most people have been at one time or another. How did you react—was it a good experience for you or bad?

Sometimes the examiner will sense that the patient has strong concerns about homosexuality but is unable to verbalize them. In such a circumstance the examiner may ask: At any time in your life has there been another man (another woman) was was important to you sexually—someone with whom you had an important relationship? The patient may find this a more comfortable and nonjudgmental question to answer.

Often it is helpful to pose theoretical questions to get an idea of the patient's feeling about homosexuality. These can be phrased in two series (for convenience I will phrase them as if to a husband):

> What do you suppose your wife would think (feel, do) if she found out you...? What would you think (do, feel) if you found out your wife...
>
> > had a homosexual experience in the past?
> > is actively homosexual now?
> > had had an extramarital sexual affair?
> > had to have a breast removed?

wanted to have anal sex?
wanted to be tied up during sex?
wanted to swap partners with another couple?
wanted to be spanked during sex?

There are an infinite number of variations which can be used to explore other sexual attitudes and feelings.

Over the last several thousand years of human history, societal attitudes toward homosexuality have varied greatly. In the recent past, it was believed that homosexuality was a mental aberration which if "cured" would result in "normal" heterosexual feelings. At the present time, many experts believe that erotic preference for individuals of the same sex simply represents an alternate life-style. Homosexuality is no longer classified as a disease.

Individual homosexuals are therefore caught in a slow and painful period of societal transition, still receiving powerful negative and punitive messages from traditional sources and, at the same time, strong underground and aboveground messages from more liberal sources. As a consequence, homosexuals often have major problems being comfortable in their sexual role and in having it accepted by others. Less often do they wish to change it to a heterosexual role.

Most terms that have been applied to homosexuals are regarded by them as derogatory and are therefore rejected. The most widely accepted terms for homosexuals seem to be "gay" for males and "gay" or "lesbian" for females. "Gay" is without question the safest term to use in 1979.

Homosexuals may have sexual dysfunctions with a same-sex partner just as heterosexuals may have with an other-sex partner. The male homosexual may therefore suffer from erective difficulty, ejaculatory incompetence, or premature ejaculation; and the female homosexual may be anorgasmic.

Although many same sex couples live together for many years, homosexual relationships in general have tended to be more often transitory than permanent. This increases the likelihood of venereal disease transmission as well as the frustration of searching for emotionally gratifying relationships. Homosexual couples develop the same problems of communication and all the other relationship problems seen in heterosexual couples.

IV. SEXUAL HISTORY TAKING WHEN THE INITIAL COMPLAINT IS NOT SPECIFICALLY SEXUAL

The female.   Among female patients there are two points in history taking which provide easy access to sexual history. These are: (1) menstrual history, which leads naturally into coital and reproductive history; and (2) family history, which leads naturally into parental and sibling relationships; relations with the same sex and opposite sex peers; and dating, courting, and petting history.

Either or both of these approaches can be used comfortably by the physician, but the menstrual history approach is more appropriate in a health survey situation.

In the following, the essential survey-type questions of the female sexual function history (as distinct from the routine gynecology-obstetric history) are marked by an asterisk. They are designed to assess the patient's sexual function and level of satisfaction at the present time.

Menstrual History Approach

When was your last period?
How many days did it last?
Do you use tampons or pads?
How many times did you change tampons on the heaviest day?
Was that a normal period?
When was the last period before that?
Was it about like your most recent period?
How often do your periods usually come?
Do you ever miss periods?
Do your breasts bother you before or during a period?
Do you have any pain or discomfort during your period?
How old were you when you had your first period?
Did your mother or anyone else explain about periods to you?
During the first year or so after your periods began, did they bother you in any way?
How old were you when you stopped growing taller?
How old were you when you began to grow breasts, hips, pubic hair?
Do you remember how you felt about going through the changes of puberty? Was that an easy or a difficult time for you?
Do you remember how old you were when you had intercourse for the first time?
What were the circumstances?
  * Are you having intercourse now? (see section on Frequency of Intercourse)
  * About how often? (per month, or per week)
  * Is that an increase or decrease from previous years?
  * Do you have any pain or discomfort when you have intercourse? (see section on Dyspareunia and Vaginismus)
  * Is intercourse pleasurable for you?
  * Are you having orgasms? (Do you reach a climax? Can you come? see section on Anorgasmia)
  * About what percent of the time do you have orgasm?

* Are you satisfied with intercourse the way it is for you now?
* Do you think your partner is satisfied with intercourse the way it is now?

Do you want to become pregnant now?

What are you using to keep from getting pregnant? (This leads into a contraceptive and reproductive history.)

The male. Obtaining a sexual history from males is somewhat less complex than the same task from females in spite of the fact that males are no less anxious about sexual matters and, in many cases, seem to be even more so than females. Most females have had some experience with physician-asked sexual questions related to menstruation and pregnancy. Most males have never been asked by a physician to describe their sexual functioning in any way at all. In addition, many if not most males in American culture are performance oriented and concerned lest they be sexually judged and found wanting. Women tend to be much more open and matter-of-fact about sexual feelings and gratification. Men tend to be more open about techniques and mechanics of sexual expression.

The technique of psychosocial history taking from men does not differ greatly from that of women, and questions are generally equally applicable. Specific coital history can begin within the genitourinary portion of systems review:

Are you having sexual intercourse now? (see section on Frequency of Intercourse)

About how often do you have intercourse (per week or per month)?

Is that an increase or a decrease from previous years?

What do you think has brought about a change in the frequency of intercourse?

At the present time, do you ever have any difficulty in getting an erection when you want it? (see section on Erective Difficulty)

Have you ever had that problem in the past?

Have you ever had a problem of coming too soon (ejaculating) before you wanted to? (see section on Premature Ejaculation)

Is that a problem for you now?

Was it ever a problem when you were a young man?

Do you ever find that your erection is all right but you are unable to come—to ejaculate?

Have you noticed any changes in your sexual feelings or your sexual functions recently?

If so, can you tell me about that?

Are you satisfied with your sexual functioning (your sex life) the way it is now?

Do you think that your partner is satisfied with things the way they are now?

V. SEXUAL HISTORY TAKING WHEN THE INITIAL COMPLAINT IS SPECIFICALLY SEXUAL

Annon has described a sexual problem history format divided into five parts:

1.   Description of the problem in the patient's own terms as much as possible. Clarify words and sexual terms used.
2.   Onset and cause of the problem. What were the time and situation in which the problem began? What has the course of the problem been; that is, what has happened over time?
3.   Patient's assessment of the cause. May be of great help in defining emotional response and attitudes of the patient to his problem. Avoid questions that include "Why?" since these tend to make people defensive.
4.   Past attempts at resolution: Professional as well as personal. Books read, nonprofessional advice received, the patient's own strategy. What has been the outcome of these attempts?
5.   Goals of the patient: What does the patient want? Patient goals may be far different than the therapist imagines. Does he/she want to save the marriage, reverse the symptoms, absolve him/herself of responsibility, punish the partner, provide data for separation or divorce, get permission for extramarital experiences? Is the goal that of the patient or of the patient's partner? Is the goal to feel "normal" or "average?"

When sexual partners are seen together, each will have a different viewpoint of the problem, its onset and course, its cause, attempts at resolution, and goals. Goals, particularly, may be quite different with as many as six different goals involved at the same time:

Partner A goal for self
Partner A goal for partner B
Partner A goal for relationship
Partner B goal for self
Partner B goal for partner A
Partner B goal for relationship

When the patient is seen alone but presents a problem which he perceives as primarily that of the partner, then history taking is distorted in another way. As the patient's insight into the problem changes, so does the history. The examiner must consider at all times where the patient is, in terms of understanding. The examiner must at all times remember that the history taken is one of both facts and feelings and that feelings are equally important.

Selected References

1. Annon JS: *The Behavioral Treatment of Sexual Problems*, vol 1: *Brief Theory*. Honolulu, Kapiolani Health Services, 1974.
2. Kaplan HS: *The New Sex Therapy: Active Treatment of Sexual Dysfunctions*. New York, Bruner/Mazel, The New York Times Book Co, 1974.
3. Masters WH, Johnson VE: *Human Sexual Inadequacy*. Boston, Little, Brown, 1970.
4. Masters WH, Johnson VE: *Human Sexual Response*. Boston, Little, Brown, 1900.

Frequency of Intercourse
MALCOLM G. FREEMAN, MD

Definition

There is no "normal" frequency of intercourse, but changes in coital frequency are of great significance in evaluating health and sexual function.

Technique

Begin by asking: Do you have a sexual partner now? Tell me something about your partner. If the patient has a partner ask: About how often are you having intercourse? per week or per month? Has there been any significant change in your frequency of intercourse in the last several years? If so, can you give me any idea as to why it has decreased (increased)? Reasons for change may include either patient or partner factors, or both. Such things as illness, physical separation, depression, alienation, sexual boredom, fatigue, work or household pressures, and fears of conception may be given as reasons for decrease. Such things as improved interpersonal relationships, relief from fear of pregnancy, a new partner, or regained health may be given as reasons for increased frequency.

If the patient responds negatively to the question of sexual intercourse, determine whether this absence of sexual activity with a partner is a change from previous habits or has been a lifelong habit. If a lifelong habit, it should be determined if this has been a voluntary choice or has been the result of other factors. Similarly, if celibacy is a change for this patient, some inquiry should be made as to the reason or reasons. The death or serious illness of a partner, divorce, separation, prolonged sexual dysfunction, or emotional incompatibility may be given as an explanation of sexual abstinence.

Background Information

Age and marital status should not be used as indicators of whether or not a patient is sexually active with a partner (partners). Sexual intercourse (implying penile-vaginal sexual connection) may not always be the most appropriate or exact term to use in order to describe an interpersonal sexual relationship. A patient may have had heterosexual and/or homosexual relationships which include oral, manual, and instrumental sexual manipulation and orgasm, or penile-anal penetration and, at least technically, still not have had intercourse. Most patients in a nonjudgmental setting do not quibble to that extreme and respond to questions about sexual experiences fairly readily and quite frankly. Never make the mistake of assuming that elderly, ill, or disabled patients are not sexually active.

The frequency of sexual intercourse varies according to opportunity, attitude, health, and age (Table 12). Coital frequency in marriage decreases fairly rapidly with advancing age but in many couples, coitus persists well into the seventies and eighties.

Table 12. Marital coitus: frequency per week as estimated by husbands and wives, 1972.*

	Husbands			Wives	
Age	Mean	Median	Age	Mean	Median
18–24	3.7	3.5	18–24	3.3	3.0
25–34	2.8	3.0	25–34	2.6	2.1
35–44	2.2	2.0	35–44	2.0	2.0
45–54	1.5	1.0	45–54	1.5	1.0
55 and over	1.0	1.0	55 and over	1.0	1.0

* Morton Hunt, *Sexual Behavior in the 1970's*, Playboy Press, 1974.

Clinical Significance

It is a mistake to allow patients to feel that you regard them as abnormal or atypical in coital frequency. Couples who regularly have coitus several times per day may be as normal as couples who seek sexual connection only every few months.

The biological capacity of woman for sexual intercourse and orgasm is far greater than that of man. Her capacity for multiple (read "unlimited numbers of") orgasms is well documented. The male's capacity for coitus leading to orgasm and ejaculation is limited by the "refractory period." Although young men sometimes can have repeated orgasms at a single sitting, there is, in general, a postorgasmic period in males during which it is first difficult to develop an erection and later, after erection is possible, difficult to ejaculate. This period of time varies from minutes in younger men to one or several days in aging men. Elongation of the refractory period is a normal part of the male aging process just as increased time to attain erection, decreased firmness of erection, and reduced force of ejaculation are. None of the above is a sign of impending impotence in the aging man. Just as it takes the aging man longer to walk around the block than it did in his twenties, so is the physical evidence of his sexual arousal somewhat delayed. It is no less pleasurable or gratifying, however.

Aging in women results in some reduction in vaginal lubrication and thinning of vaginal mucosa but does not ordinarily decrease capacity for sexual performance unless postmenopausal vaginal atrophy has occurred.

The maintenance of an active partner-oriented sexual life into advancing age depends upon three factors for men:

1. An interested and interesting partner
2. A reasonably good state of general health
3. Continuance of sexual activity without interruption

An aging man whose opportunity for partner sexual relations is interrupted by separation or partner death or by illness in himself or his partner for a period of months may lose his ability to develop and maintain an erection sufficient to effect satisfactory penetration. This is a disuse phenomenon and may be roughly compared to the athlete who drops out of training. When exercise is resumed, the athlete may have a significant reduction in ability to perform. In the case of the aging man, retraining may, but sometimes does not, result in return of erective capacity.

Maintenance of active coitus in the aging woman depends upon:

1. The availability of a male partner with the physical ability to perform
2. An interested and interesting partner

3. A reasonably good state of health
4. An estrogenized vaginal epithelium
5. Sufficient natural or artificial lubricant (water-soluble surgical lubricant, moisturizing nonalcoholic skin lotion, saliva)

Patients who have a single sexual partner have less risk of venereal disease but should not be regarded as having no risk. Any patient who describes more than one sexual partner is without question a high-risk candidate for venereal diseases. The risk is based not only on the increase in partners per se but also on the fact that patients who accept short-term partners are accepting individuals who are likely themselves to have had multiple previous short-term partners and are therefore more likely to have become infected.

Selected References

1. Annon JS: *The Behavioral Treatment of Sexual Problems,* Vol 1: *Brief Theory.* Honolulu, Kapiolani Health Services, 1974.
2. Hunt M: *Sexual Behavior in the 1970's.* Chicago, Playboy Press, 1974.
3. Kaplan HS: *The New Sex Therapy: Active Treatment of Sexual Dysfunctions.* New York, Bruner/Mazel, The New York Times Book Co, 1974.
4. Masters WH, Johnson VE: *Human Sexual Inadequacy.* Boston, Little, Brown, 1970.
5. Masters WH, Johnson VE: *Human Sexual Response.* Boston, Little, Brown, 1966.

Masturbation

MALCOLM G. FREEMAN, MD

Definition

The induction of sexually pleasurable sensations in self or another person by means of physical or psychic stimuli, usually deliberate. Often, but not necessarily, carried to the point of orgasm. Also called autoeroticism, onanism, self-gratification, self-abuse, jacking-off, and a host of other slang terms. When performed by partners upon each other, it is called mutual masturbation. Masturbation implies something other than genital to genital contact.

The sensory stimuli can be tactile, thermal, visual, auditory, gustatory, proprioceptive, and olfactory. The psychic stimuli often involve dream, fantasy, and memory.

Technique

Until recently, active self-induction of sexual pleasure was so heavily discouraged by persons in positions of authority that many individuals feel great guilt and perceive masturbation as a problem, a weakness, or a perversity. Masturbation in one form or another is an almost universal activity among men and is probably equally so among women.

While taking a history of masturbation, the physician should be nonthreatening, accepting, reassuring, and permission giving. The following questions should be asked of men: When did you first learn about masturbation? During your high school and college years did you have other sexual outlets besides masturbation? Since your marriage, has your frequency of masturbation increased, decreased, or stayed about the same? Approximately how often are you masturbating to orgasm at the present time?

For women, self-masturbation is even more guilt-laden than for males, since traditionally in American culture women have had less freedom to express their sexuality. As a consequence, some women avoid direct and obvious self-stimulation (that is, genital stroking, etc.) but still make heavy use of sensuous fabrics, scents, lotions, touch, massage, tight or loose clothing, and daydreams for self-gratification and to excite others sexually. Some women may be reluctant to identify these as masturbatory activities but will readily admit that such stimuli are sensually pleasurable and enjoyed.

Direct sexual self-stimulation, is, nevertheless, common among women. When problems of sexual functioning are present, data on masturbation are an essential part of the history. Questioning should proceed from the more general toward the specific: Can you describe for me situations that you find particularly pleasurable in a physical sense—things that feel good to your body?

Often the patient is uncertain or reluctant to offer anything. Examples such as a long, hot bath, a steak dinner with wine, the use of bath powder or body lotion, and back rubs can be suggested by the physician as sensual experiences, and the patient is encouraged to think in terms of body pleasures. What kinds of things can you think of that make you feel sexually exciting or excited?

Some people can have orgasms during sexual daydreams or fantasies: Do you remember having had fantasies or daydreams that made you become excited? Have you ever had an orgasm while you were dreaming or having a fantasy?

Some women are able to have orgasm just by touching or stroking their breasts: Is touching your breasts sexually exciting for you? Have you ever been able to have orgasm in that way? Have you ever been able to have orgasm by rubbing, touching, or stroking any part of your body? your female organs? your clitoris? Have you ever used an electric vibrator to give you sexual pleasure?

If such a line of questions discloses that the patient regularly or irregularly enjoys self-stimulation, then some questions as to technique should be asked. Many women who masturbate by genital stimulation avoid direct clitoral stroking because the clitoris is exquisitely sensitive. More commonly, a finger alongside the clitoris or on the labia minora is employed. Most women do not employ intravaginal instruments for self-stimulation, although some women whose sexual experiences have all been penis-oriented do so.

Background Information

There is no normal frequency of masturbation for males or females. In males, masturbation, like coitus, is usually followed by a refractory period of variable length depending on age, habit, or strength of sexual stimuli. Masturbatory frequency is likewise dictated by levels of sexual tension, opportunity, absence of distractions, habit, or strength of sexual stimuli. Frequencies varying from several times per day to never are all considered normal.

In females the absence of a physiologic postorgasmic refractory period increases the possibility of multiple occurrences within a limited time frame. Some women regularly attain more than a dozen self-induced orgasms per day without any known deleterious effect. Among prostitutes repeated sexual experiences in the course of their work often induce high levels of sexual tension but may not result in multiple orgasms with concomitant relief of pelvic congestion. Relief of pelvic congestion may be subsequently obtained with orgasm by masturbation or by orgasmic coitus with a desired partner. Masturbation to orgasm has also been used by women to relieve the pelvic congestion of menstruation.

During times of sexual activity, women without serious sexual inhibitions rarely reject and almost always encourage direct and indirect sexual stimulation of themselves by an accepted partner and readily stimulate the accepted partner by many of the means at their disposal. Mutual masturbation in some form is therefore so common as to become a rule in satisfactory sexual relationships.

Clinical Significance

A masturbatory history in men is useful under at least four circumstances:

1. To establish that the typical adolescent development of sexual tension and subsequent gratification has developed, and to determine the individual's emotional response to his own emerging overt sexuality
2. To document the patient's continuing ability to attain erection and ejaculation (that is, absence of structural damage)
3. To give evidence of persisting libido
4. To determine if a postmasturbatory refractory period is contributing to coital erective difficulty or ejaculatory incompetence

Additionally, a masturbatory history may give important insights into the patient's sexual fantasy life.

A masturbatory history in women is also useful for other reasons:

1. To give some indication of a patient's range of sexual experiences and responses
2. To add data about her concepts of sexuality and of herself as a sexual person
3. To give evidence of persisting libido
4. To define some of the specific stimuli the patient finds pleasurable

Encouragement of masturbation in women has been used as a technique by which a previously anorgasmic woman can learn what orgasm is like and what sorts of stimuli she finds most gratifying. By accepting permission to experiment with self-gratification, some anorgasmic women whose prior training and conditioning do not restrict such activity will be able to identify the orgasmic goal they seek. Thereafter, their coital efforts to reach orgasm have the advantage of a clearly defined and experienced goal. The female masturbatory history may therefore give important background information upon which to base a future therapy program.

Selected References

1. Annon JS: *The Behavioral Treatment of Sexual Problems*, Vol 1: *Brief Theory*. Honolulu, Kapiolani Health Services, 1974.
2. Kaplan HS: *The New Sex Therapy: Active Treatment of Sexual Dysfunctions*. New York, Bruner/Mazel, The New York Times Book Co, 1974.

3. Masters WH, Johnson VE: *Human Sexual Inadequacy.* Boston, Little, Brown, 1970.
4. Masters WH, Johnson VE: *Human Sexual Response.* Boston, Little, Brown, 1966.

Premature Ejaculation
MALCOLM G. FREEMAN, MD

Definition

Inability of the male to control the ejaculatory process during intravaginal containment long enough to satisfy his female partner in at least 50% of coital opportunities. This definition, patterned after that of Masters and Johnson, breaks down when the female partner is persistently anorgasmic. Premature ejaculation has been variously defined by others as ejaculation after less than 30 seconds of vaginal containment, less than 1 minute, etc. Each definition leaves something to be desired.

Technique

When you were having intercourse fairly regularly, about how long would it last? How long was it usually from the time you put your penis in until you would climax (come, have orgasm)? The typical answer for a premature ejaculator is considerably less than 2 minutes unless the patient had a prior orgasm by masturbation or coitus. Was there ever a time when you climaxed before you got your penis in? Can you tell me about that time, what were the circumstances? What's the longest time you could have intercourse without ejaculating? Can you tell me about that?

Is your partner able to have orgasm during intercourse? If she can't come during intercourse, do you ever use your hand or mouth or a vibrator to help her come? Is that before or after intercourse?

Do you feel that you have any control over when you'll come? Would you like to be able to last longer? Has your partner ever said that she would like intercourse to last longer? The factor of control is important to introduce, both in terms of history and for future therapy. Characteristically, premature ejaculators describe themselves as lacking control.

Have you tried anything to make you last longer? What kinds of things have you tried? Premature ejaculators usually attempt a variety of strategies to delay ejaculation. These range from intellectual distraction and self-induced pain to topical anesthetic agents. Other destructive strategies include deliberately avoiding foreplay to reduce levels of sexual excitation, avoiding touch by the partner, reduced vigor of thrusting during coitus. The female partner often retaliates with violent efforts to reach orgasm before her male partner ejaculates. This means that she often attempts to make strong pelvic thrusting movements while his actions are designed to minimize friction and excitation. Thus both partners have the same goal (prolongation of coitus until both have orgasm) but are trying to achieve this goal by diametrically opposite means. The sexual act is therefore likely to end in failure and frustration.

Background Information

Couples with the problem of premature ejaculation rarely require detailed questioning to elicit a history. When given a sympathetic and nonjudgmental listener, they will readily relate a history so classic as to be repeated with minimal variations in almost every case. Once the examiner is familiar with the usual sequence of events in a sexual partnership frustrated by premature ejaculation, it requires little perception to recognize the story.

Often the female partner is the complainant. Her complaint usually begins with her dissatisfaction with their usual pattern of lovemaking highlighted by inadequate foreplay, her infrequent orgasm, frequent postcoital pelvic congestion, and increasing frustration. This pattern has led to decreased coital frequency, recrimination, degeneration of their interpersonal relationship, and often the development of secondary impotence on the part of her husband.

The man is more likely to be a complainant if he is college educated. He is more likely to express concern if he feels to some degree responsible for his partner's gratification or lack of it. This seems to be largely a cultural phenomenon.

A decrease in the frequency of coitus significantly increases the severity of premature ejaculation because of increased sexual tension levels. In the same manner, a period of separation or a new or more exciting partner increases the severity of premature ejaculation.

Clinical Significance

Premature ejaculation is certainly the most common male sexual dysfunction. It is most common in young men. As men age, some of those who have had premature ejaculation learn ejaculatory control. The cooperation of a warm, sympathetic partner facilitates this learning process.

A man with pronounced premature ejaculation, if sufficiently excited or anxious, may ejaculate at the sight, sound, or touch of a woman. Sometimes, in a situation in which sexual performance is expected of him, he may ejaculate at his own touch. Ejaculation has become a reflex phenomenon as voluntary control has been lost or never learned. In terms of the sexual response cycle, excitation leads to ejaculation with a minimal intervening plateau phase.

Premature ejaculators have no specific personality type or psychic pathology. Classical psychoanalysis as a therapy for premature ejaculation is reported by Helen Singer Kaplan to be minimally successful, although other forms of psychotherapy may be useful in helping the premature ejaculator cope with the emotional problems engendered by his dysfunction. Premature ejaculation is believed to be a learned response and is therefore treated in uncomplicated cases by retraining for ejaculatory control.

Premature ejaculators fall into two major groups. Those born before 1930 or so often had their early sexual experiences with prostitutes. In this setting, sexual performance is male-gratification-oriented, and the customer who performs quickly wins approval from the prostitute and her other clients. Among men born after 1930, early experiences were less often with prostitutes but were commonly enacted in situations where urgency and risk of discovery and disapproval from authorities were important (drive-in movies, automobile back seats, living room sofas). Again, sexual experiences were primarily male-gratification-oriented, and couples encouraged themselves to perform quickly.

In addition, men with premature ejaculation commonly have a history of premarital petting to orgasm by rubbing against their partner while fully clothed and of the use of coitus interruptus as a form of contraception; again, these are male-gratification situations.

Not uncommonly, the man with premature ejaculation presents with a complaint of secondary impotence. The experience of being unable to exert ejaculatory control, repeated frustrating coitus, an unhappy complaining wife, reduced sexual stimuli, and a degenerating marital relationship all contribute to a sense of sexual and marital inadequacy. The most common sexual counseling situation encountered is that of an anorgasmic wife with a premature ejaculator husband who may or may not be secondarily impotent.

Selected References

1. Annon JS: *The Behavioral Treatment of Sexual Problems,* Vol 1: *Brief Theory.* Honolulu, Kapiolani Health Services, 1974.
2. Kaplan HS: *The New Sex Therapy: Active Treatment of Sexual Dysfunctions.* New York, Bruner/Mazel, The New York Times Book Co, 1974.
3. Masters WH, Johnson VE: *Human Sexual Inadequacy.* Boston, Little, Brown, 1970.
4. Masters WH, Johnson VE: *Human Sexual Response.* Boston, Little, Brown, 1966.

Ejaculatory Incompetence
MALCOLM G. FREEMAN, MD

Definition

Inability to ejaculate after achieving erection.

Technique

Begin by asking: Do you ever find that your erection is all right but you are unable to come—to ejaculate? When did you first notice that? Does it happen all the time or just sometimes? Have you noticed any relationship to how long it has been since the last time you ejaculated? Are you taking any drugs or medicines at the present time that you started before this problem began? Can you remember anything going on in your marriage—any problems that began about the same time as this problem?

Background Information

Ejaculatory incompetence is regarded by many as a form of impotence. Ejaculation is brought about by both the sympathetic and parasympathetic nervous system. The ejaculatory center is probably located in the lumbar region of the spinal cord. Initially, the sympathetic division causes muscle contractions that deliver the semen to the urethra. Then the parasympathetic system causes clonic spasms of the muscles surrounding the urethra with subsequent expulsion of the fluid.

Clinical Significance

It is relatively uncommon but has been described under several circumstances:

1. As a part of the male refractory period. After male orgasm and ejaculation occur, there is a period of time when it is difficult for a man to regain an erection. After erection is attainable, there is a second phase during which ejaculation is difficult or impossible and requires very prolonged penile stroking. With advancing age, the second phase lengthens in time.

2. With advancing age the need to end coitus with ejaculation decreases. The patient may interpret this as failing powers or impending impotence when it is simply a change due to aging which diminishes gratification very little.

3. The same general categories of pharmacologic agents that may contribute to erective difficulty may in some cases retard ejaculation.

4. Some men who consciously restrain ejaculation for a period of time (to avoid conception, or for other reasons) may retrain themselves and thereafter have difficulty ejaculating when they wish to do so.

5. Occasionally, emotionally traumatic events (discovery by children, discovery by the sexual partner's husband) have been reported to inhibit the subsequent ability to ejaculate.

Selected References

1. Annon JS: *The Behavioral Treatment of Sexual Problems,* Vol 1: *Brief Theory.* Honolulu, Kapiolani Health Services, 1974.

2. Kaplan HS: *The New Sex Therapy: Active Treatment of Sexual Dysfunctions.* New York, Bruner/Mazel, The New York Times Book Co, 1974.

3. Masters WH, Johnson VE: *Human Sexual Inadequacy.* Boston, Little, Brown, 1970.

4. Masters WH, Johnson VE: *Human Sexual Response.* Boston, Little, Brown, 1966.

Erective Difficulty (Impotence)
MALCOLM G. FREEMAN, MD

Definition

Inability to develop or sustain a penile erection for sufficient time to accomplish sexual connection and ejaculation. The term "impotence," like "frigidity," is judgmental and disparaging and probably should be avoided by physicians. It is, however, in common usage.

True impotence is classified as primary or secondary, psychic or physical.

1. *Primary.* Failure to have ever sustained penile erection for a time sufficient to accomplish intromission, whether the partner is male or female, whether the orifice is vagina, mouth, or anus.
2. *Secondary.* Failure to accomplish erection sufficient for penile intromission for at least 75% of sexual opportunities, regardless of partner's sex or the orifice (assumes at least one successful previous intromission).

The ability to successfully masturbate, have nocturnal emissions, and morning erections do not invalidate the diagnosis of impotence or erective difficulty. These abilities commonly persist in psychogenic impotence and often disappear in organic impotence.

Technique

Ask: At the present time, do you ever have any difficulty in getting an erection when you want it? If so, when? Have you ever had this happen in the past?

If the patient answers affirmatively, a series of questions should be asked to define the circumstances under which erective difficulties occur:

How often do you have difficulty with erections?
Do you tend to lose an erection too soon or is it difficult to get an erection from the beginning?

How long have you noticed this?

Does it occur each time you want to have intercourse or is it just sometimes?

Does the problem seem to be getting worse, better, or staying the same?

Do you have difficulty getting an erection when you masturbate, or is it only when you are about to have intercourse?

Do you ever wake up in the morning with an erection?

Have you noticed any change in your interest in or your reaction to sexual thoughts or to sexy books or pictures?

Can you remember the first time you ever noticed any difficulty with erections? At that time, what else was happening in your life, at work, or in your marriage?

Are you taking any drugs or medicines regularly? Do you use any drugs from time to time? pot, speed, LSD, or anything?

Can you give me an idea about how much alcohol you ordinarily drink in a week's time?

When would you say was the last time that you had too much to drink?

What kind of an effect has this difficulty with erections had on your marriage (with your social life)?

What kind of a reaction did your partner (wife) have to this problem? How did you feel about that? How have things been between the two of you lately?

Background Information

Inability to achieve and sustain penile erection under appropriate circumstances or when desired by the patient is an important complaint. The physician must indicate to the patient that his complaint is accepted as important while avoiding any suggestion that the nature of the complaint devalues the complainant or that the impotence is "serious." As in all sexual history taking, a matter-of-fact, nonjudgmental approach is both reassuring for the patient and most productive for the physician. Sometimes the questioner finds himself taking a history of male impotence from the involved female partner if she is the presenting complainant. The questions may differ slightly in form but not in content.

The patient's initial complaint of impotence must be evaluated carefully rather than being accepted on face value alone. Not uncommonly, a patient may complain of impotence when the actual problem is one of the following:

1. Loss of libido
2. Ejaculatory incompetence
3. Premature ejaculation

4. Disinterest in a partner
5. Change in quality or quantity of sexual performance from one level to some lesser level
6. Decrease in volume or force of ejaculate
7. Increase in the length of the postcoital refractory period
8. Sexual exhaustion
9. Normal changes of aging
10. Unwillingness or inability to meet the sexual needs or desires of a real or proposed partner
11. Anxieties about penile size

Examiners must be alert to these possibilities.

Clinical Significance

Probably 90% of impotence is of psychic rather than physical origin. The following points help to differentiate psychic from physical causes.

Psychogenic	*Organic*
Acute onset	Insidious onset
Temporal relationship to specific stress	None
	Persistent, progressively worsening
Selective, intermittent, transient	Progressive waning of sexual interest and desire (absence of spontaneous erections and use of other outlets)
Potential to respond erotically (masturbation, morning erection, erotic desire in sexual situations)	

Physical causes of secondary impotence fall into three major categories:

1. General debilitating diseases. Men who are seriously ill or debilitated may lose the ability to develop or sustain erections.
2. Neurologic and/or vascular diseases. Whether these conditions are central or peripheral may have a significant impact on potency.
3. Pharmacologic. Included particularly are antihypertensive agents, psychotropic drugs, antiulcer therapy, and estrogens.

Some men who consult physicians for psychic erective problems may have had tranquilizers prescribed which potentiate the problem rather than diminish it.

The two most common events related to the development of secondary impotence are episodes of acute alcoholic intoxication and a history of premature ejaculation. Most men have had erective failure occasionally. It is more often attributable to emotional or intellectual fatigue than to physical fatigue. The typical male response to such an experience is a feeling of regret coupled with self-accepted rationalization of fatigue or distraction as a cause, with no significant threat to future sexual function. The dysfunctional male is apt to view an isolated episode of erective failure as a portent of future impotence and to begin to respond with high levels of anxiety about his ability to perform. Soon it is performance anxiety and fear of failure that distract him from pleasure and sexual gratification and result in impotence.

In the male virgin who has significant insecurity about his ability to play a male sexual role, intolerable levels of anxiety about his ability to perform may lead to primary impotence. Such insecurity may arise from absence of an adequate male role model, excessive maternal domination, adolescent homosexual experiences, excessive religious orthodoxy, lack of encouragement and reassurance, or previous humiliating experiences.

Selected References

1. Annon JS: *The Behavioral Treatment of Sexual Problems, Vol 1: Brief Theory.* Honolulu, Kapiolani Health Services, 1974.
2. Kaplan HS: *The New Sex Therapy: Active Treatment of Sexual Dysfunctions.* New York, Bruner/Mazel, The New York Times Book Co, 1974.
3. Masters WH, Johnson VE: *Human Sexual Inadequacy.* Boston, Little, Brown, 1970.
4. Masters WH, Johnson VE: *Human Sexual Response.* Boston, Little, Brown, 1966.
5. Cooper AJ, Ismail AAA, Smith CG, et al: Androgen functions in "psychogenic" and "constitutional" types of impotence. *Br Med J* 3:17–20, 1970.

Frigidity
MALCOLM G. FREEMAN, MD

Definition

Frigidity is a lay term implying lack of sexual responsiveness. The word "frigid" is usually applied to a woman in a judgmental way by another person. The terms "cold" and "indifferent" are more often applied to men.

Technique

In response to questions about a woman's satisfaction with her own sexuality or her partner's satisfaction, she may indicate that the word "frigid" has been used to describe her sexual responses and attitudes. Avoid the word "frigid." It has no medical meaning and is, moreover, deprecatory and disparaging. If used by the patient, ask instead for a precise description of her complaint: I don't know what that word means. It means a lot of different things to different people. Can you tell me exactly what "frigidity" means to you?

Background Information

Problems sometimes included within this term are the following:

1. Lack of factual knowledge
2. Shyness
3. Poor body image
4. Rejection of an unwanted lover or an unacceptable sexual practice
5. Lack of willingness to experiment or try new sexual experiences
6. A difference in sexual needs between partners
7. Sexual or social inexperience
8. Primary anorgasmia

9. Secondary anorgasmia
10. Situational anorgasmia
11. Random anorgasmia
12. Anger or failure to communicate with partner leading to sexual rejection
13. Insufficient lubrication
14. Dyspareunia
15. Vaginismus
16. Sexual anesthesia
17. Loss of libido
18. Fear of pregnancy
19. Emotional reaction to a previous rape
20. Sexual aversion

The examiner should explore with the patient her complaint and assess how much of the problem is the patient's failure to achieve her own expectations, to achieve her sexual partner's expectations, or to achieve some other authority's expectations. Are the expectations in fact realistic? Does the failure to achieve expectation represent an inability, an unwillingness, a disagreement about goals, an absence of information, or an absence of permission?

The withholding or dispensing of sexual favors or nurturing (tenderness, warmth, touching, cuddling, holding, grooming, caressing) is a traditional barometer of interpersonal closeness and of sexual partners' satisfaction with one another. In a sexual relationship, manipulation of sexual favors is used both to make war and to make peace. Displeasure with a partner's responsiveness leads to anger, frustration, and anxiety. Anger and anxiety often lead to name calling: thus, "frigidity" or coldness. Most if not all of the above problems also occur among male partners, and the cold, indifferent, or sexually nonassertive man is a relatively common female complaint.

Women or men can be said to be sexually aversive when they actively avoid sexual expression or experience. Sometimes this avoidance is accompanied by denial of sexual feelings, by anxiety, or by anger. Sexual aversion represents one end of a spectrum of sexual responsiveness. The other extreme is characterized by sexual interest, pleasure, and excitement from sexual gratification. The great majority of men and women are found at the interest, pleasure, and excitement end of the spectrum. Excessive sexual interest, eg, "Don Juanism" in men or "nymphomania" in women, is associated with a continuing unsuccessful search for sexual gratification.

It is not known how much natural biological variation in amount of sexual interest exists among human beings. The impact of culture on sexual interest and on the freedom to express sexual feelings is so enormous that most decrease in sexual interest is probably the result of cultural inhibitions. In general, when we (and lower animals as well) enjoy and are gratified by an experience or feeling, we seek to repeat that experience. When an experience or feeling has been painful or frustrating we seek to avoid it.

Sexual aversion may be a way of life or it may be in response to a situation. The expression of sexual feelings that have been blocked by circumstance or by inhibition may be handled by denial or sublimation, giving the individual a neutral or disinterested (uninvolved) posture. A disinterest or aversion to sexual expression is an important symptom justifying further investigation.

Clinical Significance

Both men and women who are not demonstrative or overtly affectionate may actually yearn for a warmer and more intimate relationship. Often it is found that such individuals lack a satisfactory role model upon which to pattern themselves and as a consequence have had no practice or experience in a close and nurturing interpersonal relationship. Sometimes previous sexual or social experiences have been so unsatisfactory that an individual avoids the risk of intimacy in order to avoid the risk of further hurt. The application of a disparaging label further alienates the individual.

Properly defined, the problem can be analyzed for its constituent elements and these, in turn, further explored.

Selected References

1. Annon JS: *The Behavioral Treatment of Sexual Problems, Vol 1: Brief Theory.* Honolulu, Kapiolani Health Services, 1974.
2. Kaplan HS: *The New Sex Therapy: Active Treatment of Sexual Dysfunctions.* New York, Bruner/Mazel, The New York Times Book Co, 1974.
3. Masters WH, Johnson VE: *Human Sexual Inadequacy.* Boston, Little, Brown, 1970.
4. Masters WH, Johnson VE: *Human Sexual Response.* Boston, Little, Brown, 1966.

Anorgasmia

MALCOLM G. FREEMAN, MD

Definition

In women, the inability to achieve orgasm. There are three different types of anorgasmia:

1. *Primary anorgasmia.* Never having achieved orgasm under any circumstance, heterosexual or homosexual, with or without a partner.
2. *Situational anorgasmia.* Inability to achieve orgasm regularly in one or more desired sexual circumstances, by means of penile, oral, manual, or other stimulation. Such a patient may be orgasmic with masturbation and not with penile-vaginal coitus (or vice versa). She may be orgasmic in a homosexual relationship but not in a heterosexual one (or vice versa).
3. *Random anorgasmia.* Ability to respond fully at some times but not at others, in an unpredictable fashion. Many women are orgasmic in only a portion of coital opportunities; however, one woman may be satisfied to be orgasmic in 40% of coital experiences while another may be frustrated when she achieves orgasm in only 75% of opportunities. Another form of random anorgasmia involves the woman who has been regularly orgasmic in the past and has now ceased to be. This should more properly be called "secondary anorgasmia."

Technique

After the fact of coitus and the approximate frequency have been described the examiner can begin to determine patient satisfaction: Is sexual intercourse pleasurable for you? Do you enjoy it? If not, what do you find unsatisfying about it?

In addition to anorgasmia, possible answers include coitus too frequent or too infrequent, insufficient foreplay, pain on penile insertion or deep thrusting, dissatisfaction with the partner, a feeling of being used, too rapid ejaculation, or insufficient closeness and tenderness during the resolution phase of sexual excitement: Are you having orgasm when you have intercourse? Approximately what percentage of the time? Is that frequency of orgasm satisfactory to you? Even if the frequency of orgasm is far below 100%, if the patient expresses satisfaction with her present level, then there is usually no need for the physician to pursue the matter further.

If the patient says that she is orgasmic at some times but not at others and that this is not satisfactory, then the physician should inquire more deeply. Under what circumstances have you been orgasmic in the past? Can you tell what sorts of things make it easy for you to have orgasm, and when it's going to be difficult for you?

If the patient had previously been orgasmic and has now ceased to be, search for a temporal reference and then try to relate important physical, pharmacologic, emotional, social, or interpersonal events: Do you remember when it began to be hard for you to reach orgasm? Was anything in particular happening in your life along about that time? Did you change birth-control methods, get sick, have a serious fight with your husband—anything like that? Do you remember what else was going on in your life at that time? As in any history taking, it is helpful to ask the patient for her own insights: Do you have any idea what made it difficult for you to have orgasms along about that time? Often when directly asked, patients will volunteer meaningful observations and perceptions that otherwise might be missed.

Background Information

Orgasms among women vary. One may be a simple physical release no more complicated than that of the typical man. More commonly, it is a physical response prepared by an elaborate and complex list of sexual values (expectations) which must be met satisfactorily before the woman is fully responsive. Many, if not most, of these sexual values have never been consciously defined by the woman to herself, much less to someone else. Among sexual therapists, much history taking is aimed at defining the woman's sexual value system.

Orgasm in men usually occurs rather early in adolescence with so-called wet dreams and masturbation. Among women, even though many sexually exciting experiences (dreams, fantasies, kissing, caressing) may have occurred during adolescence and young adulthood, orgasm has often not occurred. It is common for women to be orgasmic only after coitus has become a well-established pattern. Presumably this is related to acceptance of her sexual role, a sense of comfort and confidence in her partner and in the relationship, as well as some experience and learning on her part.

In a woman who has failed to achieve orgasm within a self-determined expected range of time and experience, an unwarranted lack of self-confidence and doubt about her womanhood sometimes begin to appear. Coupled with this is often confusion about what orgasm is and what it feels like.

Clinical Significance

In American society, orgasm for the man has been a way of keeping score. A man may view his female partner's absence of orgasm (that is, "success") as a reflection on his ability as a lover. He may react to this with feelings of guilt at having deprived his partner of orgasm or with feelings that there is something wrong with her or the relationship ("she's frigid"). These feelings are an additional burden for the woman and for the relationship to bear.

For a woman to be maximally sexually responsive, her personal sexual values must be met. Most female sexual dysfunctions are related to an unfulfilled or an unrealistic and nonserving sexual value system. The sexual value system is composed of biophysical and psychosocial factors. Biophysical factors include such things as health, fatigue, warmth, comfort, sight, sound, odor, taste, and touch. Psychosocial factors include such things as respect, tenderness, acceptance, anger, approval, disgust, conditioning, and learned values. For example, one woman might find the idea of a sexual relationship with a tall, dark, hairy, bearded, silent stevedore exciting while another would be unexcited unless her partner was a fair-haired, loquacious, clean-shaven college professor. This, however, is a gross oversimplification of a complex and ever-changing state of conscious and unconscious attitude and need.

Sometimes learned sexual values are nonserving. For example, a young woman may have learned from her mother that all young men are only interested in taking sexual advantage of her. As a consequence, she finds it hard to be trusting and open in social contact with men and loses opportunities to establish a gratifying relationship.

In a woman who is anorgasmic, the examiner must carefully explore sexual values as well as experiences in order to determine which values are unfulfilled, unrealistic, or nonserving. The examiner must also determine how much nonthreatening opportunity to learn to be orgasmic the patient has had. When there is significant pressure on the patient (either self-induced or received from her partner) to be orgasmic and therefore "normal" and "really sexy," it is difficult for her to be fully and un-self-consciously sexually responsive. Her lack of orgasmic response may be self-interpreted as reducing her value as a person and implying that she is less feminine or less of a "real woman" than others. Such feelings may result in both anxiety and depression.

When a woman's regular sexual partner is impotent or ejaculates prematurely, she may react with anger and hostility or with exaggerated self-doubt about her own sexual identity and capacity as a satisfactory sexual partner. Many such women, therefore, become insecure about themselves as well as about their partners. Sometimes women who are anorgasmic deny their own responsibility and ascribe their lack of sexual responsiveness entirely to their partner's inadequacies. To some extent, this may be real, but all persons must accept ultimate responsibility for their own sexual gratification. When patients ascribe all of a sexual problem to their partner and accept no responsibility themselves, then both understanding and solution of the real problem are thwarted.

Many patients, in a conscious or unconscious effort to define which partner is at fault, go outside of the marriage (partnership) and try another sexual partner. Sometimes this extramarital sexual relationship serves simply as an experiment designed to clarify who is at fault in the partnership. Sometimes the relationship serves to achieve gratification not found in the marriage. It seldom solves the original problem.

A clear distinction must be made between a gratifying and enjoyable sexual experience and orgasm (which is only one form of sexual gratification). Many women report that sexual intercourse may be pleasurable, enjoyable, desired, and gratifying even when no orgasm occurs. Orgasm provides dramatic and sudden relief from sexual tension, myotonia, and vascular engorgement, but nonorgasmic coitus at lesser levels of sexual tension may still provide opportunities for closeness, tenderness, excitement, touching, holding, and caressing that are significantly rewarding. When sexual tension is close to orgasmic levels but orgasm is not obtained, unrelieved pelvic vascular engorgement often leads to prolonged pelvic congestion. Congestion plus unfulfilled expectations for orgasmic release and pleasure make the coital experience frustrating. Even if orgasm has been achieved, the coital experience may be unsatisfying if the patient's expectations for tenderness and foreplay were not met.

Selected References

1.   Annon JS: *The Behavioral Treatment of Sexual Problems, Vol 1: Brief Theory.* Honolulu, Kapiolani Health Services, 1974.
2.   Kaplan HS: *The New Sex Therapy: Active Treatment of Sexual Dysfunctions.* New York, Bruner/Mazel, The New York Times Book Co, 1974.
3.   Masters WH, Johnson VE: *Human Sexual Inadequacy.* Boston, Little, Brown, 1970.
4.   Masters WH, Johnson VE: *Human Sexual Response.* Boston, Little, Brown, 1966.

Dyspareunia and Vaginismus
MALCOLM G. FREEMAN, MD

Definition

Dyspareunia is painful or uncomfortable sexual intercourse. The term is usually applied to women, although under some circumstances intercourse may be painful for men.

Vaginismus is one cause of dyspareunia. Vaginismus is an involuntary spastic contraction of the superficial muscles of the perineum. This results in temporary narrowing of the vaginal opening and pain on attempted insertion of an object into the vagina. In susceptible individuals, the involuntary contraction is precipitated by any real or threatened vaginal invasion and is relieved by cessation of attempted invasion.

Technique

Ask: Do you ever have pain or discomfort when you have sexual intercourse? If the answer is yes, try to establish a temporal relationship. Is that a problem for you now? Does it bother you all the time or just sometimes? Under what circumstances did you have pain? Was it only in a particular position or at a particular time of the month (your menstrual cycle)? What makes the pain worse? Is there anything you or your partner can do to avoid it or make it better? Has it ever made you stop having intercourse or made you avoid intercourse?

Does it hurt when you first start (when he first puts his penis in, when the penis is being inserted) or is it a pain that you feel on deep thrusting (when he pushes deep inside you, when he hits something inside)? This is a critical question because it helps to differentiate problems of superficial penetration (such as vaginismus, too rigid a hymen, absence of lubrication, atrophic vaginal epithelium, vaginitis, or introital scarring) from problems of deep penetration (such as a prolapsed ovary in the cul de sac, pelvic inflammatory disease, endometriosis, retroverted uterus, pelvic peritonitis, or universal joint syndrome).

Questions of lubrication can be resolved by asking: Do you find that you lubricate (get wet) easily when you get sexually excited? Do you ever seem to be too dry? Does dryness seem to be part of the problem?, Have you used any kind of artificial lubricant? Lack of lubrication may be secondary to dyspareunia since repeated pain on attempted intercourse interferes with sexual excitement and lubrication. Even when no organic cause for dyspareunia exists, absence of sufficient sexual excitement at the initiation of penile thrusting results in deficient lubrication which causes pain, thereby decreasing excitement and lubrication further. A vicious cycle is set up. Absence of sufficient excitement also sometimes causes pain on deep penetration because the upper vagina does not undergo its characteristic ballooning.

Atrophic vaginitis as a cause of dyspareunia occurs in women who have been surgically castrated or who are postmenopausal and have no estrogen supplementation to restore the vaginal epithelium to its normal thick resilient status. How long has it been since you had a menstrual period? Have you been given any hormone treatment since your surgery (since your periods stopped)?

Do you have any pain or discomfort that lasts after intercourse is finished or does it quit hurting as soon as you stop? Do you have any discharge, burning or itching around your vulva (privates, female organs)? Do you seem to be swollen?

When pain is only on deep penetration and is random rather than frequent or consistent, it suggests that the penis has thrust against an ovary temporarily lodged in the cul de sac. When pain is consistent in coital positions of deep penetration, questions related to deep pelvic pathology arise.

Background Information

Pain on intercourse should be considered organic until proved otherwise. It cannot be evaluated without a concomitant physical examination. The examiner should attempt to reproduce the patient's pain during the examination. Often it is precisely located, and a specific site can be identified exactly.

The examiner's willingness to accept the pain source as physical is very reassuring to the patient, who will often then freely describe the psychic overlay which makes her dyspareunia so troublesome. The psychophysiologic interplay between pain, sexual excitement, and lubrication can then be easily explored by the patient and physician together. Dyspareunia is a situation in which history taking, examination, reassurance, patient education, and specific treatment proceed so rapidly and are so intermingled that it is difficult to separate them.

Clinical Significance

An excessively large male organ is rarely a cause for dyspareunia. In the presence of adequate levels of sexual excitement, the mature vagina dilates in depth and diameter to accommodate almost any erect penis. The presence of an object (penis, finger) in the vagina further increases vaginal capacity. An excessively long penis increases the possible length of stroke, but as penile length increases, rigidity decreases somewhat and the penis becomes more limber. This may be a disadvantage since the shaft may bend in the midst of thrusting.

Coital vaginal lacerations both anterior and posterior to the cervix in the vaginal fornices have been described, and rarely such a patient may present to the emergency room with vaginal bleeding. It is my personal impression that these are more often due to excessive coital vigor than to excessive penile length. In such cases, the use of foreign objects in the vagina must be ruled out.

The normal premenopausal vagina in a sexually excited adult woman is a resilient structure and (with the exception of occasional minor superficial mucosal tears) not easily damaged by a wide range of sexual experiences. Pain on intercourse, therefore, suggests that some other non-physiologic process is underway.

It is often possible to relieve dyspareunia on deep penetration by a change in coital position if the primary cause of pain seems temporarily or permanently inaccessible. After some experimentation early in the relationship, most couples adopt two or perhaps three coital positions as their usual pattern and seldom experiment much more. The most commonly used position (man above woman, female thighs flexed) allows deep penile penetration and increases the chance of pain in susceptible individuals. Often a simple position change (woman supine, thighs extended and together with man's thighs outside; or woman above) will alter the relationship enough to relieve pain on deep penetration.

The following differential diagnosis is useful when interviewing a patient with pain on coitus:

1. Vaginismus
2. Rigid hymen
3. Recently lacerated hymen
4. Perineal scarring (episiotomy, trauma)
5. Bartholin abscess or cyst
6. Vaginitis
7. Vulvitis
8. Atrophic vaginitis
9. Direct clitoral manipulation
10. Inadequate lubrication
11. Allergic or topical sensitivity reaction

12. Radiation vaginitis
13. Traumatic lacerations of uterine supports
14. Pelvic inflammatory disease and/or abscess
15. Endometriosis
16. Postsurgical
17. Prolapsed ovary

Vaginismus is commonly encountered in the gynecologic examining room when a young, inexperienced, frightened, or previously traumatized woman is approached for examination. Her typical response to the approach of an examining finger is to pull her knees together, lift her hips, slide to the upper end of the examining table, and cry out in alarm. Even when the patient has been reassured and intellectually accepts the idea of pelvic examination, she may not have mastered the painful involuntary spastic contraction of superficial perineal muscles. Usually recognition and acceptance of her vaginismus on the part of the examiner coupled with reassurance and a nonforcing attitude will help the patient regain voluntary control of her perineal muscles.

Vaginismus is one important cause of unconsummated marriage (other causes include primary impotence, imperforate hymen, and vaginal atresia). The response of a frightened, inexperienced, fatigued virginal bride to an assertive but inexperienced and anxious groom may be similar to the above experience in the gynecologist's examining room. Fortunately, in most cases rest, increasing self-confidence, some patience, and a natural buildup of sexual excitement combine to make most young brides both physically and intellectually enthusiastic for coitus. In a small minority, initially painful attempts at coitus are so discouraging that physician assistance will be necessary.

Coital vaginismus is also seen among unmarried young women who are beginning coitus. In my experience, a suggestion by some previous physician that the patient's vagina may be narrow or small often has reinforced her belief that coitus will be painful or impossible. This is usually the result of a previous physician's failure to recognize vaginismus in the examining room or failure to allow for the reduced caliber of the virgin vagina. Many unnecessary hymenectomies are performed for unrecognized vaginismus.

Young women with vaginismus often have a history of inability to insert vaginal tampons and often have never inspected their own vulva with a mirror or never inserted a finger in their own vaginas.

Selected References

1. Annon JS: *The Behavioral Treatment of Sexual Problems, Vol 1: Brief Theory.* Honolulu, Kapiolani Health Services, 1974.

2. Kaplan HS: *The New Sex Therapy: Active Treatment of Sexual Dysfunctions.* New York, Bruner/Mazel, The New York Times Book Co, 1974.
3. Masters WH, Johnson VE: *Human Sexual Inadequacy.* Boston, Little, Brown, 1970.
4. Masters WH, Johnson VE: *Human Sexual Response.* Boston, Little, Brown, 1966.

BREAST

78. Breast Lump

R. WALDO POWELL, MD
CONSTANTINE DROULIAS, MD

Definition

A lump or a mass in the breast is an area of texture different from the surrounding tissue.

Technique

Begin by asking: What bothers you most about your breast? Ask the patient to point to the spot with one finger, then ask specific questions in order to fully characterize the lump: its duration, manner of discovery, size change and relationship to menses and pain or tenderness associated with menses. Continue with more general questions related to:

1. Her menstrual status (age at menarche, age at menopause, spontaneous or artificial menopause)
2. Number of pregnancies and children and ages at which the patient became pregnant.
3. History and duration of breast feeding (both children and patient)
4. Family history of breast cancer (include age of diagnosis)
5. Previous breast problems and treatment
6. Other symptoms related to the lump, such as nipple and skin changes or axillary masses
7. History of trauma and infections

8. Medications, especially hormones, antihypertensive and anti-depressive drugs

Background Information

Cancer of the breast is the most common cancer in white women over 40 years of age. Almost 7% of all women will develop cancer of the breast in their lifetime. Several findings about cancer are now substantiated.

1. It is more common in outer than inner quadrants. In about 70% of the patients, it occurs in the upper outer quadrant and central portion of the breast, 20% in the medial portion, and 10% in the outer lower quadrant tail of the breast, and periphery of the breast.
2. It is more common in women whose first child was born after age 30 and/or who have borne no children.
3. It is bilateral (simultaneous or nonsimultaneous) in over 10% of cases.
4. The male to female ratio is slightly lower than 1:100.
5. There is a fivefold increase among those with a family history of breast cancer.
6. Although no common causative factor has become evident, etiologic factors being investigated in the laboratory, particularly in mice, include hormonal mechanisms, viral agents, and immunologic processes.
7. It is more common in the left side than the right side.

There is a high-risk group of patients who are prone to develop cancer of the breast. Such a patient would be a white woman, over 40 years of age, living in the Western world, and who has a mother or sister with history of breast cancer.

Clinical Significance

About 85–90% of all breast lumps in the female fall into one of the following.

1. Fibrocystic disease. Over 60%. It is commonly bilateral and associated with pain or tenderness, or both. These symptoms are usually more severe in the premenstrual period.
2. Cancer. Under 10%. Usually solitary, unilateral.
3. Fibroadenoma: About 15%. It occurs usually in young women, is painless, and may be multiple.

4. Miscellaneous. Around 15%. Lesions included here are intraductal papilloma, duct ectasia, lipomas, angiomas, fibromas, hematomas or hematocysts, foreign body granulomas, fat necrosis, galactocele, inflammatory lesions or abscesses. In men, about 90% or more of breast lumps are due to gynecomastia, less than 10% to cancer. Other benign breast lesions are extremely rare.

Selected References

1. Leis HP Jr: *Diagnosis and Treatment of Breast Lesions.* New York, Medical Examination Publishing Co, 1970.
2. Rush BF Jr: Breast, in Schwartz I (ed in chief), Hume DM, et al (eds): *Principles of Surgery.* New York, McGraw-Hill, 1969.
3. Haagensen CD: *Diseases of the Breast,* ed 2. Philadelphia, WB Saunders, 1971, p 101.
4. Savlov E: Breast cancer, in Rubin P (ed): *Clinical Oncology for Medical Students,* ed 4. New York, University of Rochester, American Cancer Society, 1974.

79. Breast Pain

R. WALDO POWELL, MD
CONSTANTINE DROULIAS, MD

Definition

A sensation of aching, pulling, drawing, burning, or stinging in one or both breasts due to functional or pathologic conditions of the breast or due to other extrinsic causes.

Technique

Begin by asking whether the pain is unilateral or bilateral, localized in a certain area or diffuse. If localized, ask the patient to point out the spot with one finger and to clarify the type of pain, possible radiation to

other areas of the breast or the body, whether it is continuous or intermittent, and any relationship to her menstrual period. Consider traumatic
causes such as oral manipulation during sexual activity, exercises, sports,
or change of job requiring use of one arm more than the other. Is the patient under any unusual physical or mental stress? Is she taking birth
control pills? The inability to sleep on her abdomen is a good indicator of
the true severity of the symptoms. The evaluation of breast pain and
tenderness is completed with a careful breast examination.

Background Information

Innervation of the breast is provided by somatic sensory nerves and
automatic (sympathetic) motor nerves (Fig 7). Parasympathetic fibers do
not exist in the breast.

The supraclavicular nerves (somatic) supply sensory fibers for the
innervation of the upper cutaneous parts of the breast, while the lateral
(IV–VI) and medial (II–IV) branches of the intercostal nerves supply the
lower cutaneous parts and the mammary gland. Sympathetic motor fibers
destined for the smooth muscles of areola, nipple, and wall of the vessels
travel along with all the above-mentioned nerves and then follow the

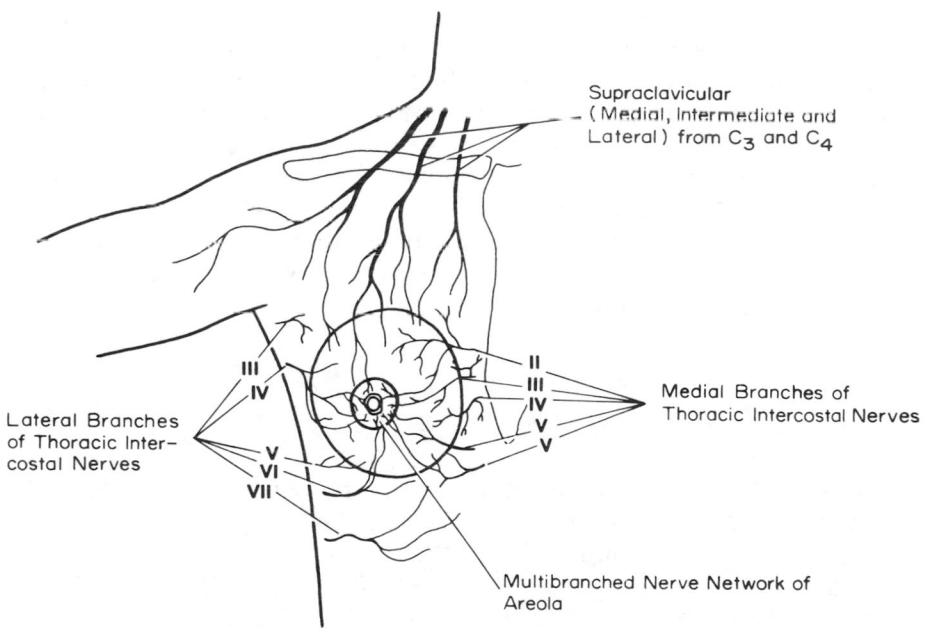

Figure 7. Innervation of the breast.

arteries of the breast. The postganglionic sympathetic fibers stem from the ganglia of the paraverterbral upper thoracic sympathetic chain.

In breast disease, pain is experienced in the breast itself, but because of the kind of innervation described above, it may also radiate to the side of the chest or to the back (along the intercostal nerve trunks), above the scapula or the medial side of the arm (along the intercostobrachial nerve), and to the neck (along the supraclavicular nerves).

For 3 to 4 days before the onset of the menstrual cycle, the blood flow to the breast increases significantly. During this time, some women can experience variable degrees of tension, tightness, fullness, heaviness, and breast pain, symptoms that disappear after menstruation.

Clinical Significance

Normal cyclical pain and tenderness are commonly bilateral, but more pronounced in one breast, and are among the most common complaints. In diffuse fibrocystic disease, pain and tenderness are common and bilateral. They are often the main symptoms that cause the patient to seek medical aid. Most benign neoplasms are painless. Cysts that grow rapidly are usually painful and tender. Contrary to the general belief, pain does not always denote benign disease. Egan, in gathering mammographic data at Emory University for the past 12 years, found that unilateral breast pain (especially of stinging, burning, or pulling type) is the second most common complaint in breast cancer. Pain is four times more common than the next complaint of nipple discharge. Tenderness is rare in breast cancer. If no apparent cause for the pain is found by history, physical examination, and x-rays of the breast, the patient can be reassured that no evidence of a serious problem exists. This statement, along with the assurance that her symptoms will very likely clear up within one to two menstrual cycles will usually be all that is required. However, a burning or stinging pain rather than tenderness warrants repeat examinations in one to two months.

Selected References

1.   Corry DC: Pain in carcinoma of the breast. *Lancet* 1:274–276, 1952.
2.   Egan RL: *Priorities in Managing Breast Problems: Roundtable Discussion in "Patient Care,"* April 1975, pp 20–83.
3.   Haagensen DC: *Diseases of the Breast,* ed 2. Philadelphia, WB Saunders, 1971, p 101.
4.   Leis HP Jr: *Diagnosis and Treatment of Breast Lesions.* New York, Medical Examination Publishing Co, 1970.

5. Pack GT, Ariel IM: *Tumors of the Breast, Chest, and Esophagus.* New York, Paul B Hoeber, 1960, vol 4.
6. River L, et al: Carcinoma of the breast: The diagnostic significance of pain. *Am J Surg* 82:733, 1951.
7. Vorherr H: *The Breast: Morphology, Physiology, and Lactation.* New York, Academic Press, 1974, pp 20–70.

80. Nipple Discharge

R. WALDO POWELL, MD
CONSTANTINE DROULIAS, MD

Definition

The passage of liquid material through the nipple either spontaneously or after stripping.

Technique

Spontaneous discharge is apparent from the stain of the drainage on clothing. Factors to consider are the association of the discharge with other symptoms, such as mass, pain, skin, or nipple changes, and with menses, the type and duration of discharge, whether it is continuous or intermittent, and current drug intake. Nonspontaneous discharge is elicited by the examiner, as described in section 78, Breast Lump.

Background Information

There are seven basic types of nipple discharge:

1. *Milky.* Thin, white, skimmed-milk-type.
2. *Grumose.* Thick, sticky discharge of varied color; may be white, yellow, gray, green, or brown. If brown, may appear bloody but no red cells are visible on microscopic examination.

3. *Purulent.* Thick, creamy matter, which under the microscope resembles pus.
4. *Watery.* Rare and thin, colorless.
5. *Serous.* Faintly yellow, thin, clear secretion that dries as a yellow stain on the patient's clothing.
6. *Serosanguineous.* A thin, clear discharge with a pink tinge, showing red blood cells microscopically.
7. *Bloody.* Usually brownish, but may resemble frank blood.

Clinical Significance

Nipple discharge is the third most important symptom in breast disease. It is due to benign disease in the majority of cases but it may herald cancer. To be significant, nipple discharge must be spontaneous or accompanied by a mass.

Physiologic. Physiologic nipple discharge is milky during lactation and from multiple milk sinus openings. It is the most common type of nonpathologic discharge. Physiologic lactation is not considered abnormal unless it continues for 12 months or longer after cessation of nursing or after termination of the last pregnancy.

Abnormal lactation. Continuation of milk secretion long after breastfeeding has stopped occurs occasionally from continuous stimulation by suckling, after trauma, pituitary necrosis or adenoma, hypothyroidism, after intake of medications such as phenothiazines, reserpine, methyldopa, or oral contraceptives. Three syndromes have been described in connection with this rare type of milky discharge: Chiari-Frommel, Forbes-Albright, Del Castillo. The cause is unknown but Relkin postulates that the basic abnormality is an increased output of prolactin.

Grumose discharge. Duct ectasia or comedomastitis, the advanced state of which is called "plasma cell mastitis," is seen usually in multiparous or parous patients at or near the menopause. Palpation reveals the characteristic wormlike feeling under the areola. In advanced stages, inflammatory changes and fibrosis result in a tumorlike mass (plasma cell mastitis), which closely mimics carcinoma. Water and serous discharges are also present in duct ectasia. Serosanguineous bloody discharge with or without a small mass underneath the areola is commonly due to intraductal papilloma. When associated with a mass greater than 1 cm in diameter, this type of discharge is highly suggestive of a malignancy.

Selected References

1. Leis HP Jr: *Diagnosis and Treatment of Breast Lesions.* New York, Medical Examination Publishing Co, 1970.
2. Haagensen CD: *Diseases of the Breast,* ed 2. Philadelphia, WB Saunders, 1971, p 101.
3. Powell RW: *Priorities in Managing Breast Problems: Roundtable Discussion in "Patient Care,"* April 1975, pp 20–83.
4. Relkin R: Galactorrhea: A review. *NY State J Med* 65:2800–2807, 1965.
5. Vorherr H: *The Breast. Morphology, Physiology, and Lactation.* New York, Academic Press, 1974.

SKIN

81. The Dermatological History

PEARON G. LANG, MD

Definition

The dermatological history serves four purposes: (1) it allows the clinician to establish that the patient has a complaint in reference to the skin; (2) it helps uncover important etiological and aggravating factors; (3) it aids in eliminating certain diseases on the physician's list of differential diagnoses; and (4) it determines the presence of associated systemic symptoms.

Technique

Although important, for the dermatological patient the history should not take precedence over the physical exam.

If the patient has a cutaneous complaint, the clinician should initially inquire only about the location and distribution of the cutaneous disorder. After completely examining the skin, one may take a more efficient, intelligent, and relevant history. Moreover, with this approach one can avoid being misled and biased.

For the patient with cutaneous disease, the following inquiries are an essential part of the dermatological history:

1. Age, race, sex, and occupation of the patient
2. Original appearance of the skin eruption or lesion
3. Duration of any eruption or lesion
4. Associated cutaneous symptoms
5. History of previous treatment
6. History of stress and psychological upheaval
7. Associated systemic symptoms
8. History of seasonal exacerbations
9. Aggravating environmental factors
10. Aggravating hormonal factors
11. Drug history
12. Family history
13. Previous experience with the same disease

In screening for dermatological disease, the following questions should be asked:

Has there been a change in the color or texture of the skin?

Has there been a change in the growth, texture, color, distribution, or strength of the scalp and body hair?

Has there been a change in the color, thickness, attachment, or growth rate of the nails?

Has there been hemorrhage into the skin?

Have there been any new growths?

Is there an area that has ulcerated, bled, or will not heal?

Has there been a "rash" in the recent past or is one now present? If the "rash" is not present now, was the patient seen by a physician and told what he had?

Has there been itching or burning of the skin in the absence of a rash?

Are there any new pigmented lesions?

Has there been a sudden change in the size or color of a mole?

Has there been any change or discomfort in the eyes, mouth, or genitalia?

Clinical Significance

The history should help to: (1) eliminate certain diseases which are being considered; (2) discover those factors which influence the disease process, and (3) ascertain if the skin changes are reflecting or associated with systemic disease.

The age, race, sex, and occupation of the patient may help to eliminate certain diseases in the differential diagnosis. For example, a tumor on the face of a child is less apt to be a basal cell carcinoma than in the case of a 60-year-old farmer.

Information about the original appearance and duration of the eruption or lesion is especially significant if the disease has been altered by scratching or treatment. A rapidly growing crater-form lesion of the face is more apt to be a keratoacanthoma than a squamous cell carcinoma.

Although symptoms such as pruritus, pain, and burning are subjective complaints, they may help distinguish between two disease processes. For example, bullous pemphigoid and dermatitis herpetiformis are both vesiculobullous diseases that are at times hard to differentiate. The presence of burning and itching in such a case would favor dermatitis herpetiformis.

A history of previous treatment is important because: (1) the morphology and distribution of the lesions may have been altered, rendering the diagnosis more difficult; (2) the original eruption may have been replaced by or perpetuated by a contact dermatitis from some over-the-counter preparation; (3) past therapeutic efforts may have been ineffective, and repetition of an ineffective treatment program will waste time and money.

In many dermatological conditions (eg, eczema, psoriasis, urticaria), stress and psychological upheaval may aggravate or even precipitate the disease process.

Extensive cutaneous disease may lead to a variety of systemic complications or be an expression of systemic disease. An older patient with exfoliative erythrodermatitis may develop high output congestive heart failure and thus may complain of orthopnea or dyspnea. A patient with cutaneous lupus erythematosus may complain of arthritis or chest pain which is positional or pleuritic.

Mobility and world travel require consideration of diseases which are not endemic to the area in which the patient resides. Recent travel out of the country or to a different region of the United States might provide a clue to cutaneous leishmaniasis or coccidiomycosis.

Seasonal exacerbations are typical of certain dermatological diseases. A history revealing seasonal variation will not only help the clinician know what aggravates the disease process but will also give him insights concerning proper management. For example, some lupus erythematosus patients are photosensitive and experience more disease activity in the spring and summer. Thus, regular use of a sunscreen during these seasons would be mandatory.

Environmental and other aggravating factors should be sought and eliminated if possible. Inquire about the patient's hobbies, job, social habits, and diet. A patient's hives could be due to a certain food ingested. The man with hand dermatitis will not improve the condition if he washes his hands with defatting soaps. The patient with porphyria cutanea tarda should restrict alcohol intake.

Hormonal changes may either aggravate or alleviate many skin conditions. A history of a flare in the disease at mid-cycle or premenstrually may lead to a diagnosis. For example, progesterone dermatitis typically begins after ovulation and improves with menstruation; thus, hormonal manipulation may be indicated.

A history of drug ingestion, both prescription and nonprescription, is important (see section 113, Current and Past Medications). Drug eruptions may mimic almost any disease and drugs may aggravate a preexisting skin disease. Beta-blockers appear to aggravate psoriasis, and aspirin can aggravate urticaria. Moreover, it often is not the drug itself but a preservative or the dye in the tablet coating that is the culprit.

A family history of similar dermatological conditions may provide insight into a genetic etiology of the disease, help the patient better understand the disease, and help the clinician decide if other family members need to be examined. A positive family history may also indicate a common source outbreak. With scabies, the entire family may need to be treated before the patient will be cured.

Total duration of the dermatological disease should be determined since chronic skin disease may have significant psychologic, physical, and economic impact.

Selected References

1. Fitzpatrick TB, Arndt KA, Clark WH Jr, et al (eds): *Dermatology in General Medicine.* New York, McGraw-Hill, 1971, pp 11–12.
2. Rook A, Wilkinson DS, Ebling FJG (eds): *Textbook of Dermatology.* Philadelphia, FA Davis Co, 1968, pp 24–26.
3. Moschella SL, Pillsbury DM, Hurley HJ Jr (eds): *Dermatology.* Philadelphia, WB Saunders, 1975, pp 114–118.

82. Itching

HIRAM M . STURM, MD

Definition

A distinct and disagreeable cutaneous dysesthesia also called pruritus, which an individual often attempts to relieve with voluntary or involuntary scratching.

Technique

The patient is simply asked if he has been bothered by itching. If so, further questions are indicated: Is it anatomically diffuse or localized (scalp, genital area, clothing contact areas, flexural or extensor areas of the extremities)? How bad is it? (Severe pruritus typically interferes with sleep patterns and is associated with excoriations.) What is the duration of the pruritus? Are there any temporal relationships? Has there been any associated rash, new medication, or past allergic history? Is the occurrence seasonal, such as winter and fall only? Are there associated signs and symptoms? (respiratory, gastrointestinal, genitourinary, lymphadenopathy, skin color changes such as flush or pallor).

Background Information

The sensation of itching is carried by fine unmyelinated C nerve fiber endings located in the subepidermal area of the skin and transmitted to the thalamus and sensory cortex via the lateral spinothalamic tract. These same pathways are also involved in the transmission of other cutaneous sensations, including hot and cold, pain, and tactility. Controversy remains, however, concerning whether itching is a subthreshold pain sensation or a totally separate sensation. Itching is presumed to be induced by the action of chemical mediators, such as histamines, proteases, and kinins, on the peripheral cutaneous nerve filaments. In cholestatic jaundice, the itching results from excess skin content of the free dihydroxy bile acid derivatives, deoxycholate and chenodeoxycholate. Vasodilation typically exacerbates pruritus and may partially relate to worsening with hot or relief with cold showers or baths. Pruritus is a subjective complaint and the itch threshold varies widely with alterations in the patient's perceptual and psychological state. Psychogenic factors may exacerbate pruritus whether or not associated with increased vascular dilation or with sweating. Similarly, asteatotic (dry) skin may primarily or secondarily precipitate or aggravate itching. This phenomenon is exaggerated in the dehydrated climate of winter or with excessive air conditioning.

Clinical Significance

Itching may be associated either with primary skin disorders or systemic diseases, or with neither (essential pruritus). Dermatoses most commonly encountered with intensive pruritus include dermatitis herpetiformis, lichen planus, lichen simplex chronicus (circumscribed, lichenified plaque of pruritic skin), atopic dermatitis, contact dermatitis, urticaria, scabies, insect bites, and pediculosis. In many cases the pruritus may be related to previous physician or patient therapies with drying agents, medicaments, and soaps. Pruritus may also be related to skin dehydration subsequent to low humidity in winter heating systems or summer air conditioning, leading to excessive scaliness and dryness. If a physician is ever tempted to append a label of "psychogenic pruritus" to a patient's complaint of pruritus, every other possible cause of pruritus should be excluded. Constant reevaluation must be made, lest a serious, treatable etiology be recognized belatedly. Pruritus associated with systemic diseases may occur with no skin lesions, with skin lesions due only to excoriations, or with skin lesions directly related to the primary disease. Diabetes mellitus is probably the most common systemic disorder presenting with isolated pruritus. Biliary cirrhosis and other types of cholestatic jaundice are also typically associated with pruritus. Rarer conditions, such as mastocytosis (urticaria pigmentosa) display erythematous, urticarial, pruritic skin lesions.

Pruritus may also be an early symptom or may even precede the onset of Hodgkin's disease, leukemia, and polycythemia rubra vera, as well as intestinal parasitosis, carcinoid syndrome, hyperthyroidism, mycosis fungoides, multiple myeloma, and carcinoma with liver metastasis. Severe pruritus is also typical of patients with chronic renal failure and/or advancing secondary hyperparathyroidism and may represent a major indication for parathyroidectomy, dialysis, or both. Innumerable other systemic illnesses, covered in the references, are less frequently associated with pruritus.

Patients may seek emergency help for intense pruritus with no rash. The clinician often prescribes mild antihistaminic therapy and overlooks the history of recently prescribed antibiotic or other medication. This story is typical of patients subsequently admitted with life-threatening acute drug eruptions. Full consideration must be given to immediately discontinuing any new drug in patients who present with acute pruritus in the absence of rash since pruritus may be a prodromal symptom of serious drug allergy.

Selected References

1. Rook A, Wilkinson DS, Ebling FJG (eds): *Textbook of Dermatology,* ed 2. Oxford, Blackwell Scientific Publication, 1972.
2. Domonkos AN; *Andrews' Diseases of the Skin,* ed 6. Philadelphia, WB Saunders, 1971, pp 61–76.
3. Varad DP: Pruritus induced by crude bile and purified bile acids: Experimental production or pruritus in human skin. *Arch Dermatol* 109:678–681, 1974.
4. Demis DJ, Dobson RL, McGuire J: *Clinical Dermatology.* Hagertown, Md, Harper and Row, 1977, vol 4, sect 29-2, pp 1–3.

83. Change in Mole

J. THOMAS APGAR, MD

Definition

Mole is the common name given to a pigmented nevocellular nevus. A change in mole refers to any color changes, irregular growth, itching, pain, crusting, bleeding, or inflammation of a preexisting pigmented nevus. Also included in this definition is the recent onset and rapid growth of a deeply pigmented lesion. It should be noted that pigmented nevi may be speckled or nearly flesh-colored, particularly in the head and neck region.

Technique

Ask: Do you have any moles that bother you? Do you have any dark spots on your skin that have changed to shades of red, white, or blue? Are there any new, rapidly growing, dark blue black spots? Do you have a large tan or black birth mark that has changed recently?

Although nonspecific, these questions may indicate an early change in the natural history of malignant melanoma. Ask more specific questions if the above history is positive. These would include the time of onset of the pigmented lesion; the duration and location of the new growth; the presence of itching, bleeding, or crusting; the presence of an irregular border or a white color at the border (halo effect); and the occurrence of multiple new dark moles over the trunk. Also ask if any dark spots have appeared on the palms or soles (particularly in the black patient), mouth, fingernails, or toenails. Although the occurrence is rare, ask about a family pedigree for malignant moles, particularly in a young patient with many new and irregular-size moles over the back or trunk.

Background Information

Pigmentary changes in the skin can be attributed to the presence of carotene, carotenoids, heavy metals such as gold or silver, hemosiderin, or melanin. Hemosiderin and melanin are mainly responsible for the brown black appearance of a superficial skin lesion, or the blue black coloration of a deep dermal lesion (Tindall effect). Vascular phenomena that produce color changes are transient except when red blood cells are extravasated into the tissue and hemosiderin leads to a pigmentary change (bruise).

Melanocytes contribute to normal pigmentation of the skin and may give rise to melanomas. Melanocytes are derived from neural crest cells and rest along the dermal-epidermal junction in a usual ratio of 1:10 with basal cells. Melanin is produced from tyrosine and dopamine precursors, and is packaged in the form of melanosomes inside the melanocyte. According to recent studies with radioactive dopa, human melanin pigment is probably a co-polymer of dopa-quinone, indole 5,6-quinone, and indole 5,6-quinone 2-carboxylic acid. The melanocyte may discharge its prepackaged melanin into 1 of 30 to 35 epidermal keratinocytes. This transfer within the melanocyte-keratinocyte unit accounts for much of the normal skin color and for certain pigmentary changes such as tanning. In the skin of caucasians, small melanin granules are aggregated in lysosomal membranes in the lower epidermis. In the skin of negroid or Oriental individuals, single and large melanin granules reside in keratinocytes throughout all layers of the epidermis.

Nevus cells are the usual subepidermal cellular constituent of common moles or nevi. They may become malignant and give rise to melanomas. Nevus cells are probably derived embryonically from neural crest tissue and may represent an intermediary form of Schwann cell or melanocyte. Nevus cells probably contain incompletely formed or packaged melanin. They may also engulf melanin particles, much in the fashion of macrophages.

Melanomas may thus arise from malignant melanocytes or malignant nevus cells. Clinically, less than 30% of melanomas arise in preexisting moles. Exceptions include patients with congenital dermal nevi such as "bathing trunk" nevi. Reportedly 2% to 45% of giant congenital melanocytic bathing trunk nevi may develop into a malignant melanoma by the third or fourth decade. However, most melanomas occur as de novo lesions.

Most recent authors classify malignant melanomas into three major forms: lentigo maligna melanoma, superficial spreading melanoma, and nodular melanoma. *Lentigo maligna melanoma* usually occurs in older whites and is located almost exclusively in sun-damaged areas of the face and neck. *Superficial spreading melanoma* is the most common type of melanoma and has a latent period of 5–15 years before beginning invasive growth. Diagnostic clues are irregular borders and irregular colors of blue, gray, white, or red developing in a tan, black, or brown lesion. This type of melanoma occurs mainly on the backs of men and women, and on the calves of women. *Nodular melanoma* may have a rapid onset. It may occur de novo, or as the vertical growth phase of a preexisting superficial spreading melanoma. A rarer fourth type of lesion, the acral-lentigenous melanoma, may occur on the palms, soles or nailbeds.

The etiology of melanoma is unclear, but in some instances there is a strong relationship to ultraviolet solar irradiation. The value of long-term use of sunscreen lotions in patients with a predisposition to melanoma remains to be proven.

Clinical Significance

Melanoma should be suspected in any patient with a history of recent onset or change in a raised, pigmented cutaneous lesion. Other causes of pigmented lesions include various types of nevi, benign seborrheic keratoses, lentigines (age or "liver" spots), freckles, and pigmented basal cell carcinomas. Table 13 provides a differential diagnosis of these lesions. A sudden onset of a black or brown band in the fingernail or toenail in a white patient may represent subungual melanoma. Long-standing pigmented nail bands may be a normal finding in black patients. A history of a black spot in the mouth could indicate melanoma but may also be noted with oral varices, mucous retention cysts, or dental amalgam tattoos.

A suspicion of widespread metastatic melanoma should be aroused by a history of diffuse hyperpigmentation of the skin or of darkening of the urine upon standing or light exposure (melanogenuria). Patients who have unexplained pulmonary, gastrointestinal, or central nervous system symptoms require careful questioning about moles since these regions are common metastatic sites of malignant melanomas.

Table 13. Differential diagnosis of pigmented skin lesions.

Lesion	Average Age of Onset (yr)	Major Location	Margin or Surface	Color	Comments
Seborrheic keratosis	40–70	Trunk, head, and neck	Wartlike, greasy, "stuck-on" appearance	Brown, yellow, or occasionally black	A most common benign lesion often mistaken for a mole or melanoma
Pigmented nevus (mole)	5–35	Anywhere, but majority on sun-exposed areas of trunk, arms, or face	Smooth or papular; sometimes normal skin markings and regular border	Brown, black, speckled, or flesh-colored	Orderliness of color, surface, and margins; most are less than 1 cm diameter
Lentigo, freckle	5–60	Sun-exposed areas	Smooth or flat (nonpalpable)	Brown or black	Common in children; known as "age spots" or "liver spots" in the elderly
Dermatofibroma	25–55	Lower extremities	Dimpled or fixed, may be slightly raised	Brown, purple, or red brown	Palpation between thumb and finger reveals a deep (or dermal) fixation of the lesion
Pigmented basal cell carcinoma	40–60	Head and upper trunk	Waxy, smooth, or ulcerated; often with specks of brown or black and telangiectatic vessels	Brown, black, yellow, or speckled	When compared to melanoma, this lesion may be more common in the brown-eyed as opposed to the blue-eyed patient

Lentigo maligna melanoma	65–75	Head, neck, and arms (sun-exposed areas)	Irregular, raised or flat	Irregular, brown or black	Often grows slowly for many years in the elderly patient, and irregular color changes or palpable areas indicate malignant degeneration
Superficial spreading melanoma	50–60	Posterior trunk in males and females; posterior legs in females	Irregular margin, often with a notch, or white border, and noticeable loss of surface markings	Shades of red, white, or blue occurring in a brown or black lesion	Usually slow radial or horizontal growth until invasion of the dermis occurs (vertical growth phase)
Nodular melanoma	40–50	All body surface areas	Palpable, large nodule with loss of skin markings	Usually black or blue black	Characterized by a rapid period of growth and invasion of deeper skin layers (vertical growth phase)

Early detection and treatment of melanoma carries an excellent prognosis with 90–100% six-year survival rates. This is especially for lentigo maligna melanomas and superficial spreading melanomas less than 0.76 mm deep (Clark's level I and II). In contrast, metastases are common and prognosis is much poorer when detection is delayed and dermal or subcutaneous involvement occurs. For example, the five-year survival rate for nodular melanoma greater than 1.25 mm deep is 10–14%.

Selected References

1. Kopf AW, Bart RS, Rodriguez-Sains RS: Malignant melanoma: A review. *J Dermatol Surg Oncol* 3(1):41–125, 1977.
2. Mihm MC Jr, Clark WH, From L: The clinical diagnosis, classification, and histogenetic concepts of the early stages of cutaneous malignant melanoma. *N Engl J Med* 284:1078–1082, 1974.
3. Mihm MC Jr, Fitzpatrick TB: Early detection of malignant melanoma. *Cancer* 37(1):597–603, 1976.
4. Clark WH, From L, Bernardino EA, et al: The histogenesis and biologic behavior of primary human malignant melanomas of the skin. *Cancer Res* 29:705–726, 1969.
5. Clark WH, Reimer RR, Greene M, et al: The origin of familial malignant melanomas from heritable melanocytic lesions. *Arch Derm* 114(5):732–738, 1978.
6. Mishima Y: Melanocytic and nevocytic malignant melanomas: Cellular and subcellular differentiation. *Cancer* 20:632–649, 1967.

84. Skin Cancer

J. THOMAS APGAR, MD

Definition

Primary skin cancer is a malignant neoplasm arising in the epidermis or main surface layer of the skin. The two most common tumors are basal cell epithelioma (BCE) and squamous cell carcinoma (SCC). Precancers in this group are nonmalignant lesions which may evolve toward malignancy following a latent period: a common example is the actinic keratosis (AK).

This section does not include tumors of pigment cells (melanoma), skin appendages, dermal structures, or subcutaneous fat. Also not included are metastatic tumors arising from noncutaneous sites.

Technique

Direct the history toward primary skin cancer rather than "age spots," "cysts," "growths," "moles," or "fatty tumors." Ask the patient directly: Have you had a sun damaged spot or skin cancer removed by a doctor? Is there a family history of skin cancer? Do you have any red, scaly, crusted spots or waxy yellow growths on your skin that will not go away? Also inquire about nonhealing of traumatized skin sites using such questions as: Is there a shaving nick or scar that has not healed? Do you have an ulcer or sore which has not healed (ie, leg ulcer)? Do you have an old burn or x-ray scar that is growing or bleeding?

If the history for skin cancer is positive or suspicious, proceed with additional questions concerning the age of onset, location, environmental exposure history, and record of previous treatment.

Determine if the patient had multiple skin cancers occurring before the age of 40. Inquire if the location of a skin cancer was characterized anatomically by frequent sun exposure. Ask about environmental exposure to x-rays, radium, coal tars, paraffin oil, soot, pitch, and arsenic. The following questions may be of further help: Are you regularly outdoors in the sun (ie, farming, sailing, gardening)? Do you sunburn easily? Did your ancestors have fair complexions, blue eyes, or a Celtic background? Have you ever had prolonged x-ray therapy for ringworm, severe acne, or previous skin cancer? Do you work around radium or coal tar products of any type?

Arsenic contact may be detected by asking about prolonged exposure to desert, spring, or artesian well water, insecticides, rodent poison, herbicides, copper-ore smelting occupations, and remedies such as Fowler's or Donovan's solution. Fowler's and Donovan's solutions were used in the past for the therapy of asthma, rheumatism, cancer, syphilis, and psoriasis. Record any data concerning previous treatment of skin cancer by surgery, x-ray, or local chemotherapy. Note whether recurrences have been documented and treated.

Background Information

Basal cell epithelioma arises from the lower germative cell layer of the epidermis. Squamous cell carcinoma usually arises from a more mature and higher level of the epidermis known as the stratum spinosum. Actinic keratoses often show atypical and dysplastic cell changes of both layers.

Prolonged ultraviolet light exposure is a major factor in the development of SCC and AK, and to a lesser extent, BCE. It is estimated that a latent period of 10–25 years occurs before significant sun damage results in malignant changes in epidermal cells. Biochemical effects of ultraviolet light interacting with the skin include epidermal cell proliferation, DNA damage, depression of DNA and RNA synthesis, short-term inhibition of cell mitoses, and with severe sunburn, cell death. C_4-cyclobutane dimers of thymidine and cytosine occur within the DNA molecule with alteration of its physical properties. Cross-linkage of proteins to DNA may further lead to unstable high-energy free radicals and destruction of the cell membrane.

The solar spectrum of light energy reaching the earth's surface at sea level begins at 290 nm. The most damaging and presumably the most carcinogenic rays are between 290 and 320 nm, the so-called sunburn range. There is some additional damage to the dermis and epidermis by light from 3,300 to 7,000 (long ultraviolet light spectrum), a process called photoaugmentation. As the sun nears its nadir and the angle of incidence on the atmosphere decreases, sunlight is relatively filtered by the ozone layer. In contrast, the most damaging sunrays occur when the sun's light is most perpendicular to the ozone layer, particularly between the hours of 10 AM and 2 PM during the months of June, July, August, and September. As one approaches the equator, this effect becomes intensified. Controversy exists concerning the effects of supersonic transports, aerosol propellants, and urban pollutants on the ozone layer.

Clinical Significance

Primary skin cancer is common, and constitutes approximately 50% of all new cases of cancer diagnosed yearly. It is definitely more common in patients with Celtic background, fair complexion, blue eyes, red hair, or in patients with little melanin pigmentation. The black patient has skin cancer less frequently, and then it is often confined to the palms, soles, or relatively nonpigmented sites.

Primary skin cancer rarely has a high mortality but may have a great morbidity, particularly if the original tumor is incompletely removed. Local infiltration and tissue destruction may follow inadequate therapy whether it be irradiation or electrodesiccation and currettage. BCE of the head and neck rarely metastasizes. SCC arising in an actinic keratosis (precancerous atypia) metastasizes in less than 0.1–5% of cases. This contrasts with those squamous cell carcinomas which arise in nonsunlight exposed areas. For example, SCC arising in burn scars or the anogenital region may metastasize in 25–60% of cases, respectively. An exception to this trend is carcinoma of the lower lip which arises in an area of solar exposure, yet has a rate of metastasis approximating 30–35%. SCC is locally invasive in about 10–12% of cases.

Approximately 70% of SCC and 90% of BCE occur in the head and neck region. The maximal light exposure areas are the rims of the ears, posterior neck, nose, cheeks, and lower lip. Less exposed areas include the periorbital area, nasolabial fold, anterior neck, and upper lip. Basal cell carcinomas often occur in head and neck areas that are not those of maximal light exposure.

Single or multiple skin cancers occurring before the age of 40 should initiate a search for genodermatoses. Examples include xeroderma pigmentosa and the basal cell nevus syndrome. Xeroderma pigmentosa is characterized by autosomal recessive inheritance, skin photosensitivity, photophobia, and occasionally mental retardation, microcephaly, and sensorineural deafness. The basal cell nevus syndrome is manifest by dominant inheritance, multiple superficial plaquelike BCE, bony abnormalities, dentigenous cysts, pits on the palms and soles, and renal resistance to the effects of parathyroid hormone.

SCC may occur in the lesions of benign cutaneous disorders. Examples include burn scars, radiodermatitis, chronic leg ulcers, lupus erythematosus, lupus vulgaris, fistulous tracts from osteomyelitis, and granuloma inguinale.

Skin cancer may on occasion be an indicator of internal malignancy. Bowen's disease (in situ or intraepidermal SCC) arising in nonsolar exposed areas may be associated with tumors of the larynx, esophagus, stomach, breast, bladder, prostate, kidney, or reticuloendothelial system. Skin cancer may also occur in immunosuppressed hosts such as renal transplant patients receiving steroid and antimetabolite therapy.

Careful and long-term follow-up is clearly indicated for patients with a history of skin cancer. Twenty to fifty percent of patients with one skin cancer may develop new carcinomas in less than two years. In addition, prompt recognition and management of tumor recurrences helps prevent local invasion and its high associated morbidity.

Prevention of prolonged sun damage is best accomplished by the combined use of para-amino benzoic acid (PABA) and benzophenone sunscreens, or by similar blocking agents which afford a high index of topical protection against sun rays (2,900 to 7,000 A).

Selected References

1. Chernosky ME: Squamous cell and basal cell carcinomas: Preliminary study of 3817 primary skin cancers. *South Med J* 71:802–803, 1978.
2. Andrade R, Gumport SL, Popkin GL: *Cancer of the Skin: Biology, Diagnosis, Management.* Philadelphia, WB Saunders, 1976, vol 2.

3. Stoll HL Jr: Squamous cell carcinoma, in Fitzpatrick TB, Arndt KA, Clark WH Jr, et al (eds): *Dermatology in General Medicine,* New York, McGraw-Hill, 1971, pp 407–425.
4. VanScott EJ: Basal cell carcinoma, in Fitzpatrick TB, Arndt KA, Clark WH Jr, et al (eds): *Dermatology in General Medicine.* New York, McGraw-Hill, 1971, pp 466–472.
5. Braverman IM: Cancer, in Braverman IM (ed): *Skin Signs of Systemic Disease.* Philadelphia, WB Saunders, 1970, pp 38–53.
6. Bergstrasser PR, Halprin KM: Multiple sequential skin cancers: The risk of skin cancer in patients with previous skin cancer. *Arch Derm* 111:995–996, 1975.

NEUROLOGICAL SYSTEM

85. Headaches

PATRICK A. GRIFFITH, MD
H. KENNETH WALKER, MD

Definition

Pain or discomfort in the upper half of the head, from the brow up.

Technique

Begin in a nondirective open-ended fashion. Ask: Do you ever have problems with headaches? If the answer is yes, then ask: Tell me about your headaches. Extract as much spontaneous information as possible from the patient before becoming more directive. Be especially observant for clues that will give you insight into the emotional status of the patient.

At the end of the spontaneous part of the history, decide which of two groups the patient falls into: (1) The headache is acute and severe, occurring in a patient who has never had this type of headache before. (2) The headache is chronic and recurrent with onset some time in the past.

In the directed part of the history, get more information using the following seven specific questions:

1. Type of pain: Family history of similar type headache; prodromata (warning); more specific description of quality of pain, ie, pounding, squeezing like a hatband that is too tight, dull like a toothache.

2. Location of pain: Unilateral or bilateral; frontal, occipital, hemicranial or vertex, or generalized.

3. Radiation of pain: To the neck, eyes, shoulders, occiput.

4. Worsening (precipitating factors) or improvement of pain: Coughing; sneezing; straining at stool; birth control pills; emotional trauma; specific modes of relief, ie, cool, quiet dark room, sleep.

5. Duration and frequency of pain: Hours, days, weeks, or months; time-intensity curve of the pain relative to rapid or gradual buildup of discomfort; specific comment about recurrence.

6. Associated symptoms: Nausea, vomiting, diplopia, blurred vision, visual obscuration, focal neurologic deficits, parasthesias, weakness, seizures or unconsciousness, stiffness or soreness of neck (meningismus), fever or other symptoms of systemic infections. Concentrate here if the headache falls into the first group. Problems such as meningitis, subarachnoid hemorrhage, brain tumor, or pseudotumor cerebri may be the cause of these associated symptoms.

7. Time of day of onset, age at previous onsets, hospitalizations: Use of narcotics, past drug therapy, postoperative or intramuscular, including efficacy.

Background Information

Intracranial pain-sensitive structures include the intracranial venous sinuses and their tributaries, the dural arteries (anterior and middle meningeal arteries), the cerebral arteries of the circle of Willis, and portions of the dura mater at the base of the brain. As a generalization, pain originating above the tentorium projects in the fifth cranial nerve and is referred to the frontal, temporal, and parietal areas. Pain originating in the posterior fossa is carried in the ninth nerve and upper cervical nerves and is referred to the occipital area.

The following four mechanisms can produce headache (see reference 1):

1. Traction on the veins and displacement of the venous sinuses
2. Traction on or distention of the meningeal arteries and the large arteries at the base of the brain
3. Inflammation of or pressure by masses on any of the pain-sensitive structures
4. Spasm of cranial and cervical muscles

Migraine headache is one type of headache in which something is known of the pathophysiology. There is initially a release of amines due to unknown stimuli. The amines cause vasoconstriction of large arteries supplying various areas of the brain, thereby causing ischemia in the arterial territory. This ischemia is the cause of various preheadache symptoms or prodromata. The particular symptoms are visual (usually), motor, or sensory, depending upon the territory that is ischemic. The vasoconstriction in turn causes release of vasoactive substances that produce vasodilation of pain-sensitive intracranial arteries, thus the headache. In summary, there is an initial vasoconstriction that produces the prodromal neurological symptoms, followed by vasodilation producing the headache.

The headache caused by masses such as brain tumor is due to local traction by the tumor on adjacent pain-sensitive structures or distant traction caused by displacement of the brain. The Valsalva maneuvers cause an increase in the central venous pressure and thereby a distention of vessels that exacerbates the brain tumor headache. The redistribution of body fluids with a shift from dependent portions that occurs with the recumbent posture presumably increases the brain edema slightly at night, which in turn causes more traction and thus increases the headache. The patient perceives this increased pain upon awakening. Upon resuming the upright posture, the fluid once again begins to accumulate in the dependent areas of the body, and the headache decreases. Inflammation such as meningitis produces headache by direct involvement of pain-sensitive structures.

Clinical Significance

A careful and thorough history is crucial in formulating hypotheses regarding the etiology of headaches in a particular patient. The physical examination should be quite thorough, with special attention to the following:

Vital signs
General: Tenderness or ropiness on the temporal arteries; pressure tenderness over the sinuses; bruits over the orbits, head, neck, or supraclavicular fossa; nuchal rigidity.
Neurologic: Fluctuating mental status; aphasia or dysarthria; anosmia, papilledema or ophthalmoplegia; asymmetric reflexes or Babinski sign; ataxia of gait or dysmetria of limbs.

After gathering and analyzing the historical, physical, and appropriate laboratory data, fit the patient into one of the following etiologic categories:

1. Life-threatening headaches can be caused by potentially reversible problems such as meningitis, brain abscess, tumors, subdural hematomas, subarachnoid hemorrhage, or arteriovenous malformations. These etiologies usually fall into the first group of headaches in the technique section: an acute severe headache with a relatively short history. The prototype is the sudden onset of a severe headache in a patient who seldom complains of one. Associated symptoms and signs are the key to diagnosis. Certain features are often present in headaches due to inflammation or masses such as tumors, although they are by no means pathognomonic. The headache becomes suddenly more intense with a Valsalva maneuver (which raises intracranial pressure by decreasing venous outflow from the cranium) such as coughing, sneezing, bending over, urinating, or straining at stool. The best way to get this history is to ask the patient: Does coughing make your headache better? An indignant denial gives a validity to the answer not possessed by an affirmative answer to the question: Does coughing make your headache worse? The headache is often more severe upon awakening and becomes more tolerable as the day progresses (intracranial pressure is probably higher with the recumbent position due to a redistribution of fluid that accumulates in dependent parts with an upright posture). This characteristic of headaches caused by masses contrasts to tension headaches, which are often not present upon awakening. They have an onset during the day and increase in severity as both the day and the patient's perceptions of troubles progress.

2. Tension headaches, or muscle contraction headaches, are usually located occipitally or radiate around the head in a hatband distribution. Patients will often describe them as being present for many years and remaining unchanged despite all sorts of medications. Clearly recognizable but often denied emotional stress such as marital discord and occupational difficulties exacerbate them. The patients are chronically depressed or anxious.

3. Migraine headaches are recurrent and often fairly stereotyped in any one patient. The onset is hemicranial, occurring sometimes on one side, sometimes on the other. About 10% have prodromal aura of visual (by far the most common), motor, sensory, or rarely ophthalmoplegic symptoms. A positive family history of similar headaches is fairly common. The pain is described as throbbing or pounding. Onset in adolescence or early adulthood is common.

4. Cluster migraine (Horton's histamine cephalgia) is unilateral, brief (usually under one hour), exceptionally intense, and often awakens the patient from sleep. The pain is burning or boring and is so severe patients have contemplated suicide. The headaches occur in clusters over a period of weeks or months, followed by remissions that may last for years.

Most headaches will not fit clearly into any of the categories described above. The clinician must use common sense and let the patient know there is no current evidence for a serious etiology. Aspirin, reassurance, and an open invitation to return is the best one can do in these cases.

Selected References

1. Dalessio DJ (ed): *Wolff's Headache and Other Head Pain,* ed 3. New York, Oxford University Press, 1972.
2. Friedman AF: Headache, in Baker AB, Baker LH (eds): *Clinical Neurology.* New York, Harper and Row, 1975, vol 2, chap 13.
3. Fisher CM: Headache in cerebrovascular disease, in Vinken PJ, Bruyn GW (eds): *Handbook of Clinical Neurology: Headaches and Cranial Neuralgias.* Amsterdam, North-Holland Publishing Co, 1968, vol 5.
4. Graham JR: Seven common headache profiles: Symposium on headache: Its mechanism, diagnosis and management. *Neurology* 13(3):16–23, pt 2, 1963.
5. Diamond S (ed): *Current Concepts of Headache. Postgrad Med* 56(3): 55–185.

---

86. Epileptic Seizures

H. KENNETH WALKER, MD

Definition

The following definitions are discriminative.

Epileptic seizure: An attack of cerebral origin resulting from excessive discharge of a hyperexcitable neuronal population.

Epilepsy: Recurrent epileptic seizures.

Seizure: Any attack of cerebral origin no matter what the cause.

Convulsion: Involuntary contraction of the body musculature. Can be of epileptic etiology or caused by a variety of nonepileptic conditions.

Technique

The history is crucial for the diagnosis and characterization of epileptic seizure disorders. Begin with a nondirective question such as: Tell me what happened to you. Or: Tell me about your seizures. Extract all the spontaneous information possible from the patient, then ask more specific questions. Use the same procedure with observers. The following topics need to be covered:

1. Onset of seizure: The initial manifestation of the seizure: What is the very first thing that occurs? Can you predict when you are about to have a seizure? Do you have any warning? The purpose is to discover if the onset is focal or if the first manifestation is a generalized convulsion and unconsciousness. Some manifestations of focal onset are:

a. Sensory:
Unpleasant odor or taste
Focal sensory or visceral sensory sensations, such as prickling, numbness, formication, or abdominal pain
Auditory: whistle, ringing, chirping
Visual: nonformed shapes, colors, or movements
Psychical: illusions, hallucinations

b. Motor:
Repetitive contraction of an extremity or corner of the mouth
Automatic movements such as throwing arm up, stroking, patting
Verbal: a cry or stereotyped phrases or mutterings

2. The seizure (ictal phase): A description of the seizure itself; the pattern of the seizure. There are three types:

a. Focal onset followed by other focal manifestations without a generalized convulsion and unconsciousness: may be motor, sensory, or a combination. Example: a jerking right hand followed by jerking of shoulder, hip, face, and leg—all on the right side. This type is the so-called Jacksonian march. Sensory focal seizures can march in a similar fashion.

b. Focal onset followed by generalized convulsions with unconsciousness: There will be a focal onset with or without other subsequent focal manifestations and then a generalization of the convulsion as described below.

c. Generalized epileptic convulsion: May or may not be preceded by focal manifestation(s). The most common form is characterized by a generalized tonic phase of sustained muscular contraction followed by a clonic ("jerking") phase. Autonomic manifestations such as bladder (more common) or bowel incontinence, or both, often occur.

Note that the terms "generalized seizure" and "grand mal seizure" are not synonymous. A grand mal seizure is an epileptic convulsion due to a particular form of epilepsy, grand mal epilepsy. This specific type of epilepsy has particular EEG characteristics. A generalized seizure is a generalized epileptic convulsion that involves the entire body and can be produced by a number of causes: grand mal epilepsy, metabolic derangements such as hypoglycemia, focal seizures which secondarily generalize, and others. In other words, generalized seizure is a generic term that includes *all* causes of generalized epilepsy, while grand mal is a specific term referring to a generalized seizure seen in a particular and fairly rare form of epilepsy.

3. Postictal phase: After the last tonic contraction of a generalized seizure, there is usually a 2–10 minute phase of gradual return to consciousness. At times a generalized seizure is followed by a focal neurologic paralysis of function that may last up to 24 hours. This postictal paralysis is known as "Todd's paralysis." Hemiparesis is common, but other focal deficits such as aphasia or visual field deficits can also be seen. This postictal deficit usually can be interpreted to mean that the seizure originated in the cortical structures serving the area of the deficit. Historical evidence for postictal focal deficits should be carefully searched for, since the clinician is then able to classify the seizure as focal, even though the clinical presentation was generalized.

4. Interval between seizures: Investigate the usual length of this period, how variable it is, and whether it has been changing; the influence of medication should be obtained. Inquire carefully about the presence or absence of any neurologic symptoms during the interval.

5. The age of onset, whether or not the seizure pattern has changed, frequency of seizures, and medication history: Inquire about head or birth trauma history and other common seizure etiologies such as stroke, cardiac valvular dysfunction, or arrhythmia.

Background Information

The pathophysiology of epilepsy is not yet clear. What follows is a simplification of a scheme that seems reasonable and which can be applied in a useful way to clinical medicine. This scheme divides seizures into two groups: seizures generalized from the start (centrencephalic seizures) and seizures not generalized from the start (focal seizures). This division fits both clinical and pathophysiologic findings.

1. Centrencephalic seizures (seizures generalized from the start): This group includes grand mal and petit mal epilepsy and seizures due to various metabolic derangements: hypoosmolarity (hyponatremia), hyperosmolarity (hypernatremia), hypoglycemia, hypocalcemia, drug withdrawal, and others. Experimentally these seizures are characterized electroencephalographically by generalized synchronous and bilaterally symmetrical convulsive waves that affect the entire scalp. Clinically there are convulsions which involve the entire body. This is in distinct contrast to focal seizures, where the EEG manifestations are localized on the scalp

and motor activity which, if present, involves a specific group of muscles. "Generalized from the start" means that there is never a focal motor or focal electrical component to this group of seizures. Focal seizures can become generalized as will be discussed later, but they have a focal beginning and only later become generalized.

These generalized seizures are postulated to arise from a group of "pacemaker" subcortical neurons in the rostral or thalamic portion of the reticular activating system. The reason or stimulus for the epileptic discharge of these neurons is unknown but presumably relates to a biochemical or electrophysiological abnormality, since gross or microscopic pathologic lesions have never been discovered. This abnormal discharge spreads to or "invades" the cortex bilaterally, producing unconsciousness. The caudal portion of the reticular activating system in the pons and medulla is thus removed from cortical influences and proceeds to produce tonic-clonic convulsions. Thus the two cardinal features of a generalized seizure, unconsciousness and motor convulsions, are explained.

This postulated pathophysiological mechanism fits many of the clinical and experimental features of seizures generalized from the start. Certain types of seizures in infants and children do not fit so readily into this model (see reference 6).

2. Focal epilepsy (partial epilepsy, seizures beginning locally): This group includes all seizures produced by focal pathological lesions such as tumors, infections, or scars. There are two principal differences between this group and the preceding one:

a. The seizures of focal epilepsy originate in the cortex of the cerebral hemispheres, whereas centrencephalic seizures are thought to begin in subcortical structures.

b. Focal seizures, as the name implies, have a focal origin which is reflected both in the clinical and EEG manifestations. (Apparent exceptions to this statement are discussed below.) Centrencephalic seizures begin with generalized clinical and EEG manifestations.

Focal lesions produce epileptic discharges by injuring a group of cortical neurons in such a fashion that they periodically become hyperexcitable and produce an abnormal electrical discharge. This discharge can spread in two ways:

1. To surrounding cortical areas. A good example is the Jacksonian march. A group of cells on the motor cortex, eg, in the hand area, begin an abnormal discharge which then spreads to the contiguous cortex. The initial clinical manifestation is convulsive movements of the hand, followed by a spread up to the face and down to the hip and leg. Local propagation is very slow, from 1 mm/sec to 1 mm/min, like a "drop of oil."

2. To remote areas of the brain by virtue of large fiber connecting systems. The more important of these include the connections between the cortex and brainstem reticular formation and between the cortex and hippocampus. Spread of the abnormal electrical discharge is more rapid through these circuits.

Thus a focal seizure begins with an abnormal electrical discharge by a local group of cortical neurons. The initial manifestation of the seizure depends upon the anatomical location of these neurons and their connections with other cortical and subcortical structures. Classically there will be a local manifestation such as convulsive movements of the hand. Then the seizure activity spreads to contiguous cortex, producing a succession of further clinical manifestations, eg, convulsive movements of the head and leg. There are then two possibilities that can occur:

1. The seizure can stop at any point in this progression. (See reference 9 for a discussion of what is known of inhibitory mechanisms.) In this event the seizure has remained focal, with the clinical manifestations relegated to those portions of the body served by the involved cortex. The level of consciousness has not been altered.

2. The seizure can proceed to produce unconsciousness and generalized convulsions. The postulated mechanism of this "secondary generalization" of what began as a focal seizure is that the abnormal discharge comes in contact with a large fiber system that enables it to spread to subcortical areas. More specifically, the spread is via corticothalamic projection systems to the reticular activating system in the thalamus. At this point the same series of events occur as described under centrencephalic seizures. The rostral reticular system is activated and the entire cortex is invaded, with the production of unconsciousness. The caudal reticular system is removed from the cortical influences and consequently produces generalized tonic-clonic movements.

The location of the cortical focus determines the particular clinical manifestations, whether or not generalization occurs, and the time interval between the onset of the focal seizure and the secondary generalization. If a seizure originates in a cortical sector that has sparse connections with other areas, it will tend to remain focal. The opportunities for generalization are much greater if the sector has rich and diffuse connections with other cortical and subcortical areas. In fact, generalization may occur so rapidly that neither the patient nor observers discern an initial focal manifestation. In this latter circumstance the clinician has great difficulty in classifying a particular seizure as a centrencephalic seizure or as a focal seizure.

The international classification of epileptic seizures is as follows:*

* Abstracted from: Gastaut H: Clinical and electroencephalographical classification of epileptic seizures. *Epilepsia* 11:102–113, 1970.

I. Partial seizures (seizures beginning locally)
  A. Partial seizures with elementary symptomatology (generally without impairment of consciousness)
    1. With motor symptoms (includes Jacksonian seizures)
    2. With special sensory or somatosensory symptoms
    3. With autonomic symptoms
    4. Compound forms
  B. Partial seizures with complex symptomatology (generally with impairment of consciousness) (temporal lobe or psychomotor seizures)
    1. With impairment of consciousness only
    2. With cognitive symptomatology
    3. With affective symptomatology
    4. With "psychosensory" symptomatology
    5. With "psychomotor" symptomatology (automatisms)
    6. Compound forms
  C. Partial seizures secondarily generalized

II. Generalized seizures (bilaterally symmetrical and without local onset)
    1. Absences (petit mal)
    2. Bilateral massive epileptic myoclonus
    3. Infantile spasms
    4. Clonic seizures
    5. Tonic seizures
    6. Tonic-clonic seizures (grand mal)
    7. Atonic seizures
    8. Akinetic seizures

III. Unilateral seizures (or predominantly)

IV. Unclassified epileptic seizures (due to incomplete data)

The international classification of the epilepsies is as follows:*

I. Generalized epilepsies
  A. Primary generalized epilepsies (includes petit mal and grand mal seizures)
  B. Secondary generalized epilepsies
  C. Undetermined generalized epilepsies

* Abstracted from: Merils JK: Proposal for an International classification of the epilepsies. *Epilepsia* 11:114–119, 1970.

II. Partial (focal, local) epilepsies (includes Jacksonian, temporal lobe, and psychomotor seizures)

III. Unclassifiable epilepsies

Clinical Significance

The clinical value in fitting a patient into one of the two groups described above is that focal seizures are caused by anatomical lesions, while seizures generalized from the start are caused by metabolic or unknown but presumed nonanatomic lesions (grand mal and petit mal).

The specific cause of focal seizures, such as neoplasm or scar, must be ascertained with a reasonable degree of certainty.

Seizures with onset during adulthood that are clinically generalized from the start, that is, neither the patient nor observer is aware of any initial focal manifestations, fall into one of these two groups:

1. Centrencephalic seizures from both pathophysiologic and clinical standpoints. Grand mal and petit mal epilepsy have their onset very rarely after age 30, so for all practical purposes they need not figure in the differential diagnosis. Other etiologies are: alcohol and barbiturate withdrawal; abnormal osmolarity (hyponatremia, hypernatremia); hypoxia; hypocalcemia; hypomagnesemia. Note that laboratory testing can rule out the large majority of these causes very simply. The only group that cannot be ruled out so easily is alcohol and barbiturate withdrawal. In many patient populations this group forms a large percentage of seizure patients. The most helpful diagnostic points in diagnosing alcohol withdrawal seizures are a history of heavy alcohol intake with a generalized seizure(s) occurring 12–72 hours after cessation of drinking, and a nonfocal EEG. These findings are quite suggestive of alcohol withdrawal seizures provided the history, physical, and laboratory examinations otherwise support the diagnosis.

2. Seizures that are clinically generalized from the start but pathophysiologically fit into partial epilepsy. The anatomical location of the focus is such that neither patient nor observers are aware of focal manifestations. If the EEG suggests focal cerebral disease, then the patient without further ado fits into the partial epilepsy group. If alcohol withdrawal can be satisfactorily ruled out, often a difficult task, then for purposes of a diagnostic work-up the patient should fall into the focal epilepsy group. As a generalization any adult with onset of generalized seizures should be in the focal epilepsy group until proved otherwise.

Selected References

1. Babb RR, Eckman PB: Abdominal epilepsy. *JAMA* 222:65–66, 1972.
2. Carney LR: Seizures after the age of sixty. *Practitioner* 217:74–81, 1976.

3. Celesia GC: Modern concepts of status epilepticus. *JAMA* 235:1571–1574, 1976.
4. Daly DD: Ictal clinical manifestations of complex partial seizures. *Adv Neurol* 11:57–83, 1975.
5. Earnest MP, Yarnell PR: Seizure admissions to a city hospital: The role of alcohol. *Epilepsia* 17:387–393, 1976.
6. Gastaut H, Broughton R (eds): *Epileptic Seizures*. Springfield, Ill, Charles C Thomas, 1972.
7. Gastaut H, Fischer-Williams M: The physiopathology of epileptic seizures, in Field J, Magoun HW, Hall VE (eds): *Handbook of Physiology*. Baltimore, Williams and Wilkins, 1959, vol 1, pp 329–363.
8. Hecker A, Andermann F, Rodin EA: Spitting automatism in temporal lobe seizures. *Epilepsia* 13:767–772, 1972.
9. Jasper HH, Ward AA Jr, Pope AB (eds): *Basic Mechanisms of the Epilepsies*. Boston, Little, Brown, 1969.
10. Lawall J: Psychiatric presentations of seizure disorders. *Am J Psych* 133:321–323, 1970.
11. Lende RA, Popp AJ: Sensory Jacksonian seizures. *J Neurosurg* 44:706–711, 1976.
12. Maguire F, Courjon J: Somatosensory epilepsy: A review of 127 cases. *Brain* 101:307–332, 1978.
13. Parsonage M: The differential diagnosis of seizures. *J R Coll Phys Lond* 7:213–234, 1973.
14. Racine R: Kindling: The first decade. *Neurosurgery* 3:234–252, 1978.
15. Victor M: Alcoholism, in Baker AB, Baker LH (eds): *Clinical Neurology*. New York, Harper and Row, 1975, vol 2, chap 22.
16. Victor M: The pathophysiology of alcoholic epilepsy. *Res Publ Assoc Res Nerv Ment Dis* 46:431–454, 1968.
17. Walker AE: Man and his temporal lobes. *Surg Neurol* 1:69–79, 1973.
18. Wells CE: Nonconvulsive status epilepticus (letter). *JAMA* 236:820, 1976.
19. Wilkinson HA: Epileptic pain. An uncommon manifestation with localizing value. *Neurology* 23:518–520, 1973.

87. Episodic Neurological Symptoms

H. KENNETH WALKER, MD

Definition

Recurrent transient episodes of neurological dysfunction lasting minutes to hours and followed by a complete return to the premorbid state. Any one or any combination of the following symptoms are likely: unconsciousness, localized motor or sensory deficits, visual dysfunction such as monocular or binocular blindness or diplopia, tonic-clonic motor activity, bladder or bowel incontinence, or both, headache. However, any neurological symptom can be present. Common causes include epileptic seizures, syncope, migraine headache, and transient ischemic attacks.

Technique

Episodic neurological problems usually come to light during the present illness or review of specific organ systems that precede this data base section. For example, the patient will describe transient blindness when queried about that symptom under visual dysfunction. On rare occasions the interviewer will not discover these symptoms until a question is asked such as: Do you ever have any problems that come and go, such as falling out, eye problems, weakness, or funny feelings?

The initial goal in characterizing such episodes is to get the exact order in which the symptoms occur and to be certain that no symptom is omitted. Begin by getting the patient's spontaneous account. The best starting point is the very first symptom that occurs. A good way to draw this from the patient is to ask: How do you know when you are about to have one of these attacks? Do you have any warning beforehand? If you are driving a car, does anything let you know you are about to have an attack in time to pull off to the side of the road?

After this starting point, ask the patient to recount the succeeding symptoms in temporal sequence. During this phase simply get the patient's account without asking about specific symptoms.

Next take each symptom in order of occurrence and ask the patient to describe each one in detail; often the patient will remember other symptoms not mentioned previously. After the patient's description, ask specific questions appropriate to that symptom.

Now you can ask about specific symptoms not mentioned. Be careful to ask first a general question: Did you have any trouble with your vision during the attack? Then proceed to a more specific question: Did you have double vision?

Some idea of the duration of each symptom is important, as well as the total length of the attack. Sometimes symptoms will persist for hours, eg, a postictal or Todd's paralysis after a focal seizure. Seek out other postictal symptoms such as headache, confusion, or aphasia. If a symptom begins in one area of the body and then spreads to other areas, ask the patient to indicate the speed of the spread with a hand. The date of the first attack and the frequency should be clearly pinpointed. Find out if the attacks are repeated without variation or whether there has been change in the pattern over time.

Some of the more frequently occurring symptoms are given below:

1. Cerebral cortex: aphasia, confusion, unconsciousness
2. Cranial nerves (including cortical projections):
   I: Distasteful odor
   II: Monocular blindness, visual field deficit (usually homonymous hemianopsia but can be more restricted), blurring of vision
   III, IV, VI: Diplopia
   V: Paresthesias
   VII: Weakness
   VIII: Tinnitus, vertigo
3. Extremities: Weakness, abnormal sensations
   Autonomic: Bladder or bowel incontinence, or both
4. Common postictal symptoms or signs include:
   Confusion or lethargy
   Aphasia
   Hemiparesis
   Headache

Background Information

The pathophysiology of migraine, seizures, and syncope is given in sections 85, 86, and 51. Transient ischemic attacks (TIAs) are evanescent focal neurological deficits that usually last a few minutes and rarely for 1 to 2 hours. They are caused by ischemia insufficient to cause infarction of a focal area. The specific symptoms and signs depend upon the particular vessel(s) affected. For clinical purposes it is sufficient to divide the arterial supply into the carotid or anterior circulation and the vertebrobasilar or posterior circulation. Symptoms commonly seen with anterior circulation TIAs include monocular blindness ("amaurosis fugax" or fleeting blindness) and aphasia (when the dominant hemisphere is involved). Posterior circulation symptoms include diplopia, crossed symptoms (one side of face and opposite side of body), and dysarthria. Some symptoms are common to both circulations: weakness, dizziness, numbness.

The pathophysiology of TIAs is not settled. Three factors are felt to be involved in most TIAs:

1. Atherosclerosis
2. Individual arterial anatomy, especially collateral circulation
3. A triggering mechanism such as decreased cardiac output due to dysrhythmias; blood abnormalities such as increased viscosity; microemboli released from atherosclerotic plaques such as cholesterol crystals; local factors such as head movements

As a result of interaction of the factors listed above and perhaps others that are unknown, a particular area of the brain becomes ischemic before other areas, and focal symptoms occur.

Clinical Significance

It is quite important and often difficult to distinguish among TIAs, seizures, hemiplegic migraine, and syncope. The history is of crucial importance in making this distinction, supplemented by the physical and laboratory findings.

When focal seizures produce motor convulsions, there is no problem in separating them. Autonomic phenomena such as incontinence are seen most often in seizures. Initial symptoms (or aura) such as a bad odor or taste (seen in uncinate seizures), "automatic" phenomena (a stereotyped gesture such as throwing up a hand), or a cry usually indicate focal seizures. Focal seizures often begin with "positive" phenomena such as tonic-clonic movements and can be followed by a postictal paralysis; TIAs often begin with a paralysis. Sensory seizures are more difficult to separate from TIAs. Certain symptoms point squarely toward TIAs: monocular blindness, "crossed" symptoms or signs, diplopia.

Hemiplegic migraine often ends with a severe hemicranial headache and usually begins earlier in life than TIAs. Many times there is a positive family history.

Selected References

1. Karp H: Cerebral vascular disease and neurologic manifestations of cardiovascular disease, in Hurst JW (ed in chief): *The Heart,* ed 4. New York, McGraw-Hill, 1978, chap 105, pp 1889–1905.

2. Toole JR, Cole M: Ischemic cerebrovascular disease, in Baker AB, Baker LH (eds): *Clinical Neurology.* New York, Harper and Row, 1975, vol 1, chap 10.

88. Pain and Sensory Perversions

NETTLETON S. PAYNE, MD

Definition

Pain is an unpleasant sensory experience that most often accompanies bodily injury and serves to warn the individual of harm in order that protective measures may be taken.

Sensory perversions can be divided into paresthesias and dysesthesias. Paresthesias are spontaneous, abnormal sensations. They may be tactile, thermal, or painful and periodic or constant. Dysesthesias are painful irradiating sensations consistently elicited by nonpainful cutaneous stimuli such as a light touch or a gentle stroke. Synonyms are hyperpathia and hyperalgesia. The induced sensation will often outlast the stimulus by seconds or minutes and frequently results in a complaint of intense burning. Paresthesias and dysesthesias must be considered phenomena distinct from symptoms implying sensory loss such as numbness, and from painful conditions described as aching, throbbing, or itching.

A sensory perversion always indicates disease of neural tissue in contrast to most pain, which implies the normal response of nocioceptive nerve fibers and their central connections to trauma or other pathological processes.

Technique

Painful sensations are the most common problem that brings the patient to the physician. The pain may not be associated with obvious structural abnormality. The physician's goal is to *localize* and *characterize* the abnormal sensation(s).

To define the anatomical limits of the sensory experience, begin by asking the patient to outline the afflicted region by using one finger. This task may be difficult because the patient often interprets the abnormal sensation as afflicting a wide region of the body. To determine the central area, and perhaps the site of origin of the pain may require persistence on the part of the physician. If the pain or sensory perversion is associated with numbness the task is made easier by having the individual map out this hypesthetic region.

If dysesthesias are present, the examiner may accurately determine the afflicted area by using a wisp of cotton to touch the skin.

Suggest words such as sharp, stabbing, aching, throbbing, burning, shooting to the patient during the history taking. Some pains are constant and rarely aggravated by movement, positions during sleep, or by other physical or emotional stress, while other pains are not. Therefore, it is important to ask the patient what makes the pain worse, what makes the pain better, how long it lasts, and whether it is more severe at the onset or gradually lessens, or vice versa.

Background Information

The concept that cutaneous sensation is composed of two distinctive and divisible components was first put forth by Henry Head early in the twentieth century. He described these components as epicritic, or discriminative; and protopathic, or noxious sensation. He further stated that if the epicritic senses, including tactile localization and fine grades of tactile and temperature discrimination, are selectively removed in a particular region, the protopathic senses in that region, including pain and temperature, cannot be accurately localized and furthermore take on that excessively unpleasant spreading or irradiating quality characteristic of dysesthesias. Subsequent investigators in neurophysiology have shown that distinct types of sensory axon indeed do exist in all cutaneous nerves, separable on the basis of conduction velocity and axon diameter. The receptors of the large axons, designated A-alpha and A-beta with axon diameters of 6–14 micra, respond to light touch or hair displacement at extremely low threshold and have rapid nerve conduction times. Smaller sized axons, termed A-delta (myelinated) and C (unmyelinated) fibers with diameters under 4 micra and with slower conduction times, convey the entire spectrum of cutaneous sensibility with a broad range of thresholds. Among this group exist those axons whose terminals respond only to high thresholds of tissue-damaging stimuli.

Centrally, the large and small axons send terminals to distinct laminae in the dorsal gray of the spinal cord. Among the group of smaller axons, those conducting solely nociceptive, or pain, information terminate in lamina I, lamina IV, and V. These laminae generate sensory projections distinct from those conveying "epicritic" sensation. At all levels of spinal cord and brain, the tracts and systems responsible for perception of the most severe forms of pain (visceral, perversions) are located medial to the other sensory projections and are anatomically and physiologically not separable from other systems in the reticular formation.

In 1965, Melzack and Wall posed a gating mechanism in the dorsal gray matter of the spinal cord wherein the substantia gelatinosa, after activation by the large axons, would inhibit those neurons conveying pain sensations. Thus, large fiber input would serve to shut off pain. Recent anatomical and physiologic studies have failed to confirm the existence of the gate as conceived by Melzack and Wall. It is now accepted that modulation of nociceptive activity occurs at many levels within the brain including certain areas in the reticular and limbic systems. Endogenous morphine-like compounds (endorphines, encephalins) have been found in high concentrations only in those areas that are active in the processing of pain information.

Clinical evidence indicates that some disorders which selectively damage the larger axons or that cause loss of myelin will often result in paresthesias and dysesthesias over those cutaneous areas deprived of this larger fiber innervation, whereas those disorders that selectively damage the smallest sensory fibers result in selective anesthesia for pain and temperature, without sensory perversions and with preservation of discriminative touch. Structural changes causing nerve or nerve root compression and toxic or metabolic disease-inducing neuropathy are commonly encountered conditions that tend to damage the larger axons or their myelin sheaths. These conditions often include paresthesias and dysesthesias among their symptoms and signs.

Clinical Significance

Pain, while most often a warning sign of acute injury or disease, may become persistent in disorders in which it is not possible to effectively treat the cause of pain. Severe degenerative spine disease, rheumatoid arthritis, and terminal cancers are examples of disorders that often result in this type of pain. The pain is no longer useful and becomes a large portion of the patient's disability. These most difficult types of pain to treat often lead to drug dependency, searches for miracle cures, and inappropriate surgical procedures. Patient management in the setting of a pain clinic staffed by a variety of specialists with particular interest in chronic pain is often beneficial.

Pain may be localized to a known anatomical structure or it may be *referred* from a more distant site over common neural pathways. Examples of the latter include sciatic nerve pain found in association with herniation of a lumbar intervertebral disk, or medial upper extremity pain in angina pectoris.

Sensory perversions commonly occur in disorders of peripheral nerve and nerve roots, usually in association with other symptoms and signs of dysfunction such as weakness, pain, and the loss of feeling. This constellation of symptoms and signs together with their anatomical distribution will usually guide the clinician toward those special studies that will pinpoint the origin and etiology of the disturbance. If a certain nerve can be implicated, then nerve conduction studies may be applied to find the exact locus of the disturbance. Other diagnostic studies include myelography or computerized axial tomography of the spine, which may demonstrate involvement of the spinal cord, nerve roots, or their rami in the region of the spine.

Certain painful disorders are so characteristic that they are considered distinct clinical syndromes. These include: (1) causalgia, (2) posttraumatic sympathetic dystrophy, (3) postherpetic neuralgia, (4) phantom pain, and (5) tic douloureux.

Causalgia is the sensation of burning pain or hyperpathia that involves the upper or lower extremity following partial injury to the median, ulnar or sciatic nerve. The pain is most pronounced in the digits, palm of the hand, or sole of the foot. Trophic changes occur. The skin becomes shiny and glossy smooth and may be scaly or discolored. Sudomotor (sweating) and vasomotor abnormalities are usually present. There may be profuse sweating of the palms or soles associated with emotional stress. At rest the involved limb is warmer or cooler than the normal one. The dysesthesias may become so intense that the patient cannot bear contact with clothing or drafts of air. The extremity is kept constantly protected and immobile, often wrapped in a cloth or moistened with lukewarm or cool water. The patient often finds that the pain is aggravated by heat, noise, and emotional stress.

Posttraumatic sympathetic dystrophy with pain and trophic changes similar to causalgia occurs after blunt trauma to an extremity and does not have an associated injury to a major peripheral nerve. Its pathogenesis is not understood.

Postherpetic neuralgia is a constant aching burning pain which develops following an attack of herpes zoster (shingles), and which may be accompanied by severe dysesthesias. It develops in the dermatomal distribution of the involved nerves. Following the infection, small scars may be found marking the site of the vesicles, a physical finding most helpful in cases where the diagnosis is otherwise obscure.

Phantom limb or phantom body pain is the paresthesia in an area of complete sensory loss which may occur following amputation of a limb, avulsion of the brachial plexus, or spinal cord injury. Sensations of burning, tingling, severe crushing pressure, or a feeling of streaming fire are often reported by the patient. The distal portion of the missing or denervated limb is felt to be in a clenched fist position, or in the position that it was in immediately prior to amputation. Gradually, over several years, the phantom becomes less vivid, the imagined extremity smaller, and the pain less severe. Only 10% or less of individuals have a long-term intolerable phantom pain.

Trigeminal neuralgia (tic douloureux) is hemifacial paroxysmal pain of extreme intensity confined to the distribution of the trigeminal nerve (see section 198). The pain is provoked by various sensory stimuli including facial movements and light touch, and is not associated with hypesthesia, hypalgesia, dysesthesias, or other neurologic deficits.

The pathology of trigeminal neuralgia appears to involve the sensory root entry zone of the fifth cranial nerve. Tumors, bony and dural abnormalities, aberrant blood vessels, and sclerotic plaques of demyelination alter the microanatomy of the fifth nerve and may result in abnormal electrical discharges within the central nervous system. Animal investigation (cat) of trigeminal neuralgia has demonstrated that fiber degeneration and synaptic reorganization occur in brainstem nuclei following injury to the peripheral nerve and may provide the substrate for a seizurelike discharge within the brainstem somatic sensory column. The severity of the pain of trigeminal neuralgia suggests that there is a recruitment of many axons, possibly through reverberating circuits. Such circuits may develop as the result of cross-talk between axons partially bared of their myelin or by reflection of axonal discharges at loci of abrupt changes of axon diameter. While the exact mechanism of trigeminal neuralgia remains unknown, it appears at present that both peripheral nerve and central synaptic abnormality share the responsibility for this painful condition.

The pain of trigeminal neuralgia is limited to the distribution of the involved divisions of the fifth cranial nerve. On rare occasion this pain may be referred to or involve the distribution of the seventh, ninth and tenth cranial nerves or the occipital nerve. Any single paroxysm is hemifacial. The paroxysms of pain associated with trigeminal neuralgia are acute and lancinating or lightninglike. The pain may occur as a single shock or in repeated bursts separated by seconds or minutes. Light touch over facial trigger zones located around the mouth, cheek, and eye may precipitate acute tic pain. The pain lasts seconds to minutes and is often set off by a blast of cold or hot air, shaving, combing the hair, or similar stimulus. The patient often guards the face, and may not speak, eat, or shave to prevent a paroxysm of pain. A weight loss of 30 lbs. or more during symptomatic periods is not unusual. The paroxysm of pain may come so often as to be considered "tic status." As the sharp pain subsides, the patient may experience aching in the distribution of the lancinating pain. Surprisingly, even during periods of severe symptoms, sleep is only rarely interrupted.

Recognition of trigeminal neuralgia is important for two reasons: (1) it is vital not to misdiagnose a lesion such as a tumor that is masquerading as tic; (2) 95% of the cases of tic can be successfully treated. Medical management with carbamazine or phenytoin is effective in 60–80% of individuals. In patients who fail to respond to medical management, surgical therapy directed at removal of structures causing abnormal nerve root compression may be safely accomplished using microneurosurgical techniques without resulting in sensory deficit. In those instances where the patient's general condition will not tolerate open surgery, a percutaneous radiofrequency approach to the sensory root is performed. This results in pain relief and a partial sensory deficit in the portion of the fifth nerve involved, with pain relief in 96% of patients.

On rare occasions, sensory perversions may be caused by brain lesions. In these instances, wide regions or even an entire side of the body may be involved, to the extent that the slightest cutaneous stimulation will result in a massive assault of pain and discomfort. This condition, usually the sequelae of a cerebral vascular accident, is popularly termed the thalamic syndrome and is habitually blamed on a lesion in that structure.

Neurosurgical experience with a variety of pain-relieving procedures, including lateral spinothalamic tractotomy and central stimulation, indicates that central pain may be generated within multisynaptic medial systems, activated by nociceptive input and projecting into the reticular core of the brainstem. Lesions at any level that interrupt the lateral spinothalamic tract (or its thalamic terminus) but spare those more medial systems may result in central pain.

Selected References

1.   Head H: *Studies in Neurology*. London, Oxford University Press, 1970, vol 1.
2.   Kerr FWL: Neuroanatomical substrates of nocioception in the spinal cord: Review article. *Pain* 1:325–356, 1975.
3.   Mitchell SW: *Injuries of Nerves and Their Consequences*. Philadelphia, JB Lippincott, 1972.
4.   Pagni CA: Place of stereotactic technique in surgery for pain. *Adv Neurol* 4:699–706, 1974.

89. Weakness

H. KENNETH WALKER, MD

Definition

Weakness: (1) A feeling of weariness, tiredness, lassitude, or malaise that is a frequent symptomatic concomitant of all systemic illnesses. Similar complaints when heard from otherwise healthy people are suggestive of emotional problems such as depression. (2) A decrease or less than normal function of muscles, best analyzed in terms of these muscle groups:

a. Lower extremities: distal, proximal (including pelvic girdle)
b. Upper extremities: distal, proximal (including shoulder girdle)
c. Trunk
d. Head
e. Respiration

Fatigability: Used specifically here to mean weakness that occurs in a progressive fashion as muscles perform work, that is, weakness with exertion.

Technique

The complaint of weakness is present in a large number of patients. The meaning usually appears to be so vague or varied as to be worthless. But weakness can be the earliest or only manifestation of important disease processes. Examples include early corticospinal dysfunction, myasthenia, myopathies, and the neuropathies that accompany cancer, diabetes, and other diseases. The symptom of weakness can be best used when the clinician forms a clear concept of what patients may be saying when they use the word. The two most frequent categories are given in the definition above. These two categories can usually be separated from each other fairly easily by the history.

There are two cardinal principles to taking a history for weakness:

1. The history should be focused upon the patient's daily activities.
2. Weakness is analyzed in terms of the body segment involved: distal, proximal, trunk, and face. This is useful for two reasons:
   a. Segmental dysfunction instantly places a patient complaining of weakness into the category of having a discrete disease of the neuromuscular system.
   b. Most disorders affecting this system have a characteristic distribution of dysfunction.

The patient will usually volunteer the complaint of weakness. If not, ask about it. In many cases asking about "weakness" is less productive than asking specific questions about activities such as walking, housecleaning, and keeping up with peers. A patient who denies difficulties when asked about weakness will often give positive data when asked these specific questions.

In a systematic fashion inquire about the common problems patients with weakness will notice with the segments listed above. Start with a nondirective question (Do you have trouble with your feet?) then use a directive one if necessary (Do you trip over rugs?). Add questions based upon the patient's daily activities to your questions about each segment (see section 115). The common segmental difficulties are given below. Note that other types of dysfunction, such as ataxia, can also interfere with some of these activities (eg, typing). So be sure to get a description of the exact problem the patient has with these activities.

Lower Extremities
    Distal: Tripping over rugs, carpets, curbs, cords
    Proximal: Getting up from chairs, getting off commode, stepping on bus platforms
Upper Extremities
    Distal: Opening jars, shaking hands, using screwdriver, writing, playing piano, typing
    Proximal: Lifting arm over shoulders, as in fixing hair
Trunk: Getting up from lying position
Head: Pursing lips as in kissing or whistling; keeping soap out of eyes while taking shower; specific cranial nerve functions, especially speech, swallowing, and extraocular movement
Respiration: Breathlessness

The mode of onset and progression of the weakness are quite important. Careful history taking can reveal progression from one segment to another over a period of time. Illnesses preceding the onset of weakness, such as febrile illnesses, must be asked about, as well as familial history. Many congenital disorders of weakness are sex-linked or dominant. If the patient is an adult, the examination needs to include careful questioning related to muscle strength during childhood and adolescence. Athletic activities, especially when compared with peers, can form a productive part of this inquiry.

Fatigability is used here to mean the onset of weakness with exertion. Compare it with the amount of exertion that produced fatigability before the onset of weakness. Comparison with peers is helpful in young people.

Observe the patient as you take the history and as the patient walks. (See section 205 for clues that observation can furnish.) Facial appearance can be helpful, eg, myotonic dystrophy patients have frontal balding; apathy; temporal and masseter hollowing; ptosis—all adding up to a characteristic and unforgettable facial appearance.

Other symptoms important in the characterization of weakness include muscle pain at rest, muscle pain on exertion, cramps, and urine color (myoglobinuria, hemoglobinuria).

Background Information

Bilaterally symmetrical segmental weakness can be caused by diseases of muscles, the myoneural junction, peripheral nerves, spinal roots, and less commonly by afflictions of the spinal cord and central nervous system. The background information is covered in sections 204 and 205.

Clinical Significance

In many cases weakness is the earliest symptom with which the clinician is confronted in a patient with vague complaints who appears otherwise healthy. The temptation to dismiss such patients as having emotional problems is almost too great for most of us to resist. Every patient who has been admitted to our hospital in the past five years with the Guillain-Barre syndrome had been turned away from the emergency clinic at least once and often twice.

A general principle of inestimable value is that *when weakness follows a neuroanatomical distribution, it is due to organic disease.* This is why it is so important to analyze weakness in terms of body segments. In general, distal weakness is caused by neuropathies, and proximal weakness by myopathies. Inherited metabolic problems (such as enzyme deficiencies) and the muscular dystrophies have their onset in childhood or early adulthood. The inflammatory myopathies or myositides usually have a fairly rapid onset with marked weakness and, at times, pain. They are often associated with other problems such as collagen diseases.

Selected References

1.   Walton JN (ed): *Diseases of Voluntary Muscle*, ed 3. Edinburgh, Churchill Livingstone, 1974.
2.   Adams RD: Lassitude and asthenia, in Wintrobe MM, et al (eds): *Harrison's Principles of Internal Medicine*, ed 6: New York, McGraw-Hill, pp 101–105, 1970.

90. Head Trauma

ALAN S. FLEISCHER, MD

Definition

Clinically significant craniocerebral trauma consists of trauma severe enough to:

1.   Produce changes in level of consciousness ranging from temporary loss of consciousness (concussion) to deep coma.
2.   Require a surgical procedure for evacuation of a traumatic intracranial mass lesion such as an acute subdural or epidural hematoma.
3.   Produce transient or permanent neurological deficit such as hemiplegia, visual field deficit.
4.   Result in a seizure disorder.
5.   Result in a leak of cerebrospinal fluid (CSF).
6.   Produce a skull fracture.

Technique

Inquire about any past history of significant head trauma with particular attention to the following:

1.   Was there alteration of level of consciousness?
2.   Was or is there a neurological deficit (aphasia, hemiparesis, sensory loss, diminished intellectual function)?

3. Have there been any seizures? If so, did they begin shortly after the head injury or after a significant time delay?
4. What medications, specifically anticonvulsants, if any, is the patient using?
5. Is there persistent headache, vertigo, dizziness, blurred vision? The headache, particularly, should be characterized as to location, description, relationship to activities or time of day.
6. Is there pending litigation concerning the traumatic incident?

Background Information

Delayed effects of head trauma are numerous and may be severely incapacitating. Those permanent neurological deficits related to the initial injury may or may not improve or remain as fixed deficits.

Skull fracture, especially when associated with persistent CSF rhinorrhea or otorrhea, may require surgical repair to avoid repeated bouts of meningitis. Prophylactic antibiotics should not be utilized and the patient should undergo further neurosurgical evaluation.

Posttraumatic seizures are not uncommon and are directly proportional to the severity of the injury as well as the type of injury, penetrating injuries being far more likely to result in seizure. Posttraumatic seizures are of two basic types, early and delayed. Early seizures occurring within a few days to weeks following trauma are less likely to persist on a chronic basis. The most reliable factors related to the development of posttraumatic seizures include dural laceration and the extent of antegrade and retrograde amnesia associated with the traumatic event.

Posttraumatic syndrome including headache, dizziness, vertigo, and anxiety is very common and frequently related to persisting litigation concerning the injury.

Clinical Significance

Obviously persistent seizures require the utilization of prophylactic anticonvulsants. CSF leaks must be repaired. Diminished intellectual function may be related to the development of posttraumatic-communicating hydrocephalus, which may respond to a CSF shunting procedure. A CT scan will demonstrate this finding. Headache associated with the posttraumatic syndrome, the etiology of which is unknown, must be differentiated from organic headache on the basis of a chronic subdural hematoma especially if associated with focal neurological deficit or signs of increased intracranial pressure. A CT scan should be obtained.

Selected References

1.   Crockard HA, Brown FD, Calica AB, et al: Psychological conse-
     quences of experimental missile injury and the use of data analysis
     to predict survival. *J Neurosurg* 46:784–794, 1977.
2.   Miller JD: Clinical aspects of intracranial pressure volume relation-
     ships in head injuries, in McLaurin RL (ed): *Proceedings of the Sec-
     ond Chicago Symposium on Neural Trauma.* New York, Grune and
     Stratton, 1976, pp 239–245.
3.   Flamm ES, Demopoulos HB, Seligman ML, et al: Ethanol potentia-
     tion of central nervous system trauma. *J Neurosurg* 46:328, 1977.
4.   Beker DP, Miller JD, Ward JD, et al: The outcome from severe head
     injury with intensive management. *J Neurosurg* 47:491–502, 1977.
5.   Jennett WB, Bond MR: Assessment of outcome after severe brain
     damage. *Lancet* 1:1031–1034, 1975.
6.   Miller JD, Beker DP, Ward JD: Significance of intracranial hyperten-
     sion in severe head injury. *J Neurosurg* 47:503–516, 1977.

91. Muscle Cramps

CLAUDIA R. ADKISON, PhD
H. KENNETH WALKER, MD

Definition

Pain associated with a severe muscle contraction. The muscle is firm
and hard, and voluntary relaxation is impossible. The usual duration is a
few minutes. In certain problems the contraction is painless, eg, myotonia.

Technique

The occurrence of muscle cramps is pervasive—everyone has had a
"charley horse." Consequently, cramps are often regarded as trivial by
both patient and physician. However, cramps can at times be the only or

an important clue to serious disease. An example is McArdle's disease, or muscle phosphorylase deficiency. The diagnosis is all too frequently made concomitant with an episode of acute renal failure due to exertional rhabdomyolysis and myoglobinuria. Yet careful questioning almost always reveals the presence of muscle cramps noted since early childhood and often previous episodes of postexertional dark urine, the significance of which was not appreciated by physicians.

The symptom of painful muscle cramps can dominate the clinical picture, and the physician has little difficulty in getting an excellent history. But even when they appear to be trivial, a careful history needs to be taken. It is wisest to begin with open questions, since in many instances associated symptoms will be brought up by the observant patient that the physician would not have thought to ask. After the patient has described the cramps, ask more specific questions. The following points should be covered.

Time of occurrence. During rest, during use of the muscle, after exercise, nocturnal.

Precipitating factors. Exercise (determine whether mild or strenuous) meals, emotional stimuli, sensory stimuli, or nothing. The relationship of exercise to cramps is quite important and very variable, even in the same person. Prolonged exertion at times will produce no symptoms, but on other occasions milder exertion will.

Duration of cramp. Seconds to minutes, or hours (see contracture below).

Age of onset. This needs to be determined in a most careful fashion since it can lead to the suspicion of hereditary causes of cramps. Initially focus your questioning on periods of severe exercise, such as basketball games or running around the schoolyard. Then obtain the patient's judgment about quantity of exercise compared to peers; use examples such as playing football, running, and the like.

Pain. The occurrence of pain during contraction serves to separate several syndromes.

Weakness. The presence or absence of weakness either during and after cramps or as a continuously present symptom.

Myoglobinuria. The occurrence of postexertional dark discolored urine is a critical historical point. It indicates rhabdomyolysis with myoglobin being excreted in the urine, producing the potential of acute renal failure and irreversible renal damage.

Contracture. The inability to relax muscles after being held in a particular position is another historical point that helps to separate serious from nonserious causes. Holding heavy objects provides the most fruitful area of inquiry: holding a heavy iron skillet while cleaning it, gripping a bat while playing baseball, and the like. The patient finds the fingers cannot be extended after these activities but remain curled as though still holding the object. They will often tell you they have to use the other hand to straighten out their fingers. Muscle phosphorylase deficiency (McArdle's) and phosphofructokinase deficiency (Tarui's) are two examples.

Drugs. Carefully ascertain all the drugs the patient is taking, since an ever-increasing number are being implicated in the production of cramps and even muscle injury.

Family history. Although at present fairly rare, very important muscle diseases are hereditary, and a positive family history is quite important in any patient with cramps. The glycogen storage diseases are good examples.

Associated symptoms. See Table 14 for some diseases that have cramps as one manifestation. A good rule is to do a careful and complete review of systems and then examine all the positive findings for evidence of diseases such as hypothyroidism that may produce cramps.

Table 14. A partial list of causes of muscle cramp and stiffness syndromes.

---

1. Muscle contraction disorders: muscle phosphorylase deficiency, muscle phosphofructokinase deficiency, malignant hyperthermia.
2. Muscle membrane disorders (myotonia): hyperkalemic periodic paralysis, myotonic dystrophy, myotonia congenita.
3. Peripheral nerve disorders: tetany (due to hypocalcemia, hypomagnesemia, or alkalosis), clofibrate, ordinary muscle cramps ("charley horse"), lower motor neuron disease, myxedema, salt depletion or diuretic therapy, pregnancy, uremia, renal dialysis, pseudomyotonia of grip in C-7 root lesion, hemifacial spasm.
4. Central nervous system disorders: tetanus, strychnine poisoning, stiff-man syndrome, continuous rigidity due to spinal cord lesions, tonic spasms in multiple sclerosis, "painful legs and moving toes," alcohol spasms, acute dystonic reactions to phenothiazines and butyrophenones.

Modified from Layzer. The level of origin of some of the syndromes have not been completely identified, and some operate at several levels.

Background Information

The skeletal muscles of the body consist of elongate bundles of muscle cells or fibers bound together by fibrous connective tissue. The fibers are the functional units of the muscle; they attach at each end to the muscle tendons and usually function in voluntary movement in response to stimulation by motor nerves.

A muscle fiber is a long, multinucleate, cylindrical cell whose complex structural features are closely related to its function. Occupying most of the fiber's interior are the myofibrils, which are orderly bundles of myofilaments along the full length of the cell. Myosin and actin are the contractile proteins that make up the thick and thin myofilaments, respectively. The actin of the thin filaments has the regulatory proteins troponin and tropomyosin bound to it. The myosin molecules of the thick filaments contain "heads" of heavy meromyosin which project out from the filament, have ATPase activity, and form cross-bridges with actin.

Myofibrils display a banded pattern, based on the orientation of thick and thin filaments to each other. The sarcomere is the structural and functional subunit of the myofibril and is limited by two Z bands. Shortening of the sarcomeres results in muscle shortening. The structure of the sarcomere is reviewed in Fig 8.

Surrounding each myofibril like a sleeve are the longitudinal and cisternal components of the sarcoplasmic reticulum (SR). The transverse tubules, invaginations of the plasma membrane, weave among the myofibrils and are closely associated with SR cisternae at the junctions of the A and I bands along the myofibrils. Numerous mitochondria are located in the sarcoplasm between the myofibrils, along with ions, glycogen, lipids, high energy compounds (ATP and phosphocreatine), and enzymes, all of which have important roles in muscle contraction.

Muscle contraction occurs in response to the generation of action potentials in the fibers. Skeletal muscle fibers may be excited by chemical, electrical, or mechanical stimuli, but ordinary voluntary movement is the

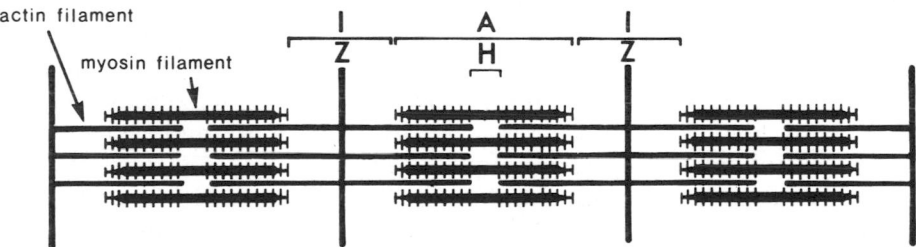

Figure 8. The longitudinal organization of the myofibril. (Modified from Huxley, HE: The mechanism of muscular contraction. *Science* 164:1356, 1969.)

result of motor innervation. A motor unit is one motor neuron and all the muscle fibers innervated by the branches of its axon. Each muscle fiber usually has one neuromuscular junction. When a motor neuron fires and releases acetylcholine at the neuromuscular junction, an action potential is generated in the sarcolemma and spreads into the fiber along the T tubules, initiating the contractile response. The small contraction resulting from one neural impulse and one depolarization is a muscle twitch. During voluntary movement, nerve fibers may fire up to 50 times per second. Since the duration of a twitch is greater than the duration of an action potential, twitches may overlap to result in smooth contraction of the muscle. As voluntary effort increases, more motor units and fibers are recruited.

Excitation of the sarcolemma is coupled with the contractile apparatus at the level of the T tubules and SR cisternae. By a mechanism which has not been clearly defined, depolarization of the T tubule (plasma membrane) causes the release of calcium ions from the adjacent terminal cisternae of the SR into the sarcoplasm around the myofibrils. Calcium binds to troponin, which is bound, in turn, to actin by tropomyosin. The Ca^{++}-troponin complex alters the actin molecule, allowing the formation of cross-linkages between actin and the myosin-ATP complex. The myosin heads bind to actin at an angle and then swivel in an energy-requiring process. The continued breaking and reforming of cross-linkages between actin and myosin at sequential sites slides the myosin filament along the actin filament, pulling the Z lines closer and shortening the sarcomere. This phenomenon is repeated in sarcomeres along the length of the myofibril.

When neural stimulation ceases, relaxation of the muscle occurs. The SR takes up calcium from the sarcoplasm by an energy-requiring active transport mechanism. Actin and myosin cross-linkages cease to occur as the concentration of calcium in the sarcoplasm decreases. If the active uptake of calcium ions by the SR is inhibited, relaxation does not take place even when there are no action potentials, and contracture or physiologic rigor is the result.

Both contraction and relaxation require energy. When a muscle is at rest and during recovery after contraction, free fatty acids from the blood are the major substrates for energy production. Glucose is used to build up the intracellular glycogen deposit. During moderate exertion when the oxygen consumption by the muscle does not exceed the supply, aerobic glycolysis is the high energy source. During extreme or prolonged exertion when the oxygen supply is inadequate, anaerobic glycolysis is possible because of abundant glycogen stores. Another source of high-energy phosphate for the synthesis of ATP during exercise is phosphocreatine. Lactic acid levels may build up both intracellularly and extracellularly during anaerobic glycoysis, and eventually may cause a decrease in pH and in enzyme activity.

Muscle spindles and the neural control of contraction via inhibitory and excitatory synopsis are discussed in section 209, Deep Tendon Reflexes.

Clinical Significance

There are numerous causes of cramps. The article by Layzer and Rowland (reference 3) is an elegant presentation and is highly recommended. The following discussion is a brief summary of some of the causes and associated findings.

Myoglobinuria. When muscles are injured, myoglobin can be released into the blood and excreted in the urine. A large variety of problems can cause rhabdomyolysis and myoglobinuria. Metabolic abnormalities are among the more common causes: alcoholic rhabdomyolysis, barbiturates, heroin, hypothermia, hyperthermia, diabetic ketoacidosis, and hypokalemia. Hereditary disorders that produce myoglobinuria include phosphorylase and phosphofructokinase deficiency. Muscle ischemia and the crush syndrome cause myoglobinuria. Severe exertion, especially in persons such as untrained military recruits, and prolonged seizures are additional causes. See references 1 and 2.

Glycogen storage diseases. Muscle phosphorylase and phosphofructokinase deficiency are the two types that produce muscle cramps, weakness, easy fatiguability of muscle, and myoglobinuria (reference 4).

Malignant hyperthermia. Occurring during general anesthesia or succinylcholine administration, this produces widespread rhabdomyolysis, severe acidosis, and renal failure in certain persons. In most cases there appears to be an inherited predisposition.

Myotonic syndromes. These can produce cramps that are not painful—a "silent cramp." These syndromes include myotonia congenita, myotonic muscular dystrophy, hyperkalemic periodic paralysis, and others.

Local tetanus. This is an important and little recognized, albeit rare, syndrome. The source of the tetanus toxin is often forgotten by patients. The hallmark is a patient who complains of cramps or severe "tightness" or "stiffness" in a muscle group that often rapidly spreads to involve the entire body. Adams terms this "recruitment spasm." This painful spasm will last some minutes and then disappear, to recur again. The muscles initially affected are those around the wound, eg, the thigh muscles near a buckshot wound to the femoral area (a personally observed case) or the forearm muscles around a porcupine quill injury site (Adams). Twitch-

Table 15. Characteristics of cramp syndromes.

Kind of Cramp	Synonyms or Examples of Disease	Provoking Factors	Painful Cramps	Continuous Stiffness at Rest	Electromyogram
Muscle Contracture	Deficiency of muscle phosphorylase or phosphofructokinase	Exertional only	Yes	No	Little or no electrical activity in muscle affected by contraction
Myotonia	Myotonia congenita, myotonic dystrophy, paramyotonia, hyperkalemic periodic paralysis, and chondrodystrophic myotonia	Delayed relaxation of voluntary contraction; percussion or electrical stimulation of muscle	No	No	Myotonic bursts after contraction, percussion or needle movement
Nerve Neuromyotonia	Pseudomyotonia, myokymia with delayed muscular relaxation, quantal squander, and armadillo syndrome	Delayed relaxation of voluntary contraction	No	Yes	Continuous electrical activity at rest; afterdischarge follows contraction; potentials range from single muscle fibers to motor units
Tetany		Spontaneous; provoked by hyperventilation or nerve compression	Usually not	No	Regularly repetitive motor-unit discharges in doublets or triplets at 15/sec
Ordinary muscle cramps		Exertional; with minor movement; in sleep	Yes	No	Irregular, high-frequency, high-voltage, profuse bursts of motor-unit potentials
Central Tetanus		Movement and emotional or sensory stimuli	Yes	Yes	Persistent normal motor-unit discharges at rest; heightened during spasm
Stiff-man syndrome		Movement and emotional or sensory stimuli	Yes	Yes	Persistent normal motor-unit discharges at rest; heightened during spasm

From Layzer RB, Rowland LP: Cramps. N Eng J Med 285(1):31–40, 1971. Modified with permission from the N Eng J Med.

ings and brief muscle spasms around the injury site then spread rapidly to contiguous muscles. The spasms initially are brought out by exertion, but then as the disease progresses they become more stimulus sensitive, to the point that, like generalized tetanus, a stimulus as slight as a gentle clap will provoke an intensely painful spreading muscle spasm (reference 5).

Thyroid disease. Both hyperthyroidism and hypothyroidism can produce muscle pain, stiffness, and cramps.

Other causes of cramps are listed in Tables 14 and 15.

Selected References

1. Rowland LP, Penn AS: Myoglobinuria. *Med Clin N Am* 56:1233–1256, 1972.
2. Rowland LP, Layzer RB: Muscular dystrophies, atrophies and related diseases, in Baker AB, Baker LH (eds): *Clinical Neurology*. New York, Harper & Row, 1978, vol 3, chap 37.
3. Layzer RB, Rowland LP: Cramps. *N Eng J Med* 285:31–40, 1971.
4. Rowland LP, Dimauro S, Bank WJ: Glycogen storage diseases of muscle: Problems in biochemical genetics. *Birth Defects* 7:43–51, 1971.
5. Struppler A, Struppler E, Adams RD: Local tetanus in man. *Arch Neurol* 8:162–178, 1963.
6. Spillane JD, Nathan PW, Kelly RE, Marsden CD: Painful legs and moving toes. *Brain* 94:541–556, 1971.

92. Stroke

H. KENNETH WALKER, MD

Definition

A neurological catastrophe of sudden onset that occurred in the past, presumably due to cerebrovascular disease.

Technique

Simply ask: Have you ever had a stroke before? If so, a good way to begin the history is to discover what the patient was doing when the stroke occurred, thus setting in motion the memory of the stroke. Let the patient relate spontaneously as much information as possible before becoming more directive in your questions.

Establish the presenting manifestation and then get all succeeding manifestations exactly in the order in which they occurred. The following information is especially pertinent:

1. What the patient was doing at the time of onset: asleep and awakened by the stroke or discovered it when awaking at usual time, occurred during strenuous exertion, or occurred while resting quietly.
2. Presenting manifestation.
3. Whether following occurred:
    a. Level of consciousness and cortical function altered: confusion, stupor, unconsciousness, aphasia.
    b. Headache: was it initially focal and then spread? how severe?
    c. Stiff neck or pain on flexion of neck.
    d. Cranial nerve symptoms: blurring of vision, blindness, visual field deficit, diplopia, ptosis, facial paralysis, tinnitus, vertigo, dysarthria.
    e. Weakness or paralysis: where did it start, where did it spread to and with what speed, did it slowly increase or was it initially maximal?
    f. Sensory symptoms (numbness, paresthesias): same questions as with weakness.
    g. Whether gait was involved.
    h. Staggering or incoordination of extremities.
    i. Seizures: if so, characterize as outlined in the section on seizures.
4. Inquire about associated symptoms that may give a clue to etiology.
    a. Chest pain.
    b. Evidence of systemic infection.
    c. Evidence of emboli to other sites: an extremity, skin, lung.
    d. Evidence of long bone fracture, especially hip, preceding the stroke.
5. Inquire as to presence or absence of possible specific etiologies:
    a. Hypertension.
    b. Chronic cardiac arrhythmia, especially atrial fibrillation.
    c. Valvular heart disease.

     d.   Myocardial infarction in recent past.

     e.   Diabetes.

     f.   Birth control pills.

6.   Establish the time course of the stroke:

     a.   Acute onset, slow improvement over days, weeks, or months to a plateau.

     b.   Slow onset and progression: In this case be especially careful to determine whether symptoms are still progressing. If so, a mass lesion is highly likely with this history.

     c.   Saltatory or stepwise progression.

7.   Establish current functional capacity.

8.   Acquire physician and hospital names so records can be obtained.

Background Information

Stroke or cerebrovascular disease ranks third as the cause of death in the United States and accounts for 50% of neurological hospital admissions and for 10–20% of all cases of sudden death. The great majority of cerebrovascular disease can be divided into cerebral thrombosis, embolism, and hemorrhage. Diseases or conditions which greatly increase susceptibility to cerebrovascular disease include hypertension, diabetes, cardiac disease (atherosclerotic heart disease, valvular disease, or chronic arrhythmias of whatever cause), and elevated serum lipids.

Cerebral thrombosis is closely related to atherosclerosis, explaining in part why the risk of stroke greatly increases in diseases that accelerate atherosclerosis such as hypertension, diabetes, and all diseases with elevated serum lipids. Atherosclerotic involvement of cerebral arteries parallels atherosclerosis elsewhere in the body, such as the coronary arteries. The vessels involved earliest and most frequently are the proximal internal carotid artery and carotid sinus in the neck, the vertebral and basilar arteries at their junction, the carotid siphon, the trifurcation of the internal carotid, the main bifurcation of the middle cerebral artery, and portions of the posterior and anterior cerebral arteries. Atherosclerotic arteries have intimal roughening, plaque formation, elongation and buckling, decreased vessel caliber due to stenosis, luminal obstruction, and dissection of the intima (see reference 22 for a full discussion). The following pathophysiologic effects help explain how atherosclerosis produces strokes (see reference 24):

1.   Decreases perfusion pressure and thereby reduces flow.

2.   Acts as a source of emboli consisting of fibrin, platelets, or cholesterol crystals.

3. Serves as a substrate upon which a thrombosis forms and occludes the lumen.

The end result of these pathologic and physiologic lesions is ischemia or frank infarction. A consideration of the pathophysiology outlined briefly above indicates the deranged physiology, and consequently the clinical picture can vary over a wide spectrum: from transient mild ischemia (the TIAs described in section 87, Episodic Neurological Symptoms) to a stuttering or saltatory progression (an "evolving stroke"), to sudden onset of complete occlusion (a stroke that is complete at onset). The point along this spectrum occupied by an individual patient is determined by a number of factors: the location of the ischemia, degree of compromise of circulation, collateral circulation, state of general circulation (perfusion pressure, viscosity, oxygen-carrying ability), metabolic demands of that part of the brain, and many others not known or incompletely understood.

Causes of cerebral thrombosis other than atherosclerosis are rare. They include principally the conditions that cause arteritis of the cerebral arteries: syphilis, tuberculous and fungal meningitis, and collagen diseases. Takayashu's disease (the aortic arch syndrome) and fibromuscular hyperplasia can cause strokes. Estrogen-containing oral contraceptives are associated with an increased incidence of thrombosis. Of special concern are women who have hypertension and migraine or other forms of vascular headache who are receiving estrogen-containing contraceptives.

Cerebral embolism is largely a manifestation of heart disease. The common diseases producing emboli are rheumatic heart disease, atherosclerotic heart disease, and bacterial endocarditis. Chronic atrial fibrillation due either to rheumatic or atherosclerotic heart disease may result in embolization. Mural thrombus forming in the left ventricle after a myocardial infarction is frequently associated with embolization. Valvular lesions of whatever etiology serve as a substrate for the development of bacterial endocarditis with the break-off of embolic particles. Other causes of cerebral emboli are rarer: atrial myxoma, air or fat emboli, pulmonary venous emboli, cardiac surgery.

Emboli of varying sizes leave the site of origin and make their way to the brain; the middle cerebral territory is most often affected. On occasion the particle will get hung up in a proximal vessel and produce a prodromal headache or other symptom before ending in a distal vessel. Most emboli announce their presence by the sudden onset of a focal neurological deficit caused by vessel occlusion with infarction of the area supplied by that vessel. Emboli are usually small and thus end in small vessels with a resultant small area of infarction that produces a discrete neurological deficit: aphasia, visual field deficit, or weakness or sensory loss of one extremity. Another consequence of the pathophysiology of emboli is that where there is one embolus there are others: therefore a picture of multiple embolic episodes often appears.

Cerebral hemorrhage is the third category of cerebrovascular disease. Hypertensive intracerebral hemorrhage and ruptured berry (or saccular) aneurysms account for the large majority of hemorrhages. Massive intracerebral hemorrhages occur in a setting of prolonged hypertension. Charcot and Bouchard and later Russel, Cole, and Yates demonstrated that patients over age 40 with prolonged hypertension have miliary or microaneurysms (or Charcot-Bouchard aneurysms) that occur on small perforating arteries. The walls of the aneurysms consist of intima and adventitia; the media is not present. The distribution roughly parallels the location of intracerebral hemorrhages in hypertensive patients: putamen 60%, thalamus 10%, pons 10%, cerebellum 10%. However, on occasion they have been found in normotensive patients. See reference 20 for a good review.

Saccular or berry aneurysms average 8–10 mm in diameter and are principally located at bifurcations of the cerebral arteries (Locksley):

Internal carotid communicating junction	25%
Anterior communicating	28%
Main branchings of middle cerebral	12%

Ruptured saccular aneurysms are the fourth cause of stroke, after thrombosis, embolus, and hypertensive intracerebral hemorrhage. The rupture occurs in the subarachnoid space, producing a neurological catastrophe that is often without localizing findings. The aneurysms can become quite large and act as a mass in producing local deficits, such as third nerve paralysis. Pathologically they do not have a muscular media; it ends at the beginning of the aneurysmal dilation. The elastic membrane between intima and media is often missing. The role of these and other developmental defects in causing what are probably congenital aneurysms is not entirely clear.

Clinical Significance

There are at least three reasons why it is valuable to take a careful history on a stroke that occurred in the past:

1. To make sure you agree that cerebrovascular disease was indeed the etiology of the stroke, and not a mass lesion that is still present. This mistaken diagnosis happens more often than one would like to contemplate.
2. In order to determine if future strokes are preventable. This statement at the moment largely applies to hypertensive patients.
3. To carefully assess the patient's functional capabilities and make plans for rehabilitation if necessary.

The clinical hallmark of a cerebrovascular lesion is abrupt onset, progressing rapidly to death or slow recovery. In contrast, the onset of mass lesions is gradual over days, weeks, months. Therefore, a patient with slowly progressive symptomatology has a mass lesion until conclusively known otherwise. Of course there are exceptions to these generalizations. Occasionally the stuttering progression of a cerebral thrombosis will be indistinguishable from a mass lesion. Certain tumors bleed into themselves and thereby in fact do have a vascular-type onset. On occasion the presenting manifestation of a tumor is a focal seizure that can mislead the clinician into suspecting vascular disease. But these cases are rare compared to the large number of cases that follow the generalizations given, and the more distant the illness the less likely one is to be misled by the rare exception, that is, the stroke patient will have improved and the mass lesion will have become worse.

Some generalizations are occasionally useful in coming to retrospective conclusions:

A. Cerebral thrombosis
   1. A history of transient attacks preceding the main stroke by seconds to 8 hours or longer occurs in 80% of cases of thrombosis and very rarely in embolism or hemorrhage. If frank TIAs have preceded the attack for weeks or months, the pathology is almost surely thrombosis.
   2. Patients often awaken and discover the deficit, or the stroke occurs shortly after arising (60% of patients in some series).
   3. A stuttering or saltatory evolution of a stroke over hours or days strongly suggests thrombosis.
   4. Lacunar infarction occurs in patients with long-standing hypertension. Recognition of lacunar infarction as the cause of a stroke is quite important because treating the hypertension will probably prevent future strokes. The clinical hallmark of lacunar infarcts is that in any one acute episode in a patient either the motor or sensory system is predominantly involved. Patients do not usually have a mixed deficit. The classical findings in the pure motor and pure sensory variety are given below.
      a. Subjective:
          A stepwise evolution of weakness or paresthesias involving face, arm, and leg occurring over a short period of time, usually up to 24 hours. In a few cases the deficit is sudden and complete.
          The level of consciousness is unimpaired.
          There is no headache.

Slurred speech in over two-thirds of patients with the pure motor variety.

b. Objective:

Mental faculties usually normal, in spite of what may appear to be a massive neurological deficit.

c. Pure motor types:

Severe dysarthria in most patients; without aphasia.

Marked hemiplegia involving face, arm, and leg.

Extensor plantar response present on the involved side of the body.

No sensory involvement; testing for pain, temperature, touch, and visual fields being completely normal.

d. Pure sensory type:

Numbness and mild sensory loss over the entire half of the body, involving face, arm, and leg.

No weakness, vertigo, diplopia, dysarthria, aphasia, visual field deficit, or nystagmus; the lumbar puncture is normal.

5. A clinical environment of evidence of atherosclerosis elsewhere, diabetes, hypertension, and elevated blood lipids suggests thrombosis.

B. Cerebral embolism

1. A clinical setting of valvular heart disease, chronic atrial fibrillation, recent myocardial infarction, or bacterial endocarditis, plus a cerebral catastrophe of sudden onset are highly suggestive of embolus. Evidence of emboli to other sites virtually assures the diagnosis. With regard to myocardial infarction there is some evidence that risk for embolic stroke can be correlated with the size of the myocardial infarction, as inferred from creatinine kinase levels (reference 23).

2. Embolism is highly likely when there is sudden onset of stroke with focal findings in a young person in whom atherosclerosis is unlikely and hypertension is not present.

C. Hypertensive intracerebral hemorrhage

1. Headache (50%) and unconsciousness *with* localizing findings in a patient with long-standing hypertension is very suggestive.

2. Usually occurs when patient is active, occurrence during sleep is rare.

3. There is no prodrome. The onset is over minutes or hours. A time span of 5–30 minutes is common, depending on the speed of bleeding.

4. Mortality is 90%; consequently patients who have survived are less likely to have had an intracerebral hemor-

rhage but are more likely to have had one of the other causes of stroke.

5. Hypertensive cerebellar hemorrhage is an important cause of strokes. The diagnosis of cerebellar hemorrhage should be entertained in every stroke occurring in a hypertensive patient because of the potential reversibility by surgery. This is in contrast to hypertensive hemorrhages located in other sites such as the cerebral cortex or thalamus, where the therapy is principally supportive. There is considerable variation in the presentation of these hemorrhages, but certain features make the diagnosis very suggestive:

a. Subjective:
The presence of long-standing hypertension.
The sudden onset of a stroke with only transient loss of consciousness, or without loss of consciousness.
Inability to stand or walk, but with intact strength in the legs.
Other less constant features such as headache, vomiting, and vertigo.

b. Objective:
Intact motor and sensory examination. This is in distinct contrast to hypertensive hemorrhages located in other sites, as they often have hemiplegia and hemianesthesia.
A disorder of eye movements. This is usually an inability or difficulty in looking to one side, but other findings (such as downward deviation of one eye) may be present.
Ataxia of limbs and inability to walk.
A midline pineal on skull x-ray, or a midline ECHO-encephalogram.
Bloody xanthochromic CSF.

D. Subarachnoid hemorrhage due to ruptured berry aneurysm

1. Abrupt onset of severe headache *without* localizing findings is the common presentation of a ruptured berry aneurysm. This clinical picture in a young patient who is normotensive is almost diagnostic.

2. Symptoms of meningeal irritation are always present if the patient can remember stiff neck or pain on flexion of neck.

A fitting conclusion for this chapter on stroke is to call the reader's attention to the reference by Brodal—a careful and thought-provoking account of his own stroke by one of the world's great neuroscientists.

Selected References

1. Brodal A: Self-observations and neuro-anatomical considerations after a stroke. *Brain* 96:675–694, 1973.
2. Brennan RW, Bergland RM: Acute cerebellar hemorrhage. *Neurology* 27:527–532, 1977.
3. Cole FJ, Yates PO: The occurrence and significance of intracerebral microaneurysms. *J Path Bact* 93:393–411, 1967.
4. Dinsdale HB: Spontaneous hemorrhage in the posterior fossa. *Arch Neurol* 10:200–217, 1964.
5. Fisher CM: A lacunar stroke: The dysarthria-clumsy hand syndrome. *Neurology* 17:614–617, 1967.
6. Fisher CM: Lacunes: Small, deep cerebral infarcts. *Neurology* 15:774–784, 1965.
7. Fisher CM: Pure sensory stroke involving face, arm, and leg. *Neurology* 15:76–80, 1965.
8. Fisher CM: The arterial lesions underlying lacunes. *Acta Neuropath* 12:1–15, 1969.
9. Fisher CM, Cole M: Homolateral ataxia and crural paresis: A vascular syndrome. *J Neurol Neurosurg Psychiat* 28:48–55, 1965.
10. Fisher CM, Curry HB: Pure motor hemiplegia of vascular origin. *Arch Neurol* 13:30–44, July 1965.
11. Fisher CM, Mohr JP, Adams RD: Cerebrovascular diseases, in Wintrobe MM, et al (eds): *Harrison's Principles of Internal Medicine,* ed 6. New York, McGraw-Hill, 1970, chap 357, pp 1727–1764.
12. Fisher CM, Picard EH, Polak A, et al: Acute hypertensive cerebellar hemorrhage: Diagnosis and surgical treatment. *J Nerv Ment Dis* 140: 38–57, 1965.
13. Freeman RE, Onofrio BM, Okazaki H, et al: Spontaneous intracerebellar hemorrhage. *Neurology* 23:84–90, 1973.
14. Karp H: Cerebral vascular disease and neurologic manifestations of cardiovascular disease, in Hurst JW (ed in chief): *The Heart,* ed 4. New York, McGraw-Hill, 1978, chap 105, pp 1889–1905.
15. Lavy S, Melamed E, Cahane E, et al: Hypertension and diabetes as risk factors in stroke patients. *Stroke* 4:751–759, 1973.
16. McKissock W, Richardson A, Walsh L: Spontaneous cerebellar hemorrhage. *Brain* 83(1):1–9, 1960.
17. Meyer JS: Stroke—past, present, and future: A personal view. *Stroke* 2:95–100, 1971.
18. Phillips LH, Whisnaut JP, Reagan TJ: Sudden death from stroke. *Stroke* 8:392–395, 1977.
19. Richter RW, Brust JC, Bruun B, et al: Frequency and course of pure motor hemiparesis. *Stroke* 8:58–60, 1977.

20. Russell RWR: How does blood pressure cause stroke? *Lancet* 2:1283–1285, 1975.
21. Russell RWR. Observations on intracerebral aneurysms. *Brain* 86:425–442, 1963.
22. Stehbens WE (ed): *Pathology of the Cerebral Blood Vessels*. St. Louis, CV Mosby, 1972.
23. Thompson PL, Robinson JS: Stroke after acute myocardial infarction: Relation to infarct size. *Br Med J* 2:457–459, 1978.
24. Toole JF, Cole M: Ischemic cerebrovascular disease, in Baker AB, Baker LH (eds): *Clinical Neurology*. New York, Harper and Row, 1975, vol 1, chap 10.
25. Utterback RA: Hemorrhagic cerebrovascular disease, in Baker AB, Baker LH (eds): *Clinical Neurology*. New York, Harper and Row, 1975, vol 1, chap 11.

93. Sleep Disorders

GERALD W. VOGEL, MD

Definition

In general there are three kinds of sleep disorders: (1) insomnias, ie, partial inability to sleep which results in daytime sleepiness; (2) hypersomnias, ie, no inability to sleep with excessive daytime sleepiness (EDS). (The term EDS is reserved for hypersomnia because daytime sleepiness is more severe in this syndrome than in insomnia); (3) dyssomnias, ie, a failure of sleep to inhibit certain phenomena which should only occur during wakefulness or should not occur at all.

The insomnias can be classified as primary or secondary. Primary insomnias are sleep reductions caused by a disturbance during sleep. Secondary insomnias are sleep reductions secondary to a waking illness. Causes of primary and secondary insomnias include the following:

Primary	*Secondary*
1. Nocturnal myoclonus	1. Drug dependencies including alcoholism
2. Central sleep apnea	

3. Circadian rhythm distur-
   bances
4. Pseudoinsomnia
5. Idiopathic insomnia

2. Depression
3. Temporary situational stress
4. Medical illness

The hypersomnias include the following:

1. Narcolepsy-cataplexy syndrome
2. Idiopathic hypersomnia
3. Upper airway sleep apnea
4. Narcolepsy-cataplexy with upper airway sleep apnea
5. Depression
6. Drug dependencies

The dyssomnias include the following:

1. Enuresis
2. Somnambulism
3. a. Parvor nocturnus (night terrors in children)
   b. Incubus (night terrors in adults)
4. Nightmares

Technique

If possible, interview both patient and bed partner of patient because the latter may have observed sleep characteristics unknown to the patient.

The distinction between insomnia and hypersomnia, both of which produce daytime sleepiness, can be made by history. Simply ask whether at night the patient sleeps too little or too much. Patients with insomnia complain of too little sleep while patients with hypersomnia complain that in spite of normal (6–9 hours) or often excessive (greater than 9 hours) nocturnal sleep duration, they are extremely sleepy during the day. Ask whether during the day the patient usually fights sleep and often uncontrollably falls asleep. These symptoms are characteristic of the EDS in the hypersomnias. In contrast, the daytime sleepiness of the insomnias is less severe and often is accompanied by an inability to sleep during the day.

In persons with a complaint of EDS without sleep reduction, a presumptive diagnosis of the specific hypersomnia syndrome can usually be made by history alone. Begin with an attempt to determine the presence or absence of the narcolepsy-cataplexy syndrome, because this is the most common cause of EDS. Ask the patient about uncontrollable daytime sleep attacks (narcolepsy) and daytime episodes of muscle weakness (cataplexy). Narcoleptic sleep attacks can vary from a few seconds to a half hour and are often precipitated by boring, monotonous situations. However they can also occur when the patient is attentive, such as during driving, eating, or even walking. In cataplexic episodes the muscle weakness may be profound and generalized, causing the patient to fall to the ground and not move; or it may be mild to moderate, eg, making the knees buckle. There is no diminution of consciousness during cataplexic attack. Cataplexy is often precipitated by strong emotion such as anger or laughter and lasts a few seconds to half a minute. It is important to note that the sleep attacks in a patient without cataplexy are not symptoms of classical narcolepsy-cataplexy syndrome. Sleep paralysis and hypnogogic hallucinations are two other symptoms that often occur in this syndrome. Together with narcolepsy and cataplexy, the four symptoms constitute the narcoleptic tetrad. Sleep paralysis occurs as the patient falls asleep and/or awakens. It is a paralysis of all voluntary muscles except those controlling eye movement and respiratory movements. The paralytic episodes, which are often frightening, usually last a few seconds to a minute. Hypnogogic hallucinations occur as the patient falls asleep, but before he is fully asleep. Often the hallucinations are combined with a perception of the patient's real surroundings (eg, a hallucinated bear coming through the wall of the patient's bedroom), as if the patient began to dream before he was fully asleep.

A final note about technique in the diagnosis of the narcolepsy-cataplexy syndrome. Patients are often so embarrassed about this disease that they are reluctant to describe their symptoms. Often they have been told that their sleep attacks indicate laziness, that their cataplexy indicates epilepsy, and that their hypnogogic hallucinations indicate insanity. For this reason, in patients with EDS it is important to be careful, persistent, and reassuring in eliciting the symptoms of the narcolepsy-cataplexy syndrome.

Patients with a complaint of EDS (including daytime sleep attacks) but without cataplexy almost certainly do not have classical narcolepsy. Furthermore, do not assume that the diagnosis of the narcolepsy-cataplexy syndrome rules out other causes of EDS. As many as 5% of EDS patients have both the narcolepsy-cataplexy syndrome and upper airway sleep apnea. Thus, continue the interview by asking about all other possible diagnoses. Ask about depression, another common cause of EDS. Although most depressed patients will admit to being depressed, sad, dejected, in low spirits, others will not recognize these feelings. Sometimes if asked, "How does the future look?," the patient's response of a bleak or dark future will be revealing. Sometimes only the interviewer's vague, intuitive hunch of depression will be present and consultation with a psychiatrist will be required for the diagnosis.

Drug dependency of a particular sort is another cause of EDS with daytime sleep. Ask patients and their close relatives to report all drugs taken (including dose and frequency) in the three months before and during the EDS. Withdrawal from chronic use of stimulants such as amphetamines and methylphenidate (Ritalin) can cause EDS.

Upper airway sleep apnea is virtually limited to males. Patients are never aware of sleep apnea. However, ask the patient and bed partner about heavy snoring and about episodes of no breathing during sleep, both of which occur in sleep apnea. In idiopathic hypersomnia, nocturnal sleep is prolonged, and daytime sleep attacks occur in the absence of cataplexy, symptoms of sleep apnea, or depression.

In patients with a complaint of insomnia, begin by asking the patient about the duration of the insomnia and how it began. Specifically determine whether the insomnia began during a situational stress, a concurrent medical illness, or in relation to starting or stopping a drug. Also inquire about the usual bedtime, its regularity, and its associated rituals or habits. Answers to these questions yield important clues about the presence of specific secondary insomnias. In this regard note the following characteristics of secondary insomnias.

Situational insomnia is brief (usually two months duration) and the patient or close relatives can relate its onset to some life stress.

Depression is among the most common causes of secondary insomnia. (Paradoxically then, depression can cause either hypersomnia or insomnia.) The insomnia of endogenous depression is usually, though not always, characterized by middle of the night awakenings and/or early morning awakenings. The insomnia of reactive depression is usually, though not always, characterized by difficulty in falling asleep. The distinction between these two kinds of depression is important because different treatments are effective for each. A thorough psychiatric history, is indicated in all patients with sleep disorders secondary to depression.

Drug dependency is another cause of secondary insomnia. Ask about all drugs taken before and during the insomnia. Obtain the dose, frequency, and duration of drug intake. Note especially that insomnia can result from the chronic use of either stimulants or hypnotics (stimulants can cause insomnia during use and hyperinsomnia during withdrawal). Abuse of caffeinated beverages, eg, cola drinks, coffee, tea, can also cause insomnia. It is also important to ask about alcohol intake since alcoholism is a common cause of insomnia.

Insomnia can also be secondary to any medical illnesses that produce pain, anxiety, discomfort. Thus a careful medical history and physical examination is required in all patients with insomnia.

If insomnia is not secondary to some waking illness, then investigate the primary insomnias. Among the latter, nocturnal myoclonus and central sleep apnea require a sleep laboratory study for confirmation. Indeed, the patient never experiences these causes of insomnia and is usually unaware of them. Ask the bed partner about repetitive muscular jerks occurring predominantly in the lower limbs (nocturnal myoclonus); and about heavy snoring and periods of no breathing (possible sleep apnea).

Patients with pseudoinsomnia complain they sleep too little when, in fact, they do not. To establish this diagnosis, ask patients whether they are tired or sleepy during the day. If these daytime symptoms are not present, the diagnosis is pseudoinsomnia. Other patients with pseudoinsomnia grossly exaggerate their sleep loss and, because of suggestibility (not sleep loss) are tired during the day. This diagnosis cannot be made by history alone but requires sleep laboratory study.

Circadian rhythm insomnias arise because the patient's endogenous sleep/wake cycle differs substantially from the 24-hour day. Ask the patient about his usual bedtime and his usual sleep time. In patients with a circadian phase shift, typically the patient cannot fall asleep until long after the conventional bedtime, but once asleep he will sleep well and have a great deal of difficulty waking up in the morning. In patients with a free-running circadian rhythm the patient has a variable 24-hour sleep/waking rhythm. In such patients sleepiness begins at different times each day, but sleep duration is usually 6–8 hours.

Last but not least, idiopathic insomnia (chronic insomnia without known primary or secondary cause) may well be the most common type of insomnia. Although its severity may be influenced by life events, idiopathic insomnia is a chronic or persistent insomnia that is not eliminated by pleasant circumstances. Most patients with this disorder have mild to moderate psychiatric problems but manage to function socially and at work. The diagnosis is made by exclusion, after history, physical examination, and sleep laboratory studies have revealed no known cause of the insomnia.

The dyssomnias are diagnosed by history. In primary enuresis (bedwetting) the child has never been dry for more than one or two weeks; in secondary enuresis he may be dry for several weeks, months, or years before enuresis begins. These distinctions are important because they have etiological and treatment implications. In particular, secondary enuresis may be a symptom of diabetes mellitus, diabetes insipidus, nocturnal epilepsy, or severe mental retardation.

Sleep walking (somnambulism) is to be distinguished from hysterical dissociative reactions. Ask about the duration of and behavior during an episode. Compared with dissociative reactions, sleep walking is shorter (maximum of a few minutes), the patient is less alert, more confused and disoriented (and hence more likely to harm himself), and his behavior is less complex and less purposeful. Occurring during sleep, night terrors are characterized by intense terror. The patient may begin the episode with a scream or cry and show terrified and confused behavior from which he is difficult to awaken. After awakening, there is little or no recall for the event. Nightmares, on the other hand, are frightening dreams, easily recalled and not accompanied by confused behavior, and from which the patient is easily awakened.

Background Information

At present the neurophysiological substrate of sleep and wakefulness is not fully understood. Current views, including some speculations, are as follows:

Wakefulness is the result of activation that originates in the reticular activating system (RAS). High activity in this system precludes sleep; low activity apparently leads to drowsiness.

Nonrapid eye movement (NREM) sleep requires low RAS activity and the activity of a sleep system that may involve the raphe nuclei in the pons, the medial forebrain area, or both.

Normal human sleep consists of the cyclic alteration of two very different kinds of sleep. The cycle, which is about 90 minutes long, begins with NREM and ends with REM sleep. The cycles are repeated throughout the night. NREM sleep consists of stages 1 through 4 increasing depth of sleep and is not accompanied by rapid eye movements. REM sleep is accompanied by rapid eye movements, and active inhibition of all voluntary muscles except those controlling eye and respiratory movements, and the experience of vivid prolonged dreams. The physiological mechanisms responsible for the alternation of NREM and REM sleep are unknown, but the pons appears to contain structures that are necessary, if not sufficient, for this alternation.

Clinical Significance

The four symptoms of the narcoleptic tetrad are manifestations of a precocious triggering of REM sleep or its dissociated components. The sleep attacks themselves are attacks of REM sleep, ie, episodes of sleep onset REM periods. Both cataplexy and sleep paralysis are dissociated manifestations of the active muscle inhibition that occurs during REM sleep. The hypnogogic hallucinations represent the dream experiences associated with REM sleep.

Causes of sleep apnea are unknown. However, it is known that apneic episodes during sleep are followed by a brief awakening. Literally hundreds of apneic episodes can occur each night in affected patients. With upper airway sleep apnea (obstruction of the upper airway airflow), sleep curtailment is greater than with central sleep apnea (temporary cessation of respiratory movement with no airway obstruction). This difference may account for the fact that EDS occurs with the former rather than the latter.

In patients with nocturnal myoclonus, bilateral or unilateral leg twitches occur during sleep every 20–40 seconds for intermittent periods lasting several minutes to 2 hours. With each twitch the patient is usually aroused for 5 to 15 seconds. Thus, several hundred twitches in a night are associated with a drastic reduction of total sleep time. The physiological relationship of myoclonus to sleep is unknown.

Since the modes of action of stimulant and hypnotic drugs are not understood, the following views are speculative. Stimulant drugs reduce total sleep time, in part perhaps, by stimulating the RAS. With prolonged use, tolerance to their stimulating effect occurs, perhaps by the development of RAS resistance to stimulation. When the stimulant drugs are withdrawn, persistent RAS resistance to endogenous stimulation prolongs nocturnal sleep and produces EDS. Hypnotic drugs may stimulate the sleep system. With prolonged use, tolerance to their sleep-promoting properties develops. Perhaps this involves the sleep system's development of resistance to stimulation. Thus, insomnia during prolonged hypnotic drug use may be caused by excessive resistance of the sleep system to stimulation. Further, when hypnotic drugs are withdrawn, the insomnia worsens because the sleep system may no longer be stimulated by the drugs. The physiological pathogenesis of the other insomnias and hypersomnias is unknown.

Although it is known that bed-wetting occurs mainly during NREM sleep, the pathogenesis of this disorder is unknown in cases without physical causes. Both sleep-walking and night terrors occur during an incomplete arousal from the deepest stages of NREM sleep. Hence, these dyssomnias are not the result or the acting out of vivid, long, complex dreams. Nightmares, on the other hand, occur during NREM sleep. However, other than this knowledge about the physiological correlates of night terrors and nightmares, their pathogenesis remains unknown.

Selected References

1. Dement W, Guilleminault C, Zarcone V: The pathologies of sleep: A case series approach, in Tower DB (ed) *The Nervous System. Vol. 2: The Clinical Neurosciences.* New York, Raven Press, 1975.
2. Kales A, Soldatos CR: Sleep disorders: Description, assessment and treatment, in Shader RI (ed): *Manual of Psychiatric Therapeutics.* Boston, Little, Brown, 1979.
3. Raskin A, Schulterbrandt JG, Reatig N, et al: Differential response to chlorpromazine, imipramine, and placebo: A study of subgroups of hospitalized depressed patients. *Arch Gen Psychiat* 23:164–173, 1970.
4. Kales A, Bixler E, Tan T, et al: Chronic hypnotic-drug use: Ineffec-

tiveness, drug-withdrawal insomnia, and dependence. *JAMA* 227: 513–517, 1975.

5. Hobson, JA: The cellular basis of sleep cycle control. *Adv Sleep Res* 1:217–250, 1974.
6. Hobson JA, McCarley RW, Wyzinski PW: Sleep cycle oscillation: Reciprocal discharge by two brainstem neuronal groups. *Science* 189: 55–58, 1975.
7. Dement W, Rechtschaffen A, Gulevich G: The nature of the narcoleptic sleep attack. *Neurology* 16:18–33, 1966.
8. Broughton RJ: Sleep disorders: Disorders of arousal? *Science* 159: 1070–1078, 1968.

HEMATOPOIETIC SYSTEM

94. Excessive Bleeding or Bruising

JULIAN JACOBS, MD

Definition

Excessive bleeding or bruising is of a degree or lasts an amount of time inconsistent with physiologic cycles, trauma, or surgical procedures.

Technique

Go from general to specific questions: Do you have any bruising or bleeding tendency that you believe is abnormal? Is it still present? Is it or was it local or diffuse? Was it spontaneous or related to trauma? Does anyone in your family have similar problems? Are you taking aspirin, "blood thinners," or other medicines?

If questioning leads you to localized bleeding, unrelated to known trauma, proceed to detailed questions:

Vaginal. If the bleeding is vaginal, ask about frequency, duration, and number of pads or tampons used each day (Are pads or tampons changed when soaked or slightly stained? Does the bleeding follow intercourse? Do you spot between periods? Are current periods different from previous ones? Had you missed any periods before the bleeding? Do you pass clots at any time during your periods?

Nasal. How long has it been present? Is it localized to one nostril or do both nostrils bleed? Does blowing your nose start it? Is it clots of blood or blood-stained mucus? Do you pick your nose? Once it starts, how long does it usually last?

Gastrointestinal or genitourinary bleeding. For rectal bleeding, ask: What color is the blood? Is it bright or dark? Are your stools red, maroon, or black? Is the blood streaking on the stool, mixed with mucus, or in clots? Do you have pain with the bleeding? Is it any time or only with bowel movements? For urinary bleeding, ask: Is the urine only red or do you pass clots? Do you have pain with it? Is blood present at beginning, end, or all through urination? For vomiting blood, ask: When was the first time? What color was it? Did you have prolonged vomiting before you vomited the blood? Did you have abdominal pain before vomiting? Do you suffer from indigestion or heartburn? Have you been told you have ulcers or liver disease? Did you get dizzy, weak, sweat, or lose consciousness?

If initial questioning points to inappropriate localized bleeding related to trauma or surgery, inquire about the following:

Dental extractions. Ask when, the type of bloody material, duration, need for transfusion, cardiovascular symptoms. Did the bleeding problem occur at the time of extraction or within 24–36 hours? Was there a period of 5–7 days without trouble before the bleeding began? How was it treated? Did a stitch stop the bleeding? Did you require transfusions? Were you taking any medications at the time, including aspirin?

Surgical procedures. Did bleeding occur at the time of surgery or later? What was the surgery? Did you need transfusions? Have you had the same problem with any surgical procedures before or since?

Trauma. What type of injury was it? Once a physician or oral surgeon treated you, did the bleeding continue? Do you know what the physician or oral surgeon did? Do you bruise or bleed more easily after trauma than normally?

Generalized spontaneous bleeding. This is the least common complaint and is related to inherited or acquired disorders that interfere with some basic aspects of the coagulation system. How long have you had this problem? Does anyone in your family have a similar problem? Is it continuous or cyclic? Have you had a recent viral infection? Is bleeding in the soft tissue, joints, nose, or mouth? Is it rectal or urinary, or is it from all those places? Have you been transfused for this? Do the skin bruises start as small dots or large bruises? Have you or has anyone in your family been checked for this by special laboratory tests?

Remember that the most valuable tool for excluding a bleeding disorder due to a coagulation factor abnormality is a careful history, personal and family, since screening laboratory studies are not sensitive enough to detect mild to moderate decrease in factor levels.

Background Information

Maintenance of hemostasis may be thought of in three categories:

1. Local vascular factors
2. Platelet number and function
3. Coagulation factors

Abnormal bleeding may occur when any of these are abnormal.

Vascular factors of a gross anatomical nature are the most common cause of abnormal bleeding. Local interruption of a vessel by trauma or disease is most frequent. More extensive vascular changes of a gross nature such as hemorrhoids or esophageal varices can be causes of localized bleeding. Microscopic vascular changes such as a vasculitis can cause bleeding into the skin. Hereditary hemorrhagic telangiectasia may be the etiology of repeated epistaxis or gastrointestinal bleeding.

Abnormalities of platelet number and function constitute the next most common cause of bleeding problems, with reduced numbers of platelets being the major cause. Platelets may be low because of abnormally rapid destruction, decreased production or sequestration in the spleen, or any combination of these. Platelets do not usually cause spontaneous bleeding problems until numbers are reduced below 30,000-40,000/cu mm unless there is an associated vasculitis or markedly elevated white blood cell count. However, platelets below 80,000-100,000/cu mm can aggravate bleeding from local lesions. Idiopathic immunologic thrombocytopenia (ITP), as well as drugs and viral infections (immunologic and/or marrow suppression mechanisms) are common causes of low platelet counts. Less common, but certainly not rare, causes are hypersplenism (sequestration), bacteremia (rapid destruction and depressed marrow production), systemic lupus erythematosus (immune mechanism with increased destruction), uremia (cause not clear). Uremia causes functional disability of platelets much more commonly than decreased numbers. Inherited functional platelet defects of clinical significance are much rarer.

Deficiencies of coagulation factors are inherited or acquired. The hemophilioid diseases are inherited deficiencies of specific coagulation factors and are diagnosed by specific assay of the factors. Factor VIII disorders, classic chromosome X-linked hemophilia and autosomal dominant von Willebrand disease account for 85–90% of these diseases. In classic hemophilia, functional procoagulant activity of the factor is decreased or absent, but immunologic testing shows a protein identical to the factor VIII antigen to be present. In von Willebrand disease, functional activity and antigen levels may both be decreased and a platelet aggregation abnormality is also present. There is current dispute whether there is a multimolecular identity for factor VIII/von Willebrand complex or whether the functional, antigenic, and von Willebrand factor activities reside in a single large protein molecule.

Factors IX and XI disorders occur in decreasing frequency, and the rest are rare. Acquired deficiencies of coagulation factors occur in liver disease most commonly, and to a much lesser degree when a systemic disease sets off a consumptive coagulopathy (disseminated intravascular coagulation), or causes an inhibitor against a factor (circulating anticoagulant).

Clinical Significance

Localized bleeding, unrelated to known trauma, is practically always due to local anatomical abnormalities:

Vaginal.   Irregular cycles and duration of menses are common at adolescence and beginning of menopause, usually related to hormonal effects on the uterus. The amount of bleeding may be normal yet frightening to an individual since the pattern is irregular. Any history of intercycle bleeding or postmenopausal bleeding, or spotting after intercourse is ominous because this may mean malignancy. Any passing of clots during menses is to be considered abnormal even if it is a long-term pattern for the patient. Pap smear and pelvic exam must be done.

Nasal.   Nasal bleeding is most commonly due to erosion of superficial veins, which is almost always the reason if the bleeding has been present since childhood. Recent onset may be due to local malignancy, platelet deficiency, or coagulation deficit. Direct examination of nose, throat, and sinuses is the first step. After local cause is excluded, hematologic investigation starts.

Gastrointestinal.   Rectal bleeding must always be investigated with proctoscopy and barium enema. The presence of hemorrhoids does not protect a patient from cancer. Melena is discussed in section 20.

Vomiting blood is practically always due to local vascular factors, although the bleeding may be aggravated by low platelets or coagulation factor deficiencies, either inherited or acquired. Screening laboratory studies to exclude the latter should always be done, particularly in patients with liver disease and in heavy alcohol consumers.

Urinary. Urinary bleeding may be due to stone, bladder, prostate, or renal disease. Coumadin toxicity commonly presents as hematuria. Coumadin decreases several vitamin-K-dependent coagulation factors. Studies to exclude a local lesion with bleeding must be done (intravenous pyelogram and/or cystoscopy).

Trauma or surgery. Inordinate bleeding after dental extraction most commonly is due to poor hemostasis because of gingival infection or inadequate surgical technique. It usually occurs within hours after surgery. Bleeding within hours after extraction that persists despite adequate suturing is almost always due to thrombocytopenia. Initial adequate hemostasis and then bleeding after 7–8 days strongly suggests a coagulation factor defect. The history of need for transfusions after dental extraction is prima facie evidence for a serious episode, and makes laboratory study mandatory prior to further extractions. Anyone who has undergone major surgery in the past without need for transfusions most likely does not have a significant inherited bleeding abnormality. However, one must still be careful to exclude an acquired disorder, if the history is strong otherwise.

Generalized and spontaneous. If bleeding is recent in onset, it is usually either due to an acquired deficit of platelets (immunologic, decreased production by abnormal marrow) or coagulation factor deficit (due to decreased production because of severe liver disease). Massive transfusion of blood with major surgical procedures can cause spontaneous bleeding because of "washout" of coagulation factors and of platelets. If the history is long-standing, it is probably one of the hemophilioid diseases. Screening laboratory studies including prothrombin time, partial thromboplastin time, examination of the peripheral blood smear, platelet count, bleeding time, clot retraction test are the initial tests. Frequently women who are slightly overweight complain of spontaneous small-sized bruising that occurs without cause and is never of an extensive nature. This is known colloquially as "devil's pinches," and even extensive testing fails to reveal a cause. Laboratory screening tests may not detect mild to moderate deficits. A strong history, personal and family, is the best screening test for a significant inherited or acquired bleeding disorder. Proceed to specific assays of factors if the history is strong and the laboratory screen is negative.

Selected References

1. Deykin D: The clinical challenge of disseminated intravascular coagulation. *N Eng J Med* 283:636–644, 1970.
2. Blood coagulation and fibrinolysis in clinical practice, in Douglas AS (ed): *Clinics in Hematology*, vol 2, pp 1–213, 1973.
3. Platelet disorders, in O'Brien JR (ed): *Clinics in Hematology* vol 1, pp 231–441, 1972.
4. Roberts HE, Cederbaum AI: The liver and blood coagulation: Physiology and pathology. *Gastroenterology* 63:297–320, 1972.
5. Mibashan RS (ed): *Seminars in Hematology: Hemostasis and Thrombosis*, July 1977 14 (3); Oct 1977 14 (4); Jan 1978 15 (1).
6. Gralnick HR, Coller BS, Shulman NR, et al: Factor VIII. *Ann Intern Med* 86:598–616, 1977.

95. Anemia

JULIAN JACOBS, MD

Definition

Anemia is defined as a reduction in the hemoglobin concentration of an individual below a population norm. One sets a lower limit of normal, below which the individual is said to be anemic. In the United States the normal figures usually accepted are $15 \pm 1g/100ml$ for the adult male, $13.5 \pm 1g/100ml$ for the female. The hematocrit can also be used, but varying intravascular plasma volume has a significant effect on this value, and most prefer the hemoglobin definition. The bell curve distribution of any biological value in a population obviously means some persons with values outside the above arbitrary numbers will not really be anemic from a physiologic standpoint.

Technique

Direct questions need to be asked, going from general to specific. The phrasing obviously depends on the socioeducational background of the patient. Have you been told you were anemic or that you had "low blood"? Is there any history of "poor iron" in the blood? Has there been a history of gastrointestinal bleeding that may have resulted in anemia? A history of multiple pregnancies, deliveries, abortions or menstrual irregularities should be sought. Those of African, Mediterranean (Greek, Italian, Spanish, Sephardic Jewish) or Oriental lineage must be questioned not only regarding anemia in their own medical history but also about anemia in relatives.

Background Information

Anemia, a decrease in hemoglobin concentration of the blood below the levels defined above may result from:

1. Inadequate RBC production
2. Acceleration of RBC destruction by random death of erythrocytes rather than age related death, taking place either within the vessels or by loss of blood from the intravascular space
3. Sequestration and destruction of RBCs in an enlarged spleen

Poetically, anemia may result from problems of production, destruction, and/or the spleen in between.

Inadequate production. This may result from "factory failure," the bone marrow itself being a victim of chemical or physical assault, both iatrogenic in origin and otherwise. Production may be abnormal through the fault of genetic dose, or be disrupted and damaged by cellular proliferation of acquired diseases, which may originate in the marrow or arrive there as metastatic disease. Abnormal production or abnormal delivery to red cells of the raw materials of hemoglobin, iron, and amino acids cause factory production failure, as do deficiencies of essential elements for the nucleus, such as B_{12} and folic acid. Factory failure also occurs from lack of fuel, erythropoietin. This protein, a product of precursors produced in the kidneys and liver and influenced by endocrine factors, is probably the fine adjustment mechanism for the hemoglobin level in a normal person. An anemia caused by any of the above mechanisms is termed "hypoproliferative anemia."

Acceleration of RBC destruction. This may be inherited or acquired. Hemoglobinopathies, resulting from inheritance of abnormal hemoglobins, may cause erythrocytes to be poorly pliable and get "hung up" and die in the microcirculation. Hereditary spherocytosis is an inherited RBC membrane defect in which the sodium, potassium, and water content of the RBC is abnormal, resulting in a spherocytic red cell that gets caught and damaged in the spleen. Another example of an acquired cause of accelerated random RBC destruction is autoimmune hemolytic anemia where antibodies damage the RBC membrane. This causes the cell to be trapped by phagocytes in the spleen and destroyed, or to rupture intra-vascularly. Viral, bacterial, and parasitic (eg, malaria) infections also may cause accelerated RBC destruction. Anemia due to acceleration of RBC destruction is called a "hemolytic anemia."

Splenic sequestration. Together with accelerated destruction of trapped normal RBCs, this may be initiated by an enlarged spleen caused by a nonhematologic disease state such as portal hypertension. Potential spaces are opened wherein the RBC is delayed in transit. Because of a relative lack of glucose in this environment, the RBC, which is totally dependent on this energy source, suffers metabolic marasmus. Its protective mecha-nisms fail because of inability to replenish energy stores, and it perishes prematurely. Abnormal RBCs are trapped by the normal size spleen, a giant lymph node with a specialized circulation. "Work hypertrophy" of the spleen may occur, potential spaces open up, and more RBCs are caught. A vicious cycle ensues, speeding the RBCs on their way to de-struction. This is called "hypersplenic anemia" (some classify this as a subdivision of hemolytic anemia). It can be due to a large spleen per se, or to a spleen that enlarges as it rids the blood of circulating elements it recognizes as abnormal. The latter may occur with particulate elements other than RBCs. An example of another abnormal element is a malarial parasite.

These mechanisms may act singly or in any combination to cause anemia. For example, chronic lymphocytic leukemia may initially cause anemia by infiltrating and disrupting the architecture of the marrow. Auto-immune hemolytic anemia may also occur to add a further mechanism. The spleen may enlarge due to infiltration of lymphocytes and by "work hypertrophy" from trapping coated RBCs, resulting in hypersplenism. In addition, infiltration in the liver and kidneys by lymphocytes may cause damage and decreased erythropoietin precursor production.

Clinical Significance

Anemia is not a diagnosis; it is a manifestation of an underlying dis-ease that causes the anemia. The etiology must be stated for anemia to become a diagnosis. Thus, even "iron deficiency anemia" is an inadequate diagnosis. The cause of the iron deficiency must be sought, identified, and corrected. Most commonly, anemia is secondary to an underlying dis-ease of the liver, kidney, endocrine system; a malignancy; an infection or an inflammatory state such as rheumatoid arthritis. The minority of anemias are due to what one would term a primary hematopoietic cause such as leukemia, primary marrow disease, or primary RBC defects.

Symptoms of anemia such as decreased exercise tolerance and stamina are referable to the cardiopulmonary system and are nonspecific. There are other causes for "pale people" than anemia. In general, patients with a chronic anemia of 7g/100ml of hemoglobin or more, and no underlying cardiovascular problem, have only minimal complaints. This is due to internal adjustments of erythrocyte metabolism that allow the decreased number of RBCs to deliver more oxygen. There is also a compensatory plasma volume increase that maintains an adequate intravascular volume.

In summary:

1. Anemia is a laboratory finding.
2. Anemia is not a diagnosis.
3. Anemia demands that you find the cause and correct it.
4. The complaints are rarely helpful in diagnosis, except in specific anemias (see sections 96 and 97).
5. Most anemias are not due to primary diseases of the hematopoietic system, but are secondary to diseases of other organ systems.

Selected References

1. Hillman RS, Finch CA: *Red Cell Manual,* ed 4. Philadelphia, FA Davis Co, 1974.
2. Garby L (ed): *Clinics in Hematology.* Philadelphia, WB Saunders, pp 575–719, 1974.

96. Pica

JULIAN JACOBS, MD

Definition

Pica is the persistent craving and ingestion of food in unusually large amounts and the craving and ingestion of inedible materials.

Technique

Collecting subjective data for pica challenges the clinician's skill in history taking perhaps more than in any other area with the exception perhaps of sexual problems. The patient commonly recognizes his appetite as bizarre and because of the practice has often been subjected to ridicule by family members or friends. General dietary questions should be the opening move: How many meals a day do you eat? What is the usual content of each meal? At what hours do you eat? Then begin to narrow down: Do you eat between meals? at bedtime? Do you have a particular fondness for any food? Only then do you ask: Do you eat an unusual amount of this food compared to your friends or relatives? Do you have a craving for a particular food that you think is unusual? What food, how frequently, and how much of it do you eat? And finally: Do you have a craving to eat anything that is usually not considered a part of a person's diet?

Notice that you should avoid words like "abnormal," "weird," and "bizarre" which contain a value judgment. Question the patient privately. As rapport increases, question him privately several times, if you seriously suspect pica.

Individuals with a poor diet, even without pica, frequently minimize their difficulty, and may fabricate a description of a diet superior to yours, probably because of the embarrassment at the inability to supply self and family with this basic need.

The patient has difficulty admitting a dietary foible that separates him from the "normal" person. It may help the patient to talk more freely if you describe previous patients with pica and its relation to iron deficiency.

Background Information

Reports in the literature have described daily ingestion of peeling paint, dirt, clay, starch, large amounts of ice, one to two jars of green olives, multiple heads of lettuce, many stalks of celery, bunches of carrots, large amounts of goober peas (peanuts), and the ashes from two packs of cigarettes. Potato chips, peppermint Life Savers, and croutons are also recorded. One woman stated she chewed 12 packs of gum weekly. In addition, at the Atlanta VA Hospital, Dr. J. E. Hardison has collected histories for daily ingestion of seven cataloupes, two boxes of saltine crackers, coffee grounds, brown paper bags, and the unprinted margin of newspapers. This listing is not complete, but gives the reader a taste of the problem of pica.

The mechanism that drives the individual to this peculiar practice is by no means clear. Some believe a large part is culturally caused by exposure to the practice resulting from false health information, religious beliefs, or incorrect dietary information.

Pica most commonly occurs in nutritional deficiency states, with iron deficiency the most common finding. Most authors believe that pica *follows* the onset of the iron deficiency. Indeed, after only a few days of iron therapy, picas of ice (pagophagia), carrots, and other materials cease. This occurs long before amelioration of any coexisting anemia or replacement of iron stores.

A pica that causes anemia is the classic lead-poisoning epidemic and iron-loading anemia occurring in children living in old housing with peeling paint. However, current data indicate that pica is likely the result of iron deficiency (usually with anemia) and not the cause of iron deficiency. Some authors still suggest malabsorption of iron resulting from chelation as the inciting factor of anemia in clay eaters.

The molecular cause-effect step is far from clear. Other heme-containing compounds are replaced with iron at faster rates than hemoglobin. Catalase, myoglobin, and mucosal cytochrome C are some examples recorded in the literature. Cytochrome oxidase levels in buccal mucosa increase within 24 hours of initiation of iron therapy in humans, and cytochrome C in rat intestinal mucosa is normal long before the hemoglobin returns to normal. While no causal connection between intestinal mucosal cytochromes and pica is proved, pagophagia amelioration and resolution of anemia in the human is similar to the studies in the rat. At least in pagophagia, the cause is iron deficiency, not necessarily iron deficiency anemia. The linking mechanism is still not clearly defined.

Clinical Significance

Pica in children may be the result of environmental elements, eg, peeling paint precipitating ingestion and resulting in iron loading anemia secondary to lead poisoning. The "milk anemia" of fat babies who demand large quantities of milk may be an iron deficiency pica and is self-perpetuating until iron therapy is given. Bizarre appetites in adults should always suggest iron deficiency even when anemia is not present, and should not be considered a cultural phenomenon until iron deficiency is excluded by a bone marrow iron stain. The patient can often date the onset of pica and thereby reveal the duration of the iron deficiency.

Strange appetites in gravid women, the pickle pica of pregnancy, if you please, may be secondary to iron deficiency. Pica occurs in both sexes. Proving iron deficiency in the pica patient is still not resolving the problem to the proper point. The cause of the iron deficiency should be found and corrected, and iron replacement therapy should be initiated. Blood loss is the cause of iron deficiency in this country, usually gastrointestinal blood loss in men and menometrorrhagia in women. However, a gastrointestinal source of bleeding must also be considered in women.

Selected References

1. de la Burde B, Reames B: Prevention of pica, the major cause of lead poisoning in children. *Am J Publ Health* 63:737–743, 1973.
2. Bronstein ES, Dollar J: Pica in pregnancy. *JAMA Georgia* 63:332–335, 1974.
3. Coltman CA Jr: Patophagia and iron lack. *JAMA* 207:513–516, 1969.
4. Coltman CA Jr: Pagophagia. *Arch Inter Med* 128:472–473, 1971.
5. Crosby WH: Food pica and iron deficiency. *Arch Intern Med* 127:960–961, 1971.
6. Crosby WH: Pica: A compulsion caused by iron deficiency. *Br J Hematol* 34:341–342, 1976.
7. Crosby WH: Pica. *JAMA* 235:2765, 1976.
8. Mengel CE, Carter WA, Horton ES: Geophagia with iron deficiency and hypokalemia. *Arch Intern Med* 114:470–474, 1964.
9. Reynolds RD, Binder HJ, Miller MB, et al: Pagophagia and iron deficiency anemia. *Ann Intern Med* 69:435–440, 1968.

97. Family History of Sickle Cell Gene Inheritance

JULIAN JACOBS, MD

Definition

The patient who gives information spontaneously or under direct questioning that he or some family member has been told that one of them has sickle cell anemia, sickle trait, or a combination of sickle hemoglobin and another "interacting" hemoglobin.

Technique

This information is acquired by questioning the patient during the review of systems in the personal history: Have you ever been told you were anemic or had "low blood"? If the answer is yes, then ask: Were you told the cause? Then specifically ask: Did anyone tell you or any of your family that you had sickle hemoglobin or "sickly red blood cells"? Did any relatives have blood problems or unexplained repeated pain episodes? Are all your brothers and sisters still living? If not, do you know the age the individual died and the cause of death? If there is any question of a positive history, laboratory investigation will resolve the problem.

Background Information

Normal hemoglobin (Hgb A) consists of four heme molecules (protoporphyrin-Fe) placed among four chains of amino acids, two alpha and two beta chains. (See reference 2 for detailed schematic structure.) Sickle hemoglobin (Hgb S) results from a mutation of a single gene that causes the substitution of a valine molecule in place of glutamine at position six of the beta chain. This single amino acid substitution causes profound alterations in the physicochemical behavior of the hemoglobin, resulting in a potential pathophysiologic sequence of events. On deoxygenation, molecules of hemoglobin S tend to form linear aggregates, and with oxygenation the process is reversed. Loss of oxygen by delivery to the tissues reduces the solubility of sickle hemoglobin. The linear aggregates of insoluble hemoglobin form rigid bundles that distort and "sickle" the RBC. X-ray diffraction patterns are typical of those obtained from highly organized fibers, all identical, with a periodicity along the fiber equal to one dimension of the Hgb molecule. Conceptually, the fibers are long tubular structures thought to consist of six filaments wound around a hollow core. The filaments are Hgb S molecules "like beads on a string." Recent work by Dykes et al, based on electron microscopy suggests an inner helical core of 4 strands surrounded by an outer helix of 10 strands in roughly hexagonal shape.

The sixth position on each beta chain is externally located on the hemoglobin molecule. Deoxygenation changes the spatial configuration of the molecules bringing the exposed regions of the Hgb S molecule into line with receptor sites on an adjacent molecule, and the molecules "stack up" because of "interlocking" sites. The beta six position may be the primary interacting site. The amount of "sickling" seen grossly depends on the propensity to "stack." Among other things, this depends on the degree of oxygenation of the Hgb, the amount of Hgb S present, and the type and quantity of other hemoglobin present. Hgb F ameliorates the stacking phenomenon. Hgb C, D, and B-thalassemia interact with Hgb S and induce stacking, but not as severely as homozygous Hgb SS.

The polymerization and fiber formation increase the internal viscosity and membrane rigidity of the deoxygenated cell containing Hgb S. These stiff, nonpliable "freakish poikilocytes" get stuck in the microvasculature at capillary crossroads and cause reversible and irreversible capillary obstruction with resultant microinfarction distal to the point of occlusion. Macroinfarction also occurs when, with continued blockade, platelet thrombus is added to the "tumble weed" mass of RBCs and activation of the coagulation system causes local clotting.

In addition to the pliability abnormality of the RBC in sickle disease (AS hemoglobin is sickle trait and not considered sickle disease), there is shortening of RBC survival with random death of cells (hemolytic process) that leads to anemia (hemolytic anemia). This is probably due to the increased mechanical fragility of the cell, as well as to loss of membrane and hemoglobin during the "sickling-unsickling" cycle, resulting in fragmentation and destruction. Hemolysis occurs either intravascularly, or in the liver of the adult patient (who has undergone autosplenectomy secondary to microinfarctions) or the spleen and liver in the child. The rate of hemolysis in any patient is constant and for practical purposes never changes.

Clinical Significance

Sickle gene inheritance is most common in individuals of African descent. However, it has also been described in Caucasians, particularly of Mediterranean Basin origin, as well as Asians. Sickle trait (AS) must never be confused with the diseases associated with S Hgb. "Trait" is a heterogeneous state that combines inheritance of a normal gene with an abnormal one.

Reports of complications associated with sickle trait are, for the most part, anecdotal and have not been studied in a controlled way. There is no evidence that life span is shortened by sickle trait. Anemia that is present in the AS patient is due to some other cause. Certain abnormalities do have a higher incidence in sickle-trait individuals than in the general population: hyposthenuria and renal hematuria (other causes must be excluded), splenic infarction at unpressured high altitude (over 7,000–10,000 feet), bacteriuria, and pyelonephritis in pregnancy.

The following dramatic complications have yet to be proved to have a significantly higher incidence in sickle trait patients than the general population: sudden death, anesthesia and postsurgical complications other than those associated with hypoxia, intravascular sickling associated with strenuous exercise, complications of pregnancy, and frequency of hospitalization.

In contrast, sickle cell diseases (SS, S-thal, SD, SS with high F) are a group of illnesses that are relatively pernicious in decreasing severity as listed. Clinical signs and symptoms are a result of the basic pathophysiologic consequences of sickling described above: obtruction of microvasculature and a hemolytic process resulting in anemia.

Crises occur in sickle diseases. Pain crisis is the most common clinical presentation, caused by hypoxic infarction of tissue. Precipitating causes are not clear. Pain is present all over: joints, bones, back, and abdomen. An acute surgical abdomen may be mimicked. Painful, swollen, hot, and tender hands and feet occur in children as the hand-foot syndrome of sickle cell dactyllus. Under severely hypoxic conditions, the AS individual may have a pain crisis.

Hemolytic anemia is invariably present in sickle diseases. The laboratory stigmata of hemolysis are reticulocytosis, indirect bilirubinemia, and decreased haptoglobin. The peripheral blood smear examination gives the answer to the experienced observer practically always in SS disease, most of the time in SC disease, and some of the time in S-thalassemia. The conclusive diagnosis of a sickle disease is proved by a properly performed hemoglobin electrophoresis, and the quantitative determination of Hgb F and A_2.

Anemic crisis with aggravation of the anemia may occur. It is my opinion that hemolytic crises due to S hemoglobin per se do not occur in sickle diseases. A hemolytic crisis is the acceleration of random red cell destruction. Inherited hemolytic disorders, of which the S hemoglobin diseases are an example, have a constant hemolytic rate that does not change. Changes in hemoglobin level in S diseases not due to blood loss occur for reasons described below. Hemolytic crises do occur in acquired hemolytic disease such as autoimmune hemolytic anemia and paroxysmal nocturnal hemoglobinuria. Aggravated hemolysis in S diseases in this country occurs most commonly because of associated Glucose 6 Phosphate Dehydrogenase (G6PD) deficiency. In children, sequestration of RBCs in the spleen and liver may mimic a hemolytic crisis because of falling hematocrit.

Anemic crisis does occur in S diseases because of bone marrow failure due to: (1) aplastic crisis, which is characterized by aggravation of anemia, reticulocytopenia, fall in serum bilirubin and a marrow that shows practically no RBC precursors. Many causes are postulated, but none proved. Treatment is transfusion with packed RBCs until spontaneous marrow recovery occurs. (2) In megaloblastic crisis: The same peripheral blood findings are present in aplastic crisis, but the marrow is classically megaloblastic. The cause is hyperutilization of folic acid for erythropoiesis. The folate is not replaced pharmacologically or by food intake; this results in a folate deficiency. This lack of intake may be due to socioeconomic factors or illness. I place all sickle disease patients on folic acid prophylactically.

Other clinical features due to chronic in situ microvascular obstruction are aseptic necrosis of articular bone (commonly the femoral head), hematuria, renal concentrating defects, priapism, leg ulcers, and pulmonary vasculature occlusion. The last may also be caused by fat and/or marrow embolization from infarcted bone. Frequently it is difficult to tell infarction secondary to thrombosis from infection. Cor pulmonale has been reported. Ischemic retinal infarcts and other ocular manifestations are common. There is an increased incidence of cerebral thrombosis.

Cardiovascular abnormalities are almost uniformly present in sickle diseases. This is probably due predominantly to the severe chronic anemia. Chronic increased cardiac output secondary to anemia, arterial oxygen unsaturation, and occlusion of pulmonary and cardiac microvasculature may all be important. More than 80% of patients have cardiac silhouette enlargement on x-rays, loud systolic ejection type murmurs that radiate over the precordium and a third heart sound. Since the chronic severe anemia is probably the primary cause of the abnormalities, it is not surprising that the diseases of SC, S-thal, SD, and SS high F, which have higher hematocrits, have a lesser incidence of serious cardiovascular disease.

Infection with pneumococcus and salmonella is increased in sickle diseases: pneumonia, bacteremia, and meningitis with the former, and osteomyelitis with the latter. Abnormalities of the reticuloendothelial system (eg, functional asplenia) and in the complement system have been described.

Some individuals recommend random screening for S Hgb in all blacks. I do not believe random population screening for sickle hemoglobin is indicated because of: lack of effective therapy; the emotional trauma caused by "reliable misinformation" concerning sickle trait versus sickle diseases; and the resultant reluctance of industry to employ or insurance companies to insure at regular rates individuals with sickle trait.

Selected References

1. Diggs LW: Sickle cell crises. *Am J Clin Pathol* 44:1–19, 1965.
2. Ranney HM: Sickle cell disease. *Blood* 39:433–439, 1972.
3. Lessin LS, Jensen WN (eds): Sickle cell symposium. *Arch Intern Med* 133:529–705, 1974.
4. O'Brien RT: Perspectives in sickle cell disease screening. *South Med J* 67:1269–1271, 1974.
5. Dykes G, Crepeau RH, Edelstein SJ: Three dimensional reconstruction of the fibres of sickle cell hemoglobin. *Nature* 272:506–510, 1978.
6. Finch JT: Editorial on work of Dykes et al. *Nature* 272:496–497, 1978.
7. Sears DA: The morbidity of sickle cell trait (review). *Am J Med* 64:1021–1036, 1978.

MUSCULOSKELETAL SYSTEM

98. Joint Stiffness

COLON WILSON, MD
JOHN A. GOLDMAN, MD

Definition

Relative immobility of the joints.

Technique

This complaint is generally volunteered by the patient; however, you might begin by asking nonspecific questions such as: Have you had any problems with your joints? Have any of your joints bothered you?

Some people do not understand what stiffness is, and speak about limbering up, getting going, tightness, difficulty in moving, and resistance. Nondirect questioning is certainly better, and questions such as, "In what way have your joints bothered you?" or, "Tell me about the problems you have had with your joints," give more meaningful information. Although nondirect questioning of a patient usually gives more relevant information, sometimes some direct questioning must also be done, ie: Do you ever feel stiff?

It is important to characterize this stiffness. Information that is needed includes:

1. Distribution (single versus multiple joints)
2. Duration (a few minutes to hours). The endpoint of stiffness is not always easy to define. Some patients will notice that their stiffness continues all day long, and thus in them it is better to ask when the stiffness begins to resolve. This will give you a time interval and end point.
3. Associated circumstances (in the morning, after sitting for a long time, ie, "jelling," or after brisk exercise).

Background Information

The reason that a person perceives stiffness is because of the inability to move the joint through its normal arc with normal muscular effort. Various types of stiffness have been investigated to better understand what causes morning stiffness. It appears that these may be due to anatomical changes within the joint or edema around the joint.

Anatomical changes. Stiffness due to anatomical changes occurs when the joint capsule has become loosened by (1) degeneration of cartilage, (2) a tear of the capsule, or (3) adhesions of tendons and tendon sheaths or joint capsular structures due to trauma or preceding inflammation.

In the case of stiffness due to degenerative disease, the joint capsule has become somewhat loosened due to thinning of the cartilage. The redundance of the capsule can be somewhat compensated by good muscle tone; hence, the stiffness occurs when muscle tone is lost, specifically in the early morning after sleeping through the night or after remaining immobile for a long time (frequently referred to as "jelling"). Characteristically this stiffness is rapidly dissipated by a brief period of exercise to restore muscle tone (less than 30 minutes).

Edema. Stiffness due to edema of the structures about the joint capsule occurs in inflammatory joint disease such as rheumatoid arthritis and the rheumatoid variants.

Stiffness due to edema of the joint capsule structures secondary to inflammation is also more pronounced after a period of rest, when the edema has collected in the connective tissue structures. It, too, is most pronounced in the early morning. Unlike the stiffness previously discussed in association with degenerative changes in the joint structures, this type of stiffness is more slowly dissipated because the edema is slowly mobilized. The usual history is of stiffness that lasts for several hours in the morning. However, arbitrarily, any stiffness that lasts longer than 30 minutes is suggestive of inflammatory synovial disease.

Clinical Significance

Joint stiffness is common. In osteoarthritis stiffness frequently persists for 5 to 10 minutes in the morning, or after a prolonged period of rest ("jelling"). Stiffness persisting for more than 30 minutes suggests rheumatoid arthritis, other inflammatory arthritides, or polymyalgia rheumatica. In these conditions, stiffness characteristically persists for one to several hours in the morning and tends to recur after periods of prolonged rest. Arbitrarily, stiffness persisting longer than 30 minutes in the morning can be significant evidence of an inflammatory rheumatic condition. Other disorders associated with stiffness include ankylosing spondylitis, systemic sclerosis, systemic infections, stiff-man syndrome, congenital mucopolysaccharoidoses such as Hurler's and Morquio's disease syndromes, ochronosis, and serum sickness.

Selected References

1. Hollander JL, McCarty DJ Jr (eds): *Arthritis and Allied Conditions.* Philadelphia, Lea and Febiger, 1971, pp 15–25.
2. Katz WA (ed): *Rheumatic Diseases: Diagnosis and Management.* Philadelphia, JB Lippincott, 1977, pp 15–16.
3. Polley HF, Hunder GG: *Rheumatologic Interviewing and Physical Examination of the Joints,* ed 2. Philadelphia, WB Saunders, 1978.
4. Scott JT (ed): *Copeman's Textbook of the Rheumatic Diseases.* London and New York, Churchill Livingstone, 1978.
5. Wright V, Johns RJ: Quantitative and qualitative analysis of joint stiffness in normal subjects and in patients with a connective tissue disease. *Ann Rheum Dis* 20:36–46, 1961.

99. Joint Pain

COLON WILSON, MD
JOHN A. GOLDMAN, MD

Definition

The experiencing of pain localized in a joint.

Technique

This complaint is usually volunteered by the patient. The nondirective questions suggested in section 98 on Joint Stiffness should be adequate to produce complaints of pain. If these questions do not elicit a positive response or if the patient complains of stiffness but does not follow with a complaint of pain, ask a specific question such as: Have you had any painful joints? If the patient answers affirmatively, characterize the pain more thoroughly.

It is better to be nondirective and ask the patient to describe the pain, but you may have to become directive and ask more specific questions such as: Is the pain steady or throbbing? Does the pain occur only with use, or does it persist at rest? If so, how long? A description of the development of pain is helpful. If it involves more than one joint, determine whether the pain pattern is one of migration or recruitment. Migratory joint pain is characterized by migration of the pain from one joint to other joints while the earlier joints resolve. In recruitment one joint begins and continues as other joints become involved. Also determine what time the pain comes, where it is located and whether there are associated precipitating circumstances.

Background Information

Pain in the joint may be due to trauma or inflammation of the structures within the joint or adjacent to it, or it may be referred from another area (eg, the adjacent shaft of the bone, or thalamic pain).

The clinician must consider all complaints of joint pain to be due to abnormalities of structures within the joint and seek objective signs to support this phenomenon. Pain in joints is a frequent complaint associated with psychosomatic illnesses; however, well-documented signs of a functional illness should precede dismissal of joint pain as psychosomatic.

Clinical Significance

Some clues to the significance of the pain can be obtained by a thorough description in the history:

1. Onset.
    a. Rapid onset (30 minutes to 4 hours) suggests gout, septic arthritis, acute rheumatic fever, or palindromic rheumatism.
    b. Gradual, insidious onset suggests a nonspecific, chronic inflammatory arthritis (eg, rheumatoid arthritis).
2. Character.
    a. Pain on motion relieved by brief periods of rest suggests degenerative joint disease.
    b. Aching pain accentuated by motion, but persisting at rest, suggests an inflammatory arthritis.
    c. Severe, excruciating, throbbing pain suggests gout or septic arthritis.

3. Time.
   a. Pain on awakening in the morning lasting greater than 30 minutes suggests an inflammatory arthritis.
   b. Low back pain at night, relieved by walking about, suggests ankylosing spondylitis or other causes of sacroiliitis.
   c. Acute arthritis that awakens the patient at night suggests gout.

4. Location.
   a. Low back pain suggests muscle sprain, disk compression, compression fractures, or spondylitis.
   b. Neck pain suggests cervical spine disease or myalgia.
   c. Plantar heel pain suggests heel spurs, rheumatoid nodules or the spondylitis group of arthritides.

5. Associated circumstances.
   a. History of preceding injury is strongly suggestive of traumatic arthritis; however, this history can be present in gouty arthritis.
   b. History of excessive activity (eg, several sets of tennis) preceding the onset of arthritis is suggestive of traumatic arthritis. In a person with preceding degenerative joint disease, the precipitating activity might be within the norm for an average person (eg, a 1-mile walk).
   c. A preceding banquet or alcoholic "spree" might suggest gout.
   d. A preceding sore throat suggests acute rheumatic fever.
   e. An associated urethritis suggests gonococcal arthritis or Reiter's syndrome.
   f. Ingestion of medication suggests allergic vasculitis and arthritis.

6. Duration.
   a. Pain that persists from a few hours to 24 hours in one joint and disappears, followed by pain in another joint (migratory) suggests rheumatic fever, but is also seen frequently in the early stages of gonococcal arthritis.
   b. Persistent pain in the original joint with eventual involvement of an increasing number of joints (recruitment) suggests a chronic inflammatory arthritis, ie, rheumatoid arthritis, spondylitis, etc.
   c. Pain present for greater than 2 weeks would make acute gout unlikely.
   d. Pain present for 6 weeks or greater would indicate chronic arthritis.

7. Measures that produce relief such as aspirin, heat, codeine, antibiotics, or rest.

Selected References

1. Hollander JL, McCarty DJ Jr (eds): *Arthritis and Allied Conditions.*
    Philadelphia, Lea and Febiger, 1971, pp 15–25.
2. Polley HF, Hunder GG: *Rheumatologic Interviewing and Physical Ex-
    amination of the Joints,* ed 2. Philadelphia, WB Saunders, 1978.
3. Scott JT (ed): *Copeman's Textbook of the Rheumatic Diseases.* Lon-
    don and New York, Churchill Livingstone, 1978.
4. Katz WA (ed): *Rheumatic Diseases: Diagnosis and Management.* Phil-
    adelphia, JB Lippincott, 1977.

100. Joint Swelling

COLON WILSON, MD
JOHN A. GOLDMAN, MD

Definition

Swelling localized in a joint.

Technique

The techniques described for taking a history of joint stiffness and
joint pain (sections 98 and 99) should be adequate to elicit this complaint. If the patient does not complain of swelling on nondirective interview, it is not necessary to specifically ask for this complaint unless the
patient complained of joint pain, joint stiffness, or both. If either of these
complaints is elicited and the complaint of swelling is not volunteered,
ask if the pain or stiffness has been associated with swelling.

If the patient gives a history of joint swelling, try to ascertain if
swelling is limited to the joint or if in actuality the complaint is one of
soft tissue swelling of the periarticular structures. The easiest way to determine if the swelling is truly joint swelling is to ask the patient to demonstrate the boundaries of the swelling. If this is not possible, attempt to
get as clear a description as possible from the patient.

In measuring the significance of the history of swelling, it is important to ask the patient if there has been redness or heat associated with the swelling. Either or both of these complaints suggests inflammation in the joint; however, they are of less significance in history taking than when they are objectively observed.

Background Information

I. True joint enlargement.
    A. Bony enlargement. In degenerative joint disease (due to aging, repeated trauma), reactive changes occur in subchondral bone leading to an increase in density of the subchondral bone and a hypertrophic ridge about the margin of the joint at the junction of the cartilage. This is often read as "spurring" on x-ray and is palpable on examination as bony widening of the joint.
    B. Synovial inflammation. The joint capsule is lined with synovium, which in the normal state is a very thin, smooth, glistening membrane. In the normal state the thin synovial membrane is not palpable. The synovium is approximately two cells thick and is composed of two cell types:
        1. Type A cells. These are phagocytic and remove debris from the joint.
        2. Type B cells. These secrete synovial fluid, which is present in the normal joint in very small amounts. This fluid lubricates the joint and is the medium through which the cartilage is nourished. When the synovial membrane becomes inflamed, it thickens due to reactive hyperplasia of the synovial cells, infiltration of the synovial membrane by inflammatory cells (first by polymorphonuclear leukocytes and later by lymphocytes and plasma cells), and proliferation of fibroblasts. As the synovium becomes thickened, it becomes palpable. With practice you will become adept at perceiving the "doughy" consistency of chronically inflamed synovium.
    C. Effusion.
        1. Noninflammatory effusion. As degenerative changes occur in the cartilage, fragments break off into the joint capsule. Concurrent with this process or as a consequence of it, there is an overproduction of synovial fluid by the synovial cells. On analysis this type of fluid has few white cells and a good mucin content.

    2.   Inflammatory effusion. When the synovial membrane becomes inflamed (whether due to the nonspecific inflammation of rheumatoid arthritis, the presence of bacteria, or the presence of crystals), the synovial cells are stimulated to an increased production of synovial fluid. In addition, the synovial membrane becomes permeable to plasma elements, and there is an exudation of these substances into the joint capsule. The polys that have infiltrated the synovial membrane also migrate into the fluid within the capsule. An analysis of the fluid in an inflammatory effusion reveals an increased number of white cells and a poor mucin content. In addition, because plasma elements may pass the inflamed synovial barrier, there is an increase in protein. Fibrinogen and other clotting factors present in the fluid will allow the fluid to clot on standing. The magnitude of inflammation of the synovium is reflected in these elements and can be estimated by quantitating them.

    3.   Hemorrhage. Hemorrhage into the joint capsule may occur secondary to trauma or to a coagulation defect that is congenital, iatrogenic, or secondary to a disease process.

II.   Periarticular swelling.

    A.   Subcutaneous tissues.

        1.   Edema. Soft tissue swelling which pits on pressure of the subcutaneous tissues about a joint may be produced by edema due to:

            a.   Increased extracellular fluid secondary to congestive heart failure, renal disease, associated with dependency.

            b.   Increased vascular permeability due to trauma.

        2.   Inflammation due to infection along fascial planes or local abscess formation.

    B.   Tenosynovitis. Tendon sheaths are lined with synovial membrane similar to that described above within the joint capsule. This tenosynovium may become inflamed and swollen, and an effusion may form due to:

        1.   Trauma. Usually severe repeated stress (eg, a brisk tennis game).

        2.   Specific infection. This is a common occurrence with gonococcal arthritis (especially the dorsum of the wrist and the ankle).

        3.   In association with chronic inflammatory joint diseases (eg, rheumatoid arthritis, systemic lupus erythematosus, gout).

C. Bursitis. There are many bursae throughout the body, situated primarily over bony prominences, to facilitate the smooth gliding of muscles and tendons. The conditions under which these may become inflamed and swollen are essentially the same as those for tenosynovitis.

D. Nodules.
1. Rheumatoid nodules. Chronic granulomatous nodules form about small vessels and may proliferate to varying sizes. These may occur anywhere in the body, but are seen more frequently in areas where pressure is common over bony prominences. A characteristic site for these nodules is over the olecranon process at the elbow.
2. Gouty tophi. Monosodium urate crystals deposit at various places in the body in patients suffering from chronic gout. These areas of deposition are seen more frequently in cartilage, subchondral bone, and tendon sheaths. Two sites that are frequently observed and palpated are the helix of the ear and the olecranon bursa.

Clinical Significance

Swelling limited to a joint can be due to:

1. Inflammation of the synovium, as in the nonspecific inflammatory arthritides, acute rheumatic fever, collagen-vascular disease, septic arthritis, or gout.
2. Effusion or hemorrhage into the joint due to inflammation or trauma. In the case of degenerative joint disease or osteoarthritis, trauma does not have to be great and may not be beyond the limits of normal use for a normal joint.
3. Local infiltration due to leukemia, myeloma, or abnormally stored products or metabolism such as amyloid.

Periarticular swelling may be due to edema secondary to venous insufficiency or fluid overload, in which case it should be painless and not tender. This type of swelling will pit on pressure. On the other hand, several types of true joint involvement are frequently associated with periarticular involvement:

1. Gout is frequently associated with a significant amount of very painful, warm, periarticular soft tissue swelling. Pitting edema may also occur with this.
2. Gonococcal arthritis is frequently associated with tenosynovitis

in the tendon sheaths adjacent to the joint involved, particularly the wrist and ankle.
3. Jaccoud's arthritis following rheumatic fever is also associated with a significant amount of periarticular involvement.
4. Trauma to a joint if very significant will also traumatize the periarticular structures and produce a significant amount of periarticular soft tissue swelling. This is most often tender, but cool.
5. In addition, tenosynovitis or bursitis due to trauma or other cause might be present in the area adjacent to a joint without actual joint involvement.

Selected References

1. Hollander JL, McCarty DJ Jr (eds): *Arthritis and Allied Conditions.* Philadelphia, Lea and Fegiber, 1971, pp 15–25.
2. Polley HF, Hunder GG: *Rheumatologic Interviewing and Physical Examination of the Joints,* ed 2. *Philadelphia,* WB Saunders, 1978.
3. Scott JT (ed): *Copeman's Textbook of the Rheumatic Diseases.* London and New York, Churchill Livingstone, 1978.
4. Katz WA (ed): *Rheumatic Diseases: Diagnosis and Management.* Philadelphia, JB Lippincott, 1977.

101. Family History of Musculoskeletal Disease

COLON WILSON, MD
JOHN A. GOLDMAN, MD

Definition

To determine if there is a history of arthritis that might be inherited.

Technique

In this case there is nothing to be gained in being nondirective in the interview. One should ask directly: Has there been any gout in your family—your father, brothers, uncles, or anyone else related to you? Follow this with: Have any of your relatives had any other type of arthritis, such as rheumatoid arthritis or ankylosing spondylitis? Should the patient state that a relative has had arthritis, one should attempt to get some clue to the type. In doing this it is important to understand a few words in the patient's glossary: "the crippling kind" usually equates to rheumatoid arthritis or one of the rheumatoid variants. Ask what joints were most affected. Peripheral joint predominance would be more consistent with rheumatoid arthritis; significant spinal involvement, with one of the spondylitides.

If there has been a significant amount of arthritis in the family, the person taking the history should diagram a family tree, which would make the chart a more useful source document.

Background Information

For many years several of the rheumatic diseases have been known to be associated with a high family incidence, eg, gout, ankylosing spondylitis, and Heberden's nodes in osteoarthritis. More recently, specific genetic markers have been demonstrated in some of these diseases and in several of the other arthritides, and the frequently noted familial clustering of rheumatoid arthritis and systemic lupus erythematosus with other autoimmune abnormalities, while not statistically significant, is attracting more attention, suggesting that these clusters should be observed more closely.

Clinical Significance

Some conditions with genetic transmission are the following:

1. Several types of familial amyloidosis are well described in the literature and their pattern of genetic transmission is well documented.

2. The genetic transmission of several enzyme defects that lead to hyperuricemia and gout has been documented. Lesch and Nyhan in 1964 reported an inherited disease in children characterized by hyperuricemia, mental retardation, choreoathetosis, and self-mutilation, with occasional gouty attacks. This disease was shown by Seegmiller and his coworkers in 1967 to be due to a complete lack of enzyme hypoxanthine-guanine phosphoribosyl-transferase (H-G PRTase), and the genetic transmission of the enzyme was shown to be X-linked. Kelly et al in 1969 documented a genetically determined partial deficiency of this same enzyme in other instances of familial gout.

   A second genetically transmitted enzyme defect was described in 1972 by Spurling et al due to an increase in the intracellular activity of the enzyme phosphoribosylpyrophosphate synthetase (PRPP).

Glycogen storage disease (type I, Von Gierke) is an autosomal recessive disease that leads to lactacidemia and ketoacidemia and decreased renal clearance of uric acid, also causing hyperuricemia and gout.

3.   In 1973 Schlosstein et al and Brewerton et al described independently an extremely high incidence of HLA-B27 in patients who have ankylosing spondylitis. The genetic determinant for this antigen is localized on an autosomal chromosome, as are the determinants for the other tissue type antigens useful in determining histocampatibility. The locus of these antigenic site determinants is closely related to genetic determinants of the immune system. Since that time a high incidence of HLA-B27 has also been demonstrated in Reiter's syndrome, psoriatic arthritis, and the spondylitis of inflammatory bowel disease (ulcerative colitis and regional enteritis).

Selected References

1.   Brewerton DA, James DCO: The histocompatibility antigen (HL-A27) and disease. *Semin Arthr Rheumatol*:4(3):191–207, 1975.

2.   Hollander JL, McCarty DJ Jr (eds): *Arthritis and Allied Conditions*, ed 8. Philadelphia, Lea and Febiger, 1972.

3.   McKusick VA: *Heritable Disorders of Connective Tissue*, ed 4. St. Louis, CV Mosby, 1972.

4.   Polley HF, Hunder GG: *Rheumatologic Interviewing and Physical Examination of the Joints*, ed 2. Philadelphia, WB Saunders, 1978.

5.   Scott JT (ed): *Copeman's Textbook of the Rheumatic Diseases*. London and New York, Churchill Livingstone, 1978.

6.   Smyth CD: Disorders associated with hyperuricemia. (Proc Sec Conf Gout: Purine Metabolism), *Arthr Rheum* 18(suppl 6):713–719, 1975.

7.   Katz WA (ed): *Rheumatic Diseases: Diagnosis and Management*. Philadelphia, JB Lippincott, 1977.

102. Previous Psychiatric Problems

JOHN B. GRIFFIN, MD

Definition

Everyone has had times of emotional stress with minor disruption of function. In this portion of the history the examiner is not seeking information concerning such minor episodes but rather significant data about psychiatric problems that may bear on the present illness. Significant psychiatric problems are those that produce important interference with the patient's daily activities. If the mental health problem is of enough severity to require hospitalization, it should be regarded as significant.

Technique

Attempt to assess whether the patient has shown a tendency toward development of emotional symptoms under stress. In particular, discover if these symptoms produced appreciable loss of function in educational, family, work, or social activities. Always inquire about the nature of any treatment the patient received for these symptoms.

In approaching this area, be specific in your questions. The question, "Have you ever had any emotional illness?" is so general that the patient may answer negatively, when with more specific questioning, different information might be given. Beginning with a definite question related to severe illness and progressing to lesser degrees of illness is often a satisfactory pattern. The patient should be asked about any hospitalization for treatment of an emotional or psychiatric illness. With some patients, it is helpful to use the term "nervous breakdown" since this is a commonly used lay phrase. In these cases, ask: Have you ever had a nervous breakdown serious enough to require your spending time in a hospital? It is not sufficient to ask whether the patient has ever been hospitalized by a psychiatrist since patients are frequently hospitalized for emotional difficulties by internists, general practitioners, and others. If the patient replies negatively, then inquire about any period of counseling by a psychiatrist, social worker, psychologist, minister, or other mental health worker. If the patient again responds negatively, ask: Have you ever experienced a time in which you felt that your emotions significantly interfered with your performance? If the patient replies affirmatively, inquire further about the details of this episode.

Do not close inquiry into this area without asking patients whether they have ever had physical symptoms for which their physician suggested an emotional etiology or for which their doctor could find no cause. A positive response to either of these questions may be the first clue that the patient reacts to stress by either hypochondriacal or psychophysiological symptoms.

Background Information

Working with Joseph Breuer, Sigmund Freud discovered that certain patients with conversion symptoms showed dramatic improvement when they were encouraged to talk freely while in a hypnotic trance. Freud later discovered that similar improvement in symptoms could be obtained if patients were allowed to free associate while not in a hypnotic trance. The patient was encouraged to discuss freely anything that came into mind during the therapeutic sessions. As Freud proceeded with these investigations, he repeatedly found that the roots of many of the emotional conflicts appeared to be found in childhood experiences. Eventually it became clear that emotional problems in the present were usually linked in an integral way to past experiences. At the present time, there are many theories of human behavior. However, whether behavior is regarded from the standpoint of a psychoanalytic model or a learning theory model, there is general consensus that past experience is a heavy determinant of current activity. Ethological experience, such as the studies of Konrad Lorenz, also provides support for the concept that early experiences are of great importance in shaping later behavior. In almost every clinical situation, it has been found useful in treatment to have a clear concept of the patient's past experience.

Clinical Significance

In assessing the significance of a positive history of previous psychiatric problems, details must be obtained concerning the treatment received by the patient. Psychiatric illness severe enough to require hospitalization suggests that the patient's susceptibility to emotional stress is greater than that of the general population. Such patients are generally regarded as having a higher statistical likelihood of further difficulty than patients without such a history. Patients who have obtained only outpatient therapy that involves counseling around a specific stress situation in their lives or counseling for the purpose of clarifying life goals should not, simply because of this counseling, be regarded as having greater likelihood of difficulty in the future. By resolving their conflicts through therapy, many of these patients have better understanding of themselves and may be even less likely to have further psychiatric difficulties than the average person.

In general, patients who receive medications during outpatient treatment can be regarded as having had a more serious emotional problem than patients who did not receive medication. It is important to know as precisely as possible what medications were taken. Many patients will know the names of the medications taken. If a major tranquilizer such as chlorpromazine (Thorazine), thioridazine (Mellaril), or trifluoperazine (Stelazine) was taken, the illness is likely to have been more severe than if a minor tranquilizer such as chlordiazepoxide hydrochloride (Librium) or diazepam (Valium) were given. If an antidepressant medication was used, one must inquire further concerning the extent of the depression, as will be outlined in section 105, Depression.

Some patients will know what their diagnosis was during past treatment. Psychotic illnesses such as schizophrenia are generally regarded as more severe than neurotic problems such as phobic or anxiety reactions.

Selected References

1. Rosenblum L: Ethology: Primate research and the evolutionary origins of human behavior, in Simons RC, Pardes H (eds): *Understanding Human Behavior in Health and Illness.* Baltimore, Williams and Wilkins, 1977, chap 8, pp 83–99.
2. Kolb LC: Predisposing and precipitating factors in mental disorder, in Kolb LC (ed): *Modern Clinical Psychiatry.* Baltimore, WB Saunders, 1977, chap 7, pp 160–194.
3. Gregory I, Smeltzer DJ: Development and dynamics, in Gregory I, Smeltzer DJ (eds): *Psychiatry: Essentials of Clinical Practice.* Boston, Little, Brown, 1977, chap 1, pp 1–14.

103. Interpersonal Relationships

JOHN B. GRIFFIN, JR., MD

Definition

Interpersonal relationships refers to reciprocal social and emotional interactions between the patient and other persons in the environment. Almost every mental disorder is accompanied by problems in this area. Frequently a basic cause of conflict with other people is the presence of some psychiatric disorder. Major areas in which these conflicts may occur include the following relationships:

1. Family
2. Social
3. Work
4. Religious
5. Sexual

Technique

Family relationships. Family relationships include those both with the spouse and with other relatives. Inquiry into this area usually begins with investigation of the marital relationship. Marital conflicts are often quite subtle. Patients frequently fail to see a relationship between their presenting symptomatology and their marital disharmony, particularly when the presenting problem is a psychophysiologic one such as asthma or peptic ulcer. At times the patient is unconsciously resisting seeing such a connection out of fear that exploration of the conflicts might lead to dissolution of the marriage.

It is often useful to start with open-ended general questions such as: Tell me about your marriage. What is your marriage like? The degree of warmth and enthusiasm with which the patient describes the marriage may be more important than the actual words. At times patients may say that the marriage is fine even when it is not because they feel uncomfortable in discussing the difficulties which are present. If anything in the patient's response indicates that there may be difficulties within the marriage, proceed to more detailed questioning. Asking the patient to describe the spouse is often a helpful beginning. If the patient lists no shortcomings of the spouse, this can be pointed out and the patient encouraged to describe even minor things that might be annoying. Even in the best of marriages there are bound to be some attributes of the spouse which are somewhat trying to the other member of the pair. If the patient indicates in some fashion that there are serious difficulties but becomes uncomfortable when inquiry is made into these areas, it is usually wise to avoid pressing the patient strongly in the initial history-gathering process. If strongly pressed, many patients will begin to deny difficulties. This will make later therapy more difficult since the patient will eventually have to admit having misled you.

However, if the patient is comfortable with describing the marital problem in detail, this should be pursued fully. The patient should be asked to describe the nature of the conflicts, feelings about the conflicts, and efforts at resolution. In gathering this information, the physician often gains important information concerning the patient's flexibility, assertiveness, independence, and insight.

In addition, the examiner should seek information about the interaction of the patient and other significant family members, particularly children and parents. Most patients do not feel threatened by direct inquiry concerning their children or parents.

If the patient's children are young, the physician often has the opportunity for preventive mental health intervention. Many mothers sense that their children have significant emotional difficulties but fail to bring these out unless the physician inquires. In some instances, these difficulties will be incidental to the patient's main complaint, at other times, significantly tied to it. In any event, if the history indicates that a child may have significant emotional problems, this difficulty can often be more easily resolved in childhood than in later years. The primary physician can then encourage early intervention that may prevent more serious later difficulties.

However, the relationship of older patients with their adult children is also of great importance. Inquire about the fit between the expectations and hopes that the parents have had for their children and actual life events. In cases where children have been a disappointment, many patients will experience considerable guilt.

Emotional ties to relatives—parents, siblings, children, grandparents —are often particularly close. Questions such as, "How do you get along with your parents?" or, "What contact do you have now with your relatives?" will often open floodgates of important information. If married patients do not spontaneously mention their relationships with in-laws, specific questions should be asked by the physician since these relationships, as evidenced by the multitude of mother-in-law jokes, are often sources of conflict.

Social relationships.   The circumstances in which the patient is living can be explored with direct questions. Information should be sought from unmarried patients about relationships with any persons with whom they share their dwellings. The patient should be asked to describe recreational activities and community involvement. The physician can then lead quite naturally into a discussion of interpersonal relationships. Many people feel that they have numerous acquaintances and superficial friends but nevertheless feel quite lonely and isolated in respect to having close friends. The patient can be asked whether the number of friends is as great as desired and whether some are persons to whom the patient can freely confide feelings.

Work relationships.   Since work is an almost universal human experience, it is not surprising that this area is an important source of stress. Gainful employment in American society is so important that its lack is almost always associated with emotional upheaval and loss of self-esteem. In this area, one must be particularly careful not to be deceived by a patient's statement that work is a problem-free area. This may be true in the patient's mind, but indirect effects of the occupation on other areas of life experience may not have been recognized. Many people are so emotionally invested in their work that they fail to see the devastating effects of their long hours and arduous schedule upon their family relationships. Physicians are particularly prone to this difficulty.

Beginning inquiry in this area with an open-ended question such as, "Tell me about your work," is usually more productive than asking direct questions that can be answered by yes or no. It is advisable to ask for more details if a patient gives only a general statement. For example, a patient who reports working in a chicken plant has not told the physician precisely what the job is. There is a vast difference between the secretary's job in the central office and the job of the person on the production line who removes the intestines. Inquiry into goals is often helpful. Asking about childhood ambitions may lead to a comparison of current status with what the patient would have preferred to become. If a person describes difficulties, either dissatisfaction with advancement, personality clashes, or a failure to see meaning in the work, this area should be explored in as much depth as the patient indicates willingness to pursue.

One should not close inquiry without asking for a specific report of the patient's work schedule. This should include information concerning total hours of work per week, amount of night work, and extent of out-of-town travel. The spouse should also be asked about the work schedule since many people tend to underestimate the amount of time they are spending at work.

Religious relationships.   Most Americans state some religious preference. More than half of all Americans are affiliated with some church organization. However, many Americans have only a superficial contact with these religious organizations. Emotional problems revolving around religious conflicts are not as frequent as those arising out of marital or work relationships. However, such conflicts do occur frequently enough to warrant some investigation of this area.

If a patient indicates no religious belief, additional questions can still be useful. One might ask whether the lack of religious belief creates any problem. The patient's response to this or a similar question will often reveal whether this area is one that should be explored further. Some patients with no religious preference are clearly choosing this course out of unconscious rebellion toward parents or from some other motivation that they do not fully understand. In these cases, the presence of the apparent conflict can be noted and later explored in more depth. For patients who do express a religious preference, inquiry into their contact with church activities can be helpful. As they describe their church contacts, it is usually easy to make an accurate estimate of the significance of religion to them and of the presence of potential conflicts. Asking if religious beliefs cause behavior that is unlike that of most others in the patient's social group or whether religious beliefs cause feelings of being different can also be revealing in terms of bringing emotional difficulties to the surface.

Many people find strong emotional support from their religious convictions. Deep religious conviction is not in itself a sign of emotional difficulty. However, if a patient's behavior is considerably different from that of most others in the religious group, the physician should inquire carefully into reasons for this discrepancy.

Sexual relationships.   Most sexual difficulties are not caused by physical problems. They are usually the result of emotional conflict. Consequently, it is of great importance to explore the feelings which the patient has toward the sexual partner. The procedures for taking a sexual history have been outlined in section 77.

Background Information

Not only has mental illness been found in all cultures that have been carefully studied, but also evidence of its existence can be found in the depths of antiquity. There were many views of the basic cause of mental disturbance, but almost all ancient theories saw it as basically being the result of something amiss within the individual. Many ancient views focused upon mental illness as the result of actions of the gods or infestation of persons by demons. Hippocrates (460–377 B.C.) suggested that madness came from the effect of various forms of bile. From that time to the present, physicians have continued to be fascinated by the effects of physical dysfunction upon mental activity. After the demonstration by

H. Noguchi of *Treponema pallidum* in the brain of patients with central nervous system syphilis, there could be little question that physical problems could be the basic etiology of major mental problems. Since that time, many psychiatric conditions have been found to have an organic etiology.

A related but somewhat different line of thought also placed the basic problem of mental illness within the patient but saw this as a problem of organization of thinking rather than as some physical defect in nervous system function. Studies of hypnosis clearly demonstrated that major changes in thinking patterns and behavior could be accomplished purely by the psychological technique of suggestion. Early work in the area of hypnosis by such people as Anton Mesmer (1734–1815), James Braid (1795–1860), Hippolyte Berheim (1840–1919), and Jean Martin Charcot (1825–1893) illustrated both that the symptoms of certain patients could be altered by suggestions and that the mind could block out awareness of posthypnotic suggestions without in any way diminishing the patient's need to follow the suggestions.

The psychoanalytic studies of Freud, Jung, Adler, and Rank have demonstrated the presence of unconscious motivation for behavior. Clinical investigation into the reasons for unconscious emotional conflicts has repeatedly led to the conclusion that interpersonal relationships play a major role in the development of personality. Relationships with parents have been found to be of particular importance in the development of basic attitudes. Harry Stack Sullivan (1892–1949) utilized astute and accurate clinical observations to focus intensively on the importance of the interpersonal relationships. His emphasis on communication processes in interpersonal behavior laid the groundwork for the present strong emphasis upon environment and interpersonal relationships as an etiology for many emotional disorders.

Present-day thinking sees the emotional state of the patient as being primarily the result of an interaction between the internal and external environment. If the internal environment is altered by physical disease such as central nervous system syphilis (general paresis) or Korsakoff's syndrome (an organic brain syndrome caused by vitamin deficiency associated with alcoholism), mental illness can occur. Similarly, a patient overwhelmed by unconscious conflicts may experience derangements in organization of thinking. Such patients show no nervous system lesions that would account for the neurotic or psychotic behavior.

Disruptions in interpersonal relationships are frequently the precipitating reasons for neurotic and psychotic behavior. Consequently, most modern thinking sees mental illness as an interaction between an internal emotional substrate different for each individual and environmental stresses.

Many modern treatment techniques including psychotherapy focus upon both resolution of internal conflicts and improvement in the patient's ability to handle interpersonal relationships. Many psychiatrists view psychotherapy as an educational process that provides increased understanding of self and enhanced ability to deal with interpersonal relationships.

Clinical Significance

In many cases, inquiry into the area of interpersonal relationships will produce evidence of considerable strength. This information in itself may be of considerable help in dealing with medical problems. For example, if a strong harmonious marriage exists, the physician can then count upon the patient's spouse to be supportive of the patient during the illness being treated. In some cases in which interpersonal conflicts are present, these conflicts may exist without significant relationship to the presenting illness. However, identification of these conflicts may make it possible for the patient to be helped by counseling at a later time. In other circumstances, elucidation of the emotional conflict may be the single most important item in the history. Little is gained by only treating physical complaints when these are actually of psychophysiologic origin. In these cases, the solution is found in dealing effectively with the emotional difficulties.

The physician must judge whether emotional conflicts are or are not a significant factor in the presenting complaints. This determination is at times made somewhat by exclusion. When the physician can find no organic etiology for physical complaints, a psychiatric consultation is frequently appropriate. However, it must be emphasized that psychological causation for a condition must not be accepted purely on the basis that nothing else can be found. There must also be clear evidence of a psychiatric disorder.

Diagnostic entities in which psychological factors are often of great importance in the production of physical illness include duodenal ulcer, ulcerative colitis, asthma, neurodermatitis, and essential hypertension.

Surveys of internists and family physicians have indicated that 25–50% of the patients whom they see in office practice come with problems that are basically of emotional origin. Some of these problems can be solved by environmental manipulation such as divorce or changing jobs. Others will require specialized psychiatric intervention.

The physician should not attempt to make decisions for the patient. Rather, the patients should be encouraged to explore all alternatives and then make their own decisions. Although the physician should be careful to allow patients to make their own decisions, the physician does have the responsibility of stating clearly to each patient the fact that psychophysiologic symptoms are coming from emotional stress. Without such a statement of the facts, the patients do not have all the information needed to fully understand their situations.

Selected References

1.   Freedman AM, Kaplan HI, Sadock BJ: The Family, in Freedman AM, et al (eds): *Modern Synopsis of Comprehensive Textbook of Psychiatry*, ed 2. Baltimore, Williams and Wilkins, 1976, sect 4.3, pp 173–186.
2.   Erikson EH: Eight ages of man, in Erikson EH (ed): *Childhood and Society*, ed 2. WW Norton, 1963, pp 247–274.
3.   Greenbaum H: Marriage, family, and parenthood. *Am J Psych* 130:1262–1264, 1973.
4.   Mumford E: The social significance of work, and studies on the stress of life events, in Simons RC, Pardes H (eds): *Understanding Human Behavior in Health and Illness*. Baltimore, Williams and Wilkins, 1977, pp 295–304.

---

104. Anxiety

JOHN B. GRIFFIN, JR., MD

Definition

Anxiety may be defined as apprehension, tension, or uneasiness that stems from the anticipation of danger, the source of which is largely unknown or unrecognized ("A Psychiatric Glossary"). It is distinguished from fear which is the emotional reaction to a real and consciously recognized threat. A person being pursued by a bear would correctly be described as feeling fear. A person in no danger who constantly is afraid that something terrible is about to happen is experiencing anxiety. Since anxiety is probably the most common symptom experienced by psychiatric patients, inquiry for its presence is extremely important.

Technique

Most patients who feel anxious will express this by saying that they feel nervous or worried. Patients usually see this condition as distressing and wish to find relief for it. In some cases, the anxiety appears in the form of phobias. For example, a patient may become phobic about driving a car following an auto accident. Often the patient recognizes that the anxiety is not realistic but, nevertheless, is unable to control it. Since the patient does not in most cases understand the unconscious roots of the anxiety, the physician should inquire carefully concerning the circumstances in which the anxiety was first felt. By noting the situations in which anxiety is most intense the physician can often gain clues regarding underlying etiology. The physician should ask how the anxiety has affected the patient's daily life routine. Finding the unconscious roots of anxiety is often a complex process requiring many visits. During the initial contacts with the patient the clinician should endeavor to determine the severity of the anxiety. It is usually of some help to ask for the patient's opinion concerning the reason for anxiety. Although the patient typically will be unable to explain the anxiety, the responses given in the attempt will help the physician estimate the degree of psychological sophistication. Psychological sophistication is a term which refers to the patient's awareness that there are reasons for feelings and that these reasons are not always consciously known. Involved in this concept is the ability to assess accurately one's own feeling state. During therapy the patient who is able to look realistically at personal motivation will be effective in uncovering unconscious conflicts.

Background Information

Anxiety is sometimes referred to as the psychological equivalent of physical pain. It is apparent that the mind has difficulty in dealing with strongly conflictual emotions. One of the mental mechanisms that the mind uses to deal with such conflicts is repression. In the process of repression, the mind simply blocks out one side of the conflicting emotions. When this act of repression is not entirely successful, the repressed material is constantly struggling to erupt into consciousness. The anxiety that is felt by the patient is often closely correlated with the amount of mental effort spent in keeping this material out of consciousness. A number of mental maneuvers, referred to as "defense mechanisms," are utilized in the effort to prevent repressed material from reaching consciousness. These mental mechanisms include such things as reaction formation, projection, rationalization, and displacement. These mental mechanisms are discussed at length in standard textbooks of psychiatry, such as reference 4 at the end of this section.

One reason that extensive utilization of defense mechanisms creates problems for patients is that such use tends to distort reality. The patient who is forced to block out one side of a conflict has created a situation that limits the ability to see all aspects of a problem. This, in turn, often makes it difficult to choose the most appropriate solution for difficulties.

Clinical Significance

Many patients who show evidence of anxiety neither seek nor desire treatment. Such persons usually regard themselves as having a nervous temperament and have no expectation of ever being different. When questioned about their anxiety, these patients usually state that they have always been nervous and that there has been no recent change in the extent of their nervousness.

Patients who require treatment for anxiety are those who have either experienced significant impairment of function and/or who are asking for relief of the internal distress associated with their anxiety. The primary physician can often treat acute conditions which have a strong environmental component. Examples might include anxiety related to job change, divorce, moving to a new location, physical illness, and financial difficulties.

Anxiety states related to long-standing emotional patterns such as those found in phobias, conversion reactions, compulsions, and personality disorders usually are best treated by referral to a mental health professional.

Selected References

1.   Freud S: The anxiety neurosis, in *Collected Papers*. New York, Basic Books, 1959, vol. 1, p 84.
2.   MacKenzie KR: The eclectic approach to the treatment of phobias. *Am J Psych* 130:1103–1106, 1973.
3.   Rosne H: Ego defense mechanisms, in Rosen H: *A Guide to Clinical Psychiatry* Miami, Mnemosyne Publishing Co, 1978, pp 73–79.
4.   Silver R: The Neuroses, in Kraft A (ed): *Psychiatry: A Concise Textbook for Primary Care Practice*. New York, Arco Publishing Co, 1977, pp 73–79.

105. Depression

JOHN B. GRIFFIN, JR., MD

Definition

Depression is a subjective experience in which a patient feels sad, unhappy, and often hopeless. The depressed patient experiences little pleasure. Suicidal thoughts are often present.

Technique

Since depression is an almost universal experience, most patients are able to respond directly to questions about it. Although some patients may not understand the term "depression," almost everyone will understand terms such as "feeling blue" or "feeling sad." At times, patients with depression may be more aware of associated physical symptoms than of the fact that they are depressed.

The physician should be alert to investigating physical symptoms that are often associated with the depressive syndrome. These include anorexia, weight loss, menstrual irregularity, difficulty with concentration, insomnia, and easy fatigability. Other complaints may include change in activity level, which may be either agitation or retardation, and feelings of guilt. When these symptoms are present, the physician should always inquire about the presence of depression.

Inquiry into life circumstances will usually elicit conditions that are of concern to the depressed patient. At times such inquiry will reveal occult depression (ie, depression that the patient does not recognize). For example, a depressed female patient might mention that her husband has been staying out late at night but deny that she is concerned about this. Although she is denying her concern about her husband, anger toward him is present on an unconscious basis and may be a highly significant cause of her depression. In detecting occult depression, it is particularly useful to have the patient describe activities that bring pleasure. One of the major characteristics of depression is loss of zest for living and a vague feeling that "nothing is worth the effort anymore."

Whenever depression exists, the interviewer should inquire concerning suicidal thoughts. At times, inexperienced interviewers are concerned about asking whether the person has thought of suicide. This concern has little basis. If the patient is deeply depressed, the possibility of suicide will certainly have been considered. There is general agreement among workers in the field of suicidology that asking a patient about suicidal thoughts carries little risk of precipitating a suicide attempt. Omission of inquiry about suicidal thoughts is far more dangerous since this could result in failure on the part of the physician to take preventive action that could save the patient's life.

Background Information

It is now known that there are definite biochemical changes that occur in the brain during depression. Frequently these biochemical changes appear to be initiated by emotionally laden events such as loss of a close friend. At other times the reasons for decreased catecholamine levels are unclear. In general, depression is associated with a decrease of brain catecholamine levels and recovery from a depression with a return of catecholamine levels to normal. Antidepressant medications appear to relieve depression by increasing brain catecholamine levels.

The subject of suicide has been carefully studied, and most major cities now have a suicide prevention center. Suicide is a major cause of death, with at least 24,000 each year in the United States.

Since a majority of persons who commit suicide have visited a physician within a few months of their deaths, physicians probably have more opportunities to prevent suicide than any other professional group. Unfortunately physicians who fail to diagnose serious depression may unwittingly furnish the patient with the means for suicide. Murphy (reference 1) found that over half the patients in the series of overdose deaths that he studied had received recent prescriptions for a lethal amount of hypnotic medication. Since about one-fourth of all suicides are by overdosing with medication, it is apparent that physicians need to be alert for evidence of suicidal potential in their patents. If even the slightest doubt about this possibility exists, the physician should either refuse to prescribe sedative hypnotics or should prescribe only small amounts. Murphy recommends that no more than 10 to 15 times the hypnotic dose be prescribed at one time (roughly a two-week supply).

Most suicides are potentially preventable. Characteristically, a person who commits suicide feels ambivalent about what is being done. The act is often carried out impulsively and, if delayed, may not take place at all. It behooves every physician to make strong efforts to prevent suicide, even to the point of involuntary hospitalization.

Clinical Significance

Depression is a very treatable illness. It can be successfully treated by a variety of measures including psychotherapy, antidepressant drugs, and electroshock therapy. It is also a potentially fatal condition. It may be a part of many physical illnesses. As mentioned above, certain physical findings are characteristically associated with depression. These include loss of appetite, loss of weight (if more than a 15-lb (6.8 kg) weight loss occurs without other cause in a three-month period, the depression is probably quite severe), difficulty with sleeping, and disturbances in menstruation. The patient's inability to sleep is often characterized by awakening in the early morning hours and then being unable to return to sleep. Menstrual disturbances are usually in the direction of sparse, irregular, or absent menstruation.

The physician is often required to make a judgment concerning the seriousness of suicidal potential. Many factors should be considered in making this judgment.

Expression of intent.   In general, it is a wise axiom that the physician always take seriously any expression of suicidal intention. If the patient mentions plans to commit suicide and is able to describe in meticulous fashion plans for carrying this out, the likelihood of suicide is much higher than if the patient has only vague ideas of "ending it all."

Method chosen.   Suicide attempts in which a method that will produce significant physical disfigurement is chosen are usually considered more serious efforts than those in which there is no such disfigurement potential. Thus, attempts by hanging, use of a gun, or jumping from a building can generally be viewed as more serious than efforts that produce little disfigurement such as slashing the wrists. The seriousness of suicide attempts by drug overdose can often be judged by the amount of medication taken and the manner in which this was carried out. If a person takes a relatively small dose of medication in circumstances in which early discovery is very likely, there is reason to suspect that the attempt was aimed more at obtaining psychological support than at actually causing death.

Impulsivity.   Suicide potential is higher in patients who are impulsive. Most people who commit suicide are ambivalent about it. Many people carry out the act with some hope that they will be prevented from actually causing their own death. The mood of a person who is considering suicide may change from suicidal to nonsuicidal in a short period of time, even a few hours. Other factors being equal, suicide is less likely if the patient will have to make considerable effort in order to obtain a drug, a gun, sleeping medication, or other materials for the suicide effort.

Consequently, removal of easy access to methods of suicide can have a protective effect.

Family history.   Many statistical studies demonstrate that a history of suicide by a close relative of the patient significantly increases risk of suicide. Thus, suicidal thoughts in a patient whose mother committed suicide would be regarded as having more serious potential, other factors being the same, than would be the case if there were no family history of suicide.

Age and sex.   Suicide is infrequent in children below the age of 12. When it does occur in children below the age of 8, it may be, in a sense, accidental since the child may not fully understand the finality of the suicidal act. In both adolescents and adults suicide is a significant cause of death. Although women attempt suicide more frequently than men, men actually commit suicide four times as often as women. In both sexes, the incidence of suicide increases with age.

Living circumstances.   Suicide is considered more likely to occur in a depressed person who has experienced a change in living circumstances which will predispose toward a life of loneliness. In general, people who are living in solitary circumstances are more serious risks for suicide than people who have companions.

Physical illness.   Twenty percent of all suicides occur in patients who have a chronic physical illness. Thus, the presence of a chronic physical illness heightens the risk of suicide.

Religion.   Patients who belong to religious groups, such as the Roman Catholic Church, which have strong teachings against suicide, have a somewhat lower rate of suicide than the general population.

Occupation.   Occupations which combine high stress with easy accessibility to materials for suicide tend to show a higher rate of suicide. For example, physicians have a higher suicide rate than the general population.

Level of depression.   Patients with severe depression are more likely to commit suicide than patients with mild depression. It should, however, be noted that a time of particular danger in depression may occur as a patient is first showing some improvement. Patients can be so depressed that they are unable to pull themselves together sufficiently to commit suicide. Then as they begin to improve, they are able to organize sufficiently to commit suicide. They may go through a phase in which they are sufficiently organized to carry out the act but still depressed enough to wish to do it even though their depression is showing improvement. Consequently, patients must be carefully watched during the early stages of improvement from a very severe depression.

Psychosis. Psychotic patients are generally considered to have an increased risk of suicide. This usually relates to their poor reality contact. In some cases, these patients may be having hallucinations which are instructing them to kill themselves.

Previous history of attempted suicide. Physicians are sometimes falsely reassured by the fact that a patient has attempted suicide unsuccessfully several times before. Unless it is very clear that the suicide efforts were quite minor and only represented efforts to gain attention, the physician should be more concerned rather than less concerned about a patient who has had previous suicide attempts. A high percentage of patients who commit suicide have attempted unsuccessfully at least once before to carry out the act.

Obviously, most patients will not be positive for all of the above items. The clinician must be aware of the presence of these factors and make a judgment of the likelihood of suicide on the basis of the overall picture. In general, the larger the number of these factors present in a single patient, the higher the risk of suicide.

Surprisingly significant numbers of physicians note the presence of depressive symptoms and then fail to institute treatment because there is a clear explanation for the depression in the patient's life situation. Fawcett has aptly stated that "the presence of a 'reason' for depression does not constitute a good reason for ignoring its presence."

Selected References

1. Murphy, G: The physician's responsibility for suicide: I, An error of commission; II, Errors of omission. *Am Intern Med* 82:301–309, 1975.
2. Flach, F: *The Secret Strength of Depression.* Philadelphia, JB Lippincott, 1974, pp 53–64.
3. Cassem NH: Depression, in Hackett T, Cassem NH (eds). *Massachusetts General Hospital Handbook of General Hospital Psychiatry.* St. Louis, CV Mosby, 1978, pp 209–225.
4. Fawcett J: Suicidal depression and physical illness. *JAMA* 219(10): 1303–1306, March 6, 1972.

106. Loss of Control

JOHN B. GRIFFIN, JR., MD

Definition

Loss of control generally refers to lack of the ability to provide conscious limitation of impulses and behavior as a result of overwhelming emotion. States of agitation such as fighting, screaming, and uncontrollable weeping are most often thought of as behaviors illustrative of loss of control. Panic reactions are included in this category, but delirium due to organic conditions is not included. Panic reactions are of two types: those in which the patient sits or lies immobile with a frightened expression, and those in which the patient wildly runs about.

Technique

It is important that the physician use terms with which the patient is familiar. Patients often refer to states of agitation as times when they were "hysterical" or "wild with rage." Panic reactions are often described as times of being "in a state of shock." The patient should be asked to describe any episodes of such behavior.

The patient should be specifically asked whether there have been any episodes of loss of control that resulted in injury to another person or in extensive property loss. Investigation of this portion of the psychiatric data base enables the physician to estimate the likelihood of future episodes of loss of control. This is especially important when there is the potential for violent behavior.

Although it is true that no one can predict with 100% accuracy the fact that a person is about to carry out a violent act, most clinicians use certain factors to make judgments regarding the likelihood of violence.

Past behavior. Perhaps the most important factor in judging potential for violence is the patient's past performance. In general, patients who have shown frequent loss of control and who have inflicted significant injuries on others must be regarded as having more potential for homicide. In one case a man had repeatedly threatened his wife and had beaten her severely on a number of occasions. Being frightened of him, the wife had him arrested on numerous occasions. She did not, however, leave him. Finally, after eight years, he killed her. In retrospect, the man had given clear evidence of his homicidal potential, and the murder could have been prevented had stronger action been taken to control him or to help the wife separate from him.

Presence of paranoid thinking. When patients feel persecuted and unable to obtain redress of fancied injustices, the likelihood of their taking violent measures to correct the situation is heightened.

Use of drugs and alcohol. In one large study, 65% of all homicides were associated with drinking on the part of the murderer. Other drugs can similarly be associated with violent outbursts. Amphetamines are especially prone to stimulate outbursts of violence. At times psychedelic drugs such as LSD may cause terrifying illusions that lead to serious violence.

Presence of psychosis. If the patient is in poor contact with reality, there is increased danger that misperception of reality might lead to violent activity. This is particularly true if the patient is hearing voices which command that someone be harmed.

Exposure to violent environment. Most clinicians feel that patients who have experienced extensive violence are more likely to resort to this themselves. This includes both patients who have been subjected to severe violence as part of their childhood rearing and those who have been reared in situations in which violence may be regarded as an acceptable response to difficulties. It is well known that parents of battered children were usually physically abused during their own childhood.

Presence of sociopathic tendencies. Patients who have been involved in criminal activities and show evidence of a sociopathic personality in general represent a higher risk for violence than the general population.

Expression of violent intentions. At times patients will directly express their intentions to commit violence. When patients are very angry, it behooves the physician to inquire whether they have considered violence as a solution to their problem. If the patient directly expresses the intention of committing violence, this expression should be taken seriously by the physician and the patient's entire life situation carefully assessed.

Background Information

Many studies have been done to judge the accuracy with which potential for violence can be assessed. Unfortunately, most of these studies demonstrate that it is very difficult to predict when a person is about to commit a violent act. Furthermore, most violence is committed by people who are not psychiatrically disturbed and who are not seeing a physician for anything that might allow the physician to prevent the violence. Statistically, the most likely person to commit murder is a member of the victim's own family. Reading of newspaper reports of crime often leads to an erroneous impression that mental patients commit many violent acts. One reason for this impression is that newspaper reporters seem invariably to consider it important that a person's status as a current or former mental patient be reported when such a person is involved in a violent act. Often these crimes tend to be more spectacular and thus more newsworthy than homicides committed within a family. The physician should not regard mental patients as being highly prone to violent acts. Rather, the physician should be alert to the possibility of violence in any patient who shows the characteristics described above.

Clinical Significance

When a physician is convinced that a patient has serious potential for homicidal activity, several courses of action are open. In most states, the physician can arrange for involuntary hospitalization of the patient for observation and diagnosis. Such involuntary hospitalization is usually for a very short period of time (24–72 hours), unless the patient is judged to have continuing evidence of potential for harm to self or others. In the latter case, involuntary hospitalization can be maintained as long as necessary for recovery.

In many instances, however, the physician will not be certain about the potential for violence and cannot take such strong measures. Nevertheless, the clinician can still proceed with efforts to prevent violence. One way of doing this is by warning the family of the possibility of violence. The family can then take precautions such as removing weapons or separating themselves from the patient. Not infrequently families ignore obvious signs of danger out of an unconscious desire to believe otherwise. In these cases, the physician can be of great assistance by helping the family to understand the need of protecting themselves against possible harm.

Selected References

1. Scott PD: Battered wives. *Br J Psych* 125:433–441, 1974.
2. Lion JR, Bachry RG, Ervin JR: Violent patients in the emergency room. *Am J Psych* 125:1706–1711, 1969.
3. Beebe JE: Evaluation and treatment of the homicidal patient, in Rosenbaum CP, Beebe JE (eds): *Psychiatric Treatment: Crisis/Clinic/Consultation.* New York, McGraw-Hill, 1975, pp 63–81.

107. Psychological Disturbances of Vegetative Function

JOHN B. GRIFFIN, JR., MD

Definition

Vegetative functions are those bodily processes most directly concerned with maintenance of life. This category encompasses nutritional, metabolic, and endocrine functions including eating, sleeping, menstruation, bowel function, bladder activity, and sexual performance.

Technique

Problems in vegetative function are so frequent that every patient with an emotional disorder should be asked about disturbances in food intake, elimination, menstruation, and sleep. What the clinician primarily investigates is a change, which may be either increase or decrease, in the patient's usual pattern.

By the time questions related to vegetative function are explored, the physician will have already sought for evidence of anxiety, depression, or interpersonal difficulties in other parts of the psychiatric data base. Then the physician determines whether there is an association between the vegetative function disturbances and emotional conflicts. In doing this, it is helpful to ask such questions as the following: Did the bodily disturbance (eg, anorexia) begin during a time of emotional stress?

Does it become worse when emotional stress increases? Does it vary in different situations?

With the exception of the sexual area (see section 77), most patients do not find it difficult to discuss problems related to their vegetative functions. Almost everyone has experienced disturbances in these bodily functions at some time in life, and there is little or no stigma in admitting these difficulties. There is usually a temporal and a quantitative relationship between the emotional symptoms and disturbances in vegetative function. Increase or decrease in emotional symptoms is often accompanied by concomitant changes in disturbances of vegetative function. Characteristically increased emotional stress is associated with increased vegetative dysfunction.

Background Information

Modern neurological research has made it much easier to understand how emotional conflicts can result in changes in vegetative function. Many, if not most, of the neuronal circuits controlling emotions appear to be centered in the limbic system of the brain. The limbic system has many pathways connecting to autonomic centers in the hypothalamus. When emotional stress leads to increased limbic system activity, there is apparent spillover of this activity into the hypothalamic areas that control autonomic function. Changes in the output of these autonomic centers pass through the autonomic nervous system to the end organs such as the bowel and bladder. Presumably the production of psychophysiologic diseases in the end organs, such as asthma, hypertension, and peptic ulcer, is the result at least in part of long-continued overactivity of central nervous system autonomic centers.

Clinical Significance

The extent to which usual vegetative function is disrupted by emotional conflict allows the clinician to make a rough judgment of the severity of the emotional disturbance. A psychiatric condition in which there is an accompanying disturbance in vegetative function is in general more severe than the same condition without such a bodily disturbance. The presence of a distinct change in vegetative function is of more significance than the direction of the change since patients with the same emotional symptoms may show opposite changes in bodily function. For example, most depressed patients have decreased appetite, but some such patients overeat, as will be described below.

Disturbances in the following vegetative function are of particular significance:

1. Appetite
2. Sleep
3. Menstruation
4. Bowel habits
5. Bladder function
6. Sexual performance

Appetite.   Food is of strong emotional significance. Infants are repeatedly comforted by being offered food. Many people associate the process of eating with feelings of security, comfort, and happiness. For some, eating can become a means of alleviating mild anxiety or depression. This tendency to eat in response to stress is thought to be a factor in some cases of obesity. Although some patients react to depression by overeating, these are usually those in whom depression is mild. The majority of patients with significant depression have distinct loss of appetite. In a somewhat similar way, an occasional patient with anxiety may react by increasing food consumption. However, the large majority of patients with moderate to severe anxiety have some degree of decrease in appetite, although characteristically this is not as marked as is seen in depression.

Sleep.   Disturbances in sleep involve difficulties in getting to sleep, staying asleep, and in quality of sleep. Difficulty falling asleep occurs in many patients who have either anxiety or depression. A pattern of insomnia which occurs primarily in depression is one in which the patient is able to fall asleep but awaken after a few hours and then is unable to return to sleep. Many patients with emotional conflicts are troubled by disturbing dreams. Such patients often complain of feeling very tired when they awaken in the morning. Some patients respond to emotional stress by withdrawal. The clinician should remember that one form of withdrawal can be sleep. A minority of patients, much more frequently in depressed patients than in anxious ones, will sleep excessively.

Menstruation.   In the presence of marked emotional stress, female patients not infrequently show a change in their menstrual pattern. Menstrual abnormalities occur in several psychiatric conditions. Patients with marked depression often show a decrease in menstruation which may progress to cessation of menstruation. Amenorrhea also occurs in the severe psychiatric disorder known as anorexia nervosa. In anorexia nervosa severe psychological conflict leads to refusal to eat. In these patients the amenorrhea is probably secondary to starvation. Amenorrhea also occurs in the condition of pseudocyesis. Pseudocyesis is a condition of false pregnancy found in certain women with marked psychological conflict involving an intense desire to become pregnant.

Bowel habits.   Changes in bowel habits are frequent in emotional disturbances. Diarrhea often occurs during anxiety states. Constipation frequently accompanies depression.

Bladder function.   Disturbances of genitourinary function are infrequent in depression. However, the presence of anxiety is often manifest by increased frequency of urination.

Sexual performance.   Sexual performance is strongly influenced by emotional stress. Impotence or frigidity are frequent complaints in states of anxiety and in depression. Resolution of emotional conflicts will frequently return sexual performance to normal (see also sections 70, Impotence, and Frigidity in 77, Introduction to the Sexual History).

The physician must be very careful to avoid accepting a psychiatric reason for disturbances in vegetative function too readily. For example, the physician must always remember that a depressed patient who becomes constipated might have a malignancy of the colon. A psychiatric etiology for vegetative disturbances should only be accepted after physical causes have been carefully ruled out and when there is a clear association between these disturbances and the patient's emotional conflicts.

Selected References

1.   MacKinnon RA, Michels R: The psychosomatic patient, in MacKinnon RA, Michels R: *The Psychiatric Interview in Clinical Practice.* Philadelphia, WB Saunders, 1971, pp 363–373.
2.   Snibbe JR, Johnson CW: Psychophysiologic Disorder, in Snibbe JR, Johnson CW: *Basic Psychopathology: A Programed Text.* New York, Spectrum Publishing Co, 1975, pp 183–196.
3.   Freedman AM, Kaplan HI, Sadock BJ: Psychophysiologic Medicine, in Freedman AM, Kaplan HI, Sadock BJ: *Modern Synopsis of Comprehensive Textbook of Psychiatry/II,* ed 2. Baltimore, Williams and Wilkins, 1976, pp 792–844.

108. Substance Abuse

JOHN B. GRIFFIN, JR., MD

Definition

As used in this discussion, substance abuse refers to excessive use of a drug in a way that is detrimental to self or to society or to both. This definition includes both physical dependence and psychological dependence. Physical dependence caused by prolonged use of a drug refers to an altered physiological state in which withdrawal symptoms develop when the drug is discontinued. Psychological dependence refers to a state of intense need to continue taking a drug in the absence of physical dependence. By these definitions alcohol is a drug which can cause both physical and psychological dependence. In this section alcohol will be considered as one of several drugs of abuse. It should be remembered, however, that the extent of alcohol-related problems in the United States is so great that alcohol is often considered in a separate category from other drugs of abuse.

Technique

Many patients who have significant substance abuse problems will report to you that they have no problems because they are themselves unaware that they are drug dependent. Consequently, it is very important to learn exactly how much and how often they take whatever substances are used. If excessive use seems likely, it is helpful to obtain an additional estimate from a friend or family member regarding this. It is important that your inquiry thoroughly cover all of the following classes of substances:

1. Opioids: heroin, morphine, meperidine
2. Hypnotics and sedatives: barbiturates, diazepam (Valium), chlordiazepoxide hydrochloride (Librium), methaqualone (Quaaludes)
3. Stimulants: amphetamine, cocaine

4.   Hallucinogens: Lysergic acid diethylamide (LSD), phencyclidine (PCP), mescaline
5.   Volatile hydrocarbons: model airplane cement, gasoline
6.   Cannabanoids: marihuana, hashish
7.   Alcohol

In most areas of the medical history, patients try to be truthful since it is obviously in the best interest of their health that they do so. In the area of substance abuse, however, there are strong pressures from social stigma and possible legal consequences that may lead to concealment. Drug and alcohol addictions are often regarded as signs of weakness. Many patients hesitate to admit anything for which they expect to be criticized.

The physician must also be aware that severe need for drugs may lead the patient to give false information at the time the history is taken. Patients in need of narcotics, for example, may feign kidney stone pain in an effort to obtain an injection. The physician should be alert to observable evidence of use of abusable substances including the following: needle-track marks on the arms and legs or areas of fatty necrosis from subcutaneous injections in opiate addicts; redness of the eyes and tachycardia in marihuana users; excitement, tachycardia, increased blood pressure, and paranoid thinking in amphetamine users; and sensory distortion such as illusions and hallucinations in patients on psychedelic drugs.

If, in the absence of these signs, the physician nevertheless suspects substance abuse, laboratory procedures can be of great help. Reliable laboratory procedures for detection of opiates, amphetamines, barbiturates, and alcohol are now available in many places. At times, a test dose of a narcotic antagonist such as naloxone is given in order to precipitate an abstinence syndrome that will be diagnostic of narcotic addiction.

Many addicts use abusable substances as a means of relieving anxiety or depression. It is often helpful to inquire whether the patient prefers "uppers" (stimulants) or "downers" (sedatives). Drug abusers who struggle primarily with depression usually prefer "uppers." Those who suffer primarily from anxiety tend to prefer "downers."

Before closing inquiry in this area the physician should try to determine the extent to which drug and alcohol use is interfering with the patient's life performance in work, family, educational, and social relationships.

Background Information

In the United States, 5–10% of the adult population is said to have a drinking problem; about 600,000 persons are addicted to heroin; and an estimated 25 million Americans have at least tried marihuana. It is apparent from these statistics that substance abuse is a significant subject for inquiry. In almost every area of medicine, the physician will come in contact with many patients whose ability to function is significantly impaired by their use of drugs and/or alcohol.

During much of its history the United States had few laws regulating the use of drugs other than alcohol. During the early 1900s laws such as the Harrison Narcotics Act of 1914 were passed which started a trend of steadily increasing governmental regulation. At present illicit drug use is considered both a legal and a medical problem. Enforcement of laws regarding drug use is carried out by several governmental agencies of which the Drug Enforcement Agency and the Food and Drug Administration are the most widely known. The governmental agencies most involved in treatment programs for substance abuse are the National Institute on Drug Abuse and the National Institute on Alcohol Abuse and Alcoholism.

Illicit use of narcotics, particularly heroin, produces a physical addiction that is extremely difficult to overcome. In the past, figures from the federal narcotics addiction hospitals indicated over 90% relapse after release. Many heroin addicts are now treated in methadone maintenance programs and therapeutic communities where results are considerably better. Although it is true that the methadone programs substitute addiction to one narcotic (methadone) for addiction to another (heroin), many studies have shown improvement in work records and decrease in criminal activities among heroin addicts who enter methadone maintenance programs.

Use of stimulants such as amphetamine do not result in physical addiction but can lead to extreme psychological dependence. Probably the drug that produces the strongest psychological dependence is cocaine. Cocaine addiction has been somewhat limited by the fact that it is quite expensive in comparison to other illicit drugs.

Barbiturates, diazepam, methaqualone, and other sedative drugs can produce a significant physical addiction. The abstinence syndrome which results when the patient is deprived of barbiturates can be quite dangerous with severe convulsions and even death. In contrast, the abstinence syndrome from narcotics, although quite painful and dramatic, is rarely fatal.

Use of psychedelic drugs such as LSD and peyote does not produce physical addiction. There may, however, be psychological dependence and an increasing body of data suggests that prolonged use can result in deterioration of mental function.

Clinical Significance

The patient who is dependent on alcohol or other substances of abuse has a very serious problem. The substance abuse may lie at the root of many physical presenting illnesses, including serious conditions such as endocarditis, cirrhosis of the liver, septicemia, hepatitis, and subdural hematoma. Even if not the primary problem bringing the patient in for treatment, substance dependency can so complicate the patient's ability to cooperate with treatment that nothing can be accomplished until the addiction is resolved. When the patient's substance abuse represents an effort to self-medicate an emotional disorder, it is important for the physician to recognize this fact. The physician must then include in the treatment plan measures to alleviate the emotional disorder.

There is now an extensive network of private, federal, and state programs that include both inpatient and outpatient capacity for treatment of drug and alcohol problems. Physicians should acquaint themselves with these agencies so that proper referral can be made. In addition, the private organization of Alcoholics Anonymous has been of great help to many alcoholics. Since many patients with drug dependence are reluctant to admit the existence of their problem, the physician must often use a skillful blend of persuasion and pressure to convince the patient that help must be sought.

Selected References

1.   Maugh TH: Marihuana: The grass may no longer be greener. *Science* 185:683–685, 775–776, 1974.
2.   Richter, RW (ed): Clinicopharmacological aspects of mind altering and addictive drugs, in *Medical Aspects of Drug Abuse*. New York, Harper and Row, 1975, pp 1–78.
3.   Roebuck, JB, Kessler, RG: Alcoholism: Definitions and incidence, in Roebuck JB, Kessler RG (eds): *The Etiology of Alcoholism*. Springfield, Ill, Charles C Thomas, 1972, pp 3–20.
4.   Brecher, EM: The narcotics: Opium, morphine, heroin, methadone, and others; alcohol, the barbiturates, the tranquilizers, and other sedatives and hypnotics; coca leaves, cocaine, the amphetamines, "speed"—and cocaine again; LSD and LSD-like drugs, in Brecher EM, et al (eds): *Licit and Illicit Drugs*. Boston, Little, Brown, 1972, pp 101–176, 245–265, 267–293, 335–375.

109. Drug Allergy

ROBERT M. FINE, MD

Definition

A history of drug allergy refers to any clinically manifest immunological response interpreted to have been a side effect of drug administration. Allergy accounts for approximately 20% of all adverse drug reactions.

Technique

Ask: Are there any medicines you think you may be allergic to? Have you ever reacted or broken out in a rash after taking any shots or tablets? Has anyone ever told you never to take a certain medicine because you were allergic to it? Is there anything you can't take? If the responses to these screening questions are suspicious, ask more specific questions: Can you take headache or cold remedies, pain medicines, sleeping tablets, tranquilizers? Can you take penicillin and sulfa?

Pursue any positive response in detail. Determine if the history is definite or questionable.

Background Information

A history of drug allergy should be further categorized into anaphylactic (immediate), accelerated, or delayed types. Anaphylactic reactions typically occur within the first 30 minutes after administration of the drug and consist of shock, severe bronchospasm, laryngeal edema, acute urticaria, or angioedema in locations such as the tongue and floor of the mouth. The crisis may be heralded by a few seconds or minutes of intense itching, extreme anxiety, dizziness, hoarseness, or choking.

Accelerated reactions more often produce urticaria or migratory angioedema, usually within the first few hours but occasionally with more delayed onsets. The pathophysiology of anaphylactic and accelerated reactions relates to sudden release of vasoactive amines (histamine) from mast cells and basophils. The release may be induced by combination of the drug or its metabolites with preformed specific antibody of the IgE type, affixed to mast cell or basophil membranes.

The *delayed type of allergic drug reaction* usually occurs 3–14 days after the drug is instituted. It has a variety of clinical manifestations including cutaneous eruptions, localized or diffuse vasculitis, and serum sickness. The pathophysiology appears related to either classic cellular delayed hypersensitivity or tissue deposition of circulating antigen-antibody complexes. Fever, myalgia, arthralgia, or pruritus may masquerade as a nonspecific viral illness.

Penicillin most frequently causes allergic drug reactions and provides a didactic model. Approximately 0.7% (up to 10% in certain populations) of patients have an allergic reaction to administered penicillin, and 5–10% of these reactions are of the anaphylactic type. Penicillin per se is not antigenic but becomes so when it or its metabolites function as low-molecular-weight haptens bound to large proteins. All penicillins contain a 6-aminopenicillanic acid nucleus. The major antigenic determinant is the benzylpenicilloyl group; minor antigenic determinants are benzylpenicillin, benzylpenilloate, benzylpenicilloate, and benzylpenicilloylamine. Major determinant skin test reagents are provided by combining the benzylpenicilloyl group with synthetic polylysines producing PPL (penicilloyl polylysine), or BPO-PL (benzylpenicilloyl polylysine). Major determinant skin test mixtures (MDM) usually contain two or more of the minor antigenic determinants. Approximately 30–50% of patients with a history of penicillin allergy react to major determinant skin testing, whereas 3–7% of patients with no history of penicillin allergy will have positive tests. A positive reaction to major determinant skin testing implies a 5–10% incidence of reactions to administered penicillin, contrasted with 0.5–1.0% reactions if the skin test is negative. A positive reaction to minor determinant skin testing implies that well over 50% of patients will have reactions to administered penicillin. Under no circumstances should a negative skin test be relied upon if only one of the two general types of antigenic test materials is used. For example, anaphylactic reactions are relatively frequent when the major determinant skin test is negative and the minor determinant skin test is positive. In addition, penicillin reactions have occurred when skin tests were negative to both major and minor determinants.

Penicillin reactions may occur in patients who have never received penicillin therapy. The initial contact and sensitization may have been through food or environmental contact with penicillin or *Penicillium* molds. Circulating IgG and IgM hemagglutinating antibodies regularly develop after penicillin therapy. These bear no causal relationship to reactions except that extremely high titers may induce Coomb's positive intravascular hemolysis. In a sensitized patient, they may also function as blocking antibodies to inhibit the immediate allergic reaction caused by IgE specific for the minor determinants.

Immunologically mediated drug reactions occur with many other antibiotics and with all other classes of therapeutic compounds, particularly analgesics, anticonvulsants, tranquilizers, sedatives, and antihypertensives. The Selected References detail the prevalence of allergic and nonallergic adverse reactions to various agents. Also cited are references listing the drugs most likely to induce reactions in specific organs such as the skin, lung, and gastrointestinal tract.

Clinical Significance

A history of penicillin allergy is obtained in approximately 5–7% of adult patients. These patients have been shown to have a ten to twenty-fold risk of reacting to administered penicillin. A patient who has previously received penicillin without incident has no less risk than a patient who has never been treated with penicillin but has likely been exposed to penicillin antigens. (It thus behooves a clinician never to write a prescription or order for penicillin without first asking the patient or screening the records for a history of penicillin allergy. This applies to all penicillin derivatives, including ampicillin, nafcillin, methicillin, oxacillin, cloxacillin, dicloxacillin, and carbenicillin.)

Certain types of ampicillin reactions are exceptions which may not indicate true penicillin sensitivity or preclude subsequent administration of penicillin. Also, cross-reactivity between penicillin and cephalosporins has been reported in 3–20% of patients. Patients with a history of penicillin allergy should also be informed of the many different foods (especially cheeses) or inhalant exposures to antigens from *Penicillium* mold.

The principles mentioned for penicillin apply to any history of allergy to any drug. For instance, a history of allergy to sulfa implies possible cross-reactivity to drugs such as sulfonylureas (chlorpropamide, tolbutamide), sulfonamide diuretics (thiazides, furosemide), or sulfa-containing vaginal or ophthalmic preparations. Similarly, allergy to procaine implies potential reactivity to related -caine derivatives such as benzocaine.

Too often a patient first manifests an anaphylactic drug reaction while waiting on the elevator, leaving the building, entering the parking lot, or driving home. Patients receiving parenteral injections of any drug should wait in the immediate environment for at least 30 minutes.

Selected References

1. Greaves MW: Recent immunopharmacological developments in immediate hypersensitivity reactions. *Acta Dermato-Venereol* 50(suppl 64):5–14, 1970.
2. Miller RR: Hospital admissions due to adverse drug reactions: A report from the Boston Collaborative Drug Surveillance Program. *Arch Intern Med* 134:219–223, 1974.
3. Shapiro S, Slone D, Lewis GP, et al: Fatal drug reactions among medical inpatients. *JAMA* 216:467–472, 1971.
4. Van Dellen RG, Gleich GJ: Penicillin skin tests as predictive and diagnostic aids in penicillin allergy. *Med Clin N Am* 54:997–1007, 1970.
5. Rudolph AH, Price EV: Penicillin reactions among patients in venereal disease clinics: A national survey. *JAMA* 223:499–501, 1973.
6. Kasik JE, Thompson JS: Allergic reactions to antibiotics. *Med Clin N Am* 54:59–73, 1970.
7. Rosenow EC III: The spectrum of drug-induced pulmonary disease. *Ann Intern Med* 77:977–991, 1972.
8. Stewart RB, Cluff LE: Gastrointestinal manifestations of adverse drug reactions. *Am J Dig Dis* 19:1–7, 1974.
9. Kauppinen K: Cutaneous reactions to drugs with special reference to severe bullous mucocutaneous eruptions and sulphonamides. *Acta Dermato-Venereol* 52(suppl 68):5–82, 1972.
10. Arndt KA, Jick H: Rates of cutaneous reactions to drugs: A report from the Boston Collaborative Drug Surveillance Program. *JAMA* 235:918–923, 1976.
11. Levantine A, Almeyda J: Drug reactions, in Rook A: *Recent Advances in Dermatology*, ed 4. Edinburgh, Churchill Livingstone, 1977, pp 351–380.

IMMUNIZATIONS

110. Past Immunizations
SUMNER E. THOMPSON III, MD, MPH

Definition

A history of immunization should include all substances injected or ingested at any time during the patient's life with the intent to provide immunity against infectious agents. This includes immunoglobulin preparations and antitoxins (passive immunization) and vaccines containing whole or portions of live or dead etiologic agents (active immunization).

The primary course of immunization in the United States is usually completed by 2 years of age. All subsequent immunizations are given either to boost and continue this acquired immunity, or to prevent or ameliorate disease after unusual exposure.

Technique

Most patients cannot give an accurate history of childhood immunizations. The following types of records provide more reliable information:

1. Pediatrician's records
2. Hospital or clinic records
3. Childhood records often stored at home with the patient's birth certificate
4. The yellow international vaccination booklet
5. Military travel or discharge records

Inquire specifically about situations arising in adult life which may have prompted immunization. For example, a traumatic injury may have led to tetanus boosters or to passive immunization with either equine or human antitoxin.

Determine which specific childhood diseases have occurred, since many induce solid immunity and obviate the need for vaccination. Unfortunately, this method may be unreliable. For example, a female patient may think she has had rubella (German measles) but may in fact have had rubeola (measles) or an enteroviral infection. Thus at times certain past illnesses cannot be clearly identified by history alone.

Background Information

The field of immunization is in flux. The practicing physician may thus find varying recommendations published simultaneously. Table 16 lists the most commonly available immunizing agents in the United States and their composition, dosage schedule, and usual duration of immunity.

A typical United States schedule for primary vaccination follows, and all patients should have received these immunizations.

Age	Agent
2 months	DPT and trivalent oral polio vaccine
4 months	DPT and trivalent oral polio vaccine
6 months	DPT and trivalent oral polio vaccine *not ne*
15months 1 year	DPT Measles (often combined in measles-mumps-rubella)
Adult +polio	DT; tetanus booster once every 10 years
5 years DPT +polio	2 yr. hemophilus influenz

Other available but less commonly indicated immunizing agents include bacille Calmette-Guérin (BCG) (tuberculosis prophylaxis), plague vaccine, epidemic typhus fever vaccine, yellow fever vaccine, and polyvalent and monovalent *Clostridium botulinum* antitoxins. These vaccines are used only in specific settings.

Types A and C meningococcal vaccine and polyvalent pneumococcal vaccine are newly developed agents in which the immunogen is capsular polysaccharide. The meningococcal vaccines are not used for routine immunization. Current recommendations for use are to curb epidemic outbreaks and as an adjunct to antibiotic prophylaxis in household contacts to a case of meningococcal disease; these agents may be of some benefit for travellers to a known epidemic area. Immunization is a single parenteral weight-adjusted dose. The pneumococcal vaccine contains polysaccharide from 14 immunotypes which together account for about 80% of disease in the United States. Routine immunization is not recommended. The vaccine should be considered in groups at high risk for pneumococcal disease, the elderly, the institutionalized, those with certain chronic diseases such as diabetes, chronic obstructive pulmonary disease, hepatic and renal dysfunction, and those with splenic dysfunction such as SS disease.

The immune serum globulins have become important adjuncts in prevention or amelioration of certain diseases. They are antibody-rich fractions of pooled plasma from normal donors containing primarily IgG

Table 16. Immunizing agents commonly available in the United States.

Agent	Composition	Dosage Schedule	Duration of Immunity
Cholera vaccine	Killed vibrios	1 dose	3 months
Diphtheria (as DPT)*	Toxoid	0.5 ml every 4–8 weeks for 3 doses; booster 1 year later	10 years or more
Hepatitis immune globulin	Human globulin	1 dose 0.01 ml/kg	About 2 months
Influenza vaccine	Killed virus (bivalent)	1 dose	Seasonal
Measles vaccine	Live attenuated strains	1 dose (after 15 months of age); no booster; do not give with Ig	Years
Mumps vaccine	Live virus	1 dose	Years
Pertussis vaccine	Killed organism	Same as DPT; not indicated in adults	Years
Poliomyelitis vaccine	Live virus, trivalent (A, B, C types)	3 oral doses 8 weeks, 8 months	Lifelong?
Rabies duck embryo vaccine	Inactive virus	14–21 daily injections plus boosters 10, 20 days	
Rabies nervous tissue vaccine	Inactive virus	14–21 daily injections plus boosters 10, 20 days	Lifelong?
Human diploid cell rabies vaccine	Inactive virus	14–21 daily injections plus boosters 10, 20 days	As yet unknown
Rabies immune globulin	Equine serum	1,000 U/40 lb	Short
Rubella vaccine	Live attenuated virus	1 dose	Lifelong?
Smallpox vaccine	Live vaccinia virus	1 dose	3 years?
Tetanus	Toxoid	Same as DPT or given as DT†	10 years or more
Tetanus immune globulin	Human globulin	1 dose 250 U	Short-lived
Typhoid vaccine	Killed bacteria	2 doses every 4 weeks	3 years?
Vaccinia immune globulin	Human globulin	0.6 ml/kg	Short

* DPT = diphtheria-pertussis-tetanus for use with children. This concentration of diphtheria vaccine may cause severe reactions in adults and should not be used.
† DT = diphtheria-tetanus for use in unimmunized adults.

(165 mg/ml) and traces of IgA and IgM. The advantages of these preparations over whole plasma include freedom from hepatitis virus, concentration of antibodies into a small volume, and stability of the refrigerated solution for years. *Short term immunity 1 month*

These preparations are given by <u>intramuscular injection</u>, since intravenous use may provoke anaphylactic reactions. Serum levels peak in about two days, and the halflife is 20–25 days. Thus protection is short–lived.

The commonly available forms of <u>passive immunizations</u> with immune serum globulins (Ig) are used in specific settings. Tetanus Ig is useful in unimmunized persons after massively contaminated wounds. Vaccinia Ig is used in cases of disseminated vaccinia following smallpox vaccination. *Hepatitis B*

Immunoglobulins for passive immunization are of two types: the most commonly available preparation, formerly called Immune Serum Globulin (ISG), is now referred to as Immunoglobulin (Ig) and is prepared from normal human serum; it contains a wide variety of antibodies at relatively low concentrations. Hyperimmune Globulin is prepared from specific donors who have recovered from specific diseases; it contains high titers of antibody against that disease. It is usually available from a few centers only in special situations, and in most instances its administration is considered experimental. Tetanus Ig is useful in unimmunized persons after massively contaminated wounds. Vaccinia Ig is used in cases of disseminated vaccinia following smallpox vaccination. Ig is useful for prophylaxis against hepatitis A, but there is controversy over its role in preventing hepatitis B. It seems to have some protective effect in preexposure prophylaxis to hepatitis B. Hyperimmune globulin to hepatitis B (HBIG) offers some protection when given before or during exposure, but may not be superior to Ig alone. In fact, there is some reason to believe Ig may be superior to HBIG in this setting since it does not prevent antibody formation, whereas HBIG may. In postexposure prophylaxis (eg, needle stick) there does not appear to be sufficient difference between Ig and HBIG to warrant use of the latter. At this time, HBIG costs approximately $200.00 for each dose.

Varicella-Zoster Immune Globulin (VZIG) has been advocated for prophylaxis in immunosuppressed or immunodeficient individuals. Supply is extremely limited and currently is only available to patients under 21 years of age within 72 hours of exposure. Mumps, rubella, and pertussis Ig are of questionable value.

Clinical Significance

There are situations in which the specifics of an immunization history are important.

1. When individuals are exposed to a disease, one may determine the need for instituting active or passive immunization. For example, an unimmunized disaster area victim may require typhoid vaccination or a man exposed to mumps might receive vaccine unless he has been vaccinated previously or has a solid history of past parotitis.

2. When a patient is suspected of having a disease that is preventable by vaccination, a history of prior vaccination is important. For example, a patient with a membranous tonsillitis is unlikely to have diphtheria if he is fully immunized.

3. When equine antitoxin therapy is being considered, a prior history of equine antitoxin suggests increased potential for an allergic reaction. Thus one would need to weigh the need for use of equine antitoxin against the risk of an allergic reaction.

4. When individuals are planning travel or residence in foreign countries, one must determine if the special immunization requirements were met.

5. When evaluating delayed hypersensitivity reactions with mumps or PPD (purified protein derivative) skin tests, a history of prior infection or vaccination is crucial.

6. When determining the immune status to rubella in pregnant women, neither a past history of definite rubella nor a past history of rubella vaccination should be relied upon when a possible exposure has occurred. The widely available hemagglutination inhibition test should be performed since the potential risk of a "rubella baby" is too great to rely on history alone.

Selected References

1. Peebles TC, Levine L, Eldred MC, et al: Tetanus toxoid emergency boosters: A reappraisal. N Eng J Med 280:575–581, 1969.
2. Brooks GF, Buchanan TM, Bennett JV: Tetanus toxoid immunization of adults: A continuing need. Ann Intern Med 73:603–606, 1970.
3. Immunization against Infectious Disease. Atlanta, DHEW, Center for Disease Control, 1973.
4. Report of the Committee on Infectious Diseases (The Red Book), ed 17. Evanston, Ill, American Academy of Pediatrics, 1974.

111. Family Pedigree and Heritable Disease Potential

LOUIS J. ELSAS II, MD

Definition

To ascertain genetic predisposition for specific diseases in a family.

Technique

To determine the genetic risk of an individual for a specific disease, one must collect family data, graph this data in the form of a pedigree, and analyze the pedigree for a pattern of inheritance. The family history must come from several sources including, in reverse order of objectivity, history, past medical records, direct physical examination, and laboratory evaluation of individuals within the pedigree. In most instances, the pedigree originates from a patient manifesting the disease (proband, index case, or propositus). The pedigree is altered as further objective information is obtained on individuals named within the pedigree. One set of symbols used in the construction of a pedigree is indicated in Fig. 9. Men and women are symbolized by squares and circles, respectively; matings by horizontal lines; offspring by vertical lines; affected individuals by closed symbols, and obligate heterozygotes by partially closed symbols. The age of each individual at the time of the pedigree construction is indicated as a subscript below each symbol and the pedigree is dated. Individuals within the pedigree are specified by their position in the pedigree as indicated by the superscript and the Roman numeral indicating their generation. Further description of an individual's specific finding is outlined below the pedigree, using the position in the pedigree as the symbol. In most instances, causes of death are included as are answers to the more traditional questions of "diabetes," "tuberculosis," or "heart disease." This detailed family history is thus documented without interfering with the emerging graphic pattern of inheritance. An example of a completed pedigree of a family with Alport's syndrome is schematized in Fig. 10. Here the closed symbols indicate that a phenotype of hearing

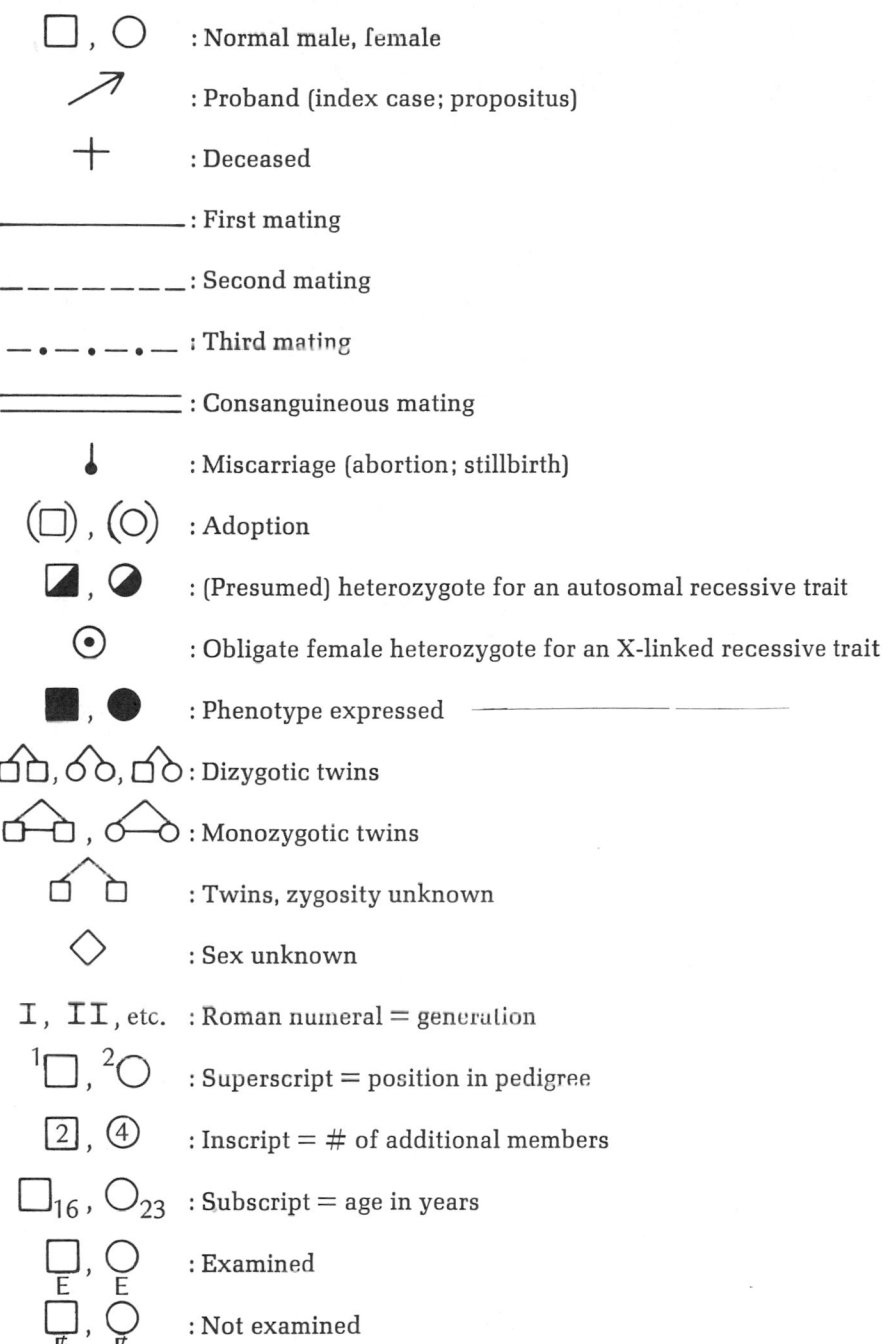

□ , ○	: Normal male, female
↗	: Proband (index case; propositus)
+	: Deceased
———————	: First mating
————————	: Second mating
—.—.—.—	: Third mating
═══════	: Consanguineous mating
↓	: Miscarriage (abortion; stillbirth)
(□) , (○)	: Adoption
◪ , ◑	: (Presumed) heterozygote for an autosomal recessive trait
⊙	: Obligate female heterozygote for an X-linked recessive trait
■ , ●	: Phenotype expressed
□□ , ◔◔ , □◔	: Dizygotic twins
◠□ , ◠○	: Monozygotic twins
□ □	: Twins, zygosity unknown
◇	: Sex unknown
I , II , etc.	: Roman numeral = generation
¹□ , ²○	: Superscript = position in pedigree
☑ , ④	: Inscript = # of additional members
□₁₆ , ○₂₃	: Subscript = age in years
□ , ○ (E)	: Examined
□ , ○ (Ɇ)	: Not examined

Figure 9.   Symbols used in the construction of a pedigree.

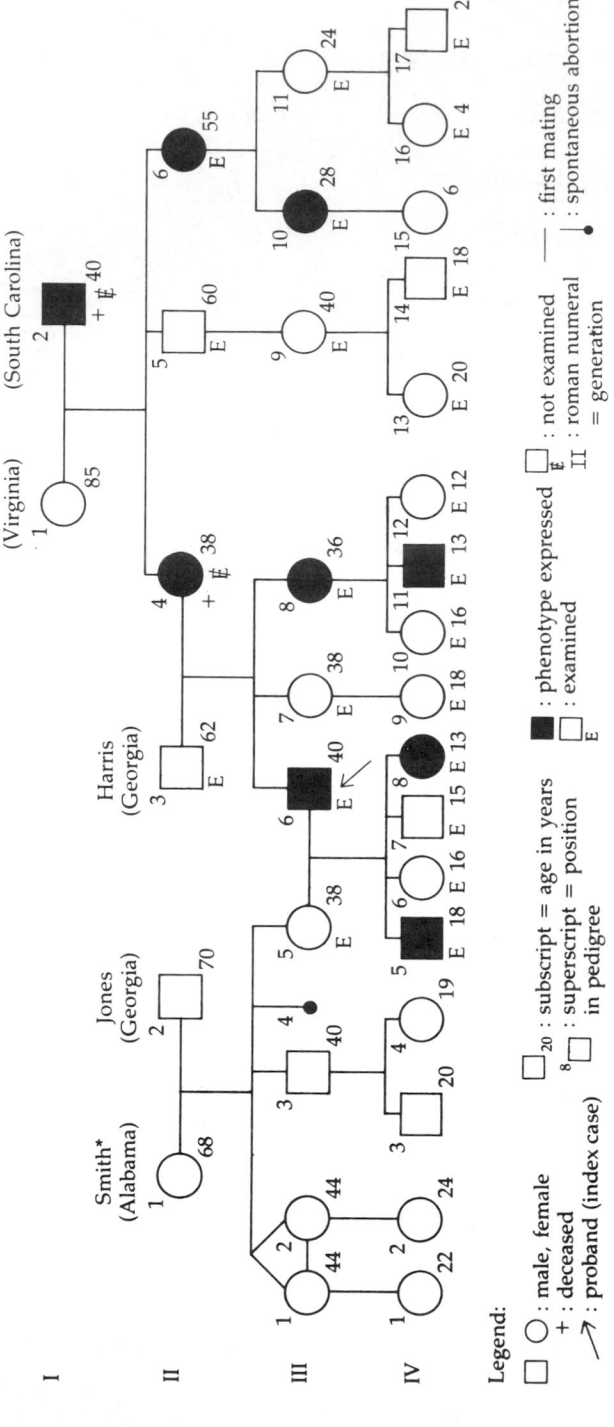

Figure 10. Example of a completed pedigree (Alport's syndrome). Patient III-6: Proband with high-frequency hearing loss, hematuria, proteinuria, azotemia and renal biopsy which demonstrated interstitial nephritis with foam cells. Patients III-8, III-10, IV-5, IV-8, IV-11: hematuria with high-frequency hearing loss. Renal biopsy not performed. Patients I-2, II-4: Died of "Bright's disease" by history only. Were hard of hearing in their early twenties.

loss and nephritis is expressed by history or by direct evaluation in four generations (I–IV). Below the pedigree, patients are designated by their position in the pedigree followed by more detailed pertinent facts (eg, III-8). An autosomal dominant pattern of inheritance is thus clear (see Background Information below). Notations of surnames and geographic origins are necessary when problems of common ancestry are relevant. Obstetrical history is important to include when analyzing the family pedigree for congenital malformations.

Background Information

Inherited human disease can be categorized broadly into three areas: (1) disorders conforming to Mendelian patterns of inheritance (monogenic); (2) disorders caused by multiple genes (polygenic) and the effects of environment (multifactorial), and (3) disorders of chromosome structure or number.

Mendelian traits are subdivided into four basic patterns of inheritance: autosomal dominant, autosomal recessive, X-linked dominant, and X-linked recessive. Recall that the normal male chromosomal pattern is XY and the normal female XX. On analysis of pedigrees, autosomal dominant patterns of inheritance demonstrate parent to offspring transmission of the expressed phenotype and thus a vertical pattern for affected individuals. On the average, half of the offspring of an affected individual are affected. The number of affected males and females is equal. Individuals not affected cannot transmit the trait. Autosomal recessive traits also have equal numbers of affected males and females; however, neither parent is affected, producing skipped generations and a horizontal pattern of affected patients. Consanguinity may be present. On the average, one in four or 25% of a sibship will be affected. In X-linked recessive traits, female heterozygotes do not express the phenotype, yet they transmit it to their hemizygous (for the X chromosome) sons. This produces an oblique pedigree pattern of affected males, likened to the move of a knight on a chessboard. Each son of a carrier female has a one in two or 50% risk of being affected, whereas each daughter has no risk for being affected but a 50% risk for being an asymptomatic carrier. In testing a pedigree for such a mode of inheritance, it is critical that an affected male's offspring be studied. The affected male parent cannot transmit the trait to his sons but must transmit the X-linked recessive gene to all of his daughters. Therefore, none of his sons can be affected but all of his daughters will be unaffected carriers. X-linked dominant patterns of inheritance look on first view like autosomal dominant traits. The difference becomes obvious only when analyzing sex ratios. In X-linked dominant traits, pedigrees will contain twice as many affected females as males. When critical matings are evaluated, affected males transmit the disorder to all of their daughters but to none of their sons. Table 17 lists a few classic examples of disease states usually conforming to the four basic patterns of Mendelian inheritance. The Selected References allow categorization of many additional diseases.

Multifactorial disorders are caused by the interaction of many genes with the environment. They do not conform to Mendelian patterns of inheritance. Common congenital anomalies such as spina bifida, pyloric stenosis, and cleft palate are examples and have known empiric recurrence risks. These recurrence risks may increase with the severity of disease expression, with the sex of the affected individual, and with the number of affected siblings within the family. Tables of empiric risk figures for specific anomalies must be used in this form of assessment.

In chromosome anomalies, the pedigree is used to analyze the obstetrical history, to identify relatedness of affected individuals, and to indicate maternal age at birth. Newer techniques of chromosome banding enable identification of many syndromes associated with transmissible chromosomal anomalies. Thus, balanced translocation or isochromosome

Table 17. Selected examples of disease states following Mendelian patterns of inheritance.

Autosomal Dominant	Autosomal Recessive	X-linked Dominant	X-linked Recessive
Adult polycystic kidney disease	Albinism	Familial hypo-phosphatemia	Fabry's disease
Alport's syndrome	Cystinuria		Classic hemo-philia
Ehlers-Danlos: Types I–III	Cystic fibrosis		Christmas disease
Facioscapulohumeral muscular dystrophy	Phenylketonuria	Xg blood group	Ehlers-Danlos (Type V)
Familial hypercholesterolemia	Ehlers-Danlos: Types IV, VI, VII		Red-green color blindness
Hypokalemic (familial) periodic paralysis	Sickle cell anemia		Duchenne muscular dystrophy
Hereditary spherocytosis	Isoniazid inactivation		
Neurofibromatosis	Wilson's disease		Retinitis pigmentosa
Hereditary angio-neurotic edema			
Huntington's chorea			

carriers may have high risks for producing unbalanced karyotypes and affected offspring. Members of the pedigree in addition to the proband may require karyotyping.

Clinical Significance

The family history and pedigree analysis can be used to provide appropriate genetic counseling to predict recurrence risks, to treat pre-symptomatic family members, and to enable potential parents to make decisions regarding reproduction. Individuals are given accurate information regarding their own prognosis and the probability of transmitting the disease to their offspring. As exemplified in Fig. 10, patients III-7, III-9, IV-9, IV-13, and IV-14 are reassured that they have not inherited this autosomal dominant gene and therefore cannot transmit the disease. On the other hand, patients IV-5, IV-8, and IV-11, who were at risk with a 50% probability, have inherited the disease. They must be medically followed for treatment of eventual renal failure and counseled at an appropriate age that they have a high risk (50%) for transmitting this disorder to their subsequent offspring. These patients then decide for themselves whether or not to take this risk for having affected children.

Selected References

1. Elsas LJ, Priest JH: Medical genetics, in Sodeman WA (ed): *Pathologic Physiology: Mechanisms of Disease*, ed 6. Philadelphia, WB Saunders, 1979.
2. Thompson JS, Thompson MW: *Genetics in Medicine*, ed 2. Philadelphia, WB Saunders, 1973.
3. McKusick VA: *Mendelian Inheritance in Man*, ed 4. Baltimore, Johns Hopkins Press, 1975.
4. Acosta PB, Elsas LJ: *Dietary Management of Inherited Metabolic Disease: Phenylketonuria, Galactosemia, Tyrosinemia, Homocystinuria, Maple Syrup Urine Disease*. Atlanta, ACELMU Publishers, 1977.

HOSPITALIZATIONS AND MEDICATIONS

112. Past Hospitalizations

STEPHEN D. CLEMENTS, JR., MD

Definition

The history of all previous hospital admissions.

Technique

Ask direct questions about any previous hospitalization, seeking the reason for and details of hospitalization, and if a prolonged stay was necessary. Record the name and location of the hospital, along with the year, reason for admission, and any surgical procedures. Patients may sometimes be reluctant to reveal past admissions to prison hospitals, alcohol programs, or psychiatric hospitals.

Background Information

Individuals often have past hospitalizations for surgical procedures such as tonsillectomy, appendectomy, and delivery. Less common reasons for hospitalization may also reveal important information.

The following style of tabulation is useful for recording the history of past hospitalizations.

Date	Location	Reason	Doctor
1974	GMH	Cervical spine fusion	
1967	GBH	Cholescystectomy (stones)	
1962	NYC	Appendectomy; intestinal obstruction	
1960	Ky	Bleeding duodenal ulcer	
1957	Ky	Hysterectomy	

Clinical Significance

Previous hospitalizations often give clues to problems that may be currently active. For instance, a long hospital stay in the early teens for fever and arthralgias suggests rheumatic fever and would be important when the patient presents 20 years later with pulmonary edema. Mitral stenosis may present in this manner. Similarly, a past history of appendectomy is of considerable importance in evaluating a patient with acute periumbilical or right lower quadrant pain.

Selected Reference

1. Morgan WL Jr, Engel GL: *The Clinical Approach to the Patient.* Philadelphia, WB Saunders, 1969, pp 185–188.

---

113. Current and Past Medications

STEPHEN D. CLEMENTS, MD
ZAFAR H. ISRAILI, PhD

Definition

A good drug use history is extremely useful in treating and evaluating patients. It is important to obtain the history of all current and past medications consumed by the patient. The value is proportional to its accuracy and completeness. Convince the patient of the importance and relevance of the questions asked about drug exposure.

Technique

Include all medications, ie, prescription drugs, proprietary formulations, home remedies, and folk medicines. Often it is relatively easy to ascertain which prescription medications the patient currently takes or has taken in the past. However, this is not so true for proprietary medications and drugs that a sympathetic friend, neighbor, or family member may have loaned or recommended to the patient.

The following procedure has been found effective in gathering drug history data and serves as a guide for interviewing patients. Ask the patient to bring a list of all prescription and nonprescription medications consumed during the 30-day period prior to the visit. The patient should be asked to bring both medications and all empty bottles, prescription numbers, and the names of the pharmacies that filled the orders. Only about half of the patients are likely to bring the information, but this request at least alerts and prepares patients for the interview about their medications.

Begin the interview with a statement such as: I would like to ask you a few questions about any medications you might have taken recently or are presently taking. A medical history checklist, such as in Table 18, may be helpful to recall current or past medications. Products often advertised should be suggested to give the patient an idea of the nature of each category of drugs. Such a checklist can help reveal products the

Table 18. Current and past medication checklist.

_____ Allergy or asthma (antihistamines, bronchodilators)
_____ Cough or cold (cough suppressants, expectorants, antihistamines)
_____ Stomach, digestion, or gas (antacids, digestion aids)
_____ Constipation (laxatives, stool softeners, mineral oil, enema)
_____ Diarrhea
_____ Headache, body ache, arthritis, menstrual pain (aspirin, aspirin combinations, aspirin substitutes)
_____ Fever
_____ Sleep or stay awake (sedatives or stimulants)
_____ Weight control (gain or loss; tonics, appetite suppressants)
_____ Nerves (tranquilizers)
_____ Motion sickness
_____ Vitamins, tonics, and mineral supplements
_____ Oral contraceptives
_____ Vaginal preparations
_____ Eye drops and ointments
_____ Ear drops
_____ Injections (insulin, liver, B_{12})
_____ Diuretics (water pills)
_____ Thyroid preparations
_____ Folk medicines and home remedies
_____ Ointments, creams, powders
_____ Heart (water pills, digitalis)
_____ Blood pressure (water pills, antihypertensives)
_____ Antibiotics
_____ Other prescribed drugs

patient may have taken, even though he did not consider them drugs. In addition to the drugs listed in Table 18, the patient should also be asked about smoking, alcohol, or other substance abuse as described in earlier sections.

Many factors may block patient response and interfere with the interview. The patient may not tell the truth, or at least not the whole truth, about individual drug habits. The patient may omit mention of alcohol, sleeping pills, sedatives, tranquilizers, oral contraceptives, adrenergic-stimulating compounds, laxatives, or water pills. Elderly patients and those with altered mental status or hypothyroidism often find it difficult to recall what medications they have taken and how often. The patient should be repeatedly questioned in different ways for recall, sometimes with the family's help.

On occasion, patients may not know what their prescribed medicines are or why they are taking them. In such circumstances, the physician should determine the size and color of the medicine, how often it is taken, and how much at a time. One can also ask whether the medicine is in the form of a capsule or a tablet, whether there is a split on the tablet ("scored"), or whether there are any identifying figures, numbers, or letters on it.

Inquire into specific drug taking habits for each medication. Patients rarely take their drugs exactly as directed on the prescription or the label; some patients do not take the drugs at all. Ask if adequate instructions were received on how to use each prescription drug.

Minor as well as major past reactions to medications (heart pounding, nausea, flashes, rashes) should be an integral part of the interview and record.

An interviewer's knowledge of the subject has a direct bearing on the reliability of the interview data. In fact, pharmacists often obtain more complete and accurate information than physicians (Stewart et al., 1977); they readily identify both prescription and nonprescription products and are likely to know the ingredients of over-the-counter preparations. It has been suggested that drug history services be considered for certain patient care programs. Such an interview should provide the physician with a copy of the patient's drug history, including prescription drugs, proprietary medications, home remedies, and folk medicines. The generic name of ingredients should be listed for each product, plus frequency of use, and the day the last dose was taken. The report should be included in the patient's permanent record.

Background Information

Approximately two-thirds of the population of the United States uses prescription drugs at one time or another. Approximately 75 million Americans take one or more drugs on a regular basis. About 3 billion prescriptions and drug orders are written in this country annually, 70–80% for nonhospitalized patients. Nonprescription drugs are consumed in enormous quantities. Over 15 million Americans take aspirin or aspirin-containing formulations; more than 10 million take drugs for high blood pressure; 10 million women use oral contraceptives; and 5 million people use mild tranquilizers. Approximately 10% of individuals in the United States take proprietary medications on a daily basis.

It is estimated that 30% of all written prescriptions are not filled. Stewart and Cluff (1972) reviewed several prospective studies and found that the percentage of patients failing to correctly take their medications ranged from 20% to 82%. Patients will often use many drugs that have not been prescribed, while not using those which are prescribed.

A drug interaction of clinical interest occurs whenever the pharmacologic effect of a therapeutically administered drug is modified by the prior or concurrent administration of another chemical substance. In this context, the term "chemical substance" includes alcohol, foods, insecticides, food additives, environmental chemical agents, as well as drugs therapeutically administered and drugs of abuse.

The problem of drug interaction is receiving more attention since both outpatients and hospitalized patients consume several drugs at a time, with or without the knowledge or approval of the clinicians. In a study of drug utilization in six hospitals, Jick et al. found that the average number of exposures was 8.4 drugs. Latiolais and Berry studied ambulatory patients and found that they took an average of 2.3 prescribed medications. Bleyer et al. showed that a group of pregnant women took an average of 8.7 medications during the last trimester of pregnancy; 80% of the drugs were taken without medical knowledge or prescription. Aspirin, thiazide diuretics, and antibiotics were used by 69%, 30%, and 16% of the patients, respectively. Stewart and Cluff (1971) studied drug utilization characteristics in a university outpatient clinic and found that the average patient had used 3.2 prescription and 2.9 nonprescription drugs within a 30-day period prior to the clinic appointment. In a group of 60 patients using prescribed drugs, 26 (43%) were taking drugs from more than one physician; the average patient had ingested 9.5 different chemicals in the month preceding the clinic visit.

The rate of adverse effects increases proportionately with the number of drugs given to the patient. Smith et al. found an adverse reaction rate of 40% in patients given 16 to 20 drugs, 7% in those given 6 to 10 drugs, and 4.2% in those receiving five drugs. One can speculate that the increase in adverse reactions is, in part, due to interactions between the drugs.

In a review of 2,422 hospitalized patients, 4.7% received interacting drug combinations. Signs of drug interaction were identified in less than 10% of these patients (Puckett and Visconti, 1971). More than half of the patients reviewed by Stewart and Cluff (1971) were taking prescription medication with a potential for interaction. About 12% of the patients had taken prescription medication that had been borrowed from friends or relatives. Almost all of the patients were also treating themselves with over-the-counter medications. The most common interaction observed in this study was duplication of agents in the same pharmacologic class as a result of taking drugs from multiple sources.

Over-the-counter drugs purchased without prescription at food stores, variety stores, newsstands, or in drug stores have assumed greater importance because of their ability to interact unfavorably with widely used prescription drugs. Hazards of self-medication include damage to the fetus during pregnancy, masking of the symptoms of a serious disease, and addiction.

The physician should thus be mindful of interactions that occur between both concurrently prescribed medications and between prescribed and nonprescribed medications. The large number of possible medication interactions described in the literature exceeds most of our memory capacities. Several good publications list the majority of reported interactions (Robinson and Sylvester, 1970; Martin, 1971; Swidler, 1971; Garb, 1973; Cohen and Armstrong, 1974; US DHEW Publication, 1974; American Pharmaceutical Association, 1976, 1978; Long, 1977; Stewart et al., 1977).

Computer-assisted programs have been developed such that pertinent information from patient records, hospitals, pharmacies, and physicians' offices can be stored for prompt retrieval and correlation.

Some of the major mechanisms of drug interactions can be summarized. The interaction of prescription drugs with other prescription or nonprescription drugs may occur at many sites in many ways, including absorption, metabolism, binding and excretion.

I. *Absorption in the gastrointestinal tract.* a. *Change in pH:* Alkalinizing agents, eg, sodium bicarbonate or citrate decrease gastric absorption and effectiveness of weakly acidic drugs such as barbiturates, sulfonamides and salicylates; they may increase absorption and toxicity of weakly basic drugs such as antihistamines, narcotic analgesics, and quinidine.

b. *Intestinal motility:* Anticholinergic drugs like scopolamine and morphine delay gastric emptying and slow absorption of orally administered drugs such as phenobarbital or phenacetin; metoclopramide stimulates gastric emptying and accelerates absorption of alcohol and phenacetin.

c. *Ionic interaction:* Aluminum hydroxide antacids complex with tetracyclines and decrease absorption.

d. *Competition for absorption:* Phenobarbital reduces the absorption of griseofulvin and warfarin.

II. *Metabolism.* a. *Enzyme induction:* Approximately 200 drugs (such as barbiturates, glutethimide, phenytoin) induce liver microsomal enzymes.

This results in increased metabolism and decreased effectiveness of other drugs such as anticoagulants, corticosteroids, digitoxin, vitamin D, antihistamines and anti-inflammatory agents. Smoking, alcohol, pesticides, and polychlorinated hydrocarbons also act as enzyme inducers.

b. *Enzyme inhibition:* Drugs such as chloramphenicol, monoamine oxidase inhibitors, and meperidine decrease metabolism and increase the activity and toxicity of other medications such as anticoagulants, phenytoin, barbiturates, and tricyclic antidepressants. Monoamine oxidase inhibitors (phenelzine, tranylcypromine, cocaine), given simultaneously with amphetamine or tyramine-rich foods (cheddar cheese, Chianti wine), can cause hypertensive crisis and even death.

Many drugs (eg, chloramphenicol, allopurinol, thyroid preparations) inhibit the metabolism of coumarins and potentiate their anticoagulant action. If the metabolism of the anticoagulant drug is inhibited by concomitant administration of another drug, the risk of hemorrhage increases. Conversely, if a patient is on chronic phenobarbital (an inducer of drug metabolism) and warfarin, sudden withdrawal of phenobarbital may precipitate a hemorrhagic episode if the daily dose of warfarin is not reduced. Coumarin derivatives should never be used without meticulously checking all other medications for potential interactions.

III. *Plasma and receptor binding site.* Many drugs are bound to plasma proteins, particularly albumin. Only the free (unbound) drug reaches the receptor to produce an effect. Important changes in drug distribution can thus arise from competition between drugs for protein-binding sites in plasma or tissues. Certain groups of drugs seem to share a limited number of common binding sites; one drug can displace another, sometimes with dramatic consequences. For example, warfarin, which is 98% bound to albumin (ie, 2% of total drug in plasma is free) can be readily displaced by phenylbutazone or clofibrate, and a reduction in binding from 98% to 96% can double the levels of free and pharmacologically active warfarin. This has roughly the same effect on the prothrombin time as doubling the administered dose of the anticoagulant.

Drugs may interact by antagonizing each other at the same or separate but physiologically related receptor sites (paired examples include atropine and cholinergic drugs, morphine and nalorphine, vitamin K and coumarins, folic acid and methotrexate, guanethidine and tricyclic antidepressants). Some drug-drug interactions at the receptor site result in potentiation of effects. For example, alcohol potentiates the sedative effect of barbiturates and the central nervous depressant effect of morphine; cocaine and desipramine potentiate the effect of amphetamine.

IV. *Excretion.* Most drugs are eliminated by the kidneys, a common site of drug interactions. Drugs may undergo passive reabsorption or active secretion in the kidneys. A decrease in excretion will potentiate the effect of the drug; an increase in excretion will reduce the effect of the drug. For drugs which are weak electrolytes, the elimination is markedly dependent upon urinary pH. Passive reabsorption can only occur in the de-ionized lipid soluble form. The degree of ionization is determined by the pH of the tubular fluid. Weak bases (pK$_a$ 7.5–10.5) like amitriptyline, amphetamines, antihistamines, imipramine, morphine, and procaine are less well reabsorbed (excreted more rapidly) in urine of low pH and better reabsorbed (excreted more slowly) in urine of high pH. Conversely, weak acids (pK$_a$ 3.0–7.5) such as nitrofurantoin, phenobarbital, salicylic acid, streptomycin, and some sulfonamides are less well reabsorbed (excreted more rapidly) at high urinary pH and better reabsorbed (excreted more slowly) at low urinary pH.

One drug may influence the excretion of another by competing for tubular secretion (dicoumarol-chlorpropamide; oxyphenbutazone-penicillin; probenecid-indomethacin). Increase in urinary output by diuretics also increases the excretion of certain drugs such as indomethacin.

Clinical Significance

A good drug use history has value in all areas of patient care. Medications may offer insight to diagnostic thoughts of other physicians who have seen the patient. For example, a history of previous digitalis therapy might suggest to the history taker that congestive heart failure has been present. However, one must exercise great caution in making this type of extrapolation without good supporting data because the diagnosis may have been incorrect, or the medication could have been used for another purpose.

Because of the possibility of drug interactions, the physician must know the patient's past medication history before altering or initiating any therapy. A thorough knowledge of drug interactions is necessary for optimal patient management. The preceding discussion (Background Information) and the Selected References should be frequently consulted.

Assorted medications alter the interpretation of laboratory tests. An excellent and extensive listing is provided in reference 20.

A patient may be prompted into recalling unwanted reactions to certain medications by simply mentioning a brand name. The drug history may thus uncover drug reactions missed by the drug allergy history. There is evidence to indicate that an individual who has experienced an adverse drug reaction in the past is more likely to have adverse reactions to unrelated drugs. This suggests that some individuals have a genetic predisposition to unusual and abnormal drug responses. Individuals who are generally allergic (hayfever, asthma, eczema, hives) are more likely to develop allergies to drugs. Sometimes a patient who is allergic to one drug may develop a cross-sensitivity to other drugs. The history of drug allergy has been covered in section 109, Drug Allergy.

Some patient problems may be due to adverse drug reactions or interactions. Caranasos et al. and McKenzie et al. report that 2–3% of all hospitalizations result directly from adverse drug reactions. In the elderly, drug reaction is one of the major causes of hospitalization. Monitoring for adverse reactions to drugs and drug-drug interactions is an integral part of good patient care.

The clinician must be aware of the habits of the patient regarding compliance. Inform the patient about the hazards of noncompliance. A detailed review of the factors which modify compliance is contained in reference 13.

Selected References

1. American Pharmaceutical Association: *Evaluations of Drug Interactions,* ed 2. Washington DC, Am Pharm Assoc, 1976, and suppl, 1978.
2. Bleyer WA, Au WYW, Lange WA, Raisz LG: Studies on the detection of adverse drug reactions in the newborn: I, Fetal exposure to maternal medications. *JAMA* 213:2046–2048, 1970.
3. Caranasos GJ, Stewart RB, Cluff LE: Drug-induced illness leading to hospitalization. *JAMA* 228:713–717, 1974.
4. Cohen SN, Armstrong MF. *Drug Interactions: A Handbook for Clinical Use.* Baltimore, Williams and Wilkins, 1974.
5. Garb S: *Undesirable Drug Interactions,* 1974–1975 rev. ed. New York, Springer Publishing Co, 1973.
6. Jick H, Miettinen OS, Shapiro S, Lewis GP, Siskind V, Sloane D: Comprehensive drug surveillance. *JAMA* 213:1455–1460, 1970.
7. Latiolais CH, Berry CC: Misuse of prescription medications by outpatients. *Drug Intell Clin Pharm* 3:270–276, 1969.
8. Long JW: *The Essential Guide to Prescription Drugs.* New York, Harper and Row, 1977.
9. Martin EW: *Hazards of Medication.* Philadelphia, Lippincott, 1971.
10. McKenzie MW, Marchall GL, Netzloff ML, et al: Adverse drug reactions leading to hospitalization in children. *J Pediatr* 89:487–490, 1976.
11. Puckett WH Jr, Visconti JA: An epidemiological study of the clinical significance of drug-drug interactions in a private community hospital. *Am J Hosp Pharm* 28:247–253, 1971.
12. Robinson DS, Sylvester D: Interaction of commonly prescribed drugs and warfarin. *Ann Intern Med* 72:853–856, 1970.
13. Sackett DL, Haynes RB: *Compliance with Therapeutic Regimens.* Baltimore and London, The Johns Hopkins University Press, 1976.
14. Smith JW, Seidl LG, Cluff LE: Studies on the epidemiology of adverse

drug reactions: V, Clinical factors influencing susceptibility. *Ann Intern Med* 65:629–640, 1966.

15. Stewart RB, Cluff LE: Studies on the epidemiology of adverse drug reactions: VI, Utilization and interactions of prescription and non-prescription drugs in outpatients. *Johns Hopkins Med J* 129:319–331, 1971.
16. Stewart RB, Cluff LE: A review of medication errors and compliance in ambulant patients. *Clin Pharmacol Ther* 13:463–468, 1972.
17. Stewart RB, Cluff LE, Philip JR: *Drug Monitoring: A Requirement for Responsible Drug Use.* Baltimore, Williams and Wilkins, 1977.
18. Swidler G: *Handbook of Drug Interactions.* New York, Wiley, 1971.
19. *Drug Interactions,* an annotated bibliography with selected excerpts, vol 1, 1967–1970 (DHEW Publication No. NIH 73-322), vol 2, 1970–1971 (DHEW Publication No. NIH 75-322). Bethesda, National Library of Medicine, 1974.
20. Young DS, Pestaner LC, Gibberman V: Effects of drugs on clinical laboratory tests. *Clin Chem* 21(5):1D–432D, 1975.

PART THREE

The Patient Profile

CHAPTER SIX

The Patient Profile

114. Occupation

LYDIA W. WHATLEY, ACSW

Definition

An adequate occupation provides remuneration according to the current minimum wage scale, is to some degree emotionally gratifying, and does not compromise reasonable standards of mental or physical health. An inadequate occupation fails to meet the above criteria.

Technique

Begin with a general question such as: What kinds of jobs have you had in recent years? This type of inquiry will lessen inhibition and provide communication space necessary for a thoughtful answer. The objective of this approach is to formulate an impression of the patient's vocational skills or absence of them.

Find out how the patient perceives his job. Is the work repetitious (dull, boring)? Are you stimulated ("turned on") by your work? Is there opportunity for interaction ("getting together") with others on the job? Are you recognized for good performance? Are your supervisors considerate and understanding? These questions enable the interviewer to gain insights into the emotional satisfaction the patient derives from his work. Some of the ways in which the absence of emotional fulfillment may be reflected in patient behavior are generalized apathy, alcohol or drug dependency, and sometimes a religiosity which gives social sanction to feelings of worthlessness.

Explore with the patient the specific tasks required on the present job. In this manner determinations can be made about the physical exertion required or mental stress created by the job. Specific questions such as, "Exactly what does a spinner do at the mill?" or, "How do you make the lift work?" will encourage descriptive information.

An impression of mental stress can be obtained by asking the following kinds of questions: Do you have frequent work-related tension headaches? (Clarify the question if necessary.) Are you under pressure? How do you feel at the end of a work day?

Background Information

Over the years there have been many suggestions and much indirect evidence linking occupation with mental and physical health. Much of this evidence has been used in efforts to establish a precise relationship between occupation and chronic disability (physical health) and occupation and mental health.

A number of studies have demonstrated an inverse relationship between the status level of occupation and the rate of prevalence of disability; that is, it has been shown that with few exceptions disability rates increase for occupations having lower earnings and requiring greater physical exertion. Not only has the occurrence of disabilities been examined, but studies have also established a relationship between the severity of disability due to certain diseases and various occupational categories. Disorders such as mental illness, visual impairment, and cardiovascular disorders account for a larger percentage of the severely disabled in the high-status work categories (professionals, managers, clerical, sales personnel), whereas musculoskeletal disorders, diabetes, digestive disorders, and hearing impairments account for a larger percentage of the severely disabled in the low-status work categories (service workers, labor workers). The occupation unknown category (including persons who are unemployed or did not report any occupation) has much higher rates of disability than either of the other occupational categories.

Studies have demonstrated relatively poorer mental health among workers in low-skill and unskilled positions than persons with higher status in occupations. There are many varying views about which variables or combinations of variables are most responsible for the general difference in mental health. Job satisfaction is the most frequently used indicator of well-being in studies of the work environment. The higher the social position or occupational status, the greater the job satisfaction. It has also been shown that the lower the job satisfaction, the higher the number of reported illnesses, that is, the higher the rate of absenteeism. Of course, one must determine whether or not the "reported illness" is due to actual illness or just an attempt to cope with an unsatisfying job situation.

The effect of unemployment on mental health is difficult to assess because of the fact that the effect of lack of money is difficult to separate from the effect of lack of a job. Much of the evidence suggests that subsequent financial difficulty rather than lack of a job is the more significant variable. Persons who find unemployment to be a very stressful situation may undergo stress-related changes in self-reported health and in physical status.

The Fair Labor Standards Act of 1938 was most recently amended in 1977 when the minimum wage was raised from $2.30 to $2.65 per hour. This amendment became effective January 1, 1978. The Fair Labor Standards Act sets minimum wage, overtime pay, equal pay, record keeping, and child labor standards. The Fair Labor Standards Act does not require the following:

Vacation, holiday, severance, or sick pay
A discharge notice or reason for discharge
Rest periods, holidays off, or vacations
Premium pay rates for weekend or holiday work
Pay raises or fringe benefits
A limit on hours of work for employees 16 years of age or older

Covered nonexempt workers are entitled to a minimum wage of not less than

Beginning January 1, 1978	$2.65 an hour
Beginning January 1, 1979	$2.90 an hour
Beginning January 1, 1980	$3.10 an hour
Beginning January 1, 1981	$3.35 an hour

and overtime at not less than one and one-half times the employee's regular rate is due after 40 hours of work in the work week. Wages which are required by the Act are due on the regular pay day for the pay period covered. Hospitals and residential care establishments may adopt, by agreement with the employees, a 14-day overtime period in lieu of the usual 7-day work week, if the employees are paid at least time and a half their regular rate for hours worked over 8 in a day or 80 in a 14-day work period.

Clinical Significance

A number of occupations such as coal mining and steel making may indicate the possibility for the development of chronic illness. In some cases a patient may be well on the way to an occupation-related chronic illness with lack of any noticeable symptoms. It is possible that after a period of time a patient may present symptoms of chronic illness. In a few cases information provided by a past data base about the patient's occupation may be helpful in determining etiology. For example, the following symptoms may present: pain in the chest, cough with little or no expectoration, dyspnea, sometimes cyanosis and fatigue after slight exertion. If the data base shows that the patient worked in a lead factory, a screen for possible lead poisoning should follow. Some conditions may require the patient to abandon an occupation due to its interference with effective treatment or full recovery. Studies indicate a higher flexibility of work schedules of high-status workers than low-status workers.

A nonoccupation status could indicate (1) inability to locate a job; (2) absence of financial need to work; (3) previous retirement; or (4) patient's desire to stop work based upon self-appraisal of disability.

Selected References

1. Wan TH, Wright A: Occupational differentials in chronic disability. *J Occupat Med* 15(6):498, 1973.
2. Kasl SV: Mental Health and work environment: An examination of the evidence. *J Occupat Med* 15(6):509–518, 1973.
3. Pender NJ: Patient identification of health information received during hospitalization. *Nurs Res* 23(6):262–267, 1974.
4. Etzwiller DD, et al: Patient education in community hospital. *Minn Med* 55(3):33–37, 1972.
5. Deutscher M: Adult work and developmental models. *Am J Orthopsychiat* 38(5):882–891, 1968.
6. Gerson LW, Skipper JK Jr: Job status and expectations of exemptions from work due to illness. *J Occupat Med* 15(8):633–634, 1973.
7. *Handy Reference Guide to the Fair Labor Standards Act*, US Department of Labor, Wage-Hour Division, WH Publication 1282, Dec 1977, pp 2–3.

115. Usual Day's Activities

DAVID D. CLARK, OTR

Definition

Usual days activities may be defined as the combination of routine activities that a person does from the time of arising one morning to the time of arising the next morning.

Technique

The technique involves interviewing the patient about his specific daily schedule and performance of usual days activities.

The objectives of using this technique are to:

1. Enable you to know and understand the patient as a unique human being.
2. Determine if the patient's life-style will change due to illness or injury.
3. Determine if the patient's usual activities may cause problems which must be solved.
4. Determine if the absence of certain activities in the patient's usual daily routine may cause future problems which may be prevented by a change in that routine.

Ask the patient to describe an ordinary day using the following questions:

1. What time do you awaken and how do you usually feel? Do you awaken by an alarm clock, another person, or just "wake up"? Do you have trouble getting out of bed? Are you stiff, sore, groggy, still sleepy, dizzy?
2. How do you manage bathroom activities? Explore the patient's ability to get in and out of the bathtub or shower. Ask: Can you reach all parts of your body? Is inability to accomplish

activities due to muscle incoordination, vision, or lack of joint flexibility?

3. How do you dress yourself? If the patient has trouble dressing, identify specifics: Are problems due to manipulation of buttons, zippers, or other closings or fasteners? Do you have trouble bending, reaching, or pulling? Do you require the assistance of another person?

4. How do you prepare meals? Do you have trouble reaching for food, dishes, or utensils from storage or work surfaces? What kind of equipment do you manage? What food preparation acts are difficult to perform (chopping, peeling, opening jars, etc.) and why?

5. How do you clean up after meals? Find out if soap, detergent, and/or other household solutions are irritating in any way. How are clean-up activities accomplished?

6. How do you do the housework? Explore the ways or difficulties encountered in housework activities: Do you move furniture? Can you reach to dust and sweep? Do cleaning supplies irritate your skin or olfactory sense? Are other members of the household responsible for helping?

7. Do you work outside of the home? Inquire about the patient's work schedule, the time involved, and the means of getting to and from work: Do you work alone or with others? Is sitting, standing, walking, or lifting involved? Is the work tiring, boring, or irritating in any way?

8. What do you do when you get home from work? Explore leisure or after-work time. Ask: Do you nap? Do you play with the children, watch television, read, play cards, or socialize with others? Do you have a drink to settle down or relax?

9. When do you go to bed? Find out the duration and the schedule of sleep: Do you always sleep at the same time or does this vary according to work schedule or to other factors?

10. Do you sleep well? Find out if the patient has insomnia, cold sweats, gets up frequently, has aches and pains or cramps.

Background Information

It is imperative that the patient feel he is being treated as a unique individual. This is accomplished best during the evaluation of the patient's usual day's activities.

By showing interest in what a person does during the day, you establish rapport with the person and gain insight into specific problem areas that may need further medical investigation. This type of approach will also enable you to plan for the type and kind of activities the patient will or will not be able to do now and in the future.

Clinical Significance

Knowledge of patients' usual activities gives a picture of their physical and mental relationship with their environment. Questions in this section provide insight into patients' personality, physical capabilities, and occupational, or environmental hazards.

Difficulty in performing a particular activity may indicate the early onset of chronic illness or potential problem areas. Trouble with joint pain or edema after performing heavy housework may indicate arthritis. Lack of sleep may indicate personality problems, pressures with interpersonal relationships, or occupational problems. Inability to manipulate clothing items or perform daily activities may be related to neuromuscular disorders. Difficulty in performing household tasks may be a clue to early vessel disease or may indicate cardiac or respiratory disease.

The usual day's activities may have to be modified if there is a functional limitation due to illness or injury. By knowing and understanding the relationship between a person's functional capacity and performance of daily activities, you can assist your patient in making necessary changes in his daily routine.

Selected References

1. Hopkins HL, Smith HD (eds): *Willard and Spackman's Occupational Therapy*, ed 5. Philadelphia, J. B. Lippincott, 1978.
2. Lansing SG, Carlsen PN: Occupational Therapy, in Valletutti. PJ, Christoplos F: Interdisciplinary Approaches to Human Services, Baltimore, University Park Press, 1977, pp 211–236.

---

116. Hobbies and Special Interests

J. GALT ALLEE, MD

Definition

A subjective item of data which describes those activities through which a person seeks pleasure and relaxation.

Technique

Ask the patient specific questions about recreational activities such as: What do you do for entertainment? Also ascertain how often the patient participates in recreational activities and if these activities have increased or decreased.

Background Information

A hobby or recreational activity requires two things. The first is interest which helps assess a person's general emotional health as well as physical health and defines better the persons personality profile. Second, it sometimes requires motor skill that demands intact neuromuscular function and to a variable degree physical stamina which assesses the adequacy of the heart, lungs, and blood vessels.

Clinical Significance

The value of taking a history of a patient's avocations falls into the following areas:

1.   It provides insight into the patient's personality.
2.   It provides a barometer to help sample the patient's mental health.
3.   It provides a tool to quantitate the patient's physical capabilities as limited by function of the heart, lungs, blood vessels, and integrity of joints and neuromuscular system.
4.   It provides clues as to certain activities which in themselves or in the environment in which they are pursued present potential hazards.
5.   It provides information with which the physician can structure realistic therapeutic goals.

Certainly there is little doubt that the patient with no outside interests is different from the person with muliple outside interests. The patient whose interest is raising rare flowers is different from the patient whose interest is sky diving. A decrease in the frequency of participation in enjoyable activities can be a barometer to the patient's mental health. One of the most common clinical problems is depression, which is often manifest from many somatic complaints. The patient with chest pain, anorexia, weight loss, insomnia, and fatigue, who has been a golfing fanatic but no longer golfs may exemplify that a great deal of the complaints are related to depression. In dealing with a population which is largely sedentary (unfortunately, the large majority of the American population), assessing someone's physical capability is extremely difficult. This information often depends upon assessing the type of recreational activity. This is particularly valuable in the patient with suspected cardiac or respiratory disease. A history of chest pain or dyspnea may be revealed by asking the quail hunter why he no longer hunts, the trout fisherman why he no longer seeks mountain streams, the gardener why he cannot stoop and weed. Information relative to peripheral vessel disease may be revealed when the deer hunter states he is unable to hunt because of severe pallor of fingers and toes on cold mornings, or the golfer who purchased a motorized cart because leg weakness and pain prevented him from walking. Recreational activities which require manual dexterity assess the integrity of joints and peripheral neuromuscular function. An example would be the woman who finds she is no longer able to crochet because of early rheumatoid arthritis, or the fly fisherman who is no longer able to tie flies because of beginning Parkinson's disease. Certain types of recreation or the environment in which they are pursued present specific hazards. The person who camps in the southeastern United States and presents with an obscure fever and rash could certainly have Rocky Mountain spotted fever; it is the recreational history that provides the hint. The parakeet raiser who presents with unexplained respiratory problems could certainly have psittacosis.

Finally, knowledge of a patient's recreational habits helps structure realistic therapeutic goals. For example, the elderly man with stable angina pectoris but severe coronary disease whose interest is sitting on the porch and reading a book is an altogether different proposition with respect to therapeutic goals than the man with the same disabilities whose interest is working and maintaining a large vegetable garden. The former patient may do very well with a therapeutic regimen based strictly on drug management of angina pectoris, whereas the latter might fare better with surgical revascularization of the coronary arteries. The young man who has asymptomatic aortic stenosis and states his recreational activities are archery, fishing, and basketball certainly should be encouraged to develop archery and fishing, which do not require vigorous physical activity, and should be discouraged from pursuing vigorous activities such as basketball. The "Type A" businessman who is burning his candle at both ends and states he has little or no recreational activities might benefit from a type of recreational activity which gives him enjoyment and helps him unwind and relax.

Although it may at first inspection seem like trivia, recreational history helps to personalize and humanize the clinician's approach to the patient; indeed it provides valuable information.

117. Nutritional History

CHERYL L. ROCK, RD, MMSc
RICHARD P. HOLM, MD

Definition

Nutrition is the process by which the human body utilizes food for the maintenance of life, for growth, for the normal functioning of every organ and tissue, and for the production of energy. Malnutrition describes a state in which a prolonged lack of one or more nutrients retards physical development or causes the appearance of specific clinical conditions. Excessive caloric intake or overconsumption of certain nutrients also adversely affects health and nutritional status.

Technique

Certain historical or physical findings indicate a detailed nutritional evaluation often via consultation with a clinical dietitian. These indications are specified in Table 19 (history) and Table 20 (physical).

Dietary or nutrient intake can be assessed by several techniques, including a detailed diet history, a 24-hour recall of intake, or a seven-day dietary record. Variables which determine the choice of method are the available time, cooperation of the patient, the patient's memory and ability to estimate quantities, and the skill and training of the interviewer.

On a practical basis the 24-hour dietary recall is most appropriate when time and patient cooperation are limited. Ask the patient to describe in detail what has been consumed on the preceding day or in the past 24-hour period. Place special attention on interviewing techniques since patients tend to respond by describing items which they believe they are expected to have eaten. For example, "What was the first thing you ate or drank after waking?" is a better question than, "What did you have for breakfast?"

Avoid focusing solely on traditional meal times and patterns, since snacks and drinks throughout the day contribute considerably to the total

Table 19. Indications for detailed nutritional evaluation from the patient history.

Area	Indicator	Possible Nutritional Implication
General	Recent weight loss or gain, appetite change, alcohol abuse	Inadequate or excessive intake of foods Food-drug interaction Vitamin, mineral deficiencies
Endocrine	Diabetes mellitus	Therapeutic diet
Eye	Night blindness, dry and scratchy eyes	Vitamin A deficiency
Ear, nose, throat	Sore tongue, sore mouth	Niacin, riboflavin, folacin, vitamin B_{12} deficiencies
Gastrointestinal	Diarrhea, vomiting, constipation	Lactose intolerance
	GI, liver, or pancreatic disease	Therapeutic diet
Cardiac	Congestive heart failure, hypertension, heart disease	Therapeutic diet Sodium, potassium intake Hyperlipoproteinemia
Genitourinary	Renal stones	Excess ascorbic acid
	Renal failure	Therapeutic diet
Gynecological	Menorrhagia	Iron deficiency
	Recent or current pregnancy	Vitamin, mineral deficiencies
	Oral contraceptive use	Vitamin deficiencies
Skin	Easy bruisability	Ascorbic acid, vitamin K deficiencies
	Pruritis	Vitamin A excess
	Yellow discoloration	Carotene excess
Neurological	Dementia, irritability, headaches, depression	Protein, vitamin deficiencies
Hematopoietic	Pica	Possibly related to iron deficiency
Skeletal	Bone and muscle pain	Ascorbic acid, vitamin D deficiencies Vitamin A excess

day's intake. If the patient has previously been instructed to adhere to a therapeutic diet, note the degree of implementation and compliance.

Food models and measuring cups and spoons may be of assistance in making patient recall of quantities more accurate. Review of the previous day's activities and cross-checking with general questions are helpful. Additional relevant information should also be collected: the presence or absence of cooking or refrigeration facilities, known food allergies, dental restrictions, dietary supplements, weight history, alcoholic bever-

Table 20. Indications for detailed nutritional evaluation from the patient physical examination.

Area	Indicator	Possible Nutritional Implication
General	Cachexia	Special nutritional support
	Obesity	Therapeutic diet
Endocrine	Goiter	Iodine deficiency
Eye	Xerophthalmia, Bitot's spots	Vitamin A deficiency
	Corneal vascularization	Riboflavin deficiency
Ear, nose, throat	Cheilosis	Niacin, riboflavin deficiencies
	Atrophic red tongue	Vitamin B_{12}, folacin, niacin, riboflavin deficiencies
	Gingivitis	Ascorbic acid deficiency
	Aphthous stomatitis	Folacin deficiency
Cardiac	Arrhythmias	Low or high serum potassium
	Cardiac enlargement and failure	Thiamin deficiency; excess sodium intake
Skin	Nasolabial seborrhea	Pyridoxine, riboflavin, niacin deficiencies
	Bilateral parotid enlargement	Protein deficiency
	Dry, pluckable, dyspigmented hair	Protein-energy malnutrition
	Sun exposed and pressure point dermatitis	Niacin deficiency
	Hyperkeratosis	Vitamin A deficiency
	Edema	Excess sodium intake; protein, thiamin deficiencies
Neurological	Dementia, ataxia, ophthalmoplegia	Thiamin deficiency
	Vibratory and position sense loss with fine motor control abnormality	Vitamin B_{12} deficiency
	Tetany, seizures	Vitamin D deficiency
	Symmetrical lower extremity peripheral neuropathy, resistant convulsions in children	Pyridoxine deficiency
Skeletal	Costochondral beading	Ascorbic acid, vitamin D deficiencies
	Epiphyseal enlargement, cranial bossing, bowed legs	Vitamin D deficiency

age consumption, laxative use, unusual food cravings, and who in the household is responsible for food preparation.

Food composition tables provide reasonable estimates of nutrients under most circumstances, although they present the total amount of nutrient without considering availability or percent absorption. Reference 6 provides extensive tables. Availability may vary for certain nutrients, and absorption is influenced by food source and other factors. For example, less than 10% of the iron from most vegetable sources is absorbed. If time is at a premium, certain short methods of evaluation may be applied. For example, if an individual consumes adequate amounts of high protein foods, it is likely that adequate pyridoxine is consumed.

Important limitations of the 24-hour dietary recall include not assessing the past history of nutritional factors, weekend or holiday meal differences, and seasonal or daily variations. Recent evidence suggests that with obese subjects retrospective dietary histories (as compared with direct measurements of food intake) are less accurate estimations than with normal weight subjects.

Background Information

Water and energy are primary requirements for metabolic processes and activity. Food energy values are usually expressed in kilocalories, although the accepted international unit of energy is the joule.* The body obtains approximately 9 kcal/g food fat, 7.1 kcal/g ingested alcohol, and 4 kcal/g food protein or carbohydrate. A common method of estimating daily caloric need is to multiply the ideal body weight by 10 to derive the basic metabolic requirement, then add 30%, 50%, or 100% to allow for sedentary, moderate, or strenuous physical activity, respectively (Table 21). During periods of tissue growth (youth, pregnancy, lactation, rapidly proliferating tumors), additional energy is required. The caloric distribution of the average American diet is 10–14% protein, 45–50% carbohydrate, and 40% fat.

The body requires nine amino acids (lysine, leucine, isoleucine, threonine, methionine, tryptophan, valine, phenylalanine, histidine) which cannot be synthesized. Since proteins differ in their composition of amino acids, nutritive quality may be described in terms of chemical score, biological value, or nitrogen balance index. With the exception of human milk, eggs contain the highest quality food protein: the amount and proportion of the essential amino acids resemble human serum albumin most closely. Eggs are thus referred to as a protein source of high biological value. Vegetables and grains supply generally lesser quality proteins, but supplementation or complementation with other foods improves utiliza-

---

* 1 kilocalorie = 4.184 kilojoules.

Table 21.   Caloric requirement calculations.

Ideal body weight (IBW)* × 10 = basal metabolic requirement (BMR)
    0.30 (sedentary activity)
BMR × 0.50 (moderate activity) = activity requirement
    1.00 (strenuous activity)
BMR + activity requirement = estimate of total daily caloric requirement
Example: 150 (IBW) × 10 = 1,500 (BMR)
        1,500 (BMR) × 0.30 (sedentary) = 450 (activity)
        1,500 (BMR) + 450 (activity) = 1,950 (caloric requirement)

---

* IBW: For adult females, allow 100 lb for the first 5 feet of height plus 5 lb for each additional inch. For adult males, allow 106 lb for the first 5 feet of height plus 6 lb for each additional inch. Subtract or add 10% for small or large frame.

tion considerably. The combination of legumes plus cereals can serve as a general guide to protein complementation in the vegetarian diet.

The National Research Council recommends a daily protein intake of 0.8 g/kg adult body weight. Unless sufficient energy is obtained from other sources (dietary carbohydrate or fat), tissue protein and dietary amino acids will be deaminated and metabolized into energy-yielding compounds and will not be available for protein synthesis.

Two polyunsaturated fatty acids, linoleic and arachidonic acid, are considered essential for the human body. Since the body is able to convert linoleic acid to arachidonic acid, the only dietary essential fatty acid is linoleic. Although essential fatty acid deficiency has not been reported in human adults on ordinary diets, deficiencies have been reported in infants fed artificial formulas and in hospitalized adult patients maintained exclusively on intravenous feeding for prolonged periods. Essential fat soluble vitamins include vitamin A, vitamin D, vitamin E, and vitamin K.

Water soluble vitamins that must be supplied by the diet are ascorbic acid (vitamin C), thiamin, riboflavin, niacin, folacin (folic acid, folate), pyridoxine (vitamin B_6), cobalamine (vitamin B_{12}), pantothenic acid, and biotin. Major mineral elements required for maintenance of life and for growth are calcium, phosphorus, magnesium, sodium, potassium, and chloride. Trace elements required by the body include fluorine, chromium, manganese, iron, cobalt, copper, zinc, selenium, molybdenum, and iodine. A number of these essential nutrients have only recently been identified as such. The probability of obtaining adequate amounts of all macro and micronutrients is greatly increased by a dietary intake consisting of a variety of foods.

Food habits are among the most persistent and deeply ingrained of cultural and familial patterns and are often most resistant to change. Religious, cultural, and personal beliefs are expressed in food choices and eating patterns.

The clinical dietitian is a valuable resource for both the diagnostic and the treatment phases of patient care. A registered dietitian is a specialist educated for a profession based on the application of food science and human nutrition and is responsible for the nutritional care of individuals and groups.

Clinical Significance

The 1968–1970 Ten-State Nutrition Survey (California, Kentucky, Louisiana, Massachusetts, Michigan, New York, South Carolina, Texas, Washington, West Virginia) documented a high prevalence of obesity and iron deficiency, particularly in low-income populations. Other nutrients noted to be low in the diets of many Americans were riboflavin, ascorbic acid, and vitamin A. Preliminary reports of the 1971–1974 Health and Nutrition Examination Survey indicate that most Americans, including low-income groups, usually obtain adequate amounts of protein from the diet.

Age groups most apt to present with malnutrition are infants, adolescents, and the elderly. The alcoholic patient is particularly susceptible to malnutrition because alcohol interferes with the absorption and utilization of several nutrients and, is often consumed in place of, rather than in addition to, nutritious foods. Obese individuals may develop deficiencies of nutrients that an excessive intake of calories does not necessarily provide.

Studies indicate that malnutrition, particularly protein-energy malnutrition, may affect from one-fourth to one-half of medical and surgical patients hospitalized for two weeks or more. This condition generally delays wound healing and reduces resistance to infection. Enteral supplementation and peripheral and central hyperalimentation can be employed to provide adequate nutritional support for patients managed with severely restricted diets or dependent on parenteral nourishment for extended periods of time.

Excessive intake of several nutrients has been demonstrated to result in serious and potentially toxic effects. Most notable of these are the fat soluble vitamins, particularly vitamins A and D, which may accumulate due to low urinary clearance rates. Massive doses of carotenoids, when not converted rapidly to vitamin A, accumulate in the body and produce yellow skin, which in itself is harmless. Hypervitaminosis-A may result in transient hydrocephalus, vomiting, fatigue, lethargy, bone or joint pain, exophthalmus, and other manifestations. Vitamin D toxicity may result in hypercalcemia, renal damage, and death. Excessive amounts of ascorbic acid, sometimes used for the prevention and treatment of the common cold, may enhance renal calculi formation, interfere with the absorption of other nutrients, and interfere with simple tests for glycosuria.

Food-drug interactions. The interactions between food and drugs fall into two general categories:

1. Drugs which impair the absorption or utilization of nutrients.
2. Foods or eating patterns which alter drug absorption or response.

Chronic use of mineral oil may reduce the absorption of lipid soluble nutrients. Chronic and excessive use of some antacids may lead to thiamin deficiency by inhibiting uptake. Hypocholesterolemic agents (for example, clofibrate) may inhibit the absorption of vitamin B_{12}, electrolytes, iron, and glucose. Stool softeners affect fat dispersion and the permeability of the lipoprotein membrane, thus promoting malabsorption of several nutrients.

Antibiotics such as neomycin, sulfonamides, and broad-spectrum antibiotics may impair utilization of folacin, vitamin B_{12}, and vitamin K. Anticonvulsant drugs (phenytoin, primidone, phenobarbital) also adversely affect folacin and vitamin B_{12} utilization. Alcohol impairs the absorption of folacin and vitamin B_{12} and the utilization of thiamin, in addition to increasing the renal excretion of magnesium. Most diuretics promote hypokalemia through excessive renal loss of potassium. Oral contraceptives impair the absorption or utilization of folacin and increase the requirement for pyridoxine, riboflavin, and ascorbic acid. Unpleasant taste sensations and alterations in taste acuity can result from many medications.

Any dietary-induced change in the gastrointestinal tract pH, osmolality, motility, and secretion may affect drug absorption and response. Interaction between food and drugs may reduce the rate of absorption.

Foods that contain pharmacologically active substances may interact with drugs: for example, ingestion of tyramine or other pressor amines (in alcoholic beverages, especially Chianti and red wine, cheese, chicken livers, chocolate, coffee, yogurt, pickled herring, and other foods) may cause hypertensive crisis in patients receiving monoamine oxidase inhibitors. Pharmacologically active substances in foods may be present as food additives or contaminants.

Therapeutic diets. Dietary management is an integral component of the treatment of numerous disorders. Adult onset diabetes mellitus or abnormal glucose tolerance usually responds favorably to a controlled diet, including weight reduction. The American Diabetes Association and the American Dietetic Association endorse a diet based on food exchange lists, which permit regularity of food intake and controlled amounts of carbohydrate. Ideally this diet should be individualized to suit the needs, preferences, and comorbid diseases of the patient. The most common caloric distribution prescribed provides 40%, 40%, and 20% of the intake from fat, carbohydrate, and protein, respectively. The American Heart Association recommends that fat contribute less than 35% of the calories for diabetics and others at risk of developing coronary atherosclerotic heart disease.

The most commonly utilized mode of treatment for the hyperlipo-proteinemias is dietary modification, including weight reduction. Specific recommendations may limit amounts of dietary carbohydrate, cholesterol, and the amount and type of dietary fat, depending on which of the lipo-protein types is predominantly elevated. Reduced intake of saturated fat and increased intake of polyunsaturated fat are generally effective in lowering the plasma cholesterol level. Cholesterol is found in both lean and fatty portions of meat and other foods derived from animals. Satu-rated fats are found in most animal products and hydrogenated vegetable products; polyunsaturated fats are most abundant in liquid oils of vege-table origin.

Dietary sodium restriction reduces blood pressure in 30–60% of pa-tients with hypertension. The average American diet provides 8–10 g of salt (3,176–3,970 mg sodium or 138 to 173 mEq sodium) per day.* Dietary sodium derives from salt added to food as a condiment, processed foods with salt or other sodium compounds added in handling, and foods with sodium of natural origin. Various levels of restriction include: 90–130 mEq (2,000–3,000 mg) sodium per day, considered a mild restriction; and 43–90 mEq (1,000–2,000 mg) sodium per day, considered a moderate re-striction. Severe restrictions of 9–22 mEq (200–500 mg) sodium per day produce a more dramatic effect, but compliance is difficult within the confines of the American mixed diet. Congestive heart failure and other chronically edematous states also usually improve with sodium restric-tion.

The value of strict dietary control in the management of peptic ulcer disease is questionable, but reduced intake of gastric irritants and acid-stimulating foods remains appropriate. High fiber diets may decrease in-traluminal pressure and discourage the development of diverticula, but they remain controversial in the treatment of colonic disorders.

Management of the patient with liver disease requires close atten-tion to dietary protein, sodium, and sources of ammonia. A protein intake of 1 g/kg body weight and an adequate caloric intake promote the re-generative processes in uncomplicated hepatitis. Excessive dietary pro-tein or high ammonia foods (for example, gelatin products, cheese) may precipitate hepatic coma in the patient with liver disease. Edema and ascites are common complications of cirrhosis; sodium restriction is use-ful in the management of fluid retention but may be complicated by hy-ponatremia unless fluid restriction is simultaneously employed.

Therapeutic diets for renal failure usually restrict protein intake to a minimum of high-quality protein. Restriction of sodium and potassium is also frequently necessary, yet an intake of at least 2,000 kcal per day

* 1 mEq sodium = 23 mg sodium = 58.5 mg salt (NaCl).

is desirable for most adults. Chronic renal failure is also associated with abnormal vitamin D metabolism and impaired calcium absorption from the gut. Phosphorus is retained in both acute and chronic conditions. Management may include reduction in phosphorus intake and the incorporation of oral phosphate-binding drugs. Dietary intake of the renal patient must be closely monitored with recommendations or restrictions individualized for the specific disorder and the status of the patient.

Lactose intolerance is associated with acquired lactase deficiency in children and adults, and it frequently follows diffuse mucosal damage or alterations in intestinal transit. Approximately two-thirds of the world's adult population exhibit low-intestinal lactase activity: American blacks have a higher prevalence than American whites. Elimination of milk and lactose-containing foods from the diet provides relief from abdominal distention and discomfort. Small servings of milk or dairy products containing small amounts of lactose (for example, hard cheese) may be tolerated.

The surgical patient may require mechanical dietary modifications or intensive nutritional support with enteral or parenteral supplementation. Neoplastic diseases are often associated with anorexia, cachexia, malabsorption, and electrolyte disturbances which indicate dietary modifications or special nutritional support.

When obesity is present, weight reduction is desirable in the management of diabetes mellitus, hypertension, hyperlipoproteinemias, degenerative joint disease, gout, and other clinical disorders. A weight reduction diet should be reduced in calories, adequate in all nutrients, and compatible with the life-style and preferences of the patient. A deficit of 500 kcal per day promotes a loss of 1 lb (0.45 kg) body weight per week: a deficit of 1,000 kcal per day promotes a weekly loss of 2 lb (0.9 kg).

Selected References

1. *Recommended Dietary Allowances,* ed 8. Washington, DC, National Academy of Sciences, 1974. (Available from: Printing and Publishing Office, National Academy of Sciences, 2101 Constitution Avenue, Washington, DC 20418.)
2. Christakis G (ed): *Nutritional Assessment in Health Programs.* Washington, DC, American Public Health Association, 1977. (Available from: American Public Health Association, 1015 Eighteenth Street, NW, Washington, DC 20036).
3. Butterworth CE, Blackburn GL: *Hospital Malnutrition and How to Assess the Nutritional Status of a Patient.* Annapolis, Nutrition Today, 1975. (Available from: Nutrition Today, 101 Ridgely Avenue, PO Box 465, Annapolis, MD 21404.)

4. Goodhart RS, Shills ME (eds): *Modern Nutrition in Health and Disease*, ed 5. Philadelphia, Lea and Febiger, 1973.

5. March DC: *Handbook: Interactions of Selected Drugs with Nutritional Status in Man*. Chicago, American Dietetic Association, 1976. (Available from: The American Dietetic Association, 430 North Michigan Avenue, Chicago, IL 60611.)

6. Adams CF: *Nutritive Value of American Foods in Common Units* (Agriculture Handbook No. 456). Washington, DC, United States Department of Agriculture, 1975. (Available from: Superintendent of Documents, US Government Printing Office, Washington, DC 20402; Stock Number 0100–03184.)

7. Nutrition misinformation and food faddism. *Nutr Rev* 32 (suppl 1): 1–73, 1974.

---

118. Education

LYDIA W. WHATLEY, ACSW

Definition

Patient education may be adequate or inadequate.

Adequate: Accumulation of usable knowledge which enables patients to understand their medical needs and function effectively in their environment.

Inadequate: Reserve of usable knowledge insufficient for understanding of medical needs and effective functioning.

Technique

Studies have shown that patients with some high school education have a much greater level of health knowledge than those who have not completed elementary school. The explanation does not lie in health education courses taught in high school but in the "general awareness" and reading skills of those with high school background. There are, however, individuals whose level of functioning defies this generalization.

Years of formal education are not the exclusive index to cognitive ability and reasoning.

Verbal skills can be a reliable indicator of intellectual functioning, making listening to patients tantamount to questioning them.

The following approaches are helpful in eliciting useful information relative to education. It should be noted that there are regional, ethnic, and many other sociocultural factors which influence self-expression. The interviewer is, therefore, alert to nuances in speech, remembering that interaction can be enriched by responding to the patient's patois.

To the patient whose communication pattern (vocabulary, grammar) suggests average or above average ability to comprehend, the questions could proceed as follows: Tell me about your school experiences. Allow the patient to first articulate according to his own interpretation, then raise specific questions for additional insights into the patient's intellectual potential such as: In what subjects did you excel during your years in school? Or: What was your favorite subject? What vocational aspirations have you had? If a course of study was abandoned or school not completed, ask why in this manner: Did health or other problems interfere with your education? Have you considered returning to school?

In patients whose responses suggest limited comprehension, care should be taken not to evaluate from an absolute standard but with consideration of the gamut of sociocultural variables: It would be helpful to know how far you were able to go in school. If the patient responds with overtones of guilt or embarrassment; give support by reassuring that this information "will help us help you." Specific questioning may further inhibit the patient who feels intellectually inferior because of academic limitations. Sensitivity on the part of the interviewer is needed; the interviewer can project, via emotional expression, caring, and understanding which will enable the patient to ventilate without loss of dignity.

Another way to obtain impressions of a patient's intellectual functioning is to engage the patient in a discussion of his medical problems. Can he recall the onset of symptoms (approximate date, reasonable description)? Can he associate symptoms with diagnosis? Does he know his diet (when applicable)? Is he familiar with his medications?

Background Information

Patient education has long been recognized as a significant factor in patient treatment. In general, the better educated a patient is about a particular illness the more effective will be the treatment. The leading causes of death to date are the chronic illnesses such as cancer, diabetes, heart disease, stroke, and respiratory and renal diseases. These are conditions which persist over a long period of time and which, consequently, call for long-term management. The major portion of management and general care is the patient's responsibility. If the patient is to properly execute self-management, he must first be well educated about the existing illness.

Studies indicate that physicians often perceive the patient with a higher academic background to have greater appreciation for knowledge about his illness. Such a patient is more likely to express his needs openly because of positive feedback from the physician. The informational needs of patients of lower academic background may be overlooked because of these patients' inability to conceptualize such needs. However, verbal deficiency does not categorically negate the patient's capacity to absorb information when given in language the patient can understand.

The effect of patient education upon patient behavior has been documented. The more a patient knows about an illness the more willing he may be to modify behavior and accept the limitations of his illness. The provision of adequate information has been shown to have direct therapeutic effects resulting in decreased patient stress and shorter periods of hospitalization. For example, patients admitted in diabetic coma decreased from an average of 500 to about 100 per year at Grady Memorial Hospital's Diabetic Day Care Center.

To promote patient cooperation, the practitioner should be concerned with (1) assessment of patient's knowledge of his illness, (2) determination of patient's educational needs based on the assessment and nature of illness, and (3) provision of necessary information in a manner which can be most easily understood and accepted by the patient.

Clinical Significance

When ordinary treatment procedures appear too complex for a patient to fully understand and properly execute, creativity in approach is necessary. This may call for literally drawing a picture to make the message clear. The effectiveness of graphic technique has been demonstrated by home dialysis training teams who successfully teach illiterate patients to operate the artificial kidney machine.

Nothing can be taken for granted. Observations of patient understanding of medical instructions reveal that there is not always a correlation between academic background and comprehension. Interest in learning about illness, anxiety level, and motivation to participate in treatment are significant variables.

Selected References

1. Reader GG, Schwartz D: Developing patients' knowledge of health. *J Am Hosp Assoc* 47:111, March 1, 1973.

2. Beier EG: Nonverbal communication: How we send emotional messages. *Psychol Today,* Oct 1974, pp 53–56.
3. Ley P, Spelman MS (eds): *Communicating with the Patient.* St. Louis, Warren H Green, 1967, pp 45–77.

119. Finances

LYDIA W. WHATLEY, ACSW

Definition

Income may be adequate or inadequate.

Adequate income is at least one-half the median household income. The term "adequate" is used in a relative rather than absolute frame of reference. It by no means reflects what is equitable or ethically desirable. Reference 1 gives the following information:

> **Money Income in 1975.** The median money income of households in the United States rose to $11,800 in 1975, an increase of about 5 percent over the revised 1974 median of $11,200. However, this increase was eroded by rising prices which resulted in a net loss in real purchasing power. After adjusting for the 9 percent rise in prices between 1974 and 1975, the 1975 median in terms of constant dollars decreased by about 3 percent below the revised 1974 median.
>
> The decline in real median household income reflects the continued sluggishness in the economy as evidenced by a decline of 2 percent in the real Gross National Product between 1974 and 1975.

Inadequate income is less than one-half the median household income. Unpublished data of May 5, 1978, from Region IV Community Services Administration indicate the poverty threshold for a nonfarm family of four to be $6,200.

Technique

1. Assure confidentiality. Explain to the patient that information given is privileged and will be used discriminately and exclusively for the patient's benefit.

2. Ask brief, unbiased questions. For example: How much money do you have coming in now? This is a nonassumptive question which seeks to determine *what* money is available, not *how* it is derived. Questions such as, "Do you have a job?" and, "What do you do for a living?" tend to convey value judgment. The work ethic is implicit in the question. Censorship of the patient's life-style or behavioral code is professionally inappropriate.

    Depending upon the patient's response, the follow-up questions should be more specific. For example: Have you worked in recent years? What kind of work have you done?

3. Reassure the patient that knowledge of the nature and permanence of his income will enable health practitioners to more accurately assess and respond to his health needs.

    Questions for explication of finances might proceed as follows: Could you give me an idea of what you spend for rent, food, and utilities each month? What do you use for transportation?

    Nondirective queries minimize interviewee resistance to probing questions and require a relaxed interval of interviewing time. Questions related to finances can be particularly anxiety provoking. The interviewer must exert conscious effort to sense the patient's feelings and given the patient interactional space to respond in his own unique way.

    Data concerning household size and composition are helpful in clarifying the financial picture. Questions must be precise in phraseology. "How many people live in your house?" is more likely to evoke an objective response than, "How many people are in your family?" The latter question allows for variances in interpretation as the patient may have unrelated persons in the home, but not regard them as members of the household. The concept of family generally connotes genetic kinship.

4. Involve the patient in evaluating his financial situation whenever possible. For example, the question, "Can you think of any ways your financial situation might be improved?" stimulates the patient's feelings of personal worth and self-determination while giving him an opportunity for meaningful participation in a significant decision affecting his health.

5. Refer to the patient's chart for additional clarification of certain data.

Background Information

Prior to the twentieth century the physician, particularly in nonurban areas, maintained an intimate relationship with the community. Revered as a healer of disease, the secular counseling and crisis intervention expected from the physician were of equal importance. Our present techno-culture does not generally afford the emotional comfort of such continuity.

The transition from a largely pastoral society to an industrial one has made health a basic commodity in the sense that medical services must be purchased in order for people to maintain the physical capacity to earn.

Industrialization has been a positive factor in bringing about national awareness of health needs; for example, an epidemic in a Utah town becomes the concern of the Center for Disease Control in Atlanta, and mass media keep the public informed.

Efforts to modulate a system that rations health services according to purchasing power rather than need resulted in the consideration of 18 national health insurance bills in the 49th Congress and President Carter's National Health Insurance plan (July 1978). Among factors inhibiting passage of such legislation are (1) the small margin between tax income and inflated costs of existing programs, (2) administrative opposition to "social programs," (3) self-fulfilling predictions of more inflation, (4) deadlock between sharply polarized views, and (5) remoteness of compromise.

It should be pointed out that national health insurance cannot be the sole answer to the problem of health care in American society where poor housing, inadequate diet, low income, and environmental pollutants contribute to ill health. Shannon and Dever cite the "profit motive" to be one of the reasons for maldistribution of health services in the urban ghetto, poverty-stricken rural areas, and Indian reservations. Some improvements have been realized in different regions of the United States primarily, according to Shannon and Dever, because of the "humanistic concerns and perceptions of decision makers" involved with some of the major health planning acts in the United States, such as the Comprehensive Health Planning Act and the Hill-Burton Hospital and Health Facilities Survey and Construction Act. In late 1973 the Health Maintenance Organization Act of 1973 was passed by Congress.

Clinical Significance

The absence of money to meet basic human needs is a recurring theme in many patient histories, necessitating concern among health practitioners with how the patient's financial inadequacies effect treatment. A diagnosis is of little functional value if the patient has no means of transportation for follow-up appointments or is without funds for prescribed diet and medications.

In an attempt to ameliorate problems in financing the costs of health care, a new division in the Department of Health, Education and Welfare named Health Care Finance Administration (HCFA) was created in 1977. Among functions of HCFA (see Fig. 11) is overseeing activity of Professional Standards Review Organization (PSRO), established in the 1972

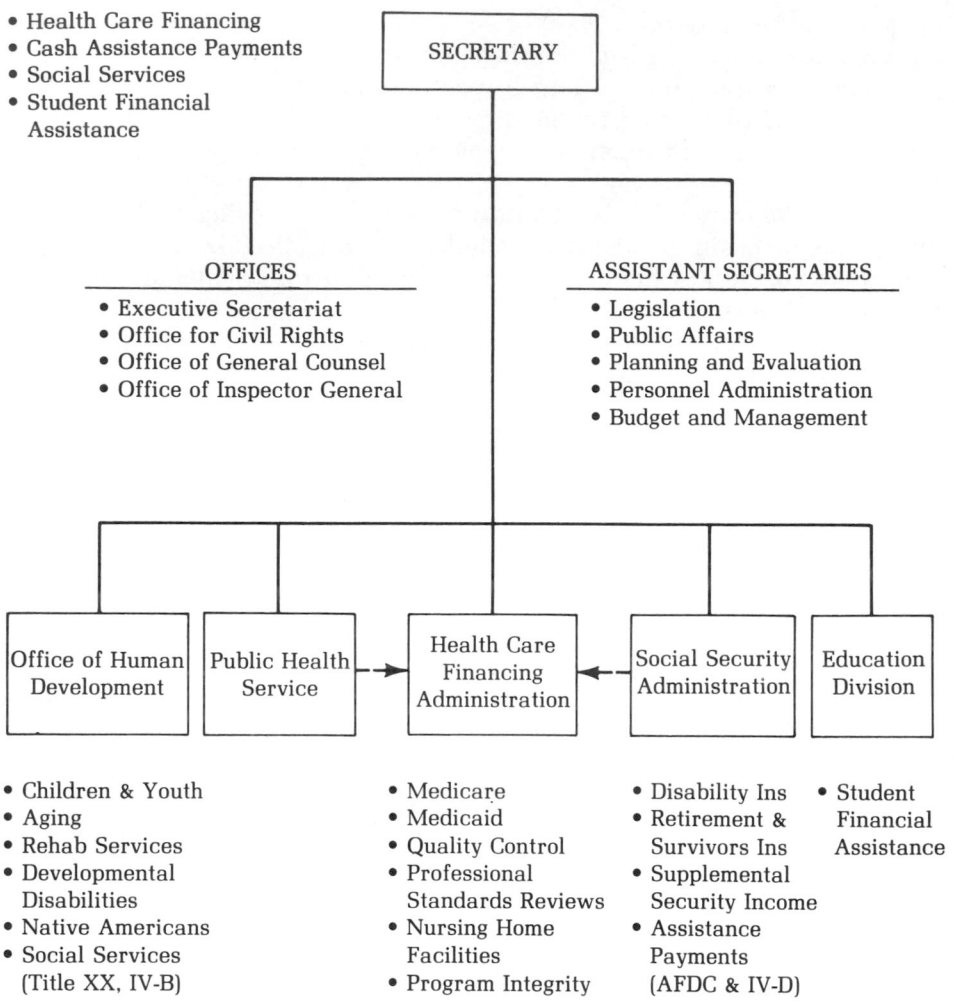

- Health Care Financing
- Cash Assistance Payments
- Social Services
- Student Financial Assistance

SECRETARY

OFFICES
- Executive Secretariat
- Office for Civil Rights
- Office of General Counsel
- Office of Inspector General

ASSISTANT SECRETARIES
- Legislation
- Public Affairs
- Planning and Evaluation
- Personnel Administration
- Budget and Management

Office of Human Development	Public Health Service	Health Care Financing Administration	Social Security Administration	Education Division

- Children & Youth
- Aging
- Rehab Services
- Developmental Disabilities
- Native Americans
- Social Services (Title XX, IV-B)

- Medicare
- Medicaid
- Quality Control
- Professional Standards Reviews
- Nursing Home Facilities
- Program Integrity

- Disability Ins
- Retirement & Survivors Ins
- Supplemental Security Income
- Assistance Payments (AFDC & IV-D)

- Student Financial Assistance

Figure 11. Department of Health, Education and Welfare: Summary of reorganization.

Amendments to the Social Security Act. The original concept of peer review was addressed to physicians, but since the implementation of the program in 1974, other disciplines such as nursing and social work have adopted standards and criteria for assessing the quality, availability, and appropriateness of patient care.

HEW's reorganization plan placed all cash payments under Social Security Administration. Former "welfare" payments are now designated as Supplemental Security Income (SSI), and Aid to Families with Dependent Children (AFDC) has also been added to the purview of Social Security Administration. They also administrate Retirement and Survivors Insurance and Disability Insurance.

Selected References

1. Household Money Income in 1975 and Selected Social and Economic Characteristics of Households, *Curr Pop Rep Ser* P-60, No. 104, March 1977.
2. Folta JR, Deck ES: *A Sociological Framework for Patient Care,* New York, John Wiley and Sons, 1966, pp 53–61.
3. Fuchs VJ: An alternative income-oriented definition, in Will RE, Vatter HG (eds): *Poverty in Affluence,* ed 2. New York, Harcourt Brace and World, 1970, p 14.
4. Fulton T: Health insurance delay may be beneficial. *NASW News* 20(9):9–12, 1975.
5. Satir V: *People Making.* Palo Alto, Calif, Science and Behavior Books, 1972, p 7.
6. Shannon GW, Dever GEA: *Health Care Delivery: Spacial Perspectives.* New York, McGraw-Hill, 1974, p 27.
7. Enright E: Concerning National Health Insurance. *CNSW Newsletter* (National Kidney Foundation) 3(4):30–33, 1978.
8. Johnson RL: Notes on the state of black America: 1978 and beyond. *Black Scholar* 9(6):42–44, 1978.
9. Legislative Update. *CNSW Newsletter* (National Kidney Foundation) 3(1):2, 1977.

PART FOUR

The Physical Examination

CHAPTER SEVEN

The Physical Examination

W. DALLAS HALL, MD

The techniques of physical examination in this text represent a part of the Defined Data Base collected on each patient. Over 100 individual physical features are tested in addition to the patient profile, history, and laboratory examinations. The physical examination items were chosen with regard to the principles of selecting any data base items, discussed in Chapter 2 on the Medical Record. The primary medical problem recorded on 3,391 consecutive hospital admissions to the Internal Medicine Service of Grady Memorial Hospital helped tailor the physical examination portion of the data base to screen for common problems in this particular population.

Cardiovascular and neurological events are the primary problems leading to hospitalization. Thus, the physical examination data base items are relatively concentrated in these areas. The prevalence of certain problems changes with time and will induce corresponding alterations in the data base.

Following is a list of equipment useful in performing the physical examination:

Medical bag	Tongue blades; cotton swabs
Stethoscope	Measuring tape (metal or cloth)
Sphygmomanometer (aneroid)	Pocket eye chart
Thermometer (oral)	A mydriatic solution
Otoscope	Sharp pin
Ophthalmoscope	Vanilla or lemon flavoring
Reflex hammer	Disposable gloves
Tuning fork (128 cps)	Lubricating jelly
Flashlight	

The logistics of performing the physical examination do not follow the anatomical aphorism "from head to toe." The sequence of examination depends more on which items are most conveniently and appropriately accomplished in various body positions. The following is one of a myriad of possible methods of procedure for a thorough physical examination on relatively alert patients.

1. Have the patient disrobe into a gown or other examination garment. If no such robe is available, leave only the pelvic underclothing intact. Cover the female chest with a towel or equivalent. Be sure that temperature, height, weight, and respiratory rate are recorded.

2. Diminish interfering noises as much as possible by closing doors or windows. Turn off any radios or television sets. Move to a separate examination room if extraneous noises remain apparent. Do not compete with such interferences. Concentration on a good physical examination is difficult and valuable time should not be wasted haphazardly.

3. Begin by having the patient sit on the side of the bed or examination table.

4. Measure the radial pulse rate and brachial blood pressure. Record any abnormality of pulse rhythm or amplitude. Simultaneously observe the nails and joints of the fingers. Make particular note of the general appearance of the patient including body habitus, hair distribution, skin abnormality, temporal or quadriceps muscle wasting, breathing pattern, and motor movements.

5. Examine the pupils, external eye structures, and visual acuity, then proceed with examination of cranial nerves III, IV, and VI by testing extraocular movements. Test cranial nerves V and VII, followed by VIII and XI.

6. Have the patient protrude the tongue and evaluate cranial nerve XII. Then examine the oral cavity with the light provided with the otoscope without attachment. Examine cranial nerves IX and X while using a tongue blade.

7. Attach an earpiece to the otoscope and examine the ears. Substitute the short attachment and examine the nasal cavity. Attach the ophthalmoscope head and lay the instrument aside.

8. Palpate the neck for adenopathy or thyroid enlargement.

9. Move behind the patient and examine the thyroid gland.

10. Examine the breast in females. Check the axillary and epitrochlear areas for adenopathy.

11. Listen over the posterior and lateral lung areas.

12. Examine the vertebral column.

13. Return to the front of the patient and check proximal and distal motor strength. Proceed to deep tendon reflex testing, beginning with the upper extremities. Check joint range of motion following each tendon reflex; include the shoulders. Screen pedal pulses and distal sensation while examining ankle reflexes.

14. Turn the lights off in the room and examine the ocular media and fundi.
15. Illuminate the room and recline the patient to approximately a 30° angle.
16. Examine the jugular venous and carotid pulsations. Listen over the carotids, eyes, and cranial vault.
17. Examine the heart.
18. Listen over the anterior lung structures.
19. Reexamine the female breast in the supine position.
20. Listen over the abdomen for bowel sounds and arterial bruits.
21. Inspect, percuss, and palpate the abdomen.
22. Examine the inguinal, femoral, and popliteal areas. Evaluate the femoral pulses. Check the range of hip motion.
23. Perform a pelvic examination in females.
24. Examine the rectum in both males and females; collect any stool for occult blood testing.
25. Have the patient stand. Repeat the pulse and blood pressure measurement.
26. Examine external male genitalia in the standing position.
27. Check Romberg and gait.
28. Observe carefully for skin disorders (pigmented moles, irritation) in each of the aforementioned areas of examination.

The sequence will provide a convenient style for the physical examination of most patients. Specific techniques are described in the subsequent sections devoted to each area. No physical examination is ever "complete." The more a patient's history suggests abnormality in an area, the more detail and special physical examination techniques should be applied toward that area.

Important and readily reversible abnormalities are rarely overt on physical examination. Consider for instance the lateral eyebrow thinning of hypothyroidism, the enlarged optic cup of glaucoma, the low cervical node of malignancy, the soft diastolic blow of aortic regurgitation, the synovial thickening of rheumatoid arthritis, the fasciculation of amyotrophic lateral sclerosis, or the tiny pigmented lesion of melanoma. Physical examination should be performed with concentration equivalent to or exceeding that of any other type of examination.

Selected References

1. Morgan WL Jr, Engel GL: *The Clinical Approach to the Patient.* Philadelphia, WB Saunders, 1969.
2. Judge RD, Zuidema GD (eds): *Methods of Clinical Examination: A Physiologic Approach,* ed 3. Boston, Little, Brown, 1974.

3. Johns RJ, Tumulty PA: The physical examination, in Harvey AM, Johns RJ, Owens AH Jr, et al (eds): *Principles and Practice of Medicine,* ed 19. New York, Appleton-Century-Crofts, 1976, pp 18–28.
4. MacBryde CM, Blacklow RS (eds): *Signs and Symptoms,* ed 5. Philadelphia, JB Lippincott, 1970.
5. DeGowin EL, DeGowin RL (eds): *Bedside Diagnostic Examination,* ed 3. New York, Macmillan, 1976.
6. Delp MH, Manning RT (eds): *Major's Physical Diagnosis,* ed 8. Philadelphia, WB Saunders, 1975.
7. Chamberlain EN, Ogilvie C (eds): *Symptoms and Signs in Clinical Medicine,* ed 9. Chicago, Year Book Medical Publishers, 1974.
8. Wolf GA Jr: *Collecting Data from Patients.* Baltimore, University Park Press, 1977.
9. Bates B: *A Guide to Physical Examination.* Philadelphia, JB Lippincott, 1974.
10. Wiener S, Nathanson M: Physical examination: Frequently observed errors. *JAMA* 236:852–855, 1976.

GENERAL

120. General Appearance

W. DALLAS HALL, MD

Definition

General appearance refers to the physical appearance of the patient. It is abnormal whenever the appearance of the patient induces the examiner to consider an underlying disease process.

Technique

A careful look at the patient is the technique utilized. The art requires both mental and visual acuity. The examiner must *deliberately* concentrate on the patient's appearance for 15–30 seconds.

Background Information

General appearance demands less data collection than any of the other represented items of data base content. Yet information gleaned from the patient appearance is particularly valuable since it is usually the first bit of objective data. Examining the general appearance of the patient may be likened to surveying the forest before walking among the trees. Writings of 50 or more years ago contain the very best descriptions relating patient appearance to disease. Osler's detailed description of the patient with typhoid fever is a classic example. The sensitivity and specificity of patient appearance have withstood the test of time. Excellent clinicians continue to use this technique with high yield. Reference 4 contains outstanding color photographs of several relatively diagnostic patient appearances.

Clinical Significance

Following are a few selected examples intended to illustrate how the general appearance of the patient may announce a problem or diagnosis.

Clothing and Paraphernalia

Heavy sweater or coat in a warm environment. Consider hypothyroidism, uremia, anemia, malnutrition, scaly dermatologic disorders.

Short sleeves or no coat in a cool environment. Consider hyperthyroidism as well as rare causes of hot, flushy sensations such as pheochromocytoma, medullary thyroid carcinoma, pancreatic and cerebellar tumors.

Cap or hat inside building. Consider scalp or hair disorder.

High neck collar. Consider thyroid enlargement.

Thin copper bracelet. Consider arthritis.

Untied shoestrings. Consider severe edema.

Toe cut out of shoe. Consider gout, osteomyelitis.

Body Size Features

Overweight. Consider diabetes or hypoventilation if weight distribution is symmetrical; Cushing's syndrome if asymmetrical.

Underweight. Consider all causes of weight loss.

Tall and lanky. Consider Marfan's syndrome, homozygous hemoglobinopathy, homocystinuria.

Short stature. Consider endocrine disorder, prepubertal steroid therapy.

Facial Features

Morose. Consider depression or apathy induced by medications.

Fidgety. Consider hyperthyroidism.

Temporal or interosseus muscle wasting. Consider all causes of weight loss, including malignancy and hyperthyroidism.

Rhythmic head bob. Consider aortic insufficiency.

Rounded facies. Consider parotid enlargement, Cushing's syndrome, pseudohypoparathyroidism.

Conjunctival irritation, rhinophyma, and puffy lacrimal or parotid areas. Consider chronic alcoholism.

Multiple facial scars. Consider trauma elsewhere such as occult rib fractures or arteriovenous fistulas.

Xanthelasma, horizontal ear crease. Consider hyperlipoproteinemia, coronary artery disease.

Exophthalmos. Consider hyperthyroidism or alcoholism if bilateral; retro-orbital tumor, aneurysm, or infection if unilateral.

Periorbital discoloration. Consider malignancy, dermatomyositis.

Dense eyebrows with excessive chin hair. Consider diabetes.

Yellow sclerae. Consider all causes of jaundice.

Orange facial discoloration. Consider all causes of hypercarotenemia.

Flushed cheeks. Consider toxic infection, mitral stenosis.

Prominent jaw, frontal bones. Consider acromegaly.

Ashen, anxious appearance. Consider hypoxia or impending circulatory collapse.

Selected References

1. Osler W: *The Principles and Practice of Medicine.* New York, D Appleton and Co, 1892, pp 2–39.
2. Cheraskin E, Ringsdorf WM Jr: *Predictive Medicine: A Study in Strategy.* Mountain View, Calif, Pacific Press Publishing Assoc, 1973.
3. Feingold M, Gellis SS: Syndrome identification and consultation. *Am J Dis Child* 121:82–83, 1971.
4. Roberts HJ: Difficult Diagnosis: *A Guide to the Interpretation of Obscure Illness.* Philadelphia, WB Saunders, 1959.

121. Temperature

See section 3.

122. Respiratory Rate and Rhythm

JAMES C. CRUTCHER, MD

Definition

Normal respiration is an automatic, seemingly effortless inspiratory expansion and expiratory contraction of the chest cage. This act of normal breathing has a relatively constant rate and inspiratory volume that together constitute normal respiratory rhythm. The accessory muscles of inspiration (sternocleidomastoid and scalenes) and expiration (abdominal) are not normally used in the resting state.

Abnormalities may occur in rate, rhythm, and in the effort of breathing. Specific abnormalities that should be looked for are as follows:

Kussmaul breathing. There is a marked increase in the inspiratory-expiratory volume occurring at a normal to slightly slowed respiratory rate. During this deep breathing, the accessory muscles of inspiration and expiration are often used.

Cheyne-Stokes breathing. This pattern is a regularly recurring stepwise increase in inspiratory volume followed by a stepwise decrease, followed by a period of no breathing (apnea). This sequence recurs in a regularly occurring pattern. The cycle is depicted in Fig 12.

502

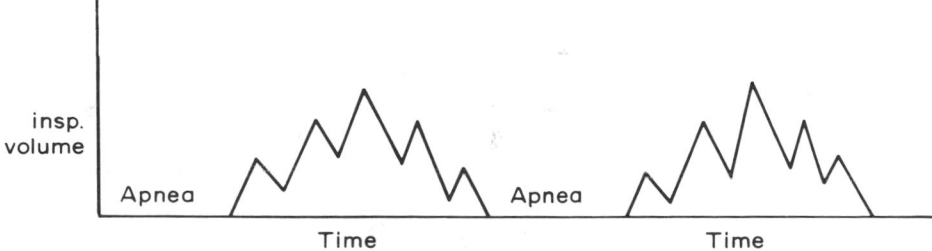

Figure 12.   Cheyne-Stokes breathing.

Biot's breathing.   This pattern is an irregular gasplike chaotic inspiratory effort that is irregular both in volume and in rate.

Sighing respiration.   During regular, normal rhythmic breathing the patient may interrupt the cycle with a deep inspiration/expiration often associated with an audible sigh.

Technique

Simple inspection of the respiratory cycle, observing rate, rhythm, inspiratory volume and effort of breathing is all that is necessary. The rate is noted by observing the frequency of the inspiratory phase since this phase is active and easy to count. Record the number of breaths per minute; this is the respiratory rate. While observing the rate, note the inspiratory expansion of the chest cage. This expansion should be the same during each cycle.

Normally, the accessory muscles of inspiration and expiration are not used. Their use should be observed and, if found, recorded as "use of accessory muscles on inspiration" and, "expiration is active with abdominal muscle contraction."

Background Information

The ventilatory system is a complex oscillating feedback control system that continuously functions at an automatic level to maintain within narrow limits the arterial pH, partial pressure of oxygen (PaO_2) and carbon dioxide ($PaCO_2$) and, indirectly, the bicarbonate stores of the body. In order to maintain this delicate balance, it is necessary to have sensors, controllers, and effectors.

I. Sensors
  A. Chemoreceptors
    1. Peripheral chemoreceptors for arterial oxygen and carbon dioxide are located in the carotid bodies. A decrease in the PaO_2 and $PaCO_2$ stimulates these sensors to send neural impulses to the medullary inspiratory center causing an increase in ventilation.
    2. Central chemoreceptors located near the ventral-lateral surface of the medulla are exquisitely sensitive to the extracellular pH of cerebrospinal fluid as well as to the partial pressure of CO_2.
  B. Stretch receptors. The major stretch receptors are located in the trachea, bronchi, lungs, and pleura. There are three major classes: (1) pulmonary stretch receptors, (2) Irritant receptors, and (3) type "J" receptors.
    1. The pulmonary stretch receptors lie within the smooth muscles of the airways and are activated by distension of the lungs. As these receptors are activated, there is a reflex slowing of the inspiratory effort and rate. The termination of inspiratory effort is classically termed the Hering-Breuer inspiratory inhibitory reflex.
    2. Irritant receptors lie between the airway epithelial cells and are susceptible to irritants, both within the inspired air and to locally released chemicals such as histamine. These irritant receptor reflexes increase the rate of inspiration.
    3. The type "J" receptors are found in the walls of the pulmonary capillaries. Distension of the capillary wall reflexly causes increase in respiratory rate.

II. Controllers
  A. Voluntary control of respiratory rate and rhythm is governed primarily by the cortex.
  B. Automatic control of respiratory rate and volume is governed within the brainstem. The three major centers for this control are the pneumotaxic center, the apneustic center, and the medullary center.
    1. The *pneumotaxic center* is the highest center in the brainstem and functions mainly in controlling the inspiratory-expiratory phasic rhythm of breathing.
    2. The *apneustic center* located below the pneumotaxic center has, as its main function, the inhibition of the inspiratory cycle. It may be the cut-off switch for normal inspiration by integrating impulses from the stretch receptors of the lung.

3. The *medullary center* is composed of two major sub-groups. One aggregation of primary inspiratory cells is located in the ventrolateral portion of the nucleus tractus solitarius and has been termed the dorsal respiratory group (DRG). The second aggregation containing both inspiratory and expiratory cells is located within the nucleus ambiguous and the nucleus retro-ambigualis. This concentration is termed the ventral respiratory group (VRG).

III. *Effectors.* Stimuli to the above mentioned respiratory centers within the brainstem in continuity with the spinal cord effect a motor response to the muscles of inspiration and initiate a respiratory cycle. Inhibition of nerve impulses to these muscles terminates the inspiratory cycle and allows for passive expiration. When working normally, the inspiratory-respiratory rhythm is maintained cycle to cycle.

Clinical Significance

It should be evident that the specific abnormalities that may result in changes in respiratory rate and rhythm are so numerous that this part of the physical examination is, indeed, a vital sign of health or disease.

Rather than remember a long list of specific disease entities, the examiner should consider which areas of the complex respiratory cycle are being stimulated in order to produce the bedside observations.

Voluntary control of ventilation can result in an increase in rate and minimal increase in volume. During the physical examination the patient may be anxious and cause an increased rate. In this situation, recheck the rate when the patient is relaxed.

The observation of a deep inspiratory-expiratory cycle associated with a sigh may be a clue to underlying chronic anxiety state. Since the patient is in a delicate balance, one deep breath may induce symptoms of respiratory alkalosis. These symptoms include a sense of unreality, dizziness, apprehension, blurring of vision, numbness around the mouth, and tingling of the fingers. Such symptoms may be quite disabling but are easily treated if identified.

Change in automatic control of respiration that results in abnormality of rate and rhythm is usually due to serious diseases. An increase in depth of inspiration associated with the use of accessory muscles as seen in Kussmaul breathing should alert the examiner to the active excitation of the peripheral and central chemoreceptors. This type of breathing is characteristic of a fall in pH in both the peripheral tissues and the central nervous system. The most common cause is a metabolic acidosis.

Increase in rate alone may be due to activation of the stretch receptors in the lung. Disorders that would stimulate these receptors would include such diseases as pneumonia, pulmonary emboli, increase in pulmonary capillary pressure, or the inhalation of an irritant.

Increase in rate and effort of breathing would suggest a combination of stimuli to stretch receptors and an associated obstruction to the movement of air within and out of the lung. Increased rate and effort are observed in patients with pulmonary emphysema, chronic bronchitis, interstitial fibrosis of the lung and asthma.

A decrease in rate to below 10 per minute may be due to depression of the medullary center secondary to sedative drugs, metabolic encephalopathy, elevation in cerebral spinal fluid pressure, elevation in cerebral spinal fluid CO_2, or intrinsic disease of the cortex or medullary center.

A decrease in rate and abnormality of rhythm typified by Biot's respiration is usually indicative if severe brainstem dysfunction due to numerous causes.

Rhythmic changes in the respiratory rate and rhythm as described in Cheyne-Stokes respiration is a very commonly observed abnormality. It is usually associated with some decrease in cardiac output as well as a decrease in cerebral blood flow due to intrinsic vascular disease of the brain. This abnormality of breathing may also be seen in elderly patients during sleep.

Weak, ineffectual, and shallow respiration may be due to inability of the neural stimulus to activate the respiratory muscles due to diseases of the central nervous system or to primary muscles diseases.

In summary, observation of the respiratory rate and rhythm is a vital sign of health and disease. An understanding of the physiologic control of respiration in the normal state allows the examiner to make vital deductions from observations of abnormality in rate, volume, and rhythm.

Selected References

1. Berger AJ, Mitchell RA, Severinghaus JW: Regulation of respiration (part one). N Eng J Med 297(2):92–97, 1977.
2. Berger AJ, Mitchell RA, Severinghaus JW: Regulation of respiration (part two). N Eng J Med 297(3):138–143, 1977.
3. Berger AJ, Mitchell RA, Severinghaus JW: Regulation of respiration (part three). N Eng J Med 297(4):194–201, 1977.
4. Kelsen SG, Altose MD, Cherniack NS: Interaction of lung volume and chemical drive on respiratory muscle EMG and respiratory timing. J Appl Physiol 42(2):287–294, 1977.
5. Cherniack NS, Fishman AP: Abnormal breathing patterns. Med Clin North Am 59(4):1–45, 1975.

123. Pulse Rate and Rhythm

I. SYLVIA CRAWLEY, MD

Definition

Pulse rate is the number of pulsations of a peripheral artery per minute. Pulse rhythm is the regularity or irregularity of the occurrence of each pulse. The terms pulse rate and pulse rhythm are not synonymous with heart rate and heart (cardiac) rhythm.

Technique

The radial pulse is the classic peripheral pulse utilized for rate and rhythm estimation. The carotid pulse is recommended for determination of arterial pulse contours. The femoral pulse is best for detection of pulsus paradoxus. Pulsus alternans is discussed in section 168.

Place one or more fingers over the radial pulse, using varying degrees of pressure. If the pulse is irregular, count for a full minute, then count the heart rate by listening over the cardiac apex. If the heart rate exceeds the pulse rate, then a pulse deficit exists. Pulse deficit implies that some cardiac contractions are too weak to transmit the impulse to the peripheral artery.

Pulse rhythms are sometimes referred to as regular or irregular. In a regular pulse, each beat occurs within the same time interval. In an irregular pulse, there is variation in the time interval between beats. The variation may occur in a predictable or unpredictable manner.

Pulse amplitude should be evaluated on a beat-to-beat basis. Variation in amplitude may not be appreciated if too much pressure is applied with the examining fingers. Determine the relationship of any variation in amplitude to the variation in rhythm. Make particular note whether normal inspiration and expiration alter pulse amplitude. When there is a decline in pulse amplitude during inspiration (ie, pulsus paradoxus), it should be quantitated as described in section 124, Blood Pressure.

Background Information

Left ventricular contraction occurs as a result of an electrical impulse in the conduction system. As diagrammed in Fig 13, this impulse normally originates in the sinoatrial (SA) node, conducts through the atria, and induces atrial contraction. The impulse then spreads through the atrioventricular (AV) node to the right then the left ventricular bundle branch (RBB, LBB) with resultant ventricular contraction. Under normal conditions, there is a constant beat-to-beat occurrence of the peripheral pulse with the heart sounds.

Constant pulse amplitude requires a constant beat-to-beat volume of blood ejected (stroke volume) by the left ventricle. A change in either force of contraction (contractility) or diastolic volume of filling of the left ventricle can directly effect stroke volume.

Regular Pulse Rhythms. Six regular rhythms include normal sinus rhythm, complete heart block, junctional tachycardia, atrial tachycardia, atrial flutter with fixed AV block, and ventricular tachycardia.

Normal sinus rhythm is regular with no variation in amplitude from beat to beat or during phases of respiration. Children and young adults have a slightly faster rate during inspiration. This is referred to as sinus arrhythmia. The JVP is normal in contour and S1 is constant in intensity. The normal sinus rate is 60–100 per minute. A rate less than 60 is called a bradycardia. If it is the result of a sinus mechanism, it is sinus bradycardia. Sinus bradycardia may occur in normal individuals (especially athletically well-trained persons) as well as disease states such as hypo-

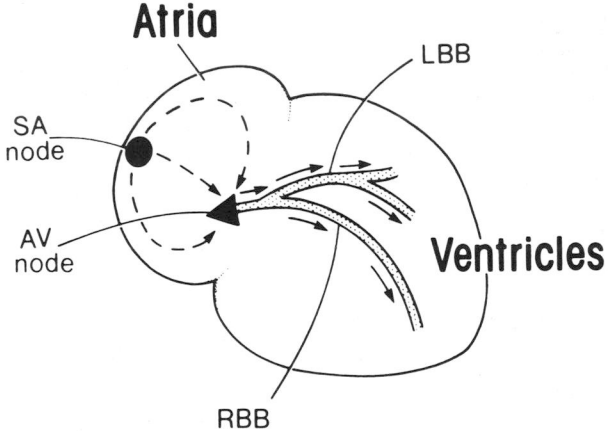

Figure 13. Normal pathway of the electrical impulse through the cardiac conduction system.

thyroidism or increased intracranial pressure. It may also result from medications such as reserpine, propranolol, clonidine, guanethidine, or methyldopa. A rate greater than 100 is called a tachycardia. If it is the result of a sinus mechanism, it is called sinus tachycardia. Sinus tachycardia occurs in normal individuals (exercise, excitement) as well as with conditions such as hyperthyroidism, pheochromocytoma, pulmonary embolism, blood loss, fever, dehydration, hypoxia, and congestive heart failure. It may also result from compounds and medications such as nicotine, amphetamines, cold remedies (ephedrine, phenylephrine, phenylpropanolamine), atropine, hydralazine, prazosin, and amitryptiline. In either sinus tachycardia or sinus bradycardia, the jugular venous pulsations will be normal and S1 will be of constant intensity.

In complete heart block, the normal SA node impulse is blocked at the AV node. The heart rhythm is thus determined by impulses originating either in the area of the AV node or junction (40–55 per minute) or in the ventricles (25–50 per minute). This results in independent activity of the atria and ventricles. The intensity of S1 will vary depending on the interval between atrial contraction and ventricular contraction. Cannon "A" waves occur in the jugular venous pulse when the atria and ventricles contract simultaneously.

In junctional tachycardia, the origin of the electrical impulse is near the AV node with conduction of the impulse to the ventricles. The impulse may also conduct backward (retrograde) to the atria. The first heart sound is constant in intensity. There are regular cannon A waves in the jugular venous pulse. The rate is usually 140–200 per minute. A regular pulse also occurs with accelerated junctional rhythms (60–100 beats per minute) not fast enough to qualify as junctional tachycardia.

In atrial tachycardia, the origin of the electrical impulse is in the atria with normal conduction through the AV node. The normal SA node impulse is usually suppressed. Atrial tachycardia usually occurs at a rate of 140–220 per minute. Sinus tachycardia in adults does not usually exceed 160 beats per minute. Cannon A waves should not be visible in the jugular venous pulsations of patients with atrial tachycardia.

In atrial flutter, the impulse originates in the atria at a rate of 280–320 per minute. Most often the AV node will only conduct every other impulse (2:1 conduction) to the ventricles, resulting in a regular pulse rate of 140–160. Atrial flutter with 2:1 block should always be considered when the pulse rate is exactly 150 per minute. Atrial flutter may also result in regular rates of 100 or 75 with fixed 3:1 or 4:1 blocks. Many patients with atrial flutter have varying degrees of block (alternating 2:1, 3:1 4:1) such that the pulse rate is irregular. Rapid atrial contractions result in continuous atrial flutter waves in the jugular venous pulse. These are most easily recognized when the AV conduction is 3:1 or 4:1.

In ventricular tachycardia, the impulse originates in the ventricular conduction system. The rate is usually between 140–200 per minute.

There is usually no conduction back to the atria. The independent SA node impulses continue without conduction to the ventricles. Since the atria and ventricles contract independently and at different rates, their relationship varies from cycle to cycle. S1 varies in intensity. Simultaneous atrial and ventricular contraction results in cannon A waves at irregular intervals. Ventricular tachycardia is the regular rhythm most likely to result in impairment of ventricular function. The abnormal sequence of contraction of the ventricles prevents appropriate emptying of the left ventricle; thus, pulse amplitude and blood pressure are depressed.

Irregular pulse rhythms. Four irregular rhythms include atrial fibrillation, premature contractions, bigeminy, and Wenckebach.

In atrial fibrillation, electrical activity of the atria is rapid, irregular, and poorly organized. Impulses conduct through the AV node in a rapid and irregular manner such that the rate and timing of ventricular contractions are unpredictable. Atrial fibrillation thus classically causes an irregularly irregular pulse. S1 varies in intensity (varying rate), and the peripheral pulse varies in amplitude. With rapid ventricular rates, there is marked shortening of diastole and reduction in ventricular filling such that some of these cycles may not produce a palpable pulse despite generation of heart sounds. Thus, atrial fibrillation is the most common cause of a pulse deficit.

In premature contractions, a regular rhythm may be interrupted by a premature beat. The premature beat may originate from an impulse in the atrium (premature atrial contraction or PAC), in the AV junction (premature nodal or junctional contraction), or in the ventricle (premature ventricular contractions, PVC, VPC). If the premature contractions interrupt a regular rhythm at constant intervals (for example, every third beat), a regularly irregular pulse occurs. If the premature contractions occur at irregular and unpredictable intervals, an irregularly irregular pulse occurs. Recall that the premature beat may or may not produce a palpable pulse. The beat following the premature beat generally has an increase in amplitude as a result of increased filling during the longer diastole. A longer (compensatory) pause is more likely when the premature beat is of ventricular origin.

Bigeminy occurs when a premature beat occurs after every sinus beat. The interval between the sinus beat and the premature beat is less than the interval between the premature beat and the next sinus beat. The pulse amplitude generated by the ectopic beat is less than that of the sinus beat. The resulting pulse rhythm is thus: strong-weak-pause; strong-weak-pause. This pattern must be differentiated from pulsus alternans where the intervals between the strong and weak beat remain the same, creating a strong-weak-strong-weak pulse sequence. Occasionally a bigeminal rhythm produces a strong beat, weak beat, and a pause so minimal that its recognition is difficult without electrocardiographic confirmation.

In Wenckebach Type I AV block, there is gradual prolongation of conduction time (PR interval) of the sinus impulse through the AV node to the ventricles until one impulse is completely blocked. This results in a pause in the pulse followed by a cycle which repeats itself.

Clinical Significance

The pulse rate is primarily of benefit in screening for arrhythmias which can be further delineated by electrocardiography. The significance of a particular rhythm disturbance is influenced by the etiologic factors in its development, the presence of heart disease, and the effect of the particular arrhythmia on cardiac function. Certain arrhythmias occur in the absence of heart disease. Atrial or ventricular ectopic beats, for example, are commonly associated with emotional stress, excessive coffee, tobacco, or alcohol. Atrial tachycardia or atrial fibrillation may occur in paroxysms in a healthy individual. However, atrial fibrillation demands a search for rheumatic mitral valve disease and thyrotoxicosis. Paroxysmal atrial tachycardia may be associated with abnormal conduction pathways between the atria and ventricles such as the WPW syndrome. Etiologies of sinus bradycardia and tachycardia have been discussed.

The presence or absence of heart disease is an important determinant in the clinical significance of arrhythmias. Atrial or ventricular ectopic beats in acute myocardial infarction may herald the onset of life-threatening arrhythmias. Atrial tachycardia or rapid atrial fibrillation is well

Table 22. Bedside differentiation of rhythm disturbances.

Rhythm	Rate	Favorable Findings
Sinus bradycardia	35–60	
Normal sinus rhythm	60–100	
Sinus tachycardia	100–160	Constant S_1
Atrial tachycardia	140–220	Normal JVP
Atrial fibrillation	100–160	Varying S_1, grossly irregular No A wave in JVP
Atrial flutter	140–160	Constant or only slight variation in S_1; flutter waves in JVP
Wenckebach type I AV block	Variable	Gradual shortening of interval with gradual decrease in S_1 followed by a pause
Complete heart block		
Ventricular escape	25–50	Varying S_1
Junctional escape	40–50	Irregular cannon A waves
Ventricular tachycardia	140–200	

tolerated when there is no heart disease, but may be life-threatening in a patient with severe valvular disease. Therapy is thus directed toward the patient with an arrhythmia, not the arrhythmia per se. In the presence of severe heart disease the bradyarrhythmias may be as poorly tolerated as the tachyarrhythmias. A sinus bradycardia may be normal and well tolerated in a young athletic adult, whereas it may aggravate severe congestive heart failure in other patients.

Arrhythmias may result from noncardiac problems. Noncardiac causes of sinus tachycardia and bradycardia are examples. Electrolyte abnormalities and medications should always be considered as a cause of arrhythmias. For example, ventricular ectopic beats or ventricular tachycardia can result from severe hypokalemia. Cardiac standstill may result from severe hyperkalemia. Large doses of psychotropic agents may cause ventricular tachycardia. Accidental digitalis poisoning may cause a variety of arrhythmias.

Rhythm status can also be valuable in assessing adequate drug effect. Digitalis is used in the treatment of atrial fibrillation to control the ventricular rate. However, heart rates are much preferable to pulse rates in patients with atrial fibrillation since pulse deficit is often present. A reduction in the resting sinus rate, occasionally even to bradycardia, is one guide to the adequacy of propranolol dosage.

Pulsus paradoxus is more commonly caused by obstructive pulmonary disease than cardiac tamponade. Pulsus paradoxus is less frequently present in chronic constrictive pericarditis than in acute pericardial tamponade. Pulsus paradoxus may also be seen in superior vena cava obstruction, severe heart failure, and rarely in cardiogenic shock.

An increase in amplitude is expected in the normal beat following an ectopic beat. When there is an obvious decrease in the amplitude of this beat, one should suspect the presence of left ventricular outflow obstruction due to obstructive cardiomyopthy such as idiopathic hypertrophic subaortic stenosis. Large pulse amplitudes are also seen in association with elevated stroke volumes such as with aortic insufficiency.

Selected References

1.   Marx HJ, Yu PN: Clinical examination of the arterial pulse. *Prog Cardiovasc Dis* 10:207–325, 1967.
2.   Bedford DE: The ancient art of feeling the pulse. *Br Heart J* 13:423–437, 1951.
3.   Harvey WP, Ronan JA Jr: Bedside diagnosis of arrhythmias. *Prog Cardiovasc Dis* 8:419–445, 1966.
4.   Shabetai R, Fowler NO, Guntherold WG: The hemodynamics of cardiac tamponade and constrictive pericarditis. *Am J Cardiol* 26:480–489, 1970.

5. Hurst JW, Schlant RC: Examination of the arteries and their pulsations, in Hurst JW (ed in chief): *The Heart*, ed 4. New York, McGraw-Hill, 1978, chap 14, pp 183–201.
6. Marriott HJL, Myerburg RJ: Recognition and treatment of cardiac arrhythmias and conduction disturbance, in Hurst JW (ed in chief): *The Heart*, ed 4. New York, McGraw-Hill, 1978, chap 46D, pp 637–694.

124. Blood Pressure

GARY L. WOLLAM, MD
ELBERT P. TUTTLE, JR., MD

Definition

Blood pressure is the force per unit of area that is exerted by blood as it flows through the circulation. The pressures generated within the different portions of the cardiovascular system vary considerably since the pressure within arteries is much greater than that within capillaries and veins. However, the general use of the term "blood pressure" refers to "arterial pressure."

Blood pressure is usually expressed in millimeters of mercury. This is the height of a column of mercury that will be supported by the pressure of the blood in the arterial circulation. The maximum arterial pressure occurs near the end of the contractile phase of the cardiac cycle (systole) and is called the systolic pressure. The minimum pressure occurs at the end of the relaxation phase (diastole) and is called the diastolic pressure. The difference between the systolic and diastolic pressures is the pulse pressure. Figure 14 is a representation of these pressures derived from an arterial pulse tracing.

Systolic and diastolic blood pressures are usually recorded as a number looking like a fraction, eg, 120/80. A normal blood pressure in an adult is in the range of 90–140 mm Hg systolic and 60–90 mm Hg diastolic. Different values apply for the pediatric age groups and can be found in reference 2.

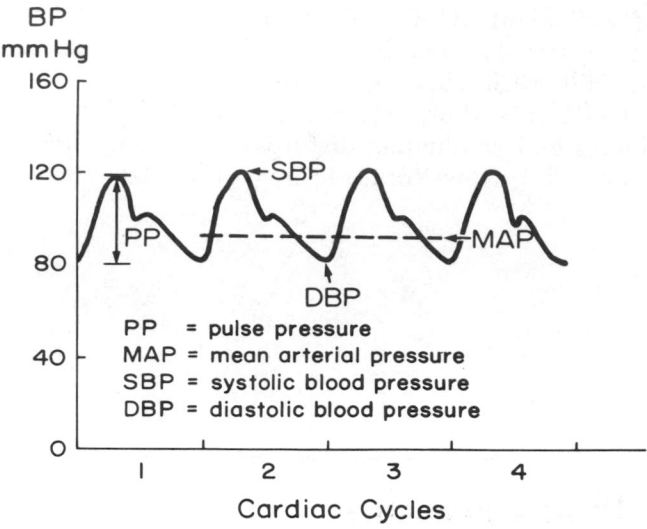

Figure 14.   Aortic pressure tracing.

The "official" definition of normotension and hypertension by the World Health Organization criteria is as follows:

Normotension: systolic < 140 and diastolic < 90 mm Hg
Hypertension: systolic > 160 and diastolic > 95 mm Hg
Borderline: any reading between these limits

Technique

Blood pressure is measured by a variety of techniques depending on the indication and the precision required. Direct intra-arterial pressure recordings provide the most accurate measurements of arterial pressure. However, arterial pressure is most commonly measured by an indirect method using a sphygmomanometer and stethoscope.

In adults with normal sized arms, blood pressure is measured using a standard or regular size sphygmomanometer cuff with an inflatable bladder approximately 13 cm in width and 23 cm in length. In order to perform this measurement accurately, the bladder width should exceed the midarm diameter by 20% and the bladder length should be adequate to encircle more than two-thirds of the arm. If the arm is too large, an obese size ("large") blood pressure cuff must be used to avoid erroneously high measurements.

The arm should be free of all clothing and other encumbrances during the measurement. The blood pressure cuff should be placed on the arm so that the distal edge is approximately one inch above the elbow. The cuff bladder should be placed over the inner aspect of the arm directly over the brachial artery, and should be snugly secured into place. The brachial artery is then located by palpation on the medial side of the antecubital area, immediately below the bottom edge of the cuff. Prior to the actual measurement, the systolic pressure should be estimated by inflating the cuff until the arterial pulse is no longer palpable. The cuff is then slowly deflated, and the pressure at which the pulse is again palpable is used to approximate systolic pressure.

The blood pressure is then measured by inflating the cuff to a pressure 30–50 mm Hg above the palpable systolic pressure. The cuff is then slowly deflated at a rate no greater than 5 mm per second. The pressure at which the first Korotkoff sound appears (the "first phase") is taken as the systolic pressure.

As the pressure continues to drop, a "muffling" of the Korotkoff sound is often noted. This is known as the "fourth phase" or "fourth phase diastolic pressure." As the cuff is deflated a little further, the Korotkoff sounds disappear completely. This is the "fifth phase" or "phase V diastolic pressure," and is stated to be the most precise index of diastolic pressure in adults by some authorities. It occurs within a few millimeters of the fourth phase in most patients and is more easily recognizable and reproducible among different observers. For this reason, the fifth phase is generally used to define the diastolic pressure. However, it is often advisable to record both phase IV and phase V since the true diastolic pressure, as determined by direct intra-arterial measurements, usually falls somewhere between the two.

In some individuals (particularly in hypertensive patients), the Korotkoff sounds transiently disappear as the cuff pressure falls. This temporary disappearance of the Korotkoff sounds is known as the "auscultatory gap." Because it occasionally extends over a pressure range of 40 mm Hg or more, the auscultatory gap can lead to serious underestimation of the systolic pressure (or overestimation of diastolic pressure). This error is avoided by estimating systolic pressure by the palpation method previously described and by continuing to listen over the artery as the mercury falls 10–20 mm below what is thought to be the final disappearance of sound.

Occasionally, the fifth phase occurs far below the expected diastolic pressure, and in a few patients, Korotkoff sounds are audible to zero. This situation is not infrequent in patients with high cardiac outputs (eg, anemia, pregnancy). In this case, record the fourth phase (muffled sound) diastolic pressure.

Normally, the systolic pressure varies with respiration and is lower on inspiration than expiration. However, an inspiratory fall in systolic pressure of more than 8 mm Hg is abnormal and is referred to as "pulsus paradoxus." This may occur in patients with obstructive airway disease such as asthma or emphysema as well as in cardiac tamponade and constrictive pericarditis. To determine if pulsus paradoxus is present, have the patient breathe normally and then deflate the cuff until the first Korotkoff sound appears. Maintain the cuff pressure at this level. If the Korotkoff sounds are audible on both inspiration and expiration at the same level of pressure, then no paradox is present. However, if the Korotkoff sounds are audible only during expiration, the cuff should be slowly deflated until the Korotkoff sounds are heard throughout the entire respiratory cycle. A difference in the systolic blood pressure (expiratory-inspiratory) of more than 8 mm Hg is indicative of pulsus paradoxus.

One cannot overemphasize the importance of proper technique in obtaining accurate and reliable blood pressure measurements. Besides taking the necessary care to ensure that the first, fourth, and fifth Korotkoff phases have been accurately identified, one must be particularly careful in choosing the proper cuff size. The use of an improperly fitting cuff, ie, a regular size cuff on an obese patient, is probably the most common source of error in measuring blood pressure. In order to assess fully the blood pressure status, a standing blood pressure should be measured as well as a supine or sitting pressure. This is particularly important in patients on antihypertensive treatment or in those in whom therapy is anticipated. Orthostatic or postural hypotension is a common side effect of antihypertensive drugs, and the presence of a baseline orthostatic reduction in pressure may alter the choice of therapy.

Background Information

Circulatory physiology. During the contraction phase of the cardiac cycle, the systolic pressure is generated when the left ventricle ejects a small volume of blood (about 75 ml) into the arterial circulation. Each cardiac contraction produces a rise in pressure because the stroke volume is ejected into a partially filled reservoir (the aorta) that has limited capacity and distensibility (compliance). The aorta and major arteries possess viscoelastic properties (ie, the distensibility is both time and pressure dependent), and they distend to accept the stroke volume as it is ejected from the left ventricle, storing energy in the process. Then, during the relaxation phase of the cardiac cycle, the stored energy is released by the elastic recoil of the aorta and large arteries, and, as a result, arterial pressure falls only gradually during diastole. This important function of the aorta and large arteries has been termed the "windkessel effect." (This label was apparently coined in 1834 by Ernest Weber of Leipzig, when he noted the functional similarity between the aorta and the windkessel or compression chamber of pump-operated fire engines.)

In fundamental terms, arterial pressure is determined by the interaction between cardiac output or blood flow and the resistance to flow, according to the equation:

Mean arterial pressure = cardiac output × total peripheral resistance

Arterial pressure is regulated within relatively narrow limits by a variety of mechanisms that act by influencing cardiac output and vascular resistance. These include viscosity, volume, humoral, neural, anatomial, and other factors. Pathophysiologic mechanisms responsible for abnormalities of pressure act by influencing either cardiac output or resistance. For example, in most cases of renovascular hypertension, the increased levels of circulating angiotensin II produce arteriolar vasoconstriction and result in an increase in total peripheral resistance, while cardiac output is variably affected. In this situation, the elevated arterial pressure is largely maintained by an increase in resistance.

The mean arterial pressure is the average blood pressure over the cardiac cycle and is approximated by the diastolic pressure plus one-third the pulse pressure:

$$MAP = DBP + 1/3 \ (SBP - DBP), \text{ or } MAP = \frac{2 \ DBP + SBP}{3}$$

Cardiac output is the product of heart rate and stroke volume ($CO = HR \times SV$). It is largely determined by the venous return to the right side of the heart and the level of autonomic regulation of heart rate and myocardial contractility. Total peripheral resistance is calculated from measurements of cardiac output and arterial pressure. It represents the summation of all vascular resistance in the peripheral circulation. For precise calculation of total peripheral resistance, the blood pressure should be expressed as central aortic pressure minus right atrial pressure. However, since right atrial pressure is a relatively small number in comparison with systemic arterial pressure, in actual practice it is frequently assumed to be zero in the calculation of total peripheral resistance.

According to Poiseuille's law, the flow (Q) in a given vessel varies directly with the pressure gradient ($P_1 - P_2$) and the fourth power of the radius (r), and inversely with the vessel length (l) and the viscosity (η) of the fluid:

$$Q = \frac{\pi \ (P_1 - P_2) \ r^4}{8 \ \eta \ l} \text{ or } R = \frac{P_1 - P_2}{Q} = \frac{8 \ \eta \ l}{\pi \ r^4}$$

Therefore, assuming that the blood viscosity and vascular length remain constant in a given individual, variations in resistance (R) will usually result from changes in the luminal diameter of the blood vessels. Since the radius is magnified to the fourth power, flow and pressure are greatly affected by relatively small structural or functional changes in vessel size.

The greatest resistance to flow in the arterial circulation occurs at the level of the arterioles, frequently referred to as the "resistance vessels." Total peripheral resistance, however, represents the summation of all resistance in the peripheral circulation. It cannot be strictly equated with arteriolar vasoconstriction because other factors such as arteriovenous shunts, collateral vessels, and structural changes within the vessel walls can also affect resistance.

Whereas the mean arterial pressure is determined by the relationship between cardiac output and total peripheral resistance, the absolute level of the systolic and diastolic pressures is influenced by factors that may not result in changes in mean blood pressure. The factors that primarily determine systolic pressure (and pulse pressure) are aortic distensibility, the volume of blood ejected from the left ventricle (stroke volume), and the velocity of ejection.

Aortic distensibility plays a major role in determining systolic pressure. Indeed, the height of the systolic pressure (and pulse pressure) generated is inversely correlated with aortic distensibility. As the aorta distends to accept the stroke volume, it absorbs part of the energy of left ventricular ejection, and the rise in systolic pressure is lessened or buffered. Therefore, the more distensible the aorta, the lower the systolic pressure, and conversely, the less distensible the aorta, the greater the systolic pressure for a given stroke volume. It should be noted that the ability of the aorta to distend reduces the work load of the myocardium, because the left ventricle is required to generate less of a pressure load to eject the stroke volume. When the aorta becomes rigid, such as in elderly patients with large vessel atherosclerosis, the work load on the myocardium is correspondingly increased because of the greater pressure load generated in ejecting the stroke volume.

The height of the systolic pressure is also correlated with the size of the stroke volume and the velocity of ejection. A larger stroke volume will result in a higher systolic pressure due to greater filling of the arterial tree. The height of the systolic pressure is also directly correlated with the velocity of left ventricular ejection. Since the aorta's ability to distend is both rate and pressure-dependent, the aorta becomes transiently less distensible, and systolic pressure rises when the velocity of ejection increases.

The factors which primarily determine diastolic pressure appear to be heart rate and total peripheral resistance. In experimental models where all other variables are held constant, an increase in either heart rate or total peripheral resistance results in a rise in systolic as well as diastolic pressure. However, the diastolic pressure rise is greater. The mechanism involved is thought to be overfilling of the arterial circulation as the result of diminished peripheral run-off of blood into the capillaries and veins. When heart rate is increased, the overfilling is presumably due to decreased time for diastolic run-off to occur. When total peripheral resistance is increased, the diminished run-off is presumably a reflection of arteriolar vasoconstriction. Although this information is largely derived from experimental models, it is interesting to note that the majority of patients with essential hypertension have an elevated total peripheral resistance as their major hemodynamic abnormality. Furthermore, hypertensives as a group have a higher mean heart rate than normotensives.

Baroreceptor reflex. The autonomic nervous system provides short-term regulation of arterial pressure by means of the baroreceptor reflex. This cardiovascular control mechanism consists of an afferent (sensory) limb, a vasomotor center in the medulla, and an efferent (effector) limb. The baroreceptors located in the carotid sinuses and aortic arch constitute the afferent limb. These pressure-sensing devices are actually stretch receptors that respond to mechanical deformation of the vessel wall. Afferent nerve fibers travel via the glossopharyngeal and vagus nerves to the vasomotor center in the medulla. Impulses are mingled here with impulses from other centers of the brain, and the efferent portion of the baroreceptor reflex flows out from the parasympathetic and sympathetic nuclei in the medulla. These efferent tracts provide innervation to the heart and peripheral circulation.

The baroreceptor reflex mechanism controls arterial pressure within a narrow range. It adjusts for postural changes by signaling the medulla to modulate sympathetic and parasympathetic outflow to the heart and peripheral vessels. For example, when a normal individual stands, gravitational pooling of blood in the lower extremities causes a reduction in venous return to the heart and results in a fall in cardiac output with a 3–10 mm drop in systolic pressure. If this sequence of events were to continue, hypotension would result. However, the fall in systolic pressure is immediately sensed by the baroreceptors, resulting in a sudden increase in sympathetic vasomotor tone. This causes arteriolar vasoconstriction that raises diastolic pressure slightly and also increases venous tone to reestablish venous return and stabilize cardiac output. Because of the slight fall in systolic pressure and the slight increase in diastolic pressure, the pulse pressure is narrowed somewhat. However, mean arterial pressure is only slightly changed (± 10 mm Hg). Heart rate is increased slightly as a result of the general increase in sympathetic neural activity.

Clinical Significance

Mortality is correlated with arterial pressure throughout much of the normotensive as well as the hypertensive range. Although cardiovascular morbidity and mortality are related to both the systolic and diastolic pressure, the correlations are actually higher for systolic than for diastolic pressure. This is true for myocardial infarction, left ventricular hypertrophy, cardiomegaly, congestive heart failure, and stroke.

Systolic hypertension is not uncommon in the hypertensive population. It may occur as isolated or "pure" systolic hypertension, in which the systolic pressure is greater than 150 mm Hg and the diastolic is below 90 mm Hg, or as predominantly systolic hypertension. In the latter instance, both systolic and diastolic pressures are elevated. However, the systolic pressure is inappropriately increased for the level of diastolic pressure according to the Koch-Weser formula, which states that systolic pressure is disproportionately increased when it exceeds two times the (diastolic pressure − 15). Thus, in a patient with a blood pressure of 200/105, the systolic pressure exceeds the "appropriate" value of 180 mm Hg or less and is therefore disproportionately elevated.

Systolic hypertension is commonly found in the older hypertensive population where the primary abnormality is impaired aortic distensibility ("rigid aorta"). It is also seen in younger patients with "borderline" or "labile" hypertension when the systolic pressure elevation is largely attributable to an increased stroke volume and mean velocity of ejection (ie, increased contractility). Coarctation of the aorta may present with predominantly systolic hypertension as a result of a reduction in the capacitance (and compliance) of the aorta above the coarctated segment. Systolic hypertension also results from large A-V fistulas and from aortic regurgitation.

One should always remember in measuring blood pressure that the reading obtained will form the basis of a clinical assessment. If the measurement is invalid, then the judgment that follows is likewise apt to be erroneous. Because of spontaneous variation in blood pressure and the variability in response to psychological factors, the last two of three consecutive readings are a more stable estimate of blood pressure than the first. Blood pressure readings on several different occasions are necessary to characterize an individual's usual blood pressure.

Selected References

1. Kirkendall WM, Burton AC, Epstein FH, et al: Recommendations for human blood pressure determination by sphygmomanometers. *Circulation* 36:980–988, 1967.
2. Report of the Task Force on Blood Pressure Control in Children. *Pediatrics* 59(suppl):797–820, 1977.
3. Wiggers CJ: *Circulatory Dynamics: Physiologic Studies.* New York, Grune and Stratton, 1952.
4. Dustan HP, Tarazi RC, Hinshaw LB: Mechanisms controlling arterial pressure, in Frohlich ED (ed): *Pathophysiology,* ed 2. Philadelphia, JB Lippincott, 1976.

5. Berne RM, Levy MN: *Cardiovascular Physiology,* ed 3. St Louis, CV Mosby, 1977.
6. Rose JC: Pressures on the millimeter of mercury. *N Eng J Med* 298:1361–1364, 1978.
7. Koch-Weser J: Correlation of pathophysiology and pharmacotherapy in primary hypertension. *Am J Cardiol* 32:499–510, 1973.
8. Ramirez EA, Pont PHG: Relation of arterial blood pressure to the transverse diameter of the heart in compensated hypertensive heart disease. *Circulation* 31:542–550, 1965.
9. Kannel WB, Gordon T, Offutt D: Left ventricular hypertrophy by electrocardiogram. *Ann Intern Med* 71:89–105, 1969.
10. George CF, Breckenridge AM, Dollery CT: Value of routine electrocardiography in hypertensive patients. *Br Heart J* 34:618–622, 1972.
11. Kannel WB, Castelli WP, McNamara PM, et al: Role of blood pressure in the development of congestive heart failure: The Framingham study. *N Eng J Med* 287:781–787, 1972.
12. Kannel WB, Gordon T, Schwartz MJ: Systolic versus diastolic blood pressure and risk of coronary heart disease: The Framingham study. *Am J Cardiol* 27:335–346, 1971.
13. Kannel WB, Wolf PA, Verter J, et al: Epidemiologic assessment of the role of blood pressure in stroke. *JAMA* 214:301–310, 1970.

125. Body Size: Height and Weight

CHERYL L. ROCK, MMSC
RICHARD P. HOLM, MD
W. DALLAS HALL, MD

Definition

Body height or length is the distance from the lowest to the highest body part. Weight is the total weight of the body.

An estimation of ideal body weight for women allows 100 lb for the first 5 feet of height plus 5 lb for each additional inch of height. For men, allow 106 lb for the first five feet of height plus 6 lb for each additional inch. Subtract or add 10% of the figure derived to adjust for small or large frame, respectively.

Technique

Height is best measured (without shoes and in the standing position) against a vertical measuring rod with a headpiece. The head should be in an upright position with eyes straight ahead and with arms by the sides. The bar of the headpiece should make contact with the scalp. Height is recorded in inches or centimeters: 1 inch is equal to 2.54 cm.

Weight is best measured (with light or no clothing and without shoes) on a beam or lever balance scale. The scale should be checked periodically for accuracy. Spring balance scales are not sufficiently accurate in assessing weight change. Patients who are unable to stand may be weighed on bed scales. Weight is recorded in pounds or kilograms: 1 kg is equal to 2.2046 lb avoirdupois.

Neither height nor weight should be obtained by asking the patient since this information is most likely inaccurate.

Background Information

Body weight represents the sum of the mass contained within four compartments of the body: cell residue or protoplasm, extracellular fluid, bone mineral, and fat. In the average adult of normal weight, the relative mass proportions of these compartments are approximately 50%, 25%, 7%, and 18%, respectively.

Protoplasm usually comprises 30–65% of the total body weight. As active tissue mass, it utilizes a major proportion of energy intake. Most investigations are directed toward identifying this component of the body since it is the major determinant of energy and nutrient needs.

Water accounts for more than half of the adult weight, averaging 60% for men and 54% for women. Of the mass of total water, one-third is found in the extracellular compartment and in the interstitial spaces. Intracellular fluid accounts for two-thirds of the body water. Extracellular water thus accounts for 20–25% of total body weight.

Bone minerals account for only a fraction of the total skeletal mass. In the living state, the entire skeletal mass may average one-sixth of the total body weight.

By definition, fat is that portion of the body obtained by ether extraction. Adipose tissue is not pure fat as it contains connective tissue, blood vessels, and cell walls. The fat content of a normal weight individual ranges between 14–30% of the total body weight and depends on sex, age, and activity. Under normal conditions, women contain a greater percentage of body fat than men. A tendency toward increased fat deposition and changes in the distribution of subcutaneous fat occur with aging. Persons who engage in regular physical activity demonstrate a lower fat content than sedentary individuals at comparable weights.

In research investigations, the body may be partitioned and described as two parts: (1) fat and (2) fat free. Early studies defined the latter portion as lean body mass, which includes a certain amount of fat (2–10%) considered essential and compatible with health. Since body fat is less dense than other body materials (0.9 g/ml at 37°C), densitometric methods may be applied to quantitate body components. A human body, with a fat content of 15.3% (of total body weight) has a density of 1.064 g/ml at 37°C. Body density is the reference method that best estimates the contribution of fat to total body weight: obese individuals have a lower body density. Body density is determined by water displacement after removal of nonvital body air. Methodological difficulties and the inconvenience of total immersion make this impractical as a common clinical procedure.

Measurements of body water and total body potassium are also applied to the determination of body composition. An estimation of body cell mass may be obtained from the potassium content of the body, since potassium is the major cation in the intracellular compartment.

Weight and height bear a close relationship to each other and to the surface area of the body. In turn, the surface area of the body bears a relationship to the heat dissipation and caloric requirements of the human. The best estimate of surface area is that provided by Gehan and George and represented mathematically by the equation:

$$\text{Surface area} = 0.02350 \times \text{height}^{0.42246} \times \text{weight}^{0.51456}$$

where weight is in kilograms, height is in centimeters, and surface area is in square meters. Approximations of the surface area from height and weight are available from normograms contained in many standard texts. Surface area in adults usually ranges 1.60–1.90 sq m.

Overweight and obesity are not synonymous terms. "Overweight" carries no direct implication with regard to fatness. "Obesity" is defined as a condition marked by excessive body fat. A body weight greater than 120% of the ideal body weight is often used clinically as an indicator of obesity. Since skeletal mass, body structure (ectomorphic, endomorphic, mesomorphic), and height influence formula estimations for relative weight, other indices are applied for comparative purposes.

Standards of reference such as tables of average weight for height are usually based on insurance company data and are not necessarily those weights most conducive to health. Epidemiologists often use the average weight for height and sex of a study population as a reference point for the sample population. The extent of prevalence of obesity in the reference population will thus influence the derivation of relative weight.

To minimize the influence of height on weight, some function of height may be incorporated into a formula. An example of this type of index is the Quetelet index (weight/height^2 × 100), where weight is in pounds and height is in inches. The Quetelet index shows a high correlation with obesity at all heights and is commonly used in population studies.

About one-half of total body fat is deposited in the subcutaneous tissue as a single sheet of tela adiposa which, in many parts of the body, is only loosely attached to the underlying tissue. The tela adiposa can be pulled up between thumb and forefinger into a fold. Since the volume of subcutaneous fat bears some relationship to the volume of inner fat, it is possible to estimate the percentage of total fat from skinfold thickness. Skinfold thickness measurement is highly correlated with other more accurate indirect measurements of body fat (for example, body density and total body water methods) and is preferred over estimates using height and weight. Skinfold measurement is a fairly simple procedure, but it must be carefully standardized with respect to a number of factors.

The diagnosis of obesity in children is more difficult because the factors that produce obesity also tend to produce linear growth. Developing an index is more complicated because weight and height must be evaluated on an age-specific basis for children. According to standards presented in pediatric growth charts (based on specific groups of children studied), childhood obesity is defined as 40% or more above the medium weight for height.

Body weights below normal commonly result from loss of mass from protoplasm, adipose tissue, and extracellular volume compartments. A relative weight more than 10% below the ideal is usually considered to be abnormal, particularly in patients under 25 years of age. Protein-energy malnutrition is designated as moderate marasmus in the patient presenting with a relative weight 60–80% of ideal, and as severe marasmus in the patient presenting with a relative weight less than 60% of ideal.

Underweight or rapid weight loss is often attributable to a loss of lean body mass with the use of protein as a metabolic fuel; adipose tissue is lost more slowly due to its higher caloric content. Edema is a common feature in protein-energy malnutrition and may give deceptively high weight readings.

Assessment of an underweight patient's lean body mass is facilitated by the use of additional indices of body composition. The arm muscle circumference is calculated from the following relationship:

Arm muscle circumference (cm) = Arm circumference (cm)
$$- [0.314 \times \text{triceps skinfold (mm)}]$$

The actual measurements are compared to standards (reference 1 provides tables). Since creatinine excretion correlates with the total lean body mass in adults, the 24-hour creatinine excretion may be compared with the expected 24-hour creatinine excretion of a normal adult of the same height. Urinary creatinine excretion for various heights has been calculated as the product of the mean daily creatinine excretion on a creatine-free and creatinine-free diet. The normal values for total urinary creatinine excretion per day are 23 mg/kg in men and 17 mg/kg in women.

Clinical Significance

Recent epidemiological data indicate that 2–6% of infants, 5–33% of adolescents, 5–15% of men, and 10–55% of women in America are obese.

The risks of obesity are both medical and social. Death rates are 1.5 times greater for the moderate to severely obese than for the thin.

Abnormal lipid metabolism and systemic arterial hypertension are related to obesity and are recognized as risk factors for coronary atherosclerotic heart disease. Significant weight reduction may reduce the level of arterial blood pressure in some hypertensive patients. Cerebrovascular events appear more prevalent in obese hypertensives than in thin ones. Gallstones are a greater problem with the obese than with the thin.

Severe obesity may cause hypoventilation and hypoxia by several mechanisms. Pulmonary function testing may reveal diminished functional residual capacity, diminished compliance, ventilation-perfusion abnormalities, and increased work of breathing. The classic Pickwickian syndrome and the recently described somnolence syndrome are associated with obesity.

Maturity onset diabetes mellitus remains the disease most clearly correlated with obesity. Reduction of weight is the most important factor in controlling adult onset diabetes. Diabetes develops more readily in the obese patient with pancreatic injury.

Degenerative joint and disk diseases are often initiated and always aggravated by excessive weight. Gout and obesity have a scientific as well as historical relationship. The risk of toxemia of pregnancy is higher in obese women. Surgical morbidity and mortality occur more often in patients with a high percent body fat.

To the individual, the sociological consequences of obesity may outweigh the medical risks. Correlations exist between certain social factors (employment, education, income, monthly rent) and obesity. The obese individual may also manifest a poor self-image, a sense of failure, and an externally passive approach to life situations.

Organic causes of obesity should be considered in overweight patients. Endocrine, neurologic, and genetic etiologies are estimated to be present in approximately 5% of obese patients. A careful history, physical, and routine chemistry profile will exclude most of the organic causes of obesity listed below:

Endocrine

Hypothyroidism
Cushing's

Stein-Leventhal
Insulinoma
Excessive insulin injections
Hypogonadal states

Neurologic

Ventromedial hypothalamic lesions (trauma, infection, tumor)
Pseudotumor cerebri
Empty sella syndrome
Hyperostosis frontalis interna

*Genetic (all predominantly characterized
by abnormal habitus and retardation)*

Prader-Willi
Albright's
Alström's
Fröhlich's
Laurence-Moon-Biedl

Dietary counseling should be provided for the obese patient. A program for weight reduction should include decreased caloric intake, increased caloric expenditure, and the development of new eating and activity habits. Carbohydrate deprivation is associated with a loss of water, sodium, and potassium, thus producing rapid weight loss in the early stages of dietary restriction. Fasting or semistarvation promotes similar fluid loss in addition to several metabolic derangements. Since loss of body fat depends ultimately on net caloric deficit, the energy-reduced diet should contain a reasonable distribution of protein, fat, and carbohydrate and serve as the basis for healthful long-term eating patterns.

Protein-energy malnutrition (adult marasmus) or adult kwashiorkor affects 25–50% of medical and surgical patients whose illness requires hospitalization for two weeks or more. In outpatients, severe underweight or malnutrition is more common in children and adult men of low-income groups.

Complicating effects of chronic protein-energy deprivation can be summarized as :

1. Depressed cell-mediated immunity with increased infection, particularly Gram-negative sepsis, pneumonia, and urinary tract infection
2. Impaired wound healing, wound infections, wound disruption, and bowel fistula
3. Decreased activity with delayed physical rehabilitation
4. Depressed ventilatory response to hypoxia

5.   Decreased response to chemotherapy for infection and cancer
6.   Delayed response in the completion of radiotherapy
7.   Increased occurrence of fluid and electrolyte problems

These patients demonstrate a fall in plasma levels of albumin, transferrin, branched-chain amino acids, cholesterol, and β-lipoprotein. Cellular immunity becomes impaired and complement activity may be inadequate.

The caloric intake of underweight or malnourished patients is an important part of medical management. When a patient is eating poorly, progressive weakness and apathy promote a decreased appetite in a self-porpetuating manner. Stress and infection increase the caloric requirement, and the presence of carcinoma may increase energy needs by 10–20%. Management should include an adequate dietary intake. A calorie-intake count for two or three days is useful. For patients who are unable to consume adequate food by mouth, nutritionally complete tube feedings and defined-formula diets are appropriate. For patients whose gastrointestinal tracts are either inadequate or nonfunctional, peripheral or intravenous hyperalimentation may be appropriate.

Altered taste sensations are often present in neoplastic diseases. Specifically, an increased taste threshold for sweet and a decreased taste threshold for bitter may be observed. Thus a higher concentration of a sweet solution is required for recognition, and meat may be reported as tasting bad or rotten. Individualized food selection and dietary patterns should be prescribed to identify acceptable food substances and to improve caloric intake.

With depression there is often a loss of appetite for food. The magnitude of weight loss may mimic severe organic diseases. Pain, fear, and anxiety may inhibit appetite. Anorexia nervosa, an eating disorder of psychological origin, is characterized by self-starvation and increased spontaneous physical activity.

Several pharmacological compounds adversely affect appetite and may cause dramatic weight loss. Drugs which may impair appetite include digitalis, anticholinergics, amphetamines, antibiotics, and gastric irritants such as salicylates, iron, and potassium salts.

Selected References

1.   Blackburn GL, Bistrian BR, Maini BS, Schlamm HT, Smith MF: Nutritional and metabolic assessment of the hospitalized patient. *J Parenteral Enteral Nutr* 1:11–22, 1977.
2.   Mann GV: The influence of obesity on health. *N Eng J Med* 291:178–185, 1974.
3.   Hamwi GJ: Therapy: Changing dietary concepts, in Danowski TS

(ed): *Diabetes Mellitus: Diagnosis and Treatment.* New York, American Diabetes Association, 1964, vol 1, pp 73–78.

4. Keys A, Grande F: Body weight, body composition and calorie status, in Goodhart RS, Shils ME (eds): *Modern Nutrition in Health and Disease,* ed 5. Philadelphia, Lea and Febiger, 1973, pp 1–27.

5. Mitchell HS, Rynbergen HJ, Anderson L, Dibble MJ: Weight control, in *Nutrition in Health and Disease,* ed 16. Philadelphia, JB Lippincott, 1976, pp 374–394.

6. Bruch H: *Eating Disorders: Obesity, Anorexia Nervosa, and the Person Within.* New York, Basic Books, 1973.

7. DuBois D, DuBois EF: The measurement of the surface area of man. *Arch Intern Med* 15:868–881, 1915.

8. Gehan EA, George SL: Estimation of human body surface area from height and weight. *Cancer Chemother Rep* 54:225–235, 1970.

9. Boren HG: Unusual causes of chronic respiratory insufficiency, in Baum GL (ed): *Textbook of Pulmonary Diseases,* ed 2. Boston, Little, Brown, 1974, pp 601–607.

10. Reisin E, Abel R, Modan M, Silverberg DS, Eliahou HE, Modan B: Effect of weight loss without salt restriction on the reduction of blood pressure in overweight hypertensive patients. *N Eng J Med* 298:1–6, 1978.

11. DeWys WD, Walters K: Abnormalities of taste sensation in cancer patients. *Cancer* 36:1888–1896, 1975.

126. Body Habitus

JOHN R. PREEDY, MD

Definition

Habitus is a latin noun meaning state or condition. Body habitus is a term which includes such considerations as physical appearance, bearing, physique, constitution, body build, and body proportions. In practice, the term is generally used to assess normal adult male or normal adult female physical appearance, as appropriate to the sex of the subject. In a more restricted application the ratio of length of limbs to the trunk is assessed.

Technique

Abnormal body habitus may occur because of virilization (in women), feminization (in men), or abnormal ratio of length of limbs to the trunk.

VIRILIZATION (OR VIRILISM)

Virilization (in women) occurs when the body habitus tends toward that of the man. The voice is deepened. There is thinning and loss of head hair. This is most marked in front (calvities frontalis, frontal balding, receding hair line). Hair appears on the upper lip, chin, cheeks, chest, breasts, and sometimes neck. Arms, legs, and back may become hairy, and existing hair may increase. Shaving or the use of depilatories may be necessary. Such increase in body hair is hirsuties. It should be noted that virilization includes hirsuties, but hirsuties can occur without virilization. Skin texture is coarsened. There is a greasy skin and acne vulgaris on face, chest, and upper back, and occasionally on upper arms. Breast areolae may be flattened in women in reproductive life. Breast size is usually not altered appreciably. Musculature is increased, particularly around the shoulders, and there is a reduction of fat deposits around the hips, giving the appearance of wider shoulders and narrower hips. The pubic hair is generally increased, and there is abdominal extension, which may reach the chest (male escutcheon). The clitoris is enlarged and may become erectile. The vulva may appear atrophic, but this is sometimes difficult to judge.

FEMINIZATION

Feminization (in men) occurs when the body habitus tends toward the female. There are fewer clinical features than in virilization, and it is therefore more difficult to detect. In addition, the clinical features vary, depending on whether the feminization has occurred before or after completion of normal puberty.

If feminization has occurred before puberty and the patient is seen in adult life, the voice remains high-pitched, the head hair is fine, and there is no recession of the hair line (that is, no valvities frontalis or frontal balding). There is scanty facial hair, and the patient rarely shaves. There is no hair on the chest, scanty axillary hair, and scanty hair on the limbs; body hair is quite fine. The skin remains fine in texture, particularly that of the face and arms. The skin lacks normal male greasiness and there is little if any acne. Musculature remains poorly developed. This is particularly obvious around the shoulders. Lack of strength may be reported. There is increased fat deposition around the hips, giving the appearance of narrow shoulders and broad hips. Pubic hair is often scanty, and the upper margin is horizontal. There is no abdominal extension of pubic hair (that is, a female escutcheon). The most striking feature is gynecomastia.

If feminization has occurred after completion of normal puberty, many of the above features are absent or difficult to detect. The voice remains low-pitched. There is no change in head hair. There is little apparent change in facial hair, but the patient may report less frequent shaving. There is no change in body hair. There is no apparent change in body musculature. Diminished strength is only occasionally reported. Occasionally there may be some accumulation of fat around the hips. Pubic hair remains unchanged. Gynecomastia is prominent and is usually the only definite clinical finding.

ABNORMAL RATIO OF LENGTHS OF LIMBS TO TRUNK

Normal ratios. In normal infancy and early childhood the trunk is longer than the limbs. As age increases, the limbs grow proportionately longer, until about age 10 the limbs and trunk are the same length. This equality continues into and through adult life.

Collection of item. The patient stands upright (if old enough). The distance between the crown of the head (highest point) and the symphysis pubis is measured. This length is the "trunk" or "upper segment." The distance between the symphysis pubis and the floor is the "leg" or "lower segment." The distance between the sternal notch and the tips of the fingers is measured with the arms stretched out laterally ("arms"). In the normal subject over age 10, all three measurements should be equal. (Sometimes in the very tall normal adult man, the "limbs" may be longer than the "trunk".)

Abnormal ratios. These may be readily detected. The trunk (in the subject over age 10) may be longer than the limbs, or conversely, the limbs may be longer than the trunk.

Background Information

Normal body habitus in the adult subject as defined above is dependent in part upon normal secretion of the appropriate hormones by the gonads at puberty. (Before puberty, the body habitus of the male and female is quite similar, that is, neutral.) It is only after puberty that the distinguishing differences appear. In fact, appropriate normal body habitus constitutes a secondary sexual character. Estrogens are principally responsible for the development of secondary sexual characteristics (including body habitus) in the female. Testosterone is principally responsible in the male. If the appropriate gonadal hormone is absent, the secondary sexual characters will tend toward the neutral (or prepubertal) state, in so far as this is possible. If there is a relative excess of hormones appropriate to the opposite sex, then virilization may be expected to occur in the female, and feminization in the male.

Clinical Significance

VIRILIZATION

The immediate cause is always an excess of androgens. The androgens may be exogenous or endogenous. Exogenous androgens may be administered therapeutically. These include anabolic agents. Excess endogenous androgens may arise from the adrenal or the ovary. Androgen-producing disorders of the adrenal include Cushing's syndrome (hyperplasia or tumor), androgen-producing adrenal tumors, congenital or acquired adrenal hyperplasia. Disorders of the ovary include Stein-Leventhal syndrome, ovarian thecomatosis, Leydig cell hyperplasia, various ovarian tumors (of which arrhenoblastoma is perhaps the best known), and cysts. Features somewhat resembling mild virilization may occur after the menopause, in which case the mechanism may be a reduction in estrogen levels proportionate to androgens.

FEMINIZATION

Since feminization is almost always associated with gynecomastia, the causes of feminization will be those of gynecomastia (q.v.).

ABNORMAL PROPORTIONS

Alterations in the ratio of length of limb to trunk may involve an increased limb to trunk ratio, or a decreased limb to trunk ratio. An increased limb to trunk ratio is seen in gonadal hormone deficiency, and is due to failure of the epiphysis of the long bones to close at the normal age. This abnormal proportion is seen in failure of testosterone secretion by the testicle in men, and failure of estrogen secretion by the ovary in women.

A decreased limb to trunk ratio is seen principally (but not exclusively) in hypothyroidism of any cause. The attainment of normal adult proportions appears to be dependent on adequate secretion of thyroid hormones during childhood. If hypothyroidism persists into the teens, then the abnormal proportion may be permanent. A decreased limb to trunk ratio is also seen in certain chondrodystrophies.

Selected References

1. Dillon RS: *Handbook of Endocrinology.* Philadelphia, Lea and Febiger, 1973, pp 469–474.
2. Kirschner MA, Bardin CW: Androgen production and metabolism in normal and virilized women. *Metabolism* 21:667, 1972.
3. Bardin CW, Lipsett MB: Testosterone and androsterone production ratio in normal women and women with idiopathic hirsuties or gonadotrophic ovaries. *J Clin Invest* 46:89, 1967.
4. Tanner JM, in Gardner LI (ed): *Endocrine and Genetic Diseases of Childhood.* Philadelphia, WB Saunders, 1975, chap 1, pp 19–59.

---

127. Hair

ALGIE C. BROWN, MD

Definition

Hair refers to the fine, cylindrical filaments growing from the skin. Hirsutism means excessive hair growth. Alopecia means too little or absent hair growth.

Technique

Observe the total body hair distribution including scalp, eyebrows, eyelashes, axillae, trunk, extremities, and pubic area. Determine if there is an abnormal quantity or quality of hair in these locations. Look for adjacent cutaneous eruptions in areas of localized hair loss. If hair is lost over portions of the scalp, determine if it is in a bifrontal distribution or localized to the occipital area where the head rests in a stuporous state. Determine if scalp hair loss is diffuse, localized or patchy, smooth or bristled.

Specialized techniques have evolved for improved objective description of the anatomical, physical, and biochemical properties of hair. These include skin biopsy to determine the presence or absence of follicles; the hair pluck technique for microscopic definition of hair cycles and filament type; scanning electron microscopic evaluation of hair surface structure; physical measurements of the hair shaft diameter; tensile strength and hair growth rate; and biochemical measurement of sulfur as a screen for the major structural amino acid, cystine. Lead, arsenic, cadmium, and other heavy metals tend to accumulate in hair as a permanent record of environmental or other exposure. Approximately 50–100 mg of clippings from the proximal shafts of scalp are sufficient for analysis if indicated. When sample size is limited, skin electron microscopy with energy-dispersive x-ray analysis can be helpful. The interested reader should consult reference 1 for a discussion of these special techniques.

Background Information

Hair is the fastest growing tissue in the body, reproducing itself every 15 hours. Normal hair grows at a rate of approximately 0.35 mm/day (10–12 mm/month) in adults and slightly faster in children. Hair growth occurs with a rapid metabolic turnover rate, characterized by a high requirement of protein. Substrate protein, however, is supplied with a low priority relative to other protein-requiring metabolic processes. The color, distribution, and number of hair follicles are genetically coded. Hormonal influences such as puberty alter follicle size and therefore the visibility of hair.

The shaft of the hair is composed of the cuticle, cortex, and medulla. The cuticle is a proteinaceous coating of scales arranged in a spiral pattern. The cortex is composed of molecules of keratin protein with an unusually high content of cystine (and some methionine) represented by a hair sulfur content of 4.52–5.15% by weight.

An average hair filament has a diameter of 0.11–0.14 mm and grows in three phases, each producing a characteristic filament. Eighty to ninety percent of hairs are in an active growth phase (anagen), lasting about three years. Approximately 1% of hairs are in a transitional or regression growth phase (catagen), lasting a few weeks. Ten to twenty percent of hairs are in a resting phase (telogen), lasting two to four months. The telogen phase is characteristic of the 50–100 hairs normally lost per day. The relative proportion of anagen or telogen hair loss is determined by microscopic examination of the follicles of 40–50 hairs obtained by the hair pluck technique. Anagen hair follicles appear as a "fan." Telogen hair follicles resemble a club or chicken drum stick. An alteration in the hair cycle is indicated if more than 34% of the follicles are telogen.

Excessive hair growth occurs idiopathically, in certain genodermatoses, as a side effect of pharmacologic agents such as minoxidil, and as an effect of androgens such as testosterone, dihydrotestosterone, α-4-androstenedione, and dehydroepiandrosterone.

Clinical Significance

Hair loss may be related to hereditary biochemical abnormalities, acquired defects in protein synthesis, localized inflammatory conditions, immunological disorders, toxic effects of drugs, and various types of physical, chemical, or thermal injury. Absence of hair may also result from a scarring process which may be acquired with lupus erythematosus or scarring alopecia of the scalp. Hereditary defects include many disorders of amino acid metabolism, abnormalities of chromosomes, and defects in development of ectoderm.

Systemic illnesses such as malnutrition cause defective hair growth and hair loss. A transient decrease in hair growth causes a constriction or pencil-pointing of the hair shaft, known as Pohl's sign. The location of this constriction in the hair shaft can date the insult, assuming 10–12 mm/month of subsequent hair growth. Similarly, the date or frequency of toxic administration of arsenic can be estimated by measuring the arsenic content of various segments of the hair shaft. Similar types of hair loss may also occur with conditions such as cirrhosis, uncontrolled diabetes, hypopituitarism, iron deficiency, hyper or hypothyroidism, hyper or hypoparathyroidism, and the postpartum state. Agents which may produce anagen or telogen hair loss would include vitamin A, arsenic, heparin, coumarins, allopurinol, gentamycin, colchicine, L-dopa, propranolol, and cytotoxic agents.

Cytotoxic agents predominantly affect actively growing (anagen) hairs and produce thinning or total hair loss, depending on the dose of drug delivered to the cell. This usually begins within the first month of therapy and may result in a spectrum of damage ranging from narrowing of the shaft to complete hair loss. It is more prominent with doxorubicin and cyclophosphamide than with methotrexate or azathioprine. Regeneration usually occurs within one to two months of tapering or discontinuing the drug. Regrowth may yield either darker or white hair depending on whether the initial injury caused stimulation or suppression of hair melanocytes.

Localized fungal infection can also cause hair loss by involvement of the cuticle and cortex or keratin of the hair shaft. This is particularly true of dermophytic involvement of the eyelashes or eyebrows such as with fungi acquired from pets, contaminated cosmetics, or epidemic *Tinea capitis* in schoolchildren.

Alopecia areata is an inherited autoimmune disorder which may frequently be associated with other autoimmune disorders such as Hashimoto's thyroiditis, pernicious anemia, idiopathic Addison's disease, diabetes mellitus, orchitis, oophoritis, vitiligo, and atopic dermatitis. Thirty-five percent of patients with alopecia areata have some form of endocrine disease.

Physical, chemical, and thermal hair injury is characterized by damage to the surface of the hair with breakage, splitting, and fracturing of the hair shaft ("paint brush hair"). This condition is generally referred to as trichorrhexis fracture and may occur as an acquired or inherited defect. Acquired trichorrhexis occurs most frequently on the scalp and genitoinguinocrural region secondary to cutaneous pruritus or external trauma to the hair shaft.

Hirsutism should be investigated for benign and malignant endocrine causes of excessive androgen activity. The androgens may be of an adrenal or ovarian source. Endocrine causes of hirsutism commonly produce associated virilization manifest by excessive muscularity, deepening of the voice, and enlargement of the clitoris. Idiopathic hirsutism sometimes has mild elevation of various androgens but never enough to cause virilization. Slight androgen excess may, however, be enough to induce a male pattern of baldness in women. This type of baldness must be differentiated from the chronic, accumulative scarring of the scalp caused by hair dye abuse. Excessive endogenous or exogenous corticosteroids may also be associated with hypertrichosis, often on the face, arms, and back. Reference 7 should be consulted for an excellent series of photographs exemplary of various diseases of hair.

Selected References

1. Brown AC: *The First Human Hair Symposium.* New York, Medcom, 1974.
2. Crounse RG, Van Scott EJ: Changes in scalp hair roots as a measure of toxicity from cancer chemotherapeutic drugs. *J Invest Derm* 35:83–90, 1960.
3. Chernosky ME, Owens DW: Trichorrhexis nodosa: Clinical and investigative studies. *Arch Derm* 94:577–585, 1966.
4. Porter PS: Genetic disorders of hair growth. *J Invest Derm* 60:493–502, 1973.
5. Preedy JRK: Endocrine investigation in hirsuties, in Brown AC (ed): *The First Human Hair Symposium,* New York, Medcom, 1974.
6. Kirschner MA, Zucker IR, Jespersen D: Idiopathic hirsutism: An ovarian abnormality. *New Engl J Med* 294:637–640, 1976.
7. Brown AC: Diseases of the hair, in Stephens GG (ed): *Continuing Education for the Family Physician.* New York, John Wiley and Sons, 1979.

128. Physical Examination of the Skin

HENRY E. JONES, MD

Definition

The skin is comprised of the surface tissue and the supportive integument. The outermost keratinized and cornefied layers are of two types: the hard keratin of the hair and nails, and the soft keratin of the general body skin. The skin is the largest organ, accounting for approximately 20% of adult body weight and having a surface area of almost 2 sq m.

Background Information

If one approaches the clinical evaluation of the patient with dermatological disease in the same manner as one approaches the patient with internal disease, it leads to a generally difficult, frustrating, and unrewarding experience. This occurs because of many factors: (1) the necessity of memorizing vast numbers of loosely related facts and diseases, (2) a complicated Latin nomenclature, (3) the relative dissociation of symptomatology and the eruption, and (4) a seemingly complex system for classification of skin diseases.

In the clinical evaluation of the skin, a clinician has the opportunity to directly visualize and examine all aspects of the healthy or diseased organ. To make full use of this advantage, dermatologists examine the skin prior to obtaining a detailed history. This approach minimizes bias which cannot otherwise be avoided if the history is taken first. Objective data always take precedence over subjective data in clinical evaluation of the skin.

When examining the skin, the clinician should make full use of his senses of sight, touch, and smell. Five technical aides are often helpful in the dermatologic exam: (1) a 10x-power magnification loop, (2) a diascopy tool (a short section of glass or transparent plastic), (3) a Wood's lamp or other black light source emitting light at 360 nm, (4) a penlight for examining the oral cavity, (5) a safety pin for estimating sensation.

Technique

After obtaining a brief history which includes the anatomical site or sites affected and the duration of the complaint, proceed with the physical exam. Explain to the patient that he needs to undress and drape so that the skin examination may be thorough. Advise the patient that you do not want to miss anything, and that a trained eye might note very subtle changes in the skin. It is often advisable to have an attendant assist during the exam.

The examination must be conducted in ample lighting, preferably natural lighting from a window or skylight. First examine the affected area(s). On occasion, the exam can be terminated at this point, but only if the diagnosis is immediately obvious to the patient and clinician and there would be no advantage in further examination. This is seldom the case, however, and one should proceed to examine the rest of the integument.

Examination with the patient sitting. Ordinarily, with the patient sitting on an examining table, one initially examines the hands and upper extremities. Much valuable information can be gleaned from careful notation of the hands. For example, red, scaling areas on the palm may be a manifestation of secondary syphilis. Periungual telangiectasia is a common finding in the collagen vascular diseases. Pits in the nail surface can be a marker for psoriasis. Subungual and periungual changes can be diagnostic of skin diseases such as lichen planus, infections, and even hereditary diseases such as tuberous sclerosis. The skin of the dorsum of the hand receives intense ultraviolet light exposure and may harbor subtle changes suggestive of skin or systemic disease. In examination of the skin of the forearm and arms, note the distensibility or elasticity of the skin as a gauge of the state of hydration.

Move from the upper extremities to the head and neck. Carefully examine the skin of the different areas of the face including forehead, eyelids, ears, nose, and lips. Examine the mucosae of the nose carefully. Examination of the lips presents an opportunity for evaluation of the mucous membranes of the buccal cavity, the teeth, the gingiva, the tongue, and the posterior pharynx. Again, one should keep in mind that there are many cutaneous and systemic diseases that have an expression in the mucosae lining the oral cavity, nose, and eye.

Next examine the hair and scalp for abnormalities, including the loss of hair or lesions of the scalp. Pay particular attention for scaling areas in the occipital region and in the otic canal as these may be common but subtle expressions of psoriasis. Note the texture, length, color, and any abnormalities of the hair. Also note the pattern and distribution of hair over the body during the rest of the physical exam, ie, normal or hirsutism.

With the patient sitting on the examining table and facing the window or other light source, next examine the expanse of skin over the chest. The skin of the infraclavicular area, when gently pinched between the thumb and first finger, is an ideal site to estimate skin turgor and thus the patient's state of hydration. In women, it is important to examine the skin of the breast, particularly the nipple region, since this may be the only area in which typical burrows of scabies can be found.

Examination with the patient prone. With the patient lying prone on the examining table, examine the skin of the posterior aspects of the body. Examine the back carefully, looking for any abnormalities of color or texture. The skin of the back of the average person above 20 years of age will contain several nevi, and each nevus should be examined carefully. See section 83, Change in Mole.

While the patient is prone, examine the posterior thighs and buttocks including the skin of the gluteal cleft and perianal area. Pay particular attention to the condition of the skin in this intertriginous area. Include the mucous membranes of the anus. It is convenient to examine the skin of the posterior aspect of the lower extremities, particularly the calf area with the patient prone.

Examination with the patient supine. Have the patient turn over and examine the lower abdomen and inguinal area, including the perineum and genitalia. Pay particular attention to the presence or absence of inguinal and femoral nodes. Note the presence or absence of urethral discharge and the condition of the mucous membranes. In men, note the presence or absence of circumcision. In women, proceed with the pelvic examination.

Next examine the anterior aspects of the lower extremities, including the thighs, knees, and pretibial area. Thyroid disease and diabetes may be first suspected by skin changes in the pretibial area.

Next, ask the patient to sit on the examining table and extend his legs. This makes it convenient to do a thorough examination of the feet. Survey the plantar surface of the feet for discrete abnormalities as well as color and texture. Examine the toenails and periungual tissue as well as the skin of the toe web spaces (particularly the third and fourth spaces which are particularly susceptible to intertrigo and dermatophytosis). The general quality of the skin, color, turgor, and the presence or absence of hair growth are additional considerations.

Even in the absence of complaints related to the skin, the cutaneous exam as outlined above should be performed regularly. Never should we pass up an opportunity to detect a subtle cutaneous sign of systemic or cutaneous disease.

Clinical Significance

All skin lesions may be classified as belonging to one of two groups: (1) primary lesions and (2) secondary lesions. The term primary lesion does not refer to the first lesion experienced and has no relationship to the history or chronology of the disease. Primary lesion refers to those changes in the fine anatomy of the skin that reflect a true and natural expression of the disease process without modification by factors external to the skin or person. In contrast, the term secondary lesion denotes an abnormality of the skin in which the anatomical lesion has been altered by external factors. Examples include excoriation from scratching, maceration from excessive moisture, or cracking from excessive dryness.

The primary lesions are 12 in number and include macule, papule, vesicle, bulla, pustule, plaque, nodule, tumor, cyst, wheal, comedone, and telangiectasia. The secondary lesions consist of scale, crust, fissure lichenification, erosion, excoriation, ulcer, scar, atrophy. Describe all cutaneous abnormalities by the appropriate primary or secondary term(s).

The configuration of each lesion and the distribution over the integument must be noted. For example, a group of vesicles on an erythematous base is suggestive of herpes simplex, whereas vesicles randomly distributed over the skin suggest a variety of diseases other than herpes simplex. Distribution is likewise important. For example, dermatitis occurring only on the back of the hands, forehead, ears, and tip of the nose strongly suggests photosensitivity. Photosensitivity may be due to many things, including systemic disease or reaction to medication.

With objective information one can usually classify the patient's disease as one of the following 10 fundamental disease groupings (see Callen et al.):

1. Macular (pigmentary) changes
2. Papulosquamous disease
3. Vesiculobullous disorders
4. Eczema dermatitis group
5. Erythema group reactions
6. Nodulotumor group
7. Disorders of the hair and nails
8. Sexually transmitted diseases
9. Cutaneous infections, infestations, and bites
10. Cutaneous manifestations of systemic disease

At this point in the examination of a patient with primary dermatologic complaints, the clinician should proceed with a detailed medical history, family history, and review of systems. This additional subjective data will occasionally indicate that a portion of the physical examination be repeated; the history may also enable one to establish a more definitive diagnosis.

Several hundred disorders involve the skin. Some affect only the skin and never the deeper tissues, ie, acne; others are cutaneous manifestations of a systemic or visceral disease. Skin disease is extremely prevalent. The 10 most prevalent skin diseases in the American population affect nearly 29 million individuals.

	Disease	Number Affected
1.	Acne	11.5 million
2.	Dermatophytosis	8.7 million
3.	Tumors	2.4 million
4.	Atopic or eczema	2.4 million
5.	Ichthyosis	1.1 million
6.	Pyoderma	1.0 million
7.	Psoriasis	0.63 million
8.	Warts	0.43 million
9.	Vitiligo	0.39 million
10.	Herpes simplex	0.35 million

In the National Ambulatory Medical Care Survey of 1975, patients having skin diseases accounted for approximately 7% of all outpatients seen. Dermatologists provide care for approximately 40% of these patients with skin disease, whereas primary physicians and various medical and surgical specialists provide medical care for the remaining 60%. Thus, all clinicians must be prepared to perform an adequate clinical examination so that the common and even rare diseases that affect the skin may be recognized and properly managed.

Selected References

1.   Callen JP, Stawiski MS, Vorrhees JJ: *Dermatology: A Teaching Manual.* Ann Arbor, University of Michigan Department of Dermatology, 1977.
2.   Johnson MLT: *Prevalence of Dermatological Disease among Persons 1–74 Years of Age: United States.* Advanced Data, HEW No. 4-1977.
3.   Fitzpatrick TB, Arndt KA, Clark WH Jr, et al (eds): *Dermatology in General Medicine.* New York, McGraw-Hill, 1971.
4.   Rook A, Wilkerson DS, Ebling JG (eds): *Textbook of Dermatology,* ed 2. Oxford, Blackwell Scientific Publications, 1972.
5.   Demis DJ, et al (eds): *Clinical Dermatology.* Hagerstown, Md, Harper and Row, 1975.
6.   The National Ambulatory Medical Care Survey: 1975 Summary. *Vital and Health Statistics,* Series 13, No. 33, DHEW Publication No. PHS 78-1784.

129. Nails

JOHN A. WARD, MD

Definition

The nails are epidermal appendages overlaying the distal phalanges of the dorsal surfaces of the fingers and toes (Fig 15). While they are derived from the skin, they possess one quality not often obvious in the skin; that is, they record metabolic events that may have occurred weeks or months previously. These metabolic derangements may be continuing up to the present. It is this quality of the nails that gives them importance in the physical examination.

Background Information

The nails form from the nail matrix and grow about 0.105–0.123 mm per day, depending on the subject's age. The usual visual adult nail is 10–15 mm in length and would thus require 3–4 months to grow out completely. A portion of the matrix can be seen through the nail plate as the lunula. Metabolic events are frequently recorded during nail growth in the form of grooves or discolorations. Thus as a paleontologist can gaze at the variation in the rings of petrified wood and deduce climatological conditions in a prehistoric forest, the clinician can recognize deranged metabolism by recording events in the nail.

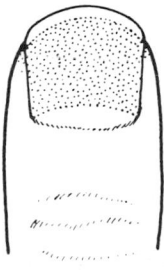

Figure 15. The normal nail. The stippled area is the normal pink nail.

Unfortunately, the nail has only a limited number of ways it is affected by deranged metabolic processes. For this reason, the nail changes in themselves are not often diagnostic of a specific condition. It is not surprising to find that a particular nail pattern has been reported in several disease states.

Terry's nails appear white to within 1 or 2 mm of the distal border where there is a distal zone of normal pink (Fig 16). The lunula may be obscured. Although Terry described these findings in hepatic cirrhosis, he noted that whiteness of the nail had been seen in chronic congestive heart failure, diabetes, pulmonary tuberculosis, rheumatoid arthritis, viral hepatitis (convalescence), disseminated sclerosis, and some forms of carcinoma.

Lindsay's nails are the "half-and-half" nail (Fig 17). The proximal portion is whitish while the distal portion is red, pink, or brown. The distal band comprises 20–60% of the nail. These nails are seen in chronic renal failure.

Mees' lines are transverse white bands parallel to the lunula occurring in the nail at the same relative position on each finger (Fig 18). They may be single or multiple. Although Mees described these changes as

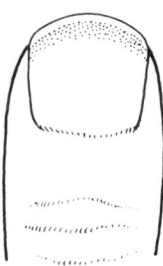

Figure 16.   Terry's nails. The lunula is obscured by a whitening of the nail. The pink color is observed only at the distal portion of the nail at the free edge.

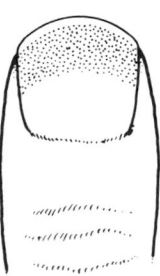

Figure 17.   The half-and-half nail. The lunula tends to be obscured.

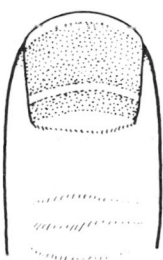

Figure 18. Mees' lines. A white band in the nail is parallel to the lunula. Such lines can be multiple exposures to incidents that produce them; with two such bands they may resemble Muehrcke's lines (see Fig 5).

occurring with arsenic intoxication, similar white lines have been seen after acute and chronic renal failure as well as other conditions such as thallium intoxication, leprosy, malaria, fluorosis, psoriasis, cardiac insufficiency, pellagra, Hodgkin's disease, pneumonia, myocardial infarction, sickle cell anemia, and infectious fevers. Drugs must be added to this list, especially cancer chemotherapeutic agents.

Muehrcke's lines are paired transverse white bands parallel to the lunula in the fingernails of patients with hypoalbuminemia, especially when the serum albumin level is below 2.2 g/100 ml (Fig 19). The conditions causing hypoalbuminemia are often associated with independent nail changes which tend to obscure Muehrcke's lines. Examples include Terry's nails in hepatic cirrhosis and Lindsay's half-and-half nails in renal failure.

Beau's lines are transverse grooves parallel to the lunula in the nail occurring on each nail at the same relative position (Fig 20). They are

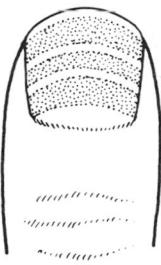

Figure 19. Muehrcke's lines. Two parallel white bands which are seen with low serum albumin.

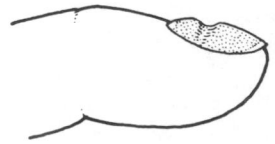

Figure 20.   Beau's lines. These are transverse grooves parallel to the lunula.

usually seen following significant infections or a severe period of illness. They may be helpful in dating a serious illness.

In onycholysis the line of separation of the nail plate from the hyponychium occurs in an irregular fashion and somewhat more proximal than usual (Fig 21). While onycholysis occurs with psoriasis and other skin diseases as well as local trauma, it is frequently a good sign of thyrotoxicosis, past or present. That is, patients who are euthyroid may still display onycholysis. The onycholysis of hyperthyroidism is most likely to occur on the ring fingers.

Koilonychia (spoon nails) appear concave rather than convex (Fig 22) and are important in that they may be associated with an anemia. They may also occur as a result of local effects on the nail from strong soaps or detergents.

Clubbing is best appreciated viewing the nail from the side and evaluating the angle the nail plate makes with the digit (Fig 23). Normally this is less than 180°. At 180° minimal clubbing is present. At greater than 180° definite clubbing is present. The base of the nail is easily depressed by the fingernail, giving the impression that the nail matrix under the cuticle is "spongy." Clubbing may be a clue to serious diseases such as chronic lung disease, certain inflammatory bowel diseases, cirrhosis, or congenital heart disease.

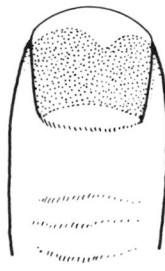

Figure 21.   Onycholysis. There is undercutting of the free edge of the nail, usually on the ring finger.

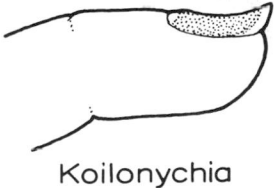

Koilonychia

Figure 22. Note the angle the surface of the nail is concave rather than convex.

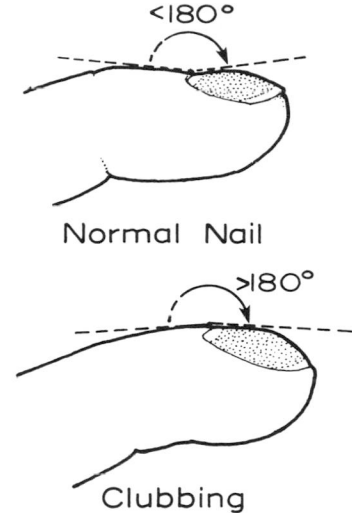

Figure 23. Note the angle the nail makes with the finger.

Splinter hemorrhages appear as small, brown or red linear streaks seen through the nail plate, usually in the more distal portion. These may represent microemboli, as seen in bacterial endocarditis. However, they are not diagnostic of bacterial endocarditis, because they may occur in up to 10% of hospital admissions. In the setting of fever and heart murmur, the occurrence of newly appearing "splinters" may be very significant.

Psoriasis is usually a condition of the skin, but the nails may also be involved. The nail may be thickened, display onycholysis, and exhibit pits in the nail plate. The typical pitting may be small enough to require closeup views of the nail. In general, nail involvement is more likely to be seen in the more severe forms of the disease.

Onychomycosis is infestation of the nails with a fungus and frequently results in a discolored nail, which appears thickened due to accumulation of subungual keratin. Cultures of the nail scrapings are necessary to identify the organism.

Blue lunulae have been reported in Wilson's disease. Slate bluish lunulae may be seen with argyria.

Red lunulae are red half-moons that have been reported in congestive heart failure.

Pigmented bands that are black have been reported in a patient with Peutz-Jegher's syndrome. Longitudinal pigmented bands have been noted with adrenal insufficiency. Transverse green bands were reported to be produced by a paronychial infection due to *Pseudomonas aeruginosa*.

Yellow nails are slow growing and are reported to occur with edema. These are thought to be related to defective lymphatic drainage.

White nails may represent leuconychia totalis, which is inherited as a simple dominant. Leuconychia punctata are white patches without known significance.

The shell nail is clubbing in reverse, that is, the angle the nail plate makes with the digit becomes more acute than obtuse. The shell nail is reported to occur with bronchiectasis.

In onychogryphosis the nail forms a hornlike structure. These nails present a problem in management and may require minor surgery.

Telangiectasia are at times visible through the nail in such conditions as hereditary hemorrhagic telangiectasia. The disease is usually evident by telangiectasia elsewhere.

A postmetabolic disorder may be observed at times (Fig 24). A band of normal pink nail growing from the lunula to a white ground glass-appearing nail may be seen signifying that the metabolic event which originally caused the whitish opacification of the nail has been corrected, and normal nail is now being formed.

The causes of distortion of shape, color, contour, or texture are not completely understood. Many varied metabolic events are recorded in similar manner in the nail structure. Most of the changes described are

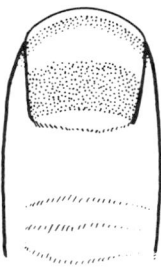

Figure 24. Postmetabolic reversible disorder. The normal nail is growing proximal to the abnormal nail.

not pathognomonic of a single condition. However, they should suggest diagnostic possibilities to the examiner. Perhaps one of the most helpful is Mees' lines. While these lines may be of diverse etiologies, they should alert the examiner to conduct proper tests to rule out arsenic intoxication. These lines may be the stimulus that produces the correct diagnostic procedures to solve a previously baffling illness and if arsenic intoxication is discovered, a life may be saved.

Selected References

1. Bean WB: Discourse on nail growth and unusual finger nails. *Trans Am Clin Climat Assoc* 74:152–167, 1963.
2. Bean WB: Nail growth: Twenty-five years' observation. *Arch Intern Med* 122:359–361, 1968.
3. Terry R: White nails in hepatic cirrhosis. *Lancet* 1:757–759, 1954.
4. Lindsay PG: The half and half nail. *J Lab Clin Med* 66:892, 1965.
5. Lindsay PG: The half and half nail. *Arch Intern Med* 119:583–587, 1967.
6. Mees RA: Een verschijnsel bij polyneuritis arsenicosa. *Nedrl T Geneesk* 1:391–396, 1919: abstr, *JAMA* 72:1337, 1919.
7. Conomy JP: A succession of Mees' lines in arsenical polyneuropathy. *Postgrad Med* 52:97–99, 1972.
8. Hudson JB, Dennis AJ: Transverse white lines in the fingernails after acute and chronic renal failure. *Arch Intern Med* 117:276–279, 1966.
9. Muehrcke RC: The fingernails in chronic hypoalbuminaemia. *Br Med J* 1:1327–1331, 1956.
10. Domonkos AN: *Diseases of the Akin Appendages in Andrews' Diseases of the Skin.* Philadelphia, WB Saunders, 1971, p 874.
11. Samman PD: The nails, in *Textbook of Dermatology.* Philadelphia, FA Davis, 1968, p 1431.
12. Anderson NP: Syndrome of spoon nails, anemia, cheilitis and dysphagia. *Arch Derm Syph* 37:816–822, 1938.
13. Lewin K: The fingernail in general disease: A macroscopic and microscopic study. *Br J Derm* 77:431–438, 1965.
14. Kilpatrick ZM: Splinter hemorrhages: Their clinical significance. *Arch Intern Med* 115:730–735, 1965.
15. Halprin KM: Afflictions of a vestigial appendage: Three disorders of free edge and lateral margins of human nail. *JAMA* 203:513, 1968.
16. Emmons CW, Binford CH, Utz JP: *Medical Mycology.* Philadelphia, Lea and Febiger, 1970, p 112.
17. Bearn AG, McKusick VA: An unusual change in the finger nails in two patients with hepatolenticular degeneration. *JAMA* 166:904–906, 1958.

18. Terry R: Red half-moons in cardiac failure. *Lancet* 3, 842–844, 1954.
19. Valero A, Sherf K: Pigmented nails in the Peutz-Jegher's syndrome. *Am J Gastroent* 43:56–58, 1965.
20. Allenby CF, Snell PH: Longitudinal pigmentation of the nails in Addison's disease. *Br Med J* 5503:1582–1583, 1966.
21. Bondy PK, Harwick HJ: Longitudinal banded pigmentation of nails following adrenalectomy. *N Eng J Med* 281:1056–1057, 1969.
22. Shellow WV, et al: Green striped nails: Chromonychia due to pseudomonas aeruginosa. *Arch Derm* 97:149–53, 1968.
23. Samman PD, White WF: The "yellow nail" syndrome. *Br J Derm* 76:153–157, 1964.
24. Harrington JF: White fingernails. *Arch Intern Med* 114:301–306, 1964.
25. Samman PD: Abnormalities of the nails. *Postgrad Med* 38:595–603, 1965.
26. Cornelius CE, Shelley WB: Shell nail syndrome associated with bronchiectasis. *Arch Derm* 96:694–695, 1967.
27. Samman PD: *The Nails in Disease,* ed 2. Springfield, Ill, Charles C Thomas, 1972.
28. Pardo-Castello V, Pardo OA: *Diseases of the Nails,* ed 3. Springfield, Ill, Charles C Thomas, 1960.

HEAD, EARS, NOSE

130. Cranial and Orbital Bruits

JOSEPH E. HARDISON, MD

Definition

Cranial and orbital bruits are sounds resulting from increased flow or obstruction to flow in the intracranial and extracranial vessels. The sounds may be systolic, primarily systolic with extension into diastole, or continuous. The sounds may arise within the cranium or be transmitted from the vessels in the neck or from valvular lesions in the heart.

Technique

The patient is asked to sit and to close both eyes. The examiner faces the patient and places the diaphragm of the stethoscope against the patient's closed eye. The pressure exerted should be firm but not painful. The patient is then asked to open the other eye (Fig 25). This maneuver helps eliminate eyelid tremor. The patient is then asked to hold his breath. Orbital bruits may be loud or faint and are often high pitched; the examiner must "tune in" as he does to hear aortic insufficiency. The skull is then auscultated with the bell or the diaphragm over the mastoid prominences, the forehead, and the lateral areas of the skull. The neck is auscultated to detect carotid bruits. Bruits which are especially loud or which arise high in the carotid may be heard over bony prominences or the orbits.

The patient may hear noises that seem to originate from within the head or ears. Patients may hear their own heartbeat, and this is usually described as a "thump, thump." If patients hear an arterial bruit, they usually describe an intermittent rhythmical hissing sound not unlike a steam locomotive climbing a hill. Venous hums are sometimes heard by a patient and are described as a continuous roaring noise. Occlusion of the internal jugular vein will eliminate this noise, thus differentiating it from arterial bruits and tinnitus.

Tinnitus is a noise that the patient hears but the physician cannot. This usually results from a problem in the ear and is described as ringing, crackling, popping, something frying, or a bunch of crickets. It is

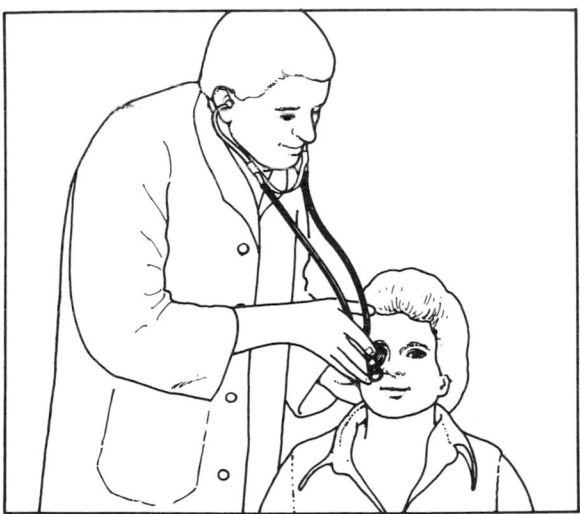

Figure 25. Technique for listening for orbital bruits.

often chaotic, irregularly intermittent, or continuous and should not be confused with arterial sounds that are coincident with the pulse.

If the patient complains of a noise which the physician cannot hear, it may be rewarding to modify the stethoscope by removing the bell and diaphragm and replacing them with another set of earpieces. Placing one set of earpieces into the examiner's ears and the other set into the patient's ears, the physician can sometimes hear the noise the patient is hearing and may be able to better localize the sound by occluding one tube of the stethoscope and then the other (Fig 26).

Background Information

The first recorded observation of a bruit in the head appears to have been made by Travers, an anatomy instructor at Guys Hospital, who noted this finding in a patient who probably had a carotid artery cavernous sinus fistula.

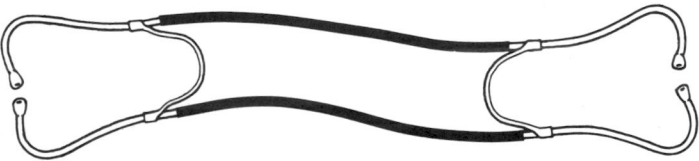

Figure 26a.   Two stethoscopes joined together so clinician and patient can listen together.

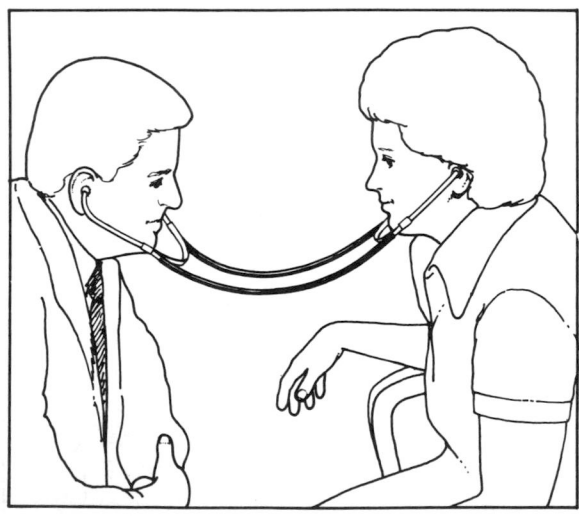

Figure 26b.   Clinician and patient listening to tinnitus or bruits together.

Since that time, many physicians have recommended auscultation of the skull and orbits as a routine part of the physical examination. Nevertheless it is often neglected, even when definitely indicated, as in patients who have seizure disorders or headaches or who complain of a noise in the head. Arterial bruits are produced by vibration of the vessel wall. This occurs as a result of turbulent or vortical blood flow. Turbulence refers to completely chaotic blood flow, and although frequently present, it is of doubtful significance in the genesis of vascular sound. The infinite directions of random eddies favor dissipation of energy to heat rather than sound. Vortical flow results from periodic swirling of blood about a local obstruction and probably produces most of the sound heard. The regular vortices impart forces directed perpendicularly to the direction of flow, which result in vibration of the vessel wall at frequencies of audible sound.

Clinical Significance

Cranial and orbital bruits are normal in infants and young children, but in the adult are always indicative of an underlying abnormality. The bruits result from conditions where flow is increased, viscosity is decreased, or there is an obstruction to flow.

The major causes of cranial and orbital bruits in the adult in probable order of frequency are:

1. Anemia
2. Atherosclerosis
3. Arteriovenous malformations
4. Vascular tumors
5. Berry aneurysms

Anemia, as a cause, is usually severe and chronic with hematocrits below 30. Bruits are especially common in patients who have both anemia and another cause for increased cardiac output. Patients on chronic hemodialysis with permanent arteriovenous shunts are in this category. Bruits resulting from atherosclerosis may or may not be associated with clinical symptoms or abnormal neurological findings. Cranial bruits are present in one-third to one-half of patients with cerebral arteriovenous malformations. These patients usually present with headaches (always on the same side), seizure disorder, or subarachnoid hemorrhage. Brain tumors may present themselves in many different ways, and a bruit is only one of many possible physical findings. A bruit resulting from a berry aneurysm is extremely unusual and indicates that the aneurysm is very large.

Cardiac murmurs such as aortic stenosis or mitral insufficiency secondary to ruptured chordae tendineae may radiate through the spine to the skull. Since these murmurs are not transmitted through the brain (soft tissue), they are not likely to be heard over the eyes.

The presence of a bruit in and of itself is therefore not an indication for brain scan or arteriography. It provides useful and important information, but the entire clinical picture must be taken into account.

Selected References

1.   McKenzie I: The intracranial bruit. *Brain* 78:350–368, 1955.
2.   Allen N, Mustian V: Origin and significance of vascular murmurs of the head and neck. *Medicine* 41:227–247, 1962.

131. Pinnae, Canals, and Drums

JOHN S. TURNER, MD

Definition

The ears—pinna, external auditory canal, and eardrum—are the sound-collection system for the body. Skin, cartilage, bone, and eardrum abnormalities may be found.

Technique

The pinna of the child under 2 years of age is pulled downward for adequate visualization of the ear canal and eardrum (Fig 27). The pinna of the adult is pulled upward and backward (Fig 28).

The external ear must be inspected carefully for nodules, growths, serious injuries, surgical scars, cysts, crusting, or fistulas. Lopears, or prominent protruding ears, are commonly seen. The pinna should be pulled firmly in all directions to determine tenderness. The tragus should be pushed on to determine tenderness.

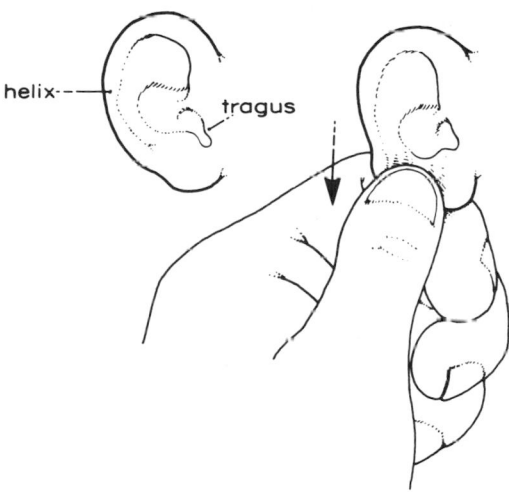

Figure 27. Examination of the ear canal and eardrum of a child under 2 years of age.

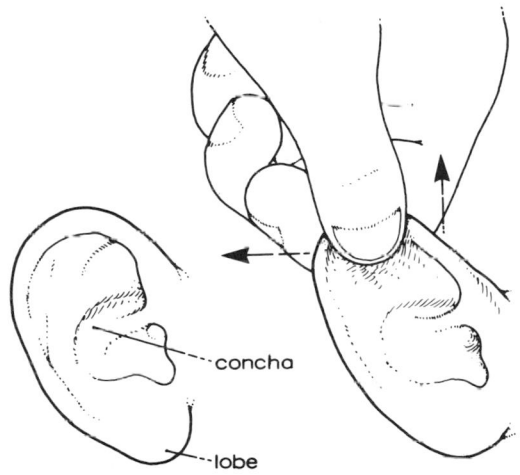

Figure 28. Examination of the ear canal and eardrum of an adult.

A good light source and a speculum that just fits the ear canal (without pain) are needed to adequately examine the canal and drum (Fig 29). Carefully inspect the ear canal, as the speculum enters. Wax is commonly seen (Figs 30 and 31). A ring wax curet may be used to remove the wax. Always keep the curet along the anterior canal wall. A syringe may be used to rinse out the wax. Never irrigate the ear canal if the patient is known to have an eardrum perforation. While inspecting the eardrum,

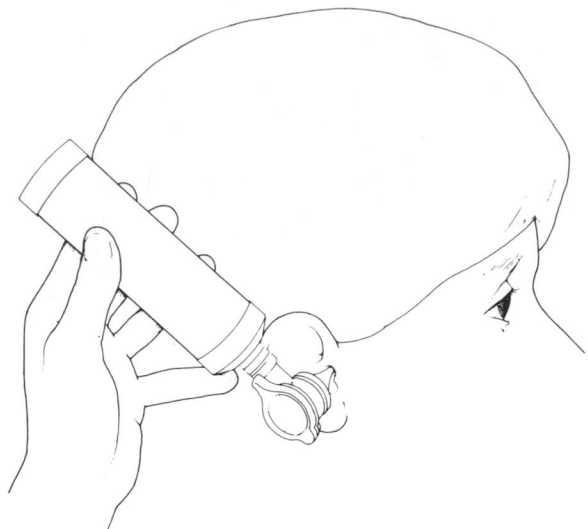

Figure 29.   Support the otoscope with the handle upward.

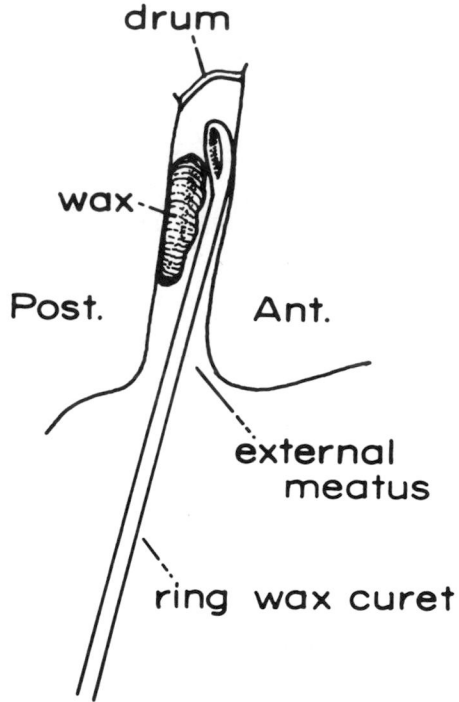

Figure 30.   A ring curet may be used to remove the wax. Always keep the curet along the anterior canal wall.

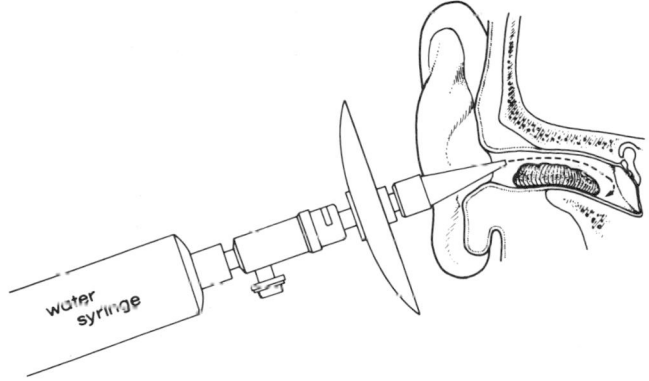

Figure 31.   A syringe may be used to rinse out the wax.

move the speculum upward, anterior and posterior, in order to visualize the entire drum surface (Fig 32).

Have the patient hold his/her nose and swallow (Toynbee maneuver), or hold the nose, close the mouth, and blow (Valsalva maneuver) to see if the eardrum moves as air pressure changes in the eustachian tube. Note changes in drum color, contour, vascularity, movement (or lack of it), perforations, distortions and scars, healed perforations, fluid meniscus or bubbles behind the drum, or retraction of the pars flaccida.

The drum is divided into quadrants for purposes of description (Fig 33).

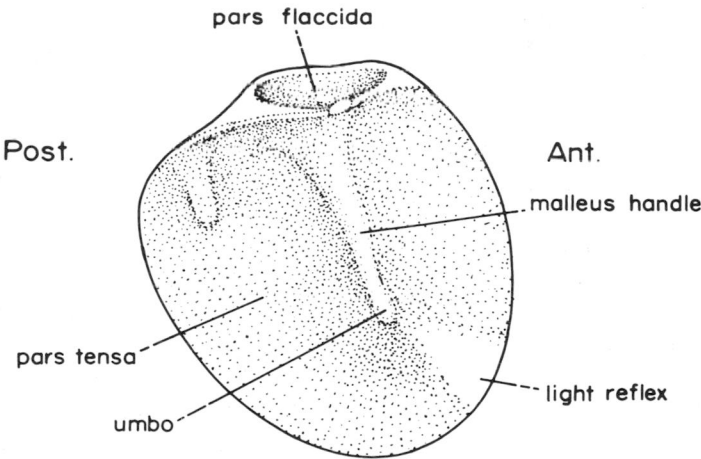

Figure 32.   Eardrum landmarks seen on a normal examination.

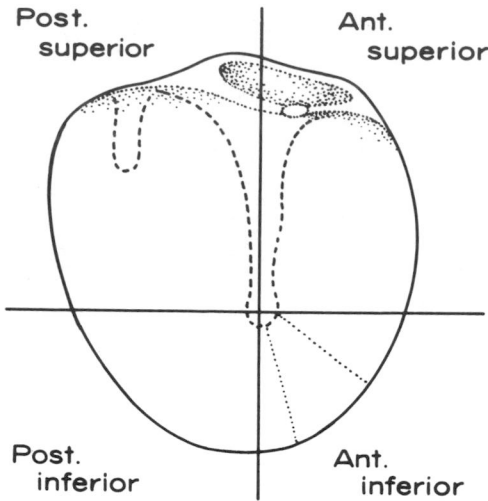

Post.
superior

Ant.
superior

Post.
inferior

Ant.
inferior

Figure 33. Quadrants of the eardrum.

Background Information

The external ear system collects sound energy for transmission into the ossicular chain (malleus, incus, and stapes) and thence to the fluids in the inner ear (cochlea). Any obstruction to the flow of energy through this system will create a hearing impairment. Proper painless cleansing of the ear canal is often necessary for adequate inspection. The canal is innervated by fibers from cranial nerves V, VII, IX, and X and thus is an exquisitely sensitive area. Patients often cough during examination of the ear because branches of the tenth nerve are stimulated (Arnold's nerve).

The skin of the pinna, canal, and drum are subject to all the disorders of the skin elsewhere in the body, and the presence of cerumen glands may lead to special problems. Wax is a normal substance and should be left undisturbed by the patient and physician unless removal is needed for accurate examination. The long tubular nature of the ear canal predisposes it to infection with saprophytic bacteria and fungi, especially if moisture is frequently present. The inner two-thirds of the ear canal is bony, the outer one-third is cartilaginous. The cartilaginous canal is freely movable and will accommodate examination instruments and speculum. The bony canal is rigid and very tender; thus the speculum should be inserted only into the cartilaginous portion. Bony protrusions often obscure adequate visualization of the drum (bulge auris and mons auris). Accurate drum visualization thus requires that the scope be angled in various directions.

The normal drum has a pale pink flesh color because of the presence of tiny vessels coursing primarily on the mucosal side.

Radial and circular fibers compose the middle layer of the drum, and after perforation from disease, the healed area lacks these fibers and usually appears as a more translucent, mobile, and flaccid area.

Negative pressure in the middle ear from eustachian tube obstruction is exceedingly common, particularly after upper respiratory infections or flying. This retracted state of the drum, with a prominent, short malleus process or increased opacity from retained fluid in the middle ear, must be searched for in each case.

Clinical Significance

Inflammation of the skin of the external ears and ear canal is very common (eczema, otitis externa, swimmer's ear). This may be caused by allergies or infection with saprophytic bacteria or sometimes yeast or fungus.

The ear canal must be carefully cleaned for adequate diagnosis. Failure to do this cleansing is often the cause of misdiagnosis of ear disease. Tenderness on moving the pinna or tragus usually indicates external canal inflammation. Canal swelling, exudate, wax, foreign bodies, or drum perforations may create a conductive hearing loss (see section 11, Difficulty Hearing or Deaf).

The upper part of the drum must be carefully inspected because retractions or perforations in this area can lead to serious ear and mastoid disease (cholesteatoma). Fluid behind the ear drum (serous otitis media) is common in children and adults. The basic cause is eustachian tube obstruction. Physical changes are subtle but must be searched for to make an accurate diagnosis: decreased movement of the drum, yel-

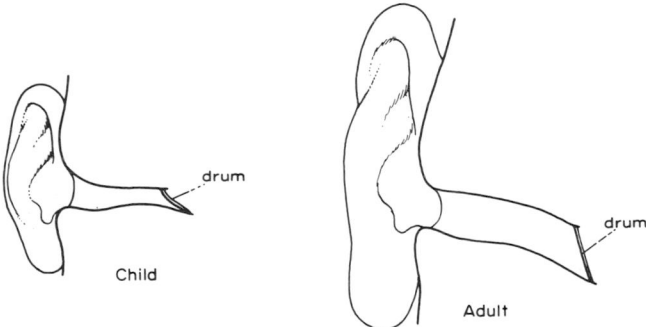

Figure 34. The eardrum of the child inclines more obliquely away from the examiner's line of vision.

lowish color, fine reticular blood vessels on the drum, prominent short process of the malleus.

The eardrum of the infant, under 2 years of age, is quite oblique to the examiner's line of vision, and the junction of canal and drum is often indistinct (Fig 34). Canal edema and inflammation may erroneously be called drum or middle ear disease.

Selected References

1. Becker W (ed): *Atlas of Otorhinolaryngology and Bronchoesophagology.* Philadelphia, WB Saunders, 1969.
2. Myers D et al: Otologic diagnosis and the treatment of deafness. *Ciba Clin Symposia* 22(2):35–69, 1970.

132. The Nose

JOHN S. TURNER, MD

Definition

The patient may complain of external or internal nose disorders. Deformities of normal contour or lesions on the skin of the nose may cause the patient to seek a medical opinion.

Internal nose (nasal cavity) complaints are the most common of all human ills (sinus trouble, hay fever, runny nose, catarrh, postnasal drip, congestion, colds, blockage, and many others).

Technique

External. Examine the nose critically by frontal and lateral inspection (Figs 35 and 36). Note the presence of humps, broadness, unusual length, drooping tips, nostril size, distortions, scars, pits, dilated vessels, skin growths, discolorations, depressions of the bridge, or deviations from a symmetrical straight contour. Palpate for the bony and cartilaginous junctions.

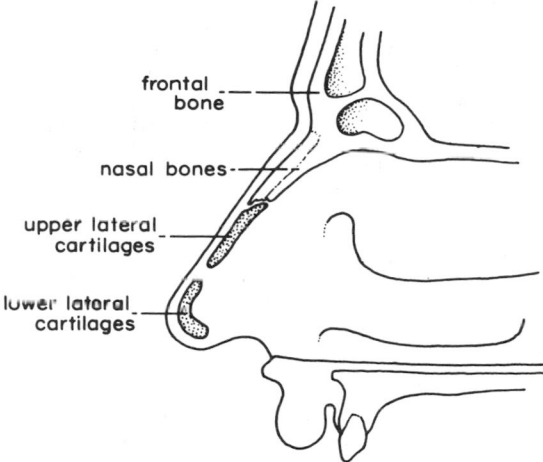

Figure 35. Cartilaginous support of the nose that permits mobility and determines contour.

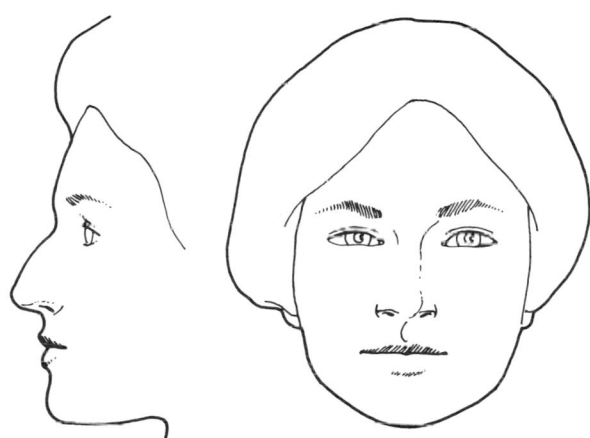

Figure 36. Straight to frontal view but hump to lateral view.

Internal. The interior nose cannot be evaluated without a nasal speculum and a headlight (Fig 37). Proper inspection and evaluation must be practiced on one's fellow students in the clinic. Caudal septal deviations or the presence of exudate or skin excoriations can be determined by careful inspection. The paranasal sinuses (maxillary and frontal) should be percussed for tenderness. A dark room should be used to see if they transilluminate light equally well (Figs 38 and 39). Examine one side and then the other.

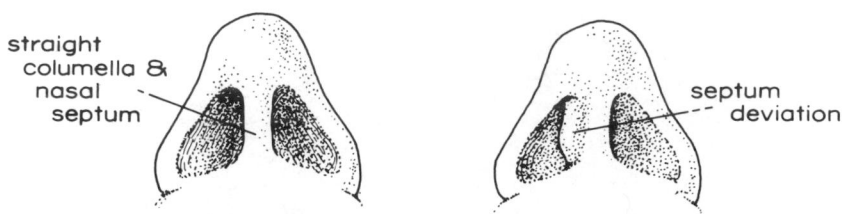

Figure 37. Inspection of the nasal septum.

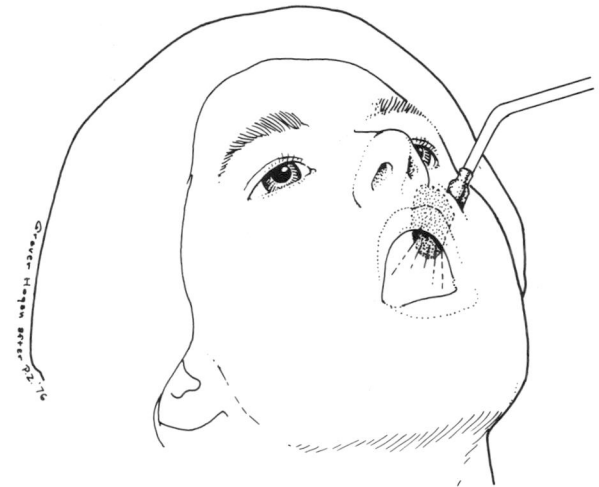

Figure 38. Transillumination of the maxillary sinus (in a dark room).

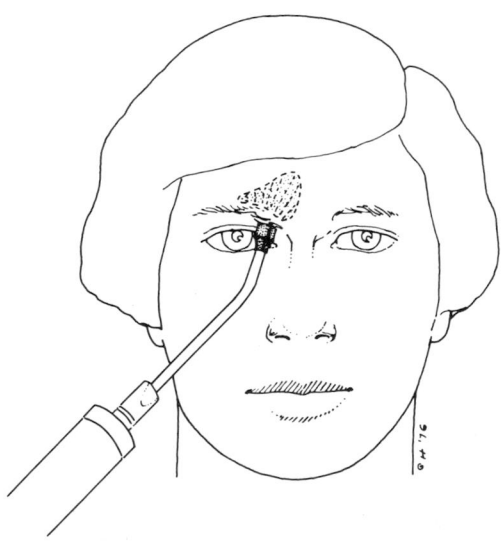

Figure 39. Transillumination of the frontal sinus (in a dark room).

Background Information

The external nose is supported by paired nasal bones, upper lateral and lower lateral cartilages, and the nasal septum. Most of the nasal skeleton is skin, subcutaneous tissue, and cartilage. The nose can therefore sustain frequent minor injuries. The skin of the nose is constantly exposed to actinic effects, and skin neoplasms are common. The internal nose is the air conditioning organ for the body. Normally it purifies, humidifies, and warms or cools the air entering the lungs. Poor nasal breathing leads to mouth breathing with secondary effects on the trachea, bronchi, and lungs. Lysozyme in the nasal mucus is bacteriocidal. Changes in nasal pH lead to decreased lysozyme and ciliary activities with subsequent nasal and sinus infection.

The frontal, maxillary (antral), and ethmoid sinuses on one side all drain into a common sulcus in the middle meatus of the nose (beneath the middle turbinate). This common drainage site leads to contiguous spread of infection, usually beginning in the maxillary and thence to the other two sinus groups.

Clinical Significance

External nose deformities often have significant psychological effects. External deformities often indicate internal nasal deformities such as a deviated nasal septum. Small skin cancers on the nose must be identified and removed before serious invasion occurs.

The cause of nasal congestion, drainage, pain, bleeding, or paranasal aching must be identified in order to treat minor infections before they

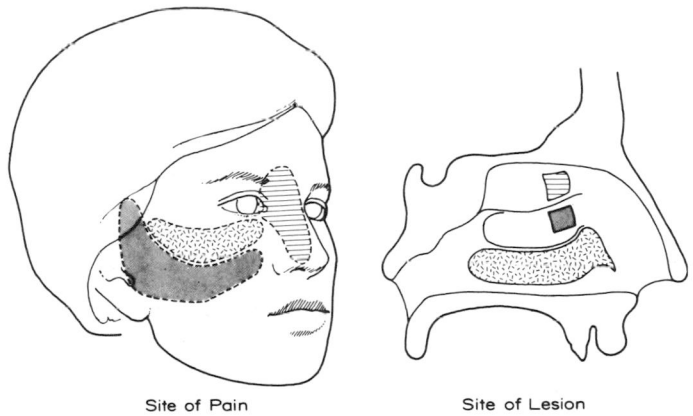

Site of Pain   Site of Lesion

Figure 40. Pain referral sites from disorders in the nasal cavity (tumor, inspection, erosion).

become major ones and to identify relatively minor causes of obstruction (hay fever) from major ones (neoplasms of the nasal turbinates, septum, sinus, or nasopharynx).

Headache may come from various sources in the nasal cavity, sinuses, or ears. Sources of pain referral are indicated in Figs 40–42.

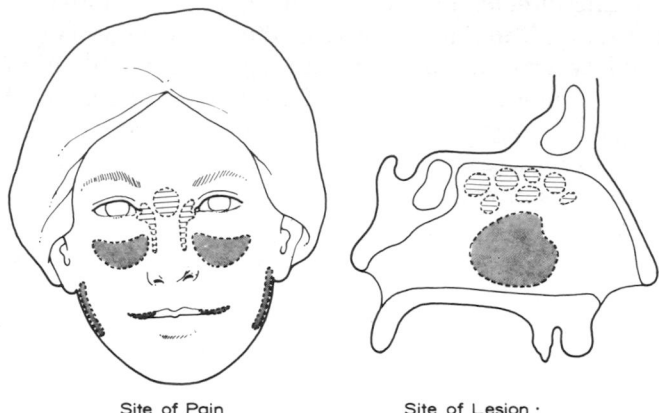

Site of Pain   Site of Lesion ·

Figure 41.   Pain referral sites from disorders in the ethmoid (striped) and maxillary (solid) sinuses.

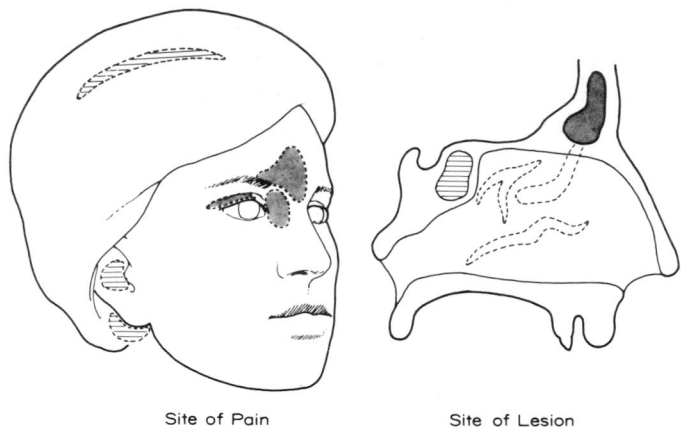

Site of Pain   Site of Lesion

Figure 42.   Pain referral sites from disorders in the frontal (solid) and sphenoid (striped) sinuses.

Selected Reference

1.   Jackson C, Jackson C (eds): *Diseases of the Nose, Throat, and Ear,* ed 2. Philadelphia, WB Saunders, 1963, pt 1.

133. External Eye Examination

FRANK C. BELL, MD

Definition

The external eye consists of conjunctivae, cornea, and sclera. The adnexal structures are lids, skin, lashes, and lacrimal glands. This section concerns detection of abnormalities of vision, external structures, and alignment of the eyes.

Technique

If the testing is done in the clinic, seat the patient comfortably and cover one eye. The patient with corrected vision should wear glasses or contact lens. The patient should then read the Snellen eye chart placed 20 feet away. After reading down the chart until the smallest line is recorded, the patient repeats the procedure for the other eye. For testing at the bedside (Fig 43), a small, pocket reading card is used. Eye charts should be properly illuminated.

After recording the central vision, determine the visual field. This is done without equipment by the method of confrontation. Cover one eye of the patient as before and instruct the patient to fixate on your nose. Place your hand behind the patient's head out of his field of view. Instruct the patient to say "now" when your hand first comes into view (Fig 44). Slowly bring your hand forward until it comes into the patient's field of view and the patient says "now." Do this in eight meridians in each eye. This is a good screening test for peripheral vision, but small defects require more sophisticated testing procedures.

Now carefully observe the external appearance of the patient's eyes, noting any asymmetry between the two sides. Note especially the prominence of the eyes, the eyelids, lashes, conjunctiva, and cornea. The undersurface of the upper lid is examined by everting the lid (Fig 45). Using your pocket flashlight, check the depth of the anterior chamber (Fig 46). In the center of each pupil is the lens. Observe the lens to see that there is no visible opacity.

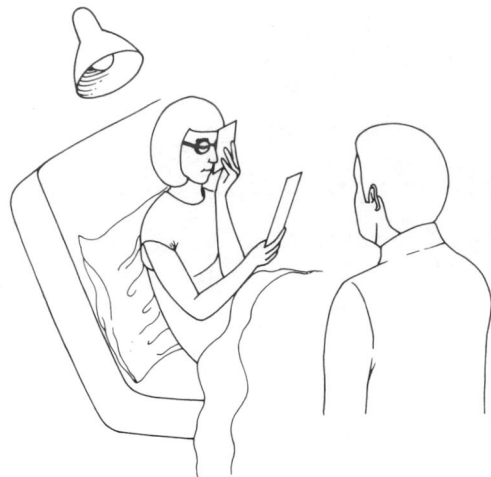

Figure 43. Testing visual acuity at the bedside. Note the pocket reading card is well illuminated and held at the proper distance. The patient reads the smallest print possible using the reading portion of her glasses (if worn) while covering the other eye.

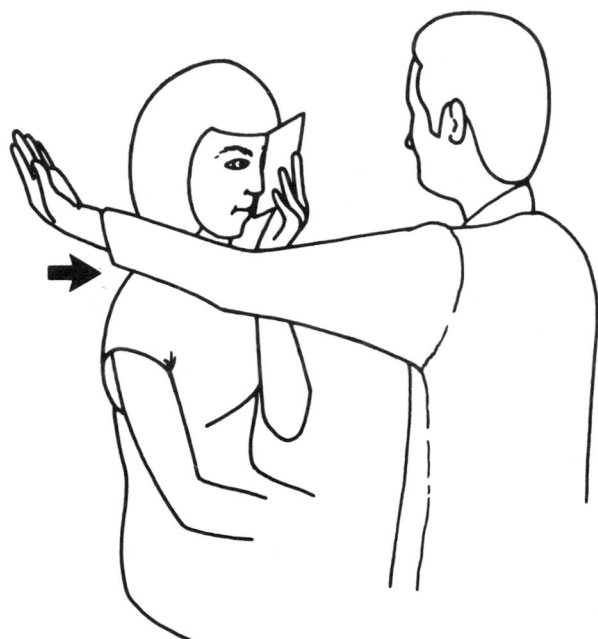

Figure 44. Testing the patient's visual field. When the patient first sees the examiner's hand, the patient says "now." By performing this test on yourself, the concept of the normal confrontation field is quickly obtained.

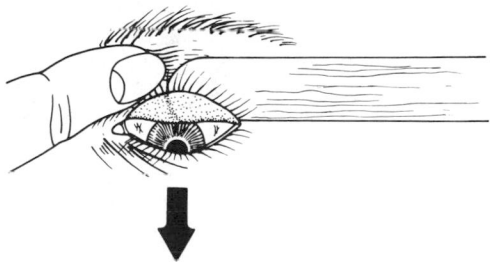

Figure 45. Everting the upper lid. A throat stick is placed in the upper lid fold and the lid is pulled upward by the lashes while the patient looks down. To reinvert the lid, have the patient look up.

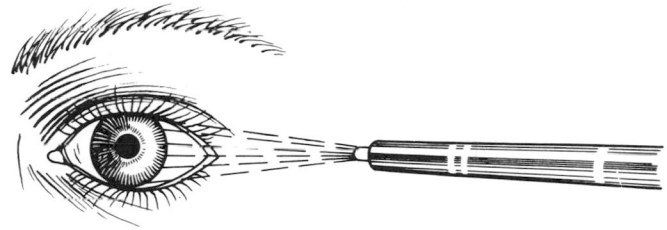

Figure 46. Checking the depth of the anterior chamber. A shadow cast by the iris when illuminated from the side suggests a shallow anterior chamber.

Note the size of both pupils. Test the constriction of each pupil to direct light and observe the normally equal constriction of the opposite pupil (the consensual reaction). Now move the pocket flashlight back and forth from one pupil to the other, being careful to shine the same quantity of light in each pupil. Observe the magnitude of pupillary constriction on each side.

Next observe the alignment of the eyes. Ask the patient to look at your pocket flashlight held approximately 2 feet away. Note the position of the light reflex on the patient's cornea (Fig 47). Note any rhythmic involuntary movements of the eyes (nystagmus). The patient is now asked to follow your flashlight from extreme right to extreme left as you observe both eyes to check horizontal gaze. At the extreme of gaze to each side, the patient follows the flashlight into up gaze and then into down gaze making an H pattern (Fig 48).

Last, the intraocular pressure should be measured. After placing one drop of an ocular anesthetic solution in the eye, the pressure in the eye is measured by the Schiotz tonometer (Fig 49).

These are the techniques that can be performed by the general physician. Additional tests available from the ophthalmologist include a

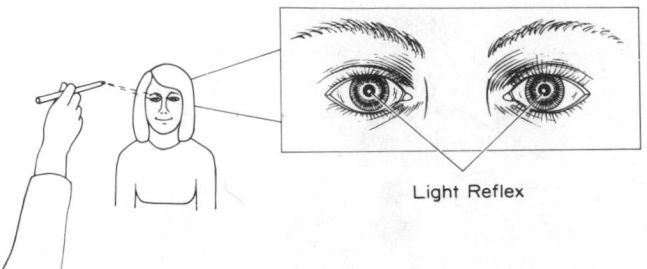

Light Reflex

Figure 47.   Observing the alignment of the eyes. The pocket flashlight is held about 2 feet from the patient and the patient looks at the light. If the visual axes of the eyes are properly aligned, the light reflex from the flashlight will be nearly centered in the patient's cornea and pupil.

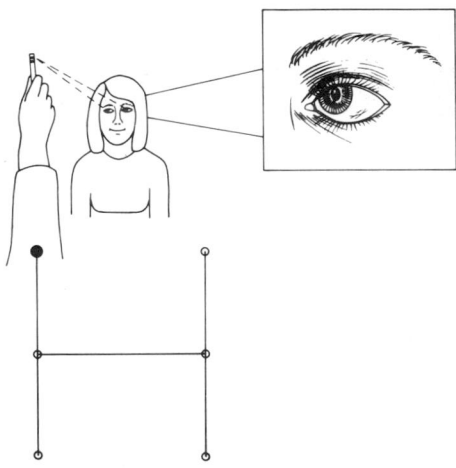

Figure 48.   Testing the extraocular muscles by having the patient look in the six cardinal directions of gaze. An H pattern is traced in the air by the examiner. Each cardinal position of gaze tests the primary action of one muscle from each eye.

slit-lamp examination, formal visual field examination, ophthalmodynamometry, and exophthalmometry. Fluorescein angiography is also performed in certain instances.

Background Information

Recording the visual acuity is the most important single part of the eye examination. Normal visual acuity is defined as 20/20. The upper number means that the patient reads the chart from a distance of 20 feet.

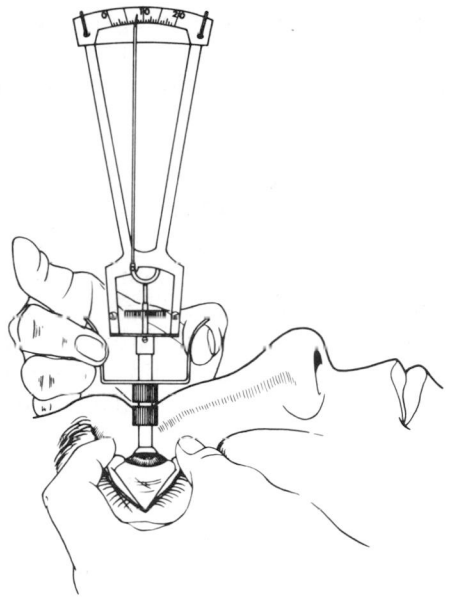

Figure 49. Measuring the intraocular pressure with the tonometer. The recumbent patient looks at the ceiling with both eyes open. After an ocular anesthetic drop is instilled, the lids are gently held apart. The tonometer is then rested on the cornea, and the reading from the scale recorded. A table converts this readily into millimeters of mercury.

The lower number indicates the distance at which a normal eye could read that size letter.

The normal visual field extends 60° nasally, 45° up, 65° down, and almost 85° laterally. Any defect indicates a malfunction in the visual system for which an explanation must be sought.

Many valuable clues to systemic disease present themselves in the external portion of the eye. The skin surrounding the eyes is very thin and delicate and is especially prone to reveal edema or metabolic deposits. The lids and lashes function to protect the eye, and any compromise of their function will quickly produce an irritated or painful eye. The lacrimal glands produce tears to lubricate the eye. Tears contain lysozyme, an enzyme that is bacteriostatic and of some help in preventing infection. On the other hand, too many tears may produce tearing, or epiphera. The conjunctiva is an excellent indicator of ocular disease, because it turns red with inflammation (conjunctivitis) from many causes. Any defect in the corneal luster is abnormal and demands further investigation.

Normally the pupils are of equal size and react equally to light shining into one eye. If the pupils are of different sizes, there must be an abnormality in the innervation or mechanical function of the iris. The pupils are innervated by the sympathetic system, which produces pupillary dilation, and by the parasympathetic system, which produces pupillary constriction. An inequality in the reaction of the pupils to the same quantity of light indicates an afferent defect, or defect in the receiving portion of the visual system.

Normally the visual axes are parallel, but the position of the eyes may vary due to congenital or acquired causes. Strabismus, which is deviation of an eye inward, outward, or upward, may be congenital or acquired. In congenital strabismus the angle of the deviation is usually the same in each direction of gaze. Acquired strabismus is frequently due to nerve paralysis and is usually not the same in each cardinal direction of gaze. Often double vision (diplopia) will result, and the abnormality will be detected during testing of the extraocular muscles. Nystagmus is produced by repetitive irregular motor impulses to the extraocular muscles.

Testing the intraocular pressure is important to detect glaucoma, or elevated intraocular pressure. Intraocular pressure is normally 10–21 mm Hg. Pressures higher than 21 may cause a pressure atrophy of the optic nerve and produce blindness. Acute glaucoma occurs from the iris blocking the outflow channels in a shallow anterior chamber (Fig 50A). Chronic open angle glaucoma is produced by diffuse resistance in the outflow channels with an anatomically normal anterior chamber and angle (Fig 50B). Acute glaucoma usually causes a painful red eye, whereas chronic open-angle glaucoma may produce no symptoms.

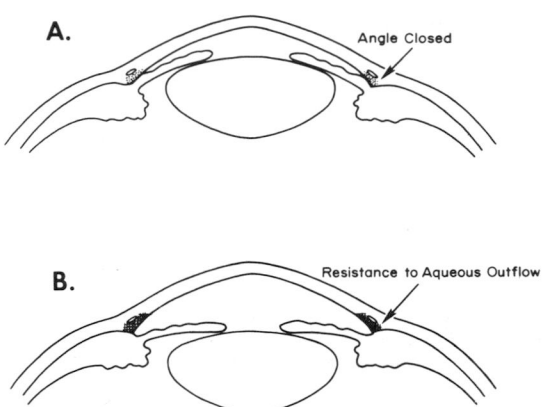

Figure 50. Anatomical explanation of two types of glaucoma. *A,* The anterior chamber is shallow and the chamber angle is closed, blocking outflow of aqueous and producing a rise in intraocular pressure. This is angle closure glaucoma. *B,* The chamber is deep and the chamber angle is open, but the aqueous drains slowly because there is resistance to outflow in the drainage structures. This is open-angle glaucoma.

Clinical Significance

Normal visual acuity is 20/20, and any lesser acuity must be explained. Inadequate motivation may cause an apparent visual disease. Very ill patients may find it difficult to read the smallest letters on the chart, particularly if the lighting is poor. The most common ocular cause of decreased visual acuity is a refractive error, and this can be corrected with glasses. An opacity in the cornea can be seen with the pocket flashlight. A cataract (opacity in the lens) is a common cause for visual decrease, and can be corrected surgically. Hemorrhage into the vitreous will decrease visual acuity, and a wide variety of retinal and optic nerve diseases may cause mild or profound loss of vision.

Visual field abnormalities may be due to ocular causes such as advanced glaucoma or retinitis pigmentosa, which produce constriction of the visual fields. A pituitary tumor typically produces bitemporal hemianopia. Cerebrovascular accidents may produce congruous (similar pattern on both sides) visual field defects.

The external examination may give a myriad of clues to ocular and systemic diseases. Prominent eyes (exophthalmos) suggest thyroid disease. Xanthelasma (Fig 51) suggests hyperlipidemia. A drooping eyelid (ptosis) suggests third nerve paralysis, myasthenia gravis, Horner's syndrome, or other causes. An acutely red, swollen, and painful lid margin may be a localized infection called a hordeolum or stye. If firm and uninflamed, a swelling on the lid margin is probably a chalazion.

Conjunctivitis is a redness and edema of the conjunctiva usually caused by acute bacterial infections. However intraocular inflammation and sometimes systemic diseases produce a similar picture. A yellow elevated plaque on the conjunctiva near the nasal margin of the cornea is a pinguecula. A pterygium occurs in the same location but contains fine surface vessels and grows out onto the corneal surface.

The cornea is normally smooth and lustrous; any defect is abnormal. The corneal epithelium may be abraded, producing a superficial defect. If there is a localized deeper corneal ulceration, a serious bacterial or viral infection may exist that should be managed by an ophthalmologist.

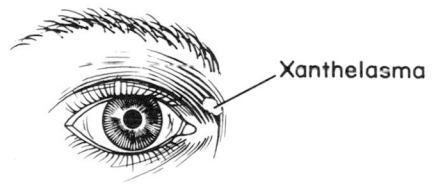

Figure 51. Xanthelasma. A flat, hard, yellow nodule present in the medial portions of both upper lids.

The normal pupillary reaction to light is a brisk and equal constriction in both eyes. Asking the patient to focus on a close object (accommodation) normally produces pupillary constriction also. In the Argyle Robertson pupil of syphilis, the pupils are smaller than usual (miotic), and unique in that they do not react to light but do react to accommodation. The Argyle Robertson pupil must be distinguished from an Adie's pupil, which is unilateral, semidilated, and sluggishly reactive to light. Horner's syndrome consists of a slightly constricted pupil which reacts to light in association with a drooping upper eyelid (ptosis) and an absence of sweating over the eye on the affected side. All of these findings are caused by an interruption in the sympathetic nerve supply to the eye. The most common causes are tumors and surgical procedures at the base of the neck. Any defect in the retina or optic nerve may produce the Marcus Gunn afferent pupillary sign. Normally each pupil constricts the same amount in response to the same quantity of light. If the pocket flashlight is moved back and forth and one pupil constricts less than the other, a defect (Marcus Gunn pupil) is present on that side.

If the visual axes are not parallel, a strabismus or squint is present. The eyes may turn in (esotropia) or out (exotropia). Strabismus develops spontaneously and asymptomatically in children, and this requires ophthalmic consultation. In adults the sudden onset of strabismus usually produces the symptom of diplopia (double vision), and most commonly is due to a paralysis of cranial nerves III, IV, or VI. A rhythmic, back-and-forth motion of both eyes is called nystagmus, and may be caused by acquired neurological disease or by poor vision since infancy.

Elevated intraocular pressure, or glaucoma, is a common cause of visual loss that can be prevented. There may be no symptoms at all until blindness occurs; hence, the testing of intraocular pressure is extremely important in a good physical examination.

Selected References

1. Newell FW, Ernest JT: *Ophthalmology: Principles and Concepts,* ed 3. St Louis, CV Mosby, 1974, pp 136–154.
2. Eye examinations, in Scheie HG, Albert DM: *Textbook of Ophthalmology,* ed 9. Philadelphia, WB Saunders Company, 1977, pp 169–198.
3. Vaughan D, Asbury T: *General Ophthalmology,* ed 7. Los Altos, Calif, Lange Medical Publications, 1977, pp 14–34.
4. Kaiden JS, Zimmerman TT, Worthen DM: Hand-held tonometers. An evaluation by medical students. *Arch Ophthal* 89:110–112, 1966.
5. Krimsky E: Simple eye tests. *Postgrad Med* 40:697–702, 1966.
6. Keeney AH: *Ocular Examination: Basis and Techniques,* ed 2. St Louis, CV Mosby, 1976.

134. The Fundus Examination

FRANK C. BELL, MD

Definition

Observing the appearance of the optic nerve, retinal vessels, surrounding retina, and macula for the presence of ocular or systemic disease.

Technique

Before beginning the examination, dilate the pupils. The vast majority of patients may be dilated safely, and the physician is urged to dilate the pupils unless a specific contraindication exists. Patients with symptoms or signs of angle closure glaucoma should not be dilated. Likewise, patients with recent head trauma or surgery should not be dilated since pupillary size is an important sign to monitor.

One drop of 1% tropicamide (Mydriacyl) or 1% cyclopentolate (Cyclogyl) in each eye produces satisfactory dilatation. Atropine may cause pupillary dilatation for up to 2 weeks and should not be used for routine funduscopic examination.

Place the patient in a comfortable position. A seated position in a semidarkened room is ideal. Remove the patient's glasses and put them in a place where they will be protected. If you wear glasses, do not remove them. Ask the patient to look straight ahead past you and instruct the patient to keep both eyes open and to blink if necessary. It is helpful for you to point out a specific object on the opposite wall for the patient to look at.

Begin by examining the fundus of the right eye. Generally you should examine the patient's right eye with your right eye, holding the ophthalmoscope with your right hand. Likewise, examine the patient's left eye with your left eye and hold the ophthalmoscope with your left hand.

Turn on the ophthalmoscope light and turn the dial to zero. Examine the ocular media (aqueous humor, lens, and vitreous) by holding the ophthalmoscope approximately 20 inches from the patient and observing through the window of the ophthalmoscope. Normally, the media are transparent and the fundus reflects a red orange glow as you shine the beam of light into the patient's line of sight. With a minimal amount of experience, you will recognize the normal red reflex and be able to see any opacities of the media, which appear as dark shadows in this red reflex. Next, slowly approach the patient's eye until you are so close as is practical, keeping the light from the ophthalmoscope shining into the pupil. It is sometimes helpful to place your hand on the patient's forehead and gently elevate the upper lid with the ball of your thumb (Fig 52). Do not bend over the patient, but keep your face vertically aligned with his. When you get close to the patient's eye, the first things you should see are some of the retinal vessels on a red orange background. These vessels may or may not be in focus. If they are not, you should turn the dial on the ophthalmoscope by trial and error until the retinal vessels are in sharp focus. Then begin a systematic observation of the fundus.

Examine the fundus in a definite sequence each time in order not to overlook anything (Fig 53). Begin by looking at the optic disk. If you cannot find the disk, follow a vessel back to its origin. Observe the disk color, margins, elevation, and shape. Also observe the size of the physiologic cup, a depression in the center of the optic disk. Compare the size of the cup to the size of the optic disk. Then note the retinal vessels as they emerge from the disk. The arteries are narrower and brighter red than the veins. The retinal vessels generally divide into four major branches from the optic disk, each supplying approximately one-fourth of the retina. Each of these should be followed as far from the disk as possible, with special attention to color, light reflexes, and points at which the arteries cross the veins. In so doing you will observe much of the retina. While you are following the vessels from the disk, be alert for hemorrhages, exudates, elevated regions, or other types of retinal pathology.

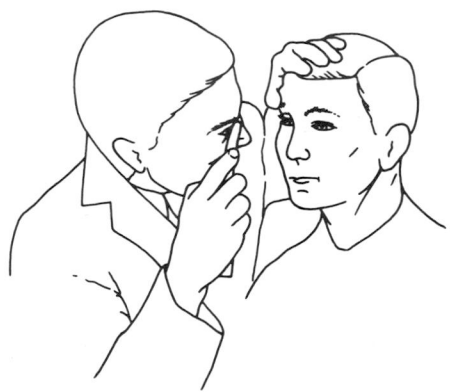

Figure 52. Examining the right eye. Correct position of patient and doctor for the examination. The doctor is looking with his right eye, holding the instrument with his right hand, and looking into the patient's right eye.

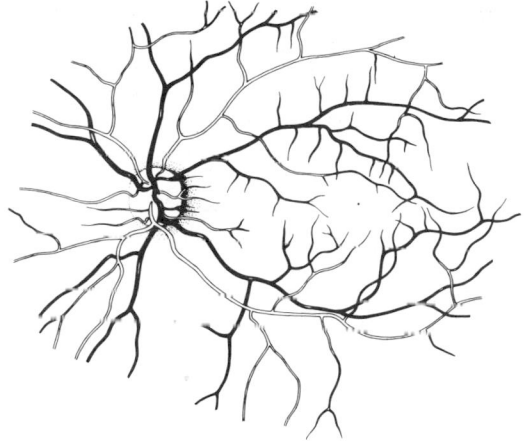

Figure 53.   Diagram of disk, vessels, and macula. There is an absence of retinal vessels in the foveal area.

The last part of the examination is the observation of the macula. The macula can be found approximately two disk diameters lateral to the optic disk. In the center of the macula is the fovea, which gives a glistening pinpoint reflex from the ophthalmoscope light. The fovea is the area of sharpest vision and is surrounded by a small area devoid of retinal blood vessels. The ophthalmoscope light seems brightest to the patient when shone there. The patient will often rapidly move the eye away when you approach the macula. You can sometimes observe the fovea best by asking the patient to look directly into the ophthalmoscope light, or by asking the patient to look at a definite object on the far wall as you search for the fovea.

Background Information

The optic disk is the visible part of the optic nerve, which is embryologically part of the central nervous system. Over 1 million axons pass through the optic disk in an area only 1.5 mm in diameter. If there is increased intracranial pressure from any cause, the optic disk will become edematous (papilledema; Fig 54); however, if there is increased pressure in the eye (glaucoma), the axons comprising the disk undergo pressure atrophy, and the central depression, or cup, becomes large in relation to the optic disk (Fig 55). A generalized death of axons in the optic nerve produces a pale white disk often compared to the color of the full moon. This is optic atrophy.

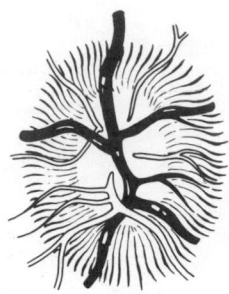

Figure 54. Papilledema. When the axons become edematous, the physiologic cup is filled and the edges of the disk are elevated above the level of the surrounding retina. The margins of the disk appear indistinct.

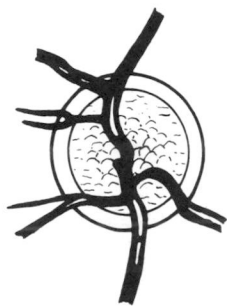

Figure 55. Glaucomatous cupping. The central depression is large in relation to the nerve head. A cup over 60% of the diameter of the disk suggests glaucoma.

The retinal vessels are branches of the central retinal artery and vein. Normally, their walls are quite transparent and what you observe as a vessel is actually the blood in the lumen of the vessel. In certain disease states, however, the vessel wall is altered. The arterioles may become sclerotic and appear in the early stages to have a widened light reflex. More advanced sclerotic arterioles, called "copper wire" arterioles, appear a dark golden brown color; even more advanced arteriolosclerosis produces a white vessel, the "silver wire" appearance. The retinal vessels are unique in the body in that whenever an arteriole crosses a venule the vessels share a common adventitial sheath. Because of this, a sclerotic arteriole will indent a venule and produce arteriovenous nicking (Fig 56). Arteriolosclerotic arteriolar changes are considered secondary to hypertensive changes, but each must be independently evaluated. Hypertension first affects retinal arterioles by producing focal narrowings (spasm) in the vessel wall. If the hypertension is severe and long-standing, the arterioles become generally constricted. In severe hypertension, papilledema may be present.

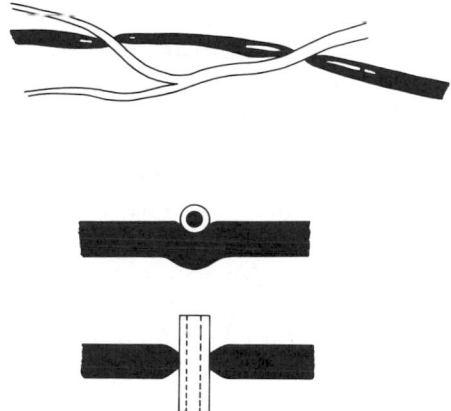

Figure 56. Arteriovenous nicking. Note the course and compression of the vein as it is crossed by the artery.

The retinal areas between blood vessels should be smooth, glistening, and of the usual red orange color. Many systemic diseases other than hypertension may produce hemorrhages or exudates. Primary ocular pathology may produce retinal masses or elevations.

At the fovea the retina is extremely thin (0.1 mm), and the smallest disturbance will decrease vision. The retinal vessels do not extend into the fovea. Foveal nourishment is provided by the choroidal circulation only.

Clinical Significance

The optic disk appearance is normally quite variable and considerable clinical experience is necessary to correctly distinguish normal from pathological. In general, far-sighted eyes will have a densely packed optic nerve which may at times give the suggestion of papilledema. Conversely, an otherwise normal near-sighted eye may have a large cupped and somewhat pale disk that may suggest glaucomatous cupping or optic atrophy. The normal nasal disk margin is usually more indistinct than the temporal margin. Venous pulsations at the disk may be present spontaneously or may be elicited with gentle finger pressure on the lid. If present, these pulsations usually indicate a normal intracranial pressure. The absence of venous pulsations indicates increased intracranial pressure only if they were previously documented to be present.

Papilledema signifies increased intracranial pressure, and may be recognized in its early stages by a blurring or feathery appearance of the disk margins. Other early signs include the presence of dilated tortuous small vessels and splinter hemorrhages along the disk margins. More pronounced papilledema produces marked elevation of the disk. Generally, posterior fossa lesions produce papilledema rather early in their course, while anterior cranial lesions produce papilledema later or not at all.

Glaucoma is a common disease, present in approximately 2% of the population over age 40. It is frequently recognized for the first time by an astute observer during a routine fundus examination. A cupped optic disk may be the only sign of glaucoma. Many patients who have absolutely no ocular complaints may be slowly going blind from glaucoma.

Arteriolosclerotic changes in the retinal vessels may give the clinician a clue to a generalized state of arteriolosclerosis. In hypertension less correlation exists between ocular vessel changes and changes in other organs of the body.

A retinal hemorrhage must always be explained. Common causes are hypertension and diabetes; however, other causes include leukemias or other blood dyscrasias, collagen diseases, or metabolic disorders. A white spot surrounded by hemorrhage is referred to as a Roth spot (Fig 57). This is classically described with septic emboli to the retina, as with endocarditis. However, there are other causes such as diabetes, blood dyscrasias, and collagen diseases.

A brown or gray spot underneath the retina may be either a benign nevus or malignant melanoma. The life of the patient may depend on the discovery of such a lesion.

An area of retinal detachment may cause difficulty in interpretation because it will appear as an elevated retina with vessels which are out of focus.

Flat white areas with pigmented borders frequently represent areas of old choroiditis, where the choroid and retinal layers have been destroyed by previous inflammation which the patient may or may not have noted.

The macular area is the area of sharpest vision, and almost any lesion there will decrease visual acuity. Common lesions are hemorrhage, edema, exudates, and rarely parasitic infestations and tumors. Most of these lesions must be further interpreted by an ophthalmologist.

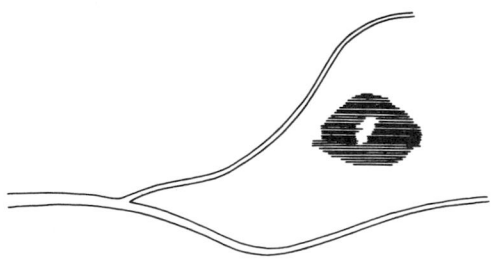

Figure 57.   Roth spot. A central white spot is surrounded by hemorrhage.

Selected References

1. Chester EM: *The Ocular Fundus in Systemic Disease.* Cleveland, Case Western Reserve University Press, 1973.
2. Vaughn D, Asbury T: *General Ophthalmology,* ed 8. Los Altos, Calif, Lange Medical Publications, 1977.
3. Gordon DM, Thomas BA (ed): *The Fundamentals of Ophthalmoscopy,* ed 2. Kalamazoo, Mich, Upjohn Co, 1973.
4. Marr WG: Ophthalmoscopic signs of cardiovascular disease. *Mod Conc Cardiovasc Dis* 31:763–768, 1962.
5. Cogan DG: Diabetic retinopathy. *N Engl J Med* 270:787–788, 1964.
6. Allen RA, Straatsma BR: Ocular involvement in leukemia and allied disorders. *Arch Ophthal* 66:490–508, 1961.

---

135. The Pupil

J. DONALD FITE, MD
H. KENNETH WALKER, MD

Definition

The normal pupil size varies 2–4 mm in diameter in bright light, to 4–8 mm in the dark. The pupils are equal in size. The pupils constrict to direct illumination (direct response) and to illumination of the opposite eye (consensual response). The pupil dilates in the dark. Both pupils constrict when the eye is focused on a near object (accommodative response). The pupil is abnormal if it fails to dilate to the dark or fails to constrict to light or accommodation.

Technique

The constriction of the pupil to light demonstrates integrity of the afferent and efferent pupillary pathways, and the dilatation of the pupil in the dark demonstrates the integrity of the ocular sympathetic pathways. The consensual response is useful in differentiating between lesions of the afferent and efferent pathways (Table 23).

Table 23.   Summary of tests of pupil function.

Test	Comment
1. Even illumination, far focus	Larger pupil abnormal
2. Red light, dark room	Smaller pupil abnormal
3. Direct and consensual response	No response to either: efferent path lesion No direct but normal consensual response: afferent path lesion
4. Swinging light	Marcus-Gunn: afferent path lesion
5. Near versus far	Response to accommodation but not to light: midbrain lesion
6. Response speed	Slow response to accommodation: tonic pupil

1. Position the patient with the face evenly illuminated and have the patient look at an object ten to twenty feet away to control the accommodative response. Measure the size of each pupil. This is best done with half circle on a ruler with 1 mm increments (Fig 58). The pupils should be equal. If they are not equal, measure them with evenly illuminated bright light (beside lamp). Under these conditions the larger pupil is abnormal, due to paralysis of the pupillary sphincter.

2. If both are equal under bright illumination, make the room as dark as you can and measure the pupil size under red light (easily done by placing the finger over the penlight). The small pupil is the abnormal one, indicating paralysis of the dilator muscle.

3. At this time the pupils should be tested individually for the direct and consensual response. With the patient fixating on a distant object, observe the amplitude and rapidity of each pupil's constriction to light. If one pupil fails to constrict, check its consensual response. Failure to constrict to both direct and consensual stimuli indicates interruption of the efferent pathways (third cranial nerve). Preservation of the consensual response indicates interruption of the afferent pathways (amaurotic pupil).

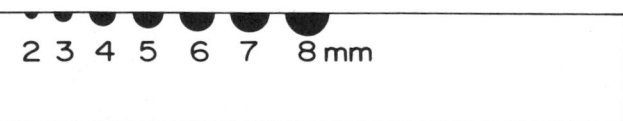

2 3 4 5 6 7 8 mm

Figure 58.   Ruler of type necessary for measuring pupils.

4. Minimal lesions affecting the afferent pathways can be detected by the swinging light test. In this maneuver the direct and consensual responses of the pupil are compared. A bright light is necessary for an accurate test. With the patient in dim illumination and fixating on a distant object, swing the light back and forth from one eye to another. Adjust the rate of the swing so that you have time to see the just-illuminated pupil constrict. This is a normal response. If the just-illuminated pupil is observed to dilate instead of constrict, the test is positive for a lesion in the afferent pathway of the eye. The test is sensitive for minimal optic nerve dysfunction. This phenomenon was first described by Marcus Gunn and carries his name.

   The swinging light test and consensual response can also be used to test the integrity of the afferent pathways of an eye in which the pupil does not function. The test is performed in the same manner as the standard swinging light test. First, illuminate the eye with the abnormal pupil and observe the pupil of the other eye. Quickly swing the light to the unilluminated eye. If the afferent pathways of the first eye are intact, the pupil of the second eye will remain the same size or constrict very slightly. However, if the afferent pathways of the first illuminated eye are not functioning, the pupil of the second eye will be seen to constrict briskly. Dr. Lawton Smith has termed this phenomenon the "reverse Marcus Gunn pupillary phenomenon."

5. If the pupils are abnormal to direct light, the response to near light must be tested. With the face evenly illuminated, measure the pupil size with the patient looking at an object 10 or more feet away. Then measure again with the patient looking at an object 18 inches from the face.

6. Does the pupil constrict briskly to light and dilate rapidly in the dark? If the response is slow or tonic, the affected pupil in light will appear larger than its mate. After prolonged stimulation to light, it will appear smaller than its mate when placed in the dark. This reaction is seen in the tonic pupil. Pharmacologic confirmation of a tonic pupil is made by putting 0.25% pilocarpine in both pupils. The affected pupil promptly constricts, while the normal pupil is unaffected.

Background Information

The afferent portion of the pupillary reflex arc begins with the rods and cones of the retina. The light reflex fibers accompany the visual fibers in the optic nerve, traverse the optic chiasm, and then part company with the visual fibers before the latter reach the lateral geniculate body. The pupillary fibers travel to the pretectal area of the midbrain where there is a synapse with the pretectal nuclei. After the synapse one group of fibers proceeds to the Edinger-Westphal nucleus, which is a part of the oculomotor or third nerve complex. The other group crosses the midline in the posterior commissure and goes to the pretectal nucleus of the opposite side. This decussation explains the consensual response: ie, the equal constriction of both pupils when the light is shone into only one eye. Pupilloconstrictor fibers arise from the Edinger-Westphal nuclei and join the oculomotor nerve. These fibers are located dorsomedially in the oculomotor nerve and may be involved early in uncal herniation, producing a dilated and fixed pupil. The preganglionic parasympathetic fibers then synapse in the ciliary ganglion. The postganglionic fibers run as the short ciliary nerves, supplying the sphincter of the iris (the pupillary light reflex) and the ciliary body (accommodation) (Fig 59).

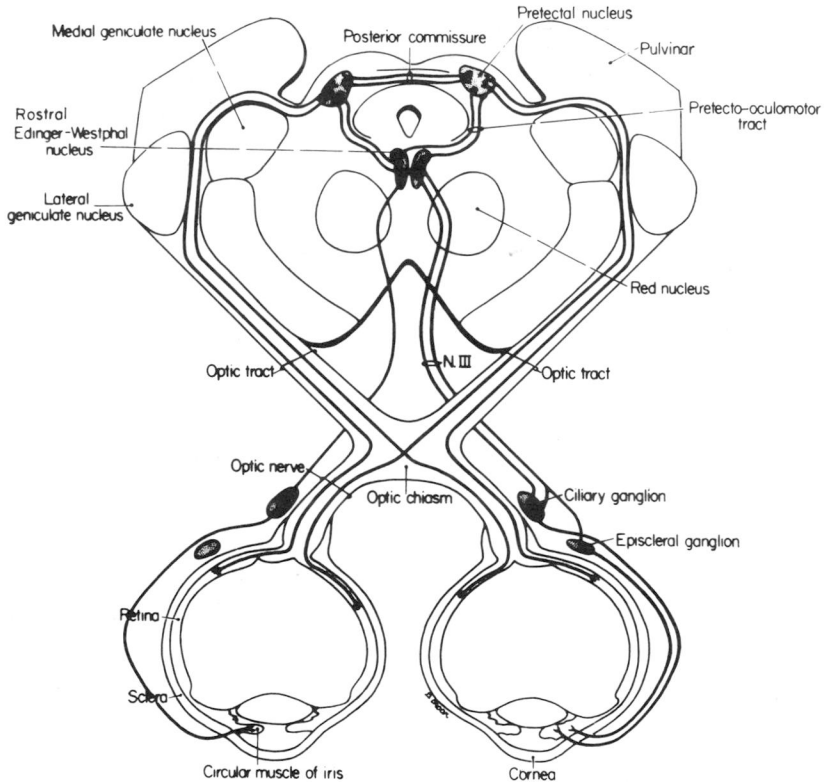

Figure 59. A diagram to illustrate the pathway for the light reflex. The cones and bipolar neurons of the retina, the first two neurons in the pathway, are not shown in the diagram. From Crosby EC, Humphrey T, Lauer EW: *Correlative Anatomy of the Nervous System,* 1962. New York, Macmillan Company, p. 236. Used with permission of the publisher.

Pupillodilation pathways are incompletely known. A variety of stimuli can produce dilation, ranging from decreased light (which would involve the cortex) to pain and severe emotions. The ciliospinal reflex is pupillary dilation produced by painful stimulation of the neck skin. The sympathetic center that the impulses ultimately reach is in the posterior part of the hypothalamus. Fibers from here descend in the lateral tegmentum of the brainstem, reaching cells of the intermediolateral cell column at C_8-Th_1. Preganglionic fibers leave these cells and synapse in the superior cervical ganglion. Postganglionic fibers then travel up the internal carotid artery, join the trigeminal nerve (ophthalmic division) in the cavernous sinus, and then reach the dilator smooth muscle fibers of the iris as the long ciliary nerves.

Fibers relating to accommodation arise in the Edinger-Westphal nucleus and are distributed with the pupilloconstrictor fibers. Note that the Edinger-Westphal nucleus and the ciliary ganglion are involved with both pupillary constriction and accommodation. Over 90% of the nuclei in both are concerned with accommodation, with only 3% being devoted to pupillary constriction. The fibers serving convergence arise in the medial rectus nucleus of the oculomotor nerve nuclei complex and then are distributed to the medial recti muscles.

The near reflex of the eye is composed of pupillary constriction, accommodation, and convergence. The anatomical substrates for these are described above.

The clinical pharmacology of the parasympathetic innervation is quite important. Acetylcholine is produced at the postganglionic nerve ending and causes a contraction of the iris sphincter, with a resulting pupillary constriction. Prostigmine and eserine interfere with the destruction of acetylcholine, thus potentiating its effects. Methacholine and pilocarpine stimulate the iris sphincter directly to bring about pupillary constriction, or miosis. Atropine blocks the action of acetylcholine, producing pupillary dilation, or mydriasis.

The sympathetic transmitter substance is norepinephrine, which is released at the nerve ending and is taken up again. Cocaine blocks reuptake, thus occasioning a buildup of the transmitter substance with consequent pupil dilation. Hydroxyamphetamine increases the release of norepinephrine, thus causing dilation. Epinephrine and phenylepinephrine produce dilation by acting directly on the muscle cells of the iris dilator muscle.

Clinical Significance

Afferent pathway lesions produce loss of the direct reflex by involvement of the retina or optic nerve. Optic neuritis and tumors compressing the optic nerve are common causes.

Parasympathetic pathway lesions can interdict the efferent outflow anywhere along its course:

1. Lesions involving the Edinger-Westphal nucleus or the fibers before they leave the brainstem are usually bilateral (in contrast to peripheral third nerve lesions, which are usually unilateral), and produce deficits of neighboring structures.

2. Uncal herniation is a common cause of a fixed and dilated pupil. An expanding supratentorial mass causes the uncus of the temporal lobe to herniate down into the tentorial notch, with resulting compression of the third nerve and other structures (see section 193, Level of Consciousness).

3. Aneurysms of the internal carotid artery are another common cause of third nerve lesions. A dilated pupil, paralysis of other third nerve functions, and pain behind the eye strongly suggests a berry aneurysm at the junction of the internal carotid and posterior communicating arteries.

4. The tonic pupil (Adie's syndrome) is a pupil that is usually large and unresponsive or very slightly responsive to light. It is called "tonic" because it constricts slowly during the near reflex and then dilates again very slowly when the stimulus is removed. In the great majority of cases it is unilateral. About half the cases have absent knee or ankle jerks. The syndrome is due to involvement of the postganglionic fibers in the ciliary ganglion. A likely explanation for the absence of the light reflex, but preservation of the near and accommodation reflexes, is that over 90% of the neurons are concerned with accommodation and near, and consequently, more of them are likely to survive when disease involves the ganglion. The disease is probably some form of a mild polyneuropathy.

Midbrain lesions involve the afferent pathway before it reaches the oculomotor nuclei. There is considerable uncertainty and disagreement about the exact mechanisms. Light-near dissociation is a common finding: the pupil constricts with near vision but does not respond with constriction to stimulus with light. This implies that in this area the fibers subserving the light reflex are separate from those of the near reflex. Argyll-Robertson pupils are thought by many to be an example of a lesion in the midbrain tectum proximal to the oculomotor nuclei (see Adams and Victor, p 177, for another opinion). The pupils are small, irregular, and do not react to light, but react normally to near. The vision is good. Dark dilation is poor. Both pupils are involved. In the past they were almost diagnostic of tertiary syphilis. Light-near dissociation can also be seen in pinealomas compressing the pretectal area (Parinaud's syndrome), in multiple sclerosis, and, rarely, in diabetes mellitus.

Sympathetic outflow lesions produce Horner's syndrome. The full-blown syndrome includes:

1. In miosis, the sympathetically-innervated pupillary dilator fibers are weak or paralyzed, leaving the parasympathetically inner-vated pupil constrictors as the dominant or only influence on pupil size. The miosis is best picked up in dim light, where in normal circumstances pupillary dilation is maximal.
2. Ptosis is the drooping of the upper eyelid with consequent nar-rowing of the palpebral fissure. Due to paralysis of Muller's muscle, a sympathetically innervated involuntary muscle helps keep the eyelid open.
3. Anhidrosis is due to involvement of the sympathetic supply to the face.

Recall that there are three neurons in the sympathetic supply to the eye and face: (1) an area in the ipsilateral posterior hypothalamus con-tains the first neuron. Fibers arising here descend to (2) the intermedio-lateral cell column C_8-Th_1 (and sometimes 1–3 segments lower), which contains the second neuron. The preganglionic fibers leave the spinal cord and synapse in (3) the superior cervical ganglion, which is the third neuron. Postganglionic fibers then travel up to supply the face and eye. Lesions at any point along this long pathway can produce Horner's syn-drome, although all three components of the syndrome are not always present. All defects are ipsilateral to the lesion.

1. Hypothalamus: miosis, ptosis, and anhidrosis. In this case the anhidrosis involves the entire ipsilateral half of the body. This can be the first sign of incipient transtentorial herniation from a mass lesion (reference 7).
2. Thalamus: thalamotomy for relief of dyskinesia has produced Horner's, as has stroke causing hemiballismus.
3. Midbrain: nuclear lesions can involve both sympathetic and parasympathetic structures, producing midposition fixed pupils. Cerebrovascular hemorrhage is a common cause.
4. Pontine lesions produce pinpoint pupils probably due both to sympathetic interruption and parasympathetic "irritation." Pon-tine hemorrhage is a common cause. Multiple sclerosis and tumors are other causes.
5. Lateral medullary or ventrolateral cervical cord lesions: a mild Horner's syndrome. Common causes include occlusion of the posterior cerebellar arteries or the basilar artery, and syringomyelia.
6. Cervical sympathetic chain: cancer of the apex of the lung

(Pancoast tumor), tuberculosis of the lung apex, aortic aneurysms or large goiter.

7. Postganglionic fibers coursing with the internal carotid artery: any lesion or trauma can involve these fibers and produce a Horner's.

One should *always* inquire about drugs—both local for the eyes and systemic—that the patient may be taking before concluding the discovered abnormality indicates disease.

Figure 60 gives the findings in some common pupillary disorders.

LIGHT		DARK		NEAR		LESION
Right	Left	Right	Left	Right	Left	
2mm	8mm	8mm	8mm	2mm	8mm	Left internal 3rd nerve paralysis
3mm	3mm	3mm	8mm	3mm	3mm	Right ocular sympathetic paralysis
4mm	4mm	4mm	4mm	2mm	2mm	Bilateral Argyll Robertson pupils
3mm	6mm	8mm	6mm	3mm	6mm	Left tonic pupil

Figure 60. Findings in some common pupillary disorders.

Selected References

1. Walsh FB, Hoyt WF: *Clinical Neuro-ophthalmology,* ed 3. Baltimore, Williams and Wilkins, 1969, vol 1, pp 470–483.
2. DeMeyer W: *Technique of the Neurologic Examination: A Programmed Text,* ed 2. New York, McGraw-Hill, 1974.
3. Hollenhorst R: The pupil in neurologic diagnosis. *Med Clin N Am* 52:871–884, 1968.
4. Zinn K: *The Pupil.* Springfield, Ill, Charles C Thomas, 1972.
5. Cogan DG: *Neurology of the Ocular Muscles,* ed 2. Springfield, Ill, Charles C Thomas, 1956.
6. Adams RD, Victor M: *Principles of Neurology.* New York, McGraw-Hill, 1977.

7. Plum F, Posner J: *The Diagnosis of Stupor and Coma*, ed 2. Philadelphia, FA Davis Co, 1972.

8. Haymaker W: *Bing's Local Diagnosis in Neurological Diseases*, ed 15. St Louis, CV Mosby, 1969.

9. Crosby EC, Humphrey T, Lauer EW: *Correlative Anatomy of the Nervous System*. New York, Macmillan, 1962.

10. Kerr FWL: The pupil. Functional anatomy and clinical correlation, in Smith JJL (ed): *Neuro-Ophthalmology: Symposium of the University of Miami and the Bascom Palmer Eye Institute*. St Louis, CV Mosby, 1968, vol 4, chap 4, pp 49–80.

11. Wirtschafter JD, Volk CR, Sawchuk RJ: Transaqueous diffusion to denervated iris sphincter muscle. A mechanism for the tonic pupil syndrome (Adie syndrome). *Ann Neurol* 4:1–5, 1978.

12. Smith JL: *The Pupil*. Available from JL Smith, MD, Bascom Palmer Eye Institute, Miami FL 33152.

ORAL CAVITY AND ASSOCIATED STRUCTURES

136. Teeth, Gums, and Oral Mucosa
WILLIAM B. WALKER, DDS

Definition

Examination of:

1. Teeth
2. Gums
3. Oral mucosa
4. Tongue
5. Parotid ducts
6. Submaxillary gland ducts
7. Lips
8. Occlusion
9. Muscles of mastication
10. Temporomandibular joint

Technique

Seat the patient in an upright position preferably with the head supported in the back much as in a dental chair. Bedridden patients present no special problem. Merely raise the bed to a 30–45° angle, and the pillow can act as a head support.

The examiner needs a good flashlight or clinical examination light, tongue blades, examination gloves, and 2-×-2 gauze sponges.

An established routine for the examination of the oral cavity is essential. A suggested routine includes examination of:

1. The ability to open and close jaws maximally and without deviation
2. The inner surfaces of the cheek
3. The mucosa of the cheek
4. The maxillary and mandibular mucobuccal folds
5. The palate
6. The tongue
7. The sublingual space
8. The gingivae
9. The teeth and their supporting structures
10. The occlusion
11. The muscles of mastication
12. The temporomandibular joint

Have the patient open and close the mouth maximally. Note any apparent restriction on the patient's ability to open freely to a distance of 4–4.5 cm and any deviation to right or left.

Gently grasp the mandibular lip between your thumb and forefinger and roll it downward. Note the difference in the appearance of the normal tissues between the dry border and the wet mucous membrane, referred to as the vermilion border.

Inspect for the presence, exact size, and position of any unusual growth or any change in the normal appearance such as white spots or leukoplakia.

If the patient is wearing dentures or partial dentures, have the patient remove the prosthesis and place it on a clean paper towel. To observe the right buccal mucosa, have the patient open only about half way. Holding the tongue blade in your left hand, gently place it just inside the patient's right buccal mucosa using your right hand to direct the flashlight or clinical light. Then move the tongue blade upward and downward several centimeters while pressing outward, thereby revealing the entire mucosa front to back and from the maxillary to the mandibular vestibule.

Direct your attention to the mucosa across from the maxillary first molar. Here lies the orifice to the parotid gland. Under normal conditions saliva may be readily expressed by gently pressing back to front bimanually with one finger on the cheek and the other opposing it intraorally. The orifice itself appears to be on a small raised mass of tissue. With the same technique, inspect the mucobuccal folds or vestibules. Have the patient tilt the head backwards as far as he can and open the mouth as wide as possible. Using your light, scan the palate from back to front. As your light passes from the soft palate onto the hard palate, the tissue will become rougher culminating in rugae, which are raised transverse projections of dense connective tissue just behind the maxillary incisors. Many investigators believe the rugae aid in speech; thus some attempt is made to reproduce them in artificial dentures.

Frequently near the midline of the hard palate you will note a bony outcropping (torus palatinus) or exostosis that resembles a small smooth pebble covered by skin. It is totally benign, fairly common, and of no concern unless complete upper dentures need to be made.

The left buccal mucosa and mucobuccal folds may be viewed by using the reverse procedures from the right.

To properly inspect the tongue, put the patient at ease and instruct him in exactly what you expect. Stand to the front right of the patient with a 2-×-2 gauze sponge in your right hand. The patient should be facing forward. Ask the patient to extend the tongue from the mouth as far as possible without forcing. Gently grasp it at the tip with a 2-×-2 gauze sponge and pull it forward and to the patient's left. Visualize the right lateral border with the aid of the clinical light. Then use your gloved left index finger to gently but firmly palpate the patient's right lateral tongue border, looking for masses, irregularities, or sore points. This is a common site for squamous cell carcinoma. Early diagnosis is crucial since currently over 50% of these lesions have metastasized by the time of diagnosis.

Many investigators feel the high incidence of carcinoma in this area is attributable to almost constant trauma as the tongue brushes past the mandibular molars in motions such as deglutition and speech.

Reversing hand roles without changing either your or the patient's position, inspect the left surface of the tongue.

To inspect the sublingual space, have the patient place the tongue in the roof of the mouth and open wide. Because of its relative protection from food, the sublingual space does not have highly keratinized epithelium. It is also not a likely site for intraoral carcinoma, but due to its abundant lymphatic drainage, cancer in this space is likely to have metastasized.

Focus your attention on the middle fold of the ventral surface of the tongue, the lingual frenum. Ordinarily, this frenum attaches about one-third of the way back from the tip of the tongue. Occasionally, however, this attachment will be almost to the tip of the tongue in children with the result that the child is "tongue-tied." The inability of the child to place the tongue in the roof of the mouth just posterior to the maxillary incisors to form the "T" sound results in early speech defects.

At the very base of the lingual frenum is the salivary caruncle, which includes the openings to the submaxillary ducts that drain the submaxillary glands and the sublingual ducts that drain the sublingual glands. Near the posterior limits of the sublingual space and near the lingual border of the mandible may be seen salivary eminences that mark the superior surfaces of the sublingual glands, the remaining portion of the gland being nestled in the lingual fossa or a shallow depression in the mandible itself.

If oral carcinoma is detected in the sublingual space, its most common site will be at the junction of the tongue with the floor of the mouth.

Figure 61 illustrates the relationship between a normal healthy tooth and its supporting structures. The tooth itself will appear white and without obvious signs of decay. The gums (gingiva) are as described, pink to red, without signs of recession from the tooth or bleeding.

Figure 62 represents a single side of one tooth and many of the ab-

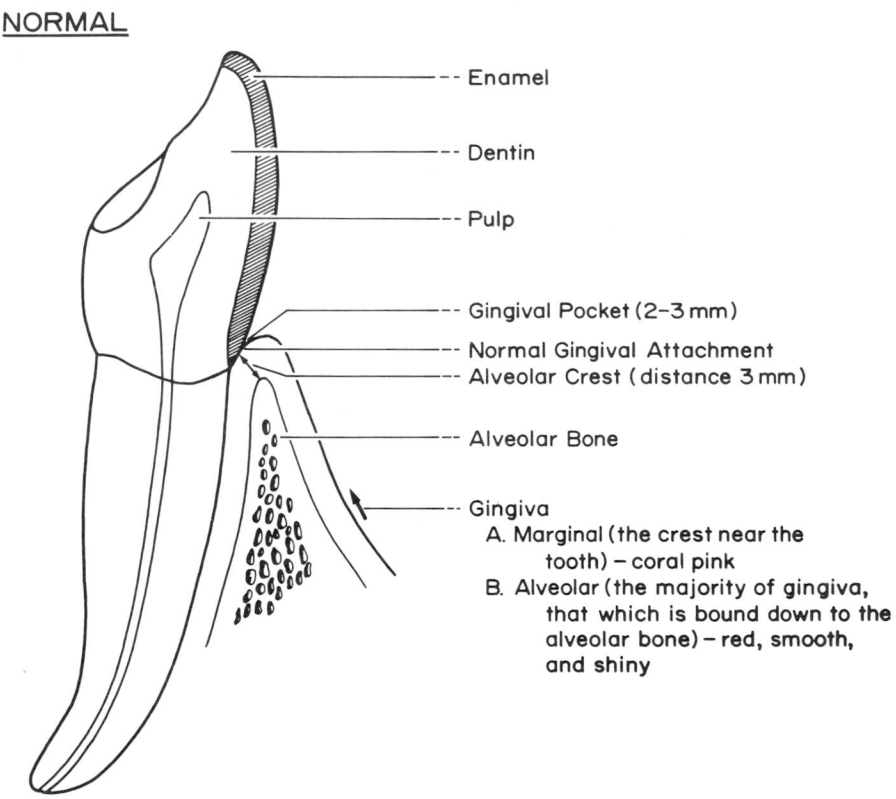

NORMAL

Enamel

Dentin

Pulp

Gingival Pocket (2–3 mm)

Normal Gingival Attachment

Alveolar Crest (distance 3 mm)

Alveolar Bone

Gingiva
A. Marginal (the crest near the tooth) – coral pink
B. Alveolar (the majority of gingiva, that which is bound down to the alveolar bone) – red, smooth, and shiny

Figure 61.   Normal tooth and gum.

normal processes which may be going on at any one time. Each tooth has four sides, and there are 32 teeth in the normal dentition.

Abnormal findings of the teeth and accompanying structures may be reflected by overt caries, receding and bleeding gums, mobility of teeth, malocclusion, and obvious physical deformities.

Have the patient open wide: with the tongue blade in your left hand, place it in the patient's right commissure and gently draw the right cheek outward, first with gentle downward pressure to allow you to inspect the mandibular gingivae and next with gentle upward pressure to reveal the maxillary gingivae. Are the teeth smooth and shiny near the attachment, or is there obvious plaque deposition near the gingiva? Note the color of the gums. A pink to red red denotes healthy tissue. Are the roots of the teeth exposed, suggesting advanced periodontal disease? Use the pad of your right index finger to exert pressure along the gingival crest from back to front. Note bleeding on pressure and in some cases frank pus extruding from between the gums and the teeth. Without varying your position, glance at the maxillary and mandibular teeth on the right. Note

ABNORMAL

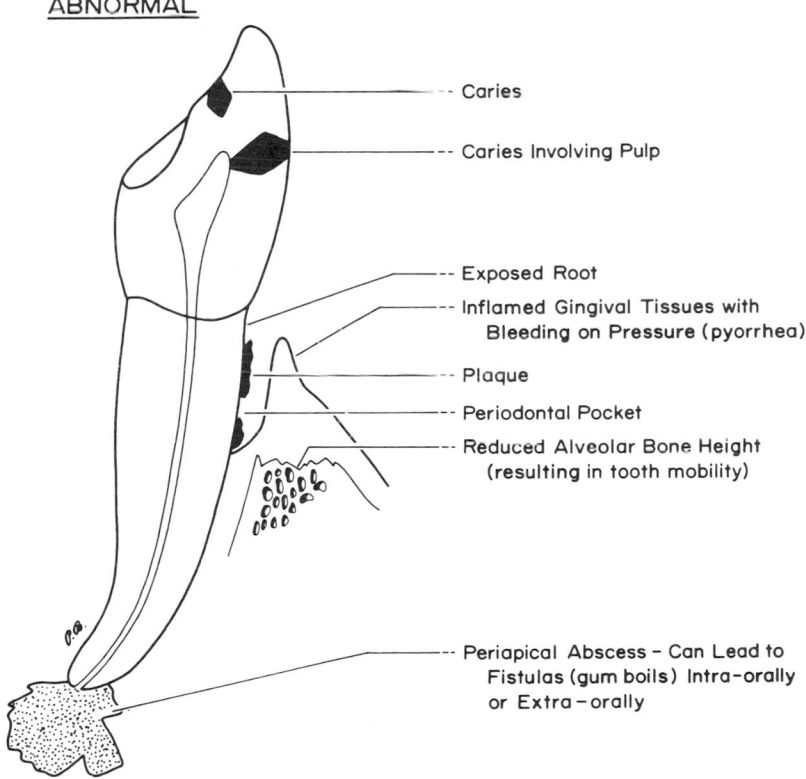

Figure 62. Potential abnormalities.

overt caries and missing teeth. Use finger pressure to test for mobility of teeth.

Switch the tongue blade to your right hand and examine the patient's gingiva and teeth on the left in the same manner.

The teeth viewed separately in each arch should number 16 if the patient is 18 years of age or older and the wisdom teeth are present. They should be in close apposition in the arch, each one lending support to the other (Fig 63).

When the mandible is closed against the maxilla and the patient's teeth interdigitate into their normal alignment, the teeth are said to be in occlusion.

The posterior upper teeth will be slightly buccal or to the outside of the lower teeth. Once again, the long axis of the roots are tilted ever so slightly to accommodate and foster this arrangement (Fig 64).

The front or anterior teeth are in a similar alignment, but more pronounced with the upper teeth extending further out over the lower teeth and further down on the outer surface. The amount of horizontal clearance is referred to as "overjet" and the amount of vertical overlap as "overbite." This occlusal relationship represents the dentition closed; ordinarily, however, we let our jaws hang loose or at rest. At this time, they are about 3 mm apart. This is referred to as the physiological rest position.

Last, have the patient close the mouth in the normal bite and "bare the teeth." Now using your tongue blade to retract either cheek, you may visualize the patient's occlusion. Obvious occlusal deformities should be noted. Many occlusal deformities can be corrected by oral surgery and orthodontic treatment.

Any discussion of the teeth and their occlusion must include a reference to the muscles of mastication and the temporomandibular joint. These three systems may be viewed separately for pure anatomical considerations but represent a finely balanced and dynamic relationship in the patient, as any clinician who has observed a case of acute gonococcal arthritis of the temporomandibular joint, a fractured mandible, or a painful abcess of a molar tooth can attest.

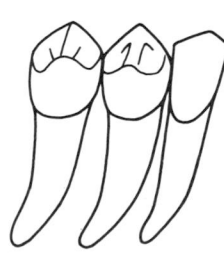

Figure 63.   The roots are slightly inclined toward the back of the mouth thereby giving a slight forward thrust to each tooth to help maintain its place in the arch.

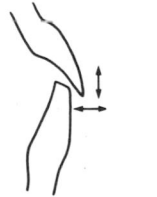 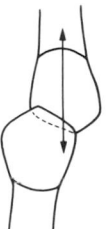

Figure 64. Normal occlusion.

An integral part of occlusion and the ability to masticate properly is bilateral symmetry of the muscles of mastication. The main group of muscles comprises the masseters, temporalis, and internal and external pterygoids. Their attachment to the mandible and the maxilla enable the patient to open and close the mouth at will.

Examine the muscles of mastication next. Face the patient directly. Note any bilateral asymmetry beginning at the midcheek area and extending to the angle of the mandible posteriorly and up to the temporal area superiorly. If asymmetry exists, the masseters and external pterygoids may be palpated bimanually.

Have the patient hold the jaw slack. Place your right gloved forefinger intraorally in the patient's right cheek. Use your left index finger and thumb extraorally opposing your right finger. Palpate the muscles in this fashion looking for lumps or masses that are not readily appreciated otherwise.

The third component of occlusion is the temporomandibular joint. With the teeth in occlusion and the muscles of mastication in contraction, the head of the condyle is in its most posterior and superior position in the glenoid fossa, which is shaped like a flattened S.

The temporomandibular joint is a very complicated joint of the ginglymoarthrodial type. It has three main movements along the glenoid fossa: downward, forward, and rotational, as the mandible opens and moves from side to side.

To examine the temporomandibular joint, face the patient once again. Turn your little fingers toward you and gently insert them into the patient's external auditory meatus. Have the patient open and close several times. You should be able to feel the heads of the condyles as they move forward and down to begin the opening movement in the glenoid fossae.

Position yourself in front of the patient's ear. Place your stethoscope approximately 7–10 mm in front of the patient's tragus of the ear and on a line to the alae of the nose. Listen carefully for signs of grating or crepitus as the patient opens and closes. The condyle head may also be palpated externally at this point.

Background Information

The skin (dry zone) of the lip has all the components of facial skin: sweat and sebaceous glands and hair. The vermilion border, on the other hand, has neither hair nor sweat glands. It is characterized by a thin, hornified epithelium which is abundant in cleidin, a transparent protein. For this reason, the underlying capillary network may be readily visualized and the lips appear either pink or red depending on the state of the capillaries.

The peculiarities of the oral cavity are unique. No other body cavity shares such a close relationship to the external environment, represents as many varied and functional anatomical entities, or contains bacterial flora in the amount or variety encountered in the normal human mouth.

The mechanical irritation of smoking, eating, and drinking alter the "normal" appearance of the oral cavity from one patient to another, and in many instances in the same patient from week to week. The warm moist contents of the mouth harbor enormous bacterial populations that immediately superimpose themselves on lesions, whether mechanical or pathological, and frequently distort the diagnostic picture by giving the lesions the appearance of being bacterial in nature. Lesions of the mouth cannot form "crusts" due to the dissolving effect of saliva, and wet-line lip lesions have different physical appearances than do dry-line lip lesions. While many lesions and abnormalities of the oral cavity are purely dental in origin and scope, many are not.

Sir William Osler was the first to refer to the mouth as the "mirror" of the body. Early signs of many of the common degenerative diseases, nutritional deficiencies, and diseases of metabolism are seen intraorally weeks and months before they are physically apparent elsewhere.

Our daily diet plus the mineral constituents of our saliva lead to the formation of dental plaque, which consists, for the most part, of bacteria with a scattering of leukocytes, macrophages, and epithelial cells contained within an amorphous ground substance matrix. The plaque is soft at first and may be brushed away with a soft toothbrush. About 2–14 days after the formation of soft plaque, the precipitation of calcium salts begin to harden the plaque until it becomes hard dental calculus.

Numerous factors contribute to the amount and quality of plaque that each patient generates; diet, pH of saliva, age, sex, and oral hygiene are but a few of the variables that are thought to influence plaque formation.

Current dental research indicates that plaque, sugar, and streptococci must all three be present and in sufficient quantities before dental caries can be initiated.

Except when masticating and swallowing, the jaws are usually in a "rest" position approximately 3 mm apart. On closing, the condyle goes to its most posterior position in the glenoid fossa, the closing muscles contract, and the teeth contact. This in itself is a complicated maneuver involving numerous neuromuscular reflexes, teeth that occlude, and conscious effort. However, this only begins the chewing motion. We only chew on one side at a time. Dentists refer to this as the "working" side involving the actual grinding. At the same time, the opposite side of the dental arch is involved in "balancing" as the lower buccal cusps sweep up to and balance against the lingual cusps of the upper molars. As this occurs, different opening and closing muscles are brought into play and each condyle head goes through different motions.

Taken quite literally, there are many components interacting to produce the chewing motions that we take for granted, and the disruption of any of these components can lead to problems. For instance, a new filling that is only 0.5 mm too high can interfere with chewing to such an extent as to make eating impossible.

Edentulous patients are a different case entirely. Dentures must closely mimic the natural dentition in terms of jaw distances on closing. If they do not, then temporomandibular joint dysfunction may result.

Clinical Significance

Oral manifestations of systemic diseases, malocclusion, and the more local aspects of dental problems (eg, caries and periodontitis) should be viewed in the proper context. That is, a normal healthy dentition functioning in a healthy oral cavity is critical to the patient's nutritional well-being. Anything that interferes with mastication at the beginning of the digestive process only makes function of the patient's other systems more difficult. Early recognition of this fact can often be the critical factor in rectifying future problems. This often falls to the physician since many patients never visit a dentist or seek dental care until it is too late both for their dentition and certain aspects of overall health.

Oral carcinoma as the primary site represents about 5% of the total incidence of carcinoma. Due to the abundant drainage of the oral cavity, early metastasis via the lymphatic and venous systems is common. The lungs and breasts are the most common areas of secondary involvement. Approximately 8,000 deaths a year are now accorded to oral cancer. The five-year cure rate is less than one-third for all cases, one of the lowest for any form of cancer. However, the number of victims surviving five years is doubled if treatment is initiated when the lesion is less than 2 cm in diameter.

Inability to open and close the mouth maximally can indicate an acute process or a chronic one. Examples of an acute process include a focal abscess involving any of the muscles of mastication or a fractured zygoma, which hinders the movement of the coronoid process of the mandible. Chronic inability to open the mouth freely can be due to ankylosis of the temporomandibular joint, or result from a formerly broken and unmanaged condyle head, or can be caused by long-standing arthritis.

Deviation of the mandible to either right or left can reveal the same type of acute or chronic processes. Local invasion of a basal or even squamous cell carcinoma or tuberculosis involving the temporomandibular joint can cause the muscles of mastication to present the same clinical picture.

The lip is the most common site of oral carcinoma, with squamous cell restricted to the lower lip in about 99% of cases and occurring more often in men than in women in the ratio 15:1. It is most commonly a result of overexposure to sunlight (actinic radiation). Fortunately, it tends not to metastasize and may be treated by a wide local excision or irradiation. Basal cell carcinoma commonly occurs on or above the maxillary lip.

The buccal mucosa is a common site for leukoplakia, defined clinically as a white patch that will not rub off (moniliasis, for instance, will rub off). It is a precancerous lesion that should be biopsied or removed. Cancer of the buccal mucosa appears most frequently in the middle third of the cheek. The vestibules are common sites for leukoplakia caused by snuff dipping.

Cancer of either the hard or soft palate is usually squamous cell, but it can be glandular. It may begin as a shallow punched-out ulcer with rolled indurated margins or it may be papillary with a wide base. Failure to detect the lesion early can lead to oral-antral or oral-nasal fistulas.

The tongue is the second most common site of oral carcinoma with the more posterior lesions generally being the most malignant ones. Unlike most other oral cancers, pain can be an early symptom. Carcinoma of the tongue may present as leukoplakia, an ulceration, or as the papillary type and may extend into the floor of the mouth. The junction of the lateral base of the tongue and the anterior tonsillar pillar is a common site for a fissure-appearing lesion which is easily missd on examination. Over 50% of all tongue cancers have metastasized by the time of detection.

Cancer in the sublingual space is often associated with leukoplakia, although this is not a common site for leukoplakia. As a general rule, the more posterior the lesion, the more malignant it is. Early metastases to the cervical lymph nodes are common.

If plaque accumulates near the gingival attachment, especially in the 3-mm normal gingival "pocket," it becomes a source of chronic irritation. This eventually leads to chronic inflammation of the gum tissues with resultant downward migration of the gum attachment. This in turn leads to a progressive loss of bone (since physiologically the height of the supporting alveolar crest bone is always 2–3 mm below the gingival attachment), deeper gum pockets, accumulation of more bacteria including anaerobic strains in deeper pockets, mobile teeth, and bleeding gums.

The common term for these signs is "pyorrhea." It may occur in only one area of the mouth or throughout the dentition; it may occur early in childhood or after approximately 40 years of slow buildup.

Periodontal pain due to chronic or acute periodontal disease is generally characterized as an ache or pressure-related ache in contrast to the "heart-throbbing" quality of a dental pulp pain or classic toothache. If allowed to encroach on the dental pulp, decay leads to pulpal necrosis with resultant death to the neurovascular component of the tooth. Necrosis of the dental pulp usually begins at the apex of the root where the foramen is small and therefore the blood supply most vulnerable. At this time, the pain is usually of the "heart-throbbing" nature characteristic of a vascular component, which is exactly the effect the necrosis is having on the vascular component of the tooth. If allowed to progress further, the necrosis results in an abscess once again at the site of the first necrosis, the apex of the root.

Accumulation of purulent exudate at the root of the tooth continues until relieved by root canal therapy or tooth extraction or until erosion of nearby bone opens a fistula, usually on the outside of the dental arch because buccal bone is thinner than lingual bone.

Sometimes the first signs of an abscess with resultant cellulitis can be a large swelling or fistula on the face near the apex of any of the teeth. This is not uncommon since frequently the apex of certain teeth are below the attachment (or above on the maxilla) of the buccinator, mentalis, mylohyoid, or other muscles, and the easiest avenue for the fistula is through subcutaneous tissue directly onto the face rather than through muscle attachments back into the oral cavity.

Occlusion, of course, is the key to mastication. Severe occlusal deformities can frequently be corrected by a combination of orthodontics and oral surgery.

Since the muscles of mastication, occlusion, and the temporomandibular joint are so closely related functionally, pathology in this area is often difficult to pinpoint. A frequent complaint involves the so-called temporomandibular joint syndrome. The patient reports pain on opening or closing the mouth and, more specifically, on chewing occurring in the general area of the external auditory meatus. Current investigators attribute this to a disruption of occlusion that causes the muscles of mastication to spasm, and they in turn exacerbate the occlusal disharmonies. This cyclic phenomenon is difficult to break and requires a combination of drugs, physical therapy, and occlusal adjustments in most cases. Certain drugs such as aspirin, the monoamine-oxidase inhibitors, compazine, stelazine, or thorazine are also capable of mimicking this particular kind of pain.

Selected References

1.   Archer WH: *Oral and Maxillofacial Surgery,* ed 5. Philadelphia, WB Saunders, 1975.
2.   Burket LW, Castigliano SG: *Oral Medicine: Diagnosis and Treatment,* ed 6. Philadelphia, JB Lippincott, 1971.
3.   Cheraskin E, Langley LL: *Dynamics of Oral Diagnosis.* Chicago, Year Book Medical Publishers, 1956.
4.   Glickman I: *Clinical Periodontology,* ed 3. Philadelphia, WB Saunders, 1964.
5.   Kerr DA, Ash MM Jr, Millard HD: *Oral Diagnosis,* ed 3. St Louis, CV Mosby, 1970.
6.   Shafer WG, Hine MK, Levy BM: *A Textbook of Oral Pathology,* ed 3. Philadelphia, WB Saunders, 1974.
7.   Sicher H: *Oral Anatomy,* ed 3. St Louis, CV Mosby, 1960.

137. Tongue

CHARLES HUGULEY, MD

Definition

This discussion refers to the anterior two-thirds of the tongue (oral tongue) visible on routine examination. The oral tongue is moist and pink with neither localized nor diffuse discoloration or ulceration. Filiform, fungiform, and circumvallate papillae are visible. There is normally a very thin "coat."

Technique

First examine the tongue within the oral cavity. Confirm the presence of all three types of lingual papillae. Check carefully for unusual size or coat. The coat is best evaluated in the posterior two-thirds of the oral tongue. Search for any areas of ulceration or discoloration. Now have the patient protrude the tongue. Briefly repeat the above examination and also evaluate the range of anterior tongue thrust. Refer to additional comments in the preceding section and in section 203, The Hypoglossal Nerve.

The most important disease of the tongue is cancer. The technique for examining the tongue for cancer is described in the preceding section.

Background Information

The oral portion of the tongue derives from the first branchial arch. The skeletal muscles of the tongue are covered by a mucous membrane containing three types of papillae in humans. Filiform papillae are the multiple small structures over most of the dorsum of the tongue. Fungiform papillae are slightly redder nearer the surface, and more numerous at the tip and margins of the tongue. Circumvallate papillae, 8–12 in number, are larger and lie at the junction of the oral and pharyngeal tongue.

The tongue functions to assist in taste, mastication, deglutition, and speech. Each type of papilla houses taste buds that convey the different tastes of sweet, sour, bitter, and salty. Specialized techniques beyond the physical examination are necessary for evaluation of taste.

Many references are made to the coat of the tongue. One interpretation of the formation of the coat is that dying stratified squamous epithelial cells become hydrated and white. The thickness of this coat is largely dependent upon the balance between the rate of production of epithelial cells and the rate at which the dead ones are worn away by activity such as eating and talking. If a disease interferes with the proliferation of cells, the hydrated dead epithelial cells of the tongue will not be replaced as fast as they wear off and there will be no coat. If cellular proliferation is normal but the usual removal processes decrease, there will be a thick coat.

Clinical Significance

In the past the tongue has been such a major object of interest that many adult patients reflexly stick out their tongues as soon as the examiner displays a flashlight or tongue blade. This focus evolved largely to determine if the coat was thick, or if the patient had a coatless, beefy-red tongue. Since the major wear comes from eating and talking, a thick coat indicates that the patient is neither eating nor talking very much and therefore must be sick. Since the patient already knows this, the observation adds little.

The standard descriptions of the tongue in pernicious anemia are that it is beefy-red, sore, and smooth with papillary atrophy. This description covers two separate developments, both rare nowadays. Inflammation of the tongue with redness and soreness may occur at any time in the deficiency of B_{12} or folic acid. It is usually transitory and seldom seen. Atrophy of the papillae with a resulting smooth tongue is a very late development. The diagnosis is nearly always made much earlier. A much more likely cause of a smooth tongue is false teeth. What is important is that if the deficiency of folic acid or vitamin B_{12} is severe enough to produce anemia, there will be no coat on the tongue, which may appear quite normal otherwise.

The tongue is severely affected by other vitamin deficiencies. These are much less common since the advent of fortified foods. When a vitamin deficiency does occur, it is very likely to be multiple. Therefore the distinction between the black tongue of niacin deficiency (pellagra) and the magenta tongue of riboflavin deficiency are not likely to be of diagnostic importance. Deficiencies of niacin, riboflavin, pyridoxine, folic acid, or vitamin B_{12}, resulting from poor diet or from the administration of antagonists, may cause a sore, beefy-red tongue without a coat. In the chronic vitamin deficiency state, the tongue may become atrophic and smooth. Chronic iron deficiency may also lead to an atrophic, smooth tongue.

The buccal mucosa may participate in an inflammatory reaction due to a vitamin deficiency. An increasingly common cause of an acutely sore and ulcerated mouth and tongue is the administration of anticancer drugs such as methotrexate, which antagonizes folic acid, or 5-fluorouracil, which directly interferes with production of DNA and therefore with the proliferation of cells.

Vitamin deficiency, particularly of riboflavin, can also cause cheilosis or fissuring at the corners of the mouth. A more common cause of cheilosis, however, is the drooling occasioned by the excessive folding at the corners of the mouth in the elderly patient with dentures and atrophy of the gums.

Patients receiving antibiotics on a chronic basis, particularly if immunocompetence is depressed by disease or immunosuppressive drugs, are particularly likely to develop moniliasis with stomatitis. It is characterized by snowy white fungal patches.

Prolonged penicillin use can lead to infection with *Aspergillus niger* and a characteristic painless brown or black "hairy" tongue with long, thickened and fused papillary tufts.

Another lead to systemic disease from examination of the tongue is macroglossia. This should be examined not only visually but also by palpation. True macroglossia will not only elevate the tongue but will bulge beneath the mandible displacing the sublingual glands. This finding may be an obvious and major clue to amyloidosis. Macroglossia may also occur in acromegaly or myxedema but is a rather unimportant finding among the many other manifestations of those diseases.

Minor abnormalities of the tongue deserve some mention. There is an anomaly of no significance in which the furrows in the tongue are deeper than usual without disturbance in the arrangement of the papillae. This is called "furrowed" or "scrotal" tongue. Another abnormality is the so-called geographic tongue in which there are areas of atrophy of the filiform papillae with normal fungiform papillae. These areas are separated by white lines of hypertrophied filiform papillae. The patches may wander or remain static. The condition usually appears early in life and is of obscure etiology. Reference 2 provides 30 excellent color photographs of various clinical disorders of the tongue.

Selected References

1. Vilter RW: Sore tongue and sore mouth, in MacBryde CM, Blacklaw RS (eds): *Signs and Symptoms,* ed 5. Philadelphia, JB Lippincott, 1970, chap 7.
2. Merril A, Kruger GO: An atlas of the tongue. *Am Fam Physician* 8(10):158–165, 1973.
3. Chosack A, Zadik D, Eidelman E: The prevalence of scrotal tongue and geographic tongue in 70,539 Israeli school children. *Comm Dent Oral Epidemiol* 2:253–257, 1974.

138. Tonsils and Pharynx

JOHN S. TURNER, MD

Definition

The palatine tonsils lie between the anterior and posterior tonsillar pillars and represent one part of a diffuse collection of lymphoid tissue in the pharynx (Waldeyer's ring).

The pharynx extends from the area behind the posterior nasal cavities and above the soft palate (nasopharynx) down to the tip of the epiglottis and mucosa lateral to the larynx (hypopharynx). This area and the nose are the most frequent sites of disease in the body.

Technique

The tongue often obstructs clear examination in this area. Ask the patient to open the mouth wide and inspect the hard and soft palate, buccal mucosa, tongue surface, teeth, and anterior tonsil pillars. Examine the anterior mouth with the tongue elevated; look for Wharton's duct openings (Figs 65 and 66). Using a flat tongue blade, depress one-half of the tongue and examine the tonsils, pillars, base of tongue, and posterior pharyngeal wall on that side (Fig 67). Repeat on the other side. A com-

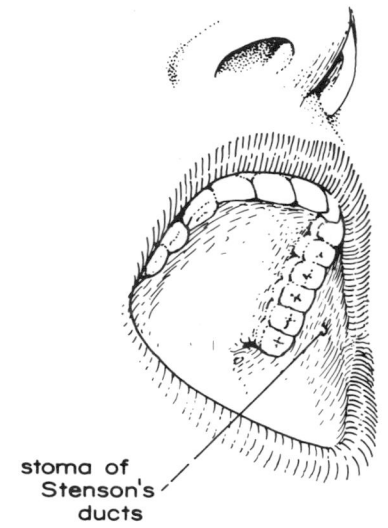

stoma of
Stenson's
ducts

Figure 65.   Stensen's duct stoma (opposite second molar).

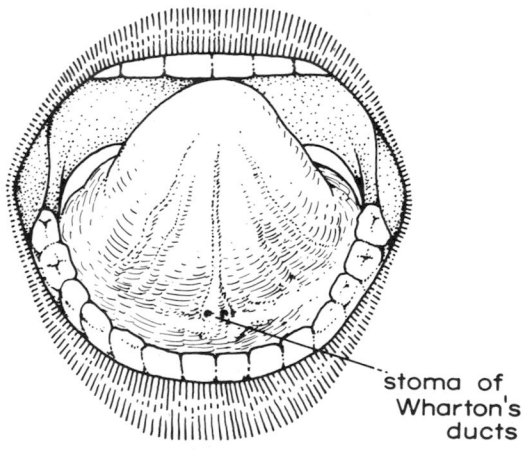

stoma of
Wharton's
ducts

Figure 66.   Wharton's duct openings.

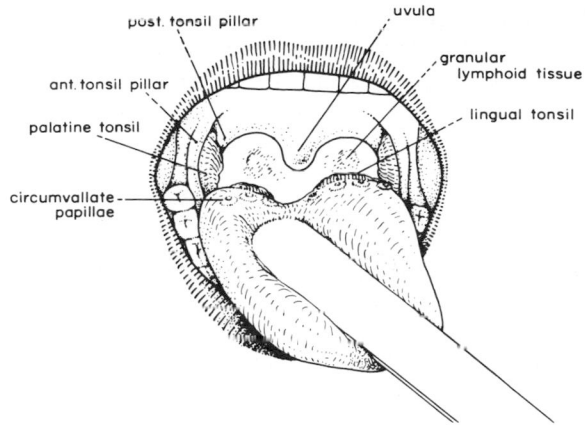

Figure 67. Place tongue blade two-thirds of way back, and press down hard (use two blades together of one blade bends).

mon mistake is to insert the blade too far posteriorly so that it gags the patient. If the blade is placed too far anteriorly, the tongue will mound up further and obstruct viewing.

If the gag reflex is excessive, ask the patient to gargle with Dyclone solution (10 cc) or lidocaine hydrochloride viscous solution (5 cc). (Do *not* use pontocaine or cocaine.) Wait five minutes and repeat the examination using a glove or a finger cot. The index finger is inserted into the mouth, and the entire tongue is palpated for masses or tenderness. The tonsil fossa is palpated for hardness, fluctuance, pulsations, and tenderness (Fig 68).

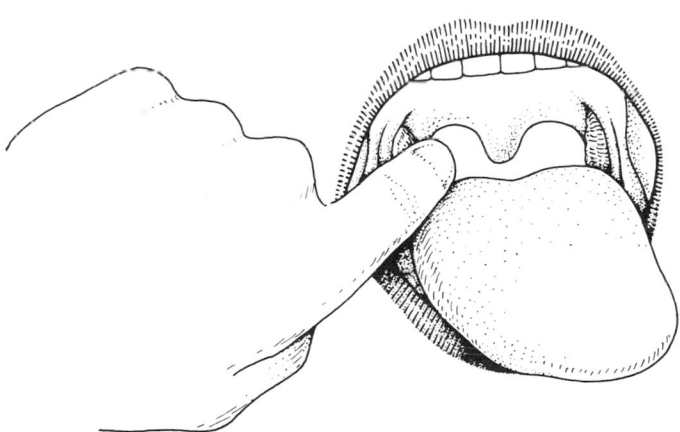

Figure 68. Palpate the tonsil fossa for hardness, fluctuance, pulsations, and tenderness.

Bimanual palpation is often helpful by placing one finger in the mouth and one under the chin. In this manner, the submaxillary gland, the sublingual area, and the floor of the mouth can be evaluated for tenderness or induration (Fig 69).

Background Information

The tonsils and other lymphoid tissue of the pharynx are considered to be a source of initial antibody formation for the body. This tissue is so diffuse that there appears to be little harm in removing the tonsils and adenoids (on posterior nasopharynx) if evidence of chronic debilitating infection exists or for any reason the tonsils have "forfeited their right of domicile." Enlargement alone is not a basis for tonsil removal unless significant impairment of respiratory physiology has developed.

Abscess around the tonsil is very common and occurs at the superior pole because the supratonsillar fossa is a loose potential space that permits pus to accumulate and spread into the soft palate.

Inflammatory ear disease develops when infection, edema, and stasis occur around the nasopharyngeal cushions (torus) or the eustachian tube. Changes in pH lead to decreased ciliary activities and ascending infection into the middle ear. Accurate anatomical, immunological, and bacterial diagnosis is needed in order to institute timely treatment of pharyngeal disease and prevent secondary ear disease.

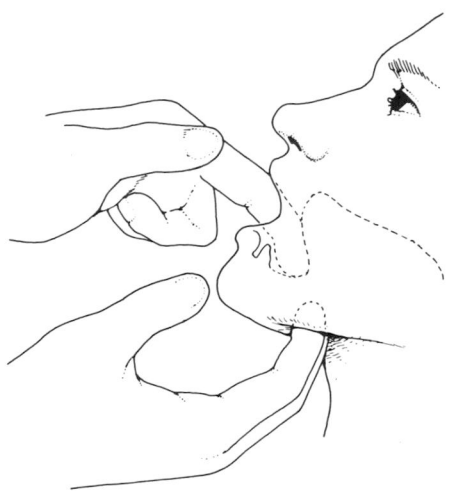

Figure 69.   Bimanual palpation is often helpful in evaluating the mouth for tenderness or induration.

Normal breathing occurs through the nose. Whenever obstruction in the nose is present (allergy, polyps, deviated nasal septum), the patient can no longer breathe properly and consequently breathes through the mouth (especially at night). The prolonged use of mouth breathing often leads to secondary "sore throat" and pharyngeal complaints, although the primary cause is nasal abnormality.

Clinical Significance

The mouth is often a mirror of disease in other parts of the body. The student must examine many hundreds of patients to determine the variations from normal. Inspection and often palpation indicate disease in the floor of the mouth, on the tongue, in the submaxillary gland, and in all areas of the pharynx.

Deep pits (crypts) in the tonsils are frequently seen with whitish material in them. This may not be abnormal since almost all patients with tonsils have these to some degree. The size of the tonsils and the presence of dilated blood vessels should be noted as possible indicators of disease. Enlargement alone may not be pathological and may be asymptomatic, but size should be noted.

Severe redness of the entire pharynx or areas of white exudate should be noted. These signs or the presence of small punched-out ulcerations may indicate bacterial or viral infection.

Enlargement of the lymph nodes in the neck are often a sign of disease in the mouth or pharynx. All areas of the pharynx must be searched carefully for a source of disease whenever an enlarged cervical node is found by palpation. An enlarged node just under the angle of the mandible is often a sign of tonsil infection or neoplasm (digastric node). Chronic infection or allergic reaction in the lymphoid tissue of the pharynx and nasopharynx are often seen associated with recurrent sinus and ear infections.

Patients with acute sore throat and an inflamed pharynx should have the tonsil area swabbed for bacterial culture (Fig 70). Patients with chronic sore throat should have a culture of the nasopharynx taken through the nose with care taken not to touch the nostrils with the swab (Fig 71).

Any granular or ulcerated area in the mouth, tongue, pharynx, or tonsil area should be watched for healing. Any lesion which does not heal in three weeks should be biopsied. Squamous cell cancer is commonly seen on the tongue, on the palate and palatine arch, and on the floor of the mouth. Almost all patients with oral cancer smoke heavily and drink alcohol regularly. Always ask about drinking and smoking and exercise a higher index of suspicion for neoplasm in patients who indulge heavily.

Obstruction in the nose with secondary poor nasal airway is a basic

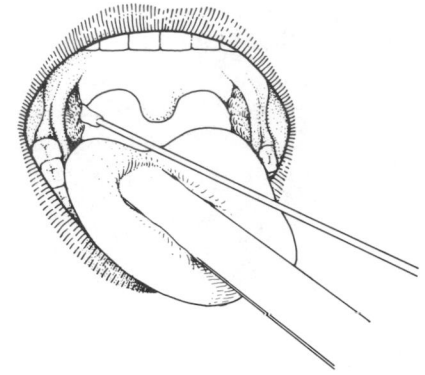

Figure 70.   Swab deep into tonsil tissue.

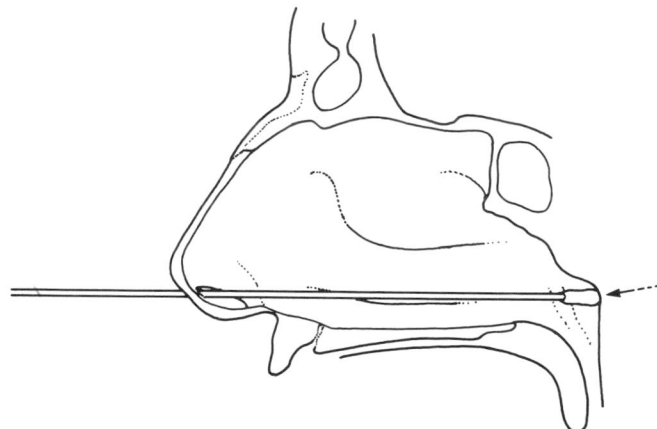

Figure 71.   Place swab low in nose along floor and go back to nasopharynx.

cause of many respiratory complaints both in the upper and lower airway. Much secondary sinusitis, sore throat, postnasal drip, recurrent laryngitis, and bronchitis develop because of nasal obstruction.

Selected Reference

1.   Jackson C, Jackson C (eds): *Diseases of the Nose, Throat, and Ear,* ed 2. Philadelphia, WB Saunders, 1963, pt 1.

139. Parotid Enlargement

MARK E. SILVERMAN, MD
W. DALLAS HALL, MD

Definition

The parotid gland(s) is considered enlarged if one (or both) is either visible or palpable.

Technique

Subtle parotid abnormalities usually go undetected by examiners who are not specifically seeking parotid enlargement as a clue to systemic disease. Enlargement is best suspected by the appearance of the patient (Fig 72). Normally there is a concave area between the superior ramus of the mandible and the anterior head of the sternocleidomastoid muscle as they near each other below the earlobe. Parotid enlargement causes swelling in this area and loss of the usual concavity. Marked bilateral parotid enlargement produces a chipmunk appearance (Fig 73), and the "moon facies" can be mistaken for those of Cushing's syndrome or pseudohypoparathyroidism. Striking enlargement usually conceals the earlobes when the patient is viewed from the front.

Enlargement of the parotid gland is confirmed by palpation. The normal parotid gland cannot be palpated. Place the thumb approximately 1 inch (2.5 cm) below the earlobe and the index finger in front of the external ear canal. Apply moderate pressure, then squeeze the thumb and index finger together. An enlarged parotid gland will "roll" between the thumb and index finger.

Background Information

The three paired salivary glands include the parotid, submaxillary, and sublingual glands. The parotid is the largest, varying in weight from 14 to 28 g. The gland is located in the parotid compartment slightly below and anterior to the ear.

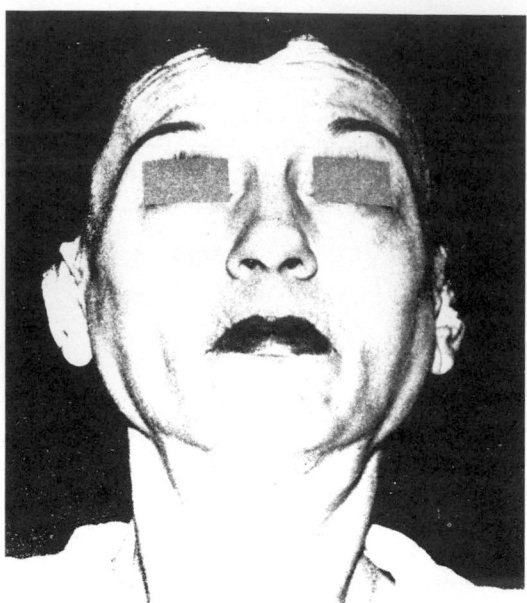

Figure 72. Parotid enlargement causing lack of concavity between mandible and sternocleidomastoid muscle. (From Hemenway WG, Allen GW: Chronic enlargement of the parotid gland: Hypertrophy and fatty infiltration. *Laryngoscope* 69:1512, 1959)

Saliva originates in terminally located acini and is delivered through Stensen's duct into the oral cavity. The entrance is visible as a small reddened area on the buccal mucosa opposite the second upper molar tooth. The parotid glands secrete about 45% of the 1,000–1,500 ml of salivary fluid that is produced daily. At rest the flow rate is less than 0.05 ml/minute. The masticatory and gustatory stimulation of eating promotes a vigorous flow of 0.5 ml/minute of saliva containing amylase, glycoproteins, immunoglobulin A, a secretory piece which joins to immunoglobulin A, lysozyme, lactoperoxidase, acid and alkaline phosphatases, nonspecific esterases, ribonucleases, kallikrein, and lactic acid dehydrogenase.

The saliva functions to lubricate for deglutition and speech, protect the mucous membrane, mechanically cleanse the oral area, buffer acidogenic microorganisms, promote and maintain tooth integrity, and provide an antibacterial and antiviral defense.

Clinical Significance

Parotid gland enlargement may be a consequence of infection; metabolic, hormonal, and nutritional alterations; foreign body; allergy to food, drugs, pollen, and catabolites of irradiation; heavy metals; tumor; sar-

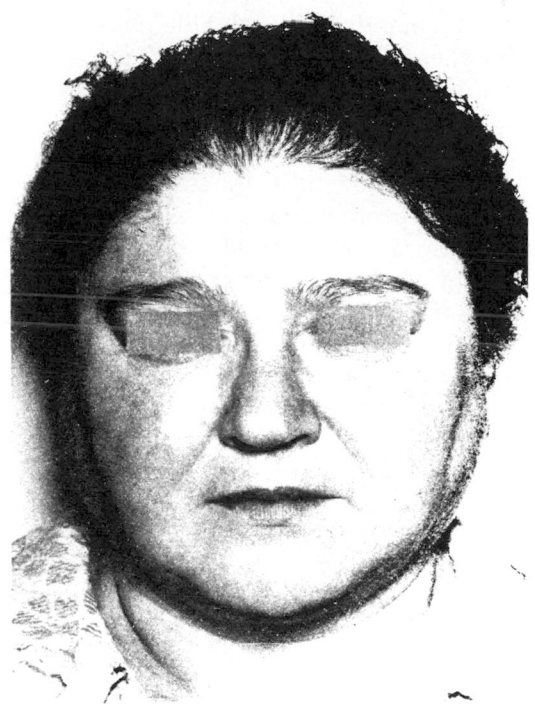

Figure 73. Rounded facies appearance of bilateral parotid enlargement. (From Hemenway WG, Allen GW: Chronic enlargement of the parotid gland: Hypertrophy and fatty infiltration. *Laryngoscope* 69:1512, 1959)

coidosis; postpartum lactation; calculi; Sjögren's syndrome; collagen disorders; dysproteinemia; ill-fitting dentures; and periodic sialorrhea. Parotid swelling has also been described in wind instrument musicians and balloon blowers. Infection, termed sialadenitis or parotitis, may occur from bacteria, particularly *Staphylococcus aureus*. Additional infectious agents include hemolytic streptococci, virus, tuberculosis, cat scratch fever, actinomycosis, histoplasmosis, tularemia, leprosy, and syphilis. Mumps virus is the most common cause of parotitis in childhood and provides lifelong immunity against infection. Since mumps is a cause of aseptic meningitis, the parotids should be carefully checked in all patients with this diagnosis. Acute parotitis is well known to follow abdominal surgery in a debilitated, dehydrated patient (postoperative parotitis).

Metabolic, hormonal, and nutritional disturbances include malnutrition, kwashiorkor, pellagra, vitamin A deficiency, liver disease, obesity, diabetes mellitus, hormonal dysregulation, hypothyroidism, mucoviscidosis, and starch ingestion. They generally cause bilateral parotid enlargement, although the glands may be asymmetric. The finding of noninflammatory parotid enlargement is sometimes a valuable clue to diabetes mellitus or alcoholic liver disease, occurring in nearly 50% of patients. Iodide, administered as potassium iodide therapy or following intravenous angiography, is a well-known cause of parotitis (iodide mumps).

Propacil (propylthiouracil), Artane (trihexyphenidyl hydrochloride), Kemadrin (procyclidine), Butazolidin (phenylbutazone), and lead or mercury intoxication can also produce parotid enlargement.

Salivary gland tumors constitute less than 3% of all tumors. Benign tumors include Warthin's tumor, hemangioma, lymphangioma, oncocytoma, monomorphic salivary adenoma, pleomorphic adenoma, mucoepidermoid tumor, and acinic cell tumor. Malignant tumors may be carcinoma in pleomorphic adenoma, adenoid cystic carcinoma, acinic cell tumor, mucoepidermoid tumor, squamous carcinoma, adenocarcinoma, undifferentiated carcinoma, lymphoma, leukemia and metastatic tumor. About 80% of salivary gland tumors occur in the parotid gland, and 80% of these are benign. Pleomorphic adenoma (mixed tumor) is by far the most common in the adult, accounting for 75% of parotid tumors, with Warthin's tumor a distant second. Some of the benign tumors tend to recur locally. Unilateral, often localized parotid enlargement should be considered tumor until thorough diagnostic procedures have ruled otherwise. Benign tumors are typically nontender, except for a pressure sensation, unless secondary infection or ductal obstruction occurs. In one series, about one-third of malignant tumors were tender. A facial nerve palsy and palpable cervical lymph nodes were ominous signs. Bilateral parotid and lacrimal gland enlargement, associated with peripheral facial nerve palsy, is very suggestive of sarcoidosis and is sometimes referred to as the Heerfordt syndrome or uveoparotid fever.

Sjögren's syndrome is a triad of keratoconjunctivitis sicca (dry eyes), arthritis, and xerostomia (dry mouth). Parotid enlargement, a systemic collagen vascular disease, and serum immunoprotein abnormalities are often present. The parotid swelling may be unilateral or bilateral and is characterized histologically by lymphocytic infiltration. Mikulicz's syndrome, an antiquated expression formerly used as a grabbag for a variety of causes of bilateral parotid enlargement, is now thought to be a less florid manifestation of Sjögren's syndrome.

Selected References

1. Cornog JL, Gray SR: Surgical and clinical pathology of salivary gland tumors, in Rankow RM, Polayes IM: *Disease of the Salivary Glands.* Philadelphia, WB Saunders, 1976, chap 5, pp 99–142.
2. Davidson D, Leibel BS, Berris B: Asymptomatic parotid gland enlargement in diabetes mellitus. *Ann Intern Med* 70:31–38, 1969.
3. Dunn EJ, Kent T, Hines J, Cohn I: Parotid Neoplasms: A report of 250 cases and review of the literature. *Ann Surg* 184:500–506, 1976.

4. Levine SB, Sampliner MD, Bennett PH, et al: Asymptomatic parotid enlargement in Pima Indians: Relationship to age, obesity, and diabetes mellitus. *Ann Intern Med* 73:571–573, 1970.
5. Mandel L: Inflammatory disorders, in Rankow RM, Polayes IM: *Diseases of the Salivary Glands.* Philadelphia, WB Saunders, 1976, chap 9, pp 202–228.
6. Rauch S, Gorlin RJ: Disease of the salivary glands, in Gorlin RJ, Goldman HM: *Toma's Oral Pathology.* St Louis, CV Mosby, 1970, vol 2, chap 22, pp 962–997.
7. Rothbell EN, Duggan JJ: Enlargement of the parotid gland in diseases of the liver. *Am J Med* 22:367–372, 1957.
8. Silverman M, Perkins RL: Bilateral parotid enlargement and starch ingestion. *Ann Intern Med* 64:842–846, 1966.
9. Wolfe SJ, Summerskill WHJ, Davidson CS: Parotid swelling, alcoholism and cirrhosis. *N Eng J Med* 256:491–495, 1957.
10. Wotman S, Mandel ID: The salivary secretions in health and disease, in Rankow RM, Polayes IM: *Diseases of the Salivary Glands.* Philadelphia, WB Saunders, 1976, chap 3, pp 32–53.

NECK

140. Neck Inspection

JOHN A. WARD, MD

Definition

Structures to be noted in the examination of the neck include the cervical lymph nodes, the salivary glands, the thyroid gland, the muscles, bones, and joints. Inspection of the arteries and veins in the neck is discussed in subsequent sections of the cardiovascular system.

Technique

Before beginning the inspection of the neck, try to obtain the best lighting possible. Sometimes adjusting the light to strike the neck obliquely produces shadows that magnify pulsatile movements, making them easier to observe. The use of a small flashlight can be profitably employed in this manner. Observe carefully for any evidence of trauma to the neck manifested by lacerations, contusions, or hematomas. If there is no history of trauma to the neck and the patient is able to sit up, inspection of the neck is more easily accomplished with the patient sitting upright.

Note the position of the trachea. If it is not in the midline, note how it is deviated from the midline.

From a position in front of the patient, note any parotid enlargement from the angle of the mandible to the earlobe. Look for any enlargement of the submaxillary salivary glands and any visible cervical lymphadenopathy.

Observe carefully the base of the neck for enlargement of the thyroid gland. Its usual position is just below the cricoid cartilage. It usually moves cephalad on swallowing. Many times nodules in the thyroid are first appreciated by inspection. If there is any anterior midline mass, instruct the patient to open the mouth and then slowly protrude the tongue. Note whether the mass moves upward. Thyroglossal duct cysts usually move cephalad on protrusion of the tongue.

Record the size, shape, and position of any mass in the neck. It is sometimes helpful to see if neck masses transilluminate with the use of a flashlight in a darkened room. Utilizing transillumination, the physician may identify cystic structures filled with clear fluids.

Examine the posterior aspect of the neck. Note any abnormality in the cervical spine, particularly straightening of the normal curvature. See if the head is held in a normal position or if it is deviated due to spasm of neck muscles. Note whether the patient flexes the cervical spine.

Inspect the skin of the neck. Acanthosis nigricans appears as a dark thickening with a verrucous surface. Pseudoxanthoma elasticum is manifested by small yellowish papules oriented along skinfolds. Note the size and position of any surgical scars on the neck and elicit specific historical data pertinent to the scars. Examine for any swelling of the skin, since edema in the neck may indicate obstruction of the superior vena cava. Record any abnormal skinfolds of the neck such as webbing of the neck.

In cases of trauma, utmost caution must be taken by the examiner to avoid neural damage.

Background Information

Embryologically the branchial clefts may not completely disappear. Residual structures may be retained in the lateral neck, particularly as small slits just below the earlobe. Some of these structures may become cystic or produce a fistula from the pharynx to the skin. If these cysts are filled with a clear fluid, they may be transilluminated.

The thyroid gland forms at the foramen caecum linguae at the base of the tongue. It then migrates caudad, coming to rest at the base of the neck. This migration of the thyroid may leave a tract that may give rise to a cystic structure, a thyroglossal duct cyst. This structure is usually in the midline. Since it arises from the base of the tongue, on protrusion of the tongue the thyroglossal duct cyst rises in the neck due to upward traction on the thyroglossal duct remnants.

Certain congenital abnormalities may be noted in the neck such as webbed neck (pterygium colli), in which the skin of the neck tends to form bilateral folds from the mandible to the shoulder. This may occur in conjunction with such syndromes as hypogonadism and congenital heart disease (Turner's syndrome, Ullrich syndrome, Noonan's syndrome).

Clinical Significance

Deviation of the trachea should be correlated with the chest x-ray. One should study the chest x-ray for causes of tracheal deviation such as masses, fibrosis, atelectasis, tension pneumothorax, or collections of pleural fluid.

Thyroid gland enlargement is often first appreciated by inspection. Refer to the section on examination of the thyroid when neck inspection reveals possible thyromegaly.

Straightening of the cervical spine may be a manifestation of rheumatoid spondylitis. Spasm of the neck muscles is called torticollis and may have several etiologies including congenital or traumatic defects in the cervical spine or musculature, compensation for a paresis of extraocular muscles, and psychogenic disorders.

Acanthosis nigricans may have serious implications because of its association with malignancies. Pseudoxanthoma elasticum is a disorder of connective tissue with systemic implications. Edema or swelling of the neck tissues may be indicative of neoplastic disease in the thorax obstructing the superior vena cava.

Stiffness of the neck may be indicative of meningeal irritation and may be an extremely early and subtle clue to meningitis or subarachnoid hemorrhage.

Parotid enlargement, cervical lymphadenopathy, and neck inspection in cardiovascular disease are discussed in separate sections.

Selected References

1. Patten BM: *Ductless Glands and Pharyngeal Derivatives in Human Embryology*, ed 3. New York, McGraw-Hill, 1968, pp 427–443.
2. Clain A (ed): The neck (excluding the thyroid gland), in Bailey H: *Demonstrations of Physical Signs in Clinical Surgery*, ed 15. Baltimore, Williams and Wilkins, 1973, pp 139–153.

3.   Morgan WL Jr, Engel GL: The approach to the physical examination, in *Clinical Approach to the Patient.* Philadelphia, WB Saunders, 1969, chap 4, pp 101–105.
4.   Robinson DW: Examination of the head and neck, in Delph MH, Manning RT (eds): *Major's Physical Diagnosis,* ed 8. Philadelphia, WB Saunders, 1975, pp 212–225.
5.   Kampmier RH, Blake TM: The neck, in *Physical Examination in Health and Disease,* ed 4. Philadelphia, FA Davis Co, 1970, chap 7, pp 245–267.

141. Carotid Bruits

JOSEPH HARDISON, MD

Definition

Carotid bruits are noises resulting from vibrations of the walls of the carotid arteries. Bruits are produced when there is partial obstruction to flow of blood or when the velocity and volume of flow are increased. Carotid bruits may be systolic, primarily systolic with extension into diastole, or continuous.

Technique

With the patient in the sitting position, the carotid arteries are palpated one at a time as described in the section on Pulses and Bruits. Auscultation is then performed while the patient is holding his breath. The bell of the stethoscope is lightly applied over the course of the carotid arteries from the base of the neck to the angle of the jaw. The supraclavicular areas are similarly auscultated to detect bruits arising from the subclavian arteries. Heart murmurs, especially aortic stenosis, may radiate into the neck, and this possibility must be considered when a bruit is heard over the carotid arteries. If a bruit is loud, a thrill may be detected with the fingertips of the examining hand. Cervical venous hums are frequently mistaken for carotid bruits, and ways to avoid this trap are described in the section 142, Cervical Venous Hum.

Background Information

Carotid artery bruits fall into two groups: innocent (cause unknown), and significant (cause known). Innocent carotid and subclavian bruits are common findings in young adults and children. The older the patient, the more likely a cause for the bruit can be found. Significant bruits may be subdivided into those due to increased flow and those due to partial obstruction of flow. Bruits caused by increased flow occur in patients with anemia, thyrotoxicosis, and arteriovenous fistulas. Partial obstruction to flow is almost always due to atherosclerosis of the carotid artery.

Bruits are loudest over the site of obstruction and are propagated for a short distance downstream but cannot be heard upstream. If a carotid artery is totally occluded, a bruit resulting from increased flow may be heard over the other carotid. In general, the louder and higher pitched bruits are more likely to be significant. This is especially true if the bruit extends into diastole. A systolic-diastolic bruit may indicate high-grade obstruction with pressure proximal to the obstruction higher than pressure distal to the obstruction in both systole and diastole. A loud, continuous bruit with bounding pulses is characteristic of a fistulous connection between the carotid artery and the internal jugular vein.

An almost pathognomonic sign of carotid artery disease is the finding of bright orange atherosclerotic emboli (Hollenhorst crystals) lodged at the bifurcation of retinal arterioles. This finding may or may not be associated with a carotid bruit on the same side. These emboli are almost certainly one cause of transient ischemic attacks, including amaurosis fugax.

Clinical Significance

Since carotid bruits may occur in normal people and be absent in patients with symptomatic obstructive carotid artery disease, it does not follow that all patients with carotid bruits need carotid arteriograms. Rather, a carotid bruit is just another physical finding, a bit of information to be used along with other information from the history and physical examination to help decide what is best for the patient. Cautious palpation of the carotid arteries, scrutiny of the eyegrounds, and careful auscultation are all important and additive in the examination of the carotid arteries and should be used along with the history in deciding if an invasive procedure or other work-up is indicated.

Selected References

1. Allen N, Mustian V: Origin and significance of vascular murmurs of the head and neck. *Medicine* 41:227–247, 1962.
2. Fowler NO, Marshall WJ: The supraclavicular bruit. *Am Heart J* 69:410–418, 1965.
3. Hollenhorst RW: Significance of bright plaques in the retinal arterioles. *JAMA* 178:23–29, 1961.
4. Ziegler DK, Zileli T, Dick A, et al: Correlation of bruits over the carotid artery with angiographically demonstrated lesions. *Neurology* 21:860–865, 1971.
5. Fields WS: The asymptomatic carotid bruit—operate or not? *Corr Cone Cerebrovase Dis* 13:1–4, 1978.

142. The Cervical Venous Hum

JOSEPH HARDISON, MD

Definition

The cervical venous hum is a continuous whining or roaring noise produced by the flow of blood through the internal jugular vein. It is loudest with the patient in the upright position, during diastole and inspiration, and may be increased by turning the head away from the side being auscultated. It is obliterated by the Valsalva maneuver, compression of the internal jugular vein, or lying down. It occurs more frequently on the right than on the left, and may be present bilaterally.

Technique

The examiner faces the patient who is sitting and, by applying light pressure with the bell of the stethoscope, auscultates the base of the neck just above the clavicle and lateral to the clavicular attachment of the sternocleidomastoid muscle. The patient is asked to hold the breath without "bearing down" or "straining." This will eliminate the noise of respiration and will prevent the patient from performing the Valsalva maneuver, which would obliterate the hum. If the examiner hears a continuous noise, the flow of blood through the internal jugular vein is interrupted by the examiner applying light pressure directly above the point of auscultation with the thumb of his free hand (Fig 74). The noise will cease if it is a venous hum, and the examiner can turn the hum off and on by alternately applying and releasing the pressure. The degree of pressure needed to compress the internal jugular vein will produce no discomfort to the patient and will be less than that needed for the examiner to compress his own radial artery.

Since an arterial bruit is loudest in systole and is unaffected by light pressure, the Valsalva maneuver, or the patient's changing position, it should not be confused with the venous hum.

Background Information

The cervical venous hum was probably first described by Laennec in 1830. It is present in 95% of children and 25–50% of adults. For reasons not entirely known, hums are rarely heard over other large veins. The effect of gravity on blood flow probably plays a part in the internal venous hum of the jugular vein. In addition, experiments have been done im-

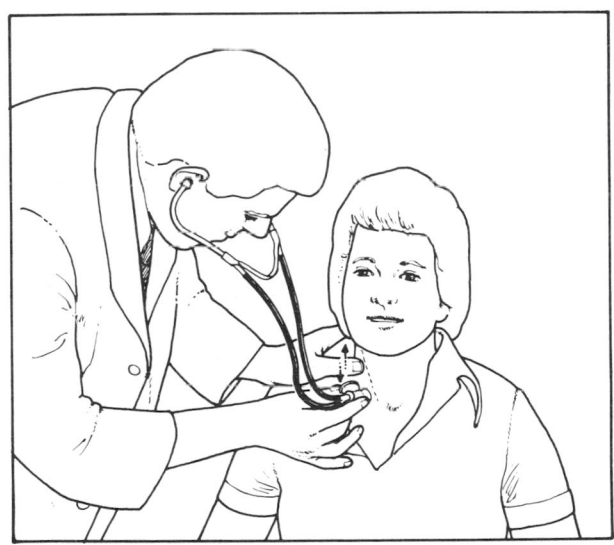

Figure 74.

plicating partial compression of the internal jugular vein by the transverse process of the atlas causing turbulent flow and thereby producing the hum.

Clinical Significance

The cervical venous hum has clinical significance in both a negative and a positive sense. Being a frequent physical finding in normal children and adults, it is often confused with the pathologic states of carotid bruit and arteriovenous fistulas or mistaken for muscle tremor or respiratory sounds. If especially loud, the hum may be heard in the first and second intercostal spaces and be misdiagnosed as a patent ductus arteriosus if heard on the left and aortic insufficiency if heard on the right. Even though present in normal people, the presence of a cervical venous hum should raise the possibility of a high output state, that is, anemia, hyperthyroidism, aortic insufficiency, intracranial and peripheral arteriovenous malformations or fistulas. These conditions are especially suspect if the hum is very loud or present in older persons. I have yet to see a patient with uncontrolled hyperthyroidism who did not have a cervical venous hum.

On the other hand, there are certain conditions that by their nature would prevent the occurrence of the venous hum: consider obstruction of the superior vena cava, constrictive pericarditis, pericardial tamponade, right ventricular failure, tricuspid insufficiency, and polycythemia vera.

In summary, the cervical venous hum is a frequent physical finding in normal people and should not be confused with pathologic states. The presence of a hum may be a clue to high output states, and the presence of a hum is evidence against significant obstruction of blood flow into the right side of the heart.

Selected References

1.   Jones FL: Frequency, characteristics and importance of the cervical venous hum in adults. *N Eng J Med* 267:656–660, 1962.
2.   Hardison JE: The cervical venous hum: A help and a hindrance. *N Eng J Med* 292:1239–1240, 1975.

143. Thyroid Examination

JOHN A. WARD, MD

Definition

The thyroid occupies a relatively superficial position in the base of the neck. This location enables the clinicians to conduct a fairly complete evaluation of the thyroid gland in most patients. By inspection, palpation, and auscultation the examiner can collect data relative to diseases and anomalies of the thyroid. The physical findings combined with laboratory measurements of thyroid functions can usually be coordinated to establish a diagnosis.

Technique

Inspection. This is best accomplished by having the patient in a sitting position with head erect. The examiner should observe the anterior neck carefully from the suprasternal notch to the floor of the mouth for any masses or thyroid enlargement. After observing the neck, have the patient swallow. It is helpful to have a cup of water available for this part of the examination as well as for palpation of the thyroid. Since the thyroid tends to move upward on swallowing, the examiner may notice the appearance of a mass or an asymmetry of the neck in the reigon of the thyroid. Note any scar in the region of the thyroid.

Palpation. For ambulatory patients or those able to sit upright the posterior approach can be used (Fig 75). The examiner stands behind the patient slightly to the left or right, whichever is convenient. With gentle palpation with the fingertips of both hands locate the thyroid cartilage, or "Adam's apple." The cartilage directly below this is the cricoid cartilage. The isthmus of the thyroid usually crosses the midline directly below the cricoid cartilage. At this point have the patient swallow by sipping water. During the act of swallowing the examiner should note that the isthmus rises cephalad under the palpating fingers. The movement of the thyroid tends to delineate it from the sternocleidomastoid

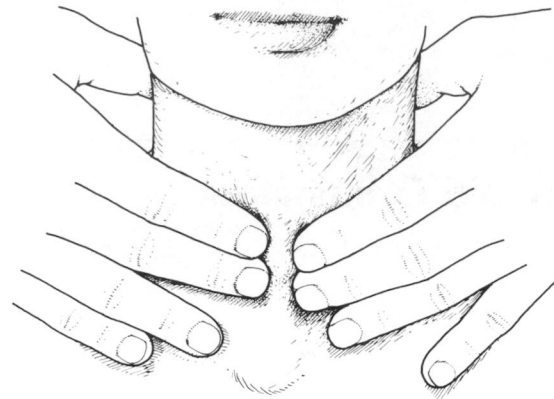

Figure 75. Posterior approach. Patient is seated with the examiner standing behind the patient.

muscles and other muscles of the neck. Gently move the palpating fingers laterally having the patient take small sips of water. In many normal patients the thyroid gland is palpable, and the examiner can palpate the right and left lobes. Continue palpating the thyroid by moving the fingers in a cephalad direction to delineate as much of the upper poles of the thyroid as possible.

Some examiners prefer an anterior approach (Fig 76). In the comatose or bed-bound patient this may be the only way to palpate the thy-

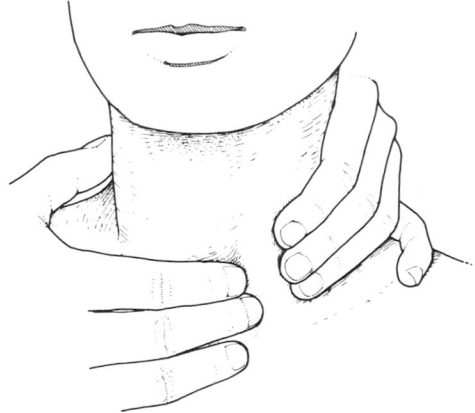

Figure 76. Anterior approach. The left lobe of the thyroid is being palpated with the examiner's right hand. The examiner's left hand is behind the neck with the fingers giving gentle counterpressure behind the sternocleidomastoid muscle.

roid. The examiner locates the cricoid cartilage and asks the patient to swallow. The thyroid isthmus is identified. The left lobe of the thyroid is gently palpated with the right hand pressing the lobe against the larynx or trachea, while the examiner uses gentle counterpressure lateral to the left sternocleidomastoid muscle with the fingers of the left hand. The right lobe of the thyroid can be against the larynx or trachea with gentle counterpressure to the area lateral to the patient's right sternocleidomastoid muscle with the other hand.

The normal thyroid gland weighs about 20–30 g and is about 6–7 cm across. Thyroidal enlargement or thyromegaly is termed goiter. Mild degrees of thyromegaly may be difficult to evaluate by physical examination alone since a considerable portion of the gland may occasionally be deeply embedded in neck structures.

During palpation note the consistency of the thyroid. Normally it should feel "fleshy" or have the consistency of muscles. With inflammatory or neoplastic processes there may be areas of varying degrees of firmness. Note whether the entire gland is firm and whether the normal anatomical contours are preserved. Also note if palpation of the gland is painful to the patient.

Note any masses palpable in the thyroid and record their size in centimeters or millimeters and their position in relation to the anatomy of the gland. A solitary nodule has a different connotation from multiple nodules. Note the consistency of any masses, recording if they feel cystic, firm, or stony hard.

If you are not able to palpate any thyroid tissue in the neck, consider the possibility of an ectopic location of thyroid tissue. The thyroid may occupy a substernal position, in which case percussion of the upper sternum may reveal a flat note rather than a relatively resonant one. Rarely the thyroid occupies a lingual position and rests at the base of the tongue. Occasionally thyroid tissue occurs in the ovary (struma ovarii) and if this tissue is oversecreting thyroid hormone, it may suppress the thyroid in the neck.

Auscultation. In hyperthyroid states you will occasionally hear a bruit in the gland. This must be distinguished from venous hums that may also be present in the hyperthyroid state. The venous hums do not usually have systolic accentuation and can be obliterated by gentle pressure to occlude venous drainage cephalad to the stethoscope.

Background Information

Embryologically the thyroid forms from the foramen caecum at the base of the tongue and migrates caudad to rest in the base of the neck. Thyroglossal cysts may form along the tract from the foramen caecum to the thyroid gland. These cysts are usually separate from the thyroid gland and move upward on protrusion of the tongue. They are usually located in the midline.

Clinical Significance

Hyperthyroidism may be produced by a diffuse hyperplasia of the thyroid gland as in Graves' disease. It can also occur with hypersecreting adenomata of the thyroid, as in toxic nodular goiter. The toxic nodule may be single or multiple. Hyperthyroidism may also be encountered in autoimmune thyroiditis, in which the gland may have areas of induration. In each of these conditions the palpatory findings of the thyroid can be quite different.

Hypothyroidism may result from pituitary failure, hypothalamic disease, or primary failure of the thyroid gland. In any case the gland may not be palpable. In some instances of primary hypothyroidism, a firm fibrotic remnant of the thyroid may be palpated.

Normal thyroid function is termed euthyroidism. Thyromegaly may occur in the setting of euthyroidism. If the gland has a smooth uniform surface it may represent a simple colloid goiter or a compensated partial defect in the synthesis of thyroid hormone. If multiple nodules are present in a euthyroid patient with an enlarged gland, the goiter is termed a nontoxic multinodular goiter.

Hashimoto's thyroiditis may present with a firm gland, sometimes described as ligneous. Usually the gland is not tender. Most often the normal anatomy of the gland is preserved. Hashimoto's thyroiditis may present with firm nodules. When involved with thyroiditis, the pyramidal lobe of the thyroid located on the isthmus may be prominent during palpation.

Subacute thyroiditis is usually painful to palpation. The gland may feel firm and may not be notably abnormal other than painful.

Neoplasms usually present as nodules within the parenchyma of the gland. These may vary from benign adenomas to carcinomas. Metastases from distant carcinomas may also present as thyroid nodules. At this point it can readily be seen that thyroid nodules require further diagnostic studies. Neoplasms of the thyroid may metastasize to regional lymph nodes. One node just over the pyramidal lobe was called the Delphian node because when it was involved, it foretold of malignancy. However, the Delphian node may be enlarged with Hashimoto's thyroiditis so that its presence may not be so dire as previously thought.

Cysts can occur in the thyroid and may present as nodules. These are frequently benign but occasionally represent cystic neoplasms.

The thyroid can be involved in systemic diseases such as sarcoid, lymphoma, and other systemic infiltrating processes. Pyogenic abscesses of the thyroid are rare, but may present with a very tender area of induration in the thyroid.

Selected References

1. Clain A: The thyroid gland, in Bailey H: *Demonstrations of Physical Signs in Clinical Surgery,* ed 15. Baltimore, Williams and Wilkins, 1973, pp 154–166.
2. Inngbar SH, Woeber KA: The thyroid gland, in Williams RG (ed): *Textbook of Endocrinology,* ed 5. Philadelphia, WB Saunders, 1974, pp 155–157.
3. Morgan WL Jr, Engel GL: The approach to the physical examination, in *Clinical Approach to the Patient.* Philadelphia, WB Saunders, 1969, pp 105–107.
4. Goss CM: The endocrine glands, in Gray H: *Anatomy of the Human Body,* ed 29. Philadelphia, Lea and Febiger, 1973, pp 1341–1344.
5. *Information for Physicians. Irradiation: Related Thyroid Cancer.* DHEW publication No. (NIH) 77–1120.

NODES

144. Lymphadenopathy

JAMES W. KELLER, MD

Definition

Lymphadenopathy refers to the presence of enlarged lymph nodes. In this section, consideration will be given only to the superficial lymph nodes where abnormalities can be detected during the physical examination. Normal superficial lymph nodes are not palpable except for occasional "shotty" inguinal-femoral nodes.

Technique

Patients are frequently unaware that they have palpably enlarged lymph nodes. When nodes are subsequently discovered, they are often referred to as "knots, swollen glands, kernels, pones, or lumps." Determine the duration of the enlarged nodes since causes of chronic adenopathy usually differ from causes of acute adenopathy. The patient may have noticed the node only recently, but it may have been there for a long period of time. Ask the patient whether the nodes are tender and if they have recently changed in size. Carefully note any systemic signs or symptoms such as fever, weight loss, night sweats, and pruritus; and any localized signs or symptoms such as sore throat, infections of the hands or feet, or a genital ulcer.

When examining for the presence of enlarged nodes, proceed cautiously. Areas of potential adenopathy are too frquently examined cursorily. Like the "new" heart murmur, a recently "negative" examination does not necessarily mean that nodes were previously absent.

Nodes in the neck are best examined by approaching the patient from behind, examining one side at a time. Carefully examine the following neck areas: occipital; postauricular; preauricular; superior, superficial, and deep cervical; submaxillary; submental; posterior cervical; and inferior deep cervical, including the supraclavicular and scalene nodes. Figure 77 illustrates the location and drainage areas of various lymph nodes in the neck.

The axilla is best examined in the sitting or recumbent position with the arm adducted and relaxed. The examiner's right hand is used to examine the patient's left axilla, and the left hand for the right axilla. The examiner's free hand may be placed on the shoulder to ensure the patient's position. Attention should be given to whether axillary nodes are high, intermediate, or low.

Epitrochlear nodes are best sought with the patient's elbow flexed to about 90°. The right epitrochlear area is approached by inserting the left hand from behind the elbow while the right hand grasps the right wrist to steady and maneuver the forearm. Examination of the left epitrochlear area is just the reverse. If the little finger of the examining hand is placed on the medial epicondyle of the humerus, the other fingers will overlie the epitrochlear area.

Inguinal nodes are found along the inguinal ligament in a horizontal plane. Femoral nodes are arranged vertically along the femoral canal below the inguinal ligament. Popliteal nodes are located behind the knee and are best examined with the patient's knee slightly flexed.

In each of the areas mentioned above, one should palpate by rolling the balls of the fingers first in a cephalad-caudad direction, then in a right to left direction. The presence of nodes should be recorded with

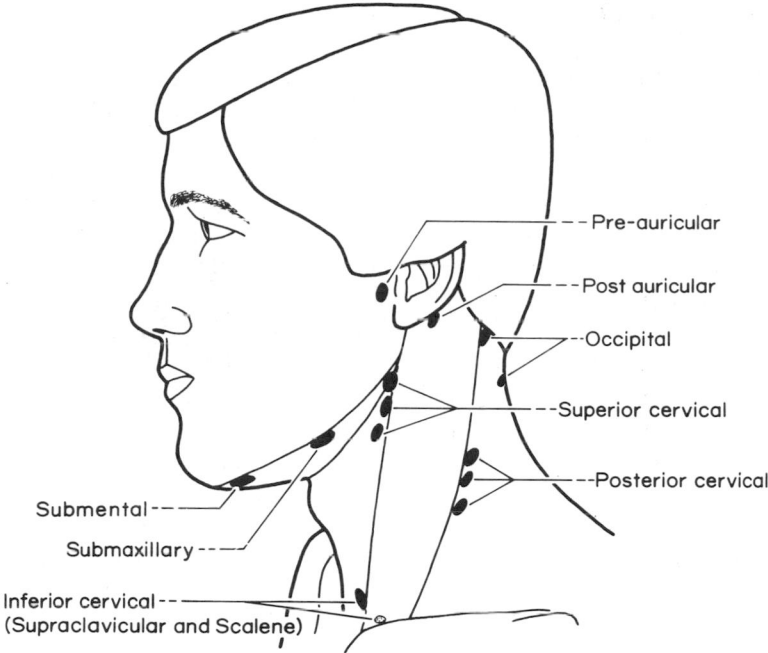

Pre-auricular

Post auricular

Occipital

Superior cervical

Posterior cervical

Submental

Submaxillary

Inferior cervical
(Supraclavicular and Scalene)

Figure 77.   Lymph node locations in the neck.

regard to location, size, tenderness, fluctuation, pulsation, and character
(matted, soft, freely movable, or fixed). Nodes less than 1 cm in perpendicular diameter are frequently referred to as "shotty" (shotlike).
Shotty nodes usually have less significance than nodes greater than 1 cm
in size.

The body contains more than 500 lymph nodes. Detection of most
requires special techniques beyond the physical examination. Mediastinal
and hilar nodes are best evaluated by standard posterior-anterior and
lateral chest films. Occasionally tomograms or gallium scans may be
helpful in certain inflammatory or neoplastic conditions. Iliac, sacral,
lumbar, and lower para-aortic nodes are best assessed by bipedal lymph-
angiography, although infusion pyelography or inferior vena cavography
are sometimes helpful. Celiac, mesenteric, splenic hilar, porta hepatis,
peripancreatic, and retrogastric nodes are not visualized with any of the
above techniques. These areas are best gauged by ultrasonography. Computerized tomographic scanning may also be useful in the upper abdominal area. The spleen is part of the lymphatic system and palpable
splenomegaly can be of considerable significance (see section 176, Spleen).

Background Information

Lymph nodes comprise the major part of the lymphatic system. They serve the important function of mounting an immune response. A great amount of new information has been accumulated on lymphocytes in the past decade. Currently lymphocytes are classified predominantly as "T" or "B" types. The T types (thymus-derived) are important for cell-mediated reactions such as delayed hypersensitivity, allograft and tumor rejection, graft versus host disease, and the production of lymphokines. The B lymphocytes (bursa equivalent) differentiate into immunoglobulin-secreting plasma cells necessary for humoral-mediated responses.

Basically, nodes consist of a connective tissue framework which houses and separates the lymphoid tissue into two general compartments: the lymph follicles and medullary sinuses. Germinal centers are within the follicles and contain primarily B cells. T cells are found predominantly in the interfollicular zones. The medullary sinuses contain mononuclear phagocytic cells such as histiocytes and monocytes. In spite of these general domains, there is ample opportunity for interaction of these cells in the node since T lymphocytes move through these different regions. In addition, each node has a blood supply, and afferent and efferent lymphatic ducts which are circuitously connected by the sinuses.

Enlargement of nodes may be due to infections, neoplastic disorders, metastatic carcinomas, hypersensitivity reactions, connective tissue diseases, endocrine-metabolic disorders, and infiltration with foreign substances. The last category is rarely a cause of superficial lymphadenopathy, but would include nodes associated with conditions such as anthracosis and silicosis.

Clinical Significance

First distinguish between generalized and regional adenopathy. Generalized adenopathy usually suggests a systemic disorder acting on lymphoid tissue. This need not imply presence of palpable nodes in every region, but usually describes nodes located above and below the diaphragm, or two or three regionally separated lymph node groups. When generalized adenopathy is present, consider the following conditions:

Infectious diseases

1. Infectious mononucleosis
2. Sarcoidosis
3. Toxoplasmosis
4. Brucellosis
5. Secondary syphilis

6.   Tuberculosis
7.   Diffuse inflammatory skin disorders

Neoplastic diseases

1.   Hodgkin's disease
2.   Non-Hodgkin's lymphoma
3.   Chronic lymphocytic leukemia
4.   Acute lymphocytic leukemia
5.   Waldenström's macroglobulinemia
6.   Blast crisis of chronic granulocytic leukemia

Hypersensitivity states and collagen vascular disease

1.   Systemic lupus erythematosus
2.   Hypersensitivity to drugs, such as diphenylhydantoin
3.   Serum sickness
4.   Rheumatoid arthritis
5.   Still's disease
6.   Dermatomyositis

Endocrine and metabolic diseases

1.   Hyperthyroidism
2.   Hypoadrenalism
3.   Hypopituitarism
4.   Lipidoses

Regional adenopathy usually suggests a localized disorder but may occur early in the course of those diseases which produce generalized adenopathy. Indeed, Hodgkin's disease frequently presents as regional adenopathy, whereas the non-Hodgkin's lymphomas usually present with several involved sites. Regional adenopathy is further considered with regard to six commonly involved areas: upper cervical, lower cervical, axillary, epitrochlear, inguinal-femoral, and popliteal.

Upper cervical adenopathy would include the following areas: occipital; postauricular; preauricular; superior, superficial, and deep cervical; submaxillary, submental, and posterior cervical. In general, lymph node enlargement in these areas usually suggests an infectious process first and a neoplastic process second. The occipital, postauricular, and posterior cervical nodes drain the scalp; the preauricular nodes drain the face and are frequently enlarged in eye problems; the high superficial and deep cervical nodes and submaxillary and submental nodes drain the pharynx and the mouth including the tongue. Accordingly, a search of the area that these nodes drain should be meticulously undertaken.

Avoid confusion of other structures with lymph nodes. In a very thin patient, one might palpate a vertebral process or a cervical rib and confuse it with a hard, fixed node. Similarly, the carotid body can be misinterpreted as a tender, high, deep cervical node unless pulsations are appreciated. Certain nodes are frequently enlarged in processes with generalized adenopathy. Classically, infectious mononucleosis causes enlargement of the posterior cervical and postauricular nodes. German measles (rubella) frequently involves postauricular nodes. Lesions of the eyelids and conjunctivae are characteristically associated with preauricular adenopathy, a combination sometimes referred to as the oculoglandular syndrome. Carcinoma of the oral cavity including the pharynx and larynx and especially tumors of Waldeyer's ring and the base of the tongue frequently metastasize to the high cervical nodes. Cancers of the anterior two-thirds of the tongue, the floor of the mouth, and the gums usually involve the submaxillary nodes.

Lower cervical nodes are located in the lower part of the neck below the level of the inferior belly of the omohyoid muscle. Enlargement of the supraclavicular or scalene nodes usually signifies a neoplastic process, so that lower cervical lymphadenopathy commands great attention. These nodes drain the head and neck area as well as the arms, mediastinum, and abdomen. Carcinomas that metastasize to these nodes include thyroid, larynx, and upper esophagus. In general, right lower cervical nodes drain the mediastinum, and left lower cervical nodes (Virchow's) drain the abdomen. However, one should not interpret this rigidly since the thoracic duct may show important anomalies, and lymphatic crossover in the mediastinum may occur. Right lower cervical adenopathy should suggest a chest x-ray for evaluation of possible mediastinal masses such as Hodgkin's disease or carcinoma of the lung. Carcinoma of the esophagus could also present as lower cervical adenopathy. Although the presence of a "Virchow node" in the lower left cervical area was once believed indicative of carcinoma of the stomach, it is now clear that this node can be enlarged with a variety of neoplasms such as from the pancreas, kidney, ovary, testicle, gallbladder, or lymphatic tissue. Likewise, the Virchow node can be enlarged in malignancies of the lung and the esophagus. In very thin patients, one must be cautious not to consider nodularity in the brachial plexus as adenopathy. Similarly, sebaceous, brachial, and dermoid cysts must be considered. Swelling in the midline usually signifies a benign or malignant thyroid disorder; thyroglossal duct cysts are also in the midline.

Axillary node enlargement is usually secondary to either infections or neoplasms which drain to this area. Infections to consider are streptococcal or staphylococcal infections of the hand or forearm, brucellosis, tularemia, cat scratch disease, and sporotrichosis. Malignancies that commonly involve axillary nodes are metastatic breast carcinoma and melanomas that have lymphatic drainage to this area.

Epitrochlear nodes are usually enlarged by infections that drain the hand and forearm. Rarely do neoplastic processes present with isolated epitrochlear adenopathy. These nodes are frequently enlarged in patients with infectious mononucleosis and non-Hodgkin's lymphomas.

Inguinal-femoral nodes drain the skin of the lower anterior abdominal wall, the genitalia, perineum, gluteal region, and lower anal canal, and most of the lower extremity. Shotty adenopathy in this region is fairly common and usually secondary to localized chronic inflammation. Certain conditions such as hernias, undescended testicles, aneurysms, and varices may masquerade as nodes in this area. Infections which commonly produce inguinal-femoral adenopathy include most of the venereal diseases, tinea, and pediculosis. Lymphogranuloma venereum may particularly cause large tender and fluctuant nodes. Isolated adenopathy secondary to neoplastic processes would include carcinoma of the genitalia and rectum as well as melanoma draining to this area. Ovarian and testicular malignancies do not usually produce enlargement of inguinal nodes.

Palpable lymphadenopathy does not necessarily imply neoplastic or life-threatening disease. Youngsters often have mild adenopathy, and it is not unusual to palpate some shotty posterior cervical nodes in young adults without apparent cause. Children of age 12 have almost twice as much lymphoid tissue as persons over age 20. Lymphoid tissue in children appears to respond promptly with impressive swelling and hyperplasia. This response is less dramatic in adults. There are 10 causes of localized or generalized adenopathy that should be considered in young adults:

1. Leukemia
2. Hodgkin's disease
3. Mononucleosis
4. Toxoplasmosis
5. Sarcoidosis
6. Tuberculosis
7. Cat scratch disease
8. Metastatic disease
9. Lupus
10. Rheumatoid arthritis

Although it is impossible to be sure what is contained in an enlarged node without biopsy, this urge should not be pursued immediately. Similarly, one should not consider adenopathy an indication for antibiotics. When biopsy is elected, it is frequently stated that a cervical node is preferable to an axillary, and that an axillary node is preferable to an inguinal. This clinical guideline acknowledges the fact that cervical nodes, especially lower cervical, are less likely to enlarge secondary to infections, whereas axillary and inguinal nodes may react to repeated trauma and trivial infections of the extremities. Biopsy of certain nodes may require a general anesthetic and can be associated with some morbidity. What some clinicians consider a "significant" small node might be difficult for a surgeon to excise since local anesthesia might distort the area. A close working relationship between clinician and surgeon is imperative.

Lymphadenopathy must be considered in the total clinical picture in making the decision concerning antibiotics or biopsy. An area of cellulitis believed secondary to a streptococcal infection in the leg with associated tender inguinal adenopathy would obviously require antibiotic treatment. A young lady with signs and symptoms of lupus with generalized adenopathy would require neither antibiotics nor biopsy. An unexplained, low, painless cervical node in a young person should prompt a thorough examination of the hypopharynx and thyroid gland, a chest x-ray to assess the mediastinum, and early biopsy if a primary tumor is not discovered. Frequently a period of observation might be warranted to collect more information and observe the behavior of a node, especially in a patient who does not appear ill.

Selected References

1. Harvey AM, Bordley J: *Differential Diagnosis*. Philadelphia, WB Saunders, 1972, chap 10, pp 361–364.
2. Slaughter DP, Majarakis JD, Southwick HW: Clinical evaluation of swellings in the neck. *Surg Clin N Am* 36:3–9, 1956.
3. Solnitzsky OC, Jeghers H: Lymphadenopathy and disorders of the lymphatic system, in MacBryde CM, Blacklow RS: *Signs and Symptoms: Applied Pathologic Physiology and Clinical Interpretation*, ed 5. Philadelphia, JB Lippincott, 1970, chap 26, pp 476–538.

CHEST

145. Chest Structure

JAMES C. CRUTCHER, MD

Definition

The configuration of the normal chest is determined by the thoracic spine, ribs, sternum, and the cartilaginous connection between the sternum and the ribs. There is variation both in the curvature of the ribs and thoracic spine so that normal variations in the A-P diameter of the chest cage are to be expected.

Abnormality of chest structure usually must be marked to be noted by the examiner. Straightening of the upper thoracic curvature, depression of the sternum, depression of the level of one shoulder compared with the other, and marked difference in the A-P diameter of one side of the chest compared with the other would constitute abnormalities of structure.

Technique

Acquisition of important information is easily done by simple inspection, using only the eyes and hands. Visual inspection of the position of both clavicles and shoulders should show relative parallelism of height. Inspection of the thoracic spine aided by digital identification of the spinous processes will usually define the expected vertical alignment and thoracic curvature. Palpation of the sternal costochondral junction along with visual inspection will usually demonstrate abnormalities such as pectus excavatum or pectus carinus.

It must be reemphasized that the major technique employed in the examination of the structure of the chest is the comparison of both sides for volume and symmetry. Variations from this normal may be significant but should be measurable. Nonmeasurable observations such as "increased A-P diameter" should be avoided.

Background Information

The primary structure of the chest is designed to facilitate ventilation, which can be accomplished only by increasing the intrathoracic volume. This increase is due to elevation of the ribs, contraction of the scalene and intercostal muscles, and descent of the diaphragm. Because of the structure of the ribs, the scalenus muscles elevate the first rib and the sternum anteriorly. This causes slight increase in A-P diameter of the chest. The lower ribs (T6–T12) expand laterally by contraction of the intercostal muscles. The diaphragm, by contracting, elevates the lower ribs superiorly and laterally as well as increasing the intrathoracic volume. Any deviation from the normal anatomical relationship of the skeletal system and the associated muscles would be expected to cause some abnormality in the inspiratory cycle of ventilation.

The relationship of the A-P diameter to the lateral diameter of the chest is approximately 0.8 to 1. The A-P diameter is measured from T8 posteriorly to the interior border of the sternum anteriorly, using the lateral chest x-ray film. The lateral measurement of the chest is measured from the interior margin of the lateral rib cage at the level of the right diaphragm, using the P-A chest x-ray.

Clinical Significance

Asymmetry of the chest cage may indicate variations of normal or significant skeletal and/or intrathoracic pathology. The difference in levels of the clavicle and shoulders may indicate abnormality of the thoracic spine (scoliosis) or volume loss on the side of the lowered shoulder. Such volume loss is usually chronic and may be due to chronic adhesive pleuritis or parenchymatous volume loss. Surgical loss of lung tissue would produce the same findings, but a surgical scar on the chest would then be the essential clue.

Abnormal depression of the sternum will cause abnormality of the cardiac silhouette by compression of the heart between the sternum and the spine. There may be accentuation of the pulmonary outflow tract. Additionally, there may be an associated flattening of the normal thoracic kyphosis, causing the "straight back syndrome." These two skeletal abnormalities, straightening of the thoracic spine and depression of the sternum (pectus excavatum), will cause abnormalities on examination of the heart. These findings include accentuated splitting of the second sound with increased intensity of the pulmonic component, parasternal ejection type systolic murmur, and occasionally systolic ejection clicks. The electrocardiogram may show incomplete right bundle branch block and minor abnormalities of the T wave over the right precordial leads. The correlation of the x-ray abnormality, auscultatory findings, and the EKG are greatly enhanced if the examiner recognizes that the patient has either pectus excavatum or straightening of the thoracic spine or both.

Selected References

1. Cherniak RM, Cherniak L: *Respiration in Health and Disease*. Philadelphia, WB Saunders, 1961, chap 1, pp 3–32; chap 4, pp 68–86.
2. Fletcher CM: The clinical diagnosis of pulmonary emphysema: An experimental study. *Proc R Soc Med* 45:577–584, 1952.
3. Forgacs P: Lung sounds. *Br J Dis Chest* 63(1):1–11, 1969.
4. Fraser RG, Paré JAP: *Diagnosis of Diseases of the Chest*. Philadelphia, WB Saunders, 1970, vol 1, chap 1–3, pp 1–156.
5. Godfrey S, Edwards RHT, Campbell R Jr: Repeatability of physical signs in airways obstruction. *Thorax* 24:4–9, 1969.
6. Nairn JR, Turner-Warwick M: Breath sounds in emphysema. *Br J Dis Chest* 63:29–37, 1969.

7. Pulmonary terms and symbols: A report of the American College of Chest Physicians and the American Thoracic Society. *Chest* 67(5): 583–593, 1975.
8. Ruth WE: Examination of the chest, in Delph MH, Manning RT (eds): *Major's Physical Diagnosis*, ed 7. Philadelphia, WB Saunders, chap 6, pp 89–116.
9. Schneider IC, Anderson A Jr: Correlation of clinical signs with ventilatory function in obstructive lung disease. *Ann Intern Med* 62:447–485, 1965.
10. Siegel JS, Schechter E: The straight back syndrome. *Am J Med* 42: 309–313, 1967.

146. Chest Motion

JAMES C. CRUTCHER, MD

Definition

Normal. The respiratory cycle is diphasic consisting of an inspiratory and expiratory phase. In the normal state, inspiration is below the conscious awareness of the patient and is caused by the automatic contraction of the muscles of inspiration: the scalenes, the intercostals, and the diaphragm. This coordinated contraction symmetrically expands the thoracic cage in the anterior-posterior, transverse, and vertical diameters. This conical expansion is bilaterally equal with the major observable increases being in the lateral expansion of the lower chest cage and the anterior movement of the sternum.

Expiration is passive and the thoracic cage returns to the preinspiratory volume by relaxation of the muscles of inspiration and the elastic recoil of the lungs.

Abnormal. In the resting state the visible use of the accessory muscles on inspiration and expiration is abnormal. Asymmetry in expansion of the thorax and inspiratory retraction are major abnormalities of motion.

Technique

Whenever possible, have the patient sit on the examining table unclothed from the waist up. Make observations separately in the inspiratory and expiratory phases of breathing during normal and forced ventilatory effort.

Inspiratory observation. Standing in front of the patient, observe for the expansion of both sides of the thorax noting the symmetry of expansion. Lateral expansion may be unilaterally or bilaterally impaired. Record whether the lateral expansion is decreased or absent, or if there is paradoxical inspiratory retraction. Observe for the use of accessory muscles of inspiration.

Moving to the side of the patient, observe for the movement of the sternum by placing one hand on the upper thoracic spine and the other hand on the main body of the sternum. Observe for the anterior-superior movement on inspiration. An anterior-superior movement of more than 45° from the horizontal should be recorded as an abnormal superior movement of the sternum.

Stand behind the patient and observe again for the lateral expansion of the chest wall. Confirm this visual observation by placing the hands firmly along the axis of the seventh intercostal space with the thumbs in apposition over the spine, the palm of the hands at the costal angle, and the fingers extended along the intercostal spaces anteriorly. On normal inspiration observe for the expansion of the interspaces and the lateral movement of the chest cage. Subtle abnormalities in this intercostal and lateral expansion may be brought out by having the patient take in a deep breath.

When chest trauma may have occurred, observe the patient in the supine position. The examiner should stand at the foot of the bed and carefully observe for inspiratory retraction of one side of the chest compared with the other and for retraction of the sternum on inspiration. This paradoxical inward movement of the chest cage on inspiration is known as a "flail" chest.

Expiratory observations. Expiration is normally passive, and there should be little discernible use of the abdominal muscles in the resting state. When abdominal musculature is used, observe carefully for contraction of the abdominal muscle just before the next inspiration. This end-expiratory contraction of the abdomen is often associated with pursing of the lips and is a discernible abnormality. Evidence of chronic active expiration may also be confirmed by looking for callous formation over the elbows or the prepatella areas of both thighs. These callouses result from the patient bending forward with elbows on the knees to facilitate both inspiration and expiration.

Background Information

The integrated function of the thoracic musculoskeletal system with the diaphragm is primarily designed for increase in intrathoracic volume to allow for inspiratory airflow to take place. This phase of breathing is always active due to the elastic recoil of the lung, the resistance of the chest wall, the subatmospheric pressure of the pleural surfaces, and the normal resistance of turbulent airflow mainly at the upper airways. In the resting state, in normal individuals, breathing is automatic and below conscious awareness.

Clinical Significance

Observation of the use of the accessory muscles of inspiration (scalenes and sternocleidomastoid) is evidence of an abnormal inspiratory effort. This abnormality may be under cortical control as seen in voluntary overventilation. It is commonly seen in patients with emphysema in which the large resting volume of the lung requires considerable inspiratory effort in order to increase the intrathoracic volume.

In airway obstructions, commonly in bronchitis or in changes in the compliance of the lung (as in various interstitial diseases), abnormal inspiratory effort is noted by use of the accessory muscles. Diseases characterized by pulmonary emboli, pneumonia, left ventricular failure, and various metabolic disorders resulting in metabolic acidosis will cause increased inspiratory motion of the chest resulting in an increase in ventilation. Use of the abdominal muscles on expiration usually indicates obstruction to airflow and/or lack of the normal elastic recoil of the lungs.

Unilateral restriction on inspiration may be secondary to rib fractures, pleuritic irritation with the spasm of intercostal muscles, organized pleural effusion resulting in adhesive pleuritis which limits the expansion of the underlying lung tissue, and unilateral obstruction to airway from a foreign body or an endobronchial tumor. At times, obstruction of a major bronchus may cause increased expansion distal to the area of obstruction because of the increased work required to inspire and expire air through a partially narrowed bronchus.

Lack of lateral excursion of the chest cage bilaterally and, at times, with paradoxical inspiratory retraction of the lower chest cage is indicative of chronic overinflation of the lung and is a common finding in far advanced emphysema. Paradoxical inspiratory collapse of the sternum or one side of the chest may be due to fracture of the ribs or chondrocostal separation resulting in a "flail" chest. An increase in the anterior-superior movement of the sternum is indicative of chronic overinflation of the lung. In summary, integration of observations of muscle contractions, amplitude and direction of chest movements, with reference to inspiration and expiration, allows the observer to make clinically significant assessments. Confirmation of these observations by more sophisticated techniques (fluoroscopy, x-ray films, pulmonary ventilation tests) may be indicated and necessary. With experience, however, such kinds of reinforcement may not be necessary. As a result, physical assessment of chest movements becomes a reliable clue to diagnosis.

Selected References

1. Cherniak RM, Cherniak L: *Respiration in Health and Disease.* Philadelphia, WB Saunders, 1961, chap 1, pp 3–32; chap 4, pp 68–86.
2. Schneider IC, Anderson A Jr: Correlation of clinical signs with ventilatory function in obstructive lung disease. *Ann Intern Med* 62:477–485, 1965.
3. Siegel JS, Schechter E: The straight back syndrome. *Am J Med* 42: 309–313, 1967.
4. Godfrey S, Edwards RHT, Campbell R Jr: Repeatability of physical signs in airways obstruction. *Thorax* 24:4–9, 1969.

---

147. Chest Auscultation

JAMES C. CRUTCHER, MD

Definition

The normal acoustical characteristic of inspiratory and expiratory breath sounds is a featureless hiss composed of random frequencies and amplitudes generated by turbulent airflow through multiple branching conduits. The site of auscultation on the chest wall will alter these sounds depending on distance from the origins and the intervening structures. For convenience of recording, there are three types of normal sounds heard:

1. Bronchial breath sounds. These sounds are heard over the trachea and major airways.

2. Vesicular. These sounds are heard over the mid third of the lower lobes, posteriorly.
3. Bronchovesicular. These sounds are intermediate and are heard between the scapula posteriorly and just below the clavicle anteriorly.

Abnormal breath sounds may be defined as finding bronchial sounds in normal areas for vesicular sounds. Increased intensity or loudness of breath sounds with normal velocity is noted as noisy breathing.

Adventitious sounds on inspiration or expiration are an abnormality. The preferred classification for these not normally heard sounds are:

1. Crackles. Discontinuous, crackling, or bubbling sounds heard almost exclusively in inspiration. Further adjectival classification adds only confusion.
2. Wheezes. These are polyphonic (musical), continuous sounds of varying harmonics. They may vary in pitch, quality, and intensity.

Technique

A defined and reproducible approach should be used in the examination of each patient. Always listen and record separately those observations made in inspiration and expiration with a normal ventilatory cycle followed by having the patient take in a deep breath and then blow it all out.

Because of the variables in chest wall thickness and the change in the variability in the lung volume, it is necessary to use patients as their own control by comparing the sounds heard on comparable areas on both sides of the chest. Time can be saved if one listens over the major lung areas. These areas are: (1) anteriorly over the midclavicular line in the second intercostal space (ICS), (2) in the midaxillary line at the fifth ICS, (3) posteriorly in the infrascapula area at the midscapula line, (4) in the midscapula area over the middle third of the lower lung fields.

Since parenchymous diseases of the lung as well as disorders of the pleura alter the transmission of breath sounds to the chest wall, one should listen primarily for alterations in airflow and the presence or absence of adventitious sounds during both phases of the ventilatory cycle. Auscultation of the chest is more precise for eliciting data on the transmission of air sounds through the conduits. The acquisition of data regarding abnormal transmission of breath sounds through the chest wall due to structural alterations within the chest area is less precise. The chest x-ray is a better source of data for determining these abnormalities. However, for continued self-education, it is advantageous to listen to the chest a second time after having seen the chest x-ray. In this manner, one can improve the technique of picking up abnormal transmission of breath sounds due to parenchymatous disease of the lung or diseases of the pleura.

Background Information

Breath sounds are generated by the flow of air through the branching conduits down to the sixth or seventh order of the bronchi. The intensity and duration of inspiratory breath sounds are dependent upon the velocity of airflow, the degree of turbulence, and the dampening effect of supporting structures that interface between the origin of the breath sounds and the area of auscultation on the chest wall. In normal subjects with normal inspiratory volume of 300–500 ml of air, breath sounds are characterized by a random collection of frequencies between 200–2000 cps and amplitude (intensity). Increase in velocity of airflow in the normal individual will increase both the intensity and the amplitude of these sounds, causing noisy breathing. Increased intensity of breath sounds with normal inspiratory flow rates would then be considered an abnormality. Such examples are illustrated by a sigh or a gasp in the normal individual.

The mechanism of the production of adventitious sounds (crackles and wheezes) remains controversial. There is general agreement, however, that the generation of these sounds from abnormal airways is in the proximal and central airways, rather than in the distal terminal bronchioles and alveoli. Flow in these areas is slow and laminar and unlikely to be heard on the chest wall.

The repetitive, staccato, sounds (crackles) heard almost exclusively in inspiration is probably due to underinflation of a pulmonary segment. The noises are generated by the opening up of previously occluded airways. Use of further adjectival descriptions such as dry, moist, sibilant, and crepitant add little information and tend to make communication from one observer to another difficult.

The polyphonic, musical sounds called wheezes are due to the turbulent airflow through narrow lumina, usually in apposition. The pitch (low or high) is dependent upon velocity of airflow and not on the size of the conduit as is commonly believed.

Transmission of breath sounds or voice generated sounds may be altered due to abnormalities or diseases of the pleura, lungs, and mediastinal structures. Breath sounds, whispered, or spoken voice should be recorded as normal, increased, or decreased. Terms such as "increased fremitus," "bronchophony," "pectoriloquy," "egophony," and "a to e" are anachronistic and confusing and should not be used.

Normal breath sounds may also be dampened by the interface of fluid between the origin of the sounds and the chest wall. This would cause dampening of the intensity. If there is both fluid and consolidation on the chest wall, one would have decreased intensity of breath sounds.

Clinical Significance

Increased intensity of inspiratory breath sounds with normal flow rates indicates increased turbulence of airflow and therefore signifies some abnormality within the airway conduction system of the lung.

Inspiratory and expiratory wheezes are due to abnormalities of airway conduction caused by apposition of the conduit wall. These wheezes can therefore be caused by anything that narrows the size of the conduit, such as bronchial constriction, mucosal edema, fluid both within the conduit and in the interstitial spaces narrowing the airways (as one would see in congestive heart failure), and infiltrative diseases of the supporting structure of the bronchi. It is evident that the finding of inspiratory or expiratory rhonchi is of low level resolution and the etiology of the narrowing of the airway requires additional information in order to resolve it more precisely.

A unilateral or focal wheeze is occasionally heard in local obstruction of a major airway, whatever the cause.

Crackles when heard are usually only in inspiration. These indicate that there is hypoinflation of the lung. In normal individuals, the dependent portion of the lung has less airflow due to the weight of the lung and blood vessels, so one may hear inspiratory crackles after the normal individual has been in the supine position for several hours.

Persistence of inspiratory crackles usually indicates some reason for hypoventilation. Clinical states characterized by inspiratory crackles and hypoinflation include left ventricular failure with retention of fluid within the interstitial areas of the lung and bronchi, diffuse interstitial diseases of the lung of many causes, and hypoventilation due to neuromuscular disorders or marked obesity. Measurement of the degree of hypoventilation is obtained by laboratory determination of arterial blood gases.

Abnormal transmission of breath sounds to the chest wall indicates abnormality of the supporting structure of the lung or diseases of the pleura. The transmission of high-frequency sounds is effectively dampened. As a result, in consolidation of the lung, moderate to low-frequency sounds are transmitted to the chest wall, and breath sounds then are usually termed bronchial. Whispered voice and spoken voice also are transmitted differently due to the frequency response of the underlying structures, and such abnormality of transmission has been historically referred to as whispered pectoriloquy or egophony. Distant breath sounds are those that are hard to hear, due either to diseases of the pleura or to distended alveoli which effectively dampen the transmission of such sounds. The usual cause of distant breath sounds in clinical practice is the presence of emphysema. Finally, the difference in intensity of breath sounds from one side of the chest to the other may indicate obstruction to airflow unilaterally. The most striking example of this would be in a pneumothorax where vesicular sounds are not heard, but the transmission of breath sounds from the normal lung are heard over the collapsed lung area, usually as a bronchial sound.

In summary, auscultation of the chest is primarily rewarding in defining abnormalities of the airways of the lung. Increased intensity with normal breathing, or the finding of adventitious sounds, both crackles and wheezes, indicate definite abnormalities of the tracheobronchial tree. Abnormal transmission of breath sounds or of the whispered or spoken voice to the chest wall indicate abnormalities of underlying structures. In the latter instance, however, the chest x-ray is a more definite source of information. For self-education, comparison of the chest x-ray with the auscultatory phenomenon should be done.

Selected References

1. Fletcher CM: The clinical diagnosis of pulmonary emphysema: An experimental study. *Proc R Soc Med* 45:577–584, 1952.

2. Forgacs P: The functional basis of pulmonary sounds. *Chest* 73(3): 399–405, 1978.

3. Godfrey S, Edwards RHT, Campbell R Jr: Repeatability of physical signs in airways obstruction. *Thorax* 24:4–9, 1969.

4. Schneider IC, Anderson A Jr: Correlation of clinical signs with ventilatory function in obstructive lung disease. *Ann Intern Med* 62:477–485, 1965.

5. Siegel JS, Schechter E: The straight back syndrome. *Am J Med* 42:309–313, 1967.

6. Nairn JR, Turner-Warwick M: Breath sounds in emphysema. *Br J Dis Chest* 63:29–37, 1969.

7. Pulmonary terms and symbols. A report of the American College of Chest Physicians and the American Thoracic Society. *Chest* 67(5):583–593, 1975.

148. Chest Percussion

JAMES C. CRUTCHER, MD

Definition

Percussion of the chest wall elicits a frequency response both felt and heard. The vibrations and sounds elicited are dependent upon the force of the percussion stroke, thickness of the chest wall, and the frequency response of the underlying structures. Normally, there are three descriptive characteristics of percussion: normal, dull, and tympanitic. In the normal individual, all three of these percussion notes can be elicited as illustrated in Fig 78.

Technique

The most common method is to use the fingers of one hand as the surface which is then struck by the second finger of the other hand. The fingers on the chest wall will interpret the vibrations while the ears will hear the frequencies. The combination of the vibratory response and the

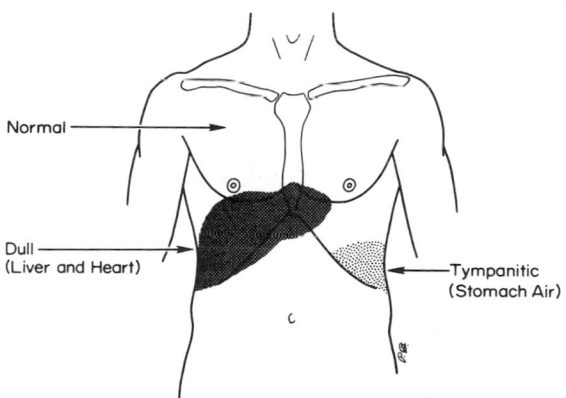

Figure 78. Findings of a percussion note varying from the normal areas constitutes the abnormality in this physical examination.

sounds will detect the significant alterations of the percussion note. Minimal experience is all that is necessary to refine this technique. Since there is so much variation in percussion note from individual to individual, percussion notes for each individual must be compared on equivalent areas on both sides of the chest.

Background Information

The increased use of the x-ray has diminished the diagnostic value of percussion of the chest. Since the percussion note only shows up abnormalities approximately 5 cm from the percussing finger, many deep-seated areas of abnormality will be missed. Thus, the finding of normal percussion does not rule out significant disorders. As a gross screening process, however, for large areas of consolidation or for massive pleural effusion, the percussion note still remains valid.

Clinical Significance

Unilateral increase in resonance may be indicative of a pneumothorax or of unilateral bullous emphysema. The loss of normal retrosternal dullness created by the heart and its replacement by a resonant note are very reliable signs of increased retrosternal airspace as seen in moderately advanced emphysema. Dullness in areas of normal resonance is reasonably accurate for determining abnormalities due to pleural effusion or for areas of consolidation within the lung.

Estimate of cardiac size is unreliable and has been replaced by palpation of the apical impulse. Estimation of the descent of the diaphragm has proven to be so significantly unreliable that, if one wishes to measure the descent of the diaphragm, it is necessary to rely on x-ray techniques (inspiratory and expiratory, P-A of the chest).

In summary, although the percussion of the chest has limited value, it is still a worthwhile technique to develop in following patients that are not easily x-rayed or as a screening procedure when there is moderately advanced pleural effusion or consolidation of the lung. It has excellent value in detecting unilateral hyperinflation and unilateral pneumothorax collapse greater than 70%.

Selected References

1. Cherniak RM, Cherniak L: *Respiration in Health and Disease*. Philadelphia, WB Saunders, 1961, chap 1, pp 3–32; chap 4, pp 68–86.
2. Fletcher CM: The clinical diagnosis of pulmonary emphysema: An experimental study. *Proc R Soc Med* 45:577–584, 1952.

3. Forgacs P: Lung sounds. *Br J Dis Chest* 63(1):1–11, 1969.
4. Fraser RG, Paré JAP: *Diagnosis of Diseases of the Chest.* Philadelphia, WB Saunders, 1970, vol 1, chap 1–3, pp 1–156.
5. Godfrey S, Edwards RHT, Campbell R Jr: Repeatability of physical signs in airways obstruction. *Thorax* 24:4–9, 1969.
6. Nairn JR, Turner-Warwick M: Breath sounds in emphysema. *Br J Dis Chest* 63:29–37, 1969.
7. Pulmonary terms and symbols: A report of the American College of Chest Physicians and the American Thoracic Society. *Chest* 67(5): 583–593, 1975.
8. Ruth WE: Examination of the chest, in Dolph MH, Manning RT (eds): *Majors Physical Diagnosis,* ed 7. Philadelphia, WB Saunders, chap 6, pp 89–116.
9. Schneider IC, Anderson A Jr: Correlation of clinical signs with ventilatory function in obstructive lung disease. *Ann Intern Med* 62:477–485, 1965.
10. Siegel JS, Schechter E: The straight back syndrome. *Am J Med* 42:309–313, 1967.

BREAST

149. Breast Mass

R. WALDO POWELL, MD
CONSTANTINE DROULIAS, MD

Definition

A true two- or three-dimensional change in a segment of the breast tissue is called mass, lump, or tumor. Nodularity, thickening, hardness, or firmness are equally important changes but are not as distinct or discrete.

Technique

Before beginning a breast examination, have the proper equipment assembled (an examining table with access from both sides and a good strong light) and an assistant to move the light from one area to another.

First position: supine (Figs 79–85). Have the patient lie with her arm abducted to 90°; one may want to put a folded sheet or towel under the shoulder. Inspect the breasts for symmetry and for subtle changes in color or texture of the skin (Fig 79). Stand on the patient's right side to examine the right breast. Using four fingers of each hand, begin palpation in the upper central portion and proceed clockwise from the superior to the medial quadrants. Palpate gently initially; with too firm pressure, a soft mass will often be missed. Repeat the maneuver, palpating more firmly (Fig 80). The next maneuver in the supine position with the arm abducted is the examination of the central portion of the breast. Very gently palpate the nipple and tissue underneath for evidence of small

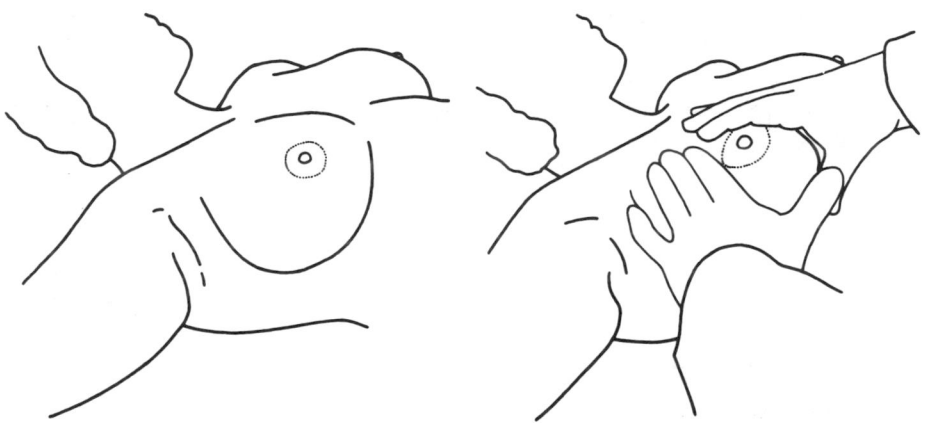

Figure 79.   Figure 80.

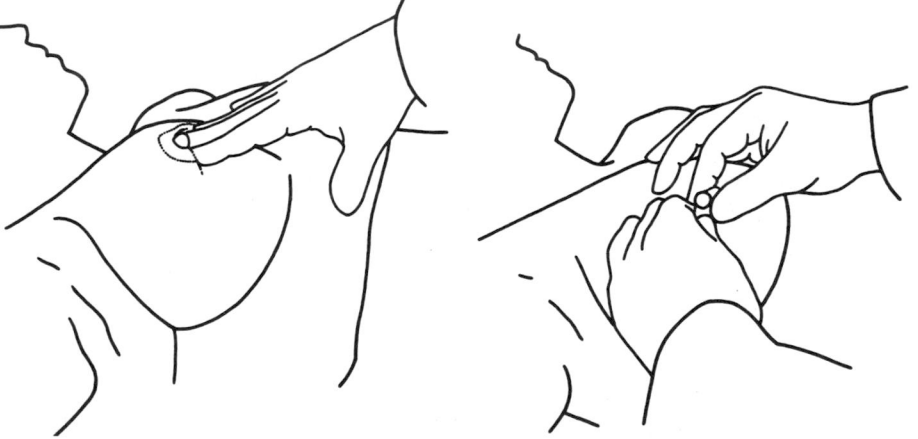

Figure 81.   Figure 82.

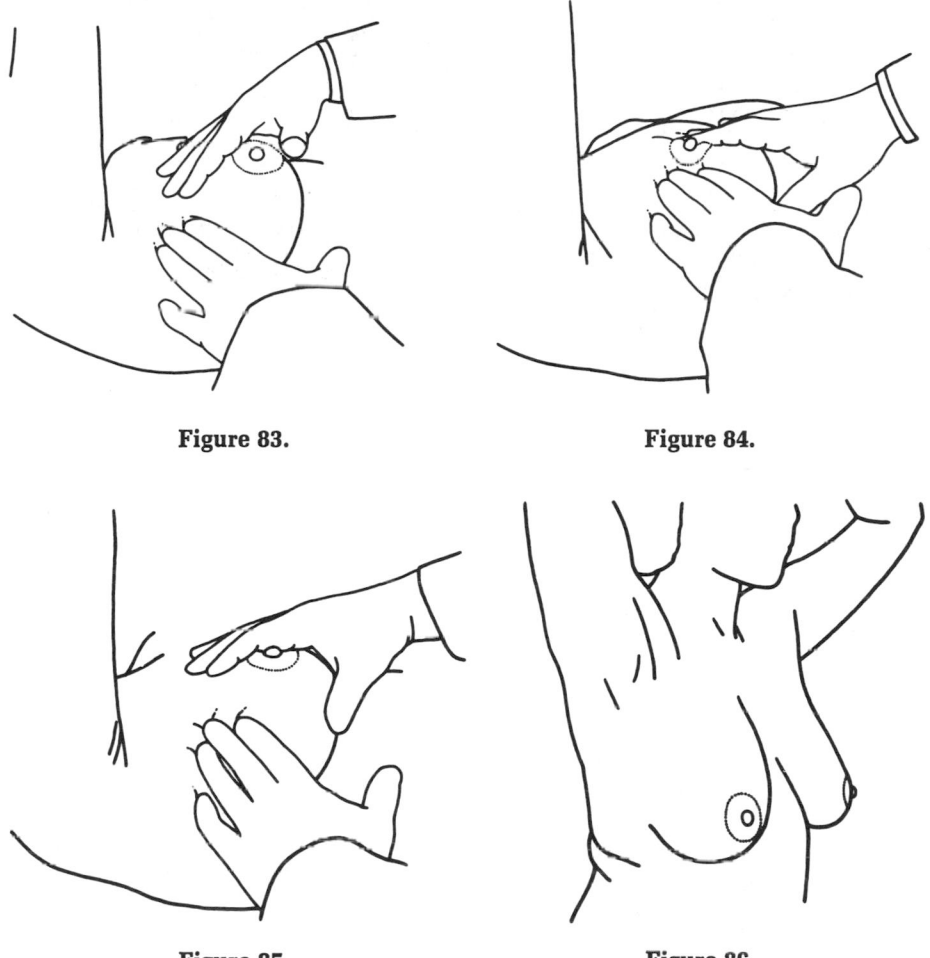

Figure 83.   Figure 84.

Figure 85.   Figure 86.

masses or duct thickening. Gently strip the nipple to check for discharge (Figs 81 and 82). Complete the examination of the right breast with patient in the supine position by having the patient rotate the arm across the chest wall. This position tends to bring the breast further across the chest wall and affords a more accurate examination of the tail of the breast (Figs 83 and 84). With the breast in this position, a small deeplying lesion that might otherwise be missed can be brought out from the intercostal spaces, trapped over a rib, and palpated readily (Fig 85). Move to the other side of the table and examine the left breast.

Second position: sitting, hands on head (Figs 86–95). Have the patient sit on the end of the table with the feet dangling, so one can get close

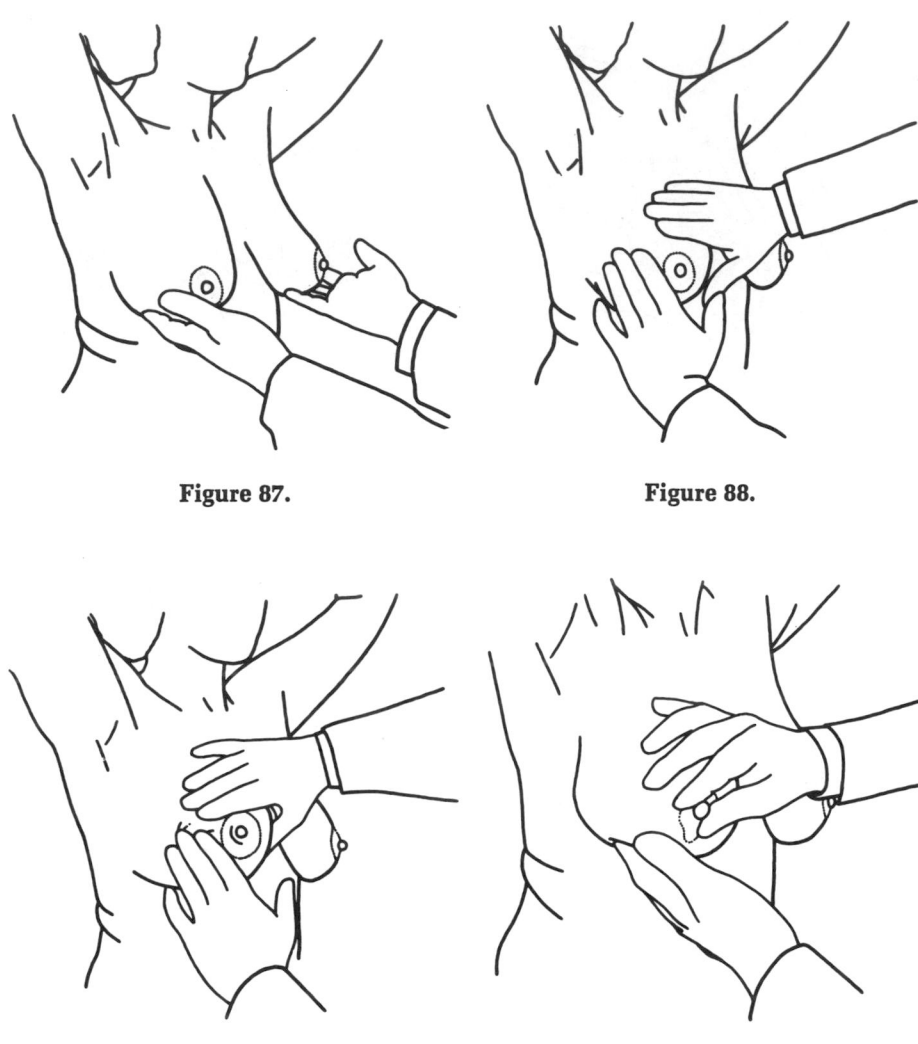

Figure 87.   Figure 88.

Figure 89.   Figure 90.

enough to have freedom of motion in examining both breasts. The hands behind the head is much more relaxing than having the patient hold the hands above the head (Fig 86). Compare the breasts for size and nipple parallelism, and check for differences in the veins of the subcutaneous tissue, skin changes, and nipple irregularities (Fig 87). Palpate the breast tissue very gently, beginning in the upper central portion; proceed clockwise about the circumference of the breast (Fig 88). Repeat the circumferential palpation of the breast, using firmer pressure to detect possible deep-lying lesions (Fig 89). Gently palpate the nipple for small, centrally located lumps or duct thickening. Check for nipple discharge by stripping

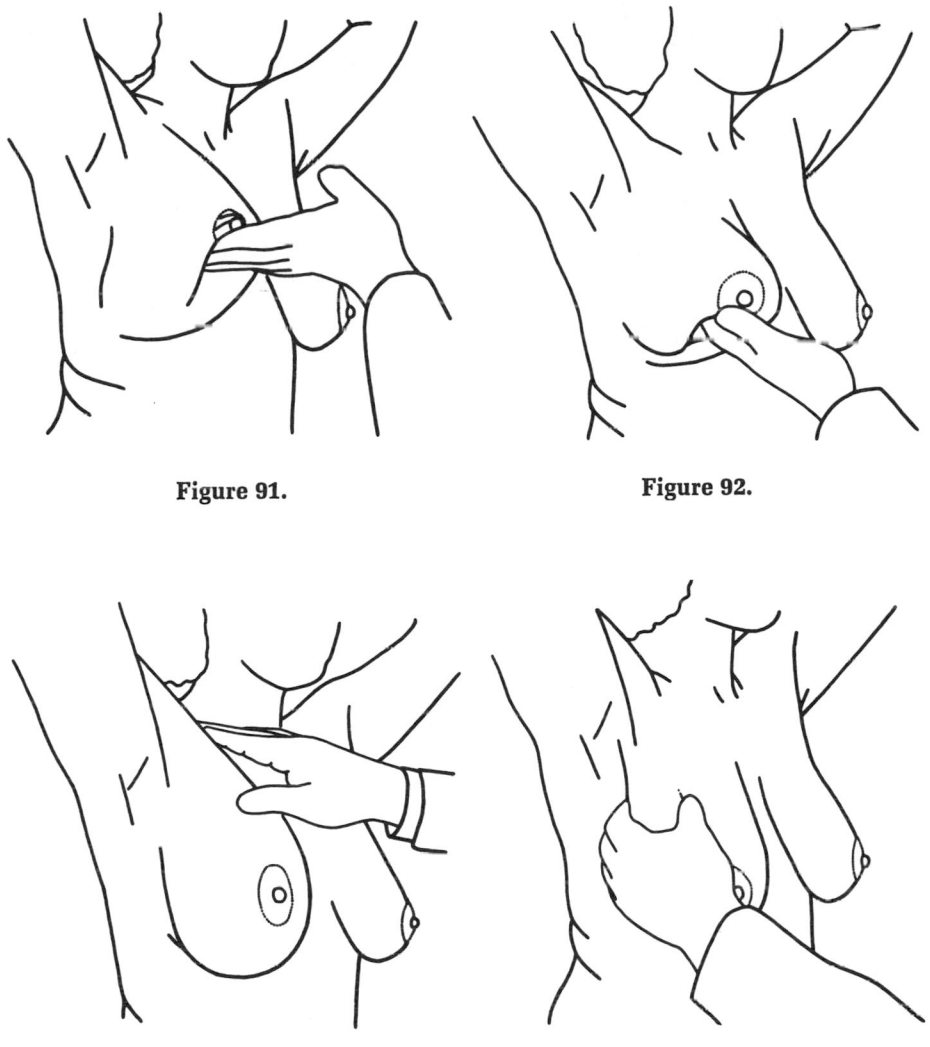

Figure 91.

Figure 92.

Figure 93.

Figure 94.

the nipple gently (Fig 90). Lift the breast with your fingertips and inspect the lower and lateral portions for subtle change in color or texture of the skin (Fig 91). Gently lift the breast tissue so that any shortening of Cooper's ligaments or flattening of the skin of the upper half of the breast may be brought out. Have the light directed at the surface of the lifted breast (Fig 92). Pull upward on the breast tissue. This gentle elevation may demonstrate nipple and skin changes such as foreshortening of the nipple or flattening of the skin (Fig 93). To conclude the examination of the right breast with the patient in the first sitting position, gently and then firmly

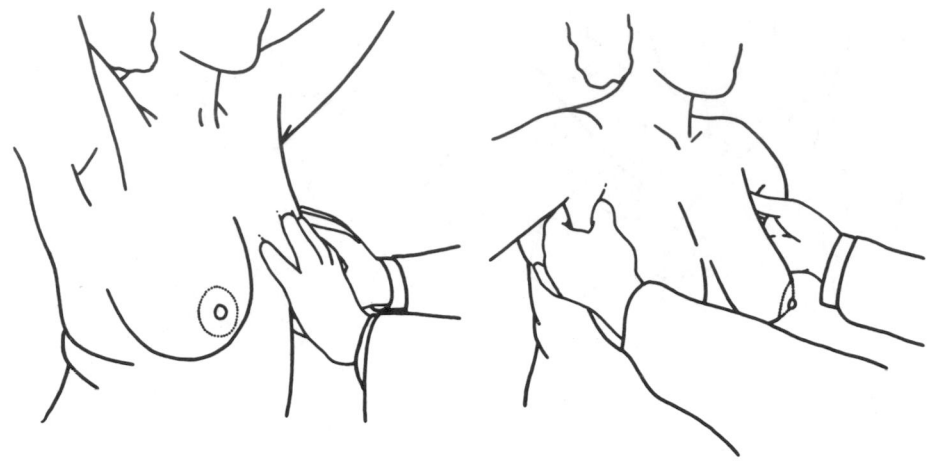

Figure 95.   Figure 96.

palpate the tail of the breast as it enters the lower portion of the axilla (Fig 94). With both the patient and the examiner maintaining the same position, the previous maneuvers for the opposite (left) breast are repeated, making certain the assistant has redirected the light (Fig 95).

Third position: sitting with pectoral muscles flexed (Fig 96). Stand directly in front of patient; check carefully to ensure flexing. Carry out frontal inspection, looking for nipple or skin abnormalities and asymmetry. Carry out all maneuvers that were done with the patient in the second position for both left and right breasts.

Fourth position: arms extended and supported while patient leans forward (Fig 97). The assistant supports the patient's hands as she leans forward. The weight of the breasts will project them from the chest wall; subtle skin changes that might otherwise be missed are detectable in this position. Occasionally, deep-seated masses can be better delineated in this position.

Fifth position: sitting relaxed (Figs 98 and 99). With the patient sitting relaxed, support her relaxed arm loosely to facilitate manipulation; palpate the axilla gently with a kneading motion. Repeat wtih opposite hand for the other axilla (Fig 98). To examine the upper portion of the axilla, rather vigorous palpation is necessary, which may cause some degree of discomfort. The examining hand is pushed upward and inward rather firmly against the chest wall so that the axillary contents are pulled inferiorly (Figs 99 and 100). Repeat with the other hand for the other axilla.

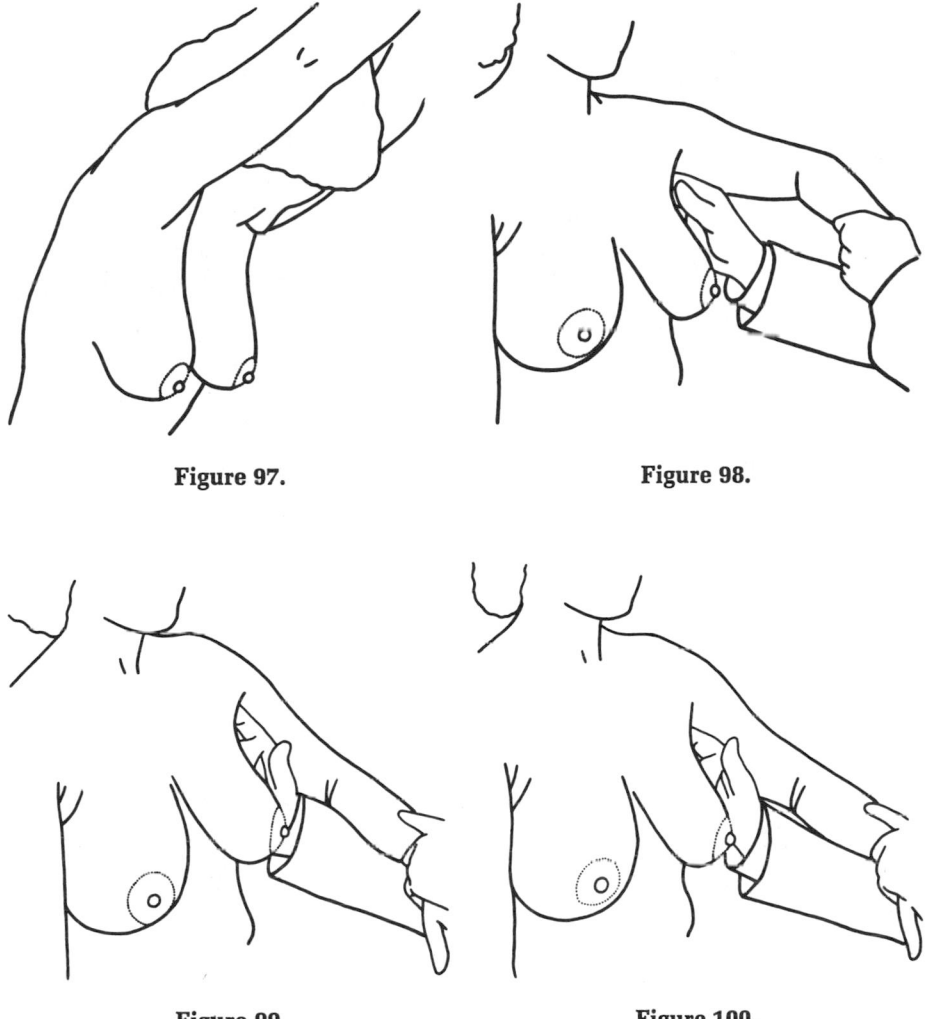

Figure 97.

Figure 98.

Figure 99.

Figure 100.

Sixth position: sitting erect (Figs 101 and 102). Gently palpate the supra-clavicular portion of the neck. The arm near the shoulder should be slightly elevated and the neck rotated toward the side of the examination. This makes deep palpation, both of the supraclavicular area and the area underneath the sternocleidomastoid muscle, more accurate. These maneuvers are repeated for the opposite supraclavicular area.

Accurate recording of the physical findings is important. A simple sketch like the one shown here can be very helpful (Fig 103). For recording tumor findings, use only centimeters; one or two dimensions of a tumor should be included. Mention should be made, if possible, of the

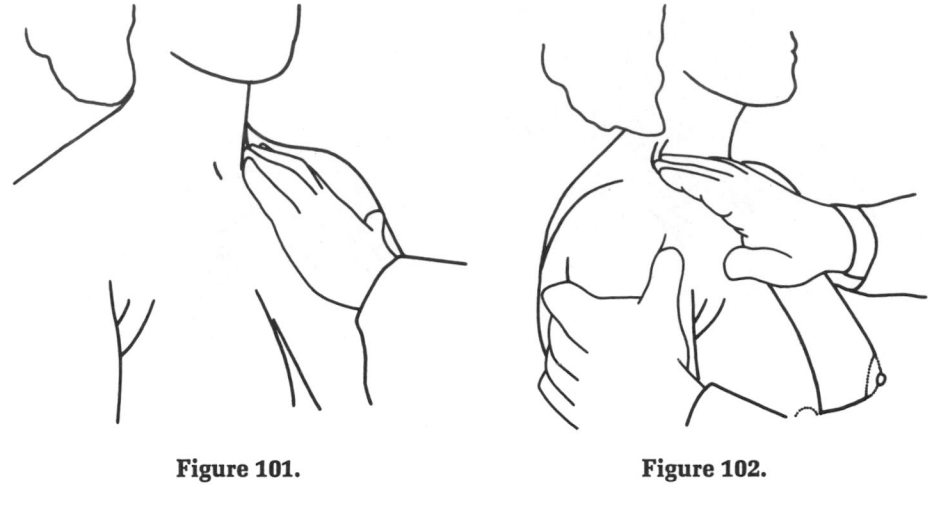

Figure 101.   Figure 102.

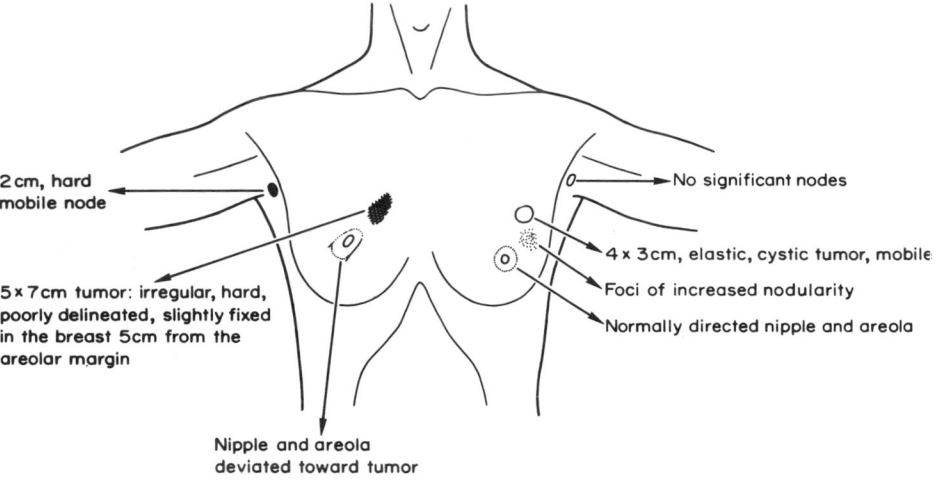

2 cm, hard
mobile node

No significant nodes

5 × 7 cm tumor: irregular, hard,
poorly delineated, slightly fixed
in the breast 5 cm from the
areolar margin

4 × 3 cm, elastic, cystic tumor, mobile

Foci of increased nodularity

Normally directed nipple and areola

Nipple and areola
deviated toward tumor

Figure 103.

distance between the tumor and the periphery of the areola as well as
the approximate depth from the skin surface. Fixation or partial fixation
of the mass to the skin or to the chest wall or to the pectoral fascia should
be noted here if this finding exists.

Background Information

The breast glandular tissue is suspended within the superficial fascia
of the anterior chest wall, extending roughly from the second to the sixth
or seventh anterior intercostal space and from the edge of the sternum

to the midaxillary line. About two-thirds of it rests upon the fascia covering the pectoralis muscle and the rest upon the fascia of the serratus anterior muscle. Toward the axilla, the axillary tail of Spence passes through an opening in the pectoral fascia, the foramen of Langer into the axilla.

The nonlactating breast weighs about 150–200 g but the lactating may weigh as much as 400–500 g. The glandular tissue is made up of 12–20 lobes which are subdivided into lobules and these in turn are composed of acini. However, overlapping of lobes ensures that no cleavage planes exist to separate one from another. The lobes are arranged like the spokes of a wheel converging on the nipple and each has a dilated ampulla just before it ends. The breast is fixed to the overlying skin and the underlying pectoral fascia by fibrous bands known as Cooper's ligaments. The glandular tissue undergoes changes from birth to old age. At birth, both female and male breasts contain a simple system of large ducts but no lobules. The ducts are lined by flattened epithelium and surrounded by collagenous tissue. With the onset of puberty, rapid growth of ductal epithelium and periductal fibrous stroma increases the size of the breast, which is quite firm. With the onset of maturity true lobules and acinar structures develop. In the male breast, lobules never develop, thus lobular carcinoma of the breast does not occur in men. In pregnancy there is marked proliferation (multiplication) of the glandular elements, which regress to normal after pregnancy and lactation. At menopause there is continuous involution or regression of breast structures with resulting loss of glandular elements and replacement with fibrous and fatty tissue.

Clinical Significance

Differential points in breast tumors:

1. Benign cyst:
   a. Size: variable.
   b. Shape: rounded, oval, or discoid.
   c. Contour: well defined.
   d. Consistency: elastic, some large ones fluctuate; when very tense, quite firm.
   e. Movability: great within the breast tissue.
   f. Tenderness: commonly present.
2. Cancer:
   a. Size: variable.
   b. Shape: nodular, irregular.
   c. Contour: ill defined, irregular (exception is the circumscribed variety, which comprises less than 10 percent).
   d. Consistency: usually wooden-hard (the papillary or medullary carcinoma may be soft).

      e.   Movability: varies with the stage of the disease from slightly limited to complete fixation of the tumor.

      f.   Tenderness: rare.

3.   Benign-fibroadenoma:

      a.   Size: variable (a large one may be cystosarcoma phylloides which is usually benign but rarely malignant).

      b.   Shape: rounded, oval, and commonly lobulated.

      c.   Contour: well-defined and often has a notch similar to the hilum of the kidney.

      d.   Consistency: quite firm to rubbery but not stony hard (unless calcified which is rarely seen in older women).

      e.   Movability: usually marked.

      f.   Tenderness: rare.

4.   Adenosis, papillomatosis, fibrous hyperplasia (all benign processes):

      a.   Size: variable.

      b.   Shape: rather diffuse but may be localized, unilateral, or bilateral; no three-dimensional lesion.

      c.   Contour: ill defined.

      d.   Consistency: the degree of firmness usually varies; some areas may be as hard as carcinoma.

      e.   Movability: limited regarding the surrounding breast tissue but not attached to the skin or chest wall.

5.   Skin changes, usually associated with the presence of a mass, may be slight or pronounced and include:

      a.   Erythema, or redness of the skin, may be seen in acute or chronic inflammatory processes of the breast and in cancer (inflammatory carcinoma or a very superficial tumor).

      b.   Edema, due to blockage of the subdermal lymphatics either by tumor cells or an inflammatory process of the breast or axilla. This edema produces the so-called peau-d'orange (French for orange peel) or pig-skin, seen most characteristically in inflammatory carcinoma.

      c.   Dilated subcutaneous veins may be seen in rapidly growing tumors both benign and malignant (eg, cystosarcomas).

      d.   Thrombophlebitis of the superficial veins of the breast (Mondor's disease).

6.   Retraction phenomena: constitute a whole series of clinical manifestations ranging from a small dimple in the skin over a tumor to shrinkage of the entire breast. They are basically due to fibrosis and shortening of Cooper's ligaments. Carcinoma is the most common cause, but inflammatory processes and fat necrosis may produce these changes.

7.   Axillary nodes: Enlarged (greater than 1 cm), rounded, firm, axillary nodes in association with a mass in the breast strongly suggest that the mass is malignant.

8.	Supraclavicular nodes: Enlargement of these nodes in the presence of a definite carcinoma suggests that the disease is advanced and inoperable.

Selected References

1.	Leis HP Jr: *Diagnosis and Treatment of Breast Lesions.* New York, Medical Examination Publishing Co, 1970.
2.	Rush BF Jr: Breast, in Schwartz, Seymour I, et al (eds): *Principles of Surgery.* New York, McGraw-Hill, 1969.
3.	Haagensen CD: *Diseases of the Breast,* ed 2. Philadelphia, WB Saunders, 1971, p 101.
4.	Powell RW: Office breast exam (roundtable discussion). *Patient Care* April 1975:59–73.
5.	Atkins, HBJ (ed): *The Treatment of Breast Cancer.* Baltimore, University Park, 1974.
6.	Bonser GW, Dossett JA, Jull JW: *Human and Experimental Breast Cancer.* Springfield, Ill, Charles C Thomas, 1961.

150. Nipple and Areola

R. WALDO POWELL, MD
CONSTANTINE DROULIAS, MD

Definition

The nipple is a conical, brownish or pink pigmented area with pigmented elevation of the skin in the center of the breast that is surrounded by a similar pigmented areola. Normally, the nipples point laterally and outward.

Technique

The technique for examining the nipple and areola is covered in section 149.

Background Information

The nipple is a conical projection in the center of the breast. The color of the nipple and surrounding areola varies with the complexion of the person but is rose pink in the young and browner during pregnancy. The pigmentation is also related to estrogens, for it is considerably more marked in younger individuals, tends to fade after menopause, and may be intensified at any age by the administration of estrogens.

Just below the surface of the nipple the milk sinuses terminate in cone-shaped ampullae and are lined with stratified squamous epithelium. In the resting breast these ampullae are filled with epithelial debris, which effectively plugs the duct openings on the nipple surface.

Both the subareolar area and the nipple contain much smooth muscle. In the subareolar area the fibers are arranged radially in concentric rings. They insert into the base of the dermis and function to contract the areola and to compress the base of the nipple in order to aid in suckling. The bulk of the nipple is made up of smooth muscle fibers arranged both longitudinally and circularly. When they contract, they make the nipple erect, smaller, and firmer, and empty the milk sinuses. The skin of the nipple is hairless and has well-developed dermal papillae. It contains large numbers of specialized sebaceous glands that are often grouped around the openings of the milk sinuses. The skin of the areola has a few hairs around its periphery and does not have well-developed dermal papillae. The skin contains three types of glands: sweat glands, specialized sebaceous glands, and not infrequently accessory mammary glands. The specialized sebaceous glands are large and superficially located, projecting as small nodules above the surface of the areola. During pregnancy and lactation they enlarge (Montgomery's glands). Their purpose is to lubricate the nipple and areola for the nursing infant. The accessory mammary glands, which are occasionally seen beneath the areola, have the same structure as normal mammary gland acini. Their miniature ducts open into small sinuses in the areolar epithelium. They secrete milk during lactation.

Clinical Significance

The most common deformity of the nipple is congenital and presents usually as fissuring or inversion. The history data will clarify this point. The second most common deformity is foreshortening or inversion due to cancer that is usually of recent onset. Many changes of the nipple and surrounding areola occur in Paget's disease. These include redness of the nipple surface, roughening and thickening, erosion with some brownish discharge, and yellowish gray crusting over the erosion. The erosion enlarges slowly but never heals. In advanced stages the entire surface of the nipple is eroded, flattened, and distorted. The areola or larger area of surrounding skin may eventually be involved.

Paget's disease of the nipple is always associated with a ductal cell carcinoma. Many nonmalignant diseases of the nipple may produce significant abnormalities. These include: (1) chronic granulomatous lesions such as syphilis or tuberculosis, (2) acute dermatitis associated with nursing or adenoma of the nipple, and (3) chronic recurring abscesses associated with duct ectasia and duct stasis.

Selected References

1. Anson BT, McVay CB: *Surgical Anatomy,* ed 5. Philadelphia, WB Saunders, 1971, pp 339–341.
2. Leis HP Jr: *Diagnosis and Treatment of Breast Lesions.* New York, Medical Examination Publishing Co, 1970.
3. Haagensen CD: *Diseases of the Breast,* ed 2. Philadelphia, WB Saunders, 1971.
4. Vorherr H: *The Breast: Morphology, Physiology and Lactation.* New York, Academic Press, 1974.

CARDIOVASCULAR SYSTEM

151. Jugular Venous Pressure

JOSEPH Z. DAVIDS, MD

Definition

The level of central venous pressure reflected by distension of the jugular veins. Normal jugular venous pressure is less than 3 cm of distension of either the internal or external jugular vein above the sternal angle of Louis. A level of distension greater than 4 cm should be regarded as abnormal. Serial determinations in the same person require that the degree of truncal elevation be recorded with the height of venous distension.

Technique

Place the patient in the supine position and elevate the trunk until maximal internal jugular venous pulsations are seen. This technique is described in the following section on Jugular Venous Pulsations. This is usually 30–60° but can be as much as 90° in patients with markedly elevated venous pressure. Relax the patient by telling him that you are going to look at the veins in the neck. Ask the patient to breathe normally and attempt to locate the internal jugular venous pulsation. Identify and mark on the patient's neck the highest point of visible pulsation. This usually occurs at the end of a normal expiration. Locate the patient's sternal angle of Louis. The distance from the highest point of visible pulsation to the sternal angle of Louis is the correct measurement for estimating the degree of neck vein distension.

Local venous obstruction or kinking of the external jugular vein at the base of the neck will cause distension of the external jugular vein independent of central venous pressure. Venous pressure is best estimated in the internal jugular vein. However, in some instances, it may be difficult to identify internal jugular venous pulsations. In that case, use the external jugular vein. Place the patient in the supine position and elevate the trunk 30–60°. Raise the chin and rotate the head slightly away from the external jugular vein being examined. Look at both sides of the neck and locate the external jugular veins. If one vein is significantly more distended than the other, choose the jugular vein that is less distended. Using your right index finger, gently press the external jugular veins at a point just above the clavicle. Maintain compression until you see the jugular vein become distended in the neck; this requires approximately 30 seconds. Suddenly withdraw compression and note the point to which the distended vein falls. This must be done immediately since the level of venous distension may fall further in several minutes. After you have marked this point on the patient's neck, the venous pressure can be estimated using the method described above.

The external jugular veins are superficial veins with valves located near their lower ends. Only when the valves are incompetent do the external jugular veins reflect the retrograde transmission of pressure and volume relationships present in the valveless internal jugular system.

Background Information

By measuring the jugular venous pressure, we are really attempting to estimate the level of central venous pressure, that is, right atrial pressure. Although the sternal angle of Louis is chosen as the reference point for measuring venous pressure, it does not have a constant relation to the midpoint of the right atrium, the true reference point for measuring venous pressure. However, in any one patient, the relationship of the sternal angle to the midpoint of the right atrium is constant. Consequently, serial estimates of venous pressure in the same patient are reliable with respect to changes in venous pressure.

The amount of venous distension is actually a gauge of venous volume and not venous pressure. There is usually a constant pressure-volume relationship in the jugular veins, implying a direct correlation between venous volume and venous pressure. However, there are circumstances in which venous volume and pressure are unrelated. As a result, patients may occasionally have markedly distended jugular veins with normal venous pressure or may have no visible venous distension with an elevated venous pressure.

Clinical Significance

Elevation of the jugular veins greater than 4 cm above the sternal angle is most commonly caused by failure of the right ventricle. Etiologies include left ventricular failure, parenchymal lung disease, pulmonary hypertension, and pulmonic stenosis. Other causes of jugular venous distension include blockade at the tricuspid valve, cardiac tamponade, constrictive pericarditis, superior vena cava obstruction, and increased blood volume.

Occasionally, a patient with mild right ventricular failure will not have an elevated jugular venous pressure on routine evaluation of the jugular veins. Performing the hepatojugular reflux test (see next section) on these patients will often reveal the elevated jugular venous pressure. Several theories have been proposed to explain why the hepatojugular reflux test will reveal an increased venous pressure in patients who have mild right ventricular failure. The most commonly accepted theory states that applying pressure to the abdomen will increase the amount of venous blood returning to the heart. A failing right ventricle will not be able to accommodate this increased volume load without an increase in central venous pressure and jugular venous distension.

Analysis of the jugular veins for purposes of measuring venous pressure can also be very helpful in detecting hypovolemia. If the neck veins are flat (nondistended) at zero truncal elevation, the patient is probably volume depleted. Serial estimates of jugular venous pressure are helpful in determining the patient's response to intravenous fluid infusion. However, measuring the jugular venous pressure will not always be a valid indicator of the volume status of the patient, since a few patients with marked volume depletion will have severe peripheral vasoconstriction with associated venoconstriction.

Selected References

1.   Hurst JW (ed in chief), Logue RB, Schlant RC, Wenger NK (eds): *The Heart,* ed 4. New York, McGraw-Hill, Inc, 1978.
2.   Burch GE, Ray CT: Mechanism of the hepatojugular reflux test in congestive heart failure. *Am Heart J* 48:373–382, 1954.
3.   Constant J: *Bedside Cardiology.* Boston, Little, Brown, 1969.

152. Jugular Venous Pulsations

JOSEPH Z. DAVIDS, MD

Definition

The normal pulsations of the internal jugular vein consist of three positive waves (A, C, and V) and two negative waves (X and Y). Abnormalities of the pulsations are manifested as either accentuations of the normal waveforms, decrease in size of the waveform, loss of the waveform, or a combination of these changes. Note the comments in the preceding section concerning the choice of internal versus external jugular vein examination.

Technique

Relax the patient by stating that you are going to look at the veins in the neck. Place the patient face up, elevating the trunk 15–30° Remove the pillow and slightly elevate the chin, avoiding rotation of the head. If the patient is uncomfortable or the neck muscles are being stretched, place a pillow under the neck. After you have properly positioned the patient, find an adequate light source for the examination. Natural daylight on the patient's neck is the best source of light. If this is not feasible or does not supply an adequate amount of light, shine a flashlight across the patient's neck. Tangentially directed light is better than direct light. Look for pulsations of the internal jugular vein by standing just behind the patient and looking down alongside the sternocleidomastoid muscle. Observe the internal jugular vein along both right and left sternocleidomastoid muscles; check for high pulsations near the earlobe. Direct your study of the pulse waves to whichever internal jugular pulse is easier to see. Venous pulsations are usually most prominent in the suprasternal notch, the supraclavicular fossa, or just below the earlobe. Routinely inspect these areas. If you are having difficulty observing the venous distension without visible waves, elevate the patient's trunk 45–90° until undulating waves can be seen. Infrequently the venous pressure is so high that undulating pulsations cannot be seen even at 90°-truncal elevation.

After identifying a pulsation in the neck, make certain that you are able to differentiate the jugular venous pulse from the carotid artery pulse. If you can see slow distinct undulating waves, then you have almost certainly identified the internal jugular venous pulse. If you cannot see distinct undulating waves, place the patient in the sitting position and reexamine the neck pulsation. Distension from the internal jugular venous pulse will decrease while that from the arterial pulse will not change. Gently compressing the pulsation below the point of observation with the index finger is also helpful. This will increase the distension of the vein above the point of compression without affecting the arterial pulse. You can also ask the patient to slowly inhale and exhale deeply while you watch the vascular pulsation. Inspiration will normally decrease venous distension and make the venous waves more prominent but will not affect arterial pulsations.

You can now begin the analysis of individual venous waves. Keep a pencil and a piece of paper within reach in order to diagram your findings. Place the stethoscope just to the left of the patient's lower sternal border and identify the heart sounds. This is necessary for proper analysis of the venous waves.

After observing venous pulsations in several patients, you should begin to recognize a cluster consisting of two almost simultaneously positive waves, a pause, and another positive wave. This cluster is followed by another pulse which is longer than the first pause at normal heart rates. The first two positive waves are the A and C waves and occur just prior to and coincident with the first heart sound. The two pauses are the negative X and Y waves and occupy systole and diastole, respectively. At heart rates below 100, diastole is longer than systole; consequently the second pause is longer than the first. At heart rates faster than 100, the two pauses will be of equal duration. The last positive wave is called the V wave and occurs in late systole.

After analyzing the jugular venous pulsations, perform the hepatojugular reflux test by applying gentle pressure with the palm of your hand over the right side of the abdomen for approximately 30 seconds while observing the jugular venous pulsations. Be sure that the patient does not strain back (Valsalva) during the abdominal pressure. In a normal person, this test will produce either minimal or no increase in the prominence of the venous pulsations.

Background Information

The internal jugular venous pulse serves as a clinical reflection of the pressure and volume changes of the right atrium and right ventricle. Since venous flow from the capillaries to the heart is nonpulsatile, the internal jugular venous waves must be produced by discontinuous filling of the right atrium and ventricle with retrograde transmission from the central veins toward the neck veins.

As previously mentioned, the normal jugular venous pulse consists of five waves: three positive, A, C, and V, and two negative, X and Y (Fig 104; Table 24). The A wave is produced by right atrial contraction in the presystolic period and is usually the largest wave seen. With the onset of atrial relaxation, the A wave descends until it is interrupted by the C wave, the second positive wave. The C wave is thought to be produced by two events: the impact of the carotid artery pulsation on the adjacent jugular vein and bulging of the tricuspid valve into the right atrium when ventricular systole occurs against a closed tricuspid valve. The C wave begins at the end of the first heart sound.

The X wave, a negative systolic wave, begins after the peak of the C wave. The initial portion of the X wave is called the X descent. The X wave is produced by a downward displacement of the tricuspid valve resulting in a fall in right atrial pressure and by atrial relaxation during systole. The trough of the X wave occurs in late systole just prior to the second heart sound. Subsequently, one normally observes a negative wave during most of systole.

The V wave is a positive wave that occurs after the X wave. It peaks shortly after the second heart sound. The V wave is produced by blood filling the right atrium during systole when the tricuspid valve is closed.

The Y wave, a negative diastolic wave, begins after the peak of the V wave, producing the initial portion of the Y wave, called the Y descent.

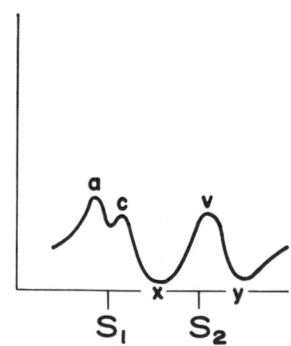

Figure 104.   Normal jugular venous pulse.

Table 24. Jugular venous pulse waveforms.

Venous Wave	Physical Exam	Physiologic Correlate	Clinical Correlate
A	Positive wave just before first heart sound	Right atrial contraction	Large A waves: tricuspid valve obstruction, pulmonic stenosis, pulmonary hypertension, IHSS, valvular aortic stenosis, pericardial effusion, constrictive pericarditis, restrictive cardiomyopathy
C	Small positive wave occurring with first heart sound	1. Impact of carotid artery pulsation on jugular vein 2. Bulging of tricuspid valve into right atrium	
X	Negative wave occupying majority of systole	1. Downward displacement of tricuspid valve 2. Right atrial relaxation during systole	Large X wave: constrictive pericarditis, restrictive cardiomyopathy, atrial septal defect Absent X wave: tricuspid regurgitation
V	Positive wave beginning in late systole and peaking just after second heart sound	Blood filling right atrium in systole against a closed tricuspid valve	Large V wave: tricuspid regurgitation, atrial septal defect
Y	Negative wave occupying majority of diastole	Opening of tricuspid valve with rapid flow of blood from right atrium to right ventricle	Small Y descent: tricuspid stenosis. Rapid Y descent: tricuspid regurgitation, constrictive pericarditis, restrictive cardiomyopathy
Cannon	Giant positive wave occurring in early systole	Right atrium contracting against a closed tricuspid valve	Regular: A-V junctional rhythm. Irregular: complete heart block, ventricular tachycardia, premature atrial and ventricular contractions

The Y wave is produced by the opening of the tricuspid valve with subsequent rapid flow of blood from the right atrium to the right ventricle. The trough of the Y wave normally occurs in early diastole. The ascending limb of the Y wave occupies a large portion of diastole and is produced by diastolic flow of blood from the peripheral veins to the right atrium and right ventricle. If the heart rate is slow with a corresponding long diastolic period, the Y wave may be followed by a small positive wave, the H wave, occurring just prior to the succeeding A wave.

If the pulse rate is less than 85 and P-Q interval is normal on ECG, all five waveforms should be visible. With faster pulse rates, analysis of the waveforms is more difficult because of fusion.

Clinical Significance

An abnormally large A wave is recognized as a large positive wave occurring just prior to the first heart sound (Fig 105). Regularly occurring large A waves imply that there is either an increase in resistance to right ventricular filling at the tricuspid valve or an abnormal compliance of the right ventricle. The major causes of increased resistance at the tricuspid valve include tricuspid stenosis, tricuspid atresia, right atrial tumor or thrombus, and Ebstein's disease. Abnormal compliance of the right ventricle is most often due to an increased afterload such as created by pulmonic stenosis or any cause of pulmonary hypertension. Large A waves can often be seen in idiopathic hypertrophic subaortic stenosis (IHSS) and occasionally in valvular aortic stenosis, without the presence of left ventricular failure. Large A waves can also be seen in pericardial effusion, constrictive pericarditis, and restrictive cardiomyopathies. An absent A wave is associated with atrial fibrillation. In patients with complete heart block, one can occasionally see A waves occurring without associated C or V waves.

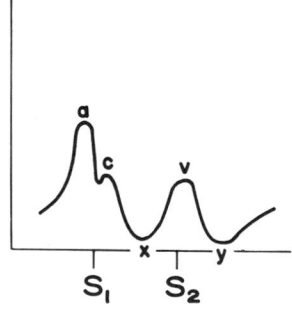

Figure 105. Giant A waves (case of pulmonic stenosis).

The major abnormality of the X wave is its obliteration in the presence of tricuspid regurgitation. Mild tricuspid regurgitation causes a prominent and early V wave that partially obliterates the X descent. As the tricuspid regurgitation increases in severity, the V wave merges with the C wave with complete obliteration of the X wave and formation of a prominent positive systolic regurgitant wave (Fig 106). In patients with mild tricuspid regurgitation, the hepatojugular reflux test may convert a normal venous pulse to one characteristic of tricuspid regurgitation. A very prominent negative X wave can occasionally be seen in patients with constrictive pericarditis or restrictive cardiomyopathy (Fig 107). The X wave is also occasionally exaggerated in cases of atrial septal defect.

As discussed above, a prominent V wave is most frequently caused by tricuspid regurgitation. This large positive systolic wave in tricuspid regurgitation is best referred to as a regurgitant wave.

Abnormalities of the Y wave may also be useful clinically. A slow Y descent is suggestive of tricuspid stenosis (Fig 108). A prominent and rapid Y descent following a regurgitant systolic wave is characteristic of tricuspid regurgitation. Constrictive pericarditis or restrictive cardiomyopathy characteristically causes a deep Y trough and a rapid Y descent without a regurgitant systolic wave (Fig 107).

As previously mentioned, inspiration will normally decrease the ap-

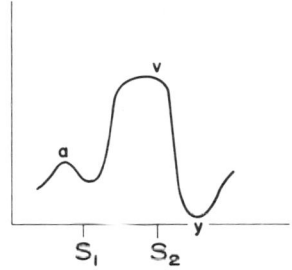

Figure 106.   Regurgitant systolic wave (case of tricuspid regurgitation).

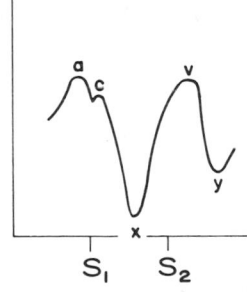

Figure 107.   Prominent X wave (case of constrictive pericarditis).

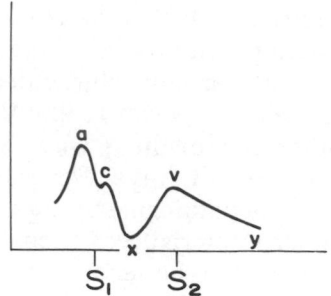

Figure 108. Slow Y descent (case of tricuspid stenosis).

parent volume of the jugular veins. However, in situations of increased venous pressure, there may be a reversal of this normal respiratory phasic pattern. Constrictive pericarditis produces an inspiratory increase in jugular venous filling. This paradoxic inspiratory increase in jugular venous pressure is known as Kussmaul's sign.

Examination of the jugular venous pulse is extremely useful in the bedside analysis of various dysrhythmias. In atrial fibrillation, there is loss of the A wave with diminution of the size of the X wave. In atrial flutter, rapid positive waves, F waves, may be visible.

Cannon waves in the jugular venous pulse are giant positive waves that occur in early systole. They are produced by the right atrium contracting during systole against a closed tricuspid valve. Regularly occurring cannon waves can be seen in patients with a junctional rhythm. Premature atrial and ventricular contractions that occur very close to the preceding beat can result in cannon waves; these cannon waves can be frequent but are not regular. Irregular cannon waves can provide the first clue to complete heart block. If irregular cannon waves are seen in a patient with a tachycardia, ventricular tachycardia is likely since there is dissociation between atrial and ventricular contractions.

Selected References

1. Hurst JW (ed in chief), Logue RB, Schlant RC, Wenger NK (eds): *The Heart,* ed 4. New York, McGraw-Hill Book Company, 1978.
2. Wood P: *Diseases of the Heart and Circulation,* ed 2. Philadelphia, JP Lippincott, 1957.
3. Benchimol A, Tippit HC: The clinical value of the jugular and hepatic pulses. *Prog Cardiovasc Dis* 10:2, 159, 1967.
4. Fowler NO: *Examination of the Heart: II, Inspection and Palpation of Venous and Arterial Pulses.* New York, American Heart Association, 1972.

153. Carotid Pulse

JOSEPH Z. DAVIDS, MD

Definition

The carotid pulse consists of a smooth and fairly rapid upstroke, a slightly sustained summit, and a downstroke that is less rapid than the upstroke.

Abnormalities involve deviations of either the pulse amplitude, the pulse contour, or a combination of amplitude and contour.

Technique

Place the patient in the supine position, elevating the trunk approximately 30°. Slightly elevate the patient's chin. Put the patient at ease by stating that you are going to feel the pulse in the neck.

Using the tips of the second and third fingers, gently palpate the carotid pulse by pressing along the medial aspect of the sternocleidomastoid muscle in the lower half of the neck. Always palpate in the lower half of the neck to avoid any possibility of inducing syncope from compressing a hypersensitive carotid sinus. Palpate both right and left carotid pulses but never palpate both carotid arteries simultaneously. Extreme caution should be exercised in patients who have a history of frequent syncope or transient neurological symptoms. After determining whether there is a difference in the right and left carotid amplitude, direct your analysis of the carotid pulse to the one which is easier to palpate.

Place the diaphragm of your stethoscope in the second left intercostal space and identify the first and second heart sounds. While listening to the heart sounds, gently compress the carotid pulse until a maximum upstroke is felt. The upstroke begins almost immediately after the first heart sound. The summit occurs approximately in the middle of systole. The downstroke begins approximately two-thirds through systole and continues throughout most of diastole.

First concentrate on the amplitude of the carotid pulse and try to decide whether it is normal, decreased, or increased. This can usually be judged only after carefully feeling 25–50 carotid pulses. If necessary, use your own carotid pulse as a control. After evaluating the pulse amplitude, direct attention to analysis of the pulse contour by evaluating its upstroke, summit, and downstroke. Concentrate on the upstroke and note whether it is normal, weak, bounding, or prolonged. Next concentrate on the summit and note if there is a single or double peak; also note if you can feel a shudder or thrill. Finally, concentrate on the downstroke of the pulse, noting whether it is normal or whether it seems too rapid. If there is a rapid fall-off, the majority of the downstroke will be complete during systole.

Different parts of the carotid upstroke can be better evaluated by applying varying amounts of pressure during compression of the pulse. For example, a pulsus bisferiens can be felt more easily with light pressure than with heavy pressure.

During routine palpation of the carotid pulse, pay particular attention to the amplitude of the pulse following any premature beat. A diminished pulse amplitude following a premature beat is suggestive of idiopathic hypertrophic subaortic stenosis.

Background Information

The amplitude and contour of the carotid pulse is a reflection of the ejection characteristics of the left ventricle and of the distensibility of the arterial vascular tree. Examination of the upstroke and summit of the carotid pulse can yield valuable information regarding left ventricular ejection.

With the onset of left ventricular systole, blood is rapidly ejected into the aorta. The aorta and large central arteries are distensible and able to transiently store a large volume of the ejected blood. As a result, blood flows into the aorta and carotid arteries at a faster rate than it flows from the aorta into the distal vasculature. After peak aortic flow is reached, the rate of blood flow to the periphery is greater than ventricular ejection into the aorta. Run-off of blood to the peripheral circulation continues during diastole.

The downstroke of the carotid pulse is a reflection of the distensibility and resistance properties of the arterial vascular tree. For example, generalized arteriosclerosis of the vascular tree will result in decreased distensibility of the vascular wall and an early and rapid run-off of blood into the peripheral circulation. Clinically, this will be manifest by a carotid pulse with a prominent upstroke and a rapidly falling downstroke. Any cause of vasodilatation and decreased peripheral resistance is associated with a carotid pulse that has a rapidly falling and early downstroke.

The upstroke of the carotid pulse typically begins approximately 80 msec after the first heart sound. This delay from the first heart sound to carotid upstroke is due to isovolumic contraction of the left ventricle plus the time required for transmission of the pulse wave to the carotid artery. The upstroke should be rapid and smooth. The summit should consist of a single peak, which is smooth and dome shaped. The descending limb of the pulse should be less rapid than the upstroke. The rate of descent slows near the second heart sound so that the fall-off is less rapid during diastole (Fig 109). The point at which there is a change in the rate of descent of the downstroke is the dicrotic notch. This notch is usually not felt, but a small wave occurring immediately after the dicrotic notch, the dicrotic wave, can occasionally be felt in normal individuals with a high cardiac output, eg, during fever, exercise, and excitement.

One can simultaneously record the carotid pulse contour with the heart sounds and ECG. This is called measurement and analysis of systolic intervals.

Clinical Significance

Abnormalities of the carotid pulse can be divided into abnormalities of the pulse amplitude and abnormalities of the pulse contour.

A hypokinetic or small, weak pulse is found in conditions which have a low stroke volume or an increased peripheral vascular resistance. Causes of a low stroke volume include any cause of low-output left ventricular failure, such as myocardial infarction, cardiomyopathy, constrictive pericarditis, cardiac tamponade, mitral regurgitation, pulmonic stenosis, tricuspid stenosis, ventricular septal defect, and atrial septal defect. Aortic stenosis classically has a small, weak carotid pulse which is due to mechanical obstruction of left ventricular outflow rather than low stroke volume. Some medications, such as propranolol, can cause a hypokinetic carotid pulse.

A hyperkinetic carotid pulse is large and bounding with a rapid and

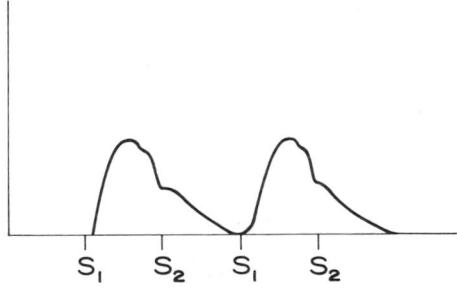

Figure 109. Normal carotid pulse contour. Note relation of upstroke and downstroke to S_1 and S_2.

high upstroke, a sharp and brief summit, and a rapid downstroke with the majority of peripheral run-off occurring during systole. A hyperkinetic pulse is caused by an increased stroke volume, decreased peripheral resistance, or decreased arterial distensibility. When the qualities of a hyperkinetic pulse become extreme, the pulse is described as "waterhammer" or "collapsing" (Fig 110). Most causes of a hyperkinetic pulse are secondary to physiologic or pathologic hyperkinetic states with an increased stroke volume. Physiologic hyperkinetic states include anxiety, exercise, fever, cigarette smoking, and pregnancy. Pathologic hyperkinetic states include thyrotoxicosis, anemia, beriberi, Paget's disease, and an idiopathic state. A large bounding pulse is present in aortic regurgitation; this hyperkinetic pulse is secondary to a combination of increased stroke volume and decreased peripheral resistance. Patent ductus arteriosus, sinus of Valsalva aneurysm, aorticopulmonary window, and arteriovenous fistulas are other etiologies of hyperkinetic pulses. The pathophysiologic mechanisms include both an increase in stroke volume and a decrease in peripheral resistance. Systemic arterial hypertension can cause decreased arterial distensibility with a resulting hyperkinetic pulse. Increasing age will also result in decreased arterial distensibility and a hyperkinetic pulse. Patients with a bradycardia who maintain a normal cardiac output have a hyperkinetic pulse secondary to increased stroke volume. This would most typically be seen in a well-trained athlete.

Abnormalities of the pulse contour include a hyperkinetic pulse, pulsus parvus et tardus, and a double-peaked pulse. Pulsus parvus et tardus describes a small pulse with a delayed upstroke and summit (Fig 111). This pulse is characteristic of moderate to severe valvular aortic stenosis; however, elderly patients with severe valvular aortic stenosis may not have this pulse abnormality because of the modifying effect of decreased arterial distensibility. In some patients with aortic stenosis, the summit of the carotid pulse may be delayed until very close to the

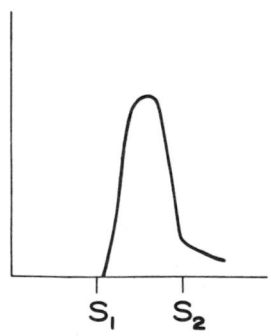

Figure 110.   Hyperkinetic carotid pulse (case of aortic regurgitation).

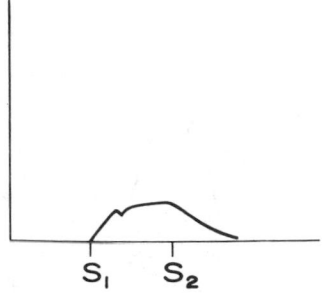

Figure 111.   Pulsus parvus et tardus (case of severe aortic stenosis).

second heart sound. Fixed-orifice subvalvular aortic stenosis can also be associated with pulsus parvus et tardus.

A double-peaked pulse is one in which two peaks are palpated. This may be secondary to a dicrotic pulse, an anacrotic pulse, or a bisferious pulse. When identifying a double-peaked pulse, the examiner must listen carefully to the heart sounds while palpating the pulse to determine whether both peaks occur during systole or whether one is in systole and one is in diastole. A dicrotic pulse occurs in early diastole, shortly after the second heart sound. As mentioned previously, a dicrotic pulse can occasionally be seen in normal individuals when the peripheral resistance is low. A dicrotic pulse palpated in the absence of fever, excitement, or exercise usually signifies severe impairment of myocardial function, primary pulmonary hypertension, constrictive pericarditis, or cardiac tamponade (Fig 112). An anacrotic pulse occurs in early systole and is found in severe aortic stenosis. This pulse abnormality is a rare physical finding. As contrasted to a bisferious pulse, the initial peak in an anacrotic pulse is smaller than the second peak.

In systole, the upstroke rises rapidly and forcefully. The initial sys-

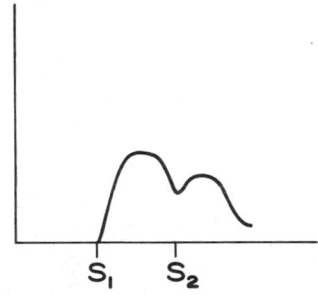

Figure 112.   Dicrotic pulse (case of severe heart failure). Note relation of dicrotic pulse to S_2.

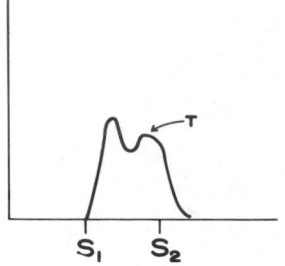

Figure 113. Pulsus bisferiens (case of idiopathic hypertrophic subaortic stenosis). Note relation of tidal wave (T) to S_2.

tolic peak is called the percussion wave; this is followed by a short dip and then a second late systolic, slowly rising peak called the tidal wave (Fig 113). At times, a bisferious pulse can be elicited by having the patient exercise. In addition, pulsus biferiens can sometimes be better appreciated at the brachial or radial rather than the carotid artery. Pulsus bisferiens is characteristic of idiopathic hypertrophic subaortic stenosis. In this entity, there is initial rapid ejection with production of the percussion wave; this is followed by a sudden decrease in left ventricular ejection as the obstruction to outflow becomes greater. The tidal wave is caused by continued ventricular ejection at a slower rate. Pulsus bisferiens can also be felt in aortic regurgitation alone, in combined aortic regurgitation and valvular aortic stenosis, in patients with anemia and other high cardiac output conditions, and in normal individuals who have a very rapid systolic ejection phase.

Another important clinical pulse abnormality is a decrease in carotid pulse amplitude following a ventricular premature beat. After a premature beat, there is increased myocardial contractility; this causes increased obstruction in idiopathic hypertrophic subaortic stenosis with a resultant decrease in pulse amplitude. This contrasts with the normal situation where pulse amplitude is either unchanged or increased following a premature beat.

Selected References

1. Hurst JW (ed in chief), Logue RB, Schlant RC, Wenger NK (eds): *The Heart,* ed 4. New York, McGraw-Hill Book Company, 1978.
2. Tavel, ME: *Clinical Phonocardiography and External Pulse Recording,* ed 2. Chicago, Year Book Medical Publishers, 1972.
3. Marx HG, Yu PN: Clinical examination of the arterial pulse, *Prog Cardiovasc Dis* 10:207–235, 1967.

4. Fowler NO: *Examination of the Heart: II, Inspection and Palpation of Venous and Arterial Pulses.* New York, American Heart Association, 1972.

154. Apex Impulse

JOSEPH Z. DAVIDS, MD

Definition

The location, amplitude, and contour of the apex impulse should be examined. The normal apex impulse is located in the fourth or fifth intercostal space medial to the left midclavicular line. It is less than 2 cm in size and is of brief duration, occupying less than two-thirds of systole. Abnormalities of the apex impulse include deviations of its size, location, force, and contour.

Technique

Place the patient in the supine position, elevating the trunk approximately 30–45°. Arrange your light source so that it shines tangentially across the left side of the patient's chest. Position yourself on the patient's right side and look tangentially across the fourth, fifth, and sixth intercostal spaces. Ask the patient to take a deep breath and then to exhale slowly as you look for a discrete area of apical movement. If necessary, ask the patient to hold the breath at a point during expiration while you look for the area of apical movement. If more than one area of movement is identified, the most lateral one is the apex impulse. If the patient has pendulous breasts, gently elevate the left breast and look for the apex impulse. If the patient has a muscular chest, a barrel-shaped chest, or an anatomical chest deformity, you may not be able to identify the apex impulse. If unable to locate the apex impulse in the left precordium, consider dextrocardia and inspect the right precordium.

Place the fingers of your right hand over the left precordium in the fourth, fifth, and sixth intercostal spaces near the midclavicular line. If unable to palpate an impulse, move your palm over to the anterior axillary line. If still unable to locate the impulse, ask the patient to roll onto the left side and attempt to palpate the apex as above. Always state in which position you identify the apex impulse because palpation in the left lateral decubitus position distorts a normal apex into appearing or feeling unduly sustained.

Having located the apex impulse, place the tips of the second, third, and fourth fingers of the right hand directly on the impulse. Palpation of the apex impulse follows along the same lines as inspection. Record the location of the apex impulse by estimating or measuring its distance from either the midsternal or midclavicular line and the intercostal space in which it is felt. Also record the approximate diameter of the apex in centimeters. State whether the impulse is of normal, increased, or diminished force; if necessary, palpate your own apex impulse for comparison.

Next, determine the duration of the apex impulse while listening to the heart sounds. Decide if the onset is with or before the first heart sound. Estimate the percentage of systole that the apex impulse occupies. The duration is an important measurement and requires concentration, patience, and experience. It may be helpful to place the bell of your stethoscope directly over the apex and watch the movement of the bell while listening to the heart sounds.

If a single tapping, nonsustained pulsation is palpated in the area previously defined as normal, then the apex impulse is normal. Often, more than a single pulsation may be detected by rolling the patient into the left lateral decubitus position. Abnormal impulses are sometimes detected by examination of the apex following 8–10 sit-ups if there is no contraindication to mildly exerting the patient. If in doubt do not exercise the patient. If a single sustained pulsation is palpated, determine whether its force is uniform throughout systole or whether there is a presystolic or late systolic accentuation or bulge.

Background Information

In a normal subject, the outward movement of the apex impulse is produced by the interventricular septum striking the anterior chest wall during systole. However, the interventricular septum rotates in the presence of either left or right ventricular hypertrophy, modifying the part of the myocardium creating the apex impulse. With marked left ventricular hypertrophy, the septum rotates to the right. As a result, contraction of the anterolateral wall of the left ventricle creates the apex impulse, and contraction of the septum causes a left parasternal impulse. On the other hand, marked right ventricular hypertrophy results in rotation of the septum to the left. Consequently, the apex impulse may result from the right ventricle.

The location of the normal apex impulse is lateral to the left sternal border, medial to the midclavicular line, and in the fourth or fifth intercostal space. It should not be more than 10 cm lateral to the midsternal line and should be less than 2 cm in diameter (a 25¢-piece is 2.4 cm in diameter). A high left hemidiaphragm, pregnancy, or chest wall abnormality can displace the apex laterally. Thus, a displaced apex impulse is not necessarily indicative of heart disease.

The normal apex impulse consists of a slight outward movement beginning with the first heart sound. This movement is produced by isovolumic contraction of the left ventricle. By the first one-third of systole, the apex impulse begins to move inward. It should return to baseline by the end of the first two-thirds of systole.

The apex impulse should be palpable in almost all normal children and young adults. It cannot be palpated in approximately 50% of older adults because of increased distance between the heart and chest wall. At times, the first heart sound can be palpated over the left precordium and mistaken for the apex impulse.

In left ventricular hypertrophy, the apex impulse may be clearly abnormal when the chest x-ray or electrocardiogram are within normal limits. In particular, a sustained apex impulse is more sensitive for detecting left ventricular hypertrophy than either its location, size, or force. Some impulses are better seen than felt; others are better felt than seen. For example, the early diastolic wave of severe mitral regurgitation or severe congestive heart failure is often better seen than felt. Both inspection and palpation are thus necessary for complete evaluation of the apex impulse.

Clinical Significance

The normal apex impulse is graphed in Fig 114. Figures in this section are sketches illustrating the various apex impulses which may be palpated. They do not represent actual recordings of apex cardiograms. The form of apex tracings varies markedly with the techniques and recording instrumentation.

Hyperkinetic circulatory conditions such as thyrotoxicosis, anemia, or anxiety can cause an apex impulse of abnormally large amplitude but normal form (Fig 115).

A sustained apex impulse is found in conditions causing left ventricular hypertrophy, severe right ventricular hypertrophy, ventricular aneurysm, and some cases of advanced coronary atherosclerotic heart disease. A sustained apex impulse is defined as one which begins with the first heart sound and lasts throughout at least two-thirds of systole (Fig 116). Increased size, increased amplitude, and displacement of the

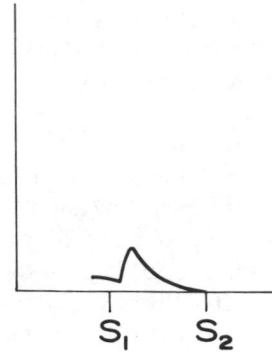

Figure 114. Normal apex impulse.

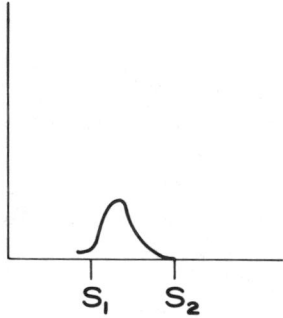

Figure 115. Hyperkinetic apex impulse (case of anemia).

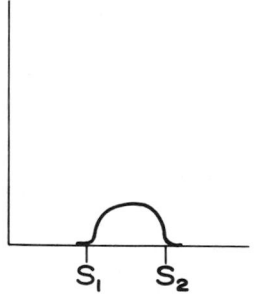

Figure 116. Sustained apex impulse (case of left ventricular hypertrophy).

apex impulse are often, but not necessarily, associated with a sustained apex impulse. However, a left ventricle that is both dilated and hypertrophied will cause a displaced, enlarged, and sustained apex impulse.

When left ventricular hypertrophy is secondary to pressure over-load, such as valvular aortic stenosis, idiopathic hypertrophic subaortic stenosis, or systemic arterial hypertension, the apex impulse may be sustained, but of normal amplitude and not displaced unless left ventricular dilation is also present. When left ventricular hypertrophy is secondary to volume overload, such as aortic regurgitation, patent ductus arteriosus, and arteriovenous fistulas, the apex impulse may be hyperdynamic, only moderately sustained, and often displaced both laterally and inferiorly (Fig 117). With long-standing or severe volume overload of the left ventricle, the apex impulse will become sustained.

A sustained apex impulse with exaggeration of its late systolic portion is called a systolic bulge (Fig 118). This is found in some patients with coronary atherosclerotic heart disease or cardiomyopathy. A systolic bulge may be felt in cases of apical ventricular aneurysm following a myocardial infarction. It may also be felt during an episode of angina pectoris or early in the course of acute myocardial infarction. In these

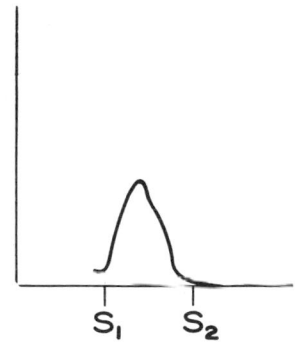

Figure 117. Hyperdynamic apex impulse (case of aortic regurgitation).

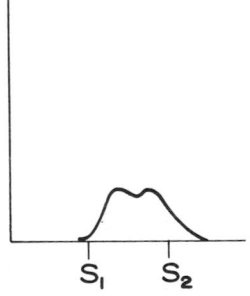

Figure 118. Sustained apex impulse with a late systolic bulge (case of ventricular aneurysm).

two conditions it may be secondary to functional paradoxic movement of the apex rather than a true anatomical aneurysm.

Another abnormality of the apex impulse is a visible or palpable presystolic component; this is analogous to the fourth heart sound (Fig 119). At times, a presystolic component will be palpable only by examining the patient in the left lateral decubitus position or postexercise. A visible or palpable presystolic component implies reduced distensibility of the left ventricle. Left atrial depolarization and contraction lead to rapid flow of blood from the left atrium into a poorly compliant left ventricle. As a result, a presystolic component may be found in any condition resulting in reduced left ventricular distensibility. A presystolic component should not be found in conditions which are associated with absent left atrial contraction, eg, atrial fibrillation. The presence of a presystolic component helps exclude hemodynamically significant mitral stenosis since blood flow from the left atrium to the left ventricle is retarded. Large and prominent presystolic components are found in 90% of patients with idiopathic hypertrophic subaortic stenosis. A presystolic component may also be found in patients with isolated aortic stenosis with a significant pressure gradient between the left ventricle and aorta. A presystolic component is often found in patients with acute myocardial infarction or during an episode of angina pectoris.

A visible or palpable early diastolic wave constitutes another abnormality of the apex impulse (Fig 120). This early diastolic wave corresponds to early rapid filling of the left ventricle and is analogous to the S₃ gallop. The early diastolic wave is most commonly felt or seen in severe mitral regurgitation and congestive heart failure of any etiology. In mitral regurgitation, this wave is secondary to a markedly increased flow of blood during early diastolic filling of the ventricle.

A bifid apex impulse consists of two positive systolic waves (Fig 121). This impulse is characteristic of but not specific for idiopathic hy-

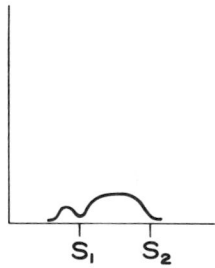

Figure 119.   Presystolic apical component followed by a sustained apex impulse (case of left ventricular hypertrophy).

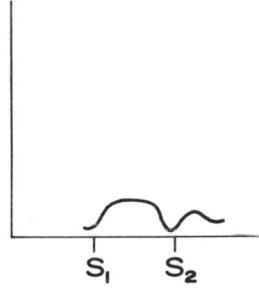

Figure 120.   Early diastolic filling wave (case of severe congestive heart failure).

pertrophic subaortic stenosis. Patients with left bundle branch block, cardiomyopathies, and left atrial myxoma may also have a bifid apex impulse. In addition, hyperkinetic states produce a bifid impulse. A systolic bulge is easily mistaken for a bifid impulse. However, the bifid apex impulse has two distinct systolic waves rather than a sustained impulse with late systolic accentuation.

When the apex impulse can be felt in constrictive pericarditis, it classically consists of retraction during most or all of systole with a plateau during diastole (Fig 122). This is known as a retracting apex impulse and can easily be mistaken for normal if systole and diastole are confused. It is thus imperative to auscultate the heart sounds while simultaneously palpating the apex. Pleuropericardial adhesions can produce a similar retracting impulse. Right ventricular hypertrophy without left ventricular enlargement produces an apical systolic retraction with a left parasternal impulse. Middle or late systolic retraction may also be seen in patients with the systolic click-murmur syndrome.

Abnormal location of the apex impulse also may be helpful in ab-

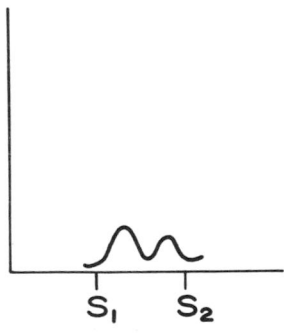

Figure 121.   Bifid apex impulse (case of anemia).

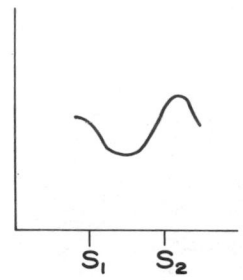

S_1 S_2

Figure 122. Systolic retraction of apex impulse with early diastolic expansion (case of constrictive pericarditis).

normalities of the lungs, especially tension pneumothorax. Prominent and leftward displacement of the apex impulse in a barrel-chested patient in acute distress suggests a right tension pneumothorax. Absence of an apex impulse in a thin-chested patient in acute distress may indicate either a left tension pneumothorax or pericardial tamponade.

Selected References

1. Hurst JW (ed in chief), Logue RB, Schlant RC, Wenger NK (eds): *The Heart,* ed 4. New York, McGraw-Hill, 1978.
2. Tavel ME: *Clinical Phonocardiography and External Pulse Recording,* ed 2. Chicago, Year Book Medical Publishers, 1972.
3. Constant J: *Bedside Cardiology.* Boston, Little, Brown, 1969.
4. Mounsey JPD: Inspection and palpation of the cardiac impulse. *Progr Cardiovasc Dis* 10:3, 187, 1967.
5. Conn RD, Cole JS: The cardiac apex impulse: Clinical and angiographic correlations. *Ann Intern Med* 75:185–191, 1971.
6. Hurst JW, Schlant RC: *Examination of the Heart: III, Inspection and Palpation of the Anterior Chest.* New York, American Heart Association, 1972.

155. Parasternal Impulse

JOSEPH Z. DAVIDS, MD

Definition

An anterior chest wall motion in the immediate vicinity of the sternum or xiphoid. Normally no impulse can be felt in this area with the exception of a very slight systolic movement in some children and thin young adults.

Technique

Place the patient in the supine position, elevating the trunk 30–45°. Place the palm of your right or left hand over the lower left sternal area, feeling for an upward movement on your palm. If no movement is felt, gently press your opposite hand over your palm and again feel for an upward movement. If no movement is felt, ask the patient to take a deep breath, exhale slowly and then hold the breath during expiration. Feel for an upward left parasternal movement. If such a movement is felt, place your stethoscope over the patient's apex, listen to the first and second heart sounds, and determine if the left parasternal impulse occurs during systole or diastole.

Next, place your palm over the right parasternal area and repeat the above maneuvers feeling for a right movement during systole.

Next, place the fingers of your right hand directly over the xiphisternum, feeling for an upward movement during systole. If such a movement is felt in this area, slide your second and third fingers under the xiphisternum, feeling for either an inferiorly or anteriorly directed movement. A pulsatile xiphisternum can be caused by either right ventricular enlargement or pulsation of the subjacent aorta. An inferiorly directed movement implies right ventricular enlargement; an anteriorly directed movement, aortic pulsation.

If you are able to palpate a left parasternal movement, four specific questions must be answered:

1. Is the impulse sustained throughout systole? This can be deter-

mined by listening to the heart sounds while palpating the parasternal impulse.

2. Is the impulse vigorous or slight?

3. Does the parasternal impulse begin with or after the onset of the apex impulse? Determine this by placing one hand on the apex impulse and the other hand on the left parasternal impulse.

4. Is the left parasternal impulse continuous with the apex impulse, or is there an area of retraction separating the left parasternal and apical impulses?

Background Information

In the normal person, there is slight retraction of the left parasternal area during systole. A very slight upward movement during systole may occasionally be felt in young children and in thin young adults in whom the apex impulse may actually be felt at the left parasternal area. Otherwise, a left parasternal impulse is an abnormal physical finding.

A left parasternal impulse may be caused by either the right ventricle, the left ventricle, or the left atrium. A right parasternal impulse may be caused by either a dilated right ventricle or right atrium striking the anterior chest wall. A xiphisternal impulse may be caused by either left atrial expansion during systole, right ventricular hypertrophy, or aortic pulsation.

The left atrium is a midline posterior structure. Expansion of the left atrium can push the right ventricle against the chest wall, creating either a parasternal or xiphisternal impulse. Comparing the onset of the parasternal impulse with the onset of the apex impulse will help differentiate whether the parasternal impulse is caused by left atrial expansion or right ventricular enlargement. A parasternal impulse secondary to left atrial expansion begins slightly after the onset of the apex impulse, whereas the impulse generated by right ventricular enlargement begins slightly before or simultaneously with the apex impulse.

Clinical Significance

A sustained left parasternal impulse is most often secondary to right ventricular hypertrophy. Pulmonary hypertension and pulmonary stenosis are common etiologies. An atrial septal defect can cause a sustained left parasternal impulse in the absence of right ventricular hypertrophy.

Right ventricular hypertrophy usually causes a left parasternal impulse that may be sustained but is not usually vigorous or marked in amplitude. Right ventricular dilatation usually produces a more vigorous and dynamic parasternal impulse. Atrial septal defect, ventricular septal defect, tricuspid regurgitation, and pulmonary regurgitation are common causes of right ventricular dilatation. In these conditions the impulse may become less dynamic in the presence of associated pulmonary hypertension.

A parasternal impulse that begins after the onset of the apex impulse is secondary to an expansile left atrium. Mitral regurgitation is a common cause. This impulse has its maximum force in late systole. When coexisting pulmonary hypertension is absent, the amount of parasternal impulse correlates with the severity of the mitral regurgitation.

A left parasternal impulse that is continuous with a sustained apex impulse may be caused by isolated left ventricular hypertrophy. A sustained apex impulse separated from a left parasternal impulse by an area of retraction is caused by biventricular enlargement or hypertrophy.

On occasion, a right parasternal impulse can be palpated. This is secondary to either right ventricular or right atrial enlargement, most often associated with severe tricuspid regurgitation.

Selected References

1. Constant J: *Bedside Cardiology.* Boston, Little, Brown, 1969.
2. Hurst JW (ed in chief), Logue RB, Schlant RC, Wenger NK (eds): *The Heart,* ed 4. New York, McGraw-Hill Book Company, 1978.
3. Hurst JW, Schlant RC: *Examination of the Heart: III, Inspection and Palpation of the Anterior Chest.* New York, American Heart Association, 1972.
4. Gillam PMS, Deliyannis AA, Mounsey JPD: The left parasternal impulse. *Br Heart J* 26:726–736, 1964.

156. Pulmonary Artery Pulsation

JOSEPH Z. DAVIDS, MD

Definition

An anterior chest wall motion in the region of the second and third left intercostal spaces near the sternum. Normally, no impulse can be felt in this area with the exception of a very slight pulsation in some children, thin adults, and patients with a hyperdynamic circulation.

Technique

Place the patient in the supine position, elevating the trunk 30–45°. Place the tips of your right second and third fingers in the second left intercostal space adjacent to the left sternal border, feeling for an outward movement. If no movement is felt, ask the patient to take a deep breath, exhale, and then hold the breath at the end of expiration. Feel again for an outward movement.

If a pulmonary artery pulsation is felt, determine if it is a brief vigorous movement or a slower and more sustained movement.

Background Information

In children and thin young adults, a pulmonary artery pulsation may be normal. Otherwise, a palpable pulmonary artery impulse is abnormal.

Assuming normal anatomy of the pulmonary artery and the ascending aorta, a pulmonary artery pulsation will usually be located in the second left intercostal space. In cases of congenitally corrected transposition of the arteries, a pulmonary artery pulsation may be felt along the right sternal border.

One may occasionally palpate the first or second heart sound in the second left intercostal space: this should not be mistaken for a pulmonary artery pulsation. A pulmonary artery pulsation will occupy a definite part of systole. A palpable or tapping first or second heart sound is very brief and coincides directly with the first or second heart sound.

Clinical Significance

A brief and vigorous pulmonary artery pulsation can be secondary to any of the following: atrial septal defect with a large left-to-right shunt, pulmonary stenosis with poststenotic dilation, or idiopathic dilation of the pulmonary artery.

A sustained and less vigorous pulmonary artery pulsation may be felt in association with secondary causes of pulmonary hypertension such as mitral stenosis or chronic pulmonary disease. It may also be noted with primary causes of pulmonary hypertension such as primary pulmonary hypertension or coarctation of the peripheral pulmonary arteries.

Selected References

1.   Eddleman EE Jr, Hughes ML, Thomas HD: Estimation of pulmonary artery pressure and pulmonary vascular resistance from ultra low frequency precordial movements (kinetocardiograms). *Am J Cardiol* 4:662–668, 1959.

2.   Hurst JW, Schlant RC: *Examination of the Heart: III, Inspection and Palpation of the Anterior Chest.* New York, American Heart Association, 1972.

157. The First Heart Sound

JOEL M. FELNER, MD

Definition

A discrete burst of auditory vibrations of varying intensity (loudness), frequency (pitch), quality, and duration. The first heart sound is produced by hemodynamic events involving the cardiac structures and coincides with contraction of the ventricles, thus defining the onset of ventricular systole and the end of mechanical diastole.

The first heart sound (S_1) consists of two major elements dependent on mitral and tricuspid closure. It coincides with the apex impulse and slightly precedes the upstroke of the carotid pulse. The first heart sound is normally audible in all four listening areas. At the second right and second left intercostal spaces it is softer than the second sound; at the cardiac apex it is louder than the second sound; at the lower left sternal border it is frequently split.

Technique

The examination should be conducted in a warm, quiet room. Place the patient in a supine position after all clothing has been removed from the chest. Explain to the patient that you are going to examine the heart. Warm your hands and stethoscope but warn the patient that your hands may be cool at first. The most comfortable and satisfactory position for most examiners is on the patient's right side. Since heart sounds may be palpable with the heel of the right hand or the finger pads, attempt to palpate the first sound initially at the cardiac apex and then over the entire precordium.

Begin auscultation with the stethoscope placed at the second right intercostal space. Listen with both the diaphragm and the bell attachments of the stethoscope. The diaphragm is best used to hear high frequency sounds such as those of S_1. It should be pressed firmly on the chest so that it produces an after-ring when removed. Continue auscultation of the first sound by sequentially listening over the second left intercostal space, the fourth left intercostal space along the left sternal border, and the cardiac apex. Follow an identical routine for every examination, passing from one part to another in a particular order. Force yourself into the habit of listening for one sound at a time. Concentrate for several cycles on the quality and intensity of the first heart sound, dismissing everything else from your mind until the sound is clearly identified and appraised.

The quality of the first sound (S_1) and its time relationship with the second sound (S_2) make it possible for the experienced observer to recognize a definite rhythm and thus easily distinguish between S_1 and S_2. At normal and slow heart rates, S_1 is the first of the paired heart sounds, following the longer diastolic period and preceding the shorter systole. These sounds can be separated by simultaneously feeling or looking at the cardiac impulse while listening; the first heart sound is synchronous with the apex impulse. When the apex impulse cannot be seen or felt, the pulsation of the carotid artery can be used as a guide; with rapid heart rates, the slight delay between the first sound and carotid pulsation may make this maneuver unsatisfactory. A finger on the carotid artery will sense the systolic thrust which is virtually coincident with the first heart sound. Use of a more distant artery for this purpose leads to error because of the time it takes the pulse wave to reach the periphery. With experience, it is possible to watch the movement of the stethoscope while listening to the heart sounds in order to time systole and diastole.

For accurate identification of the first heart sound when multiple sounds are audible, use the diaphragm and move gradually from the second right intercostal space to the fourth left intercostal space by inching along the sternal border. Then ask the patient to turn to the left lateral position. Examine the apical area while the patient is actually turning, using light pressure with the bell. Other areas of auscultation that may be helpful in certain situations include the epigastrium and first or second left intercostal spaces. Auscultation should also be performed in the sitting position, especially in emphysematous patients where sounds are quite distant or even absent in the supine position. Changing the position of the patient may accentuate sounds by bringing the heart closer to the chest wall or by accelerating blood flow due to exertion. The influence of respiration on the first heart sound should be noted. Determine whether the first sound is split and, if so, which component is loudest.

There is normal asynchrony in the closure of the mitral and tricuspid valves, with mitral closure preceding tricuspid closure by 0.02–0.03 second. This produces two audible components referred to as normal or physiologic splitting of the first heart sound. Such narrow splitting is usually best heard at the lower left sternal border with the stethoscopic diaphragm. The tricuspid component, which may increase with inspiration, is best heard in this location, but is poorly transmitted to the apical region. The mitral component, on the other hand, is best heard at the apex but in many normal individuals is intense enough to also be heard over the lower left sternal border.

Auscultation of the heart should not be performed as an isolated event. The first and second heart sounds are reference points for understanding the nature of certain pulsations. Display the heart sounds with the jugular venous pulse, the carotid pulse, the precordial movements, and with any murmurs and extra sounds heard in order to correlate the physical findings and best understand cardiac physiology and anatomy. Careful study of Fig 123 illustrates many of the points of this section concerning timing, location, and intensity of normal heart sounds.

Background Information

The genesis of the first heart sound is controversial. Two major schools of thought have emerged. The classical theory of Leatham attributes the major elements of S_1 to vibrations dependent on closure of the atrioventricular (A-V) valves. According to this theory, the two bursts of high frequency vibrations constituting S_1 can be related to mitral and tricuspid closure and therefore referred to as M_1 and T_1, respectively. This theory has come under attack by Luisada, who has pointed out a distinct time lag between the crossover of pressures in the left atrium and ventricle and the appearance of the initial major group of high frequency vibrations of S_1. Instead, they found a close relationship between the onset of the first group of high frequency vibrations and the early phase of rise of left ventricular pressure. They believe that the right side is incapable of producing the sound designated T_1. The second group of high frequency vibrations of S_1 is attributed therefore not to tricuspid closure, but rather to an additional left sided event—the ejection of blood into the root of the aorta.

The recent use of echo-phonocardiographic techniques supports the concept that S_1 consists of two major elements dependent on mitral and tricuspid closure. The first heart sound is produced by ventricular systole, which causes the initial acceleration of blood followed by a brief and sudden deceleration. The actual contact of the valve cusps is not believed to be the source of sound but rather the sudden deceleration of a mass of blood within the ventricles, associated with sudden tensing of the entire atrioventricular valve structures including the papillary muscle, chordae tendineae, valve leaflets, and valve rings, which sets the whole "cardiohemic system" into vibration with resulting vibrations in the audible range. This is supported by the fact that the first heart sound is generally audible in all four listening areas. This wide distribution is consistent

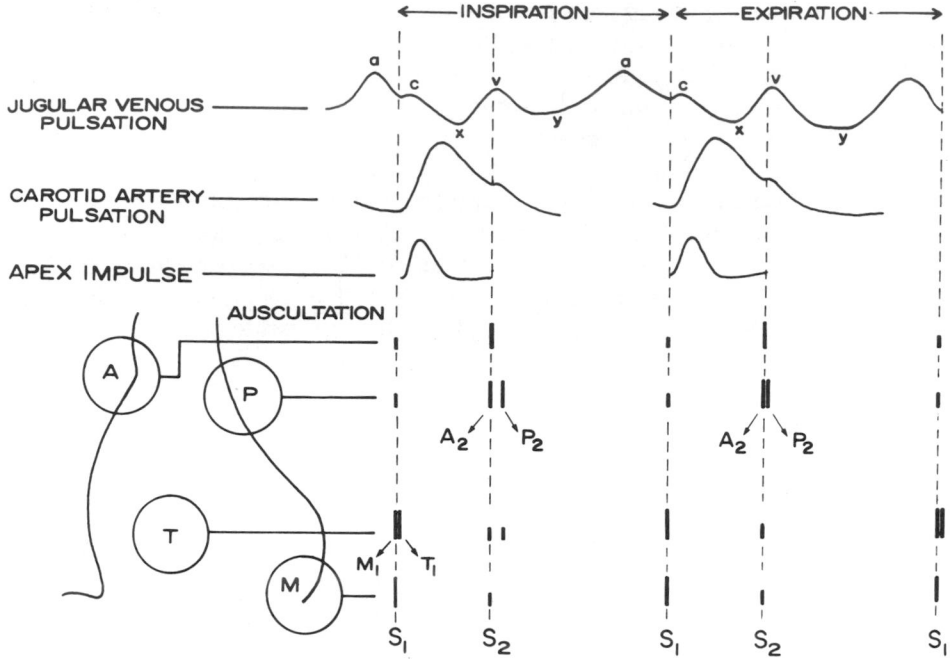

Figure 123. These graphics represent the normal cardiac pulsations and heart sounds. The *jugular venous pulsation* normally has 3 positive waves—the a, c, and v waves and 2 negative troughs—x and y troughs. The "a" wave is approximately synchronous with the first heart sound and just precedes the carotid upstroke. The "v" wave coincides approximately with the second heart sound. The normal *carotid artery pulsation* has a single positive wave during systole, followed by the dicrotic notch (about the time of the second heart sound). The *apex impulse* represents the normal brief, palpable systolic impulse occurring at the time of the first heart sound. In young normal individuals there may be a palpable early diastolic filling wave representing the rapid filling phase of ventricular diastole and corresponding to the normal third heart sound. *Auscultation* at the aortic area reveals a normal first heart sound (S_1) and second heart sound (S_2). S_2 is normally louder than S_1 in this area. At the pulmonary area there is normal inspiratory (physiologic) splitting of the second sound due to asynchronous aortic and pulmonic closure. The aortic component of the second heart sound (A_2) normally precedes the pulmonic component (P_2). At the tricuspid area there is normal splitting of the first heart sound due to asynchronous mitral and tricuspid closure. The mitral component of the first sound (M_1) normally precedes the tricuspid component (T_1). At this area, physiologic splitting of the second sound may also be appreciated. At the mitral area, the first and second heart sounds are normal. The first sound is normally louder than the second heart sound and only the aortic component of the second heart sound is normally appreciated. Occasionally a third heart sound is normal, reflecting deceleration of blood into the left ventricle during the rapid filling phase of early diastole. Children and young adults often have normal or physiologic third heart sounds.

with oscillations of the cardiohemic system produced by mass movements of blood.

The areas on the chest wall to which various acoustic events are preferentially transmitted include the second right intercostal space, the second and third left intercostal space, the fourth and fifth left intercostal space adjacent to the left sternal border, the epigastrium, and the cardiac apex. Factors responsible for this transmission include the size and position of the heart in the thorax, the presence of fluid in or fibrous thickening of the pericardium, and the position and degree of aeration of the lungs. In the region of the apex, the heart sounds are usually loud because the heart is in direct contact with the anterior wall of the thorax. In patients with thick chest walls or pulmonary emphysema, the heart sounds may be poorly heard or inaudible. They are heard more clearly if the patient bends forward or lies on the side and is examined with the lungs at the point of maximal expiration. In young persons with thin and elastic chests, the heart sounds are heard with greater intensity than in older subjects whose chest walls are thicker and stiffer. If one or both lungs are retracted by disease, the heart sounds over an area of the heart not covered by the lung will seem intensified. Before attributing abnormal heart sounds to disease of the heart, exclude such factors as these. In addition, normal heart sounds will differ considerably in the various positions. For this reason, it may be important to ausculate the patient in various positions such as supine, left lateral, sitting, and even prone.

The human auditory system is poorly suited for cardiac auscultation because of the vibratory characteristics of heart sounds. Improved auscultation can be acquired by careful training, proper use of a good stethoscope, and concentration on selected portions of the cardiac cycle. A good stethoscope must have ear tips that fit snugly, a bend in the earpieces that aligns them properly with the ear canals, double tubes 10–12 inches (25–30 cm) in length and 0.125 inch (3 mm) in internal diameter, a trumpet bell, and diaphragm that attenuates low-frequency vibrations but does not alter high-frequency vibrations. Since auscultation is deeply influenced by the noise level in the background, the examination is best carried out in a quiet room.

Hearing the components of the first heart sound depends on the ability of the ear to integrate the frequency and intensity of the vibrations making up the sound. The ear can detect two sounds separated by an interval of as little as 0.02 second. A loud sound, however, may momentarily deafen the ear with the result that an almost simultaneous faint sound may not be heard. For proper appreciation of high-pitched components of the first sound, the diaphragm of the stethoscope should be applied with sufficient pressure to leave a mark on the chest when it is removed.

The intensity and quality of the normal first heart sound will usually differ in each of the areas examined. Actually composed of three high-frequency components only two of which are appreciated clinically, the first heart sound has a booming quality and is lower-pitched, duller, and longer than the second sound. The first heart sound may be louder or fainter at the apex than the second sound, although it is usually louder and more booming. At the base, both components of the second sound are normally louder than the first sound. The first sound, however, remains lower-pitched and longer than the second sound (see next section on The Second Heart Sound). At the left sternal border, the sounds are essentially the same as those heard at the apex, but less intense. The intensity of the first sound depends upon the force of ventricular systole, sudden development of intraventricular pressure, position of the atrioventricular valves at the onset of ventricular systole, and the anatomical condition of the valves.

Clinical Significance

The first heart sound tends to be loud in young people, in patients with thin chest walls, in conditions causing vigorous left ventricular contraction, eg, exercise, and a variety of abnormal conditions (Table 25). In addition, patients with ventricular septal defect, patent ductus arteriosus, and papillary muscle dysfunction may have loud first heart sounds.

The first sound is usually soft in cases of severe aortic regurgitation, a condition which causes premature closure of the mitral valve. This and other conditions associated with a soft first sound are listed in Table 26. Ectopic beats may cause a faint first sound or no first sound at all, depending on the time relation of the atrial and ventricular contractions and the consequent variations in the position of the atrioventricular cusps at the onset of ventricular systole. When atrial fibrillation is present, the intensity of the first sound varies inversely with the duration of the preceding diastolic interval because of variable degrees of ventricular filling. Neither accentuation nor diminution of S_1 necessarily indicates heart disease.

The first sound is usually louder in subjects with a short P-Q interval on the ECG than in those with a long P-Q interval. This suggests that the

Table 25.   Increased intensity of S_1

1. Anemia
2. Thyrotoxicosis
3. Mitral stenosis
4. Systemic arterial hypertension
5. Short P-Q interval on ECG

Table 26.   Decreased intensity of S_1

---

1. Pulmonary emphysema
2. Pericardial effusion
3. Mitral regurgitation
4. Shock
5. Severe myocardial disease (eg, acute myocardial infarction)
6. First-degree heart block (prolonged P-Q interval)

---

intensity of the first sound is either related to the position of the atrioventricular valves at the onset of isometric contraction or to the speed and consequent impact of the closure. The latter is partially dependent upon the velocity of rise in the intraventricular pressure relative to atrial pressure. Although increased intensity of the first sound may be expected with shortening of the P-Q interval, this does not apply to the short P-Q interval of Wolff-Parkinson-White syndrome because the onset of ventricular contraction occurs later than is indicated by the onset of the delta wave.

The fact that the first heart sound is split may be helpful in certain disease states. For instance, a loud tricuspid component of the first heart sound may be heard in patients with Ebstein's anomaly of the tricuspid valve, right atrial myxoma, atrial septal defect, and the straight back syndrome. The mitral component of the first heart sound is extremely loud and may be heard throughout the precordium in patients with mitral stenosis. It is due to the fibrous character of the valve and/or its greater excursion during closure after the elevated left atrial pressure has kept the leaflets relatively wide apart.

A normally split first sound must be differentiated from the combination of a single first sound plus an ejection sound, which is a high-pitched, early systolic sound that follows S_1. A normally split first sound must also be differentiated from the combination of a single first sound plus a fourth heart sound, which is a low-pitched late diastolic sound that precedes S_1 (see section 160, The Fourth Heart Sound). Wide splitting of the first sound is almost always abnormal. It may be heard in right bundle branch block or in other conditions in which there is electrical delay in activation of one of the two ventricles. Examples would include ventricular ectopic beats, ventricular tachycardia, atrioventricular block with idioventricular rhythm, and left ventricular pacing. Splitting of the first sound is not characteristic of left bundle branch block because there is no significant delay in onset of left ventricular contraction. Mechanical delays in mitral closure (ie, mitral stenosis and left atrial myxoma) or tricuspid closure (ie, Ebstein's anomaly and right atrial myxoma) may cause abnormal splitting of the first heart sound.

Selected References

1. Craige E: Echocardiography in studies of the genesis of heart sounds and murmurs, in Yu P, Goodwin J (eds): *Progress in Cardiology,* vol 4. Philadelphia, Lea and Febiger, 1975.
2. Leatham A: The first and second heart sounds, in Hurst JW (ed in chief), Logue RB, Schlant RC, Wenger NK (eds): *The Heart,* ed 4. New York, McGraw-Hill, 1978, pp 237–255.
3. Levine SA, Harvey WP: *Clinical Auscultation of the Heart.* Philadelphia, WB Saunders, 1959, pp 1—97.
4. Luisada AA: *The Sounds of the Normal Heart.* St Louis, Warren H Green, 1972.
5. Luisada AA: *The Sounds of the Diseased Heart.* St Louis, Warren H Green, 1973.
6. Shah PM: Hemodynamic determinants of the first heart sound, in Leon DF, Shaver JA (eds): *Physiologic Principles of Heart Sounds and Murmurs.* New York, American Heart Assoc, 1975, pp 2–7.
7. Tavel ME: *Clinical Phonocardiography and External Pulse Recording,* ed 2. Chicago, Year Book Medical Publishers, 1972, pp 35–38.
8. Thompson ME, Shaver JA, Leon DF et al: Pathodynamics of the first heart sound, in *Physiologic Principles of Heart Sounds and Murmurs.* New York, American Heart Assoc, 1975, pp 8–18.

158. The Second Heart Sound

JOEL M. FELNER, MD

Definition

A short burst of auditory vibrations of varying intensity, frequency, quality, and duration. It is produced in part by hemodynamic events immediately following closure of the semilunar aortic and pulmonic valves. These vibrations, only two of which are usually appreciated clinically, occur at the end of ventricular contraction and indicate the onset of diastole on auscultation. The second sound is normally split on inspiration and virtually single on expiration. It is of shorter duration and higher frequency than the first heart sound.

Technique

The examination should be performed in a warm, quiet room in a manner identical to that described in the section on The First Heart Sound. First, attempt to palpate the pulmonary component of the second heart sound in the second or third left intercostal space (LICS).

Begin cardiac auscultation with the stethoscope placed at the second right intercostal space (RICS). The second sound, like the first sound, is evaluated by sequentially auscultating over the second LICS, the fourth LICS along the left sternal border, and the cardiac apex.

The quality of the second sound and its time relationships with the first sound should be determined. Concentrate for several cycles on the quality and loudness of the second heart sound, until the sound is clearly identified and appraised. The second sound, like the first, can be identified by simultaneously feeling or looking at the cardiac impulse while listening. Listen with both the diaphragm and the bell attachments of the stethoscope, using both light and firm pressure. Since the second sound has two components (A_2 and P_2), no reliable judgment about the intensity of either component can be made unless both can be heard and identified. In order to appreciate the splitting of the second sound, it may be useful to gradually move the stethoscope ("inching") from the second RICS to the fourth LICS. As with the first sound, the patient should be examined in several positions, including left lateral, sitting, and even standing.

The influence of respiration on the second sound is extremely important. The examiner will wish to note respiratory variation both during quiet breathing and at times during exaggerated breathing. The interval between the two audible components of the second heart sound normally increases on inspiration and virtually disappears on expiration. The Valsalva maneuver may be used to exaggerate splitting of the second sound. The influence of varying cardiac cycles may also exert profound influences on S_2. When the second sound is split, determine the relative loudness of the two components. The second heart sound should be correlated with other cardiac events.

Background Information

The second heart sound has two principal components. The earlier of these is labeled the aortic (A_2); the later one, the pulmonic (P_2). Rouanet, more than 140 years ago, attributed the second sound to closure of the semilunar aortic and pulmonary valves. This explanation has been generally accepted to the present time. Recent echo-phonocardiographic studies, however, have reported a discrepancy of 5–25 msc between aortic valve closure and A_2. This observation would be consistent with the hypothesis that deceleration of a column of blood in the root of the aorta at the termination of systole leads to sound-producing vibrations audible as S_2. Using similar techniques, a longer delay between pulmonary valve closure and P_2 has been found. The long interval between valve closure and sound production on the right side is attributed to the increased compliance of the pulmonary arteries. In spite of the above, some observers believe that there is an unvarying simultaneity of aortic valve closure and the initial high frequency vibrations of A_2.

The aortic valve closes earlier than the pulmonic valve because left ventricular ejection ends earlier than right ventricular ejection. During inspiration the chest expands and intrathoracic pressure drops, favoring greater venous return to the right ventricle, pooling of blood in the lungs, and decreased return to the left ventricle. The increase in right ventricular volume prolongs right-sided ejection time; the decrease in left ventricular volume reduces left-sided ejection time. An alternative explanation is that an inspiratory increase in pulmonary vascular compliance may result in a delay of P_2. This interval has been called "hangout" and its duration is a good reflection of the impedance of the vascular bed that is being injected. The net effect of expiration is to cause the pulmonary component (P_2) to occur earlier.

As a result the interval between these two sounds widens during inspiration (ie, normal inspiratory splitting of the second heart sound). During expiration, pulmonary valve closure occurs earlier as right ventricular filling, stroke volume, and ejection time decrease; the aortic component is delayed due to increased left ventricular filling, stroke volume, and ejection time. The interval between the two components is, therefore, narrowly split and may sound single to the ear.

The respiratory (physiologic) splitting of the second sound is a normal phenomenon and is usually more pronounced in children than in adults. It may become less apparent with increasing age. Although splitting is best appreciated in the third LICS adjacent to the sternum, normal subjects may exhibit splitting in the second, third, and fourth LICS along the left sternal border, or in the third and fourth RICS along the sternal border.

The components of the second sound can be heard quite widely. However, transmission to the chest wall is more restricted than in the first heart sound. Both the aortic and pulmonic components can be heard in the second RICS or the second LICS, but are most consistently heard together in the third ICS along the left sternal border. The aortic component is normally greater in intensity than the pulmonary component in most locations. The aortic component radiates widely over the chest, whereas the pulmonic component is heard mainly in the second LICS with some radiation down the left sternal border. An audible pulmonic component at the apex is rare, although it may be heard in 10% of normal children. To compare the loudness of the aortic component with that of the pulmonic component is useful, although both may be increased or decreased.

Clinical Significance

Events immediately following semilunar valve closure give rise to the two components of the second sound. With quiet respiration the aortic component (A_2) will normally precede the pulmonic component (P_2) by 0.02–0.08 second (usually 0.03–0.04) with inspiration. In younger subjects inspiratory splitting averages 0.04–0.05 second during quiet respiration. With expiration A_2 and P_2 may be superimposed and are rarely split as much as 0.04 second. If the second sound is split by greater than 0.04 second in expiration, it is usually abnormal. With inspiration, the second sound may be normally split up to 0.10 second. Therefore, wide splitting during expiration is of greater significance at the bedside in identifying underlying cardiac disease than is the absolute inspiratory increase in the A_2-P_2 interval.

Abnormally wide inspiratory splitting of the second heart sound may be due either to a delay in pulmonic valve closure or to early closure of the aortic valve. Delayed closure of the pulmonic component of S_2 may be secondary to:

1. Delayed electrical activation of the right ventricle due to right bundle branch block, left ventricular ectopic beats or paced beats, or Wolff-Parkinson-White syndrome
2. Right ventricular volume overload lesions, such as atrial septal defect, partial anomalous pulmonary venous return, congenital pulmonic regurgitation, or severe right ventricular failure
3. Right ventricular pressure overload lesions such as valvular pulmonic stenosis or primary pulmonary hypertension
4. Acute massive pulmonary embolus
5. Idiopathic dilatation of the pulmonary artery

Early closure of the aortic component of S_2 may occur in patients with decreased resistance to left ventricular outflow such as mitral regurgitation or constrictive pericarditis. Moderately large ventricular septal defects may also cause wide splitting of the second sound, but the aortic component is usually difficult to hear because of the loud holosystolic murmur.

Expiratory splitting of S_2 may occur in patients with severe congestive heart failure. The expiratory splitting usually disappears after satisfactory therapy of the heart failure. The high prevalence of expiratory splitting of S_2 in cardiomyopathy may be explained by a combination of low cardiac output, mitral regurgitation, pulmonary hypertension, right heart failure, and bundle branch block.

Audible expiratory splitting of the second sound may occur in the recumbent position in normal children, teenagers, and young adults. If these individuals sit, stand, or perform a Valsalva maneuver, however, the second sound often becomes single in expiration. In almost all patients with heart disease and auditory expiratory splitting in the recumbent position, expiratory splitting persists when the patient is in the sitting position. Thus, the finding of auditory expiratory splitting in both the recumbent and upright positions is a very sensitive screening test for heart disease.

"Fixed splitting" denotes absence of significant variation of the splitting interval with respiration such that the separation of A_2 and P_2 remains unchanged during inspiration and expiration. It is due either to the inability of the right ventricle to vary its stroke volume, causing a constant duration of systole; or to approximately equal inspiratory delay of the aortic and pulmonic components, indicating that the two ventricles share a common venous reservoir.

Atrial septal defect, either with normal or with high pulmonary vascular resistance, is the classic example of fixed splitting of the second sound. In the usual type of atrial septal defect, inspiration simultaneously delays aortic and pulmonic closure, indicating that the stroke volume of the left ventricle is increasing at the same time as the right. This inspiratory increase in left ventricular stroke volume may be related to either a transient increase in the right-to-left shunt or a transient decrease in the left-to-right shunt. In anomalous pulmonary venous return without atrial septal defect, fixed splitting is not usually seen, despite the simultaneous inspiratory delay in aortic and pulmonic closure. Respiratory splitting of the second sound returns immediately following surgical repair of an atrial septal defect, although pulmonic closure may remain delayed for weeks or months.

The Valsalva maneuver may be used to exaggerate the effect of respiration and obtain clearer separation of the components of the second sound. Patients with atrial septal defects show continuous splitting during the straining phase, and upon release the interval between the components increases by less than 0.02 second. In normal subjects, splitting is exaggerated during the release phase of the Valsalva maneuver. Variation of the cardiac cycle length (eg, R-R interval on the ECG) may also be used to evaluate splitting of S_2. Patients with atrial septal defect may show greater splitting during longer cardiac cycles. This is due to more atrial shunting and greater disparity between stroke volume of the two ventricles. In normal subjects, there is no tendency to widen the splitting with longer cycles.

Right ventricular failure may also produce fixed splitting of the second sound due to the inability of the right ventricle to further increase its stroke volume during inspiration.

Abnormally wide splitting of the second sound with normal respiratory variation is usually due to delay in the pulmonary valve closure from right heart lesions such as pure infundibular pulmonic stenosis or valvular pulmonic stenosis with intact ventricular septum. In these conditions, the pulmonic component is usually the softer of the two components and is usually not transmitted to the mitral area.

Pulmonary artery hypertension causes variable effects on splitting of the second sound. Patients with ventricular septal defects who develop pulmonary hypertension may no longer have splitting of S_2. Patients with atrial septal defects and associated pulmonary artery hypertension maintain a wide and fixed splitting of S_2. Splitting remains physiologic in patients with patent ductus arteriosus who develop pulmonary artery hypertension.

A mistaken diagnosis of abnormal splitting of the second sound must be avoided. A late systolic click, an opening snap, a third heart sound, or a pericardial knock may be incorrectly thought to represent fixed splitting of the second sound.

"Paradoxical" or reversed splitting of the second sound denotes closure of the pulmonic component before the aortic component. Splitting is then maximal on expiration and minimal or absent on inspiration. Identification of the reversed order of valve closure may be possible by judging the intensity and transmission of each component of the second sound. Often, however, the pulmonic component is as loud as the aortic component because of pulmonary hypertension from left ventricular failure. The paradoxical narrowing or disappearance of the split on inspiration is a necessary criterion for diagnosing reversed splitting by auscultation.

Paradoxical splitting is usually due to prolongation of left ventricular ejection time. This greatly delays aortic valve closure such that it follows pulmonic valve closure. The most common cause of paradoxical splitting of the second sound is left bundle branch block. Other causes of paradoxical splitting of the second sound may be due to delayed aortic closure or to early pulmonic closure (Table 27).

The loudness of each component of the second sound is proportional

Table 27.   Paradoxical splitting of S_2

Delayed aortic closure

1.   Left bundle branch block
2.   Aortic stenosis
3.   Systemic arterial hypertension
4.   Idiopathic hypertrophic subaortic stenosis
5.   Coronary atherosclerotic heart disease
6.   Severe myocardial disease
7.   Right ventricular ectopy, ectopic beats, right ventricular paced beats
8.   Patent ductus arteriosus

Early pulmonic closure

1.   Pulmonary emphysema
2.   Tricuspid regurgitation
3.   Right atrial myxoma

---

to the respective pressures in the aorta and pulmonary artery at the onset of diastole. Dilatation of the aorta or pulmonary artery may also cause accentuation of the aortic and pulmonic components, respectively. The greater radiation of the aortic component is probably due to the higher pressure in the aorta compared to the pulmonary artery. At any given level of pressure, however, the pulmonic component will be proportionately louder than the aortic component because of the closer proximity of the pulmonic valve and the pulmonary artery to the chest wall. These considerations account for the relative loudness of P_2 in young patients in whom the pulmonary arteries are quite close to the chest wall. They also account for the decreased intensity of both components of the second sound in patients with emphysema in whom both arteries are displaced from the chest wall.

The pulmonic component is considered to be abnormally loud in a subject over age 20 if it is greater than the aortic component in the second LICS or if it is audible at the cardiac apex. This may be due either to pulmonary artery hypertension or right ventricular dilatation, with part of the right ventricle assuming the position normally occupied by the left ventricle. A split second sound at the apex is, therefore, definitely abnormal. The loud P_2 commonly heard at the apex in patients with atrial septal defect, is probably due to a dilated right ventricle encroaching upon the cardiac apex.

Decreased intensity of either component of the second sound may be due to a stiff semilunar valve, decreased pressure beyond the semilunar valve, or deformity of the chest wall or lung. A decreased intensity of P_2 is most common in patients with chronic obstructive lung disease or valvular pulmonic stenosis. A decreased intensity of A_2 is most common in patients with valvular aortic stenosis.

A single second sound throughout the respiratory cycle may be normal and due to progressive delay in A_2 with age. A single second sound, however, is usually due to inability to auscultate the relatively soft pulmonary component. Such inaudibility is rare in healthy infants, children, and young adults and is uncommon even in older persons under good auscultatory conditions using a rigid stethoscopic diaphragm. Hyperinflation of the lungs is perhaps the most common cause of inability to hear pulmonary closure. All those conditions listed in Table 27 which delay A_2 may produce a single S_2 when the splitting interval becomes less than 0.02 second. Inaudibility of P_2 due to a true decrease in intensity is relatively rare, however, and suggests tetralogy of Fallot or pulmonary atresia. The pulmonic component may be inaudible in chronic right ventricular failure or may be masked by the systolic murmur in patients with aortic stenosis. Pulmonary closure is completely fused with aortic closure throughout the respiratory cycle only in Eisenmenger's syndrome with a large ventricular septal defect or in cases of single ventricle where the durations of right and left ventricular systole are virtually equal. The second sound may be single in a variety of congenital heart defects, eg, truncus arteriosus, tricuspid atresia, hypoplastic left heart syndrome, transposition of the great arteries, and, occasionally, corrected transposition of the great arteries.

Selected References

1.   Adolph RJ, Fowler NO: The second heart sound: A screening test for heart disease. *Mod Con Cardiovasc Dis* 39:91–96, 1970.
2.   Boyer SH, Chisholm AW: Physiologic splitting of the second heart sound. *Circulation* 24:180–186, 1961.
3.   Chandraratna PAN, Lopez JM, Cohen L: Echocardiographic observations on the mechanisms of the second heart sound. *Circulation* 51: 292–296, 1975.
4.   Curtiss EL, Shaver JA, Reddy PS, et al: Newer concepts in physiologic splitting of the second heart sound, in Leon DF, Shaver JA (eds): *Physiologic Principles of Heart Sounds and Murmurs.* New York, American Heart Assoc, monogr no. 46, 1975.
5.   Harris A, Sutton G: The normal second heart sound. *Br Heart J* 30: 739–742, 1968.
6.   Leatham A: Splitting of the first and second heart sounds. *Lancet* 267:607–612, 1954.
7.   Rouanet J: Analyse des bruits du coeur. Paris, Thesis No. 252, 1832.
8.   Shaver JA, O'Toole JD: The second heart sound: Newer concepts. *Mod Conc Cardiovasc Dis* 46:7–16, 1977.
9.   Tavel ME: *Clinical Phonocardiography and External Pulse Recording,* ed 2. Chicago, Year Book Medical Publishers, 1972, pp 38–41.

159. The Third Heart Sound

JOEL M. FELNER, MD

Definition

A low pitched audible vibration originating from either the left side (more commonly audible) or the right side of the heart that occurs in early diastole after the second heart sound (or in middiastole with a rapid heart rate). After the atrioventricular valves open in diastole, blood accelerates into the ventricles during the rapid filling phase. Just as it decelerates into the slow filling phase, the mitral or tricuspid apparatus (papillary muscle, chordae tendineae, and leaflets) tense and vibrate, causing the sound. The cadence of the two normal sounds plus the third (or fourth) sound is referred to as "triple rhythm," especially in the presence of a rapid heart rate.

The third sound occurs in a variety of circumstances where the common physiologic denominator is rapid ventricular filling. Children and young adults often have normal or "physiologic" third heart sounds. At times a short outward movement of the chest wall can be palpated in early diastole at the same time as this sound.

Technique

In a quiet room, turn the patient to the 30° left lateral decubitus position and locate the cardiac apex by inspection and palpation. Place the bell of the stethoscope lightly over this localized area, barely making an air seal. Since the left-sided third heart sound may be associated with a palpable or visible outward thrust of the cardiac apex, it should be detected by the combined techniques of inspection, palpation, and auscultation. The examiner best hears the right-sided S_3 using the bell of the stethoscope at the lower left sternal border with the patient supine. The apical impulse may occasionally show a systolic retraction with a right ventricular S_3.

Since third heart sounds are faint, low-pitched, and of short duration, they are best appreciated with the heart rate slightly accelerated, such as produced by turning, coughing, or lightly exercising.

The technique known as inching readily determines whether extra sounds are systolic or diastolic. The examiner moves the stethoscope inch by inch from the aortic area to the apex while focusing attention on the second heart sound. Determine whether the extra sound precedes (systolic) or follows (diastolic) the second heart sound. Both right-sided and left-sided third heart sounds occur in diastole.

Background Information

The normal third heart sound or filling sound of a child or adolescent, appearing as a manifestation of a diseased state, has been designated a ventricular or protodiastolic gallop, since three audible heart sounds occurring in rapid succession give the subjective impression of a galloping horse. The introduction of the term "gallop" is attributed to Bouillaud in 1847. Potain, however, accurately described the probable genesis and auscultatory features of gallops. The following brief description is quoted from his writings:

> One distinguishes therein three sounds, namely: two normal sounds of the heart and a superadded sound. . . . This sound is dull, much more so than the normal sound. It is a shock, a perceptible elevation; it is hardly a sound. If one applies the ear to the chest it is affected by a tactile sensation, perhaps more so than an auditory one. . . . In addition to the two normal sounds, this bruit completes the triple rhythm of the heart. It thus produces a rhythm of three sounds unequally distinct, and occasionally unequally distant, a rhythm which the ear seizes with extreme facility, provided that it had once perceived it distinctly. This is the bruit de gallop. (4)

Although usually emanating from the left ventricle, third sounds may originate in either ventricle, depending upon the location of the pathologic process and the major hemodynamic disturbances. An S_3 filling sound is best heard during tachycardia, but has the same significance at normal or slow heart rates. The usual ventricular filling sound occurs 0.14–0.16 second after the aortic component of the second sound (A_2). The precise timing is rate dependent; however, the slower the rate, the longer the interval between A_2 and the third heart sound.

The third heart sound is a diastolic event related to the end of the rapid filling phase of the ventricle. It is an exaggeration of the physiologic third heart sound commonly heard in normal subjects under 35 years of age. Whether the third heart sound is abnormal or not is judged by the context in which it occurs.

The mechanism of production and timing of the physiologic S_3 and its pathological counterpart, the ventricular gallop, has been controversial. General opinion holds that the sound is a reflection of the rapidity and volume of early diastolic filling. The traditional view presumes an imbalance between the wave of rapid left ventricular filling and the ventricle's ability to accommodate an increasing diastolic volume. Rapid stretching of the ventricular wall to its limits of distension causes acute deceleration of the blood entering the ventricle, the entire mitral apparatus, and the walls of the ventricle. The vibrations associated with this acute deceleration are manifest as the third heart sound, also referred to as the ventricular filling or gallop sound. Whether vibrations of the valve cusps or the ventricular walls are responsible for the third heart sound is a controversy that has perhaps been overplayed. It is reasonable to believe that the valve apparatus, blood, and muscular walls are all set into vibration and contribute to the sound. Different mechanisms may apply under different circumstances.

Clinical Significance

The third heart sound is frequently heard in normal children and young adults. Yet it is one of the first detectable signs of serious heart disease or cardiac decompensation in adults. It is infrequent after age 30 and virtually never seen after age 40 in the absence of circulatory overload or cardiac decompensation. The distinction between whether a third heart sound is normal or pathologic rests upon clinical grounds such as the presence or absence of other evidence of heart disease. The distinction of normal versus abnormal does not rest on its audibility, since it is generally considered an exaggeration of the normal third heart sound. Similarly, the distinction of mild versus severe left ventricular failure bears little or no relationship to whether a third heart sound is loud or soft. Factors that increase the rate of blood flow to the heart (eg, exercise, fever, elevation of the lower extremities) promote the appearance and intensity of the third heart sound. Maneuvers which decrease venous return (eg, standing) reduce the distension of the ventricle and decrease the intensity of the third heart sound. Postextrasystolic accentuation of the S_3 is well known and is related to an inability of the ventricle to accommodate to increased end-diastolic volume.

If the gallop is loudest at the cardiac apex and coincides with a palpable diastolic impulse at the cardiac apex, one can be fairly certain that it originates in the left ventricle. If it is loudest along the lower left sternal border and increases during inspiration, the gallop probably arises in the right ventricle. Occasionally left-sided gallops may be appreciated better by inspection and palpation of the cardiac apex than by auscultation; they are often associated with slight pulsus alternans.

Causes of ventricular filling sounds include:

1. Conditions associated with a high cardiac output without left ventricular decompensation (thyrotoxicosis, anemia, pregnancy, arteriovenous fistula)
2. Increased left ventricular filling in early diastole (complete heart block, left-to-right shunt, mitral regurgitation)
3. Increased right ventricular filling in early diastole (Ebstein's anomaly, tricuspid regurgitation, atrial septal defect, cor pulmonale)
4. Cardiac dilatation (frank or latent congestive heart failure from a variety of lesions such as myocarditis or cardiomyopathy)

Since a ventricular gallop implies a poor prognosis in myocardial disease, the less ominous term "third sound" or "filling sound" is more appropriate for an S_3 heard in conjunction with congenital shunts and high output states.

Most ventricular gallop sounds associated with uncontrolled congestive heart failure or mitral regurgitation persist when the patient stands. Therefore, the response of the S_3 to posture may be a useful guide to the adequacy of myocardial function. Disappearance of an S_3 after appropriate therapy usually indicates a decrease in mean left atrial pressure and an improvement in the degree of left ventricular decompensation. The prognosis is worse if the S_3 gallop rhythm persists despite therapeutic effects.

Patients with angina pectoris generally do not have an S_3 at rest. Myocardial ischemia in itself is usually not associated with an S_3 unless hemodynamic deterioration is present, such as substantial increase in left ventricular end-diastolic pressure or significant mitral regurgitation. An audible third sound in isolated mitral valve disease virtually excludes severe mitral stenosis.

Three variant forms of third heart sounds may be heard in the absence of cardiac decomposition. These include the S_3 of mitral regurgitation, the pericardial knock of constrictive pericarditis, and the tumor plop of left atrial myxoma.

In mitral regurgitation, one must distinguish between the findings in regurgitation and good ventricular function versus those with regurgitation and poor ventricular function. Patients with good ventricular function may be relatively asymptomatic despite a prominent S_3. In these cases the pathologic third heart sound is likely due to a greatly augmented diastolic flow across the mitral valve as blood rushes from the preloaded left atrium into the ventricle and then rapidly decelerates, causing the mitral apparatus to vibrate. The S_3 of mitral regurgitation usually occurs slightly earlier than the usual S_3. This is because of an elevated left atrial pressure with earlier opening of the mitral valve. This rather early S_3 can be easily confused with an opening snap or a split second sound, were it not for its low pitched and dull quality.

The pericardial knock sound is the most common auscultatory abnormality in constrictive pericarditis. A similar early third sound can rarely be heard in cardiac tamponade. The mechanism is the same for both conditions, but the sound is less consistently heard in tamponade because of the general reduction in heart sound intensity produced by pericardial effusion. The sudden deceleration (checking) of blood flow by the relatively indistensible ventricles during the stage of rapid inflow may cause the knock sound. This leads to an exaggerated filling sound (S_3) that occurs early, 0.10–0.12 second after A_2. This sound often has a higher-pitched quality than the usual S_3 filling sound. Calcification of the pericardium may influence the pitch of this sound. Since it is earlier and sharper than the usual S_3 filling sound, it must be differentiated from an opening snap of mitral stenosis or a loud P_2 of pulmonary hypertension.

A third early diastolic sound, the tumor plop, is audible in patients with left atrial myxoma. This sound probably results from the sudden checking of forward motion of the tumor on its stalk as it traverses the mitral annulus in early diastole.

Selected References

1.   Craige E: Gallop rhythm. *Progr Cardiovasc Dis.* 10:246–261, 1967.
2.   Harvey WP: Gallop sounds, clicks, snaps, whoops, honks and other sounds, in Hurst JW (ed in chief), Logue RB, Schlant RC, Wenger NK (eds): *The Heart,* ed 4. New York, McGraw-Hill, 1978, pp 255–268.
3.   Nixon PGF: The genesis of the third heart sound. *Am Heart J* 65: 712–715, 1963.
4.   Potain C: Du bruit de galop. *Gars d'Hop* 53:529–531, 1880.
5.   Rushmer RF: *Cardiovascular Dynamics,* ed 4. Philadelphia, WB Saunders, 1976, p 411.
6.   Shah PM, Gramiak R, Kramer DH, et al: Determinants of atrial (S4) and ventricular (S3) gallop sounds in primary myocardial disease. *N Engl J Med* 278: 753–758, 1968.
7.   Shah PH, Jackson D: Third heart sound and summation gallop, in Leon DF, Shaver JA (eds): *Physiologic Principles of Heart Sounds and Murmurs.* New York, American Heart Assoc, 1975, pp 79–84.

160. The Fourth Heart Sound

JOEL M. FELNER, MD

Definition

A low-pitched, audible vibration that occurs when atrial systole leads to a disproportionate rise in pressure in the ventricle in late diastole (presystole) shortly before the first heart sound. The fourth heart sound (atrial sound or S_4), like the third heart sound, is also a filling sound, and may also originate from the right or left side of the heart. It occurs after the mitral or tricuspid valve has reopened in response to atrial contraction. Its pathogenesis is incompletely understood, but its significance in terms of disturbed physiology is an indicator of an alteration in ventricular compliance. A short outward movement of the chest wall can frequently be palpated in late diastole at the same time as this sound.

Technique

The fourth heart sound (S$_4$) may originate from either the left side or right side of the heart. The left-sided fourth heart sound is usually best heard at the cardiac apex with the patient in the 30° left lateral decubitus position. Using the bell of the stethoscope, the examiner applies light pressure as described in the section 159, The Third Heart Sound. One can occasionally hear an S$_4$ over the entire precordium. The visible and palpable counterpart of the fourth heart sound, the presystolic precordial (A) wave impulse, is also most prominent at the cardiac apex with the patient in the 30° left lateral decubitus position. Careful inspection of the precordium with the naked eye or observing the movements of a wooden stick taped over the cardiac apex best demonstrates any precordial movements that correlate with gallop sounds heard with the stethoscope.

Using the bell of the stethoscope, the examiner usually hears the right-sided fourth heart sound best at the lower left sternal border toward the base of the heart with the patient supine. The right-sided S$_4$ occurs slightly earlier in diastole than the left-sided S$_4$ and often correlates with prominent or even giant jugular A waves and a sustained outward movement in the left parasternal area. Respiration, postural change, exercise, cycle length, and pharmacologic maneuvers can modify the right-sided and left-sided fourth heart sounds. In general, inspiration produces a prompt increase in the intensity of the right-sided fourth heart sound. Inspiration usually either decreases or does not change the intensity of a left-sided fourth heart sound.

Background Information

At the end of diastole (presystole) atrial contraction occurs, causing rapid blood flow into the ventricles. If the ventricle is less compliant than normal, rapid deceleration of blood occurs and causes low frequency vibrations, the fourth heart sound, analogous to those occurring with an S$_3$. It is not yet clear if an audible S$_4$ invariably implies heart disease, especially in the older patient. A fourth heart sound is rarely, if ever, audible under normal circumstances in individuals under 50 years of age because of its low pitch and intensity. When the fourth heart sound appears as a manifestation of a diseased state, it is audible.

The pathologic fourth heart sound is frequently referred to as a presystolic or atrial gallop. The term S$_4$ (atrial) gallop describes a tripling of the heart sounds resembling the canter of a horse. As with the S$_3$, tensing of the chordae tendineae and papillary muscles with early valve closure probably generates the S$_4$, which results chiefly from vibrations set up within the ventricular walls. The vibrations occur as the ventricular chambers expand with the rapid inflow and rapid deceleration of blood secondary to enhanced atrial contraction injecting blood into a relatively nondistensible ventricle. The relation of the S_4 to the P wave of the ECG, its simultaneous occurrence with the A (presystolic) wave of the apical impulse, and its failure to occur in the presence of atrial fibrillation support an atrial origin.

The left-sided fourth heart sound is closely associated with and synchronous with a brisk outward movement palpable over the precordium at the time of a vigorous atrial contraction. The brisk outward movement reflects left ventricular motion in response to a vigorous left atrial contraction. This movement provides evidence that the audible vibrations of the S_4 partially emanate from within the ventricle itself. The presence of a palpable presystolic atrial impulse in an adult patient indicates that the left ventricle has a reduced distensibility. It also indicates that the atrial kick in the left ventricular pressure tracing will be enlarged and that the left ventricular end-diastolic pressure (LVEDP) will be elevated.

Clinical Significance

Present controversy concerns the clinical usefulness of an audible S_4 (atrial) gallop. Some authors maintain that it is so common in individuals 50–80 years of age that it has little diagnostic value. Others adhere to the classical view that it is of considerable merit as an indicator of ventricular malfunction. Although inaudible fourth heart sounds may be routinely recorded graphically, audible fourth heart sounds in adults usually imply underlying pathology. If the S_4 is coupled with palpation of a large apical presystolic (atrial or A) wave, it is clearly hemodynamically significant. This may be a useful sign to help differentiate cardiac from noncardiac origins of chest pain.

The atrial gallop sound may occur with or without clinical evidence of cardiac decompensation. Atrial gallops usually occur in conditions associated with systolic overloading of either ventricle, with increased ventricular end-diastolic pressure and in conditions causing impairment in ventricular distensibility. The left-sided S_4 is a frequent finding in patients with systemic arterial hypertension, severe aortic stenosis, cardiomyopathy, and coronary artery disease manifested by acute myocardial infarction, angina pectoris, or chronic ischemic heart disease. It is unusual not to hear an S_4 in patients who are in sinus rhythm and have had a prior myocardial infarction or in patients who have idiopathic hypertrophic subaortic stenosis (IHSS). On the other hand, an S_4 is virtually always absent in isolated mitral stenosis or in the presence of a prosthetic atrioventricular (A-V) valve. Contrary to popular belief, no consistent correlation exists between the presence of an S_4 and the magnitude of the pressure gradient across the aortic valve in patients with valvular aortic stenosis. A right-sided S₄ may be prominent in patients with severe pulmonic stenosis, massive pulmonary embolus, chronic cor pulmonale, or pulmonary artery hypertension.

The fourth heart sound is also heard when there is a delay in A-V conduction such as with a prolonged P-Q interval on the ECG and especially second-degree heart block. It is unusually prevalent in high output states (eg, thyrotoxicosis, anemia, and arteriovenous fistulas). A fourth heart sound is commonly heard in patients with acute mitral regurgitation. An audible S₄ is an exceptional finding in the normal heart of patients under 50 years of age except in the presence of A-V block.

Auscultation alone is an inaccurate means to ascertain the presence of an S₄ since it typically occurs in a frequency range of about 20–30 Hz, an area in which human hearing is relatively insensitive. The apparently high prevalence with which S₄s are thought to be heard might be attributable to similar paired sounds such as physiologic splitting of the first heart sound (S₁) or an S₁ followed by an ejection click. S₄ may occasionally be confused with the presystolic murmur of mitral stenosis. Certain auscultatory features assist in distinguishing the S₄ from similar sounds near S₁. A split S₁ and an ejection click are both high pitched, widely radiating, well heard in the standing position, and easily heard with the diaphragm chest piece. On the other hand, the S₄ is low pitched, usually localized to the apex, best heard in the recumbent position, and often less audible with the diaphragm than with the bell.

In addition, the production of the S₄ is favored by factors that increase resistance to ventricular filling; these factors can be reversed by decreasing ventricular end-diastolic tension and pressure, eg, decreasing venous return or decreasing the force of atrial contraction. Thus, the left-sided S₄ may decrease in intensity and merge with S₁ during the straining phase of the Valsalva maneuver, during sitting or standing, or during carotid sinus pressure. Conversely, the S₄ increases in intensity and moves away from S₁ during increased ventricular end-diastolic tension and pressure induced by handgrip. The right-sided S₄ becomes louder and more widely separated from S₁ during inspiration.

Both atrial (S₄) and ventricular (S₃) gallops may occur in the same patient, because normal ventricular filling takes place in two separate diastolic time periods (an early passive diastolic filling and a late atrial filling). These are separated by a period when little ventricular filling occurs. The simultaneous presence of both the third and fourth heart sounds together with the cadence of the two normal heart sounds is termed "quadruple rhythm." Tachycardia, premature occurrence of atrial systole, or delay in early diastolic filling can result in superimposition of the early and late periods of ventricular filling. This often results in a critical rate of flow sufficient to produce a filling sound known as the summation gallop. A summation gallop does not necessarily signify left ventricular disease, especially if heard during extreme tachycardia, defined as a ventricular rate in excess of 140 beats per minute. With moderate tachycardia, however, a summation gallop may represent accentuation of either the third or fourth heart sound, or both. A summation gallop may thus occur in the setting of moderate tachycardia and ventricular dysfunction. Thus an accurate interpretation of the summation gallop requires consideration of its setting. It may occur in normal individuals with extreme tachycardia and a prolonged P-Q interval. If the heart rate slows, it is possible to separate the S_4 from the S_3, neither of which is as loud as the summation gallop. When both S_4 and S_3 occur in close proximity, a rumble that simulates mitral stenosis may be heard.

Additional sounds other than S_3 and S_4 may also be noted in patients with atrial flutter or other forms of A-V block. These sounds occur in diastole and are probably due to blood flow into the ventricle from the atrial contractions superimposed on the otherwise silent phase of rapid passive filling. These sounds have been referred to as "augmented atrial gallops."

Selected References

1. Fowler NO, Adolph RJ: Fourth sound gallop or split first sound. *Am J Cardiol* 30:441–444, 1972.
2. Craig E: The fourth heart sound, in Leon DF, Shaver JA (eds): *Physiologic Principles of Heart Sounds and Murmurs*. New York, American Heart Assoc, 1975. pp 74–78.
3. Harvey WP, Stapleton J: Clinical aspects of gallop rhythm with particular reference to diastolic gallops. *Circulation* 18:1017–1020, 1958.
4. Spodick DH, Quarry VM: Prevalence of the fourth heart sound by phonocardiography in the absence of cardiac disease. *Am Heart J* 87:11–15, 1974.
5. Tabatznik B: The genesis and clinical importance of the atrial and ventricular diastolic gallop, in Segal BL (ed): *The Theory and Practice of Auscultation*. Philadelphia, FA Davis, 1964, pp 126–143.
6. Tavel ME: The fourth sound: A premature requiem? *Circulation* 49: 4–8, 1974.

161. Clicks

CHARLES W. WICKLIFFE, MD

Definition

A click is a high-frequency sound heard at some time during the cardiac cycle. Clicks may be systolic or diastolic in timing and cardiac or extracardiac in origin. A click is an abnormal sound but may or may not indicate the presence of heart disease.

Technique

Clicks are heard using the stethoscope during auscultation of the heart. Because of their high frequency, clicks are best heard with the diaphragm of the stethoscope. Aortic and pulmonic clicks are most prominent along the upper right and left sternal border. Mitral and tricuspid clicks are loudest along the lower left sternal border and at the apex. The first step in identifying a click is to distinguish it from the normal heart sounds and determine its timing in the cardiac cycle. This is best accomplished by simultaneously auscultating the heart and palpating the carotid artery pulsation to clearly identify the first (S_1) and second (S_2) heart sounds. If the click falls between S_1 and S_2, it is systolic; if it occurs after S_2 and before S_1, it is diastolic. Systolic clicks may be further characterized by their location in systole, that is, early, mid, or late systolic clicks.

Once the timing of the click is ascertained, its response to respiration, postural change, Valsalva maneuver, or various pharmacologic agents, such as amyl nitrite or phenylephrine should be evaluated.

Background Information

Although clicks can be heard throughout the cardiac cycle, the majority occur in systole. Systolic clicks are classified as ejection or nonejection clicks.

Systolic ejection clicks occur in early systole and may result from either the abrupt opening of the semilunar valves or the rapid distension of the proximal aorta or pulmonary artery at the onset of ejection. Systolic ejection clicks may be aortic or pulmonic in origin. The two are difficult to differentiate. In fact, it is frequently difficult to even separate a systolic ejection click from a split first heart sound or an atrial gallop sound (S_4) followed closely by S_1.

Aortic ejection clicks are usually best heard with the diaphragm in the second right intercostal space or at the apex, whereas pulmonic ejection clicks are maximal in the second left intercostal space and left sternal border. Pulmonic ejection clicks frequently decrease in intensity or merge with the first heart sound during inspiration, whereas aortic ejection clicks are not affected by respiration. Both aortic and pulmonic ejection clicks usually occur immediately before or coincident with the initial carotid upstroke; however, a significant delay in the onset of the click suggests a pulmonic origin.

Systolic nonejection clicks are most commonly produced by the mitral or tricuspid valve apparatus. These clicks usually occur in mid to late systole and appear to be related to tensing of the chordae tendineae or valve leaflets when mitral or tricuspid valve prolapse is present. These clicks are often multiple and are quite variable in their timing, being very responsive to changes in ventricular volume induced by posture or pharmacologic agents. Originally these nonejection clicks were thought to be extracardiac, but Barlow and subsequently others have clearly demonstrated their cardiac origin. Mitral and tricuspid clicks usually move to an earlier position in systole in response to maneuvers which decrease left ventricular volume, such as standing or amyl nitrite. They move to a later position in systole in response to maneuvers such as squatting or to agents such as phenylephrine which increase ventricular volume.

Clinical Significance

Systolic ejection clicks may be heard in patients with dilatation of the aorta or pulmonary artery. Dilatation of the aorta or pulmonary artery is usually associated with semilunar valve stenosis or insufficiency, bicuspid aortic or pulmonic valves, increased flow across the valve, idiopathic dilatation of the pulmonary artery, or with pulmonary or systemic arterial hypertension. Occasionally, systolic ejection clicks are heard in patients with no detectable cardiovascular abnormality.

Aortic ejection clicks are commonly heard in patients with valvular aortic stenosis; they are distinctly unusual in supravalvular or subvalvular aortic stenosis. The mere presence of an aortic ejection click bears little relationship to the presence or absence of aortic stenosis. In patients with known aortic stenosis, the presence of a click is not related to the pressure gradient across the stenotic valve. However, the absence of a click in this setting may indicate a thickened, calcified, or immobile aortic valve.

Pulmonic ejection clicks are clinically quite useful. The more severe the pulmonic stenosis, the softer and earlier the pulmonic ejection click. This is presumably because of a decreasing pulmonary artery pressure as the stenosis becomes more severe.

Systolic nonejection clicks are usually associated with abnormalities in the mitral or tricuspid valve apparatus, resulting in systolic valvular prolapse. Prolapse of the mitral valve is quite common and may be idiopathic in origin or associated with mild rheumatic mitral valve disease, primary connective tissue abnormalities (myxomatous degeneration of Marfan's or Reed's syndrome), or associated with papillary muscle dysfunction due to coronary atherosclerotic heart disease. Mitral prolapse is also frequently found in children with atrial septal defects and occasionally has a familial distribution. The prevalence of tricuspid valve prolapse is unknown, but probably occurs commonly in association with mitral valve prolapse.

Less common causes of systolic nonejection clicks are complete heart block, ventricular aneurysm, pericarditis, Ebstein's anomaly, postmitral commissurotomy, and the presence of prosthetic valves or transvenous pacemakers.

Diastolic clicks are frequently extracardiac in origin, although they are routinely heard in patients with prosthetic mitral and tricuspid valves. The opening snap of mitral or tricuspid stenosis is a "diastolic click," as is the "pericardial knock" of constrictive pericarditis. Clicks with variable timing are frequently heard with pneumomediastinum (Hammond's "crunch"), pneumopericardium, or pneumothorax.

Selected References

1. Tavel ME: *Clinical Phonocardiography and External Pulse Recording,* ed 2. Chicago, Year Book Medical Publishers, 1972.
2. Hurst JW (ed in chief), Logue RB, Schlant RC, Wenger NK (eds): *The Heart,* ed 3. New York, McGraw-Hill, 1974.
3. Whitaker AV, Shaver JA, Gray S, et al: Sound-pressure correlates of the aortic ejection sound. *Circulation* 39:475–486, 1969.
4. Gamboa R, Hugenholtz PG, Nadas AS: Accuracy of the phonocardiogram in assessing severity of aortic and pulmonic stenosis. *Circulation* 30:35–46, 1964.
5. Barlow JB, Bosman CK, Pocock WA, et al: Late systolic murmur and non-ejection ("mid-late") systolic clicks. *Br Heart J* 30:203–218, 1968.

6. Nutter DO, Wickliffe CW, Gilbert CA, et al: Pathophysiology of idiopathic mitral valve prolapse. *Circulation* 52:297–305, 1975.
7. Fontana ME, Wooley CF, Leighton RF, et al: Postural changes in left ventricular and mitral valvular dynamics in the systolic click—late systolic murmur syndrome. *Circulation* 51:165–173, 1975.
8. Mathey DG, Decoodt PR, Allen HN, et al: The determinants of onset of mitral valve prolapse in the systolic click—late systolic murmur syndrome. *Circulation* 53:872–878, 1976.
9. Towne W: Mitral valve prolapse (review), parts I and II. *J Continuing Educ Cardiol* Jan, April, 1978.

162. Systolic Murmurs

I. SYLVIA CRAWLEY, MD

Definition

A systolic murmur is a sound of some duration occurring during systolic and lasting longer than the first or second sound.

An organic systolic murmur is a systolic murmur originating at the site of altered anatomy of the cardiovascular structures, including cardiac valves, cardiac chambers, atrial or ventricular septum, great vessels, pulmonary arteries or veins, and systemic arteries or veins.

Nonorganic systolic murmurs imply no known anatomical cardiac defects. They may or may not be associated with physiological conditions (anemia, pregnancy, etc.) which alter blood flow or ventricular function, and are sometimes referred to as either functional or innocent murmurs.

A continuous murmur is a sound that begins in systole and continues through the second sound into diastole.

Technique

If possible, the environment should be optimal with a quiet room, comfortable patient, and physician. Always approach the patient from the same side (right recommended). The stethoscope should be in good repair, and the earpieces should fit properly and be free of obstruction.

Identification of systole and diastole is the first step and may be done in one of two ways: by identification of systole simultaneously with the carotid pulse or by identification of the interval between the first and second heart sounds. The second sound is normally louder than the first at the second intercostal space to the right of the sternum.

Concentrate on systole and diastole separately. Begin with the patient supine; use the diaphragm, both with light and heavy pressure, in each area: second right intercostal space (2RICS), second left intercostal space (2LICS), left lower sternal border (LLSB), and apex. Then place the patient in the left lateral decubitus position (approximately 35° oblique) with his left arm out about 90° from the chest with the left hand under the head and the right arm resting on the right side. First use the diaphragm, again with light to heavy pressure, at the apex. Concentrate especially on systole. Then use the bell with light pressure at the apex impulse. Concentrate especially on diastole. Next have the patient sit on the side of the bed or examining table, leaning forward with held breath. Use the diaphragm with firm pressure first at the left sternal border (3LICS and 4LICS) and then at the right sternal border (3RICS and 4RICS). Concentrate on diastole. While the patient stands, listen at the apex with the diaphragm; concentrate on systole.

Any detected murmur requires that the examiner further seek the answer to five questions which often require additional techniques:

1. Is the murmur systolic, diastolic, or continuous? The first step in auscultation must always be the definition of the first and second sounds, systole and diastole.

2. What is the area of maximum intensity and area of radiation? This is best done by scanning the precordium from the apex to LLSB to 2LICS to 2RICS to right lower sternal border, using the bell or diaphragm previously determined as best for systolic murmurs. If a murmur is louder with light pressure of the diaphragm, use the bell for better definition of medium- to low-frequency sounds; firm pressure of the diaphragm is best for detection and analysis of high-frequency sounds. Having determined the precordial area of maximum intensity, listen over the neck and supra- and infraclavicular areas bilaterally, into the left axilla, over the lung fields bilaterally anterior and posterior, and over the spine cephalad and caudad. If the murmur is detected in any of these areas, determine its intensity in relation to the maximum intensity observed over the precordium. This can determine if the murmur is radiating toward or away from the precordium.

3. What is the grade of maximum intensity? Levine's classification is recommended: Grade I is heard only after a few seconds of auscultation; grade II is the faintest murmur heard immediately upon auscultation; grade V is heard with the edge of the stethoscope near but not touching the chest wall; grade VI is heard with the stethoscope near but not touching the chest wall. Grades III and IV are intermediate. Generally, if the

murmur is associated with a palpable thrill, it is considered to be at least grade IV.

4. What is the frequency characteristic and pattern of intensity? Frequency characteristics are generally classified as high, medium, or low. A few murmurs are pure sounds and are musical. Occasionally other descriptive terms are useful: harsh, blowing, rumbling. The pattern of intensity of a murmur may be constant, crescendo, decrescendo, or crescendo-decrescendo. The crescendo-decrescendo pattern is usually referred to as an ejection murmur (also called diamond-shaped or kite-shaped). Determine the onset and termination of the murmur as precisely as possible.

5. What are the effects of various maneuvers on the murmur? The effect of normal respiration, sitting, and standing on the presence and intensity of a murmur is always observed. For example, an apical systolic murmur may be heard only in the standing position; a diastolic murmur along the left sternal border may be heard only in the sitting or prone positions. The effect of standing and squatting on a systolic murmur should always be observed. The change in intensity of a systolic murmur in the cycle following a premature beat (or in the cycle following a long diastolic interval in atrial fibrillation) can be useful. Following a premature beat, the systolic murmurs of valvular aortic stenosis and idiopathic hypertrophic subaortic stenosis increase in intensity, the systolic murmur of rheumatic mitral regurgitation does not change, and the systolic murmur of papillary muscle dysfunction decreases in intensity.

The Valsalva maneuver, handgrip, and administration of pharmacologic agents including amyl nitrite and phenylephrine are useful in selected instances. When a continuous murmur is heard, particularly if maximum in the first, second, or third intercostal spaces right or left sternal border, the effect of compression of neck veins and rotation of the head should be determined to exclude transmission from an innocent venous hum.

Of all the parameters by which a murmur is analyzed, its time of occurrence (systolic or diastolic) in the cardiac cycle and the precordial area of maximal intensity are easiest to learn. More practice is required to assess the pattern of intensity and the accurate timing of onset and termination.

Background Information

The determinants of cardiovascular sound include not only characteristics of the human auditory system but also physical properties of sound production and transmission. Sound may be defined physiologically as the effect produced on the auditory system of vibrations of the air or other medium. The audible frequency (vibrations or cycles per second) of sound is limited to the range between 15,000 and 20,000 cycles per second (cps). The sensitivity of the auditory system is maximal between 1,000 and 2,000 cps but the usual range of cardiovascular sounds is below 1,000 cps. Since loudness of sound is determined not only by magnitude and frequency of the vibrations, cardiovascular sounds of low frequency are perceived as less loud sounds. Most heart murmurs are not pure tones (containing sound of only one amplitude in frequency); thus the word "murmur" connotes noise rather than pure tones. Those murmurs referred to as musical are more nearly pure tones.

The mechanism(s) of production of murmurs is not well understood. Many theories have been postulated including turbulence, vortex shedding, jet impact, and periodic wake fluctuations. No one theory seems to explain the production of all murmurs. It is, however, practical to review Leatham's classification of the production of murmurs:

1. High rates of flow (through normal or abnormal valves)
2. Forward flow through constricted or irregular valves or into a dilated vessel
3. Backward flow through a regurgitant valve, septal defect, or patent arteriosus
4. Occasional loose structures that can vibrate

In general, a murmur is transmitted from its point of origin to the direction of blood flow. From a three-dimensional view it is probably loudest at the point of origin; however, "surface" auscultation limits this. Thus the area of maximal intensity is frequently along the path of transmission, that is, aortic stenosis to the right base, mitral stenosis to the apex. High-frequency components transmit further and thus can result in a change in the quality of the murmur. A classic example of this is valvular aortic stenosis where the harsh medium-frequency murmur in the second right intercostal space may transmit only high-frequency components to the apex. Low-frequency sounds transmit poorly. Thus the diastolic rumble of mitral stenosis may be heard only at a very localized area at the apex impulse. The loudness of a murmur may be understood to have little correlation with the degree of abnormality when it is understood that not only orifice size and blood flow velocity but also transmission capabilities of intervening structures are major determinants.

Clinical Significance

Systolic murmurs may be early, mid, late or holosystolic. Holosystolic and late systolic murmurs almost always signify some abnormality of cardiac anatomy or function. Early and midsystolic murmurs may be innocent, organic, or functional (with or without heart disease).

Early systolic murmurs begin just after the first heart sound and end in midsystole. They may have a crescendo-decrescendo, decrescendo, or constant pattern.

The early systolic ejection murmur is crescendo-decrescendo with peak intensity before midsystole. This murmur may be an innocent one occurring in children and young adults in whom the murmur is of maximum intensity at the left sternal border, usually in the second or third intercostal space. Its innocence must be carefully separated from mild forms of organic systolic ejection murmurs (aortic and pulmonic stenosis) by normal splitting of the second sound, no systolic ejection click, normal deep jugular venous pulsations, normal carotid pulse, no ECG abnormality, and normal pulmonary artery pulsations on fluoroscopy. A similar early systolic ejection murmur may also occur in any age patient as a function of increased right or left ventricular stroke volume, as may occur in anemia, fever, thyrotoxicosis, complete heart block, atrial septal defect, and aortic insufficiency.

The innocent bruit of adolescents and young adults is loudest in the supraclavicular area but may radiate well into the precordial area. It is usually early systolic and its intensity may vary with change in position of the head and neck.

The vibratory murmur (Still's murmur), an innocent murmur heard in children, disappears in adolescence. It has a vibratory or buzzing quality, varied markedly with respiration and position, and is usually of maximal intensity between the apex and LLSB. The physical examination, electrocardiogram and chest x-ray are typically normal.

Midsystolic murmurs begin after the first sound and end before the second sound. They are crescendo-decrescendo with peak intensity at mid or late systole. They most often reflect pathophysiology of several categories:

1. Right or left ventricular outflow obstruction
    a. Valvular stenosis
    b. Subvalvular stenosis
    c. Supravalvular stenosis
2. Mitral valve apparatus abnormality associated with varying degrees of mitral regurgitation
    a. Mitral valve prolapse
    b. Papillary muscle dysfunction

The murmur of valvular pulmonic stenosis is of maximum intensity at the 2LICS with radiation to the left infraclavicular area. It is associated with increased splitting of the second sound with a diminished intensity of the pulmonic component, a systolic ejection click, prominent A waves in the venous pulse, and a normal carotid pulse. Fluoroscopy reveals increased pulsation of the left pulmonary artery and diminished pulsation of the right pulmonary artery. The murmur of atrial septal defect is similar but may be recognized by the associated persistent splitting of the second sound and increased pulsations of both pulmonary arteries on fluoroscopy.

The murmur of valvular aortic stenosis is usually of maximum intensity at the 2RICS (occasionally at apex). It radiates to the right infraclavicular area and may be associated with an ejection click (frequently best heard at the apex), an atrial gallop at apex, delayed carotid upstroke, and normal or paradoxical splitting of the second sound with decreased intensity of the aortic component. An associated murmur of aortic regurgitation and aortic valve calcification on fluoroscopy aid in diagnosis.

The severity of valvular stenosis (aortic or pulmonic) may be reflected in the time of peak intensity, that is, the more severe the stenosis, the later in systole peak intensity may occur. With severe forms of valvular stenosis, the murmurs may appear holosystolic.

The murmur of idiopathic hypertropic subaortic stenosis may be of maximum intensity from the LLSB to the apex and may be associated with a prominent audible and palpable atrial gallop at apex and rapid carotid upstroke with bifid peak. The murmur increases in intensity with standing or during the Valsalva maneuver; it diminishes with squatting. The peak intensity is usually during midsystole.

Mitral valve prolapse (click-murmur syndrome of Barlow) may produce a mid, late, or holosystolic murmur. It is of maximum intensity at the apex, often introduced by a systolic nonejection click. With standing, the onset of the murmur occurs earlier in systole and the murmur may increase in intensity; with squatting, the onset occurs later in systole and the murmur may diminish in intensity. The murmur is occasionally heard only in the standing position.

Papillary muscle dysfunction may produce an early, mid, late, or holosystolic murmur. It is most often midsystolic and of maximum intensity at the apex; it may radiate into the axilla. Frequently there are associated atrial and ventricular gallop sounds, accentuation of the first heart sound, and an ectopic precordial impulse. The murmur may be present only during episodes of angina, or may persist for days in the setting of acute myocardial infarction.

Late systolic murmurs (Fig 124) may be crescendo-decrescendo or crescendo, most frequently occur at the apex, and are the result of abnormal function of the mitral valve apparatus, that is, papillary muscle dysfunction or mitral valve prolapse with characteristics as previously described.

Holosystolic murmurs (Fig 125) begin with the first heart sound, end with the second heart sound, and usually have a constant pattern of in-

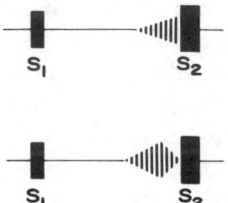

MITRAL REGURGITATION DUE TO:
MITRAL VALVE PROLAPSE
PAPILLARY MUSCLE DYSFUNCTION

Figure 124. Late systolic murmurs may be crescendo-decrescendo or crescendo, most frequently occur at the apex, and are the result of abnormal function of the mitral valve apparatus.

tensity (some may be crescendo-decrescendo). Holosystolic murmurs may represent:

1. Atrioventricular valve incompetence
   a. Mitral regurgitation (rheumatic, papillary muscle dysfunction, mitral valve prolapse, or chordal rupture)
   b. Tricuspid regurgitation
2. Ventricular septal defect

The murmur of rheumatic mitral regurgitation is of maximum intensity at the apex with radiation into the axilla. Its pattern of intensity is

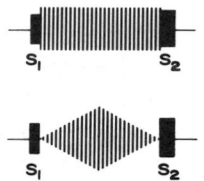

MITRAL REGURGITATION DUE TO:
RHEUMATIC
PAPILLARY MUSCLE DYSFUNCTION
MITRAL VALVE PROLAPSE
CHORDAL RUPTURE
TRICUSPID REGURGITATION
VENTRICULAR SEPTAL DEFECT

Figure 125. Holosystolic murmurs begin with the first heart sound, end with the second heart sound, and usually have a constant pattern of intensity, although certain ones may be crescendo-decrescendo.

usually constant with high-frequency sound characteristics frequently described as "blowing." Depending on severity, the remainder of the physical examination may be normal or there may be an associated ventricular gallop, functional diastolic rumble, atrial fibrillation, and diffuse sustained apex impulse. The murmur diminishes in intensity with standing and increases with squatting.

The murmurs of papillary muscle dysfunction or mitral valve prolapse may be holosystolic, thus making the differential from rheumatic mitral regurgitation difficult. The clinical setting and certain bedside maneuvers may be helpful. For example, the holosystolic murmur present only during an episode of angina favors papillary muscle dysfunction, while a holosystolic murmur that changes with squatting to mid or late systolic with a nonejection systolic click favors mitral valve prolapse.

Acute severe mitral insufficiency as is produced by chordal rupture produces a holosystolic murmur which may be crescendo-decrescendo with peak intensity in midsystole. A normal carotid upstroke and frequently associated atrial and ventricular gallops aid in its distinction from valvular aortic stenosis, which it may simulate if the mitral incompetence is primarily of the posterior leaflet resulting in radiation of the murmur from the apex to the 2 RICS. In contrast, if the mitral incompetence is primarily of the anterior mitral leaflet, it will radiate into the axilla and to the spine cephalad and caudad (caution: valvular aortic stenosis may rarely have this radiation pattern).

The murmur of tricuspid regurgitation is of maximum intensity at the LLSB with little radiation; however, with marked right ventricular dilatation, it may radiate toward the apex and mimic the sound of mitral regurgitation. It usually consists of high-frequency sounds with a constant pattern of intensity. The increased intensity in inspiration (Carvello's sign) is not always present. Prominent V waves in the jugular venous pulse aid in recognition of tricuspid regurgitation. It is most commonly due to right ventricular dilatation secondary to pulmonary hypertension. Rheumatic involvement of the tricuspid valve does occur, usually in association with other rheumatic valvular disease. A less common form of tricuspid regurgitation, involvement of the tricuspid valve by bacterial endocarditis may produce a murmur of different quality: harsh, medium-to-low frequency, with crescendo-decrescendo accentuation.

The murmur of ventricular septal defect is of maximum intensity at the left sternal border (third to fourth intercostal spaces) with little radiation; it is frequently associated with a thrill. The murmur may be high frequency with constant intensity, or harsh with a crescendo-decrescendo pattern. With a small left to right shunt, there are no other abnormal physical findings; however, with moderate defects there is a functional mitral rumble, increased splitting of the second heart sound, and evidence of increased pulmonary blood flow on chest x-ray.

Continuous murmurs. A continuous murmur (Fig 126) may begin during any part of systole and end during any part of diastole; however, it must be continuous through the second sound. It may be louder during systole, diastole, or around S_2. Continuous murmurs may be innocent or organic.

The most common continuous murmur is the innocent venous hum. It can be appreciated in most children and in many adults; it is best heard in the neck near the sternoclavicular joint with the patient sitting, head rotated to the opposite side and slightly extended; pressure over the jugular veins will obliterate it; in the supine position it may be absent or diminished in intensity. Diastolic accentuation of intensity is characteristic. Although more common on the right side of the neck, it does occur on the left, and since the venous hum can radiate inferiorly (as far as the 3ICS) it may be confused with the continuous murmur of patent ductus arteriosus which is loudest in the second intercostal space to the left of the sternum with peak intensity around the second sound, and is not affected by change in position or by compression of jugular veins.

The mammary souffle is an innocent continuous murmur which occurs during pregnancy; it is heard in the 2RICS or 2LICS (occasionally LLSB) and can be obliterated by pressure over the chest wall at the site; maximal intensity is usually in systole.

There are several communications between the systemic and lesser circulation resulting in continuous murmurs of which the patent ductus arteriosus is the most common. Less common causes include coronary arteriovenous fistula, aortic septal defect, rupture of aortic sinus of Valsalva aneurysm into the right heart, and others. The site of maximum intensity is of help in localizing the defect.

Peripheral arteriovenous fistulas, congenital or acquired, also result in continuous murmurs. These murmurs if in the upper extremities may radiate to the precordium. The continuous murmur of the arteriovenous fistula in the upper extremity utilized in chronic hemodialysis may radiate in its entirety or in part to the precordium (especially from the left arm) and simulate a systolic, diastolic, or continuous murmur originating elsewhere. For example, the diastolic component may be heard over the precordium to the left sternal border and be interpreted as a murmur of

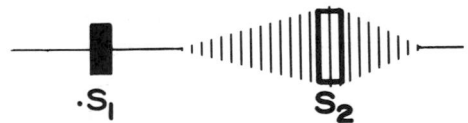

$\cdot S_1$ S_2

PATENT DUCTUS ARTERIOSUS

Figure 126. A continuous murmur may begin during any part of systole and end during any part of diastole; however, it must be continuous through the second sound.

aortic regurgitation. Transient obliteration of the fistula by pressure on the brachial artery just proximal to the fistula will obliterate the murmur.

Pericardial rub. Although this noise does not originate within the cardiac chambers or vessels, by definition it can be classified as a murmur. It usually has very typical sound characteristics, but occasionally may be confused with other murmurs.

Typically the pericardial rub (Fig 127) is a rough, scratchy sound with three phases: ventricular systole, ventricular diastole, and atrial systole. It is usually of maximal intensity at the LLSB and may be appreciated only when listening with the diaphragm (firm pressure) with the patient sitting and leaning forward in held expiration. There may be respiratory variation in intensity. There may be an associated thrill. Most frequently all three components are present when the patient is in sinus rhythm.

Since a pericardial rub is specific for some form of pericardial disease, reliability in its recognition is important. When two or all three of the components are present with the typical scratchy sound, it can be confidently recognized. When only the ventricular systolic component is present, a systolic murmur of other etiology may be stimulated. Respiratory and positional variation and the typical scratchy sound characteristics may be helpful. If it cannot be specifically defined initially, it should be called a systolic murmur. Repetitive auscultation may reveal other components of the rub. Less frequently an isolated ventricular diastolic component of a pericardial rub may simulate a murmur of semilunar valve insufficiency. The latter, however, is of higher frequency and begins with the aortic or pulmonic component of the second sound, while the ventricular diastolic component of a pericardial rub has scratchy sound characteristics and begins after the second sound.

Reliable detection and analysis of murmurs require skill in data collection and knowledge of cardiovascular anatomy and physiology to analyze the

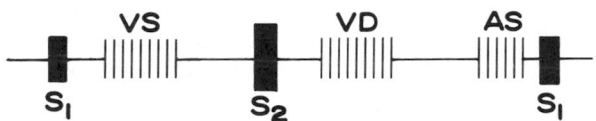

VS = VENTRICULAR SYSTOLE
VD = VENTRICULAR DIASTOLE
AS = ATRIAL SYSTOLE

Figure 127. The pericardial rub is a rough, scratchy sound with three phases: ventricular systole, ventricular diastole, and atrial systole.

collected data. The primary objective is to determine the significance of a murmur. The mere presence of a murmur does not necessarily mean heart disease. If the murmur does represent heart disease, it does not necessarily mean serious heart disease. The entire data base must be utilized in determining the significance of a murmur to appreciate the potential relationship of the murmur to other problems. For example, fever and anemia may correlate etiologically with a new systolic murmur of mitral or tricuspid regurgitation due to bacterial endocarditis.

Initial problem definition of a murmur must be quite carefully stated. It is better, for example, to define the problem simply as systolic murmur rather than to incorrectly define the problem as aortic stenosis when the initial data are inconclusive to localize its source. Once the problem is erroneously defined, the clinician's mind may become closed to other possibilities. This prejudice can carry over to subsequent physicians caring for the patient. In a patient who has no cardiovascular symptoms and whose cardiovascular examination is otherwise normal, it behooves the clinician to make a judgment as to the likelihood of a murmur reflecting some anatomical pathology. In this situation the extreme in either direction may be catastrophic. If the murmur is actually innocent and is considered organic, the patient is for life considered to have organic heart disease. On the other hand, if the murmur is actually organic and is called innocent, appropriate antibiotic prophylaxis, follow-up, and patient education are neglected.

Selected References

1. Perloff JK: Systolic, diastolic and continuous murmur, in Hurst JW (ed in chief), Logue RB, Schlant RC, Wenger NK (eds): The Heart, ed 4. New York, McGraw-Hill, 1978, pp 268–287.
2. Hurst JW, Schlant RC: Principles of auscultation, in Hurst JW (ed in chief), Logue RB, Schlant RC, Wegner NK (eds): The Heart, ed 4. New York, McGraw-Hill, 1978, pp 226–237.
3. Crawley IS, Morris DC, Silverman BD: Valvular heart disease, in Hurst JW (ed in chief), Logue RB, Schlant RC, Wenger NK (eds): The Heart, ed 4. New York, McGraw-Hill, 1978, pp 992–1081.
4. Report of the Third Bethesda Conference of the Committee on Standardized Terminology of the American College of Cardiology and the American Heart Association: Glossary of cardiologic terms related to physical diagnosis and history. Am J Cardiol 20:285–286, 1967.
5. Sacks AH, Tickner EG, Macdonald IB: Criteria for the onset of vascular murmurs. Circ Res 29:249–256, 1971.
6. Levine SA: Notes on the gradation of the intensity of cardiac murmurs. JAMA 177:261, 1961.
7. Leatham A: Auscultation of the heart. Lancet 2:757–765, 1958.

8. Bedford E: Cardiology in the days of Laennec: The story of auscultation of the heart. *Br Heart J* 34:1193–1198, 1972.

9. Pennock RS, Kawai N, Segal BL: Physiologic and pharmacologic aids in cardiac auscultation, in Fowler NO (guest ed), Brest AN (ed in chief): *Diagnostic Methods in Cardiology: Cardiovascular Clinics.* Philadelphia, FA Davis, 1975, vol 6, pp 25–39.

10. Perloff JK: *The Clinical Recognition of Congenital Heart Disease: Innocent Murmurs.* Philadelphia, WB Saunders, 1970, pp 6–13.

11. Reichek N, Shelburne JC, Perloff JK: Clinical aspects of rheumatic valvular disease. *Prog Cardiovasc Dis* 15:491–537, 1973.

12. Epstein SE, Henry WL, Clark CE, et al: Asymmetric septal hypertrophy. *Ann Intern Med* 81:650–680, 1974.

13. Perloff JK: Clinical recognition of aortic stenosis: The physical signs and differential diagnosis of the various forms of obstruction to left ventricular outflow. *Prog Cardiovasc Dis* 10:323–352, 1968.

14. Ronan JA, Steelman RB, DeLeon AC, et al: The clinical diagnosis of acute severe mitral insufficiency. *Am J Cariol* 27:284–290, 1971.

15. Jeresaty RM: Mitral valve prolapse-click syndrome. *Prog Cardiovasc Dis* 15:623–652, 1973.

16. Cheng TO: Some new observations on the syndrome of papillary muscle dysfunction. *Am J Med* 47:924–945, 1969.

17. Spodick DH: Pericardial rub. *Am J Cardiol* 35:357–362, 1975.

18. Huffman T, Leighton RF, Goodwin RS, et al: Continuous murmurs associated with shunts in the acyanotic adult. *Am J Med* 49:160–169, 1970.

163. Diastolic Murmurs

I. SYLVIA CRAWLEY, MD

Definition

A diastolic murmur is a sound of some duration occurring during diastole.

An organic diastolic murmur originates at the site of altered anatomy of the cardiovascular structures including cardiac valves, cardiac chambers, atrial or ventricular septum, great vessels, pulmonary arteries or veins, systemic arteries or veins.

A functional diastolic murmur occurs as the result of alteration in physiology (blood flow or ventricular function); heart disease may or may not be present.

Technique

The principles of detection and analysis of diastolic murmurs are the same as those described in the previous section on systolic murmurs. Special attention to auscultatory technique is essential for the detection of murmurs of aortic regurgitation and mitral stenosis.

Auscultation at the left and right sternal borders with the patient sitting forward with relaxed held breath is often required for detection of a murmur of aortic regurgitation. Since it is a high frequency sound, the diaphragm of the stethoscope must be applied with very firm pressure. Occasionally it may be necessary to auscultate at these areas with the patient prone with relaxed held expiration. The murmur may be accentuated by bedside maneuvers such as handgrip or squatting, which increase systemic blood pressure.

The murmur of mitral stenosis is best heard with the patient in the left lateral decubitus position. The bell of the stethoscope should be applied with just enough pressure to make contact with the skin. Listen directly over as well as adjacent to the apex impulse. Bedside maneuvers that result in an increase in flow often accentuate the murmur. Auscultation just after the patient has performed sit-ups (increased cardiac output) or squatted (increased venous return) may thus aid in detection.

Background Information

See previous section.

Clinical Significance

Diastolic murmurs may be early, mid, mid with late diastolic accentuation, late, or holodiastolic. The early and holodiastolic murmurs are usually high frequency and almost always signify heart disease. The mid and late diastolic murmurs are lower frequency rumbles and may be organic or functional.

Early diastolic murmurs (Fig 128) begin with the second heart sound,

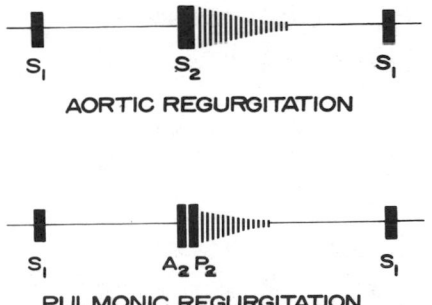

Figure 128. Early diastolic murmurs begin with the second heart sound, are usually of high frequency, decrescendo, blowing quality, and are the result of semilunar valve insufficiency.

are usually of high frequency, decrescendo, and of blowing quality. They result from semilunar valve insufficiency.

The murmur of aortic regurgitation begins with the aortic component of the second sound. It is of high frequency and is decrescendo for a variable duration of diastole. The murmur is usually of maximum intensity at the LLSB but occasionally may be maximum at the right lower sternal border, especially in etiologies involving the aortic root. A moderate degree of aortic regurgitation is associated with a rapid carotid upstroke with bifid peak, hyperdynamic peripheral pulses, and a wide pulse pressure. An early systolic ejection murmur as a function of increased stroke volume is frequently present and should not be called aortic stenosis without additional data.

The murmur of pulmonic regurgitation begins with the pulmonic component of the second sound and is decrescendo. If the etiology is acquired (most common), it is also high frequency. The most common etiology is pulmonary hypertension. The rare congenital form of pulmonic regurgitation produces a medium-frequency, harsh, early diastolic murmur.

Mid and late diastolic murmurs (Fig 129) are low frequency rumbles. They begin after S₂ (0.10–0.15 sec) and are decrescendo in pattern; late diastole may be clear, or the murmur may crescendo in late diastole (presystolic). They originate at the tricuspid or mitral valve, and may be organic (normal to decreased flow through a narrowed valve) or functional (increased flow through a normal valve). Due to their low-frequency characteristics, diastolic rumbles radiate poorly and are heard in a localized area.

The tricuspid rumble is best heard at the left lower sternal border and may be noted in patients with tricuspid stenosis, right atrial myxoma, or Ebstein's anomaly. A functional tricuspid rumble may result from an atrial septal defect or tricuspid regurgitation.

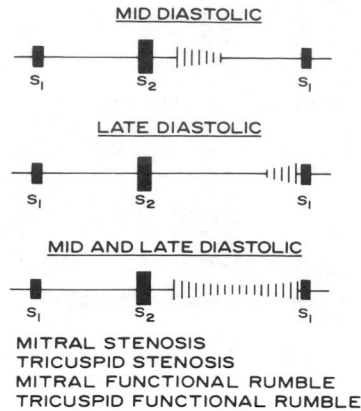

Figure 129. Mid and late diastolic murmurs are low frequency (rumble), begin after S$_2$ (0.10–0.15 sec), decrescendo in pattern; late diastole may be clear, or the murmur may be crescendo in late diastole (presystolic).

The mitral rumble most commonly results from mitral stenosis and is associated with a loud S$_1$ and opening snap. Less common causes of an organic mitral rumble include left atrial myxoma, cor triatriatum, and localized left atrioventricular groove pericardial construction. A functional mitral rumble may result from mitral regurgitation, ventricular septal defect, patent ductus arteriosus, aortic regurgitation, or complete heart block.

A diastolic rumble must be differentiated from similar sounds sometimes created by a summation gallop. This is most likely to occur with rapid heart rates or prolongation of the PR interval; it may be recognized by transiently slowing the heart rate.

Diastolic murmurs must be clinically correlated with other patient findings. Aortic regurgitation may correlate with chest pain (aortic dissection), fever and anemia (bacterial endocarditis), syphilis (aortitis with aortic valvular deformity), or rheumatic fever (aortic valvular deformity). Mitral stenosis must be carefully sought in a patient with atrial fibrillation, hemoptysis, or evidence of peripheral emboli.

Selected References

1. Perloff JK: Systolic, diastolic and continuous murmurs, in Hurst JW (ed in chief), Logue RB, Schlant RC, Wenger NK (eds): *The Heart*, ed 4. New York, McGraw-Hill, 1978, pp 268–287.

2. IIurst JW, Schlant RC: Principles of auscultation, in Hurst JW (ed in chief), Logue RB, Schlant RC, Wenger NK (eds): *The Heart*, ed 4. New York, McGraw-Hill, 1978, pp 226–237.
3. Pennock RS, Kawai N, Segal BL: Physiologic and pharmacologic aids in cardiac auscultation, in Fowler NO (guest ed), Brest AN (ed in chief): *Diagnostic Methods in Cardiology: Cardiovascular Clinics*, Philadelphia, FA Davis, 1975, vol 6, no. 3, pp 25–39.
4. Reicheck N, Shelburne JC, Perloff JK: Clinical aspects of rheumatic valvular disease. *Prog Cardiovasc Dis* 15:491–537, 1973.
5. Crawley IS, Morris DC, Silverman BD: Valvular heart disease, in Hurst JW (ed in chief), Logue RB, Schlant RC, Wenger NK (eds): *The Heart*, ed 4. New York, McGraw-Hill, 1978, pp 992–1081.

164. Edema

ELBERT P. TUTTLE, JR., MD

Definition

Edema is a physically detectable excess of fluid in the interstitial spaces of the body. Any detectable edema is abnormal and is due either to abnormality of environment or to pathologic physiology in the organism. The opposite of edema is interstitial fluid volume depletion, most often seen in conjunction with extracellular fluid volume depletion or total body sodium deficit.

Technique

The history of edema is best elicited by inquiry about "swelling." Increase of volume or swelling may be local, multicentric or diffuse, symmetric or asymmetric. The most common location and description of edema is "swelling of the feet." The old-fashioned term for this condition, still occasionally used by older patients, is "dropsy." To elicit a history of edema the line of questioning should be as follows:

Question: Have you had any swelling anywhere?

Answer: Yes

Question: Where?

Answer: (Location given)

Question: Is it more noticeable at any particular time of day?

Answer: After I've been on my feet all day or in the morning when I wake up.

Answer: No

Question: Are you sure? perhaps in your feet and ankles? swelling of your abdomen? puffiness around your eyes? swelling of your hands and fingers?

Other questions elicit information concerning the severity of edema: Did your shoes get too tight? Have you had to loosen your belt or get a larger clothes size? Did you have trouble getting the rings off your fingers? Were you unable to see the whites of your eyes in the mirror in the morning? Have you ever been given diuretic pills or 'water pills' to help make you pass more urine (water)?

Other questions may shed light on the cause of the edema: Is the swelling related to your menstrual periods? Is the swelling on one side more than the other? Have you ever been told you had heart disease, lung disease, glandular disease, liver disease, or kidney disease? Do you wear garters, a tight girdle, a corset, or strap boots? Do you have periods of emotional upset associated with your swelling? Have you or any members of your immediate family ever had diabetes? Have you ever had vein trouble in your legs?

Background Information

Relatively powerful physiologic control mechanisms allow the normal human being to maintain homeostatic balance between interstitial fluid volume deficit (dehydration) and excess (edema), despite wide variation in intake of the essential constituents of interstitial fluid, that is, sodium and water. The interstitial fluid volume is regulated by a dynamic set of feedback controls in which the fluid volume and pressure are determined by the pressure and flow of blood in the capillaries, the pressure of fluid in the interstitial space, and the protein osmotic (oncotic) pressures on either side of the capillary membrane. These are the components of Starling's Law of the Capillary. Two additional determinants of edema formation are the permeability of the capillary membrane to proteins and the flow of lymph from the tissues. Edema forms when the movement of fluid out of the bloodstream exceeds the return flow into the bloodstream and the fluid thus lost from the plasma has already been accumulated or is replaced by the retention of salt and water by the kidneys.

There are three major physiologic explanations for edema:

1.   Elevated hydrostatic pressure of blood flowing in the capillaries
2.   Reduced oncotic (colloid osmotic) pressure in the plasma
3.   Blockage of lymphatic flow

Elevated capillary hydrostatic pressure may arise from the expansion of blood (plasma) volume, increased central venous pressure or resistance in the veins draining the tissue, or increased delivery of arterial pressure to the capillary bed. Reduced plasma colloid osmotic pressure is primarily the result of reduced serum albumin concentration. This may result from inadequate hepatic synthesis of albumin, from increased destruction of albumin, or from loss of albumin from the kidney or intestine. Reduced plasma oncotic pressure may occasionally be a result of dilution of serum proteins from an excess volume of plasma water. Lymph flow removes tissue fluid transudates. Blockage may result from surgical or traumatic disruption of the lymphatics, parasitic or microbiological infestation of the lymphatics, or underactivity of the muscle pump such as with stasis during immobilization.

Clinical Significance

A history of edema may be of trivial or ponderous import. Edema occurring as an accompaniment of quiet standing or regular menstrual cycles may have no medical significance. Similarly, mild leg edema is commonly noted in massively obese individuals in the absence of other pathologic signs. On the other hand, a history of edema as noticed by the patient, either intermittently or constantly, may point toward heart, lung, kidney, liver, endocrine, nutritional, neoplastic, immunologic, or protozoal disease. The interpretation must be based on an understanding of the basic determinants of interstitial fluid dynamics and the role they play. History of peripheral edema per se, unless massive, has little consequence with regard to performance of body functions. The significance of edema depends upon what caused it, what else occurred simultaneously, and what its consequences were. For example, history of edema about the eyes in conjunction with history of bloody urine, elevated blood pressure, and shortness of breath may be the clue to acute hemorrhagic glomerulonephritis. Edema of the eyelids, swelling of the abdomen, and foamy urine may signify the nephrotic syndrome. Unilateral leg edema with purplish discoloration on standing suggests underlying chronic venous insufficiency.

There are so many elements of the circulatory tree which may by their malfunction result in a history of edema that a systematic inquiry into clues to malfunction of heart, lungs, kidneys, liver, pancreas, adrenal, and thyroid, as well as into dietetic, microbiological, neoplastic, and genetic influences must be initiated. A physician who can provide a complete and precise differential diagnosis, therapy, and prognosis of edema may be certified to have a broad understanding of internal medicine.

Selected References

1.   Starling EH: On the absorption of fluids from the connective tissue spaces. *J Physiol* 19:312–326, 1895–1896.
2.   Guyton AC, Cowley AW, Coleman TG, et al: Regulation of interstitial fluid volume and pressure. *Adv Exp Med Biol* 33:111–118, 1972.
3.   Braunwald E: Edema, in Thorn GW, et al (eds): *Harrison's Principles of Internal Medicine,* ed 8. New York, McGraw-Hill, 1977, sect 32, pp 176–182.

165. Thrombophlebitis

W. DALLAS HALL, MD

Definition

Thrombophlebitis refers to venous inflammation with secondary thrombosis of the involved vein. It is most commonly noted in the deep veins of the leg and superficial veins of the arm.

Technique

Most deep calf vein thromboses are clinically silent and cannot be detected by routine history, physical, or laboratory examination. Special techniques have thus evolved for identification of asymptomatic cases. These include transcutaneous detection of the sounds generated by augmented venous flow after muscle compression (Doppler ultrasonic), detection of changes in electrical resistance accompanying respiration-mediated changes in blood flow (impedance plethysmography), and leg photoscanning to identify fibrinogen incorporation into areas of fresh thrombus formation (^{125}I-labeled fibrinogen scanning).

The clinician should be able to detect most symptomatic and some asymptomatic cases of calf vein thrombophlebitis. Calf circumference should be determined in all suspect cases or suspicious settings. This is best measured as the maximum circumference while standing relaxed with the feet 30 cm apart. A significant difference between the two sides is 1.5 cm in males and 1.2 cm in females. The majority of patients with acute symptomatic unilateral thrombophlebitis have differences in excess of these values.

The examiner should also compare the skin temperature in the two calves since active phlebitis may create local warmth. Occasionally a short segment ("cord") of thrombosed vein may be palpable deep between the gastrocnemius muscles. "Cords" are more easily palpable in local superficial veins, particularly in infusion phlebitis related to indwelling intravenous catheters or irritating chemical, acidic, or hyperosmolar infusions.

Pain is a prominent feature of muscular, synovial, or vascular leg disease and various tests have been suggested to help identify the specific etiology. Homans' test (dorsiflexion sign) is most popularly used to detect irritability of the posterior leg muscles through which inflamed or thrombosed veins course. A popular clinical misconception is that calf pain is the endpoint of the test; however, Homans clearly stated that "discomfort need have no part in this reaction." A positive sign is when dorsiflexion of the foot on the affected side is less complete or is met with more resistance than on the unaffected side. Resistance to dorsiflexion may also be manifested by involuntary flexion of the knee.

The Lowenberg cuff test is another helpful clinical maneuver for detection of calf vein thrombosis. Wrap a blood pressure cuff around the thigh just above the knee, taking care not to pinch the skin behind the knee. Close the valve and inflate the cuff gradually to 180 mm Hg. Ask the patient to tell you of any unusual discomfort. Minimal discomfort immediately under the cuff is common. Spontaneous complaint of calf pain at 20–80 mm Hg (that is, above venous pressure) is highly suggestive of local venous disease, particularly if 150–180 mm Hg contralateral thigh pressure is well tolerated.

Other symptoms and signs include Moses' test (calf pain greater with anteroposterior than side-to-side palpation), localized leg pain on coughing (Lawrence's sign), and tenderness to touch in the sole of the foot (Owane's sign).

Background Information

The deep veins of the lower leg include the paired anterior tibial, posterior tibial, and peroneal veins that course alongside the tibia and fibula through the soleus and gastrocnemius muscles. Those veins join to form the deep popliteal vein behind the knee. The popliteal vein then drains into the superficial and common femoral vein onto the external iliac vein, inferior vena cava, right heart chambers, and pulmonary arteries.

The superficial veins of the lower leg include the long (greater) and short (lesser) saphenous. The long saphenous vein is usually visible just inside the medial malleolus of the foot. It courses superficially up the leg until joining the common femoral vein near the inguinal ligament. The short saphenous vein is often visible just outside the lateral malleolus of the foot. It courses up the lateral leg to join the popliteal vein behind the knee.

On quiet standing, the venous presure approaches 120 cm H_2O in the lower leg veins. This is reduced to 20 cm H_2O during walking. The high dependent venous pressure accounts for blood flows of only 4.0 and 0.5 cm/second in the saphenous and deep leg veins, respectively. This is quite slow when one considers that venous flow in the inferior vena cava is approximately 7.0 cm/second. Venous return up the leg is assisted by muscular contractions that squeeze blood far enough up the veins to be trapped by bicuspid venous valves, then spurted upward again by the next muscular contraction. These valves are typically present in both superficial and deep leg veins as far proximally as the external iliac vein.

Venous stasis and slow flow accelerate thrombus formation. It is therefore not surprising that various "hypercoagulable" clinical states are associated with thrombosis of the deep leg or other low flow systemic veins. Thrombosis is further accelerated by either traumatic or inflammatory injury to the venous endothelium such that platelet aggregation and fibrin formation are enhanced.

Since thrombosis in the calf veins is usually asymptomatic, an astute clinician should be aware of its potential presence given appropriately suspicious clinical settings. Examples would include:

1. Any recent leg trauma
   a. Fractures of the tibia, fibula, femur, or hip
   b. Soft tissue leg injuries
   c. Ankle sprains
2. Venous stasis and relative leg muscle immobility
   a. Bed confinement
   b. Postoperative
   c. Postpartum
   d. Varicose veins or chronic venous insufficiency
   e. Long car, truck, or bus trips, high strap boots, prolonged TV viewing with crossed legs
3. Certain drugs
   a. Postdiuresis

    b.   Corticosteroids

    c.   Estrogen-containing oral contraceptives, particularly high-dose

4.   Malignancy

Clinical Significance

There are at least four reasons why it is important to determine if a patient does or does not have thrombophlebitis. These include the threat and prophylaxis of pulmonary embolism, the risk of septicemia, the use of certain drugs other than anticoagulants, and the occasional detection of other primary disease processes.

Threat and prophylaxis of pulmonary embolism. Deep vein thrombophlebitis requires hospitalization and anticoagulation to prevent morbidity and mortality from associated pulmonary embolism. The efficacy of anticoagulant therapy in this setting was clearly demonstrated in control studies done many years ago. Evidence is not convincing that anticoagulant therapy is of benefit in phlebitis clearly isolated to superficial veins of the arm or saphenous system of the leg. However, there are communicating leg veins between the superficial and deep venous system, and the examiner bears the responsibility for determining that the aforementioned signs of deep phlebitis are absent.

Septicemia. Pelvic thrombophlebitis and thrombophlebitis associated with indwelling intravenous catheters are a surprisingly frequent source of septicemia. Recognition of either requires careful evaluation of the patient for evidence of bloodstream infection.

Other drug considerations. Thrombophlebitis and pulmonary embolism are more frequent in recently diuresed patients. One should therefore use therapeutic discretion in planning diuretic therapy for patients who belong to any of the previously described "suspicious clinical settings." In addition, patients receiving corticosteroid therapy are more susceptible to phlebitis. The same is true for women taking estrogen-containing oral contraceptives; other family planning measures should be substituted for such therapy in the presence of spontaneous thrombophlebitis.

Detection of other disease processes. Thrombophlebitis that is either recurrent, located in unusual veins (subclavian, jugular), or migratory to various superficial veins may be the first sign of an underlying disease process such as occult malignancy or systemic lupus erythematosus.

Selected References

1. Homans J: Diseases of the veins. *N Engl J Med* 231:51–60, 1944.
2. Damon A, McFarland RA: Differences in calf circumference as a diagnostic guide to thrombophlebitis. *JAMA* 153:622–625, 1953.
3. Lowenberg RI: Early diagnosis of phlebothrombosis with aid of a new clinical test. *JAMA* 155:1566–1570, 1954.
4. Richards KL, Armstrong JD Jr, Tikoff G, et al: Noninvasive diagnosis of deep vein thrombosis. *Arch Intern Med* 136:1091–1096, 1976.
5. Wessler S: Prevention of venous thromboembolism by low-dose heparin. A 1976 status report. *Mod Conc Cardiovasc Dis* 45:105–109, 1976.

---

166. Clubbing (Acropachy)

P. BAILEY FRANCIS, MD

Definition

A painless enlargement of the terminal segment of one or more fingers or toes characterized by edema and proliferation of connective tissue, especially of the nail bed.

Technique

Although clubbing is frequently presented to the student of physical diagnosis as a simple observation to make and pictorial illustrations include only the most obvious, extreme examples, the diagnosis of early or questionable clubbing is difficult even for experienced observers. Numerous complex micrometric measurements that have been advocated to diagnose clubbing are of little use to the average clinician and will not be considered further. Early clubbing is often best appreciated in the thumb or index finger. The best single clinical index of clubbing is the "profile sign." If the normal distal segment of a finger is viewed laterally, an angle of alout 160° will be seen between the plane of the proximal nail plate and that of the skin overlying the nail bed. This is called the profile angle. In mild, early clubbing, this angle will increase toward 180° at which time the concavity of the profile angle will disappear. As clubbing progresses, the angle becomes greater than 180° due to further elevation of the proximal nail plate, the proximal end of which may then be seen as a horizontal ridge paralleling the eponychial border.

In addition to the profile sign, other signs that may be present include fluctuation and vertical mobility of the nail plate imparting a spongy character to the nail bed when pressure is applied; an increased curvature of the nail in one or both horizontal planes; an increase in the size of the eponychium tending to obscure the lunula; and a smooth, shiny appearance to the skin of the eponychium with a loss of the small skin creases normally present. More severe clubbing produces a progressive increase in the volume of the distal digit best described by the German expression *Trommelschlägelfinger* (drumstick finger). Do not confuse simple curving or breaking of the nail, in which the profile angle is normal, with true clubbing.

If clubbing is found, the patient should be asked if or how long he has been aware of it and whether other members of the family also have clubbing. If the clubbing is a recent development, the patient should be asked about pain or swelling in the distal extremities. The patient may also be able to describe having to clip or file the nails more frequently.

Background Information

The first description of clubbing has usually been credited to Hippocrates, although some authors credit Caelius Aurelianus with an earlier description. In 1897, Samuel West wrote, "Clubbing is one of those phenomena with which we are all so familiar that we appear to know more about it than we really do." Unfortunately, this statement is applicable even today.

Pathologically, clubbing is characterized by a proliferation and less dense organization, suggesting edema, of the connective tissue of the nail bed. It is often accompanied by increased numbers of extravasated small lymphocytes and dilatation and thickening of the walls of small blood vessels of the distal digit. Digital blood flow studies have generally shown an abnormally increased flow of blood to the distal digits in acquired clubbing and normal flow in hereditary clubbing.

Patients with clubbing may be separated into several major clinical groupings. Acquired clubbing may be present alone or in association with secondary hypertrophic osteoarthropathy (HO) in a variety of illnesses. Acquired clubbing is also associated with idiopathic hypertrophic osteoarthropathy (pachydermoperiostosis), which is often familial. Finally, clubbing may be hereditary and unassociated with other diseases (hereditary acropachy).

Although the exact pathogenesis has not been elucidated, almost all of the diseases associated with acquired clubbing and secondary HO affect organs within the distribution of the vagus and occasionally the glossopharyngeal nerves. Cases of carcinomas of the lung are reported to have had regression of clubbing and secondary HO after section of the vagus nerve or its branches to the involved lung, which would suggest that a common reflex arc is involved. Acquired clubbing is infrequently accompanied by secondary HO. It may be associated with long-standing severe arterial hypoxemia and is usually accompanied by cyanosis, especially if a right-to-left shunt mechanism is responsible for all or a large part of the hypoxemia. A possible explanation might be the existence of a circulating vasodilator substance that directly reaches the systemic circulation through the shunt or shunts.

Clinical Significance

Acquired clubbing often with secondary HO may be seen in gastrointestinal diseases (carcinomas of the nasopharynx, esophagus, and stomach, achalasia, regional enteritis), pulmonary diseases (carcinoma of the lung, lung abcess, fibrosing alveolitis, bronchiectasis, pleural mesothelioma), and miscellaneous diseases including bacterial endocarditis. The rapid appearance of clubbing and secondary HO over a period of months in an older patient suggests carcinoma, usually lung, and may be present with tumors too small to be clinically recognizable at the time. Clubbing is rare in chronic obstructive lung disease, and its presence should suggest the diagnosis of carcinoma of the lung. Acquired clubbing is rarely associated with secondary HO but occurs in cyanotic congenital heart disease and cirrhosis of the liver.

Clubbing that gradually appears around the time of puberty in association with HO and marked thickening of the skin, especially of the face and forehead, suggests pachydermoperiostosis. Other family members may also be affected. Thickening of the skin is rarely seen in secondary HO. Simple clubbing without HO or skin changes occurring in several members of a family is characteristic of hereditary acropachy. Rarely, clubbing may be associated with certain anomalies of the aorta and may occur unilaterally in an upper extremity, or it may be unidigital following trauma to a finger or to the nerves supplying it.

Selected References

1.   Locke EA: Secondary hypertrophic osteoarthropathy and its relation to simple club-fingers. *Arch Intern Med* 15:659–713, 1915.
2.   Mendlowitz M: Clubbing and hypertrophic osteoarthropathy. *Medicine* 21:269–306, 1942.

3. Vogl A, Goldfischer S: Pachydermoperiostosis. *Am J Med* 33:166–187, 1962.
4. Fischer DS, Singer DH, Feldman SM. Clubbing: A review, with emphasis on hereditary acropachy. *Medicine* 43:459–479, 1964.

167. Cyanosis

P. BAILEY FRANCIS, MD

Definition

A bluish coloration of the skin and mucous membranes.

Technique

The areas of the body where cyanosis is most likely to be seen are the tongue, lips, conjunctiva, ears, nose, cheeks, hands, and feet. Care must be taken to examine the patient in the presence of adequate lighting, preferably daylight through a large window. It is important not to confuse the localized bluish color that occurs normally due to veins underlying the mucous membranes, especially the underside of the tongue, with the generalized bluish discoloration of cyanosis.

If cyanosis is judged to be present, note whether the patient or the patient's family is aware of it, whether it began suddenly or gradually and how long it has been present. If the patient is otherwise relatively asymptomatic, he should be asked about a family history of cyanosis and about any recent drug ingestion or chemical exposure. The shade of skin color (reddish blue, gray blue) should be recorded as well as its distribution; that is, central (generalized), peripheral (distal extremities), differential (upper and lower torso), or localized (an isolated extremity).

Background Information

The usual coloration imparted to the skin and mucous membranes arises from the blood in the underlying capillaries and small venules and is modified by skin thickness, extravascular skin pigmentation related to race or sun exposure, and the adequacy of blood flow to the surface. Classic central cyanosis results from an abnormally large amount of unsaturated hemoglobin in the arterial and capillary blood. The threshold for detection of cyanosis has been found to be about 5 gm unsaturated hemoglobin per 100 ml of blood. This type of cyanosis is related to severe hypoxemia in most patients and becomes visible at arterial oxygen saturations below 75–85%. Anemic patients with total hemoglobin concentrations of less than 7 gm/100 ml may be severely hypoxemic without becoming cyanotic. Conversely, some patients with polycythemia may have more than 5 gm/100 ml unsaturated hemoglobin and manifest cyanosis without being severely hypoxemic.

Abnormal hemoglobins may also cause central cyanosis. Methemoglobin differs from hemoglobin in that the iron atom is in the ferric rather than the ferrous state. Methemoglobinemia may be congenital or acquired. The acquired form usually results from drugs or chemicals with oxidant potential. Methemoglobinemia is a reversible process. Sulfhemoglobin is an irreversible modification of hemoglobin also related to drugs or chemicals. Only 1.5 gm/100 ml of methemoglobin or 0.5 gm/100 ml of sulfhemoglobin are required to produce cyanosis. Peripheral cyanosis results from an abnormal amount of reduced hemoglobin in peripheral capillaries and small venules as a result of slowing of blood flow leading to an excessive amount of oxygen extraction by the tissues. Localized cyanosis is commonly caused by obstruction of the flow of blood either into or out of a certain area of the body.

Clinical Significance

Central cyanosis in children is usually related to congenital heart disease or methemoglobinemia, the former often accompanied by clubbing of fingers. In adults, central cyanosis, frequently associated with dyspnea and chest pain, may be sudden in onset as occurs in acute pulmonary embolism, pneumothorax, acute pulmonary edema, or the aspiration of a large foreign body that obstructs the upper airway (the "cafe coronary"). Cyanosis appearing over a period of one or two days under similar circumstances may indicate pneumonia or atelectasis. More chronic cyanosis is seen in severe lung disorders such as chronic bronchitis and emphysema, idiopathic pulmonary fibrosis, pulmonary arteriovenous fistula, various hypoventilatory states such as massive obesity, and congenital heart disease with a reversed shunt. Asymptomatic cyanotic adults should be suspected of having methemoglobinemia or sulfhemoglobinemia.

Peripheral cyanosis associated with cold, clammy extremities is often seen in shock. Intermittent cyanosis and pain in the hands on cold exposure suggest Raynaud's phenomenon or disease. Persistent cyanosis limited to the hands in a young woman suggests acrocyanosis. Differential cyanosis may be seen in patients who have a patent ductus arteriosus with a reversed shunt. Localized cyanosis, usually of one extremity, suggests arterial thromboembolism or venous stasis.

Cyanosis must be differentiated from the deep red discoloration of polycythemia, the slate blue gray discoloration of argyria and bismuth poisoning, and the more brownish discoloration of hemochromatosis and Addison's disease.

Selected References

1. Lundsgaard C, van Slyke DD: Cyanosis. *Medicine* 2:1–76, 1923.
2. Jaffe ER, Heller P: Methemoglobinemia in man. *Prog Hemat* 4:48–71, 1964.
3. Blount SG Jr: Cyanosis: Pathophysiology and differential diagnosis. *Prog Cardiovasc Dis* 13:595–605, 1971.

168. Pulsus Alternans

JOEL M. FELNER, MD

Definition

Pulsus alternans is a characteristic pulse pattern in which the beats occur at constant intervals but with a regular alternation of strong and weak ventricular systoles. This results in alternation of a larger and smaller pulse whereby the smaller pulse occurs approximately midway between two larger ones. "Total" alternans is the ultimate expression of pulsus alternans and occurs when weak contractions fail to either open the aortic valve or to eject the volume of blood sufficient to produce a palpable pulse. Pulsus alternans is not due to an arrhythmia and is independent of respiratory influences.

Several varieties may be distinguished. When pulsus alternans is associated with alternation of other cardiac events, such as alternation in intensity of the heart sounds or heart murmurs, this is referred to as "cardiac" alternans. Cardiac alternans may involve diastole as well as systole and either the left ventricle or right ventricle. When left ventricular pulsus alternans occurs simultaneously with alternating contractility of the right ventricle and pulmonary artery, "concordant" alternans is present. When cardiac alternans affects the left ventricle and right ventricle independently, it is referred to as "discordant" alternans.

Alternation in the electrical manifestations of cardiac action showing on the electrocardiogram is referred to as "electrical" alternans. It too is not due to an arrhythmia and is independent of respiratory influences.

Technique

Palpation of the femoral artery and less often the radial artery may disclose that alternate pulses vary in amplitude. Pulsus alternans is easier to identify in a peripheral artery than in the aorta or carotid artery because of the greater pulse pressure in distal arteries. Have the patient hold his breath while you feel the pulse to make certain that the alternation of pulse intensity is independent of respiration. Be certain that the pulse is regular, since alternation of the strength of cardiac beats commonly results from bigeminal rhythm. Rarely, pulsus alternans may feel slightly irregular because of a delay in sensing the weaker beat.

The most sensitive method to discover even slight degrees of pulsus alternans is careful auscultation of the brachial blood pressure. As the pressure is lowered in the sphygmomanometer, you should routinely observe whether each successive Korotkoff sound (at a given pressure level) is heard with equal intensity. As the cuff pressure is slowly deflated in patients with mild alternans, all Korotkoff sounds are audible at the systolic blood pressure, but the sounds alternate in loudness. In severe cases, when the cuff pressure is raised above the systolic blood pressure and then lowered very slowly, only the strongest of the two alternating beats may be audible for a range of 2–10 mm Hg or more. As the cuff pressure is lowered further, the frequency of the sounds may suddenly double as the weaker beats also become audible. When pulsus alternans is prominent, it may be confirmed and quantitated by the use of the sphygmomanometer.

Pulsus alternans may be induced or exaggerated by maneuvers that decrease venous return (such as standing) or by exercise. In most instances the weaker beats are only subtly less intense than the strong beats. Occasionally the weak beats may be so small that they transfer no palpable pulse to the periphery. This is referred to as "total" alternans and occurs when weak contractions fail either to open the aortic valve or to eject the volume of blood sufficient to produce a palpable pulse.

It is important to differentiate pulsus alternans from other causes of beat to beat alternation of the pulse. These include bigeminal rhythm, postextrasystolic ventricular beats, and tachypnea where the respiratory rate is exactly one-half the pulse rate. Differentiation between pulsus alternans and pulsus bigeminus (due to one ventricular extrasystole following each conducted sinus beat) can be made at a glance from an electrocardiogram or bedside monitor. In addition, pulsus alternans may be distinguished from the strong and weak beats of ventricular bigeminy by noting that the weak beat in pulsus alternans is closer to the succeeding beat than to the preceding beat. The weak beat of a bigeminal pulse is distinctly closer to the preceding normal beat since it is premature.

Background Information

Pulsus alternans is more justifiably regarded as a coupling of weak and supernormal beats rather than of weak and normal beats. Traube first described pulsus alternans in 1872. Since pulsus alternans is associated with normal rhythm, alternating strength of the arterial pulse must be due to alternation in cardiac output. The two primary mechanisms proposed for mechanical (pulsus) alternans are alternating ventricular end-diastolic length and tension and alternating contractile states. The exact mechanism remains controversial, however, and either or both of the above may be responsible under varying conditions. It is generally attributed to a corresponding alternation in the strength of left ventricular contraction resulting in alternation in the amount of blood ejected into the peripheral artery.

Two theories have been proposed to explain the alternation in the amount of blood ejected into the peripheral artery. Either or both may be responsible under different circumstances. The first and classical hemodynamic theory is based on Starling's Law of the Heart. It maintains that alternation in left ventricular end-diastolic volume, pressure or fiber length is responsible for the alternating contractile force. Increased end-diastolic volume (increased preload) leads to increased fiber length preceding the more powerful beats. A larger end-diastolic volume results in a larger stroke volume and a higher systolic pressure than would have been produced by a smaller end-diastolic volume. For a given heart rate and aortic impedance, a larger than normal stroke volume will also elevate aortic pressure. The following systole encounters this elevated afterload and, for a given end-diastolic volume and contractility, requires longer to develop an intraventricular pressure sufficient to cause each action. This produces a decrease in stroke volume. The subsequent decreased afterload allows the next systole to quickly reach the diastolic pressure and eject a large stroke volume again.

The second or myocardial theory attributes alternation in the strength of cardiac contraction to disease or fatigue of many cardiac fibers. Primary alternation in contractility of the whole or only part of the heart occurs in the absence of changes in ventricular diastolic volume. Most of the fibers respond during the strong beat while the others are refractory. During the weak beat, which usually originates from a shorter end-diastolic fiber length, fewer fibers contract. Accordingly, variation in the basic inotropic state of the myocardium is due to a decrease in the number of contracting myocardial units every other beat. This leads to incomplete recovery or persistent refractoriness of myocardial cellular elements in the alternate diastolic intervals.

Pulsus alternans occurs when the continuous level of myocardial contractility is such that at a given heart rate, stroke volume and aortic pressure, there is inadequate time for diastole after the strong beat. Alternation in the ventricular end-diastolic volume (Starling's mechanism) and alternation in quantity of contractile fibers without end-diastolic volume or pressure change (myocardial theory) may act separately or synergistically. Alternation in cardiac cycle length and time available for ventricular filling or relaxation also influence these basic mechanisms.

Observations from various noninvasive studies appear to bear out the above physiologic mechanisms. After a strong beat there is a prolonged isovolumic relaxation. With a total diastole of constant length, the diastolic filling period shortens proportionately. At a given level of contractility, this smaller end-diastolic volume produces a decreased stroke volume of a weak beat by this Frank-Starling mechanism. The weak beat leaves an elevated end-systolic volume, longer diastolic filling period, and resultant large end-diastolic volume to produce a strong beat and continue the cycle. Echocardiography has demonstrated alternation in: (1) amplitude of systolic excursion of the left ventricle, posterior wall and interventricular septum; (2) magnitude of end-systolic left ventricular internal diameter (which is larger in diameter during the weaker beats); (3) duration of left ventricular and right ventricular ejection; (4) duration of left ventricular and right ventricular preejection periods (longer in the beats whose maximum posterior wall velocity is decidedly more depressed than in the beat following a longer diastolic filling period). Alternation of diastolic blood flow across the mitral valve has been detected using the Doppler ultrasonic flow meter catheter. Together with the echocardiographic findings, this suggests that mechanical alternans may involve diastole as well as systole. There are also data indicating the existence in some instances of discordant mechanical alternans; the occurrence of beats showing strong left ventricular systole and weak right ventricular systole alternating with beats exhibiting weak left ventricular systole and strong right ventricular systole. Mechanical alternans therefore could affect either the left or right ventricle independently. This is referred to as "discordant" alternans and occurs most often in patients with patchy involvement of the myocardium, such as is seen in ischemic heart disease.

Clinical Significance

Pulsus alternans is almost always a manifestation of myocardial damage. When found with slow heart rates, this is invariably the case, whereas with higher heart rates, in particular 120 and more, it is occasionally encountered in individuals without any other sign of cardiac disease.

Pulsus alternans is a valuable sign of left ventricular failure. In general, it has been noted in etiologies of heart failure such as systemic arterial hypertension, coronary artery disease, aortic valve disease, or cardiomyopathy. Recall that alternans may also affect the right side of the heart, although less frequently. This may occur either with isolated left heart disease or with primary right heart disease such as idiopathic pulmonary hypertension or pulmonary embolism. It has also been described in acute myocardial infarction.

Pulsus alternans is usually associated with a ventricular filling sound or gallop (S_3) at the cardiac apex. It is a particularly valuable physical finding in clinical setting where the ventricular gallop cannot be heard or felt. Pulsus alternans may also be associated with alternation of other cardiac events that depend on left ventricular contraction. For example, alternation in intensity of the heart sounds or heart murmurs, such as may occur with aortic stenosis, may be present. This is occasionally referred to as "cardiac" alternans. The murmur may be faint one cycle and loud the next. Alternation of the left ventricular contractile force is not always transmitted clearly to the peripheral pulse. Alternans of only the left ventricle is rather common in patients with severe aortic stenosis even without clinical signs of cardiac decompensation. Infrequently, cardiac alternans and pulsus alternans are associated with electrical alternans manifest in the electrocardiogram. Pulsus alternans may disappear with either improvement or worsening of congestive heart failure. If pulsus alternans is present at rest, it may be abolished by exercise if the increased venous return predominates over the effect of myocardial stress. Pulsus alternans may first become apparent during exercise if left ventricular failure is precipitated. It has been shown that this state of ventricular decompensation is reversible. Appropriate therapeutic interventions may include: (1) minimizing afterload which will reduce the pressure load on the heart while maintaining an increased cardiac output and permitting optimal coronary perfusion; (2) slowing tachycardias; (3) optimizing right atrial pressure; and (4) increasing left ventricular contractility.

In apparently normal individuals, pulsus alternans may be transiently manifest during or following paroxysmal tachycardia or following a ventricular ectopic beat. In these circumstances it does not necessarily signify left ventricular dysfunction. A dysfunctioning left ventricle, however, is more likely to exhibit pulsus alternans following a ventricular ectopic beat. Persistent pulsus alternans is associated with severe left ventricular disease and presumably occurs on the basis of the previously outlined myocardial theory. Alternation following ventricular ectopy without ventricular dysfunction appears to be due mainly to the Starling mechanism.

Selected References

1. Cohn KE, Sandler H, Hancock EW: Mechanisms of pulsus alternans. *Circulation* 46:372–380, 1967.
2. D'Cruz I, Cohen HC, Prabhu R, et al: Echocardiography in mechanical alternans with a note on the findings in discordant alternans within the left ventricle. *Circulation* 54:97–102, 1976.
3. Schlant RC, Felner JM: The arterial pulse-clinical manifestations, in Harvey WP (ed): *Current Problems in Cardiology*, vol 2, no. 5, pp 1–50, 1977.
4. Guidry OF, Glass DD: Pulsus alternans: Its therapeutic implications. *South Med J* 70:62–66, 1977.
5. Lopez-Sendon J, Coma-Canella I, Jadrague LM, et al: Pulmonary pulsus alternans in acute myocardial infarction. *Am J Cardiol* 42: 577–582, 1978.
6. Mitchell JH, Sarnoff SJ, Sonnenblick EH: The dynamics of pulsus alternans: Alternating end-diastolic fiber length as a causative factor. *J Clin Invest* 42:55–63, 1963.
7. Noble RJ, Nutter DO: The demonstration of alternating contractile state in pulsus alternans. *J Clin Invest* 49:1166–1177, 1970.
8. Parmley WW, Tomoda H, Fujimura S, et al: Relation between pulsus alternans and transient occlusion of left anterior descending coronary artery. *Cardiovasc Res* 6:709–715, 1972.
9. Spodick DH, Pierre JR: Pulsus alternans: Physiologic study by noninvasive techniques. *Am Heart J* 80:766–777, 1970.

169. Peripheral Pulses and Bruits

ROBERT B. SMITH III, MD

Definition

Assessment of pulses and detection of bruits in arteries of the peripheral vascular system.

Technique

Carotid artery (Fig 130).   The carotid pulse is palpated from the patient's side or back by pressing directly posteriorly toward the transverse processes of the cervical vertebrae along the medial border of the sternocleiodomastoid muscle. The fingertips are placed in the groove just lateral to the trachea in the lower third of the neck. It is important that the carotid pulses be palpated one side at a time, since bilateral carotid compression may produce cerebral ischemia and syncope. Care should be taken not to massage the area of the carotid bulb with the patient in the upright position, lest a hypersensitive carotid sinus reflex be evoked with resultant bradycardia and hypotension. In addition, vigorous pressure on the carotid bulb could conceivably result in atheromatous embolization of the cerebral circulation if the carotid were involved by an ulcerated, atheromatous plaque. Auscultation should be performed along the course of the carotid to detect any bruits that might be present. The location of maximum intensity of the bruit should be noted, as well as the pitch and duration of the sound. It is necessary to have the patient hold the breath during auscultation to eliminate the harsh sounds of tracheal breathing which can mask a low-pitched carotid bruit.

Brachial artery (Fig 131).   To examine the right brachial artery, the examiner supports the patient's right forearm in his right hand, with the subject's upper arm abducted, the elbow slightly flexed, and the forearm externally rotated. The examiner's left hand is then curled over the anterior aspect of the elbow to palpate along the course of the artery just medial to the biceps tendon and lateral to the medial epicondyle of the

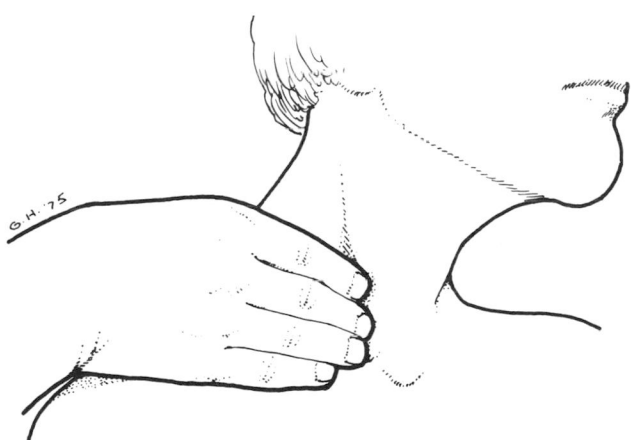

Figure 130.   Carotid artery.

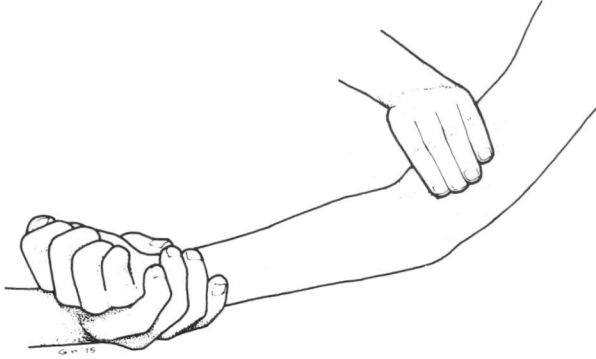

Figure 131.   Brachial artery.

humerus. The position of the hands should be switched when examining the opposite limb.

Radial artery (Fig. 132).   The patient's forearm should be supported in one of the examiner's hands and his other hand used to palpate along the radial-volar aspect of the subject's forearm at the wrist. This can best be done by curling the fingers around the distal radius from the dorsal toward the volar aspect, with the tips of the first, second, and third fingers aligned longitudinally over the course of the artery.

Abdominal aorta (Fig 133).   The abdominal aorta is an upper abdominal, retroperitoneal structure which is best palpated by applying firm pressure with the flattened fingers of both hands to indent the epigastrium toward the vertebral column. For this examination, it is essential that the sub-

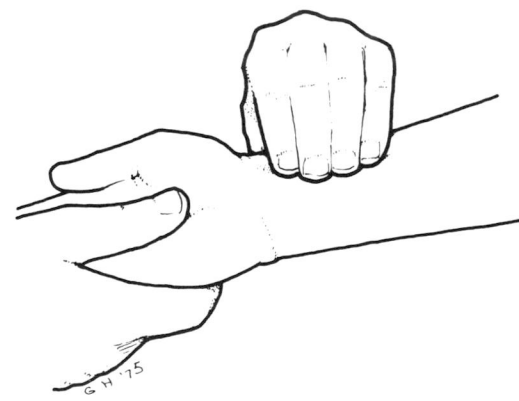

Figure 132.   Radial artery.

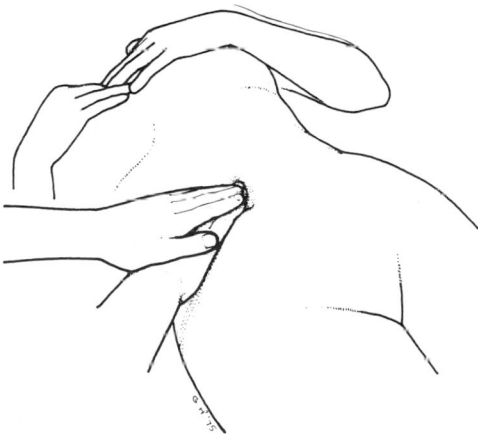

Figure 133. Abdominal aorta.

ject's abdominal muscles be completely relaxed; such relaxation can be encouraged by having the subject flex the hips and by providing a pillow to support the head. In extremely obese individuals or in those with massive abdominal musculature, it may be impossible to detect any aortic pulsation. Auscultation should be performed over the aorta and along both iliac vessels into the lower abdominal quadrants.

Femoral artery (Fig 134). The common femoral artery emerges into the upper thigh from beneath the inguinal ligament one-third of the distance

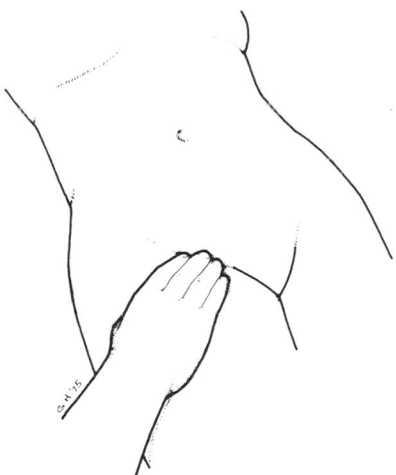

Figure 134. Femoral artery.

from the pubis to the anterior superior iliac spine. It is best palpated with the examiner standing on the ipsilateral side of the patient and the fingertips of the examining hand pressed firmly into the groin. Auscultation should be performed in this area, as well.

Popliteal artery (Fig 135).   The popliteal artery passes vertically through the deep portion of the popliteal space just lateral to the midplane. It may be difficult or impossible to palpate in obese or very muscular individuals. Generally this pulse is felt most conveniently with the patient in the supine position and the examiner's hands encircling and supporting the knee from each side. The pulse is detected by pressing deeply into the popliteal space with the supporting fingertips. Since complete relaxation of the muscles is essential to this examination, the patient should be instructed to let the leg "go limp" and to allow the examiner to provide all the support needed.

Posterior tibial artery (Fig 136).   This vessel lies just posterior to the medial malleolus. It can be felt most readily by curling the fingers of the examining hand anteriorly around the ankle, indenting the soft tissues in the space between the medial malleolus and the Achilles tendon, above the calcaneus. The thumb is applied to the opposite side of the ankle in a grasping fashion to provide stability. Again, obesity or edema may prevent successful detection of the pulse at this location.

Dorsalis pedis artery (Fig 137).   With the patient in the recumbent position and the ankle relaxed, the examiner stands at the foot of the examining table and places the fingertips transversely across the dorsum of the forefoot near the ankle. The artery usually lies near the center of the long axis of the foot, lateral to the extensor hallucis tendon, but it may be

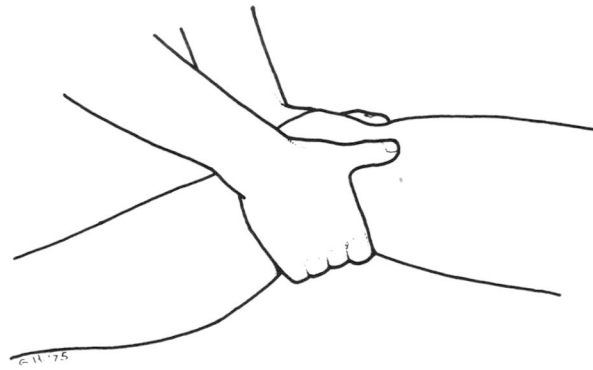

Figure 135.   Popliteal artery.

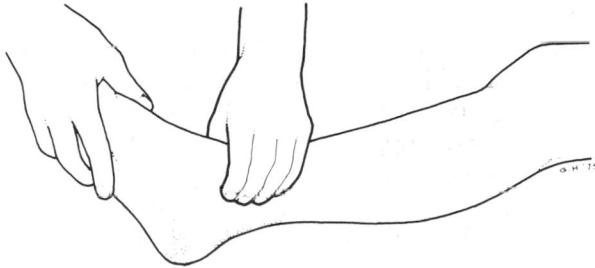

Figure 136.   Posterior tibial artery.

aberrant in location and often requires some searching. This pulse is congenitally absent in approximately 10% of individuals.

Background Information

Careful assessment and accurate recording of arterial pulsations at several standard locations is an essential part of any complete physical examination. Since examiners vary in the sensitivity of their fingertips, considerable practice may be necessary to develop the skills of locating peripheral pulses and estimating the magnitude of arterial expansion. The intensity of peripheral pulses is graded on a scale of 0 to 4+: 0 indicates no pulse palpable; 1+ means a pulse is detectable, but faint; 2+ suggests a stronger pulse, but is still somewhat diminished in intensity; 3+ is a normal pulsation; and 4+ indicates a bounding or very forceful

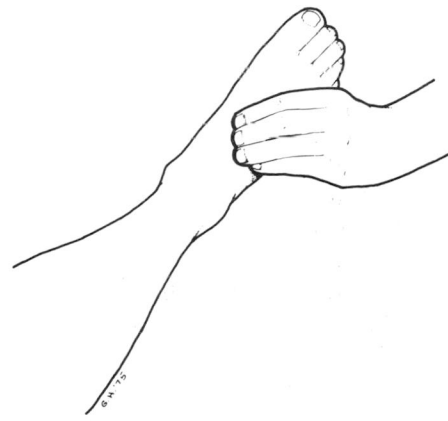

Figure 137.   Dorsalis pedis artery.

pulse. The subject should be examined in a warm environment, since extremities exposed in a cool room react with vasoconstriction and reduced peripheral pulses. If possible, the examining table or patient's bed should be so arranged that it is convenient for the examiner to stand on the patient's right side to examine the pulses on that side of the body and then to move to the left side to complete the examination.

The student examiner must be alert to the possibility that the pulse he feels may be due to digital artery pulsations in his own fingertips; this source of confusion can be eliminated by comparing the pulse in question to his own radial pulse or to the patient's cardiac sounds as determined by auscultation over the precordium. In general, it is inadvisable to use the thumb in palpating for peripheral pulses. The thumb carries a greater likelihood of confusion with the examiner's own pulse and generally has less discriminating sensation than the fingers. Frequently, inspection will be an aid to pulse location. The examiner may be able to see the skin rise and fall with each pulsation along the course of an extremity artery, particularly if a bright light is aimed tangentially across the surface of the skin.

When each artery is palpated, attention should be given to factors other than the character of the pulse wave. The examiner should note the size of the vessel in relation to expected normal for the subject's age and sex. In addition, the thickness and hardness of the vessel wall should be noted, as well as any evidence of tenderness, nodularity, or tortuosity of the vessel.

Auscultation for bruits should be performed with the diaphragm of the stethoscope placed over the carotid, brachial, and femoral arteries, as well as the abdominal aorta and its major branches. It is preferable to develop a habit of listening for bruits after examining the pulse at each location in order to avoid overlooking a significant lesion. Bruits are rushing sounds heard over large and medium-sized arteries as a result of vibration in the vessel wall caused by turbulent blood flow. The sound may originate from a local narrowing or dilation of the vessel itself, or it may be transmitted along the artery from a more proximal lesion in the vascular system. The intensity and duration of the bruit relate to the degree of vessel wall distortion. In general, bruits are not audible until an artery is approximately 50% occluded. The sound increases in pitch as the lumen becomes more narrowed to a critical size. Thereafter, the sound may no longer be detectable as the volume of blood flow becomes greatly reduced. Excessive pressure with the stethoscope may produce or intensify a bruit by indentation of the vessel wall.

Occasionally, bruits are audible over the upper abdomen in young, healthy individuals. These sounds apparently originate from tortuous vessels and are of no clinical significance; if the subject has a normal blood pressure and is free of abdominal symptoms, such findings may be disregarded.

Frequently the examiner will detect a "thrill" or palpable vibratory sensation over a vessel in which a loud bruit is audible. The thrill is indicative of marked turbulence in local blood flow and suggests significant vascular pathology. If a thrill is noted during examination of the pulses, it should be recorded in the appropriate space on the data base.

Clinical Significance

Diminished or absent pulses in the various arteries examined may be indicative of impaired blood flow due to a variety of conditions, including: (1) congenital abnormalities (coarctation of the aorta, anomalous peripheral arteries); (2) intrinsic arterial disease (atherosclerosis, thrombosis, arteritis); (3) vasospastic disorders (Raynaud's phenomenon, ergot poisoning); or (4) involvement of the vessel by extrinsic compression (thoracic outlet syndrome, trauma, neoplasms). The resultant alteration of pulses, with or without accompanying bruits, may be indicative of either acute or chronic changes in a given patient. The vascular history, together with associated physical findings such as skin color, temperature, and neuromotor status of the extremity should help to elucidate these points. More refined diagnostic techniques such as the Doppler ultrasound instrument, plasma volume analysis, and arteriography may be required to evaluate abnormalities suspected from the physical examination. In this regard, it is important to understand that significant arterial occlusive disease of the lower extremities may exist in a patient who has almost normal peripheral pulses in the resting state, since collateral circulation can produce pulsatile flow in the peripheral arterial bed in some patients. If such an individual is instructed to exercise to the point of claudication, however, pulses distal to the major vascular occlusion will diminish or disappear.

Significant widening of an artery to the examining fingers may be the best clue to an otherwise silent arterial aneurysm. The wary examiner will not be misled by tortuosity of the vessel giving a false impression of increased diameter. Careful palpation may also reveal the rock-hard vessel wall of calcified atherosclerosis, the harsh systolic thrill of a tight arterial stenosis, or the continuous thrill of a peripheral arteriovenous fistula. In the latter condition, auscultation should confirm a continuous, or machinerylike, murmur with systolic accentuation.

Much valuable information can be gained from examination of the peripheral pulses in addition to the status of the arterial system itself. The attentive examiner may detect variations in the rate, rhythmicity, intensity, and contour of the pulse wave that yield insight into a variety of disease states. The rapid, thready pulse of hypovolemic shock is a well-known clinical sign, as is the rapid, snapping pulse characteristic of thyrotoxicosis, and the collapsing, "water-hammer" pulse of aortic insufficiency. Also read the sections on Pulse Rate and Rhythm, and Carotid Pulse.

Selected References

1.   Fairbairn JF II, Juergens JL, Spittell JA Jr: *Peripheral Vascular Diseases*, ed 4. Philadelphia, WB Saunders, 1972.
2.   Linton RR: *Atlas of Vascular Surgery*. Philadelphia, WB Saunders, 1973.
3.   Edwards EA, Levine HD: Peripheral vascular murmurs: Mechanism of production and diagnostic significance. *Arch Intern Med* 90:284–300, 1952.

ABDOMEN

170. Inspection

J. RICHARD AMERSON, MD
WILLIAM J. MILLIKAN, MD

Definition

Visual observation of the abdomen in the course of a medical examination. Abnormalities encountered on inspection of the abdomen and flank areas may provide important clues to the diagnosis of abdominal wall and intraperitoneal disease processes.

Technique

Adequate inspection requires that the examiner be able to see all of the abdomen and that the patient be relaxed. Good lighting is mandatory.

The patient is positioned supine on an examining table or bed, large enough for comfort, with a small pillow or folded sheet placed beneath the knees to relax the abdominal musculature (Fig 138). Drapes should be placed high enough to allow full vision of the xiphoid process and low enough to expose the inguinal rings. The patient's arms are relaxed at the side, *not* folded above or behind the head. Instruct the patient to breathe quietly and to relax.

Observe the general contour of the entire abdomen first before inspecting specific areas. Notice whether the abdomen is flat, scaphoid, or

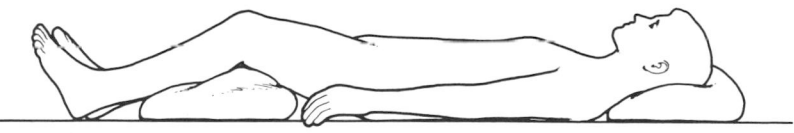

Figure 138. Position of patient for examination of the abdomen.

protuberant. If the abdomen is distended, does it appear to be secondary to obesity, fluid, or gas? Remember that adipose tissue can distend the abdominal wall not only external to the musculofascial layers, but also from within by adiposity of the omentum and viscera.

Is the usually invisible venous pattern of the abdominal wall prominent and does it appear to drain to a periumbilical caput medusae or to dilated veins on the chest wall?

Normal respiration results in abdominal wall movement toward the spine during expiration. When the patient breathes quietly, does the abdominal wall move evenly and freely, or does the patient or the disease process maintain it in a fixed position? If any area of the abdominal wall fails to move symmetrically with respiration, make a mental note to palpate that region carefully later for evidence of mass, spasm, or guarding.

If the patient is distended, can loops of bowel be seen through the abdominal wall? Can peristaltic waves be identified in the dilated loops?

Any visible protuberance or mass should be noted. If a mass is present, ask the patient when the mass was first noted and if there is any associated discomfort or tenderness. Determine if there has been any increase or decrease in the size of the mass and over what period of time the change in size has occurred.

All incision scars over the abdominal wall should be noted, and the examiner should inquire about each: What type of operation was done through this incision?

When inspecting specific areas of the abdomen, be systematic and describe findings in relation to quadrants of the abdomen areas diagrammed (Fig 139). Start with the upper quadrant, which covers the liver, gallbladder, hepatic flexure of the colon, duodenum, and right kidney. A liver that is enlarged may move downward into the abdomen on inspiration and be visible as a fullness. The markedly enlarged gallbladder frequently can be seen protruding from beneath the costal margin as a globular mass, a more distinct lump than the liver. Although pancreatic pseudocysts generally present in the epigastrium, these collections of pancreatic juice can also present in the right upper quadrant as a fullness or a discrete protrusion.

The epigastrium is the most frequent area of the abdomen where inspection will reveal an abnormal finding. In asthenic individuals, lesions of the stomach, pancreas, transverse colon, and abdominal aorta can be

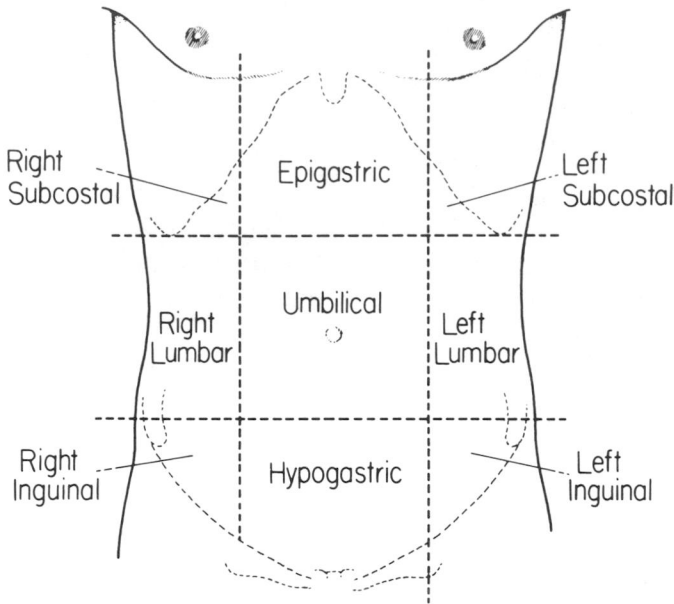

Figure 139.   Anatomical areas of the anterior abdominal wall.

seen in the epigastrium. Acute gastric dilatation will be observed as a
fullness of the epigastrium, whereas cancer of the stomach, pancreas, or
transverse colon may be seen as a definitive mass. Pancreatic pseudocysts
may mimic acute gastric dilatation, but usually can be differentiated because the epigastrium immediately below the xiphoid process is not tensely
distended. Aneurysms of the abdominal aorta may be visible as a pulsatile
midline structure lifting the abdominal wall with each heartbeat.

Splenic enlargement is difficult to differentiate from lesions of the
splenic flexure of the colon since either may present as a fullness in the
left upper quadrant during inspiration. In a similar manner, fullness in
the right lower quadrant caused by an appendiceal abscess is difficult
to distinguish on inspection from cecal carcinoma.

Lesions that can be appreciated by inspection in the left lower quadrant include cancer and inflammatory lesions of the sigmoid colon.
Ovarian cysts can ascend from the true pelvis and be observed in either
the right or left lower quadrant. Patients with acute urinary retention
and a distended urinary bladder may have an observable midline suprapubic mass that may be distinguished from ovarian lesions by pelvic
examination.

When visually examining the abdomen, have the patient cough or raise
the head and shoulders from the examining table to increase intraabdominal pressure. In this manner, bulging may be produced in a diastasis of

the rectus muscles, or through hernia sites in the inguinal, umbilical, rectus sheath (spigelian), and linea alba regions.

The normal umbilicus is inverted. Ascitic fluid or an umbilical hernia can evert the umbilicus and be seen as a protruding sac. Bluish discoloration of the umbilicus (Cullen's sign) caused by intraperitoneal blood may be the only sign of a ruptured ectopic pregnancy.

Bilateral bulging of the flanks is easily seen with large amounts of ascites, but unilateral fullness can be seen with polycystic kidney or hypernephroma. Retroperitoneal bleeding may be manifest as a bluish gray discoloration of the flanks (Gray-Turner sign).

Background Information

Before the development of diagnostic radiology, inspection and the other cardinal steps of physical examination were the only tools available for physicians to diagnose abdominal maladies. In the early decades of this century, weeks of teaching in medical schools were spent on the skills related to abdominal inspection alone. Students of physical diagnosis were allowed to go to the prepared patient and to observe only. No history could be taken and no "laying on of hands" was allowed. As diagnostic procedures have become more sophisticated (and more invasive and expensive) emphasis on the development of physical examination skills, unfortunately, has diminished. Today it is not unusual for physicians to consult one another because of an abnormal x-ray or laboratory test, rather than for elucidation of an abnormal finding on physical examination. Patients seldom complain any longer about the lack of thoroughness of the laboratory/x-ray work-up; they do complain, however, that the physician has hardly examined them.

Inspection of the abdomen is never sufficient in itself for a complete assessment of the patient, but it is an important component with the other steps of physical examination and the related history. Like the astute cardiologist who can frequently diagnose an abnormal heart problem from the patient's history and an inspection of the precordium, the surgeon with experience will often be able to anticipate what his hand will feel just from the history and visual inspection of the abdomen.

"What's within can be seen from without" is classically demonstrated in patients with end-stage liver disease. Jaundice, muscle wasting, spider angiomata, and ascites, when coupled with the history of heavy ethanol abuse, establish the diagnosis of cirrhosis. Having thus established the diagnosis with inspection, palpation, percussion, and auscultation are relegated to the level of detection of additional disease or findings not consistent with cirrhosis.

Clinical Significance

The contour of the abdomen must be related to subsequent findings on further examination including palpation and auscultation. The distended appearing abdomen may represent obesity, gaseous distension of the intestines, or ascitic fluid accumulation. Large intraabdominal masses such as ovarian cysts, intrauterine pregnancy, or retroperitoneal lesions may be the underlying problem in the patient with a distended or protuberant abdomen.

Incision scars are helpful in determining the type of past intraabdominal operative or surgical procedures. However, the presence of a right lower quadrant incision does not verify that an appendectomy has been performed unless confirmed by the patient. This is true of other abdominal incision scars usually associated with various intraabdominal operative procedures.

Dilated veins over the flank areas or around the umbilicus are usually associated with portal system hypertension.

Visible peristalsing loops of small bowel may be noted in patients with a thin abdominal wall or in patients with partial to complete bowel obstruction. Bulging in the flank areas or in the anterior abdominal area with the patient coughing or performing the Valsalva maneuver may demonstrate areas of fascial weakness and abdominal hernial defects.

Selected References

1. Bailey H: *Demonstrations of Physical Signs in Clinical Surgery*, ed 15. Baltimore, Williams and Wilkins, 1973.
2. Cope Z: *The Early Diagnosis of the Acute Abdomen*, ed 14. London, Oxford University Press, 1972.

171. Auscultation: Bowel Sounds, Bruits, and Rubs

J. RICHARD AMERSON, MD
WILLIAM J. MILLIKAN, MD

Definition

Normal bowel physiology produces sounds that are altered or rendered inaudible by disease. Inflammation of serosal surfaces can produce an audible sound (rub), just as intravascular pathology can alter arterial blood flow resulting in turbulence that can be heard with a stethoscope (bruit).

Technique

The patient is made comfortable in the supine position and instructed to breathe quietly. As the second step in examination of the abdomen following inspection, auscultation gently performed can do much to place the patient at ease and to dispel the fear that the examiner is going to inflict pain. In patients with acute abdominal pain who cannot lie supine, auscultation can be carried out in the lateral position. It is crucial that the examiner listen for a sufficient time to perform an adequate assessment of bowel sounds. In patients with hypoactive or absent bowel sounds, the examiner should listen for three full minutes and stipulate the duration, ie: "No bowel sounds heard after three minutes."

Auscultation should be performed over several areas of the abdomen with the diaphragm of the stethoscope, starting in an area away from any point of pain. Listen with the patient breathing normally and also with the patient holding his breath in midinspiration. Use a stethoscope with a head sufficiently heavy to maintain good contact with the abdominal wall as it rises and falls with respiration. The fingers of the examiner should rest lightly on the stethoscope. By gradually increasing the pressure on the diaphragm, the examiner can often "fool" the malingering patient who guards spontaneously when palpation is carried out. Suddenly releasing pressure on the diaphragm after slowly pressing down will serve to elicit rebound tenderness, if it is present, and thereby provide preliminary information for later palpation of the same area.

Auscultation for abdominal bruits is the second phase of complete auscultation of the abdomen. Bruits are systolic "swishing" sounds that may be detected over the aorta and each of the major intraabdominal arterial branches. Listen over the aorta, the celiac axis, both renal arteries, and along both iliac arteries. Like heart sounds, bruits of the abdomen can only be appreciated in a quiet environment; it may be necessary to have the subject hold his breath for a moment at each location while you listen in order to eliminate the confusion created by transmitted breath sounds.

Rubs are caused by friction between inflamed serosal surfaces usually related to the motion imparted by respiratory effort. The most common intraabdominal rub is heard over the liver in patients with hepatic abscess or tumor (see section 174).

Background Information

Familiarity with normal bowel sounds is required for the student to appreciate the subtleties produced by pathologic states affecting the bowel. Experience must be obtained by auscultating the normal abdomen in the fasting and postprandial states. Normal peristalsis produces intermittent, slowly repeating, "chuckling" sounds (borborygmi). The sound is produced by contraction and relaxation of bowel segments, peristalsis, the movement of bowel contents, and gas.

Abnormal bowel sounds or complete absence of bowel sounds characterize mechanical bowel obstruction and functional bowel obstruction (ileus). Early mechanical obstruction, without compromise of the vascular supply to the bowel, produces hyperactive, rushing bowel sounds which correspond to the increased peristaltic waves proximal to the point of mechanical obstruction. In patients with colicky pain due to intestinal obstruction, periods of hypoactive sounds may alternate with hyperactive rushes during intermittent periods of increased peristalsis. Late mechanical obstruction is signaled by infrequent, high-pitched tinkling or metallic sounds.

Paralytic ileus is a failure of peristalsis and is the normal physiologic response to laparotomy, inflammation, or other trauma. Intestinal paralysis is also seen in a wide variety of medical disorders, including pneumonia, congestive heart failure, and uremia, and usually presents no problem unless abdominal distension becomes marked. In the clinical setting, it may be impossible to differentiate ileus from mechanical obstruction by physical examination, except on the basis of auscultatory findings. The patient with ileus usually has few, if any, bowel sounds, as opposed to the patient with mechanical obstruction who may have frequent auscultatory rushes. The differential diagnosis becomes difficult when, because of increasing dilatation from mechanical obstruction, vascular compromise ensues and peristalsis ceases. Usually the mechanical obstruction that has progressed to ischemic paralysis (no bowel sounds) produces a degree of abdominal pain and tenderness not seen in paralytic ileus. Radiologic studies of the abdomen help to make this differentiation more reliable.

Systolic bruits are not uncommon in thin patients and may be heard over the epigastrium. Loud bruits are related to arterial flow through vessels with plaque formation causing varying degrees of turbulence of blood flow within the vessel. Systolic and diastolic bruits, to-and-fro sounds, or machinery-like murmurs, are abnormal and strongly suggest an arteriovenous communication.

Rubs are infrequent auscultatory findings but may be heard with respiratory motion in the upper abdomen as inflamed peritoneal surfaces glide back and forth against one another.

Clinical Significance

The presence of normal peristalsis is helpful in the assessment of other abdominal findings. Absence of peristalsis is seen not only with ileus, which can accompany a broad spectrum of medical as well as surgical disorders, but also with peritoneal irritation (chemical or bacterial peritonitis). Absent bowels sounds in the presence of abdominal tenderness require surgical consultation to rule out an active intraabdominal process, eg, ruptured viscus, appendicitis, or chemical or bacterial peritonitis. Hyperactive bowel sounds occur normally in the postprandial state and also in patients with diarrhea due to dietary indiscretion or to gastroenteritis. Acute intestinal ischemia is characterized by hyperperistalsis early, progressing quickly to a silent abdomen as ileus develops.

Abdominal bruits may be asymptomatic incidental findings, but should be conscientiously investigated in patients with elevated diastolic blood pressure (renal artery stenosis), acute or chronic abdominal pain (celiac or superior mesenteric artery insufficiency), or decreased femoral artery pulses (atherosclerotic occlusive disease). Bruits over the liver can be detected in patients with angiomas and infrequently in patients with hepatoma or cirrhosis. Continuous abdominal bruits connote arteriovenous fistulas that usually occur as a consequence of trauma or tumor but that may develop spontaneously or as a developmental anomaly.

Abdominal rubs are infrequently heard over the liver or spleen and imply abscess, tumor, or infarct.

Selected References

1.   Bailey H: *Demonstrations of Physical Signs in Clinical Surgery*, ed 15. Baltimore, Williams and Wilkins, 1973.
2.   Cope Z: *The Early Diagnosis of the Acute Abdomen*, ed 14. London, Oxford University Press, 1972.

---

172. Palpation: Pain and Tenderness; Masses

WILLIAM J. MILLIKAN, MD
J. RICHARD AMERSON, MD

Definition

Abdominal pain (the patient's complaint) and abdominal tenderness (the sign) comprise a complex that covers the entire spectrum of intraabdominal pathology plus multiple extraabdominal disorders. On physical examination, palpation is the most informative method to elucidate abdominal pain complaints. Identification and characterization of abdominal masses constitute the second major aim of abdominal palpation.

Technique

Successful palpation of the abdomen requires that the patient be as relaxed as possible and that he cooperate in the the examination insofar as possible. The subject's urinary bladder should be empty. Take the history first; talk to the patient and place him at ease, explaining that you will be careful to minimize discomfort. Position the patient supine with a pillow beneath the knees to aid in relaxation of the abdominal musculature. Inspection and auscultation, as described in sections 170 and 171, should be performed prior to palpation and may provide useful preliminary information as the examiner begins this portion of the examination. These steps are particularly helpful in patients with acute abdominal pain where deep palpation is frequently impossible.

Begin palpation in the area of the abdomen furthest removed from the location of pain described by the patient. Systematically palpate the entire abdomen with the flattened fingertips of one hand, applying very gentle pressure (Fig 140). Light pressure of this type infrequently elicits guarding and will help to place the patient at ease. Areas of superficial tenderness or prominent masses should become apparent at this time and can be delineated on the abdominal skin. Tenderness will be evident by the patient's verbal response, facial grimacing, or withdrawal efforts. Localization of parietal peritoneal irritation can be aided by having the patient cough or by the examiner shaking the subject's abdomen gently from side to side. The patient may be able to localize the site of maximal tenderness with a single finger after such motion of the abdominal viscera. Having examined the entire abdomen by quadrants with superficial pressure, repeat the examination with deeper palpation. Figure 141 depicts the two-hand technique preferred by many examiners for deep indentation of the abdominal wall. Again, save the area of pain until the last. Describe any tenderness encountered by its location in the abdomen (quadrant), the depth of palpation required to produce it (superficial or deep), and the intensity of the patient's reaction (mild to marked).

"Guarding" is voluntary muscular contraction and is a normal response to elicited pain; "spasm" is an involuntary rigidity of the abdominal wall in reaction to peritoneal irritation or neural stimulation. "Rebound tenderness" is elicited when the examiner suddenly withdraws the palpating hand from deep pressure, and the patient gives indication of sudden worsening of his discomfort. Beginning examiners may mistakenly interpret the patient's response as rebound tenderness because they either

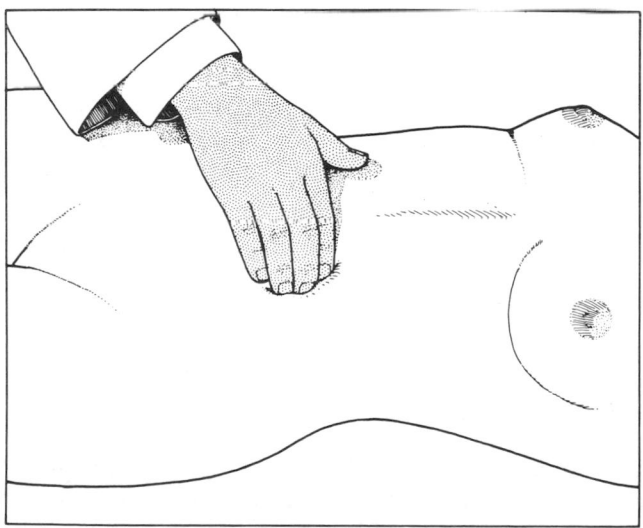

Figure 140.   One-handed superficial palpation.

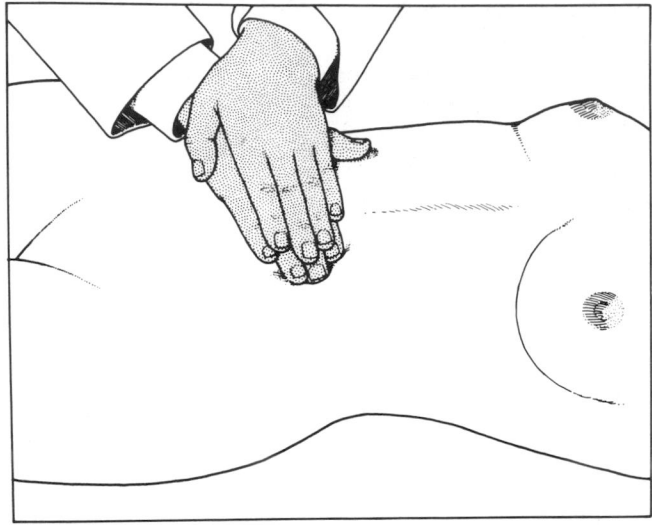

Figure 141. Two-handed deep palpation.

palpate deeper before releasing the hand or jerk the hand away suddenly and startle the patient. There is no need to raise the examining hand into the air in an exaggerated maneuver; quickly but smoothly lifting the hand an inch above the abdominal wall will suffice to test for rebound tenderness. The patient may describe accentuation of pain away from the area of direct examination, "referred tenderness," or away from the area of rebound testing, "referred rebound tenderness."

Superficial and deep palpation may lead to detection of masses at the time of systematic abdominal examination. Any mass detected should be assessed regarding its size, texture, contour, mobility, or fixation to the abdominal wall or intraperitoneal structures. Location of the mass in the various quadrants of the abdomen allows one to correlate it with organs that are located within that quadrant. The presence of bruits over the mass and whether the mass is pulsatile or transmits a pulsation should also be determined. On palpation, the presence of pain or tenderness associated with the described mass should also be evaluated.

Background Information

Abdominal pain and tenderness. Pain is the most frequent abdominal complaint and may be a manifestation of inflammation, neoplasm, or dysfunctional states of each intraabdominal or retroperitoneal organ. The distribution and pattern of pain is a function of the innervation of each organ and requires appreciation of the embryologic development of each system. Enlargement of the liver, eg, hepatitis and congestive heart failure, stretches the hepatic capsule and results in a constant dull pain that differs from the intermittent colicky pain of an inflamed gallbladder contracting against an obstructed cystic duct. Similarly, an acutely or chronically enlarged spleen (spherocytosis, portal hypertension, infectious mononucleosis) presents with a constant "dragging" discomfort, whereas a ruptured spleen (trauma) may cause no abdominal discomfort except during physical examination.

The pathophysiology of abdominal pain requires an appreciation of the dynamic aspects of the disease process, as exemplified by appendicitis. Early appendicitis frequently causes periumbilical discomfort first because the innervation of the appendix and cecum embryologically is midline (visceral pain). As the peritoneum around the inflamed appendix becomes involved, the pain migrates to the right lower quadrant (somatic pain). If rupture occurs, bacterial invasion of the peritoneum results in generalized abdominal pain and tenderness (diffuse peritonitis).

Retroperitoneal lesions can cause abdominal pain as they impinge upon the peritoneum, retroperitoneal nerves, or other pain-sensitive organs (expanding aneurysm), or as they involve these structures in an inflammatory response (perinephric abscess, pyelonephritis).

The pain caused by hepatic or splenic capsular stretching is mechanically different from that which is due to bowel dysfunction. Bowel pain is caused by: (1) distension or (2) forceful contractions against an obstruction (colic). Patients with ulcerative colitis and toxic megacolon complain of vague constant discomfort, usually over the markedly dilated segment of nonobstructed colon. This is in contrast to the patient who is obstructed by a carcinoma of the sigmoid colon and complains of an intermittent, sharp, rushing pain which corresponds to peristaltic waves. The latter patient may also have a markedly dilated cecum, which is usually painless but may be tender on examination.

The pain of pancreatitis exemplifies local inflammation, wherein the patient describes deep epigastric aching with referral to the back. Pancreatitis may also present, however, as referred pain with left subscapular or, less frequently, left subdeltoid discomfort.

Masses.   An abdominal mass may be a normal intraabdominal organ or structure, an inflammatory or neoplastic extension of an intraabdominal or retroperitoneal organ, a neoplastic growth originating outside the abdomen, or a developmental anomaly. To differentiate abnormal masses from normal intraabdominal structures may be very difficult and frequently requires careful and often repeated examinations.

Normal structures are commonly misinterpreted by the inexperienced examiner. Although the liver edge is palpable and the spleen not palpable in most patients, the lower pole of the kidney may be mistaken as a perihepatic mass or enlarged spleen in thin patients. In similar fashion, both a normal stool-filled cecum and sigmoid colon are frequently mistaken for a pathologic mass, especially in thin patients with decreased abdominal muscle tone. The normal aorta and sacral promontory are easily palpated in thin, aged patients and in young women.

Tendinous insertions of the rectus muscle can mimic an upper quadrant intraabdominal mass. A full urinary bladder may be palpated as a dome-shaped suprapubic mass and confused with other pelvic or intraabdominal structures.

Clinical Significance

Abdominal pain and tenderness.   Abdominal pain and tenderness may be the presenting complaint not only in disorders of the abdomen but also in disease processes of the cardiothoracic, musculoskeletal, and neurologic systems. The discomfort can be acute or chronic in duration.

With full appreciation that abdominal pain may be a symptom of intraperitoneal, retroperitoneal, or extraabdominal (systemic) disease, and that the historical evolution and quality of the pain may be more important in its elucidation than the properties of tenderness the examiner elicits, much can be learned by careful examination of the abdomen. Although the term "surgical abdomen" is frequently used, more frequently than not, the term connotes the summation of the surgeon's interpretation of the history and physical examination. The exception is the patient with a boardlike abdomen, who has perforated a duodenal ulcer. The abdomen is rigid, and palpation, per se, is impossible.

The remainder of abdominal signs are much more subjective. As stated above, what appears as classical "rebound" to the medical student may be dismissed as "guarding" by the more experienced examiner. Right lower lobe pneumonia can produce a classical appendicitis pain pattern that is especially difficult to elicit historically in young children and older patients. Angina pectoris occasionally presents as right upper quadrant pain, mimicking biliary colic; pericarditis can present with epigastric abdominal pain not unlike pancreatitis or peptic ulcer disease. In female patients, a very careful history and pelvic examination are required to rule out inflammatory and neoplastic processes of the ovaries, fallopian tubes, and uterus. Pyelonephritis, especially if chronic, can confuse the examiner with abdominal tenderness. Careful history and examination of the entire patient, coupled with pertinent laboratory examination, should lead to the correct extraabdominal pathology.

Disorders of each intraabdominal organ produce abdominal pain which is localized by the patient to the quadrant overlying the affected organ. Cholecystitis and cholangitis cause right upper quadrant pain and tenderness, as do acute hepatitis and active peptic ulcer disease involving the duodenum. Pancreatitis produces epigastric pain that is usually lessened by sitting up, while the pain of gastritis is unaffected by position. Active hemolysis can result in splenic pain and tenderness not dissimilar to the left upper quadrant findings seen with traumatic splenic rupture. Periumbilical pain and tenderness can be deceiving because appendicitis and right colon disorders are initially referred to this area in addition to disorders of the entire small bowel. Frequently, however, appendicitis will produce right lower quadrant tenderness before the point of maximal pain migrates. Diverticulitis and functional disorders of the sigmoid colon may cause fluctuating left lower quadrant pain that is similar to left urethral colic, and pyelonephritis. Infraumbilical and suprapubic pain may be caused by any intraabdominal organ as well as by disorders of the bladder, uterus, ovaries, and prostate.

Clinical findings of localized or generalized peritoneal irritation, or organ enlargement, lead to an assumption of intraabdominal pathology. Such an assumption should be suspect, however, until a thorough history, physical examination, and pertinent laboratory studies establish that abdominal pain is not a manifestation of systemic disease.

Masses. The examiner must become trained to think of deep anatomy in relation to the overlying areas of the abdominal wall and to consider the most common lesions first in differential diagnosis. Primary hepatic neoplasms are uncommon; metastases to the liver are common. Cysts and abscesses of the liver may also present as right upper quadrant masses. During the last decade, hepatic adenomas in young women taking oral contraceptives have been added to the differential diagnoses of right upper quadrant masses. Masses of the liver are distinguishable from an enlarged palpable gallbladder seen in patients with obstructive jaundice (Courvoisier's sign) when the edge of the liver can be identified separately, or when the mass is cystic in character. Epigastric masses generally arise from the stomach, pancreas, transverse colon, or abdominal aorta. Whereas the rock-hard, fixed carcinoma of the stomach is easily palpable in the patient who is invariably wasted from his disease, pseudocysts of the pancreas are usually firm, smooth, and not sharply defined from surrounding structures. Pseudocysts occur in the midline, but must also be considered in differential diagnosis of right upper quadrant and left upper quadrant masses because the collection can dissect retroperitoneally behind the duodenum or the splenic flexure of the colon. Neoplasms of the transverse colon can present as epigastric masses, especially if the gastrocolic ligament is involved and shortened by the process.

Splenomegaly is the most common left upper quadrant mass and must be differentiated from neoplasms of the splenic flexure and left kidney. As stated above, pseudocysts can present as left upper quadrant masses as well.

Lesions (neoplasms, inflammatory lesions) involving the sigmoid colon constitute the most common cause of an abnormal left lower quadrant mass. Sigmoid volvulus, which results from a redundant sigmoid colon twisting on its mesentery, may demonstrate signs of intestinal obstruction, with abdominal distension and a mass arising from the left lower quadrant.

Retroperitoneal pathology can produce masses in any quadrant. Although lymphoma can arise from the stomach, it more commonly presents as a diffuse, rubbery-firm supraumbilical mass originating in the retroperitoneum. Aneurysms of the abdominal aorta are generally encountered in the supraumbilical area where an expansile pulsation can be appreciated. Aneurysms of the iliac vessels arising out of the pelvis in the right or left lower quadrants sometimes can be palpated in these patients; sometimes they are best defined as a pulsatile mass on rectal examination.

Selected References

1. Bailey H: *Demonstrations of physical signs in clinical surgery,* ed 15. Baltimore, Williams and Wilkins Company, 1973.
2. Cope Z: *The Early Diagnosis of the acute abdomen,* ed 14. London, Oxford University Press, 1972.

173. Ascites

THEODORE HERSH, MD
HORACIO JINICH, MD

Definition

The presence of fluid within the peritoneal cavity.

Technique

During physical examination of the abdomen, use the techniques of inspection, palpation, and percussion to detect the presence of fluid, gas, or masses in the abdomen. This is of particular importance in the patient who has complained of abdominal "swelling." The external contour of the abdomen changes when a significant accumulation of intraabdominal fluid has occurred. In the upright patient with ascites, the fluid sinks toward the lower abdomen, while in the supine position it tends to form a fluid level with bulging in the flanks; with the patient in a lateral position, the fluid flows to the lower side. Percussion of the ascitic patient in the supine position elicits dullness in the upper borders of the flanks. The area of dullness shifts when the patient rolls to a lateral position, with the dullness found in the dependent side and tympany present on the superior side as the gas-containing loops of bowel float upward in the fluid medium. When the patient is turned to the supine position again, tympany is found in the center of the abdomen, with the flanks again having a dull percussion note, thus confirming "shifting dullness."

A second method to test for free fluid during the physical examination is the demonstration of a "fluid wave." With another examiner's hand or the patient's own hand indenting the midabdomen, tap one flank and palpate the opposite flank for arrival of a fluid wave (Fig 142). Still another physical finding indicative of ascites is the ballottement solid organs such as the liver or spleen which, when pushed downward by a thrust of the examining hand, tend to float back up and bump the hand

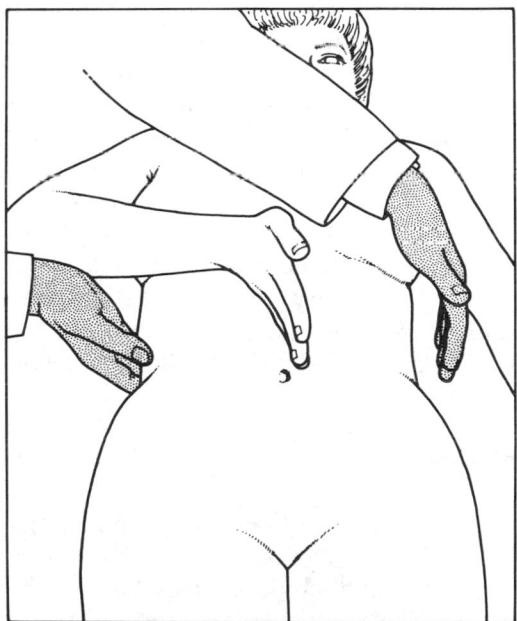

Figure 142. Testing for abdominal fluid wave. Indentation of the abdominal wall by third hand prevents transmission of the impulse via the subcutaneous adipose tissue.

as it is held in place on the abdominal wall. Progressively increasing amounts of ascites can be documented by sequential measurement of the abdominal girth and recording an increase in the circumference at the level of the umbilicus. A peritoneal tap with aspiration of fluid for examination confirms the presence of ascites and may help suggest an etiology of the fluid. Such a paracentesis is performed to analyze the peritoneal fluid for color, presence of blood or fat, specific gravity, cellular content of erythrocytes and leukocytes, chemical determination of protein, sugar, LDH (lactic dehydrogenase), cholesterol, triglycerides, and amylase, and for bacterial culture and cytologic examination as deemed necessary by the clinical data.

Background Information

Ascites occurs when there is an imbalance of factors that favors the flow of fluid from the vascular compartment over factors that maintain vascular volume or when there is exudation of fluid through infection or malignant implantation on the peritoneum. Normally, the higher pressure at the anteriolar end of the capillary allows passage of fluid without protein into the pericapillary space, while reabsorption takes place at the venous end of the capillary where the hydrostatic pressure is lower than both the osmotic pressure and extravascular tissue pressure. Ascites is most common in cirrhosis of the liver where there is portal venous hypertension and hypoalbuminemia. These factors increase the filtration pressure at the capillary level with transudation of fluid, while the low albumin levels decrease the vascular osmotic pressure. In addition to increase in portal venous pressure and decrease in colloid osmotic pressure, ascites may result from excess hepatic lymph formation with extravasation into the peritoneal cavity from renal retention of sodium and water, and from decreased permeability of splanchnic lymphatics and subperitoneal capillaries as a result of inflammatory and neoplastic processes. Bile ascites results from leakage of bile into the peritoneum, while pancreatic ascites follows rupture of a pancreatic duct or pancreatic pseudocyst.

Clinical Significance

It is important to determine the type of fluid present in the peritoneum to establish an etiology. The color and other characteristics (serous, cloudy, bloody, purulent, and chylous) can be readily appreciated following a paracentesis. The protein concentration and specific gravity of the ascites have been employed to classify the fluid as an exudate or a transudate. The former is likely when the protein concentration is over 3 gm/100 ml or when the specific gravity is above 1.016. Diseases associated with transudates include cirrhosis, Budd-Chiari syndrome, constrictive pericarditis, congestive heart failure, inferior vena caval obstruction, vasculitis, and hypoalbuminemia syndromes. Exudates are common in bacterial peritonitis, metastatic disease to the periotoneum, myxedema, and pancreatic ascites. A high content of amylase in the fluid is diagnostic of pancreatic ascites. Bloody ascites, common in carcinomatosis and tuberculous peritonitis, is also found following hemorrhagic pancreatitis, hepatic vein thrombosis, and abdominal trauma. Extravasated bile causes bile ascites following biliary tract surgery or trauma. Chylous ascites results from accumulation of lipid-rich lymph in various conditions, including lymphoma and other neoplastic diseases affecting intraabdominal, retroperitoneal, or thoracic lymph nodes. Chylous ascites may also occur with inflammatory lesions or following trauma. As a rare cause, congenital disorders of lymphatics (lymphangiectasia) may produce chylous ascites.

Selected References

1. Conn HO: The rational management of ascites, in Popper H, Schaffner F (eds): *Progress in Liver Diseases,* New York, Grune and Stratton, 1972, vol 4, pp 269–288.
2. Atkinson M, Losowsky MS: Plasma colloid oncotic pressure in relation to the formation of ascites and edema in liver disease. *Clin Sci* 22:383–390, 1962.
3. Shear L, Ching S, Gabuzda G: Compartmentalization of ascites and edema in patients with hepatic cirrhosis. *New Eng J Med* 282:1391–1396, 1970.
4. Kelley ML, Butt HR: Chylous ascites: An analysis of its etiology. *Gastroenterology* 39:161–170, 1960.
5. Sanchez RE, Mahour G, Brennan L, et al: Chylous ascites in children. *Surgery* 69:183–188, 1971.
6. Conn HO, Fessel M: Spontaneous bacterial peritonitis in cirrhosis: Variations on a theme. *Medicine* 50:161–197, 1971.

174. Liver: Auscultation

JOSEPH E. HARDISON, MD

Definition

Diseases of the liver may result in the production of auscultatory phenomena if: (1) portal vein hypertension is produced, (2) arterial blood flow is increased or partially obstructed, or (3) the liver is involved by inflammatory processes. These conditions result in the production of an abdominal venous hum, an hepatic arterial bruit, or an hepatic friction rub.

Technique

The patient is examined in the supine position.

Abdominal venous hum. The abdomen is carefully inspected for the presence of dilated superficial veins or a caput medusae (varicose veins radiating from the umbilicus). If present, these are lightly palpated for the presence of a thrill. If a thrill is present, a venous hum is present. If the thrill is absent, a venous hum may or may not be present. Finally, a hum may be present when dilated veins are not seen. The hum is listened for by using light pressure with bell or diaphragm of the stethoscope. If detected, the hum can be obliterated by increasing the pressure of the stethoscope or by compressing the veins with the free hand. The abdominal venous hum, like the cervical venous hum, is a continuous roaring or whining noise, which may be localized to the abdomen or may radiate into the chest. Unlike the cervical venous hum, the response of the abdominal venous hum to change in position, respiration, cardiac cycle, or the Valsalva maneuver is unpredictable. For instance, the Valsalva maneuver obliterates the cervical venous hum but may increase or decrease the abdominal venous hum. It is essential that the abdominal venous hum not be confused with respiratory noises and bowel sounds. The problem of respiratory noises is solved by having the patient hold his breath. Bowel sounds can be quite confusing, but usually can be distinguished by their tinkling, changing, and intermittent qualities.

Hepatic arterial bruit. The abdomen is examined by palpation and per-cussion to determine liver size, location, and configuration. The liver is then auscultated using moderately firm pressure with either the bell or the diaphragm of the stethoscope. An arterial bruit may be confined to systole or be systolic with extension into diastole or be continuous. There are many causes of abdominal arterial bruits, and it is difficult if not im-possible to be sure the bruit is coming from the liver. However, if the liver is large and the stethoscope is placed directly over it and the bruit is not heard at locations away from the liver, the odds are greatly in favor of the bruit coming from the arterial blood flow to or within the liver.

Hepatic friction rub. The patient is examined for size, location, and configuration of the liver. Light pressure of the examining hand is used to feel a thrill over the liver which is related to respiration. If felt, a fric-tion rub will be heard, but a rub more often is heard and not felt. An hepatic friction rub sounds close to the ear and is very similar to the sound produced by forcibly rubbing the thumb and forefinger together close to the ear. If the rub is being produced by movement of the liver, the rub will usually be confined to the abdomen and will not radiate into the chest. Likewise a friction rub caused by movement of the pleura will not be heard over the liver.

Background Information

Abdominal venous hum. The abdominal venous hum results from con-ditions which cause portal vein hypertension. Collateral venous channels are opened between the portal and the systemic venous channels, and the resultant flow of blood from the high pressure portal system to the lower pressure systemic system in some way results in the hum. If the patient has portal hypertension and abdominal venous hum resulting from a congenitally atrophic liver and patent umbilical vein, the condition is called the Cruveilhier-Baumgarten disease. If the portal hypertension and venous hum result from cirrhosis of the liver or other causes, the condi-tion is known as the Cruveilhier-Baumgarten syndrome. The number of reported cases in which cirrhosis is absent is very small.

Hepatic arterial bruit. Hepatic arterial bruits result from conditions which cause increased arterial flow to the liver, arteriovenous shunting in the liver, or partial obstruction to arterial flow. Primary and metastatic tumors of the liver receive their blood supply almost exclusively from the hepatic artery, and arterial flow in these conditions is increased. Alcoholic hepa-titis and cirrhosis of the liver are associated with increased arterial blood flow to the liver and intrahepatic arteriovenous shunts. Arterial bruits have been described in all of these conditions. Cancer and cirrhosis in addition to increased flow may cause bruits by partial obstruction of arterial flow by regenerating or cancerous nodules.

Hepatic friction rub. The liver because of its dual blood supply of hepatic artery and portal vein rarely develops an infarction large enough to produce a rub. Therefore, most hepatic rubs result from inflammation of the liver or contiguous structures, the commonest causes being infection and cancer, either primary or metastatic.

Clinical Significance

Abdominal venous hum. The presence of an abdominal venous hum is virtually diagnostic of portal vein hypertension which statistically is secondary to cirrhosis of the liver. If the venous hum radiates or is confined to the chest, it may be mistaken for or obscure a murmur of cardiac origin.

Hepatic arterial bruit. An hepatic bruit is indicative of alcoholic hepatitis or primary or metastatic cancer. Though reported to occur in cirrhosis of the liver, it is rare without associated alcoholic hepatitis. An abdominal venous hum and an hepatic arterial bruit in the same patient would suggest cirrhosis of the liver with alcoholic hepatitis or cancer.

Hepatic friction rub. A friction rub over the liver is indicative of cancer in the liver with inflammatory changes or infection in or adjacent to the liver. If detected in a young woman, the examiner should consider gonococcal peritonitis of the upper abdomen (Fitz-Hugh-Curtis syndrome). An hepatic rub and bruit in the same patient usually indicates cancer in the liver. An hepatic rub, bruit, and abdominal venous hum would suggest that a patient with cirrhosis had developed a hepatoma.

Auscultation of the abdomen is often neglected but can provide as much or more useful information to the examiner as can be obtained from listening to the lungs.

Selected References

1. Cheng TO, Sutton GC, Sutton DC: Cruveilhier-Baumgarten syndrome. *Am J Med* 17:143–150, 1954.
2. Clain D, Wartnaby K, Sherlock S: Abdominal arterial murmurs in liver disease. *Lancet* 2:516–519, 1966.
3. Fred HL, Brown GR: The hepatic friction rub. *New Eng J Med* 266:554–555, 1962.

175. Liver: Size and Shape

HORACIO JINICH, MD
THEODORE HERSH, MD

Definition

Evaluation of size, shape, and consistency of the liver by physical examination.

Technique

The determination of the size, shape, and consistency of the liver by physical examination can be accomplished by percussion and palpation. In the normal individual, the liver is usually not palpable below the costal margin. The size of the liver must be estimated by percussion and should be reported at three locations: anterior axillary line, midclavicular line, and midline. This can easily be determined because the liver is in close proximity to the chest wall anteriorly and laterally. Dullness of the liver begins above the inferior lung border and can be followed by percussion from above downward until the tympanitic note of bowel gas is encountered. The lower border of dullness is difficult to ascertain when the liver is small or when there is distension of the abdomen by either gas-filled loops of bowel or ascites. In evaluating the inferior level of liver dullness, the examiner should percuss from right iliac fossa upward. A tympanitic note is obtained until liver dullness occurs. The span of liver dullness from the upper to lower border is normally about 11–12 cm in the midclavicular line.

Hepatic enlargement usually occurs in a downward direction so that palpation of the lower edge is essential to establish presence of hepatomegaly. Because a well-developed right rectus muscle hinders palpation, the examiner tries to obtain relaxation of the abdominal wall by flexing the patient's knees or placing a pillow beneath the knees. The examiner's hand is placed on the right lower quadrant with the fingers pointing toward the left axilla. Everytime the patient expires, the examiner's palpating hand is moved closer to the right costal margin. Eventually the edge of the enlarged liver will be felt during inspiration, the examining hand riding over the edge of the liver as it descends. In examination of very muscular or obese individuals, the two-handed palpation technique, using the second hand to apply additional pressure, may be helpful to detect the liver edge. Since the patient may experience a twinge of pain as the liver edge is flipped, he should be reassured that the discomfort will be only momentary in duration and that it is of no untoward significance. The consistency of the organ and the degree of tenderness should be noted. The examiner can also record whether the liver edge is sharp, blunt, irregular, or nodular. The rest of the lower border of the liver can be defined by palpating from the right side to the left and making an outline with a skinned pencil. Attention is then directed to the upper surface of the liver by percussing in the right midaxillary line at about the third or fourth interspace; as noted the examiner then works downward until the resonance is supplanted by dullness to indicate the upper border. Gentle fist percussion of the liver area as shown in Fig 143 may be used to test for hepatic area tenderness. Auscultation of the liver should also be performed during this part of the examination.

Background Information

As noted, the normal liver is not palpable. The only exceptions are: (1) During infancy and perhaps until the end of the third year, the liver may extend 1–4 cm below the costal margin. (2) In thin adults, the edge

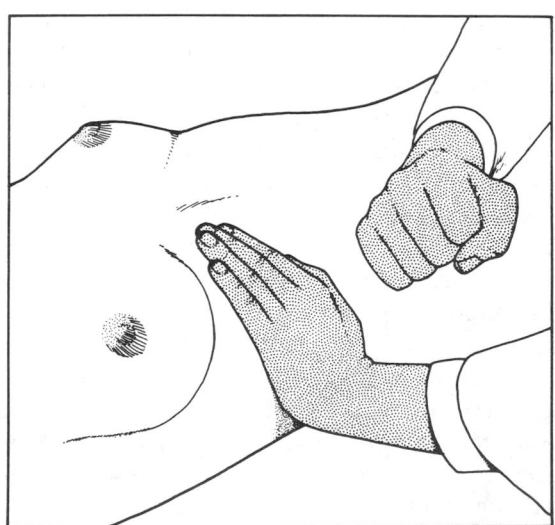

Figure 143.   Gentle fist percussion of the examiner's hand placed over the lower rib cage may elicit liver tenderness.

of the liver can be felt 1–2 cm below the costal margin during quiet breathing, and up to 5 cm during deep inspiration. (3) In patients with pulmonary emphysema, right-sided pleural effusion, or visceroptosis, the liver lies in a lower position than normal so that the edge may be palpable several centimeters below the usual level. Hepatomegaly will not be established in these cases if care is not taken to determine the upper limits of hepatic dullness through careful percussion of the upper surface of the organ. In addition, the examiner must be aware of the possibility of congenital anomalies, such as a prominent Riedel's lobe or even situs inversus, which may result in confused physical findings.

Clinical Significance

Enlargement of the liver (hepatomegaly) usually occurs downward as determined by both percussion and palpation. When necessary, verification can be obtained by a liver scan or ultrasound examination. Enlargement of the liver occurs with disorders causing congestion of the liver such as heart failure, constrictive pericarditis, and hepatic vein thrombosis. In addition, invasion of the liver by metastatic lesions, leukemic infiltration, and amyloid deposition cause significant enlargement. Alcoholic, diabetic, or obese individuals may have a large liver from fatty metamorphosis. The icteric patient with viral or alcoholic hepatitis may also show hepatomegaly. The liver edge is smooth and may be tender in all these conditions. Primary hepatic tumors, hepatomas, often complicate chronic disease of the liver, and bruits may be heard over the enlarged liver. In amebic abscess and hydatid cyst of the liver, enlargement may occur in the upper part of the organ. A small liver is present in advanced cirrhosis; in cases with fulminant hepatitis, daily percussion of the liver will often reveal an actual decrease in the size as the disease progresses. Tenderness evoked by fist percussion over the liver may indicate inflammation, intrahepatic abscess, subphrenic infection, or gallbladder disease.

Selected References

1. Peternel WW, Schaffer JW, Schiff L: Clinical evaluation of liver size and hepatic scintiscan. *Am J Dig Dis* 11:346–350, 1966.
2. Naftalin J, Leevy CM: Clinical evaluation of liver size. *Am J Dig Dis* 8:236–243, 1963.
3. Castell DO, O'Brien KD, Muench H, et al: Estimation of liver size by percussion in normal individuals. *Ann Intern Med* 70:1183–1189, 1969.

176. Spleen

JOSEPH E. HARDISON, MD

Definition

The spleen is part of the reticuloendothelial system and may be considered the body's largest "lymph node." It is a soft, freely movable organ situated posteriorly in the left upper abdomen, between the fundus of the stomach and the diaphragm. The normal spleen is rarely palpable on physical examination. In the adult it is approximately 12 cm in length, 7 cm in breadth, and 3 cm in thickness. The normal spleen is larger in whites than in blacks, averaging 93–120 gm in whites and 75–114 gm in blacks. The spleen decreases in size with old age. A wide variety of diseases may cause an enlarged and palpable spleen.

Technique

The patient is asked to lie on the bed face up with knees flexed and the soles of the feet resting on the bed. (If a patient is asked to lie down or on the back, chances are about even that the patient will lie prone rather than supine. Asking the patient to lie face up usually works.) The abdomen is examined by the clinician standing on the patient's right.

Inspection. The patient is asked to take a deep breath through the mouth, and the left upper quadrant is observed for development of fullness or the appearance of a mass.

Palpation. The examiner palpates the left upper quadrant of the abdomen just below the costal margin with the fingers of the right hand while the patient takes a deep breath. If the spleen is not felt, the examiner should palpate lower in the abdomen toward the iliac crest until satisfied he has not been feeling "on top of a greatly enlarged spleen." If the spleen is not felt by this method, the examiner can use the left hand to exert pressure upward on the patient's left flank and perform a bimanual examination using the right hand as before. The patient may further aid in the examination by placing the left fist beneath the left flank, which may push the spleen more anteriorly during inspiration, making it easier to palpate.

If the spleen is not palpated by these maneuvers, the patient may be asked to turn on the side facing the examiner. This will place the patient's right side down. The patient is asked to flex the right leg and to arrange the arms comfortably, out of the way of the examiner. Bimanual palpation is again utilized in an attempt to palpate the spleen (Fig 144).

If the examiner feels the spleen, he should record the number of centimeters the spleen descends beneath the left costal margin on full inspiration.

Percussion. The patient is asked to lie supine as before, and the examiner standing on the patient's right uses the right middle finger to percuss the left middle finger, which is applied to the patient's lowest left intercostal space in the anterior axillary line. If the spleen is normal in size, a resonant note is produced and the resonance persists with full inspiration. If the spleen is enlarged, a change in the percussion note from resonant to dull may occur during full inspiration (positive splenic

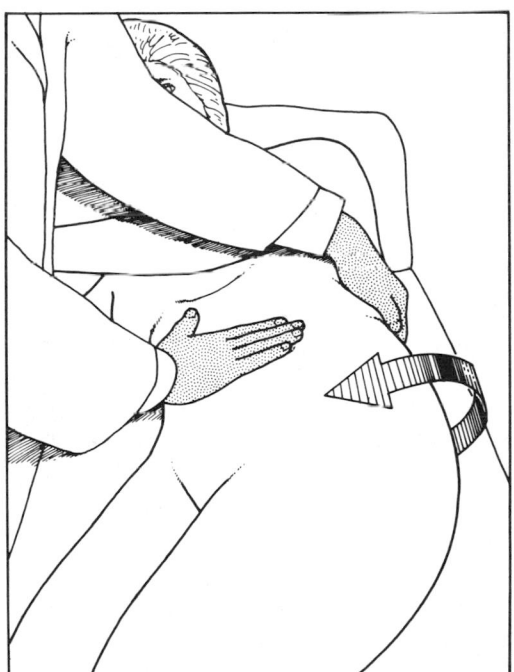

Figure 144. Bimanual palpation of the spleen with the patient turned toward the examiner.

percussion sign), and this sign may be present when the spleen cannot be felt. If the spleen is greatly enlarged, the percussion note may be dull in inspiration and and expiration.

Auscultation. With the patient supine the examiner listens over an enlarged spleen with the diaphragm or the bell of the stethoscope for the presence of a friction rub or bruit. These findings are rarely if ever present in a normal size spleen. If a friction rub is present, there may be an associated thrill. A bruit, if present, may be systolic, systolic and diastolic, or continuous.

Background Information

Like hearing the diastolic rumble of mitral stenosis or the faint murmur of aortic insufficiency, feeling the enlarged spleen that everyone else has missed can give you a great sense of satisfaction and gain for you the instant respect and envy of your peers. After all, there are spleen feelers and then there are Spleen Feelers! Detecting an enlarged spleen can be very important in many clinical situations, and persistence in mastering the techniques of palpation and percussion is very important.

It is probably not true that the spleen has to be enlarged threefold before becoming palpable. Forty percent enlargement as measured radiographically has been detected by palpation. Utilization of percussion to detect splenic enlargement was considered inaccurate until Castell correlated positive splenic percussion signs with radioisotope scans of the spleen and found this a reliable technique. I found positive splenic percussion signs in 10 patients in whom I could not palpate the spleen. The spleen scan documented splenomegaly in 9 of these patients. A false positive sign may occur with a full stomach or feces in the colon. Other masses that may be mistaken for a large spleen include a large left lobe of the liver, carcinoma of the splenic flexure of the colon and a pancreatic pseudocyst.

A palpable spleen does not always mean an underlying disease can be found. McIntyre and Ebaugh detected palpable spleens in 2.86% of 2,200 college freshmen. Thirty percent of these students continued to have palpable spleens three years later without evidence of an underlying disease.

Clinical Significance

Inspection. If the spleen is seen on inspiration, it can always be palpated.

Palpation.   The spleen is of greatest importance to the examiner when it is enlarged. It may be decreased in size as in old age, or it may be absent due to surgery or autosplenectomy as a result of multiple infarcts occurring in sickle cell anemia, but the examiner cannot detect a small or absent spleen on physical examination. If the spleen is absent, Howell-Jolly bodies will always be present on the peripheral blood smear.

The disease causing splenomegaly is rarely confined to the spleen but is usually the manifestation of a systemic process. The causes of splenomegaly are legion. When the differential diagnoses includes more than five causes, it is probably not worth trying to remember them. Broad major categories include:

1.   Myeloproliferative diseases
2.   Hodgkin's and non-Hodgkin's lymphoma
3.   Infections (bacterial, viral, or fungal)
4.   Portal hypertension of any cause
5.   Diseases associated with hemolysis
6.   Trauma (subcapsular hematoma)
7.   Diseases of unknown etiology (eg, sarcoid and amyloid)

The enlarged spleen may have secondary importance by causing sequestration or destruction of platelets or white and red blood cells (hypersplenism).

Percussion.   A positive splenic percussion sign is a reliable sign of splenic enlargement whether or not the spleen is palpable.

Auscultation.   (1) Friction rub: This is indicative of a splenic infarct which usually occurs in massively enlarged spleens in which the blood supply is inadequate. Friction rubs may also result from embolic phenomena or infection in or adjacent to the spleen. (2) Bruits: Greatly enlarged spleens may cause an increase in cardiac output by up to one-third. The increased flow to the spleen may produce enough turbulence to result in a bruit.

An enlarged spleen may be the clue that cinches the diagnosis or places everything in a different perspective. If a serious question or controversy should arise, a radioisotope scan of the spleen is a reliable indicator of spleen size as is computerized axial tomography.

Selected References

1.   McIntyre OR, Ebaugh FG: Palpable spleens in college freshmen. *Ann Intern Med* 66:301–306, 1967.
2.   Castell DO: The spleen percussion sign: A useful diagnostic technique. *Ann Intern Med* 67:1265–1267, 1967.

177. Inguinal Canal

J. RICHARD AMERSON, MD
EUGENE DAVIDSON, MD

Definition

The lower abdomen where abdominal muscular and fascial layers are attached is an area of potential weakness. Passage through the region by the vas deferens and spermatic vessels in a man and by the round ligament in a woman make the area more vulnerable to hernia protrusions. Inguinal hernias may be congenital, exiting along the spermatic cord structures as "indirect hernias," or may occur due to weakness of the transversalis fascia producing "direct hernias."

Technique

A history of pain, swelling, or presence of a mass in the groin is significant. Specific questions need to be asked: How long have you noticed the discomfort (swelling, mass, pain)? Does standing or activity such as lifting intensify or evoke the pain? Does coughing or sneezing or exertion make the lump more prominent? Will lying down relieve the symptoms or make the swelling disappear? Can you push the mass back in with your hand? Have you ever had difficulty pushing the swelling back into the abdomen? Have you ever had a hernia or operation on the other side of your groin? In children, specifically in infants, the parents' history may be the only positive feature of the examination.

Examination of the inguinal region is best performed in both men and women with the patient standing and the physician seated on a stool facing the patient. Observation of the groin in oblique light with the patient quiet and then actively coughing may reveal a bulge or abnormal motion. Scrotal masses may also be noted by inspection and palpation. Carefully observe whether any bulge observed is above (inguinal hernia) or below (femoral hernia) the inguinal ligament crease. The examiner should then stand behind and to the side of the patient with the fingers lightly applied to the groin as shown in Fig 145. The left hand is used on

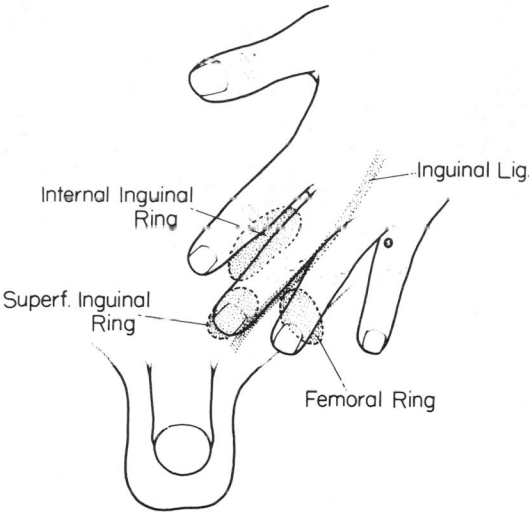

Internal Inguinal Ring

Inguinal Lig.

Superf. Inguinal Ring

Femoral Ring

Figure 145.   Placement of hand when examining for a hernia.

the patient's left side and the right hand on the right side. With the fingers placed over the femoral region, the internal inguinal ring, and the external inguinal ring (Fig 145), have the patient cough. A palpable bulge or impulse located in any one of these areas may indicate the presence of a hernia. The examiner should then return to the sitting position. In the man, the scrotum on either side can be inverted with the examining index finger entering the inguinal canal along the course of the cord structures. The size of the external ring can be ascertained by palpation just lateral to the pubic tubercle. Again, with the patient coughing, hernial bulges can be felt either against the side of the examining finger (direct hernia) or at the tip of the finger as it approaches the internal inguinal ring (indirect hernia). Large, indirect inguinal hernias may extend all the way into the scrotum giving the gross appearance of a hydrocele. Transillumination of the scrotal mass in a darkened room will aid in differentiating a hydrocele from an intrascrotal, indirect inguinal hernia.

Any mass found on inguinal examination should be gently pressed with the examining finger in an attempt to reduce the hernia and thereby cause the contents of the sac to return to the peritoneal cavity. Incarcerated hernias may be reduced more easily with the patient in the recumbent position on the examining table. Mild sedation may be necessary to provide sufficient muscle relaxation to allow for reduction. Any hernial mass that is tender to palpation or associated with symptoms of nausea and vomiting should be considered possibly strangulated (compromised vascularity of entrapped bowel), and no attempt should be made to reduce it manually. This condition represents an acute surgical emergency.

Background Information

Indirect inguinal hernias are due to a persistence of the processus vaginalis through the internal inguinal ring for a varying distance along the course of the spermatic cord or round ligament. This protrusion of peritoneum constitutes the so-called hernial sac. The hernia does not become detectable, however, until intraabdominal fat, fluid, or a viscus enters the sac. The processus vaginalis is always located anterior and medial to the structures of the spermatic cord. With time, pressure applied by the intraabdominal contents of the sac causes enlargement of the sac and dilatation of the internal inguinal ring. After prolonged enlargement, the transversalis fascia, which is the primary support of the posterior inguinal canal, becomes attenuated.

A direct inguinal hernia develops medial to the internal inguinal ring. The posterior wall weakens as the transversalis fascia thins and a bulge results. These hernias are rarely found in the scrotum. Hernias with both direct and indirect components occur. Femoral hernias, which exit from the retroperitoneal space via the femoral canal, can on occasion be confused with inguinal canal hernias.

Clinical Significance

Indirect inguinal hernias not only may cause discomfort and pain but also may lead to severe problems requiring urgent or emergency surgery to prevent or correct life-threatening complications. An incarcerated hernia represents entrapped viscera (usually small bowel or omentum) that cannot be easily reduced into the peritoneal cavity through the inguinal ring by gentle pressure on the hernia mass. Although the vascularity of the incarcerated bowel may not be compromised, the patient develops intestinal obstruction. This requires early surgical release of the entrapped bowel and repair of the hernial defect. Prolonged entrapment of bowel in the hernia sac by a tight inguinal ring leads to edema of the bowel, subsequent venous occlusion, arterial congestion, and finally gangrenous changes in the involved bowel wall and mesentery. Such strangulated hernias result not only in intestinal obstruction but also in bowel perforation, septicemia, and vascular collapse. Rapid resuscitation and surgical intervention with resection of the compromised segment of bowel are required to prevent ensuing complications that may lead to fatal outcome. The old adage, "One should never let the sun rise or set without surgery to relieve an intestinal obstruction," applies also to the patient with an incarcerated or strangulated hernia.

Selected References

1. Anson BJ, McVay CB: *Surgical Anatomy,* ed 5. Philadelphia, WB Saunders, 1971.
2. Madden JL, Nahim S, Agorogiannis AB: The anatomy and repair of inguinal hernias. *Surg Clin N Am* 51:1269–1292, 1971.
3. Condon RE, Nyhus LM: Complications of groin hernia and of hernia repair. *Surg Clin N Am* 51:1325–1336, 1971.
4. Bailey H: *Demonstrations of Physical Signs in Clinical Surgery,* ed 15. Baltimore, Williams and Wilkins, 1973.

MALE GENITALIA

178. External Male Genitalia

DAVID P. O'BRIEN III, MD

Definition

Inspection and palpation of the external genitalia including the penis, scrotum, scrotal contents, and urethra.

Technique

Inspection and palpation of the external genitalia are best performed with the patient standing disrobed in front of the seated examiner. A visual scanning of the hair distribution and general appearance of the penis and scrotum is made. Large scrotal masses, undescended testes, and the inguinal bulges of hernia are frequently apparent on inspection. If the patient is uncircumcised, the prepuce should be retracted so that the entire glans can be inspected. Palpation of the penile shaft including both corpora cavernosa and corpus spongiosum should be carried out. The urethral meatus should be visualized and spread by the examiner's thumbs. The entire pendulous urethra can be palpated without difficulty and the urethra followed through the scrotum and into the perineum. Palpation of the scrotum and its contents will reveal the presence, size, position, and shape of the testicles. The normal testicle is oval, smooth, firm, and mildly tender to palpation. The testicle is easily separated from the epididymis, which lies posteriorly and slightly medial to the testicle. The epididymis varies from individual to individual in how closely and firmly it is fixed to the testicle. Masses in the scrotum should be transilluminated in a dark room with a fiberoptic light source. An undescended testicle may be located in the inguinal or abdominal region, and palpation of these areas is imperative (see section 177, Inguinal Canal). The course of the spermatic cord can easily be followed to the internal inguinal ring by palpation. The vas deferens is felt in the scrotum by first encircling the cord with the fingers and thumb and allowing small amounts of cord tissue to pass between the thumb and second or third fingers until the thick cordlike vas is felt.

Background Information and Clinical Significance

Only experience and practice provide expertise in examining the genitalia, especially the scrotal contents of normal subjects. Even the experienced examiner, however, will use exploratory surgery for definitive diagnosis in many cases. As noted in section 68, Male Genital Lesions, many abnormalities will be apparent on inspection, eg, large scrotal masses, hypospadias, and epispadias. However, early penile carcinomas or condylomata may reside unnoticed in the coronal sulcus unless the foreskin is retracted. The inability to retract the foreskin, as in phimosis, may cause both hygienic problems and voiding symptoms. Examination of the urethral meatus may reveal stenosis or other lesions such as condylomata. In Peyronie's disease palpation of the corpora reveals the characteristic dense, fibrous plaque. Often the thickened periurethral fibrosis of urethral stricture disease can be felt in either the penile shaft or in the perineum.

Scrotal masses are the most difficult lesions to differentiate by inspection and palpation. Varicoceles usually occur on the left in postpubertal men and have a "bag of worms" feel. They should disappear or become less apparent with the patient in the recumbent position. Hydroceles of the spermatic cord or testicles are cystic and readily transilluminate light. With a hydrocele the testicle is frequently poorly felt except perhaps posteriorly. The testes may be small following mumps orchitis or in hypogonadal states. Masses located within the testes are usually tumors and require surgical evaluation. Epididymitis is the most common inflammatory disease in the scrotum and is occasionally difficult to distinguish from testicular tumors or testicular torsion. Epididymitis is favored over testicular torsion in the presence of concomitant urinary infection, prostatitis, funiculitis, inflammation of the spermatic cord, or a toxic clinical state. Acute surgical exploration is reommended when the diagnosis of testicular torsion versus epididymitis is in question. If the differentiation between testicular tumor and epididymitis is difficult, a brief trial period of appropriate antibiotic therapy (urine culture and sensitivity when possible) may be instituted. With resolution of the scrotal mass and symptoms, epididymitis is the likely source. Without resolution, surgical exploration is mandatory.

Lesions of the spermatic cord are usually either inflammatory or cystic. Spermatoceles are usually small structures that occur in the spermatic cord above the testicle. The diagnosis can be made when transillumination reveals a cystic mass and aspiration yields viable spermatozoa.

Selected References

1. Campbell MF, Harrison JH: *Urology,* ed 3. Philadelphia, WB Saunders, 1970.
2. Karafin L, Kendal AR: *Urology.* Hagerstown, Md, Harper and Row, 1973.

FEMALE GENITALIA

179. Pelvic Examination

JOHN D. THOMPSON, MD

Definition

To collect information about the following:

1. Lower abdomen and external genitalia
2. Vagina
3. Cervix, including cervical cytology
4. Uterus
5. Adnexa

Technique

After entering the examining room and assuring the patient's comfort, the physician should wash his hands. The patient should be placed on an examining table with her feet in stirrups (with the shoes left on). If a patient cannot be moved, the examination may be done in bed; however, this is usually not as satisfactory. Always instruct the patient to void before the examination is done.

The pelvic examination usually begins by inspection and gentle palpation of the lower abdomen for masses, tenderness, distension, hernias, and incisions. Note should also be made of the pubic hair and its distribution as well as the amount and distribution of facial and axillary hair.

The physician should assure the patient that the pelvic examination will be done as gently as possible. A glove should be placed on the left hand. The left hand should be used for examining the vagina since evaluation of the left side of the pelvis is easier with the left hand in the vagina. The left side of the pelvis is ordinarily more difficult to evaluate because the sigmoid colon is usually located on the left. Also, the strongest hand should be on the patient's lower abdomen, and for most people the strongest hand is the right hand.

An excellent light should be shining over the examiner's shoulder for adequate illumination of the external gentalia. With the index and middle fingers of the left hand, the external genitalia are inspected and palpated. Any lesion such as a warty growth, a mass, an ulcer, or anything else must be examined carefully. The size of the clitoris and the development of labia minora and majora should be noted. The skin between the posterior vaginal fourchette and the anus (perineal body) should be inspected. Inspection of the anus and perianal area should also be done.

The area of the Bartholin glands in the lower portion of the labia may be palpated between the thumb and index fingers of the left hand by placing the index finger just inside the vaginal introitus. Ordinarily, normal Bartholin glands cannot be felt and are not tender. Also, one does not usually see the orifice of the Bartholin gland duct.

The fingers are then inserted along the anterior vaginal wall to the base of the bladder and with firm pressure directed toward the symphysis; the fingers are then brought down against the urethra. While the urethra is being stripped from above down, the examiner should watch for the appearance of pus at the external urethral meatus. Note any tenderness or induration of paraurethral tissue or glands.

With the same two fingers, gently press downward on the posterior perineum and ask the patient to strain down and cough. This part of the examination will allow a determination of relaxation and support of the vaginal introitus, the vaginal walls, and the uterus. The presence of a urethrocele, cystocele, rectocele, enterocele, and uterine descensus or the loss of urine from the bladder through the urethra may be detected. Ordinarily, the cervix will not be visible when the patient strains down.

With two fingers in the vagina, one may also palpate the medial border of the levator muscles. These muscles are usually not tender when palpated. Some impression of the strength and competence of these muscles may be obtained by asking the patient to squeeze them tightly around the examiner's finger in the vagina. The patient may be helped to identify these muscles if she is reminded that these are the same muscles which are used to stop the flow of urine in midstream.

The bivalve speculum should now be inserted. It should be comfortably warm and moistened with water only. It should be inserted over two fingers depressing the posterior perineum along the posterior vaginal wall. The anterior vaginal wall is more sensitive. Therefore, the tip of the speculum should be directed away from the anterior vaginal wall. The bivalve speculum is then opened so that the cervix may be completely visualized. It is important to use a speculum of proper size. A thin, narrow speculum may be used for young girls and older women. Most adult parous women can be examined satisfactorily with a medium-size Graves' speculum. Only occasionally will it be necessary to use a large speculum.

A cervical cytology smear should be taken. There are several techniques for obtaining specimens for cytologic examination. It is wise to use the technique advised by the cytologist who will read the smear. Patients should be advised not to douche or have intercourse for at least two days before the cytology smear is made.

Inspect the cervix carefully. Look for erosion, eversion, cysts, polyps, lacerations, ulcerations, cervical enlargement, bleeding, and menstrual discharge. Special diagnostic procedures such as Schiller's (iodine) stain, cervical biopsy, endocervical scrape, colposcopy, and cervical and uterine sounding may be necessary. The direction in which the cervix points may give some clue to the position of the uterine corpus. For example, if the cervix points anteriorly, toward the bladder, the body of the uterus will usually be found retroverted in the cul-de-sac.

Remove the speculum slowly and completely inspect the vaginal walls. Inspect for evidence of vaginitis, vaginal discharge, foreign bodies, and other lesions.

The bimanual examination should be done next. Lubricate the fingers of the examining hand. The cervix is felt with two fingers of the left hand in the vagina. Note the location and consistency of the cervix. An especially soft cervix (? pregnancy) or an especially hard cervix (? cancer) should both be noted. Then place the right hand on the patient's lower abdomen immediately above the symphysis. The uterus is usually palpated as a pear-shaped organ in the midline and anterior. It may be lifted with the vaginal fingers for greater ease of palpation. Ordinarily it is firm, smooth, movable, and nontender. Notations should be made of any abnormality in its size, shape, symmetry, consistency, or mobility.

The adnexal region is that which surrounds the uterus and contains the fallopian tubes, ovaries, rectosigmoid, small intestine, bladder, ureters, vessels, nerves. In a thin, relaxed patient, it is usually possible to palpate normal ovaries in the adnexal region lateral and posterior to the uterus. In some patients, it may be difficult to feel normal ovaries. Examine the adnexal region for masses and tenderness. If a mass is felt, carefully note its size, location, consistency, contour, mobility, associated tenderness. Also note the presence of induration tissue in the adnexa.

Repeat the bimanual examination with the middle finger of the left hand placed in the rectum. It is extremely important that this examination be done gently. The tip of the middle finger should be well lubricated and placed against the anal orifice. Ask the patient to strain down. When she strains, only gentle pressure will be needed to insert the middle finger to its full length. With the patient straining, the anal sphincter will be more dilated and insertion of the finger will cause less discomfort.

The pelvic examination is not complete unless a bimanual examination has been done with the finger in the rectum. This part of the examination allows for a better examination of the pelvis because the rectal finger can reach beyond the posterior vaginal fornix and can therefore palpate the uterosacral ligaments, the paracervical tissue, the broad ligaments, the ovaries, the pelvic side walls. As the finger is withdrawn, the entire circumference of the rectum should be felt. Feces which are adherent to the glove covering the rectal finger should be inspected for evidence of mucus and fresh or old blood.

While the bimanual examination is being done, palpation of the bladder may also be carried out. A mass, abnormal induration, or tenderness and other findings should be noted. If there is an impression that the bimanual examination is not adequate because of constipated stool in the rectum and lower colon, the patient should be instructed to take an enema and return for another examination.

Occasionally an examination of the vagina with the patient in the knee-chest position is necessary. The vagina is naturally distended with air in this position. The vaginal walls can then be inspected better. Pelvic examination with the patient standing is not often necessary but may be done for a more complete examination of vaginal wall relaxation, uterine descensus or prolapse, and to evaluate stress incontinence.

Background Information

See Figs 146–149.

Clinical Significance

A pelvic examination must be done for the data base of a female patient to be complete. Pelvic examination does not harm the patient, and its omission can be responsible for failure to make potentially fatal diagnoses. For example, the complete gynecologic examination includes the sites from which over 50% of all malignancies develop in the female (breast, cervix, endometrium, ovary, rectum, bladder, vulva). Only in patients with vaginal bleeding in the third trimester of pregnancy should

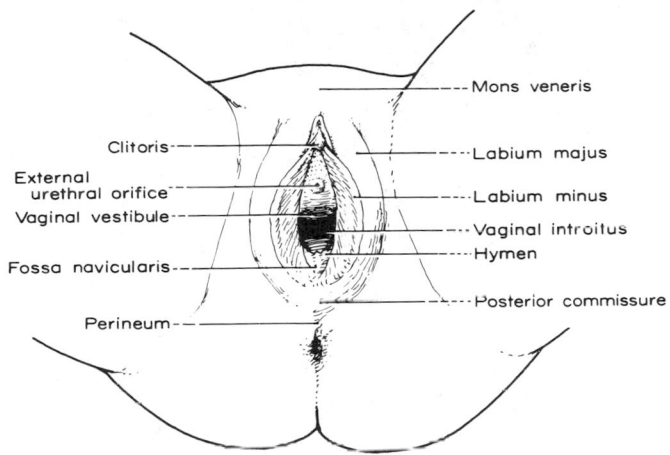

Figure 146.   External genitalia. (Modified and redrawn from F. K. Beller et al., *Gynecology*, N.Y., Springer-Verlag, 1974.) Use with permission of the publisher.

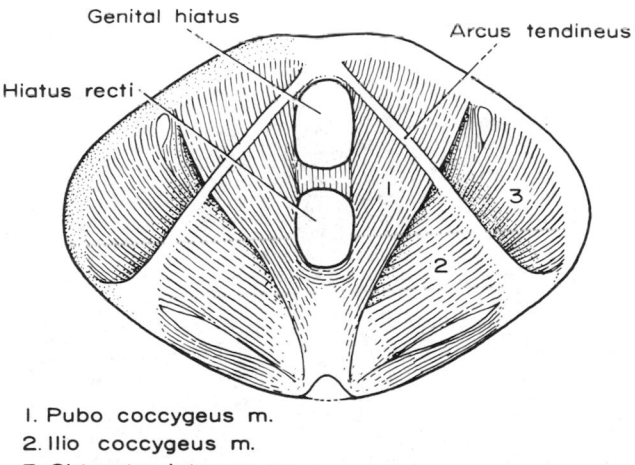

1. Pubo coccygeus m.
2. Ilio coccygeus m.
3. Obturator internus m

Figure 147.   Pelvic diaphragm.

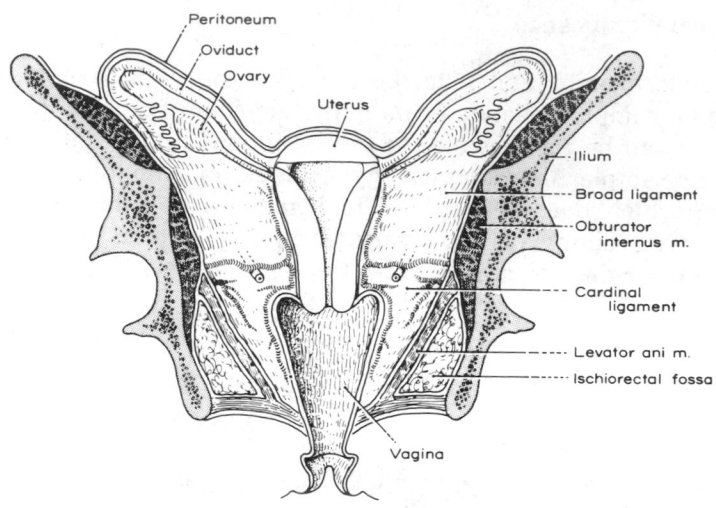

Figure 148. Frontal section of female pelvis. (Modified and redrawn from F. K. Beller et al., *Gynecology*, New York, Springer-Verlag, 1974.) Used with permission of the publisher.

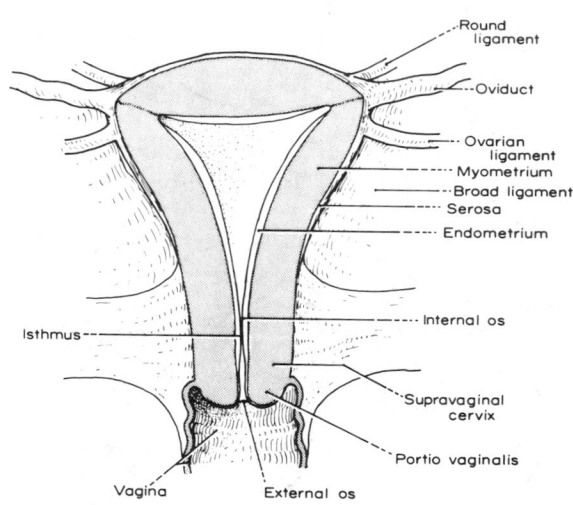

Figure 149. Frontal section of the uterus. (Modified and redrawn from F. K. Beller et al., *Gynecology*, New York, Springer-Verlag, 1974.) Used with permission of the publisher.

the pelvic examination be done in the operating room so that a Caesarean section can be performed immediately if a placenta previa is found and a hemorrhage occurs.

Gynecology patients must be made comfortable during the examination, and the examination must be conducted in a gentle manner. This is true for every patient and for every examination but is especially important for the patient having her first gynecologic examination. Some patients are embarrassed to undress and afraid of the examination. Patients must be undressed for an adequate examination, but proper draping prevents unnecessary exposure. Also remember that some patients have painful pelvic conditions.

If it is not possible to find the problem without hurting the patient, hurting her will not help. No patient enjoys a gynecologic examination. However, if the examination is properly explained and gently conducted with proper attention to the patient's comfort, adequate and accurate information can usually be obtained. Only under very unusual circumstances is it necessary to resort to pelvic examination under anesthesia.

Never omit the pelvic examination because a patient is menstruating. Menstruation is not a contraindication to the pelvic examination, nor will the patient be harmed by the examination. If a patient calls to make an appointment for her yearly gynecologic examination and Pap smear, the appointment should be given for a time when she is not menstruating, simply because the Pap smear is somewhat more accurate in the absence of menstrual blood. Do not be guilty of writing on a patient's chart, "Pelvic deferred, patient menstruating."

Selected References

1. Novak ER, Jones GS, Jones HW: *Novak's Textbook of Gynecology*, ed 9. Baltimore, Williams and Wilkins, 1975.
2. Beller FK, et al: *Gynecology: A Textbook for Students.* New York, Springer-Verlag, 1974.

180. Rectal Examination

HORACIO JINICH, MD
THEODORE HERSH, MD

Definition

Inspection and digital examination of the rectum; inspection can also be accomplished by inserting instruments of varying lengths (anoscope, proctoscope, colonoscope).

Technique

The most adequate position for a rectal examination is the left lateral decubitus. The gluteal areas should be as close as possible to the edge of the bed or examining table, the dorsum in semipronation position, the right hip and knee in forced flexion, and the left hip and knee in slight flexion. Other useful positions include the pectoral and the one which is obtained at the proctologic table. The latter is only used when planning to go on with a proctosigmoidoscopic examination following the rectal examination. However, the position which may allow the most complete rectal examination is the dorsal decubitus with the knees in flexion and, if possible, with the pelvis raised with the help of a pillow. The finger is inserted into the rectum between the legs, and with the other hand it is possible to perform a simultaneous palpation of the abdomen. On occasion it may be possible to feel masses that have been inaccessible in other examining positions.

The palpation of the perianal area should precede the digital examination of the rectum. This should never be omitted as it may reveal the presence of fistulous tracts, which are felt as strings located in the direction of the anus. The digital examination of the rectum should be done meticulously. The introduction of an adequately lubricated gloved finger should be gentle and slow, having the finger's transverse diameter parallel to the anterior posterior diameter of the anus. Once inside the rectal cavity, the inexperienced physician may make the mistake of only flexing and extending the distal phalanx, and if the physician does not feel an abnormality may conclude that the examination is negative. Pathological processes of the rectum, with the exception of foreign bodies, are necessarily related to the walls of the organ and should be palpated in a systematic manner. We recommend the following method:

First palpate the posterior wall, noticing the existence of the levator and piriformis muscles in the high postural lateral wall and also the mobility and sensitivity of the coccyx. Then palpate in the anterior aspect, the prostate in the male and the uterine cervix in the female. The prostate is an easily palpated anterior structure. Identify two smooth lateral lobes separated by a central grove. Note size, consistency, tenderness and nodules. Slide the finger along the rectal mucosa feeling for masses. If a tumor is present, note the exact location. Luminal narrowing may also be felt. Finally, instruct the patient to strain since this maneuver facilitates the palpation of tumors which descend into the rectum and become accessible to palpation. Do not confuse the cervix with an intrarectal tumor. Identify the cervix before proceeding to search for abnormalities in the rectum. A tumor might be missed if the finger moves upward after introduction into the rectum. It is therefore preferable to introduce the finger as high as possible without touching the walls of the rectum, and with a moderate flexion of the phalanx move it down slowly against the walls of the rectum. This procedure should be repeated in each of the cardinal points. It is then less likely to miss a tumor or any other lesion.

Once the examination is finished, wipe the glove onto gauze and observe the characteristics of the stool or the secretion on the examining digit. A guaiac test for occult blood should always be performed on this sample. A high percentage of carcinoma of the rectum may be uncovered by rectal palpation. When these lesions are small, they are noted as small elevations on the wall or as nodules with an indurated base. When their central portion becomes ulcerated, it is possible to feel a superficial depression of the raised borders, and the base is usually indurated. Anytime a rectal tumor is palpated, determine its proximal border and the proportion of the entire circumference of the rectum that is involved, whether it has an annular or tubular shape, whether it is ulcerated, or whether it has a cauliflower contour. Also determine whether it is fixed to the surrounding structures and its distance from the anus. Adenomatous polyps are felt as pedunculated or sessile tumors that are occasionally lobulated and are moderately firm. On the other hand, villous adenomas are soft and velvety and on occasion are jellylike; fronds can appear on the examining digit or on the proctoscope. Like other malignant tumors, they bleed easily on palpation.

Clinical Significance

The rectal examination is an extremely important part of the physical examination and should never be omitted. The inspection of the perianal area can furnish important information because fistulous openings, hemorrhoids, granulomata, dermatitis, tumors, ulcers, and protrusions can be seen and felt. Anoscopic and proctoscopic examination after the rectal examination will confirm the lesion that has been palpated. The rectal examination allows inspection of the stool and the testing for presence of occult blood. Prostatic nodules, hypertrophy, and malignancy can be discovered.

Selected References

1.   Jackman JR: The importance and technique of proctoscopy. *Dis Colon Rectum* 2:139–148, 1959.
2.   Earnest DL: Diseases of the anus, in Sleisenger MH, Fordtran JS (eds): *Gastrointestinal Disease.* Philadelphia, WB Saunders, 1973, pp 1541–1559.

181. Prostate

DAVID P. O'BRIEN III, MD

Definition

The normal adult prostate gland is almond shaped with a weight of approximately 20–25 gm. Abnormal findings on rectal examination include areas of firmness, either localized (nodules) or generalized. Bogginess and asymmetry may also be noted.

Technique

The reader should review the techniques described in section 180, Rectal Examination. The prostate gland is located anteriorly and the examiner should be able to palpate two relatively firm lobes with a distinct furrow (sulcus) between and lateral to each lobe. During the rectal examination in men, the index finger should be extended superiorly across the top of the prostate, sweeping laterally across each lobe to check for palpable nodule(s) or localized areas of softness, induration, or tenderness. The seminal vesicles may be felt as V-shaped extensions in the superolateral area.

Background Information

The normal prostate gland has five lobes: anterior, posterior, lateral (two), and middle. The middle and two lateral lobes are most prominent.

The four major conditions that affect the prostate gland are prostatic hypertrophy, nodule formation, prostatitis, and prostate cancer.

Hypertrophy of the prostate occurs primarily in the medial and lateral lobes. It involves smooth muscle, connective tissue, and glandular elements of the normal gland. It often begins in the periurethral glands where the urethra traverses the prostate. Accordingly, symptoms of lower urinary tract obstruction may occur relatively early in the clinical course of prostatic hypertrophy.

Prostatic nodules may be palpated in any portion of the prostate. True nodules must be distinguished from rectal mucosal lesions and may be due to benign prostatic hypertrophy (BPH), palpable prostatic calculi, or adenocarcinoma of the prostate. With few exceptions, it is mandatory to biopsy all prostatic nodules because the etiology of a nodule cannot be otherwise determined.

Prostatitis may be acute or chronic, bacterial or abacterial. Abacterial prostatitis is sometimes referred to as prostatosis. Acute bacterial prostatitis is accompanied by irritative urinary symptoms such as dysuria, frequency, and urgency. Fever may be significant. Prostatic examination should be limited to making the diagnosis. In this setting, prostatic massage may lead to considerable morbidity, including septicemia. Prostatitis may be evaluated by the three-glass test as described in the section on Hematuria. Urine cultures will be positive in acute bacterial prostatitis.

Chronic prostatitis may be associated with a mild urethritis causing early morning secretions in the urethra. Glass 1 of the three-glass test may be cloudy and contain mucous threads. Glass 3 (collected after prostatic massage) may contain clear evidence of pus cells not present in the previous samples. Massage should be gentle from the lateral toward the median lobe, and down the middle.

Adenocarcinoma of the prostate typically begins in the posterior lobe. The gland may be large, asymmetrical, or hard; or the cancer may be too small to palpate. Occasionally, there will be induration of a lateral lobe with obliteration of the lateral sulcus. The location of most malignancies of the prostate is such that urethral compression and symptoms of lower tract obstruction may be relatively late in the clinical course. Obstructive symptoms, however, can occur in a short time, whereas the symptoms of BPH are usually noted to be more insidious when a careful history is taken. Moreover, serum acid phosphatase usually remains within normal limits in the absence of extension or metastasis of the malignancy. Careful rectal examination of the prostate is mandatory for early detection of prostate cancer.

Clinical Significance

The clinical significance of careful examination of the prostate gland is highlighted by the observation that approximately one-third of men above age 60 will have some symptoms or findings referable to the prostate.

Prostatic carcinoma represents 10% of all noncutaneous malignancies in men, occurring in 10% of those above the age of 60. Prostatic carcinoma is found in up to 50% of autopsy specimens in men above the age of 80 who died of other causes. Sixty to seventy percent of cases show local extension or distinct metastases. Hence, early diagnosis and treatment are imperative and are best facilitated by obtaining a biopsy early in the course of suspected abnormalities of the prostate.

Selected References

1. Harrison JH, Gittes RF, Perlmutter AD, et al (eds): *Campbell's Urology*, ed 4. Philadelphia, WB Saunders, 1979, vol 2.
2. Flocks RH, Scott WW (eds): *The Urologic Clinics of North America: The Prostate.* Philadelphia, WB Saunders, 1975, vol 2, no. 1.
3. Boxer RJ: Adenocarcinoma of the prostate gland. *Urol Surv* 27:75–94, 1977.
4. Murphy GP: Prostate cancer: Progress and change. *Cancer* 28:104–115, 1978.
5. Murphy GP (ed): *Prostatic Cancer.* Littleton, MA, PSG Publishing Co, 1979.

182. Stool Guaiac

THEODORE HERSH, MD
HORACIO JINICH, MD

Definition

A test to detect occult blood in stool.

Technique

As part of the physical examination, evaluation of the rectum by digital examination includes the observation of the stool on the gloved examining finger and testing this specimen for occult blood. If there is no stool, the examiner must request that a sample of stool be brought in to the laboratory or office and see that it is properly tested. The specimen or rectal mucus can also be tested at the time of proctoscopic examination. A number of reagents are available for detection of occult gastrointestinal bleeding, but the guaiac reagent is clinically the most suitable. Various tests utilizing guaiac are available, including a saturated guaiac reagent, a dilute tincture of guaiac reagent, and the guaiac impregnated papers (Hemoccult). The most common techniques are outlined below:

Guaiac: modified filter paper method

1. Apply small particles of feces to a piece of filter paper with a wooden applicator.
2. Add 3 drops glacial acetic acid.
3. Add 3 drops 4% alcoholic solution of guaiac.
4. Add 3 drops 3% hydrogen peroxide.
5. A positive test shows appearance of blue color within 1 minute; rapidity with which color develops and its intensity is graded from trace to 4+ positive.

Hemoccult slide or tape

1. Apply a thin smear of stool specimen to the front of the slide or to the tape, both of which have been commercially impregnated with guaiac.
2. Two drops of the developing solution (hydrogen peroxide) provided are then applied to the side opposite where stool was applied.
3. The resulting color is read within 30 seconds; any trace of blue color reflects a positive reaction for occult blood.

It is preferable to test fresh samples of stool with the guaiac reaction since storing tends to yield higher numbers of false-positive reactions. Hemoccult can be employed for fresh or stored specimens (the patient can bring in or mail the Hemoccult slide), since storing does not result in false-positive reactions (see reference 4). The Hemoccult test is one-fourth as sensitive as the other tests for occult fecal blood but is virtually free from false-positive reactions, even on an unrestricted diet.

Background Information

Tests to detect occult blood in stool rely on indicators changing color by a chemical reaction between the reagent and a product in the blood. In the guaiac reaction, hemolyzed erythrocytes in the stool release hemoglobin which reacts with guaiac to yield a greenish blue color. The test depends on the oxidation of a phenolic compound, alpha-guaiaconic acid, to a quinone structure which yields the blue dye. Hemoglobin exerts a peroxidaselike activity which facilitates the oxidation of the phenolic compound with the addition of the hydrogen peroxide. Hematin of the hemoglobin molecule probably exerts the peroxidase activity since it is chemically similar in structure to peroxidase.

False-positive reactions occur when the patient ingests foods with peroxidaselike activity such as turnips, horseradish, and meat. In addition, various drugs such as aspirin, indomethacin, and phenylbutazone and oral iron preparations may cause irritation to the mucosa of the gastrointestinal tract and consequently positive stool guaiac tests.

Clinical Significance

A positive test for occult bleeding into the gastrointestinal tract must be confirmed and thus repeated on subsequent days. Particularly if iron deficiency anemia is not concurrently present, it is paramount to establish occult gastrointestinal bleeding. The repeat studies may be conducted with the patient on a meat-free diet, while drugs which may cause bleeding, such as aspirin and alcohol, should be omitted during the repeat testing period. Once occult bleeding has been ascertained, and particularly if the patient has evidence of iron deficiency anemia, a careful search for a bleeding lesion in the gastrointestinal tract is performed. Cancer of the colon is the most frequent lesion presenting as occult bleeding, and various studies screening asymptomatic subjects have uncovered cases of carcinoma of the colon. Proctoscopic examination is followed by radiologic studies of the upper and lower intestinal tract. Peroral aspiration of gastric juice is accomplished to check on the esophagus and stomach as the sites of bleeding. The gastric secretion may be similarly tested. Endoscopic studies, such as esophagogastroscopy or colonoscopy, may be clinically indicated from the history, physical examination, or radiologic studies. Care must be taken to study the cecum carefully since a neoplasm in this area often presents with occult bleeding. Radiologically, the cecum is more difficult to evaluate than the remainder of the colon.

When all studies are unrevealing and the patient continues to have positive stools, as well as decrease in hematocrit or hemoglobin levels, special diagnostic studies need be pursued in an attempt to uncover the site and source of bleeding. The fluorescein string test or an intubation study of the small intestine can be performed to localize the site of bleeding. The latter is preferable, particularly when the patient's red blood cells have been previously chromated with a radioactive marker. Concurrently, stools are tested with guaiac reagents and for radioactivity to ascertain if blood continues to ooze into the gastrointestinal tract. The aspirate taken from various levels of the intestinal tract as the tube progresses distally can be tested for occult blood and for the presence of radioactivity. At that point the progress of the tube is halted and barium can be introduced through the tube to investigate this area radiologically. The tube in place can serve as a marker for the surgeon exploring the patient for bleeding of unknown origin. Angiography may be helpful in cases of occult bleeding by demonstrating vascular lesions or tumors. Laparotomy is occasionally a last resort to the diagnostic workup of persistently positive stools for blood.

Selected References

1. Irons GV, Kirsner JB: Routine chemical tests of the stool for occult blood: An evaluation, *Am J Med Sci* 249:247–260, 1965.
2. Pittman FE: The fluorescein string test: An analysis of its use and relationship to barium studies of the upper gastrointestinal tract in 122 cases of gastrointestinal tract hemorrhage. *Ann Intern Med* 60: 418–429, 1964.

3. Siemsen JK, Hill LD, Pillow RP, et al: The diagnosis of gastrointestinal bleeding site by the use of radiochromate-tagged red cells. *Bull Mason Clin* 13:111, 1959.
4. Ostrow JD, Mulvaney CA, Hansell JR, et al: Sensitivity and reproducibility of chemical tests for fecal occult blood with an emphasis on false positive reactions. *Am J Dig Dis* 18:930–940, 1973.

MUSCULOSKELETAL

183. The Musculoskeletal Examination

COLON WILSON, MD
STEPHEN B. MILLER, MD

Definition

Table 28 lists abnormalities that may be discovered in the musculoskeletal system. If abnormalities are detected in the musculoskeletal examination, there are several questions that the examiner should keep in mind while collecting and recording the data:

1. Is the problem a local one or are many areas involved?
2. Is the problem symmetrical?
3. Is the functional abnormality due to:
    a. a defect in the forces acting on the joint?
    b. a defect in the fulcrum (joint) itself?
4. Are there systemic manifestations, eg, rash, fever.

Technique

In examining the musculoskeletal system it is important to keep the concept of function in mind. Note any gross abnormalities of mechanical function beginning with the initial introduction to the patient. Continue to observe for such problems throughout the interview and the examination.

On a screening examination of a patient who has no musculoskeletal complaints and in whom no gross abnormalities have been noted in the

Table 28.   Summary of information sought on musculoskeletal examination.

1. Skin
   a. Color change
   b. Consistency
   c. Sweating or coldness
   d. Eruptions
   e. Ulcerations
2. Heat
3. Swelling
   a. Soft tissue swelling
      (1) Synovial thickening
      (2) Periarticular swelling
      (3) Nodules
      (4) Effusion
4. Wasting (atrophy, dystrophy, spasm, contracture)
5. Tenderness to palpation and pain on motion
6. Crepitation
7. Deformity
   a. Abnormal angulation
   b. Subluxation
8. Limitation of motion
9. Stability
10. Abnormalities of trunk and spine
    a. Scoliosis
    b. Kyphosis
    c. Limitation of motion
       1. Flexion (most easily documented by measuring lengthening)
       2. Lateral flexion
       3. Rotation
11. Ambulation
    a. Ability to ambulate with or without aids
    b. Gait

interview and general physical examination, it is adequate to inspect the extremities and trunk for observable abnormalities and to ask the patient to perform a complete active range of motion with each joint or set of joints.

If the patient presents complaints in the musculoskeletal system or if an abnormality has been observed, it is important to do a thorough musculoskeletal examination, not only to delineate the extent of gross abnormalities, but to look closely for subtle abnormalities.

To perform an examination of the muscles, bones, and joints, use the classic techniques of inspection and palpation and manipulation.

1. Divide the musculoskeletal system into functional parts: With

practice the examiner will establish an order of approach, but for the beginner it is perhaps better to begin distally with the upper extremity, working proximally through the shoulder. Then beginning with the temporomandibular joint, pass on to the cervical spine, the thoracic spine, the lumbar and sacral spine, and the sacroiliac joints. Finally, in the lower extremity, again begin distally with the foot and proceed proximally through the hip.

2. Use the opposite side for comparisons: By using the opposite side for comparison, it is easier to spot subtle differences as well as identify symmetrical problems. If there is any question, use your own anatomy as a control.

3. Glean the maximum information from observation: Concentrating on one area at a time, inspect the area for discoloration (eg, ecchymoses, redness), soft tissue swelling, bony enlargement, wasting, and deformity (abnormal angulation, subluxation). While noting these changes, attempt to determine whether they are limited to the joint or whether they involve the surrounding structures (eg, tendons, muscles, bursae).

4. Observe the patient's eyes while palpating the joints and the surrounding structures: A patient's expression of pain depends on many factors. For this reason the verbalization of pain often does not correlate directly with the magnitude of the pain. The most objective indicator of the magnitude of tenderness produced by pressure on palpation is involuntary muscle movements about the eyes. Therefore, the examiner should observe the patient's eyes while palpating the joints and surrounding structures. With practice the examiner will become skilled in evaluating the magnitude of pain produced by the examination and will be able to do a skillful evaluation without producing excessive discomfort to the patient. Note areas of tenderness to pressure, and if possible identify the anatomical structures over which the tenderness is localized.

One should also note areas of enlargement while palpating the joints and surrounding structures. By noting carefully the consistency of the enlargement and its boundaries, one can decide whether this is due to bony widening, thickening of the synovial lining of the joint, soft tissue swelling of the structure surrounding the joint, an effusion into the joint capsule, or nodular formation, which might be located in a tendon sheath, subcutaneous tissue, or other structures about the joint.

While palpating the joints, note areas of increased warmth (heat). A method for doing this which will help even the most inexperienced to perceive subtle increases in heat is to choose the most heat-sensitive portion of the hand (usually the dorsum of the fingers) and, beginning proximally, lightly pass this part of your hand over all portions of the patient's extremity several times. As you proceed from proximal to distal the skin temperature gradually cools. If you find an area becoming slightly warmer, this represents increased heat.

5. Have the patient perform active movements through an entire

range of motion for each joint: Defects in function can be most rapidly perceived by having the patient perform active functions with each region of the musculoskeletal system. This reduces examination time and helps the examiner to identify areas in which there is poor function for more careful evaluation.

6. Manipulate the joint through a passive range of motion only if the patient is unable to actively perform a full range of motion, or if there is obvious pain on active motion. In passively manipulating a joint, note whether there is a reduction in the range of motion, whether there is pain on motion, and whether there is crepitus produced when the joint is moved. Note also whether the joint is stable or whether abnormal movements may be produced.

    I. Upper extremity
       A. Hands and wrists
          1. Observe and palpate both hands and wrists noting areas of color change, enlargement, and temperature change (described elsewhere). Also note deformities if present (contractures, subluxations, abnormal angulations). Look carefully for nail and cuticular abnormalities, triggering along the flexor tendon sheaths, and atrophy of thenar or hypothenar eminences. Ask the patient to make a tight fist with both hands. Ask the patient to grasp a small object such as a finger. If the patient is capable of making a tight fist and grasping a small object with no observable abnormality, then a passive manipulation of the metacarpal phalangeal joints and proximal and distal interphalangeal joints need not be made; however, should an abnormality be detected, a passive examination of range of motion of each of the joints should be performed.
             a. *Normal range of motion*
                (1) Distal interphalangeal joint (digits 2–5): 0–80° of flexion
                (2) Proximal interphalangeal joint (digits 2–5): 0–120° of flexion
                (3) Interphalangeal joint of the thumb: 35° hyperextension, 90° flexion
                (4) Metacarpal–phalangeal joints (digits 2–5): 30° hyperextension, 90° flexion
                (5) Metacarpal–phalangeal joint of the thumb: 0–70° of flexion
          2. To examine range of motion of the wrist, ask the patient to assume an attitude with the elbows flexed and the forearms parallel to the floor, and then to press

the palms of the hands and then the dorsum of the hands as closely together as possible producing an angulation at the wrist. The wrist can normally be dorsiflexed to 70° and palmar flexion should be possible to approximately 80 or 90°. Ask the patient to deviate the hand ulnarward; this should be possible to 50–60°. Finally ask the patient to deviate both hands radialward; this should be possible to approximately 20°.

B. Elbow

1. Observe and palpate both elbows and over the olecranon process, again noting areas of color change and enlargement. Be careful to observe for synovial thickening or effusion both in the joint itself and in the area of the olecranon bursa. Observe for subcutaneous nodules over the olecranon process. Ask the patient to fully extend both elbows and to fully flex them. The position of full extension is designated as 0° and flexion should be performed well to 160° in the normal state.

2. The range of motion in the radiohumeral joints is then tested by asking the patient to fully pronate and fully supinate both hands. In the normal state the palm of the hand should be able to be placed flat on a table in pronation and the dorsum of the hand flat on the table in supination.

C. Shoulder

1. The examination of the shoulder is best performed with the patient sitting or standing in such a position that the examiner can move freely about the patient's body. Range of motion of the shoulder should be examined with and without manual fixation of the shoulder.

2. The shoulder mechanism is a complicated system where several joints act in concert. The physician should be familiar with the anatomy of the shoulder and of the contiguous structures which act together. These include the glenohumeral joint, the acromioclavicular joint, the sternoclavicular joint, the gliding tissue space between the scapula and thorax, the shoulder capsule or rotator cuff, and the subacromial bursa.

3. The sternoclavicular joint, the acromioclavicular joint, the scapulae, and shoulders are inspected for enlargement, wasting, and color change. Carefully palpate

these areas, then the shoulder joints around the margin of the shoulder capsule. If swelling or tenderness is encountered, it is important to attempt to localize the responsible structure. This is most easily done by referring to an atlas on the anatomy of the shoulder.

4. Forward flexion is then checked by asking the patient to flex the shoulders fully frontward. This should be possible to 90° or parallel to the floor when the patient is standing or sitting erect. Ask the patient to rotate and to continue to flex the shoulders, placing both hands together over the head with arms parallel to and against the ears. This should be possible in the normal state to 180°. Ask the patient to abduct both shoulders which should again be possible to 90°, and to rotate and further abduct the shoulders touching both hands together over the head with the upper arms tightly pressed against the ears.

5. Ask the patient to clasp both hands behind the occiput to check for external rotation. Ask the patient to spread both elbows wide apart then to release the handclasp but maintain the flexion of the elbows and touch the elbows together in front of the head.

6. The patient is then asked to elevate both shoulders as if shrugging them. In this instance it is difficult to describe specific angles and motion, but the examiner will gain experience in detecting abnormalities.

D. Temporomandibular joint:

1. The temporomandibular joints are inspected and palpated as described previously for other joints. Continue to palpate the temporomandibular joints while asking the patient to open and close the mouth and to move the jaw from side to side.

2. Again it is very difficult to describe a specific range of motions, but experience will help in detecting abnormalities. Listen for crepitation while the motion is being performed.

II. Spine

A. Cervical spine

1. Inspect the cervical spine for loss of the normal lordotic curve. Palpate for local areas of tenderness and crepitation.

2. After inspecting and palpating the cervical spine, ask the patient to put his chin on the chest to check flexion, to put first the right ear on the right shoulder and the left ear on the left shoulder for lateral flexion, and to

extend the neck as far as possible by looking back over the ceiling as far as possible.

    3.   Rotation is then checked by asking the patient to put his chin on the right shoulder and then the left shoulder.

B.   Thoracic and lumbar spine

    1.   Examine the thoracic and lumbar spine together. Examine the back and palpate for areas of muscle spasm and tenderness. Lightly percuss over the spinous processes throughout the spine to check further for tenderness. Observe the patient both standing and sitting from behind and from the side to check for kyphosis (an abnormal forward flexed position) and scoliosis (an abnormal curvature of the spine on one side or the other). The presence of scoliosis can best be judged by determining if a list is present. If the first thoracic vertebra is not centered over the sacrum the patient is said to have a list. This can easily be measured by dropping a perpendicular from the first thoracic vertebra and measuring how far to the right or left of the gluteal fold it falls. If a list is demonstrated scoliosis must be present. Also observe whether the lumbar lordosis is present in increased amount or abnormally absent.

    2.   Check for forward flexion in the sitting position by asking the patient to place his nose on the knee, and in the standing position by asking the patient to touch the toes. Ask the patient to hyperextend the spine as much as possible to check for lateral flexion by asking the patient to pass his hand straight down the thigh, first on the right and then on the left maintaining the hips straight. Maintaining the pelvic girdle in a fixed position, ask the patient to rotate the shoulders first to the right and then to the left to check for rotation with the patient standing, check for a pelvic tilt by placing your hands on the iliac crests and observing if these are parallel. Angles of motion can be estimated from an imaginary line passing straight up through the spine, perpendicular to the floor or to the table. It is very difficult to measure these accurately or to list accurate normal measurements. The most accurate parameter of measurement is the amount of lengthening of the spine in forward flexion. The normal spine should lengthen $\geqslant 2$ inches in the thoracic area and $\geqslant 3$ inches in the lumbar area on forward flexion.

     3.   Costovertebral joint motion can be measured by plac-
ing the hands with fingers spread on the thorax and
asking the patient to inspire and expire fully. If there
is an abnormality, an accurate measurement of chest
expansion at the nipple line should be recorded as
a baseline.

C.   Straight leg raising tests

     1.   Ask the patient to lie with the spine on the table and
to relax completely. With the knee fully extended,
first one leg and then the other is slowly lifted and
flexed at the hip. This produces stretch on the sciatic
nerve.

     2.   If this maneuver produces pain in the hip or low back
with radiation in the sciatic area, the test is considered positive for nerve root irritation.

     3.   The angle of elevation of leg from the table at the
point where pain is produced should be recorded.

D.   Sacroiliac joints

     1.   The sacroiliac joints are examined by palpation and
by light fist percussion for tenderness. Other maneuvers which might produce pain in a sacroiliac joint
when inflammation is present are:

         a.   Compression of the iliac crests: This is performed
by asking the patient to lie on his side, placing
firm downward pressure on the upper iliac crest.
If pain is produced by this maneuver in a sacroiliac joint, this can aid diagnosis; but the absence
of pain does not rule out involvement of the
sacroiliac joint.

         b.   Jarring the sacroiliac joint: The patient is asked
to lie on his side, facing the examiner. The
inferior leg is flexed at the hip and knee, and the
upper leg is fully extended. Place your hand on
the upper iliac crest and produce a sharp jar on
the patient's flexed knee with the palm of your
hand. Again, pain in a sacroiliac joint is considered a positive test, but a negative test does not
rule out a possible involvement of a sacroiliac
joint.

         c.   Passive hyperextension of the lower extremity:
Ask the patient to move close to the edge of the
examining table in the supine position. With the
patient fully relaxed the examiner supports a
lower extremity and slowly allows this to passively hyperextend over the side of the examining table.

III. Lower extremity
    A. Foot and ankle
        1. The feet are inspected for abnormal coloration and localized areas of swelling. Note should be taken of skin lesions about the feet and toes. Palpate and record arterial pulsations (dorsalis pedis and posterior tibial). In addition, observe for a lowering of the longitudinal arch (pes planus, or flat foot), an abnormal elevation of the longitudinal arch (pes cavus), an abnormal angulation of the first metatarsophalangeal joint (hallux valgus), hammertoe or cockup deformities of the toes, and the formation of callus in bursae over pressure areas. Ask the patient to perform flexion and extension of the toes actively. If there appears to be an abnormality, each toe must be passively put through a range of motion. Mobility of the midtarsal joints is measured by grasping the foot with both hands and gently rotating the hands in opposite directions.

        2. Examine the ankle for discoloration and swelling and palpate for tenderness, swelling, effusion, and crepitus on range of motion.

        3. Ask the patient to dorsiflex the ankles (this should be possible to approximately 20°) and to plantar-flex the ankles (this should be possible to approximately 45°). Then ask the patient to invert (supinate) the ankle, which should be possible to 30°, and to evert (pronate) the ankle, which should be possible to 20°.

        4. Ask the patient to stand and to walk. Note attitudes of pronation or supination and toeing in and toeing out with walking.

    B. Knee
        1. The knee, the largest joint in the body, is a compound condylar joint. The specific anatomy of the knee should be reviewed. Inspect the knees for discoloration, swelling, and deformities and note whether they are laterally angulated (genu varum) or medially angulated (genu valgum). In addition, note a backward bowing of the knee (genu recurvatum) and a lack of full extension of the knee (flexion contracture). The abnormalities mentioned on inspection up to this point are best noted with the patient standing and weight-bearing.

        2. The remainder of the examination of the knees is best done with the patient supine. Look for atrophy of the

quadriceps muscles and observe the contour of the knees. In palpating a knee that appears swollen attempt to identify the structures producing the enlargement.

a. Synovial thickening, as in chronic synovitis, produces a swelling of doughy consistency: this can best be perceived as a thickening of the synovial edge as it reflects in the suprapatellar pouch. It is noted as a longitudinal ridge approximately 1.5–2 inches above the upper border of the patella.

b. Fluid or effusion in the knee is perceived in two fashions:

(1) Use the left hand to compress the reflection of the joint capsule beneath the quadriceps tendon and the fingers of the left hand cupped around the lateral margin of the joint to compress the fluid if present beneath the patella. Then use the right hand to exert downward pressure on the patella, producing a ballottement and a click as the patella strikes the femoral condyles.

(2) Small amounts of fluid can be perceived by producing pressure on the lateral surface of the joint in a stroking fashion to express fluid if present to the medial portion of the joint. Pressure is then placed on the medial portion of the joint to produce a fluid bulge as the fluid is expressed back into the lateral portion. This same maneuver can be performed by stroking the medial surface to express the fluid and producing pressure on the lateral surface to produce the bulge on the medial surface.

c. With the left hand held firmly over the patella ask the patient to slowly flex and extend the knee. In performing this maneuver note the angles of extension and flexion and whether or not crepitus is present as the joint moves. Extension should be full to 180° or 0° and flexion should be possible to 130°. If there is a limitation in this range, then these motions should be performed passively by the examiner with the patient relaxed in order to delineate the cause of the limitation.

  d. Stability of the knee should be determined by the following maneuvers:

   (1) Lateral stability is checked by asking the patient to fully extend the knee grasping the inside lower end of the femur with the left hand and the tibia just above the ankle with the right hand. Attempt to adduct the tibia on the femur in a rocking motion. In the normal state this is not possible. To test for medial stability grasp the outer lower end of the femur with the left hand and the tibia just above the ankle with the right hand. Attempt to abduct the tibia on the femur on a rocking motion. In the normal state this is not possible. The angles to which the tibia can be abducted or adducted should be estimated or accurately measured using a goniometer.

   (2) Drawer sign: Integrity of the cruciate ligaments is measured by asking the patient to flex the knee to 90°. Holding the femur in a fixed position, attempt to pull and push the tibia forward and backward on the femur. Normally one should have very little motion on this maneuver; ability to pull the tibia forward on the femur indicates a defect in the anterior cruciate; whereas the ability to push the tibia back on the femur indicates a defect in the posterior cruciate.

C. Hip

  1. The hip is a ball-and-socket joint and consequently capable of complex motions of flexion, extension, abduction, adduction, and rotation. There are a number of specialized tests performed about the hip to delineate specific abnormalities. These will not be discussed exhaustively in this section. Should an abnormality be observed in the standard routine examination, you might refer to a good orthopedic or rheumatology textbook, such as those listed in Selected References. The patient is observed in a standing position for a tilt of the pelvis, as noted above in the spinal examination. A tilt may be due to disease of the hip or to inequality in the length of the legs. The gait is observed to detect a limp which might be secondary to pain in the hips, or limitation

of motion due to structural damage to the joint itself or to the musculature and innervation about the joint.

2. Ask the patient to lie supine on the table and to actively flex first one hip and then the other with the opposite hip fully extended. Flexion with the knee straight should be possible to 90° and with the knee bent, to 120° or greater.

3. Tests for abduction of the hip are easier to perform passively. Place the left hand on the crest of the ilium and grasp the right leg with the right hand. Gradually abduct the leg as far as possible without producing motion of the pelvis. Abduction should be possible to 40° or greater. Perform the same maneuver on the left leg.

4. Rotation may be measured with both the knee and the hip flexed at 90°. The opposite leg should be fully extended. Internal rotation is measured by moving the ankle outward, which should be possible to 40°. External rotation is measured by moving the ankle inward, which should be possible to 45° or greater. Rotation of the hip may also be measured with the patient lying prone on the table and the hip fully extended. In this case the knee on the side being measured should be flexed to 90° and fully extended on the opposite side.

5. Flexion contracture of the hip is detected by flexing the opposite hip until the lumbar lordosis is flattened on the table. Ask the patient to cooperate in this examination by holding the flexed knee. The leg on the side of the hip being examined is then slowly lowered to the table. If a contracture exists, this maneuver cannot be performed completely.

6. Hyperextension of the hip can be checked by asking the patient to lie prone on the table and slowly lifting the leg being examined; this should be possible to 15° or greater.

Background Information

The musculoskeletal system is composed of muscles, bones, joints, and the other connective tissue components that join these structures. Taken as a whole, the musculoskeletal system is the mechanism by which the body performs all mechanical functions. Each joint is designed to per-

Table 29. Common problems in the musculoskeletal system.

I. Inflammatory arthritis (eg, rheumatoid arthritis, rheumatoid variants)
   1. Observation and palpation
      a. Redness (may not be present if inflammation is mild)
      b. Swelling due to synovial thickening (may be inflammatory effusion)
      c. Heat
      d. Tenderness
   2. Functional
      a. Limitation of motion due to pain
      b. Additional data if problem has been present for a long time (as in the nonspecific inflammatory arthritides such as rheumatoid arthritis)
         1. Observation and palpation (deformity due to subluxation may be present)
         2. Functional
            a. Motion may be limited
               1. Due to fibrous contractures of the periarticular soft tissues
               2. Due to joint destruction
            b. Joint may be unstable due to
               1. Destruction of cartilage and bone
               2. Rupture of tendon(s)
II. Degenerative joint disease (osteoarthritis)
   1. Observation and palpation
      a. Redness and increased warmth may be present if joint is secondarily inflamed due to trauma
      b. No palpable synovial thickening
      c. Effusion may be present
      d. Bony enlargement at joint margins
      e. Heberden's nodes on distal interphalangeal joints of fingers
      f. Tenderness frequently over tendon insertions and bursae about joints
   2. Functional
      a. Pain on motion
      b. Palpable crepitus on passive motion
      c. Instability frequently due to loss of cartilage and loosening of capsule
III. Traumatic arthritis
   1. Observation and palpation
      a. May be ecchymosis
      b. Soft tissue swelling (depending on severity of trauma may involve periarticular tissue or may be limited to effusion within joint capsule)
      c. Tenderness to pressure
   2. Functional
      a. Motion limited due to pain
      b. Instability if trauma sufficient to tear tendon(s) or joint capsule
IV. Primary muscle disease
   1. Observation and palpation
      a. Swelling of muscles may be present
      b. Tenderness to pressure over body of muscle may be present
   2. Functional
      Impairment of function due to muscle weakness; in the case of inflammatory muscle disease (polymyositis or dermatomyositis) weakness more pronounced proximally than distally

form a specific set of motions, and there is a complicated system of muscles, tendons, bursae, etc., to produce and facilitate delivery of the mechanical forces acting around the fulcrum (the joint) to effect the desired function. An abnormality in any of these structures will produce a malfunction.

Clinical Significance

Some of the most common problems in the musculoskeletal system as well as some characteristics that are helpful in arriving at a correct diagnosis are listed in Table 29.

Selected References

1. Anson BJ: *An Atlas of Human Anatomy,* ed 2. Philadelphia, WB Saunders, 1963.
2. Anson BJ, Maddock WG: *Callander's Surgical Anatomy,* ed 4. Philadelphia, WB Saunders, 1971.
3. Boyle JA, Buchanan WW: *Clinical Rheumatology.* New York, JB Lippincott, 1971.
4. Golding DN: *A Synopsis of Rheumatic Diseases,* ed 2. Chicago, Year Book Medical Publishers, 1974.
5. Goss CM (ed): *Gray's Anatomy of the Human Body,* ed 29. Philadelphia, Lea and Febiger, 1973.
6. Grant JCB, Basmajian JV: *Method of Anatomy by Regions: Descriptive and Deductive,* ed 7. Baltimore, Williams and Wilkins, 1965.
7. Hollander JL, McCarty DJ Jr (eds): *Arthritis and Allied Conditions,* ed 8. Philadelphia, Lea and Febiger, 1972.
8. Jaffe IIL: *Metabolic Degenerative and Inflammatory Diseases of Bones and Joints.* Philadelphia, Lea and Febiger, 1972.
9. Polley HF, Hunder GG: *Rheumatologic Interviewing and Physical Examination of the Joints,* ed 2. Philadelphia, WB Saunders, 1978.
10. Scott JT (ed): *Copeman's Textbook of the Rheumatic Diseases.* London and New York, Churchill Livingstone, 1978.
11. Katz WA (ed): Rheumatic Diseases: Diagnosis and Management. Philadelphia, JB Lippincott, 1977.

NEUROLOGICAL AND PSYCHIATRIC

Introduction to the Mental Status Examination

H. KENNETH WALKER, MD

The analysis of consciousness provides priceless clinical information. Each clinician needs a workable simple classification of consciousness and its disorders that can be taken to the bedside. One such classification is given in Fig 150. It is modified from suggestions made by Plum (reference 1).

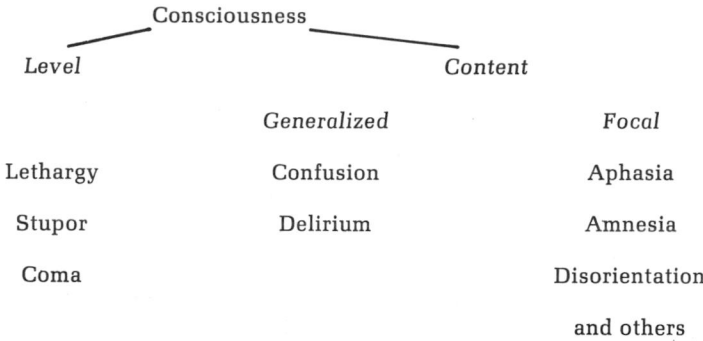

Figure 150. Organic disorders of consciousness.

The level of consciousness refers to the wakefulness or alertness of the individual and is related to brainstem structures (see Level of Consciousness). The content of consciousness refers to all other aspects of consciousness (language, creativity, judgment, reasoning). These are cortical functions. The brainstem and cortical components of consciousness are both necessary for a normal mental status.

Disorders of consciousness can be divided into those that predominantly affect the level of consciousness and those that affect the content of consciousness. This division is useful from the standpoint of analyzing

810

the disorders, but the clinician should remember that many disorders of consciousness manifest disturbances in both spheres of consciousness.

The level of consciousness is discussed in section 193. It may be divided into normal, lethargy, stupor, and coma. Conditions that commonly produce these states include mass lesions, cortical depressive drugs, and metabolic encephalopathies. They all act by interfering with the function of the reticular activating system in the brainstem.

Disorders of the content of consciousness interfere with cortical function. Examples of focal disorders include aphasia and parietal lobe problems and problems in areas such as memory, judgment, abstraction, and orientation.

The confusional-delirious states have many characteristics of both types of disorders mentioned above in that they usually have disturbances of the level of consciousness as well as a generalized disturbance of the content of consciousness. Confused patients cannot think quickly or clearly, are disoriented to varying degrees, and are bewildered. Delirium ("to rave") is characterized by vigilance, disorientation, hallucinations, delusions, noisy agitation, and at times frenzied excitement. Delirium tremens is seen in alcoholic withdrawal. Both confusional and delirious states are attended often by disturbances of the level of consciousness. There are many causes of these states: alcohol and drug withdrawal, systemic infections, and others.

Selected References

1. Plum F, Posner J: *Diagnosis of Stupor and Coma,* ed 2. Philadelphia, FA Davis, 1972.
2. Plum F: Organic disturbances of consciousness, in Critchley M, O'Leary J, Jennett B (eds): *Scientific Foundations of Neurology.* Philadelphia, FA Davis, 1972.
3. Lipowski ZJ: Delirium: Clouding of consciousness and confusion. *J Nerv Ment Dis* 145:227–255, 1967.
4. Engel G, Romano J: Delirium: A syndrome of cerebral insufficiency. *J Chron Dis* 9:260–277, 1959.

184. Appearance, Affect, and Motor Behavior

JOHN B. GRIFFIN, JR., MD

Definition

Appearance refers to those qualities of the patient that can be comprehended by external observation. Affect refers to the patient's overall emotional tone. Motor behavior refers to the patient's movements, both voluntary and involuntary.

Technique

The presence of mental illness is often associated with observable external changes in the patient. The physician can learn to make quick estimates regarding the presence of mental illness by making careful observations while taking a history and doing a physical examination. The clinician should systematically note the patient's appearance, affect, and motor behavior.

Appearance. Everyone, often quite unconsciously, forms some estimate of other people by virtue of their appearance. However, the physician who consciously takes note of appearance and behavior can often gain information quite rapidly that otherwise would take a long time to acquire. In medical and surgical specialties, clinicians often speak of acquiring a "feel" for the degree of illness in the patient. Pediatric clinicians at times will hospitalize an infant who does not have striking laboratory or physical examination signs of illness because the infant "really looks sick." More often than not, these clinical hunches based on overall appearance turn out to be correct and the infant truly has a serious malady.

When evaluating the appearance of the patient, the physician should first observe whether the patient's dress is appropriate. Many psychotic patients lose interest in their appearance as their illness progresses. They may come in with mismatched, disheveled, dirty clothing. Often as they improve in therapy, one can use improvement in their appearance as a barometer of their progress. Other patients with emotional problems may dress in a garish fashion. Female patients may wear too much makeup or clothing that is overly tight or revealing. One guideline for judging such unusual appearance is whether another person walking casually down the street would be inclined to regard the patient's appearance as unusual.

Abnormalities in vital signs observed during the physical examination can also be indicative of emotional stress. For example, tachycardia, elevated blood pressure, and increased respiratory rate are often associated with anxiety.

Sweating, vocal tremor, and overly rapid speech should be noticed by the examiner. When present, these phenomena also suggest the presence of anxiety.

Affect. The physician determines the patient's affect by careful observation of behavior in the clinical setting. The examiner should look specifically for the following emotional states:

1. Anxiety
2. Anger
3. Depression
4. Elation
5. Inappropriateness
6. Flatness
7. La belle indifférence
8. Lability

Almost everyone is familiar with many external demonstrations of a person's internal emotional state, or affect. A patient who is anxious will frequently show such mannerisms as wringing the hands, biting the nails, drumming the fingers on the chair, rhythmic movements of the legs, tremor of the voice, and other signs mentioned above under Appearance. A patient showing these signs often will comment on feeling anxious. If not, it is usually helpful to inquire whether the patient is feeling anxious.

The emotion of anger may be indicated by irritability, frowning, hostile remarks, and passive-aggressive behavior. Passive-aggressive behavior directed toward the clinician is behavior that expresses anger in indirect rather than overt ways. This may seriously compromise treatment since it can involve such things as cancelling appointments and failure to follow directions.

The clinician should also look for evidence of depression. Patients who are depressed typically appear sad. There is usually an air of hopelessness in their complaints. They show little zest for living and complain of finding little satisfaction from their daily activities. Other signs are described in section 105, Depression. At times, depression causes a general slowing of patient responses. In retarded depression there is marked decrease in movement. These patients may take several minutes to respond to questions. In agitated depression, patients may find it impossible to sit still and often pace restlessly back and forth. Crying is also an external sign of depression. If a patient begins to weep during a session, the clinician should ask what thoughts are present at that time. If the patient is unable to answer because of weeping, the clinician should sit quietly until the patient regains control. Admonitions that the patient should not cry or that things are not really as bad as the patient thinks are usually unsuccessful in helping the patient feel better. Such comments tend to cause the patient to feel that the physician does not understand how wretched the patient's situation is.

Patients who show elation are overly exuberant. They frequently talk rapidly and jump from one thought to another with little or no pause. Elation is more than simply feeling good. Patients who are elated typically have an element of denial in their elation. For example, the patient may actually be facing a serious problem such as loss of job and yet will talk as if this is of no importance. Patients who are showing elation often have difficulty seeing possible ill effects of proposed actions. Not infrequently, they will have grandiose plans which have little chance of success. Whereas the person who is highly anxious may have a quiet, short laugh often with little relationship to the content of what is being said, the person who is elated is much more likely to laugh loudly or be boisterous. The anxious patient tends to show a frequent, rather self-conscious, and almost apologetic laugh as opposed to the louder, longer laugh of the elated patient. Elation is seen in such illnesses as manic-depressive psychosis and certain types of schizophrenia.

At times the most striking thing about the affect of a patient is its lack of appropriateness. This is particularly seen in schizophrenic patients. One patient, while describing the death of her mother, punctuated the description with laughter. Often this laughter is not associated with appropriate facial changes. The patient may speak in a sad voice or show little emotion but nevertheless, experience laughter that seems to have no logical relationship to the remarks being made. In judging the appropriateness of affect, it is important to pay careful attention to whether the affect shown is congruent with the statements being uttered. Sometimes affect may be appropriate to the words being uttered but inappropriate to the circumstances. This may be seen in cases where the patient is angry with the clinician for things unrelated to the clinical situation. For example, paranoid patients may be angry with the physician because they feel the physician is about to take advantage of them; such anger is based not on the true situation but on their paranoid projections.

The affect of the patient may appear flat. Flatness of affect refers to sameness of emotional tone. At times this is also accompanied by lack of the usual emotional intonation in speech. Flatness of affect is most frequently seen in schizophrenic patients. Although the patient internally may be feeling severe emotional conflicts, the externalized evidence of that feeling tone is obscured by a quality of dullness or flatness.

Patients who have conversion reactions usually show la belle indifférence, which refers to an indifference or lack of concern about disabilities. For example, a patient who has inability to move the legs due to a conversion reaction will not show the obvious concern that would be expected from an organically caused paralysis. Although the patient with la belle indifférence may describe concern about the "paralysis" or other conversion reaction, external evidence of anxiety or depression is not evident because the "paralysis" is serving an unconscious function by providing at least a partial solution to some psychological conflict.

Lability of affect is also seen at times. This often occurs in organic brain syndromes. Lability of affect refers to very rapid shifts in mood without stimuli sufficient to explain the shift. For example, such patients may fly into a rage with little warning.

Motor behavior. In addition to the patient's general appearance and affect, it is important that the clinician observe the amount and quality of motor activity shown. The clinician should observe whether motor activity is increased, decreased, or inappropriate. Patients who are highly anxious or agitated may be unable to remain quietly in their seat. They may rock back and forth in their chair or pace around the room. At the other end of the spectrum is the extreme inactivity of the catatonic patient who sits staring ahead without movement. Catatonic patients will often show waxy flexibility (cerea flexibilitas) in which a limb can be passively moved and will stay in the position in which it is placed. The limb may remain for long periods in positions that would ordinarily be extremely tiring or even painful for the patient.

Overt signs of emotional stress such as tremors of the hands, facial tics, chain smoking, and tapping of the foot are readily detected and should be appropriately noted.

Psychiatric patients who are on high doses of certain medications such as the phenothiazines will often show a pill-rolling tremor of their fingers and thumb. This pill-rolling tremor is similar to that seen in parkinsonism. Patients on high doses of phenothiazine medications may also show a rather fixed facial expression, drowsiness, and a decrease in spontaneous movement.

Background Information

Autonomic effects associated with strong emotion have been prominently studied for many years. Cannon's work describing emotional states as preparation for either fight or flight was among the pioneering efforts that demonstrated such changes as increased respiratory rate, pulse rate, and blood pressure in the presence of strong emotion. The use of polygraph methodology in lie detection is based on the measurement of such physiologic changes in the presence of emotion. During the physical examination, the clinician has the opportunity to observe many of these physiologic changes in patients who are experiencing emotional stress.

Among lower animals, vocal communication is much less than in humans. Consequently, these animals depend heavily upon nonverbal means of conveying information. The predominance of speech in human communication has at times led to such emphasis on verbal transmission of information that relatively little attention has been paid to the nonverbal area.

Modern studies of human communication have demonstrated that nonverbal behavior is a very important supplement to spoken words. They have delineated in great detail the many nuances of nonverbal behavior. Experienced clinicians are well aware that how a patient sits or stands, the tone of voice, personal hygiene, facial expression, and other easily observable items of appearance and behavior at times give even more information about the patient's internal feeling state than the patient's actual words.

Clinical Significance

Accurate evaluation of appearance, affect, and motor behavior requires alertness and skill on the part of the clinician. These observations are very cost-effective in the sense that they require little additional time from the physician. These observations can often be made while the physician is in the process of collecting information related to other parts of the data base.

Changes in appearance often accurately reflect changes in internal emotional state. The clinician should investigate any marked changes from one visit to another in appearance, affect, or motor behavior.

Patients are not always able to describe their own emotional state. At other times they are acutely aware of what they are feeling but are hesitant to bring it up. If the physician is alert enough to comment on some of the physical and behavioral findings suggestive of emotional conflict, patients often find it much easier to discuss these difficulties. The skills needed for making these observations are relatively easy to learn. However, the physician must remember to make these observations as a routine part of a systematic approach to patients.

Selected References

1. Hill D: Nonverbal behavior in mental illness. *Br J Psychiat* 124:221–230, 1974.
2. Moldofsky H: A psychophysiological study of multiple tics. *Arch Gen Psychiat* 25:79–87, 1971.
3. Roeske, NA: Motor behavior, in Roeske NA (ed): *Examination of the Personality*. Philadelphia, Lea and Febiger, 1072, pp 53 60.
4. Morris D: Nonverbal leakage, gestures, in Morris D (ed): *Manwatching: A Field Guide to Human Behavior*. New York, Harry Abrams, 1977, pp 106–111.
5. Morris D: Gestures, in Morris D (ed): *Manwatching: A Field Guide to Human Behavior*. New York, Harry Abrams, 1977, pp 24–52.

185. General Intellectual Function

JOHN B. GRIFFIN, JR., MD

Definition

Intellectual function refers to the patient's capacity to comprehend facts and propositions, to understand relationships among data, and to reason logically from evidence.

Technique

In the process of collecting the basic medical data base, the physician can usually make a reasonable estimate of whether the patient's current intellectual functions appear compatible with educational background and past performance. However, in cases of mental illness, intellectual impairment may be so subtle that the physician will need specific data to make a determination.

Several simple procedures can obtain a quick estimate of general intellectual function. The patient can be asked to describe current events, to list the last five presidents, to name four large cities, and to give the names of the governor, mayor, and United States senators from their area. Most patients can at least name the last three presidents. Many lower socioeconomic patients do not know their senators. Similarly, patients can be asked to read a few short paragraphs and then to describe in their own words what the story was about. A good source for such brief stories is the "Life in These United States" section of *Reader's Digest*. Patients can also be asked to write a short paragraph about a subject of interest to them. This should be examined both for grammatical construction and content. Limitations in formal education will, of course, need to be taken into consideration in estimating general intellectual function. If patients comment on difficulty which they may be having when examined in this area, the examiner should inquire about the patient's opinions regarding the reason for their difficulty. Organically impaired patients are often very distressed concerning their failure to perform and state they could have done the tasks easily in the past. They often express puzzlement concerning their inability to function.

Background Information

In 1904, Alfred Binet and Theodore Simon developed a formal test instrument to measure intelligence levels among French children. There are now a wide variety of psychological test instruments that give not only accurate estimates of intellectual function but also detailed information regarding which intellectual functions are specifically impaired. The Stanford-Binet test, the Wechsler Adult Intelligence Scale, and the Peabody Picture Vocabulary Test are among the most widely used. All of these tests pose problems of increasing difficulty for the subject. The subject's score is usually compared with the average score obtained by persons of the patient's age group. The Stanford-Binet test was originally standardized with children and adolescents and is still used extensively for this age group. The children's form of the Wechsler Adult Intelligence Scale is known as the Wechsler Intelligence Scale for Children. The Wechsler intelligence scales are divided into 10 subtests that allow comparison of the patient's function for 10 different tests. Five of the tests are grouped together as the verbal portion of the test. The remaining 5 subtests are known as the performance subtests. The patient obtains a verbal IQ, a performance IQ, and a full-scale IQ. If there is a 20-point or greater difference between verbal and performance IQ scores, this is generally regarded as significant and warrants further investigation for cause. Both emotional and organic neurological difficulty disorder can result in such discrepancy in scores. The Peabody Picture Vocabulary Test is useful in testing patients with limited formal education, since it involves identifying a series of pictures and does not require that the patient be able to read.

Piaget has extensively studied the stages through which children pass in the development of intelligence. Other authors have carefully studied changes in intelligence with advanced age. There is some tendency toward decreased intelligence scores with advanced age, but there is great variability in this.

Clinical Significance

Both organic difficulty and emotional stress can influence performance in this area. Patients with impairment of intellectual function resulting from organic difficulties usually show evidence of organic impairment in other sections of the mental status examination such as memory orientation and attention span. Patients whose decrease in intellectual function is the result of emotional difficulties usually show additional evidence of anxiety, such as tremor of the voice and hands. Such patients often comment that they are anxious while they are performing the tests of intellectual function requested by the examiner. Patients with severe emotional illness such as psychosis frequently become so preoccupied with their problems that they no longer listen to television or read newspapers. They will often explain their difficulty in describing current events by saying that they have been too upset to pay attention to things beyond their immediate difficulties. The procedures outlined above under Technique are rough screening devices. When marked intellectual impairment exists, the patient should usually be referred for detailed psychological testing such as that described under Background Information.

Selected References

1. Piaget J: *The Psychology of Intelligence.* Totowa, NJ, Littlefield, Adams, 1966, pp 3–17, 53–86.
2. Roeske NA: Intellectual function, in Roeske NA (ed): *Examination of the Personality.* Philadelphia, Lea and Febiger, 1972, pp 77–82.
3. Wechsler D: *The Range of Human Capabilities.* Baltimore, Williams and Wilkins, 1952, pp 9–50, 137–155.
4. Strub RL, Black FW: Higher cognitive functions, in Strub RL, Black FW (eds): *The Mental Status Examination in Neurology.* Philadelphia, FA Davis, 1977, pp 107–118.

186. Attention Span

JOHN B. GRIFFIN, JR., MD

Definition

Attention span refers to the capacity of an individual to maintain concentration upon a single procedure or set of procedures over a period of time.

Technique

As a part of the mental status examination, the patient is asked to perform serial subtraction. This is usually done by asking the patient to begin with 100 and to subtract 7, then to subtract 7 from the answer. The patient continues this process of subtracting 7 from each new answer until 0 is reached. Most patients understand that they should repeat the answers verbally, but some patients who are quite concrete in their thinking will sit silently during the subtracting process and not give the answer to the examiner unless they are specifically asked to do the process verbally. In using this technique, it is important to be aware of the educational level of the patient. Patients of subnormal IQ or patients who have gone no higher than third grade in school may not be able to perform this task. If they are unable to subtract 7 from 100 serially, an alternate technique is to ask that they serially subtract 3 from 100. The examiner should write down each response, marking those that are correct and those that are incorrect. This will allow the examiner to obtain an accurate impression of the degree of difficulty that the patient has experienced.

This portion of the mental status examination is often somewhat threatening to the patient. Patients with paranoid tendencies will often be suspicious about what is being tested by this procedure. If a patient indicates discomfort with the procedure, the examiner should identify this feeling for the patient and discuss the anxiety. Many times the patient will ask why this is being done. The best response to such inquiries is to be as honest as possible. Usually patients are somewhat reassured by an explanation that this is a measure of concentrating ability and that many things can affect this ability, including such things as practice with calculations, education, physical illness, or emotional distress. Some patients will state that they can do it if they are allowed to use pencil and paper. This is not permissible as it destroys a major part of the effectiveness of the procedure in measuring the ability to hold an item in short-term memory while carrying out another complex mental operation.

Background Information

Serial subtraction from 100 gives information concerning several mental activities. Primary among these is attention span, or ability to concentrate. In the serial subtraction of 7 from 100, a double mental maneuver is required of the patient. Not only must the calculation be performed but also the answer from the preceding calculation must be held in memory while the patient is initiating the next subtraction. The most frequent reason for interference with this procedure is the presence of emotional distress. Typically, anxiety creates mental pressure for thought about the anxiety-provoking situation. These extraneous thoughts tend to cause patients to forget the last answer when they begin the new procedure of trying to subtract from it. Anxiety for similar reasons can also interfere with the calculation process itself. In these cases, the patient may carry out the subtraction process but make many errors while doing so. Patients with organic difficulty such as traumatic brain injury may also have difficulty with serial subtraction of 7 from 100. However, in contrast to patients who have interference from emotional causes, brain-injured patients will usually show many other areas of intellectual impairment. If patients are having obvious difficulty but seem unaware of their problem, questions should be asked to ascertain if the patients realize that they are making mistakes. If they are unaware of having difficulty, this may reflect either psychologically motivated denial or confabulation. In the former, patients are so threatened by the prospect of failure that their minds block out or repress this fact. In confabulation, patients invent answers to questions when they do not know the answer. They are quite susceptible to examiner suggestions regarding the answers which they give. In the so-called string test, the examiner acts as if an imaginary string is being tied and asks patients questions as if a real string were there. Confabulation is usually found in organic brain syndromes such as Korsakoff's syndrome seen in alcoholism. Emotionally disturbed patients may perform perfectly well in orientation, memory, reading, writing, spelling, and fund of general information but have difficulty in serial subtraction of 7 from 100 as a somewhat isolated finding.

Clinical Significance

The ability to maintain attention is an important mental function, subject to interference from a wide variety of factors. Physical illness such as fever or a severe headache makes concentration quite difficult. Similarly, emotional preoccupation reduces ability to maintain attention.

Most patients should be able to perform serial subtraction of 7 or 3 from 100 without significant difficulty. Some patients may make one error from carelessness. When the physician finds several errors in attention span, an explanation for the impairment must be found. Serious problems such as alcoholism, drug abuse, depression, anxiety states, and neurological disease can be overlooked unless careful scrutiny in the area of attention span is carried out.

Selected References

1.   Milstein V, Small JG, Small F: The subtraction of serial sevens test in psychiatric patients. *Arch Gen Psychiat* 26:439–441, 1972.
2.   Melges, FT: Mental status examination, in Rosenbaum CP, Beebe JE (eds): *Psychiatric Treatment Crisis/Clinic/Consultation.* New York, McGraw-Hill, 1975, pp 532–536.
3.   Hayman M: Two minute clinical test for measurement of intellectual impairment in psychiatric disorders. *Arch Neurol Psychiat* 47:454–464, 1942.

187. Judgment

JOHN B. GRIFFIN, JR., MD

Definition

Judgment as used in the mental status examination refers to the patient's capacity for understanding situations and relationships and for making logical decisions based on this understanding. This concept includes the patient's ability to use common sense in life situations.

Serious defects in judgment constitute such a threat to the patient's well-being that vigorous steps should be taken to reverse the defects or, if that is impossible, to protect the patient from carrying out harmful decisions.

Technique

Two general aspects of judgment are considered. One is judgment for personal matters; this involves whether or not the patient is logical and practical in handling general activities. The second item is judgment for nonpersonal matters; this involves such things as the patient's ability to differentiate between similar concepts or to see similarities between related concepts.

If adequate information concerning judgment for personal matters has been obtained in other parts of the history, no further exploration may be needed. If there is reason to suspect poor judgment, one should focus on one area of apparent bad judgment and ask the patient to explain how the difficulty arose. What is being looked for here is evidence that patients are misperceiving reality or are not able to foresee obvious consequences of their actions. Patients with organic brain difficulty, such as that following head trauma, may show gross inappropriateness and be unaware of the social consequences of their actions. For example, one such patient became so angry with his wife for forgetting his cigarette lighter that he slapped her in the face in the clinic waiting room. When judgment is impaired to this extent, it is almost impossible to overlook. However, other difficulties in judgment may be more subtle. A patient with manic-depressive psychosis may develop grandiose schemes for investments that initially sound plausible but on careful examination are clearly unrealistic. In cases where it is difficult to be sure whether a patient's judgment is truly impaired, it is often helpful to obtain the spouse's or parents' opinion of the reality or unreality of the patient's proposals.

One of the clues to impairment of judgment relates to the patient's own awareness of this impairment. Patients with organic brain injury are often completely unaware that they are showing poor judgment. Patients with neurotic emotional illness who show impairment of judgment may be quite aware that they have made mistakes and berate themselves for this. Patients with psychosis and distortion of reality may be aware of past mistakes but show little insight in using past experience to guide them in the present.

Judgment for nonpersonal items is usually evaluated by giving patients several similar concepts and asking that they differentiate between these. Patients may be asked to give the difference between a lie and a mistake, a midget and a child, idleness and laziness, poverty and misery, character and reputation. Educational background must clearly be taken into consideration here. Obviously patients cannot be expected to differentiate between two items if they are unfamiliar with one of the words. For patients of limited intellectual and educational ability, similar items can be made quite simple such as giving the difference between an orange and an apple or explaining how an airplane and a car are similar and how they are different. Most patients should be able to differentiate between at least three out of four concepts if the concepts presented are compatible with the patient's intellectual and educational ability.

Background Information

One of the most striking findings in psychiatric illness is impairment of judgment. Patients with psychosis or severe organic impairment of brain function have been observed from antiquity to behave in unpredictable ways. They frequently ignore social customs in a manner that makes their behavior objectionable for those around them. In ancient times, such persons were frequently imprisoned or cast out of the main community.

Careful study of patients with markedly impaired judgment has usually demonstrated that these patients suffer from distortion of their informational input concerning the world around them. These distortions may be quite gross as in the hallucinations of psychotic patients or more subtle as in the organically impaired patients who have lost the ability to respond to the usual social cues. Some organic patients also have marked difficulty with judgment because their impairment of memory is so great that they cannot maintain awareness of acceptable social behavior standards. An additional factor that complicates the judgment of organically impaired patients is lability of emotions. These patients sometimes become quite impulsive and unable to control rapid shifts of emotion even though they have some awareness that their behavior is unacceptable.

Clinical Significance

Gross impairment of judgment suggests organic difficulty or severe psychosis. When very striking, this may be so prominent as to be the primary reason for the patient's evaluation. The more subtle difficulties in judgment for personal problems may represent a minor or early organic impairment. When this is true, judgment for nonpersonal items will often show some impairment. A change in judgmental ability will usually have been noticed by significant persons in the patient's life situation. Patients who are showing impairment of judgment as the result of neurotic conflicts may show this repeatedly in their personal lives, such as the case of a woman who divorces her alcoholic husband then marries another alcoholic man. Such patients will usually have no difficulty with nonpersonal items of judgment. Similarly, patients with psychosis may show gross distortions of judgment for personal situations but have no major difficulty with judgment for nonpersonal items unless their psychosis has proceeded to the point of marked disorganization. Evaluating the patient's plans for the future is often a very useful way of estimating small degrees of impairment in personal judgment. In estimating judgment for nonpersonal items, the important thing is whether or not the patient understands the general concept involved. For example, a patient may state that the difference between a lie and a mistake is that a lie is deliberate and a mistake is accidental. While this answer would not cover all of the differences, such as the fact that a lie is a written or verbal communication and a mistake may occur outside the context of verbal communication, it does, nevertheless, get at the basic difference and is sufficient to be counted as correct.

Selected References

1.   Roeske NA: Judgment and insight, in Roeske NA (ed): *Examination of the Personality.* Philadelphia, Lea and Febiger, 1972, pp 83–86.
2.   Kolb, LC: Examination of the patient, in Kolb LC (ed): *Modern Clinical Psychiatry.* Baltimore, WB Saunders, 1977, pp 208–238.
3.   Gregory I, Smeltzer DJ: Record of psychiatric examination, in *Psychiatry: Essentials of Clinical Practice.* Boston, Little, Brown, 1977, pp 34–41.

188. Abstraction

JOHN B. GRIFFIN, JR., MD

Definition

Abstraction refers to the patient's capacity for understanding concepts which are not expressed concretely. The patient must understand that the meaning of an abstract statement is not found in the literal interpretations of the words but by the suggestion of a likeness between the literal and actual meanings. For example, a statement such as "Don't cross your bridges before you come to them," is impossible if taken literally. Giving abstract meaning is the only way for one to make sense of the statement. Thus the statement is a colorful way of saying, "Don't worry unnecessarily."

Technique

In attempting to measure abstraction, one focuses upon whether the patient is able to see a second meaning beyond literal words. Abstraction is usually measured by asking the patient to interpret proverbs. Some patients of very limited educational background or lower intelligence may have difficulty understanding the basic concept of an abstraction. The examiner begins repeating several proverbs until one is found that the patient has heard before. Some proverbs which are widely known include the following: "Don't cry over spilt milk," "A stitch in time saves nine," "An apple a day keeps the doctor away." After the patient responds that a proverb is familiar, the physician asks for its meaning. The examiner should focus upon whether the patient can respond to the proverb only in terms of the literal words or whether the patient understands the underlying meaning of the proverb. A literal interpretation of the proverb, "An apple a day keeps the doctor away," might be, "If you eat an apple every day, the doctor won't come to your house." Most patients are able to interpret proverbs which they have heard before. In the most severe cases of impairment, however, even familiar proverbs are either not interpreted or are interpreted literally. After the patient has responded to a familiar proverb, a proverb should be given which the patient has not heard before. Examples of less well-known proverbs are the following: "A rolling stone gathers no moss," "The apple falls near its tree," "The tongue is the enemy of the neck," "The squeaking wheel gets the grease." Usual interpretations of these proverbs are as follows: "The apple falls near its tree" means that people tend to live lives like those of their parents. "The squeaking wheel gets the grease" means that people who let a problem be known get some response to the problem. "A rolling stone gathers no moss" has two interpretations that are equally widespread. People who tend to be passive in their general life orientation often give this interpretation: "If one does not put roots down, he does not accomplish anything." People who have a more aggressive outlook toward life will often interpret this as meaning: "You will become bogged down and not accomplish anything if you don't keep moving." "The tongue is the enemy of the neck" is usually interpreted as meaning: "What you say can get you into trouble." From the literal standpoint, this proverb is very difficult to interpret and, consequently, it is quite useful in picking up difficulties in abstraction. A considerable number of patients with difficulty in abstraction can interpret a proverb that they have heard before because at some point someone has told them what it means, and they remember the explanation. However, these patients have difficulty interpreting proverbs that they have not heard.

Background Information

Eugen Blueler was one of the pioneer workers in studying and defining the ways in which psychotic thinking differed from normal thinking. In the early studies, it was soon apparent that one striking difference lay in the strong tendency of psychotic patients to respond to statements in a literal fashion. Statements with an abstract or second meaning were often wholly or partially misunderstood by the patient. Although there is wide agreement that this finding occurs in psychotic patients, the etiology for this finding is still unclear. Some workers have theorized that psychotic persons have great difficulty in organizing their world in a meaningful way and are emotionally driven toward simple solutions. Hence, such patients would take the simple, literal interpretation and might even block out awareness of deeper meaning. Whatever the cause, it is a very striking clinical finding.

Clinical Significance

For the vast majority of patients, there should be no impairment in abstraction. Patients who show impairment should be evaluated in terms of other parts of the mental status examination to find an explanation for this impairment. Patients with organic brain injury tend to have limitation of their ability to perform abstractions and also will usually show other mental impairment such as defects in memory, orientation, general intellectual function, and attention span. Such patients may comment that in the past they could interpret the proverb, but since the injury or other illness they have been unable to do this. Most patients with neurotic difficulties do not show impairment in this area, although they will frequently show a tendency to interpret the proverbs in light of their own personal situation. For example, the proverb "The apple falls near its tree" may be interpreted by a patient as follows: "I'm making the same mistakes in life that my father made." Patients with schizophrenia frequently are concrete and will show a limitation in their ability to interpret these proverbs. They tend to interpret proverbs in a literal fashion. However, patients with schizophrenia typically do not show impairment in orientation or memory.

Selected References

1. Carson RC: Proverb interpretation in acutely schizophrenic patients. *J Nerv Ment Dis* 135:556–564, 1962.
2. Harrow M, Tucker G, Adler D: Concrete and idiosyncratic thinking in acute schizophrenic patients. *Arch Gen Psych* 26:433–438, 1972.

189. Delusions, Hallucinations, and Illusions
JOHN B. GRIFFIN, JR., MD

Definition

Delusions, hallucinations, and illusions are among the most serious and significant symptoms of psychiatric patients. A delusion is defined as "a false belief out of keeping with the individual's level of knowledge and his cultural group. The belief results from unconscious needs and is maintained against logical argument and despite objective contradictory evidence" (*Psychiatric Glossary*). An hallucination is "a false sensory perception in the absence of an actual external stimulus" (*Psychiatric Glossary*). For example, a patient may hear voices or see persons when no one is there. An illusion is similar to an hallucination but is "the misinterpretation of a real experience" (*Psychiatric Glossary*). For example, the patient may see a chair and perceive it as a lion about to attack. In contrast, an hallucination occurs when there is no external sensory stimulus. In the above example, if a patient in an empty room saw a lion about to attack, this would be an hallucination as opposed to an illusion.

Technique

Hallucinatory experiences are in general quite disturbing to patients. Frequently, patients will mention hallucinations as the primary complaint. In such cases, it is a relatively simple matter to inquire concerning the exact nature of the experiences, the frequency, duration, and situations in which they most frequently occur.

However, hallucinations are recognized widely as serious evidence of "being crazy." Consequently, many patients will attempt to conceal the existence of these experiences. In such situations, the examiner can sometimes lead the patient gradually into a discussion of these phenomena with questions such as: Have you ever had any supernatural experience? Have you ever thought that you had extrasensory perception (ESP)? Have you ever had a vision? seen a ghost? or thought you saw a monster? Have you ever thought you heard or saw something and later found out there was nothing really there?

Some patients will deny any phenomena in this area but give some objective evidence of such experiences. During the interview, the patient may at times stop talking and appear lost in thought as if listening to something. At other times, a patient may suddenly laugh without apparent reason. At such times it is appropriate for the examiner to inquire whether the patient is hearing voices.

Background Information

Hallucinatory experiences have been a source of fascination for many centuries. The attitude of society toward individuals having these experiences has varied. In some cultures such individuals have been regarded with awe and even reverence. However, hallucinations with their accompanying distortion of reality are basically maladaptive. Individuals having these experiences have usually been rejected by society. In modern times hallucinations are generally considered clear evidence of severe emotional disturbance by both law and professional personnel.

Hallucinations occur in many different situations. Not all of these situations are indicative of severe emotional disorder. For example, hypnagogic hallucinations sometimes occur as people are falling asleep. Experiences where the person is in a stage of semiconsciousness between sleep and full wakefulness are not indicative of pathology. Similarly, hypnopompic hallucinations occur as a person is awakening from sleep and are not indicative of pathology. Marked sensory deprivation regularly produces hallucinatory experiences. Delirium from any of many medical causes can result in hallucinations. Effects of drugs, particularly amphetamines and psychedelic drugs, are frequent causes of hallucinations. Intense religious experiences may result in visions, not always indicative of mental disorder, particularly if these visions are characteristically found in other members of the particular religious group. Although hallucinations can occur in all psychotic states, the most frequent psychotic condition in which they occur is schizophrenia. Delusions and illusions can also occur in most of the circumstances described above. Delusions are particularly associated with paranoid thinking in which patients feel that some person or group is seeking to harm or take advantage of them. Delirium tremens, associated with excessive alcohol use, is a frequent cause of delusions, illusions, and hallucinations.

Clinical Significance

In organic psychoses such as those caused by drugs, delirium from medical illnesses, and organic brain syndrome associated with advanced age, visual hallucinations tend to be more prominent than auditory hallucinations. In addition, the visual hallucinations in such organic syndromes tend to be much more vivid than those with functional psychosis. For example, one patient with hallucinations caused by ingestion of amphetamines described an imaginary man sitting in a chair in front of her in minute detail, even giving the color and pattern of his tie.

Hallucinations with organic conditions tend to be more pronounced during night hours when external sensory input is decreased because of darkness. Hallucinations with functional psychotic conditions such as schizophrenia occur with approximately equal incidence in both daytime and night hours. In schizophrenia, auditory hallucinations are much more frequent than visual experiences. When visual hallucinations do occur in schizophrenia, they almost always occur in combination with hallucinations involving some other sensory modality. For example, schizophrenic patients with visual hallucinations may also have the sensation that a part of their body is missing or has grown much larger or smaller than it was before. Other hallucinations may involve feeling that their stomach is rotting or their heart is gradually stopping. Hallucinations can involve any of the senses. Hallucinations of smell, taste, and touch occur but are less frequent than those of sight and sound. Auditory hallucinations, particularly in the functional psychoses such as schizophrenia, usually have emotional content. The patient often hears threatening voices or commands to perform some act that would be upsetting.

The clinician must be careful to avoid overdiagnosing hallucinations, delusions, and illusions. Many patients have had times when they thought that they heard someone call their name, but actually no one had spoken, or they had been alone in a house and heard creaking noises that they feared might be a prowler. These common experiences do not indicate pathology. To make the diagnosis of hallucinations, delusions, and illusions, the experience should be a clear-cut and definite one.

When a definite diagnosis of illusions, hallucinations, or delusions is made, these phenomena indicate serious mental problems. Consequently, a careful and detailed exploration of the reasons for these phenomena is a prime responsibility of the clinician.

Selected References

1. Taylor MA: Schneiderian first-rank symptoms and clinical prognostic features in schizophrenia. *Arch Gen Psychiat* 26:64–67, 1972.
2. Goodwin DW, Alderson P, Rosenthan R: Clinical significance of hallucinations in psychiatric disorders. *Arch Gen Psychiat* 24:76–80, 1971.
3. Kolb LC: Psychopathology, in Kolb LC (ed): *Modern Clinical Psychiatry*. Baltimore, WB Saunders, 1977, pp 134–146.

190. Associations of Thought

JOHN B. GRIFFIN, JR., MD

Definition

Associations of thought, often referred to simply as associations, is a term which refers to the interconnections between successive items in thinking. Usual thought patterns progress in orderly sequence through a single topic area, arriving at some conclusion or end point. One of the characteristic findings in schizophrenia is a loosening of this process. In this looseness of association, the patient tends to move from subject to subject with only tenuous connections between the successive categories.

Technique

In severe looseness of association the diagnosis is obvious. The patient may speak in such disconnected sentences that the examiner can make no real sense out of what is being said. In the most severe cases, the patient may speak in a word salad in which words and phrases are jumbled with no apparent logical order or coherent meaning.

Many patients, however, present very subtle looseness of association. Some of these patients have learned to mask their looseness of association by speaking very little. In this way, they use people around them to structure their speech and avoid the appearance of looseness. In order to diagnose the subtle forms of looseness of association, the physician must persuade the patient to talk spontaneously. If the patient only responds to questions from the examiner, it will often be impossible to make the diagnosis. Often the examiner can evaluate this best by asking the patient to discuss some nonthreatening area of interest such as travel or a hobby. If the examiner's comments are primarily facilitative remarks such as, "Tell me more about that," or, "Yes, and then?" the patient will often reveal a tendency to drift rapidly from subject to subject.

Looseness of association is similar to the phenomenon seen in mentally healthy people who introduce a change of topic by saying, "Pardon me, but I would like to change the subject," except that the schizophrenic patient repeatedly changes subjects without any such introductory remarks and without apparent indication for change of subject. Usually the patient is unaware of doing this.

Background Information

Eugen Bleuler was among the pioneer workers who delineated the basic thought disorders in schizophrenia. The famous four "A's" of schizophrenia, autism, ambivalence, flatness of affect, and looseness of association, have been considered cardinal symptoms of the condition for many years. The neurological arrangement of the human brain is apparently such that thought processes involve many interrelated neuronal loops. The interconnections of the neuronal systems presumably lead to an orderly sequence of thinking. For reasons that are unclear, this orderly sequence tends to be disrupted in schizophrenia. In ordinary conversation, one person makes a comment, which leads to a response from the second person, which in turn generates a response from the first person, leading to an easily recognized progression in the exploration of the topic under consideration. Conversations with schizophrenic individuals often leave the other person somewhat off balance. The responses of the schizophrenic individual tend to be off target from the response expected by the other person.

It has often been said that madness is close to genius. Perhaps the saying had its origin in the fact that some schizophrenic persons are capable of brilliant originality. The looseness of association that the schizophrenic person experiences may be in part responsible for some of the creativity that surfaces at times. This looseness of association may make it possible for a few schizophrenic individuals to break out of customary thought patterns and see new relationships in a very remarkable way. For schizophrenics of high artistic or intellectual capacity this may lead to productivity widely acclaimed as genius.

However, in most situations, looseness of association is quite maladaptive. When two or more persons must work together for the accomplishment of a single goal, looseness of association on the part of one or more of the members of the group makes communication very difficult and can sharply curtail productivity.

Clinical Significance

Schizophrenia occurs in both mild and severe forms. Many schizophrenic people never see a psychiatrist and, although they are often viewed by peers and family as eccentric and difficult, are not regarded as having a serious psychiatric illness. Whether or not a schizophrenic person experiences a breakdown or decompensation probably depends both on the basic severity of the illness in the individual and on the degree of environmental stress to which the individual is subjected.

Looseness of association as a single isolated finding should not be considered indicative of serious psychiatric illness. Indeed, this phenomenon seen in participants on TV talk shows is often considered interesting and humorous. This symptom, however, should serve as a warning signal to the clinician. Combined with other findings of schizophrenia, it helps make the diagnosis. As an isolated finding, it alerts the physician to the possibility that the patient under sufficient stress could develop significant emotional disturbance. This knowledge can help the clinician to intervene early during times when the patient's life circumstances cause severe emotional stress.

Selected References

1. Meadow A, Greenblatt M, Solomon HC: Looseness of association and impairment in abstraction in schizophrenics. *J Nerv Ment Dis* 118: 27–35, 1953.
2. Roeske NA, Assue C: Thought process and content, in Roeske NA (ed): *Examination of the Personality*, Philadelphia, Lea and Febiger, 1972, pp 68–76.
3. Gregory I, Smeltzer DJ: Schizophrenic and paranoid disorders, in Gregory I, Smeltzer DJ (eds): *Psychiatry: Essentials of Clinical Practice*. Boston, Little, Brown, 1977, pp 175–190.

191. Orientation

E. STEPHEN PURDOM, MD

Definition

The individual's acquaintance with time, place, person, and situation. Disorientation is deficient knowledge of one or more of these areas.

Technique

A rapid screening test initiates your introduction to the patient. When you walk into the room, introduce yourself and pause, giving the patient an opportunity to introduce himself. As you begin to make notes of the history, pretend ignorance of the date and let the patient give it. When the patient tells you where he lives, ask about the geographic location with respect to the hospital. The answer to the question, "Why are you here?" in the initial phase of the interview provides an assessment of the patient's knowledge of the situation. Knowledge of the situation is perhaps the most sensitive index of orientation. Answers to these questions need to be obtained for other reasons, so this method saves time. Another advantage is that the patient does not perceive that there is a double purpose to these questions, avoiding the offense sometimes taken when questions are asked to obviously determine orientation.

A more complete survey of orientation must be done if disorientation is suspected on the basis of screening questions or from inaccuracies that come to light during the general history. Before beginning, inform yourself regarding certain aspects of the patient's life. Look at the records and obtain the following information:

1. Profession or employment
2. Marital status and number of children or siblings
3. Birth date and, if available, birthplace and residence
4. Prior hospitalizations, date, and locations
5. Any other bits of past or present information that may be used as a "conversation piece" during the patient interview in order to assess aspects of orientation

When available a prior interview with friends or relatives will yield information regarding the presence of disorientation. If the patient is indeed disoriented, a thorough history from the family becomes essential. The above information may then be inserted in conversation with the patient to assess recent and remote memory.

Orientation to immediate place may be easily assessed by nudging the patient to talk about the hospital room or ward area. You might, for example, ask where certain personal belongings are kept or where the bathroom is located. Such questions may uncover the fact that the patient has the delusion of being at home and not in a hospital.

The more subtle aspects of orientation to place should be pursued when one suspects cortical dysfunction, but not as part of a routine physical examination. These include:

1. Ability to draw and follow routes; that is, ask the patient to draw a map of how to go from the nursing station or elevator to his room.
2. Observe the patient on the hospital ward to see if he is able to find his way without difficulty.
3. Patients should be able to point out principal cities on a map of their native country.
4. Ask the patient to estimate distances to objects or places.

Background Information

The neural substrate for memory serves as the foundation for normal orientation (see section 192, Memory). The hippocampus and the medial thalamic nuclei are essential for the recording of passing events and for their accurate registration in a time frame. Focal destruction of these areas produces disorientation by making impossible the registration of passing daily events in memory and also by producing a retrograde amnesia for more remote events.

Metabolic encephalopathies produce similar disorders of registration and recall without focal disease. They produce confusion as to time, place, person, and situation, which are aspects of the content of consciousness. They also often produce stupor and delirium. Metabolic encephalopathies impair to a variable extent more subtle aspects of cortical function such as language, abstraction, and judgment.

Normal orientation is a very complex integrative process that requires the unhampered function of many multisynaptic systems in the cortex and brainstem. The parietal and temporal lobes are involved in many aspects of spatial and time orientation. The reticular formation in the brainstem is essential for normal consciousness (see section 193, Level of Consciousness). Many ascending reticular formation axons terminate in medial thalamic zones. When these latter areas are activated, they influence extensive areas of cortex and limbic structures in various ways depending upon stimulus parameters and physiologic state of the cortex. This polysynaptic reticulothalamic apparatus is known to be differentially sensitive to certain metabolic toxins and depressive pharmacologic agents when compared to the lemniscal and corticospinal systems.

It is likely that many aspects of disorientation as defined in this section are a clinical sign of structural or biochemical impairment of the reticular and thalamic integrative systems. Very discrete forms of spatial disorientation can be seen with lesions of the parietal lobe.

Clinical Significance

From the above discussion it is obvious that disorientation may appear in a variety of clinical states including cerebral mass lesions, meningitis, subarachnoid hemorrhage, and metabolic disorders. To assess its significance in any clinical situation, one must carefully note the presence or absence of "fellow travelers" such as focal neurologic signs, nuchal rigidity, or laboratory evidence of metabolic disorders.

In many clinical situations laboratory evidence of metabolic disease merely identifies its presence and not its severity. Hepatic failure, for example, may occasionally be associated with relatively mild changes in serum enzymes in spite of a rapidly deteriorating mental state. The mental state is a far more reliable index of ominous portent.

The presence of focal neurologic signs or focal seizures in a disoriented patient often indicates the presence of an intracranial mass lesion. Since the more severe metabolic disorders (anoxia, hypoglycemia, hepatic encephalopathy) may have such abnormalities as focal seizures, mild hemiparesis, or asymmetric reflexes, the clinician must, by experience, develop judgment in deciding which patient needs special neurologic investigation and which patient may be safely managed simply as a metabolic disorder.

Selected Reference

1. Plum F, Posner JB: *The Diagnosis of Stupor and Coma,* ed 2. Philadelphia, FA Davis, 1972.

192. Memory

H. KENNETH WALKER, MD

Definition

Memory can be divided into several modalities: verbal, visual, motor, olfactory, and gustatory. Verbal memory is usually the only one tested at the bedside. The level of consciousness and speech must be normal for valid testing. Remote and recent memory and immediate recall are tested (Table 30). Rough guidelines for normal memory at the bedside are:

Table 30. Bedside memory evaluation.

Remote memory

1. Date and place of birth.
2. Names of siblings.
3. Residence history.
4. Employment history.
5. Marriage: date, place, wife's maiden name.
6. Names of children.
7. Personal involvement in events such as World Wars, Depression of the 1930s.
8. Residence address, length of residence, telephone number.

Recent memory (the ability to learn new material)

1. Hospital: length of stay, how brought, special tests, special procedures, x-rays.
2. Three unrelated data: city, color, object such as hat or bicycle. The three data are given to the patient who is told he will be asked to repeat them later. Proceed with other portions of the examination, and 5–10 minutes later ask the patient to repeat the data.

Immediate recall

1. Seven digits forward.
2. Five digits backward.
3. Repeat a sentence such as, "One thing a nation must have to become rich and great is a large, secure supply of wood."

1. Remote memory. The patient can recall in some detail the personal manifestations of events such as the World Wars or the Depression; give dates of birth and marriage, names of siblings and children, locations where lived, employment history, residence address, telephone number.

2. Recent memory. The patient can recall length of stay in hospital and how brought to hospital; events of hospital stay such as x-rays, special tests, and procedures; can remember three unrelated data such as name of a city, a color, and an object.

3. Immediate recall. The patient can repeat seven digits forward and five backward; repeat a sentence of 15–20 words.

The individual with abnormal memory can have deficits in all areas indicated above.

Technique

The type of formal bedside memory testing given above is rarely necessary as a screening procedure but becomes necessary when relatives indicate memory difficulties are present or if the examiner uncovers suggestions of memory deficits when taking the present illness, past history, and review of systems. Begin by telling the patient that this part of the evaluation involves memory testing and that it will be necessary to pay careful attention to your questions and instructions. On many occasions the examiner will need to use tact and diplomacy. Much of the examination need not take the guise of formal memory testing since questions such as age, address, and most of the other data in the recent and remote categories are necessary anyway. Consider the patient's age, educational level, and environment in posing the questions. Table 30 lists suggestions for use in memory testing. The examiner obviously must be able to verify the data.

If significant deficits are uncovered, the examiner can test for confabulation, a characteristic sometimes seen in patients with Wernicke-Korsakoff's syndrome (see below). The patient will fabricate or "pseudo-remember" past events in response to questions by the examiner. Use questions such as: Do you remember seeing me in the grocery store last week? Didn't I see you at John's birthday party? Weren't you on the *Today* show last week? Be neutral in tone of voice and manner when asking these questions.

The tests given above are principally evaluations of verbal memory. Visual memory, which is predominantly a function of the nondominant parietal lobe, can be tested at the bedside as follows:

1. Place several objects such as a key, comb, dime, on the table and cover each with a sheet of paper after the patient has seen their location. Then ask the patient to point to the paper covering any one of the objects.

2. Carry several 2 × 2 pictures of individuals and show one or two to the patient. A few minutes later ask the patient to pick it from among the other pictures.

Background Information

The word memory has a wide variety of meanings, ranging from its implications in psychoanalysis to kinesthetic memory—such as remembering how to ride a bicycle or play a certain piece on the piano—to visual, olfactory, tactile, and verbal memories. Verbal memory is the aspect of memory most useful in clinical neurology. It is conventionally divided into three aspects, all of which can be easily tested at the bedside and can be correlated in a useful fashion with the neuroanatomy and neuropathology of memory.

Immediate recall is the ability to reproduce with total accuracy at least five digits forward and backward immediately after being given the digits. This type of activity does not test memory storage, since it is accessed too soon after receiving it. The duration of this stage of memory is probably seconds. The reticular activating system and its functions of maintaining alertness and attention is probably the anatomical substrate. Only a small part of the information is ultimately stored. The capacity for immediate recall is quite limited. New information replaces old in a continuous sequence. A good example of this is remembering a new telephone number from the directory just long enough to dial it, then forgetting the number even before the party answers!

Recent memory is the ability to learn new material. Psychologists call it consolidation. It refers to the selection of a certain small portion of the data continuously being received by the nervous system for the purposes of storage. The time of storage lasts minutes to perhaps years, and the capacity is quite large—all in distinct contrast to the seconds and limited storage capacity of the immediate recall mechanism. The hippocampal–diencephalic structures appears to be the neuroanatomical substrate:

1. Surgical removal of the hippocampus or destruction by a disease process leaves the patient with the ability to remember former events and with a normal IQ, but unable to remember new facts for more than a few minutes at a time. The lesions are usually bilateral. See reports by Scoville and Milner.

2. The medial dorsal nuclei of thalamus are the most consistent neuropathological finding in Wernicke-Korsakoff patients with a memory deficit (Victor, Adams, and Collins). The patient is unable to remember events occurring a short time previously. There are also deficits in remote memories in this syndrome.

3. Lesions involving the mammillary bodies, fornix, and cingulum

may produce memory deficits; but the evidence is not conclusive. This is principally due to the fact that lesions seen pathologically are rarely restricted to one or two structures but are usually quite extensive.

An example of memory deficit is the case of a 47-year-old physician with bilateral surgical resection of the uncus, amygdala, and anterior hippocampus (Scoville and Milner). He could give minute details of early life and medical training. His IQ was 122. He was alert and responsive, but unable to learn the name of the hospital or the examiner, could not recognize his own drawings, and could not recall any events following the operation.

A patient with Korsakoff's psychosis when told his nearest relative had died was shocked and distressed, but a few minutes later remembered neither the examiner nor the news (Victor). In another patient with Korsakoff's reported by Victor, remote memory was also affected: the patient was a 40-year-old woman who thought she was in Ireland; actually she had emigrated from Ireland at age 19 and raised four children.

The articles by McEntee et al., Ziegler et al., and McEntee review the questions about the relationship of specific anatomical structures in the diencephalic-limbic area to recent memory. The article by Benson is an excellent and practical review of the clinical and pathological aspects of memory. The follow-up report by Penfield and Mathieson gives a glimpse into the history of the clinical evolution of concepts of the hippocampus and memory, as does the reminiscence by Brenda Milner of her association with Penfield.

Remote memory, or the ability to retrieve previously learned material, is a function of the cortex. Capacity may be unlimited and storage permanent. Wilder Penfield's fascinating results with electrode stimulation of various areas of the cortex gave the first insights into this field. Fairly restricted lesions can produce special types of memory dysfunction. The loss of spatial memory and memory for faces in nondominant parietal lobe lesions are examples.

The mechanisms which form new memories, the locations of memories, and the interactions of various cortical areas with regard to memory are all completely unknown at present. Memory ultimately comes about from the cortical integration of remembered sights, sounds, smells, and tactile sensation. A good illustration of the complexity and richness of memory comes from Vladimir Nabokov's *Speak, Memory: An Autobiography Revisited.**

> The beginning of my first term in Cambridge was inauspicious. Late in the afternoon of a dull and damp October day, with the sense of indulging in some weird theatricals, I put on my newly acquired, dark-bluish academic

* Quoted from *Speak, Memory: An Autobiography Revisited* by Vladimir Nabokov, New York, GP Putnam's Sons, 1966, with permission from the author.

gown and black square cap for my first formal visit to E. Harrison, my college tutor. I went up a flight of stairs and knocked on a massive door that stood slightly ajar. "Come in," said a distant voice with hollow abruptness. I crossed a waiting room of sorts and entered my tutor's study. The brown dusk had forestalled me. There was no light in the study save for the glow of a large fireplace near which a dim figure sat in a dimmer chair. I advanced saying: "My name is —" and stepped into the tea things that stood on the rug beside Mr. Harrison's low wicker armchair. With a grunt, he bent sideways from his seat to right the pot, and then scooped up and dumped back into it the wet black mess of tea leaves it had disgorged.

Nabokov revisited his tutor many years later:

The dull day had dwindled to a pale yellow streak in the gray west when, acting upon an impulse, I decided to visit my old tutor. Like a sleepwalker, I mounted the familiar steps and automatically knocked on the half-open door bearing his name. In a voice that was a jot less abrupt, and a trifle more hollow, he bade me come in. "I wonder if you remember me..." I started to say, as I crossed the dim room to where he sat near a comfortable fire. "Let me see," he said, slowly turning around in his low chair, "I do not quite seem..." There was a dismal crunch, a fatal clatter: I had stepped into the tea things that stood at the foot of his wicker chair. "Oh, yes, of course," he said, "I know who you are."

Clinical Significance

There are several conditions in which memory defects can be out of proportion to other defects:

1. Wernicke-Korsakoff syndrome. A condition caused by thiamine deficiency in alcoholic patients. Hemorrhagic necrotic lesions are seen in the walls of the third ventricle and periaqueductal region and floor of the fourth ventricle. The Wernicke portion refers to the ophthalmoplegia, nystagmus, and cerebellar ataxia that accompany the Korsakoff's psychosis, which refers to the memory deficit and state of confusion seen in these patients. The great majority of patients have both portions of this syndrome (see reference 19).
2. Vascular or neoplastic lesions of the medial parts of the temporal lobe. Infarction bilaterally of the hippocampus, fornix, and mammillary bodies due to occlusion of branches of the posterior cerebral arteries (see reference 20). Neoplasms can involve these areas and produce a similar clinical picture (see reference 3).
3. Herpes simplex encephalitis. The orbital portions of the frontal and medial surfaces of the temporal lobes are often extensively

damaged. A residual memory deficit far out of proportion to other deficits is often seen.

4. Traumatic amnesias. A period of retrograde amnesia (RA) applies to events prior to the injury and another period of amnesia, posttraumatic amnesia (PTA), applies to events afterward. These periods are of variable length.

5. Transient global amnesia. A sudden temporary loss of memory lasting a few hours and usually occurring in a patient in whom one suspects cerebral atherosclerosis (age, disease elsewhere). The episodes are transient with complete memory functioning returning. No other neurological abnormalities are present. They may represent transient ischemic attacks involving structures associated with memory; however, there is no conclusive evidence that this is the case (see references 4 and 6).

6. Alzheimer's dementia (senile dementia). On occasion patients early in the course of this disease have deficits in memory out of proportion to other deficits. Pathologically cases may show extensive involvement of the hippocampus.

Table 31.   Neurologic diseases that may produce the Amnesic Korsakoff's Syndrome.

---

1. Amnesic syndrome of sudden onset—usually with gradual but incomplete recovery
   a. Bilateral hippocampal infarction due to atherosclerotic-thrombotic or embolic occlusion of the posterior cerebral arteries or their inferior temporal branches
   b. Trauma to the diencephalic or inferomedial temporal regions
   c. Spontaneous subarachnoid hemorrhage (mechanism not understood)
   d. Carbon monoxide poisoning and other hypoxic states (rare)
2. Amnesia of sudden onset and transitory duration
   a. Temporal lobe seizures
   b. Postconcussive states
   c. "Transient global amnesia"
3. Amnesic syndrome of subacute onset with varying degrees of recovery, usually leaving permanent residue
   a. Wernicke-Korsakoff disease
   b. Inclusion-body (herpes simplex) encephalitis
   c. Tuberculous and other forms of meningitis characterized by a granulomatous exudate at the base of the brain
4. Slowly progressive amnesic states
   a. Tumors involving the floor and walls of the third ventricle
   b. Alzheimer's disease and other degenerative disorders with disproportionate affection of the inferomedial portions of the temporal lobes

---

From *Principles of Neurology* by R. D. Adams and M. Victor. Copyright © 1977 by McGraw-Hill Book Company, New York. Used with permission of McGraw-Hill Book Company.

7. Anoxic amnesia. Recovery from cardiac arrest in some patients leaves an amnesic state very similar to Korsakoff's psychosis. Improvement is gradual and variable. See Benson.

8. Migraine headaches. On rare occasions these can involve the hippocampal-diencephalic structures bilaterally and produce a short-lived amnesia very similar to that seen in the entities described above.

Table 31 summarizes the clinical aspects of Korsakoff-like amnesia.

Selected References

1. Adams RD: The anatomy of memory mechanisms in the human brain, in Talland GA, Waugh NC (eds): *Pathology of Memory.* New York, Academic Press, 1969, pp 91–106.

2. Adams RD, Victor M: *Principles of Neurology.* New York, McGraw-Hill, 1977, pp 277–278.

3. Angelergues R: Memory disorders in neurological disease, in Vinken PG, Bruyn GW (eds): *Handbook of Clinical Neurology.* Amsterdam, North-Holland Publishing Co, 1969, vol 3, pp 268–292.

4. Benson DF: Amnesia. *South Med J* 71:1221–1227, 1978.

5. DeJong RN: The hippocampus and its role in memory. *J Neurol Sci* 19:73–83, 1973.

6. Fisher CM, Adams RD: Transient global amnesia. *Acta Neurol Scand* 40(Suppl 9):1–83, 1964.

7. Karp H: Dementia in adults, in Baker AB, Baker LH (eds): *Clinical Neurology.* New York, Harper and Row, 1978, vol 2, chap 27.

8. McEntee WJ: Hippocampal-fornix-mamillary circuit and memory (letter). *Arch Neurol* 35:618, 1978.

9. McEntee WJ, Biber MP, Perl DP, Benson DF: Diencephalic amnesia: A reappraisal. *J Neurol Neurosurg Psychiat* 39:436–441, 1976.

10. Milner B: Wilder Penfield: His legacy to neurology: Memory mechanisms. *Canad Med Assoc J* 116:1374–1376, 1977.

11. Nabokov V: *Speak, Memory: An Autobiography Revisited.* New York, GP Putnam's Sons, 1966.

12. Ojemann RG: Correlations between specific human brain lesions and memory changes: A critical survey of the literature. *Bull Neurosci Res Program* 22:77–145, 1964.

13. Patten BM: The ancient art of memory. *Arch Neurol* 26:25–31, 1972.

14. Patten BM: Modality specific memory disorders in man. *Acta Neurol Scand* 48:69–86,1972.

15. Penfield W, Mathieson G: Memory: Autopsy findings and comments

on the role of hippocampus in experiential recall. *Arch Neurol* 31: 145–154, 1974.

16. Scoville WB, Milner B: Loss of recent memory after bilateral hippocampal lesions. *J Neurol Neurosurg Psychiat* 20:11–21, 1957.
17. Symonds C: Disorders of memory. *Brain* 89:625–644, 1966.
18. Victor M: Observations on the amnestic syndrome in man and its anatomical basis, in Brazier MAB (ed): *RNA and Brain Function: Memory and Learning*. Berkeley and Los Angeles, University of California Press, 1964, vol 2, pp 311–337.
19. Victor M, Adams RD, Collins GH (eds): *The Wernicke-Korsakoff Syndrome*. Philadelphia, FA Davis, 1971.
20. Victor M, Angevine J, Mancall E, et al: Memory loss with lesions of hippocampal formation. *Arch Neurol* 5:244–263, 1961.
21. Ziegler DK, Kaufman A, Marshall HE: Abrupt memory loss associated with thalamic tumor. *Arch Neurol* 34:545–548, 1977.

---

193. Level of Consciousness

H. KENNETH WALKER, MD

Definition

The degree of "wakefulness," "awareness," or "alertness," determined by brainstem structures (diencephalon, midbrain, and pons). This does *not* refer to the content of consciousness.

Normal: Difficult to satisfactorily define. A decent working definition is a state of wakefulness, alertness, or responsiveness to stimuli comparable to that of the examiner.

Lethargy: Severe drowsiness. The patient can be aroused by moderate stimuli and will make appropriate verbal and motor responses and then drift back to sleep.

Stupor: Only vigorous and severe stimuli by a persistent examiner can arouse the patient from this state of unresponsiveness. Painful stimuli provoke grimacing, eye opening, or various voluntary responses of one sort or another. The patient immediately returns to the stuporous state when stimuli cease.

Coma: Unarousable unresponsiveness. Painful stimuli provoke no responses or only reflex responses.

Technique

There is usually little difficulty in distinguishing among the levels of consciousness. Conversation and observation during history taking rapidly establish the level of consciousness. Inattention, yawning, drowsiness —all point to lethargy and are in distinct contrast to the patient who is alert, brisk in verbal responses, and attentive.

Stuporous and comatose patients must have a very careful examination, especially with reference to respiration, spontaneous movements, and ocular signs. The following is a brief summary of some salient features. The references by Plum and Posner and by Fisher are unsurpassed. An outline of the examination is given in Table 32.

OBSERVATION

This important phase of the examination should start immediately after the clinician makes sure that no immediate life-threatening emergency such as airway obstruction or shock is at hand. Many clinicians fall into the habit of going to the bedside and immediately grabbing and shaking the patient. The best information is obtained by starting with perhaps 10 minutes of observation with the examiner standing quietly by the bedside with a notebook in which to record the findings. Begin with a general survey of the patient, looking with especial care for signs of trauma, infection, or abnormalities of any sort. Then proceed in a systematic fashion with the scheme outlined below.

Respiratory rhythm. The pattern of respiration provides valuable information about the location of the dysfunction along the neuraxis and, when observed over a period of time, can give some indication as to whether the dysfunction is remaining in the same location, regressing by moving rostrally, or progressing with rostrocaudal deterioration. Table 33 lists some of the classic patterns along with the sites of dysfunction.

Table 32. Examination procedure in comatose patients.

---

1. Observation
    a. Respiratory rhythm
    b. Position in bed
    c. Spontaneous movements
2. Reaction to graded stimuli
3. Ocular and extraocular muscle functioning
4. Remainder of examination

Table 33.   Respiratory patterns.*

Pattern	Site of Dysfunction
Cheyne-Stokes: A regular waxing and waning alternating with periods of apnea.	Cerebral hemispheres bilaterally, extending down into the diencephalon.
Central neurogenic hyperventilation: Deep, rapid respirations at a rate of 24 or more per minute.	Middle of midbrain to middle of pons, due to involvement of paramedian reticular system.
Apneustic respiration: Many varieties. Apneusis is a prolonged inspiratory "cramp," a pause at the height of inspiration. These end-inspiratory pauses often alternate with expiratory pauses and other irregularities. Of great localizing value in that it indicates involvement of the automatic respiratory control mechanisms located in the pons.	Lower pontine tegmentum around where the trigeminal root emerges.
Ataxic breathing: Completely unpredictable breathing. Random sequences of shallow and deep respiration in no discernible pattern.	Dorsomedial medulla.

* See references 4 and 5.

References to Plum provide further information. The reader is cautioned that what is observed at the bedside often will not fit into the stereotypes.

Position in bed.   Compare the position to that seen in natural sleep. Note the arrangement of the trunk and limbs with respect to each other and to the bedcovers. A comfortable looking patient curled up in bed with the sheet carefully pulled over the head for protection from the light will be in no deeper than a light stupor. Gentle curvature of the body may indicate a hemiparesis. Note the position of the jaws: trismus or tightly clenched jaws indicate a bilateral corticospinal lesion above the level of the trigeminal nucleus in the midpons; slack jaws, lips, and cheeks (the "O" sign) indicate that the fifth and seventh nuclei are not functioning. "Fisting" (saulingfaust) of the thumb lying in the palm tightly embraced by the fingers suggests hypoxia.

Spontaneous movements.   "Voluntary" type reflexes indicate light stupor at the worst. These include such movements as the "modesty reflex," pulling up the bedcovers, turning in bed, or crossing the legs.
    Seizure activity should be suspected if there is repetitive movement

of one or more parts of the body. Common sites include eyelids, corners of lips, fingers (especially the thumb), and feet. These sites have large areas of representation on the cortex, which probably explains why they are more frequently the locus of seizure activity.

Myoclonus, a sudden gross twitching of one or more muscles, is seen in metabolic problems such as hypoxia, uremia, and hypoglycemia. The facial and proximal limb musculature are commonly involved.

Many other varieties of complex movements can be seen in comatose or stuporous patients. Document these movements carefully since they indicate the integrity of various neuroanatomical pathways and over time can give clues to progression or regression of the lesion.

REACTION TO STIMULI

Proceed to this section only after thorough observation. The "wakefulness" or ease, degree, and duration of arousal is being tested, that is, you are directly assessing the functioning of the brainstem structures responsible for level of consciousness. You are titrating the level of consciousness; therefore graded stimuli are used, beginning with the least possible stimulus (the whispered name of the patient) and proceeding to painful stimuli (deep pain). Recording of the data is essential: indicate the stimulus, the site, the response, and the duration of the response. Suggested stimuli appear in Table 34.

Table 34.   Graded stimuli.

---

1. Voice
    a. Whispered last name: "Mr. Jones"
    b. Whispered given name: "Tom"
    c. Calling name with increasing loudness
    d. Interrogation: "Tom?" "Do you hurt?"
    e. Shouted commands: "Look!"
2. Tactile and painful stimuli
    a. Blow air on the cheek
    b. Pat the cheek
    c. Rub the hand
    d. Shake the shoulder
    e. Tickle the inside of a nostril with cotton
    f. Pinch the skin on the medial aspect of the elbow and knee
    g. Squeeze a pectoral or biceps muscle
    h. Pinch the Achilles tendon
    i. Press on nail bed
    j. Squeeze a testicle
    k. Irrigate the ears with ice water

Postural reflexes may occur spontaneously or in response to stimuli. They may be bilateral or unilateral. The two most common are:

1. Decorticate posture
   a. Upper extremity: adduction with flexion of arm, wrist, and fingers
   b. Lower extremity: extension, internal rotation, and plantar flexion at ankle
   c. Level of dysfunction: cerebral hemispheres or internal capsules and rostral cerebral peduncles
2. Decerebrate posture
   a. Upper extremity: rigid extension, arms adducted and internally rotated
   b. Lower extremity: rigid extension at knees, ankles plantar flexed
   c. Neck may extend and opisthotonos may be present
   d. Level of dysfunction: rostral to midpons; the vestibular nuclei must be intact to have this reflex

Adduction, flexion, or extension when occurring in response to a stimulus are involuntary movements until proved otherwise. Abduction is usually voluntary.

OCULAR AND EXTRAOCULAR MUSCLE FUNCTIONING

A review of the ocular signs in coma is beyond the scope of this section. Some of the principal features that should be observed and carefully evaluated are:

1. Blink. The activity of the brainstem structures involved in wakefulness, the reticular system, is closely linked to blink. Thus preserved blink indicates that the rostral reticular system is functioning.
2. Palpebral fissures. Lesions involving the seventh and third nerves can produce widening or narrowing (ptosis) of the fissures. See sections 197 (third nerve) and 199 (seventh nerve).
3. Pupils. See section 135 (The Pupil) and references.
4. Extraocular muscles. See section 197 (third, fourth, and sixth nerves).

REMAINDER OF EXAMINATION

The rest of the neurological examination and the general physical examination focuses upon obtaining further information about the level and degree of dysfunction of the neurological system and seeking etiologic clues.

Background Information

Stimulation of brainstem structures in the lightly anesthetized cat causes "activation" of the EEG, producing EEG and behavioral changes that are quite similar to those seen in humans when drowsiness is replaced by alertness or wakefulness. The structures that produce these functional changes begin at the root entry of the trigeminal nerve in the midpons and extend rostrally through the midbrain up to include the posterior hypothalamus, the thalamic intralaminar nuclei, and the septal nuclei. These structures collectively are known as the ascending reticular activating system (ARAS). The part that begins in the middle of the pons and goes through the midbrain is the upper portion of the recticular formation. Since the reticular formation as an anatomical entity ends in the midbrain, the more rostral portions of the ARAS in the thalamus and hypothalamus are not part of the reticular formation but certainly correspond to it functionally. The reticular formation is located in the periventricular areas of the midbrain, pons, and medulla. The ARAS receives input from all sensory systems, and efferent connections are extensive. Views on the functional organization of the reticular formation are in a state of almost day-to-day flux (see Reference 2 for a summary).

The ARAS maintains a certain level of consciousness by way of extensive cortical projections, in Plum's words, "maintaining the hemispheric tone required for the conscious state." In turn the cortex sends efferents to the ARAS; consequently, there is some measure of feedback control. The cortex can thus alert the ARAS to be on the lookout for a specific stimulus, e.g., a certain sound. When that sound is perceived by the ARAS through its input from the acoustic system, the cortex is "alerted," that is, wakefulness and attention increase.

The level of consciousness of the cortex therefore closely relates to the ARAS. Both the cortex and the ARAS must be intact to have a normal level of consciousness. Anatomic-pathologic studies have indicated one or more of the following conditions are necessary for a disease to interfere with the level of consciousness:

1. It must involve both cerebral hemispheres
2. It must involve the ARAS as follows (Plum):
   a. Occupy both sides of the midline
   b. Be located between the trigeminal root entry zone in the midpons and the posterior diencephalon
   c. Be abruptly acquired or fairly large in extent

Clinical Significance

Metabolic diseases and mass lesions are common causes of disorders of the level of consciousness. Metabolic diseases can produce stupor or coma by affecting the neuronal metabolism of the cortex or brainstem, or both. They include:

1. Diseases of other organs such as hepatic encephalopathy, uremia, diabetes (including hypoglycemia)
2. Diseases which produce hypoxia directly or by causing ischemia: pulmonary disease, cardiac disease, anemia, large or small vessel disease, hyperviscosity syndromes
3. Poisons: sedative drugs, acid poisons (paraldehyde, methyl alcohol), enzyme inhibitors (heavy metals, organic phosphates)
4. Acid-base and electrolyte abnormalities: acidosis, alkalosis, hyper and hypocalcemia, hyper and hypomagnesemia
5. Infections: meningitis, encephalitis
6. Primary neurological diseases: Alzheimer's, lipid storage diseases

See Plum and Posner for a complete classification. These conditions produce dysfunction of the neuraxis at many different levels, usually in a bilaterally symmetrical distribution. Motor abnormalities such as asterixis and myoclonus are common.

Mass lesions, such as tumors or intracerebral hemorrhages, may be divided into supratentorial and subtentorial groups. Supratentorial masses alter the level of consciousness by secondarily involving the ARAS in the brainstem. Dysfunction is brought about by various combinations of direct pressure, cerebral edema, and vascular compression, producing displacement and disruption of the brainstem. Uncal herniation is a common finding in supratentorial lesions. The expanding cortex shoves the uncus of the temporal lobe into the tentorial notch, the space between the tentorium and the brainstem. There is resulting compression of the brainstem and other structures in the notch, notably the third cranial nerve and the posterior cerebral artery. Signs include (Fig 151):

1. Ipsilateral widely dilated and eventually fixed pupil with paralysis of other third nerve functions. This produces a laterally deviated eye (if the sixth nerve is intact) and a drooping eyelid
2. Impaired level of consciousness: drowsiness progressing to stupor, then coma
3. Contralateral homonymous hemianopsia occasionally due to compression of the posterior cerebral artery
4. Ipsilateral hemiparesis occasionally due to compression of the contralateral cerebral penduncle against the tentorium.

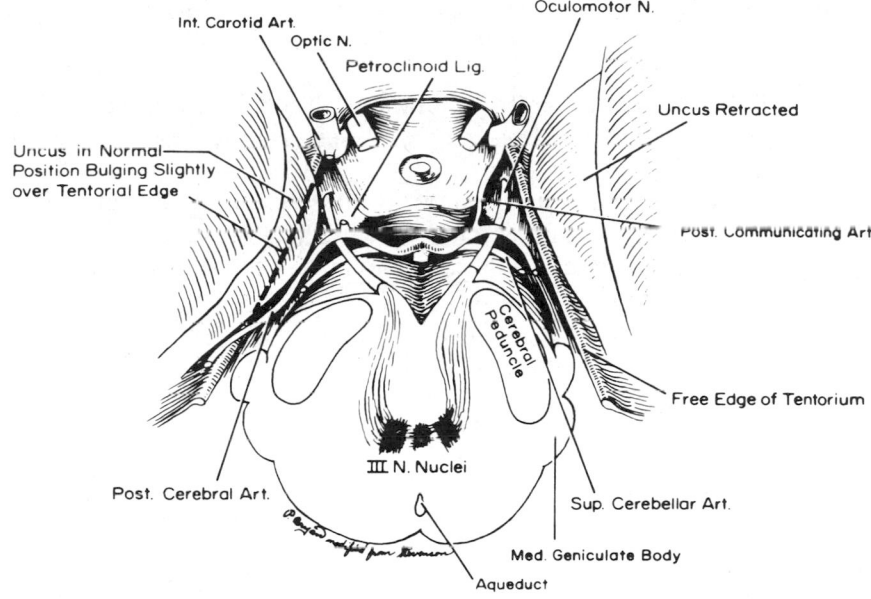

Figure 151. Relationships of structures involved in uncal herniation. (Redrawn and modified from *Clinical Neuro-Ophthalmology,* ed. 3, by FB Walsh and WF Hoyt. Copyright 1969, The Williams & Wilkins Company, Baltimore. Used with permission of publisher and author.)

Central herniation (transtentorial herniation) is another form of herniation that is caused by a downward displacement of the diencephalon and midbrain. Signs include:

1.   Drowsiness progressing to stupor and coma
2.   Respiration: yawns, sighs, occasionally Cheyne-Stokes pattern
3.   Pupils: small (1–3 mm) but responsive to light
4.   Eyes: roving or motionless but responsive to doll's head maneuver
5.   Motor: bilateral corticospinal and extrapyramidal involvement with hypertonus and abnormal plantar reflex

The important principle with regard to supratentorial effects on the neuraxis is that dysfunction occurs in an orderly rostrocaudal fashion, beginning with the cortex then sequentially involving the diencephalon, midbrain, pons, and medulla.

Subtentorial mass lesions produce stupor and coma by directly involving the ARAS.

The history is absolutely vital to the diagnosis of the causes of altered levels of consciousness. The following should be included:

1. The presenting manifestation, including whether onset was sudden (suggestive of vascular or seizure disorders) or gradual (suggestive of mass)
2. Temporal course and sequence of symptom evolution
3. Usual state of health, including when last present
4. A search for diseases or conditions that frequently cause coma:
   a. Trauma
   b. Epileptic convulsions
   c. Drugs and other poisons
   d. Cardiac disease
   e. Cerebrovascular disease
   f. Infections
   g. Cancer
5. Metabolic causes

Selected References

1. Moruzzi G, Magoun HW: Brain stem reticular formation and activation of the electroencephalogram. *Clin Neurophys* 1:455–473, 1949.
2. Brodal A: *Neurological Anatomy,* ed 2. New York, Oxford University Press, 1969.
3. Plum F: Organic disturbances of consciousness, in Critchley M, O'Leary JL, Jennett B (eds): *Scientific Foundations of Neurology.* Philadelphia, FA Davis, 1972, pp 193–201.
4. Plum F: Neurological integration of behavioral and metabolic control of breathing, in Porter R (ed): *Ciba Foundation Symposium on Breathing: Hering-Breuer Centenary Symposium.* London, Churchill, 1970, pp 159–181.
5. Plum F, Posner JB: *The Diagnosis of Stupor and Coma,* ed 2. Philadelphia, FA Davis, 1972.
6. Fisher CM: The neurological examination of the comatose patient. *Acta Neurol Scand* 45(suppl 36):1–56, 1969.

194. Speech and Other Lateralizing Cortical Functions

H. KENNETH WALKER, MD

Definition

These functions need to be tested only when an abnormality is suspected and not as part of a routine screening examination.

	Abnormality
Speech	
1. Phonation	Dysphonia, aphonia
2. Articulation	Dysarthria, anarthria
3. Language	Dysphagia, aphasia
Other dominant hemisphere functions	
1. Right-left orientation	Right-left disorientation
2. Finger identification	Finger agnosia
3. Calculation	Acalculia
Nondominant hemisphere functions	
1. Drawing ability	Drawing apraxia
2. Topographic ability	Spatial disorientation
3. Construction	Constructional apraxia
4. Dressing	Dressing apraxia
5. Facial recognition	Prosopagnosia
6. Awareness of body and space	Neglect of part of body or space
7. Motor persistence	Motor impersistence
Bilateral hemisphere functions	
1. Motor performance	Motor apraxia
2. Handedness and other sided motor functions	None

Technique

I.   Speech. The components of speech to be tested are phonation, articulation, and language. These components need to be carefully tested only when dysfunction is suspected and not as a routine screening procedure. The order in which the tests are performed will vary. In many cases the language component, especially comprehension, will have to be tested before proceeding to other tests which require intact comprehension.

    A.   Phonation. Ask the patient to say "ahh..." as long as possible. Note whether spontaneous speech is hoarse or whispery. The vagus nerve and the larynx are being tested here (see section 201, Cranial Nerves IX and X). Also see section 206, The Cerebellum, since cerebellar dysfunction can cause abnormalities in this test.

    B.   Articulation. These tests involve the muscles and structures responsible for forming words: pharynx, tongue, teeth, and lips. Innervation is from nerves V, VII, IX, X, XI, and XII.

        The soft palate must elevate and close the nasopharynx in order to produce guttural sounds such as "gut" or "kuh." Inspect palatal elevation as the patient says "ah." Ask the patient to say "gut, gut, gut" and "kuh, kuh, kuh." Palatal closure can also be tested by stimulating the gag reflex on each side while observing the palate.

        An idea of the function of the tongue can be gotten from having the patient say "la, la, la." The lips are tested by "me, me, me." Some disorders, such as myasthenia gravis, produce easy fatigability of these structures. Some idea about strength of respiratory muscles can be obtained by having the patient rapidly count to 30.

        Test phrases and words hallowed by usage can also be used to evaluate articulation:

        Hippopotamus
        Methodist Episcopal
        Third riding artillery brigade
        Truly rural
        Constantinople is the capital of Turkey
        Magnolia Petroleum Corporation
        Peter Piper picked a peck of pickled peppers
        Round the rugged rock the ragged rascal ran

Table 35a summarizes the tests for phonation and articulation.

    C.   Language. The outline below follows that given by Geschwind.

Table 35a. Phonation and articulation.

Test	Structure
Ah	Larynx and expiratory muscles
Gut, Kuh	Pharynx
La, la, la	Tongue
Me, me, me	Lips
Words, phrases, counting	All structures

1. Spontaneous speech. Spontaneous speech is best evaluated when the patient speaks at some length. The present illness query usually elicits a statement of some length. Also use questions such as: What did you do today before coming to see me? Describe your occupation. How do you perform (a particular task the patient is known to do)? How do you make a cake?

   An important feature of many cases of aphasia is that the dysfunction can be minimal; aphasia is not an all or nothing condition. As the patient speaks, listen carefully and note:
   a. *Fluency:* Words per unit of time. Place the patient into one of three groups: fluent, normal, nonfluent.
   b. *Circumlocution:* Use of phrases such as "what you eat with" instead of fork, or "what you write with" instead of pen.
   c. *"Empty" words:* Using generalized nonspecific terms to refer to specific objects: "thing," "place," "these." The patient never gets to the "punchline" words.
   d. *Paraphasia:* A common and important finding in aphasia. Phonemic or literal paraphasia is the substitution, addition, or deletion of phonemes: fish for dish, Kenry Hissinger for Henry Kissinger. Verbal or semantic paraphasia is the use of an incorrect word: "I cleaned my fingernails with an ice pick." Neologism is applied to speech when the source word is unrecognizable. Paraphasic speech commonly combines all these types.

e. *Word-finding difficulty:* Frequent hesitation before coming up with words (especially nouns), and at times using the wrong word.

f. *Delayed response to questions:* A delay in or difficulty in answering questions.

g. *Anxiety about speech:* Many patients are aware of their problems and become agitated when confronted with tasks involving language.

h. *Perseveration:* Using the same word over and over. Example: If asked to name a pencil, the patient will say "pencil" for each succeeding object regardless of what it is.

i. Note especially the handling of small grammatical words and numbers versus the handling of nouns. Some aphasic patients will handle the small words and/or numbers with much greater ease than nouns.

2. Comprehension
   a. Spoken language
      1. Use questions that can be answered by yes or no: Do you feel well? Do you live at . . .? Is this month . . .?
      2. Ask the patient to point at body parts (nose, leg) and objects in the room (chair, picture).
      3. Have the patient perform simple activities on command: Touch your nose. Move the chair.
   b. Written language
      1. Write a few simple questions and commands on paper such as: Show me your nose. Point to a chair. Is this month . . .?

3. Repetition. Ask the patient to repeat
   a. Letters
   b. Numbers
   c. Words
   d. Sentences

4. Naming. Show objects such as: comb, key, coin, billfold, watch, crystal on watch, winding stem on watch, tie, thumb, or fingers of patient or examiner. Do this rapidly, asking the patient to name each. Many examples of minimal aphasia are brought out only after showing the objects rapidly and repeating the sequence of objects in rapid succession.

5. Writing. Use numbers, letters, words, and sentences such as these taken from a first-grade reader: We saw

the horse run. A strong wind began to blow and blow.
Test the patient's ability to write by:

    a.   Command
    b.   Dictation
    c.   Copying

II. Other dominant hemisphere functions. Note that some of these tests will have been performed previously. These tests are not necessary on routine screening examinations but only when cortical function is suspected to be impaired.

    A.   Right-left orientation. Ask the patient to demonstrate various right and left parts of own and examiner's body. Command the patient to turn first in one, then the other direction. Ask the patient to say whether specific objects in the room are to the right or left of the patient.

    B.   Finger identification. Ask the patient to hold up the index finger, then the thumb, and then to identify the examiner's fingers. Then touch the finger on one hand and ask the patient to move the same finger on the other hand.

    C.   Calculation. Give oral and written tasks involving addition and multiplication, geared to educational level of patient.

III. Nondominant hemisphere functions

    A.   Drawing ability. Ask the patient to draw various shapes: triangle, square, daisy, bicycle, clock. Test the patient's ability to do this (1) by command, (2) by copying, and (3) by choosing correct shape from several drawn by examiner.

    B.   Topographic ability. Ask the patient to:

        1.   Draw outline of USA.
        2.   Describe north-south-east-west relationship of various places in relation to each other or patient: home, famous local places, New York.
        3.   Draw map of patient's home, or tell how to get from one place to another in the home, or from home to store.

    C.   Construction. The examiner takes tongue blades and has the patient first on command and then by copying form various designs: square, triangle.

    D.   Dressing. Hand the patient a shirt or robe and observe the ability to dress.

    E.   Facial recognition. Carry several 2×2 photographs of faces. Point out two, and later ask the patient to choose them from among the others. Also obtain history regarding facial recognition from family members and ward personnel. This refers to face recognition without auditory recognition: patients with certain lesions can recognize the person when the voice is heard.

    F.   Awareness of body and space. Observe for neglect of one-half of the body or surrounding space. Determine whether awareness of defect is present.

IV.   Bilateral hemisphere functions

    A.   Motor performance ("praxis"). The ability of the patient to perform simple and complex motor actions is tested in three ways:

        1.   By command

        2.   By imitation of examiner

        3.   By manipulating an object

    Each side of the body must be tested.

        1.   Face: stick out tongue
                    blow out cheeks
                    purse lips
                    make a kiss

        2.   Hands: make fist
                    wave goodbye
                    throw a kiss
                    shake hands
                    give military salute
                    pretend to play piano
                    use a key, comb, toothbrush
                    wind watch

        3.   Feet: walk normally
                    draw circle on floor with toe
                    stamp foot
                    kick ball

    B.   Handedness or laterality of motor functions. Determine the laterality of the following functions:

        1.   Handedness: Use of pen or eating utensils.

        2.   Eyedness: Eye camera is held to. Or have patient line a finger up with a vertical line in the room: picture frame, crack in wall. Do this with both eyes open. Then close first one eye then the other. The patient will discover only one eye has lined up the finger: this is the dominant eye.

        3.   Footedness: Which foot is used to kick a ball with or hop on?

Background Information

What follows is a fairly simple and diagrammatic approach to how the cortex handles higher functions. Our current knowledge is quite incomplete. There are a number of different concepts concerning how the cortex handles language. The concept outlined here is clinically useful and can be "taken to the bedside." This outline is based upon the elegant discussions of Geschwind (reference 9). Other approaches that can be used are covered in the references.

The dominant hemisphere.   The cerebral cortex receives sensory impulses, integrates them, and produces a motor response, "speech." In the great majority of individuals this is largely a function of the left or "dominant" hemisphere.

We will trace the path of a visual stimulus from the time of reading the word "monkey" through the spoken word (Fig 152). We will begin with the word in the left visual field for the purpose of illustrating certain features of the corpus callosum. Normally, of course, the word is perceived in both visual fields.

After "monkey" is seen in the left visual field, the stimulus goes to the right visual or calcarine cortex (area 17 of Brodmann). See sections

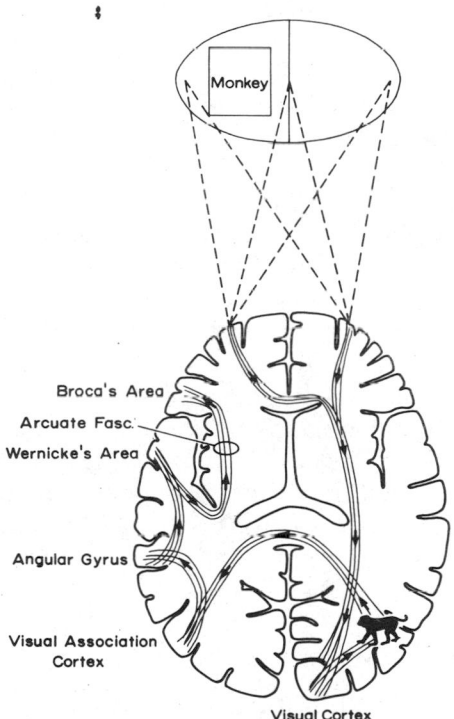

Figure 152.   Pathway taken by a visual impulse, beginning with perception of image in visual field and ending with Broca's area. For the purposes of discussion the image is shown only in the left visual field. (Adapted from *Language and the Brain*, by N. Geschwind. Copyright 1972 by Scientific American, Inc. All rights reserved. Used with permission.)

196A, Visual Acuity, and 196B, Visual Fields, for a description of the path taken. The stimulus next is transferred to a contiguous area of cortex, the visual association cortex of the parietal (areas 18 and 19 of Brodmann) and occipital lobes.

The concept of *association areas* is quite important. Current views of cerebral organization follow Flechsig's rule (reference 9). The gray matter of the cerebral cortex is composed of two types: primary cortex and association cortex. The principal primary areas include vision, hearing, sensory, and motor cortex. Each of these areas is connected only to the part of the body served (eg, retina for visual cortex) and to surrounding cortex by short U fibers. This surrounding or adjacent cortex is termed *association cortex* (Table 35b). The association cortex is connected to other association areas within the same hemisphere (intrahemispheral fibers) and to the sibling association area in the opposite hemisphere (transcallosal fibers). For example, the calcarine cortex of the right side has no direct connections with the left calcarine cortex or any other distant cortical areas. It is connected only to the retina by the visual radiation and to the adjacent visual association cortex of the occipital and parietal lobes. The visual association cortex, however, is connected to various areas in the cortex of the same hemisphere by intrahemispheric fibers, as well as the visual association cortex of the opposite hemisphere by transcallosal fibers that cross in the posterior portion (splenium) of the corpus callosum.

Similarly, there is a motor association cortex (the part dealing with the muscles of speech is Broca's area), a hearing association cortex (Wernicke's area), and a somesthetic association cortex (no eponym). These association areas have extensive distant cortical connections, quite in contrast to the absence of such connections in the case of the primary areas. The association areas of each side are connected by the corpus callosum. The visual association cortex of each side has intrahemispheric connections with the supramarginal and angular gyri of the same side, which in turn are connected to the hearing association cortex (see Fig 152). The hearing association cortex, Wernicke's area, is connected with the motor association cortex—Broca's area. The cortical integration of sensory impulses and the production of motor responses is carried out

Table 35b. Cerebral organization.

Primary Cortex	Association Area
Motor speech	Broca's area
Somesthetic	Somesthetic association area
Hearing (Heschl)	Wernicke's area
Vision	Visual association cortex
—	Supramarginal and angular gyri

through the connections of the association areas. The most prominent connection is the corpus callosum which connects each right area with its sibling on the left. The arcuate fasciculus connects Wernicke's and Broca's areas. Other connections within each hemisphere are not so anatomically discrete and have not been worked out in detail. Important clinical consequences follow the disconnection of various areas; these disconnection syndromes will be discussed later.

Let us return to the path taken by the visual stimulus "monkey." After being processed in unknown ways by the right visual association cortex, the impulse crosses through the corpus callosum to the left visual association cortex. The visual association cortex may be the place where visual images are stored. It must be admitted that this is speculative, however.

The next station is the supramarginal and angular gyri of the left parietal lobe. The supramarginal and angular gyri might be viewed as the granddaddy of the association areas, or the "association area of the association areas." They form the inferior parietal lobule (areas 39 and 40 of Brodmann). This area, which is highly developed in humans, is either rudimentary or absent in other higher mammals such as the apes. It is one of the last areas of the human brain to myelinate. Geschwind has suggested that this area is involved in connecting a sensory stimulus (here the written word monkey and perhaps the visual image monkey) with its spoken equivalent ("monkey"). This suggestion is supported by the anatomy of the connections of these gyri (the contiguity of the visual association cortex and the hearing association cortex) and by the clinical observation that discrete lesions can produce anomic aphasia. In this form of aphasia small grammatical words (articles, adverbs) are present, but the patient is bereft of nouns.

The next station is the hearing association cortex (Wernicke's area). The primary cortex and the association cortex are in the superior temporal gyrus near its posterior end. Collectively they constitute areas 41, 42, and 22 of Brodmann. Wernicke's area can be thought of as the "storehouse" of auditory associations (Geschwind). All words, at least nouns, must be processed in Wernicke's area before they are comprehended. This is apparently true of both spoken and written words and presumably is related to the fact that humans use spoken words before they learn written words. It is as if the brain has to hear the word "monkey" spoken internally before it can comprehend the word even when the word is read. This explains why comprehension for both spoken and written language is lost in lesions of Wernicke's area. One way to look at the functions of the three association areas described thus far (visual, angular-supramarginal, and hearing), is to conceive of the angular-supramarginal gyri receiving on one side the visual image of a monkey and on the other side "scanning" Wernicke's area to discover the spoken word that matches up with the visual image. Comprehension perhaps occurs when these two are matched or "associated."

Note that if the word "monkey" had been spoken instead of read as in our example, it would have gone immediately to the primary hearing cortex and thence to Wernicke's area. Presumably the angular-supramarginal gyri would have been activated then and told to "scan" the visual association cortex for the image that matched the word.

The stimulus "monkey" now goes from Wernicke's area to a portion of the motor association cortex known as Broca's area. It is located in the posterior portion of the third frontal gyrus (pars opercularis). Broca's area probably largely corresponds to Brodmann's area 44, although Mohr (reference 20) points out that it has no unique histological features. Broca's area is the association area of the primary motor cortex for speech. The question arises as to how the motor association cortex is related to the primary motor cortex. The primary motor cortex activates the individual muscles that participate in the action. Apparently, the knowledge of the sequence of muscle activation is contained in the motor association cortex. To put it another way, the "memory" or code for which muscles to activate and when to activate them is present in the motor association cortex. A lesion of the association cortex will result in inability to carry out a certain action such as walking, waving goodbye, making a fist on command, even though the strength is present. This is called *apraxia*. It is a loss of the memory of motor performance. Lesions of Broca's area will result in a loss of the memory of how to speak words. Comprehension will be intact since Wernicke's and other posterior areas are intact. The final cortical station for "monkey" is the primary motor cortex which, under the direction of Broca's area, activates the specific muscles necessary to speak the word. Table 36 summarizes the functions and locations of the language areas.

The relationship between language dominance and cerebral dominance for motor functions has been the subject of much discussion. Individuals can be characterized as to sidedness in terms of hands, eyes, ears, feet, and probably jaws also. Handedness and footedness are well correlated in right-handed (95%) but not as well correlated in left-handed (50%) individuals. Correlations between handedness and eyedness have not been clearly demonstrated. There is a problem in the definition of what constitutes handedness since many individuals have a preferred hand for a specific task: eg, writing will be done by the right hand and swinging a bat by the left. Using a battery of tests on a number of individuals, Subirana reported:

Pure right-handed	24%
Strong right-handed predominance	39%
Weak right-handed predominance	17%
Weak left-handed predominance	10%
Strong left-handed predominance	10%
Pure left-handed	0%

Area	Location	Function
Primary motor cortex	Precentral gyrus, area 4	Converts information from Broca's area into motor activity that produces speech.
Broca's area	Left third frontal gyrus, posterior portion (pars opercularis)	The motor association cortex for the face, tongue, lips, palate, pharynx, and respiration. Contains the "motor patterns" necessary to produce speech.
Arcuate fasciculus	A band of white fibers that connect Wernicke's area to Broca's area	Carries information from Wernicke's area to Broca's area.
Primary auditory cortex	Areas 41 and 42—the transverse gyri of the superior temporal convolution	Receives and analyzes auditory information.
Wernicke's area	Posterior portion of left superior temporal gyrus	The auditory association cortex. Analyzes incoming motor signals from the primary auditory cortex and probably makes sense out of them by matching incoming patterns and previously analyzed patterns stored in a memory bank. Necessary for both repetition and comprehension.
Perisylvian region	The area immediately surrounding the Sylvian fissure	Includes Broca's area, arcuate fasciculus, and Wernicke's area.
Border zone or watershed area	The area between the supply of the middle cerebral artery and the posterior cerebral-anterior cerebral arteries	Site of lesions producing the transcortical aphasias. The common denominator of these aphasias is that repetition is not disturbed, because Wernicke's area remains connected to Broca's area.
Angular gyrus and supramarginal gyrus	Form the inferior portion of the parietal lobe. They are at the confluence of auditory, somesthetic, and visual association cortices	Serve to connect the three association cortices to each other. When presented with visual information they scan Wernicke's area and arouse auditory information that matches the visual material. In a similar fashion they scan the visual association cortex when presented with auditory information.
Visual association cortex	Areas 18 and 19 of the occipital and parietal lobes just anterior to primary visual cortex	The area where primary visual information is analyzed.
Corpus callosum	Connects right and left cerebral hemispheres	Connects the sibling areas of each hemisphere.

One can easily see why there might be some confusion in the literature concerning the relationship of dominance for handedness to dominance for speech, especially since it is almost impossible to perform a battery of tests for handedness on aphasic patients.

Roberts has collected the following information from the literature with regard to aphasia and cerebral dominance for handedness: In left-handed patients, aphasia is twice as frequent with lesions of the left hemisphere as it is with lesions of the right hemisphere. If there is aphasia in a patient with a lesion of the right hemisphere, the patient is 13 times more likely to be left-handed than right-handed.

There is some evidence that there may be bilateral cortical representation for speech in left-handers but not right-handers (reference 19).

The question of determining cerebral dominance for speech is important clinically in planning neurosurgical operations and in attempting to localize the lesion in certain cases of aphasia. There is little problem in this correlation with "pure" right-handers, but progressively less correlation as the "pure" left-handed part of the spectrum is approached.

Other functions that are unique to the dominant hemisphere include:

1.   Right-left orientation
2.   Finger identification
3.   Calculation

Constructional apraxia can be seen in dominant hemisphere lesions, although it is less severe than when it occurs with nondominant hemisphere lesions.

The nondominant hemisphere. The right hemisphere has often been characterized as the "nondominant" or "minor" hemisphere or "the other side of the brain" (Bogen) in recognition of the fact that language functions in the great majority of people (whether right- or left-handed) are largely present in the left hemisphere. The uniqueness of the left hemisphere for language was discovered by Broca and Dax. Since that time, there has been much written on whether the right hemisphere has any unique functions. A view widely held for many years was that the right hemisphere was "mute and illiterate." One large problem is that it is difficult to compare performance in two patients who have similarly located lesions, one with a lesion in the left and the other with the lesion in the right hemisphere. The patient with the left hemisphere lesion often has aphasia and cannot be tested in the same way as the patient with the right hemisphere lesion.

A great stimulus to the question came in the early 1960s with a series of reports by Sperry and his colleagues on patients in whom the corpus callosum, the anterior commissure, and the hippocampal commissure had been transected in an attempt to aid in the control of intractable epilepsy.

In these patients with "split brains" it was possible to test the separate functions of the hemispheres. The following account of one of their patients, "W. J.," is taken from Pines. W. J. would obey commands such as "raise your arm" involving the right side of his body but did not obey the same commands involving the left side. When blindfolded, he could identify where he was touched on the right side but not on the left side. His left hand would do things that his right hand "deplored": one hand would pull his pants down while the other was pulling them up; on another occasion he threatened his wife with his left hand while his right hand tried to restrain the left hand. The right hemisphere was unable to do tasks which required language comprehension. These observations seemed to bear out the suspicion that the right hemisphere was mute, illiterate, and imbecilic when compared to its language endowed twin. Then one day W. J. was given the task of copying a Greek cross. The right hand was unable to do this; a few disconnected lines were drawn. But the left hand copied the outline swiftly and surely. On other occasions, W. J. could arrange colored blocks according to a diagram without any trouble with his left hand but could not even begin to do as well with his right hand. These observations suggested the right hemisphere was superior to the left in visual-spatial relationships.

Reports by other workers also suggest that the right hemisphere may be superior to the left in certain areas involving visual-spatial relationships. Below are listed some functions that may be either unique to or at least done better by the right hemisphere. The review by Joynt and Goldstein and volume 4 of the *Handbook of Clinical Neurology* summarizes the evidence for and against the idea of the right hemispheric localization of these functions.

1. Spatial orientation
   a. Extrapersonal space. Patients with lesions of the right hemisphere can neglect the left half of their visual space. There are problems with route-findings, even in familiar surroundings such as their own home, reading maps, and topographical memory. See Benton for a good review.
   b. Personal space. The left half of the body is neglected just as the left half of space. In the words of a patient of Lhermitte: "I have lost my left half." The spatial perception of body structure is disordered.
2. Construction. The right hemisphere can comprehend patterns and diagrams better than the left. Thus patients with right hemisphere lesions can have what is termed constructional apraxia: they have difficulty assembling, building, and drawing. This is probably secondary to the defect in spatial orientation described above. One way of describing some of these problems is that they deal with "part-whole" relationships. The patients cannot

see part of a pattern and deduce what the whole pattern will look like, even in a test such as the examiner drawing a part of a circle and asking the patient to complete the circle. Pattern recognition may well be one of the unique properties of the right hemisphere.

3. Clothes dressing. A prominent sign of a right hemisphere lesion can be "dressing apraxia," a severe difficulty in putting on an article of clothing or even an inability to dress. This involves perceiving the spatial relationships of a garment and relating them to the spatial structure of the body.

4. Facial recognition. The ability to recognize faces can be lost. Joynt and Goldstein report that a patient of Charcot's "misinterpreted his reflection in a mirror as another person and stepped aside to let him pass." Facial identification involves the recognition of visual-spatial patterns of faces. Some of these patients use speech or other cues to recognize people.

5. Motor persistence. Patients with right hemisphere lesions may not maintain a motor act such as keeping the eyes closed, maintaining fixation of gaze to one side, keeping mouth open, keeping the tongue protruded (Fisher). There are no good speculations as to the mechanism.

The corpus callosum. For many years the role of the corpus callosum was unknown. There were no discernible differences between patients and animals in whom it was absent or in whom it had been transected, and normals. The tongue-in-cheek suggestion was that it existed "to keep the hemispheres from sagging." But beginning in the 1950s Sperry, Myers, Gazzaniga, and others reported a series of experiments that began to shed light on the functioning of the corpus callosum and also contributed to an understanding of the abilities of each hemisphere. Myers experiments in callosum-sectioned cats and monkeys (summarized by Sperry in 1961) demonstrated that:

1. When both the corpus callosum and optic chiasm are split so that information presented to the left eye goes only to the left hemisphere and that presented to the right goes only to the right hemisphere, the animal is unable to perform with the right eye and right hemisphere tasks that were learned with the left eye and left hemisphere. There is "a complete amnesia for the visual training experienced with the first eye."

2. If only the optic chiasm is cut, tasks learned by one eye are readily performed by the other eye.

3. If the animal has the optic chiasm cut, is trained with the left eye, and the callosum then cut, both eyes still perform the task learned by one. The learning had been transferred from one hemisphere to the other via the corpus callosum. In Sperry's words (1961): "... the corpus callosum is shown to be instrumental in laying down a second set of

memory traces, or engrams, in the contralateral hemisphere—a mirror image duplicate."

Some of the dysfunctions in patients with callosal section were seen in the case of W. J. that was described earlier in this section. Gazzaniga has reported some illuminating experiments on human subjects who were tested in such a fashion that visually presented information went only to one hemisphere or the other (by showing the stimulus rapidly in either the left or right visual field):

1. When the response of the subject was to say yes if a dot appeared in the visual field, the response occurred 30 msec faster when the dot was presented to the left hemisphere. Presumably the 30 msec longer that occurred when the information was presented to the right hemisphere was at least partially due to time used for transfer across the callosum.

2. Tasks requiring verbal processing were done more quickly when the information was first presented to the left hemisphere.

3. When the task was for the subject to indicate manually if information presented was identical (AA would require a response; AB or Ab would not), both hemispheres were equally adept.

4. If the task was to indicate if letters belonged to the same class (Aa would require a response; Ab would not), the left hemisphere responded faster than the right.

5. Tasks requiring visual pattern discrimination (eg, judging which of two zigzag figures are oriented in the same direction) were done 14 msec faster by the right hemisphere than the left.

An interesting experiment by Levy, Trevarthen, and Pines with split-brain patients involved taking pictures of faces and cutting them in half, then pasting various combinations together such, as half an old man's face to half a young woman's face. This composite picture was then flashed briefly on a screen so that one-half went to the right hemisphere and the other half to the left hemisphere. After seeing the composite picture the subjects were shown the original uncut pictures and asked to pick the one seen on the screen. They invariably picked the one whose half-face had been presented to the right hemisphere, thus lending support to the clinical observation that facial recognition is a function of the right hemisphere. But if asked to *tell* which face was seen, the subjects described the half-face presented to the left hemisphere.

In summary, our knowledge of possible unique hemispheric functions and the role of the corpus callosum is presently rudimentary and much of it is speculative. The function of the corpus callosum appears to be to transfer information from one hemisphere to the other. If indeed each hemisphere has unique functions, the role of the callosum may be to make available to one hemisphere the knowledge or special abilities of the other. An example could be the interpretation of an electrocardiogram: the right hemisphere recognizes the "pattern" while the left hemisphere analyzes the information in detail. The corpus callosum enables the hemispheres to work together, each doing what it can do best. Ultimately, the information from the right hemisphere is passed to the left via the callosum, integrated with the analysis by the left hemisphere, and expressed in a "verbal package" assembled by the left hemisphere.

Clinical Significance

In this discussion of the types of aphasia, we will begin with Broca's area and proceed posteriorly.

Broca's aphasia (motor aphasia, expressive aphasia, anterior aphasia, nonfluent aphasia). Word production is sparse ("nonfluent") and words are emitted with great effort. Grammar is simplified, and sentence structure is condensed—"agrammatism." Content is largely nouns and action verbs with little use of small filler words, leading to the term "telegraphic speech." Rhythm and melody are disturbed. Writing is always abnormal. Most patients have an associated right hemiplegia due to involvement of the primary motor cortex. Repetition is quite abnormal. Auditory and visual comprehension is either intact or largely so, since the posterior speech areas are not affected. Patients become very frustrated and angry as they hear themselves speak, since self-monitoring is intact due to the fact that the posterior speech areas are spared. The lesion involves Broca's area. Bucco-facial and respiratory apraxia is present: on command the patient is unable to perform such activities as sticking out the tongue, puckering the lips, whistling, coughing, sniffing, and the like. Apraxia of the left upper extremity is present. A fascinating aspect of this type of aphasia is that many patients have intact singing, swearing, and serial speech (such as counting, months of the year, etc.) (reference 30).

Mohr (references 20 and 22) does not feel that the classical view of Broca's aphasia presented above corresponds to clinical and autopsy material. He describes two different syndromes:

1. Small lesions limited to Broca's area produce a spectrum of features. The mildest cases have a very slight disturbance in the melody of speech, in which "the mechanisms of speech are suddenly altered in such a way as to be possibly more apparent to the victim than the beholder." Severely affected patients are mute and have severe dyspraxia of both upper extremities, oral, buccal, lingual, and respiratory function. There is no agrammatism or other features of Broca's aphasia as described above, although there is some slight degree of language disorder when tested carefully. Improvement in the mute patients is rapid with the emergence of dysarthric speech that has no elements of aphasia. The lesions in these cases were small discrete infarcts produced by emboli lying at the origin

of the anterior branches of the upper division of the left middle cerebral artery.

2. Large lesions in the Sylvian region involving the operculum, including Broca's area, insula, and the adjacent cerebral cortex in the territory supplied by the upper division of the middle cerebral artery. These patients have a very different clinical picture from the one described for Broca's area infarcts. Initially there is mutism and a profound total aphasia, in contrast to mutism with very faint evidence of aphasia in the patients with lesions limited to Broca's area. Over a period of time the mutism and aphasia evolve into the classical picture of Broca's aphasia: agrammatism, telegraphic speech, and other disturbances of language and communication as described. This latter picture is present only months or years after the onset of illness. Mohr's conclusions are as follows (reference 21):

> Cases of embolic or hemorrhagic stroke affecting the anterior superior Sylvian region, including the operculum, insula, and subjacent white matter appear to produce a spectrum of deficits predicted both by lesion site and size.
>
> Broca's area appears to be but one of many regions along the Sylvian region that integrate with one another to allow speaking. The brain appears to be able to overcome Broca's area infarction, perhaps by recruitment of adjacent regions on the same side or by transcollosal pathways through the minor hemisphere. Mutism, then vocal apraxia, not a central language disorder, seem to result from Broca's area infarction.
>
> The larger disorder referred to as Broca's aphasia appears to require a much larger lesion, involving most of the upper operculum and insula. The spread of deficit into tasks other than speaking indicates a more fundamental disorder shared by all modalities of speech production and reception. The linguistic features are different from Wernicke's aphasia, and seem distinctive.
>
> The requirement that the lesion be larger than Broca's area suggests Broca's area may not be important for language function itself. It suggests that the language function mediated by the Sylvian operculum and insula might, by analogy with an orchestra, be a synergistic product of more elementary individual speech functions accomplished all along the region, and be resistant to significant persisting functional loss until enough elements have been lost that their cooperative results are no longer recognizable.

Conduction aphasia (central aphasia of Kurt Goldstein).   Three features are characteristically present in this type of aphasia (reference 1): (1) Fluent speech—though not so fluent as Wernicke's aphasia—with notable paraphasia. The paraphasia is commonly literal (fish for dish). Patients often become quite frustrated as they hear themselves speak, indicating the posterior speech areas are functioning as monitors. (2) Normal comprehension. (3) Grossly defective repetition. These three conditions must

be met to make the diagnosis. Additional common but not necessary features include: (1) Anomia of variable degree; (2) inability to read aloud
(due to repetition disturbances), although silent reading is normal in terms
of comprehension; (3) dysgraphia, varying from mild misspellings to complete agraphia; (4) buccofacial and bilateral upper limb apraxia, in the
face of mild or absent motor deficits; (5) other neurological abnormalities
including a mild right hemiparesis and hemisensory deficit.

The most common lesion lies deep to the supramarginal gyrus, in
the left anterior and inferior parietal area. This lesion interrupts the
arcuate fasciculus connecting Wernicke's and Broca's areas. A less common location is a lesion which destroys the first temporal gyrus on the
left, obliterating all of the left auditory cortex. Apraxia is associated with
the former lesion but not the latter.

*Wernicke's aphasia (receptive aphasia, sensory aphasia, fluent aphasia,
posterior aphasia).* An outpouring of words with absent comprehension
and repetition. Broca's area is running on and on without any control
from the posterior speech area of Wernicke. Since Wernicke's area is required for the comprehension of both spoken and written words, it is
understandable that comprehension—written or spoken—and repetition
are both defective. Paraphasia is common. The patient's speech is continuous and rapid—"logorrhea"—and the physician has little or no opportunity to get a word in. Such patients are usually very disruptive
influences on the wards and in the home and often have to be institutionalized. On occasion, Wernicke's aphasia may occur initially and
then evolve into a conduction aphasia. A consideration of the lesion of
Wernicke's—the posterior part of the superior temporal gyrus (auditory
association cortex)—and that described above for conduction aphasia
makes this understandable. An interesting feature of Wernicke's aphasia
is that commands involving the entire body ("stand up," "turn around")
are often intact, suggesting the right hemisphere plays a role in understanding this type of command (Table 37a).

Transcortical aphasias. 1. Isolation of speech area. A lesion that leaves
the perisylvian structures intact and connected to each other but cut off
from the rest of the cortex by extensive destruction of the entire border
zone. Since Wernicke's area is connected to Broca's area, repetition is
intact. Characteristics of a case reported by Quadfasel, Segarra, and
Geschwind are:

1.   Absent spontaneous speech and lack of comprehension.
2.   Intact repetition in addition to completion of certain phrases.
     For example, when "Roses are red..." was said to her, she
     would say "Roses are red, violets are blue, sugar is sweet, and
     so are you." She could learn new songs and sing them. She

would repeat sentences said to her in a parrotlike fashion (echo-lalia).

3.   Penmanship was intact (since Broca's area was intact) but writing was absent. For example, the patient could copy but not express ideas. Comprehension was absent because connections to other cortical areas were lacking. Written material could not be connected to Wernicke's area for verbal expression and therefore comprehension. Similarly, spoken information did not have access to the visual association area so images could not be aroused by speech.

2. Transcortical motor aphasia. Produced by a lesion in the frontal lobe anterior or superior to Broca's area. Speech is nonfluent and comprehension is relatively preserved, producing a similarity to Broca's aphasia. However, repetition is remarkably preserved: the patient can easily repeat long sentences that are phonetically and syntactically complex. Upper extremity weakness may be more pronounced proximally than distally because of the watershed distribution (reference 27).

3. Transcortical sensory aphasia. Produced by large lesions in the watershed distribution of the parietooccipitotemporal areas that destroy the connection of these areas with Wernicke's area, which again remains connected to Broca's area. Comprehension is defective as one would expect. Once again the patient can effortlessly repeat long complex sentences.

Anomic aphasia.   Fluent empty speech that is strikingly devoid of substantive words such as nouns and action verbs. Repetition is intact. Comprehension varies from intact to impaired. Most of the cases have a left angular gyrus lesion, but it is also seen in lesions in other locations—even the frontal lobe.

Pure word deafness.   These patients cannot understand the spoken word at all, although hearing is intact. They comprehend the written word normally and can read aloud without problems. Seen with bilateral temporal lobe lesions or a single deep left-sided temporal lesion that separates Wernicke's area from the primary auditory cortex. Many of these cases are seen in the recovery phase of Wernicke's aphasia.

Alexia without agraphia (pure word blindness).   Patients comprehend the spoken word normally but cannot read. They can understand letters and words traced in their palms or spelled aloud. Words are written correctly either spontaneously or to dictation, but in a few minutes the patient cannot read what he just wrote. The lesion involves the splenium of the corpus callosum plus the left visual cortex. A right homonymous hemianopsia is present. Visual information reaches the right visual cortex from the left visual field, but it cannot be transmitted across the corpus

Table 37a. Simplified aphasia summary.

Description	Fluency	Repetition	Comprehension	Lesion
Broca's Agrammatic telegraphic speech uttered with great effort and frustration.	Nonfluent	Impaired	Intact	Broca's area and perhaps much more.
Conduction Paraphasia and severe repetition disturbance, with normal comprehension	Fluent	Impaired	Intact	Lesion deep to the left supramarginal gyrus, destroying the arcuate fasciculus. Less often a lesion obliterating the first temporal gyrus.
Wernicke's Fluent paraphasic speech	Fluent	Impaired	Impaired	Posterior portion of the left superior temporal gyrus.
Transcortical aphasia 1. Isolated speech area: repetition strikingly intact—to point of echolalia—but comprehension nonexistent.	Fluent	Intact	Absent	Border zone.
2. Transcortical motor aphasia: nonfluent speech, lack of spontaneous speech, but remarkably intact repetition.	Nonfluent	Intact	Intact	In frontal lobe anterior or superior to Broca's area.
3. Transcortical sensory aphasia. Repetition intact, no comprehension.	Fluent	Intact	Absent	Border zone parietotemporooccipital lobes.
Anomic aphasia No nouns.	Fluent	Intact	Varies	Left angular gurus when marked.

				Lesion location
Pure word deafness Cannot understand the spoken word, but normal comprehension of writing.	Normal	Absent to voice	Absent to voice	Bilateral temporal lobe lesions, or deep in left posterior temporal lobe.
Alexia without agraphia Pure word blindness. Can understand spoken but not written word.	Normal	Absent to reading	Absent to reading	Left visual cortex and splenium of the corpus callosum.
Alexia with agraphia Cannot read or write. Gerstmann's syndrome often present, plus anomia.	Normal	Present to voice	Present to voice	Dominant angular gyrus.

Table 37b.   Helpful clues in aphasia localization.

Clue	Anatomical Localization	Comment
Repetition disturbed	Perisylvian speech areas	Broca's, conduction, Wernicke's.
Repetition intact	Border zone or watershed area	Transcortical aphasias.
Pronounced phonemic paraphasia	Supramarginal gyrus	Mild to moderate phonemic paraphasia seen with other lesions. Presence of buccofacial apraxia clinches supramarginal gyrus localization.
Buccofacial apraxia	Suprasylvian (frontoparietal) operculum	Often found in conduction aphasia, Broca's aphasia, and mixed aphasia where there is damage to the suprasylvian area.
Severe anomia	Inferior temporooccipital juncture	Often associated with an upper right quadranopsia.

callosum to the left visual association area and angular gyrus—which are normal. Tactile stimuli from either hand can reach these areas however, accounting for the ability to "read" words traced on the palms (this is the same route used in braille).

Alexia with agraphia.   Cannot read, write, or spell. Often associated with Gerstmann's syndrome plus anomia and constructional apraxia. These elements make up the syndrome of lesions of the dominant angular gyrus. Gerstmann's syndrome is composed of finger agnosia, right-left disorientation, acalculia, and agraphia.

Language disturbances with left thalamic hemorrhage.   Mohr et al (1975) and Reynolds et al (1978) have reported left thalamic hemorrhage associated with language disturbance. These patients had virtually intact language testing when fully alert, but often went suddenly into a state of logorrheic paraphasia resembling delirium. Repetition from dictation was intact.

Table 37a summarizes the types of aphasia. Table 37b lists a few clues helpful in anatomical localization. Figure 153 shows the location of perisylvian structures and the border zone.

Many cases of left and right hemispheric dysfunction are due to vascular lesions and neoplasms. Trauma accounts for others. In certain

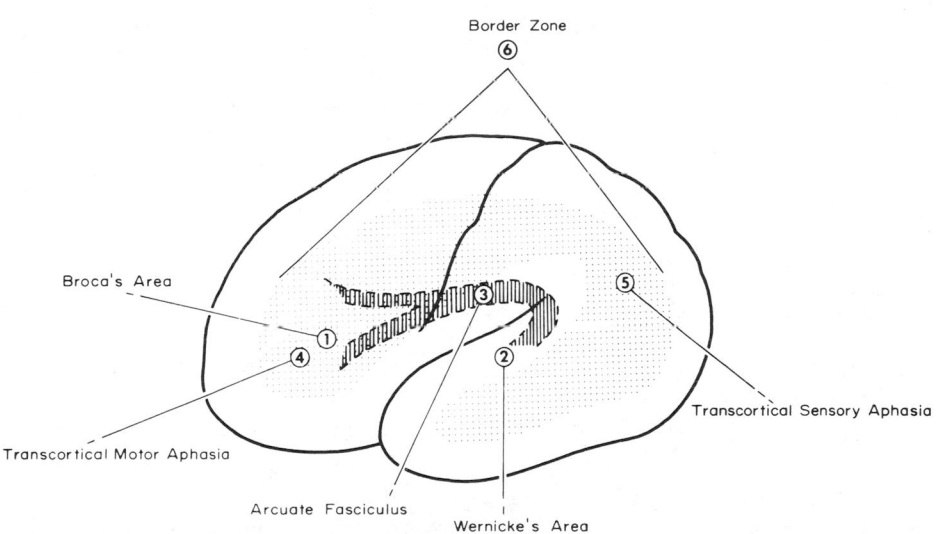

Figure 153.   Anatomy and localization of some of the aphasias. Modified from Benson DF, Geschwind N: The aphasias and related disturbances, in Baker AB, Baker LH (eds): *Clinical Neurology.* Hagerstown, Md, Harper and Row, 1977, vol 1, chap 8. Used with permission.

disease states, especially those characterized by delirium, there occur the so-called nonaphasic disorders of speech. These are separated from aphasias only with much difficulty. The reader is referred to Geschwind for a further discussion (reference 13).

Brust et al studied 850 stroke patients and discovered aphasia in 21%. Of the patients with aphasia, 32% had fluent aphasia (Wernicke's most often) and 68% had nonfluent aphasia (a mixed type most often). Hemiparesis was present in 74% of fluent aphasics and 95% of nonfluents. Homonymous hemianopsia was present in 32% of fluents and 55% of nonfluents. With regard to prognosis 32% of nonfluents and 12% of fluents died in 4–12 weeks.

The clinical significance of disorders of phonation has been given in the section on nerves IX and X. Disturbances of articulation can be caused by lesions involving nerves V, VII, IX, X, XI, and XII. These are discussed in the appropriate sections.

One disorder of articulation deserves particular mention: pseudobulbar palsy is caused by bilateral lesions involving the supranuclear corticobulbar fibers to the nuclei of the cranial nerves supplying the articulatory muscles, that is, the muscles of the face, jaws, tongue, and larynx. It is caused by any process which bilaterally interrupts the supranuclear innervation. This includes strokes affecting both sides of the brain, multiple sclerosis, and the hypertensive lacunar state. The latter two interfere with the innervation by multiple small lesions. The patients show emotional incontinence with frequent randomly occurring bouts of crying (usually) or laughter. A notable feature is progressive difficulty in using lips, jaws, tongue, and pharynx. The problem usually begins with the more complex motor actions such as speaking but ultimately involves even swallowing. As might be expected of a supranuclear disorder, the motor power is present but the patient does not know how to use the muscles.

Disorders of the minor hemisphere were included under Background Information.

Selected References

1. Benson DF, Sheremata W, Bouchard R, et al: Conduction aphasia: A clinicopathological study. *Arch Neurol* 28:339–346, 1973.
2. Benson DF, Geschwind N: The aphasias and related disturbances, in Baker AB, Baker LH (eds): *Clinical Neurology*. Hagerstown, Md, Harper and Row, 1977, vol 1, chap 8.
3. Benton AL: *Right-Left Discrimination and Finger Localization: Development and Pathology*. New York, Hoeber Medical Division, Harper and Row, 1959.
4. Benton AL: Disorders of spatial orientation, in Vinken PJ, Bruyn GW (eds): *Handbook of Clinical Neurology: Disorders of Higher Nervous*

Activity. Amsterdam, North-Holland Publishing Co, 1969, vol 3, pp 212–228.

5. Brust JC, Shafer SQ, Richter RW, Bruun B: Aphasia in acute stroke. *Stroke* 7:167–174, 1976.

6. Cohen DN, Salanga VD, Hully W, Steinberg MC, Hardy RW: Alexia without agraphia. *Neurology* 26:445–459, 1976.

7. Gazzaniga MS: One brain—two minds? *Am Scientist* 60:311–317, 1972.

8. Fischer CM: Left hemiplegia and motor impersistence. *J Nerv Ment Dis* 123:201–218, 1956.

9. Geschwind N: Disconnexion syndromes in animals and man. *Brain* 88:237–294, 585–644, 1965.

10. Geschwind N: Disturbances of language, perception, and memory, in Keefer CS, Wilkins RW (eds): *Medicine.* Boston, Little, Brown, 1970, pp 973–978.

11. Geschwind N: Language and the brain. *Sci Am* 226:76–83, 1972.

12. Geschwind N: Neurological foundations of language, in *Progress in Learning Disabilities.* New York, Grune and Stratton, 1967, pp 182–198.

13. Geschwind N: Nonaphasic disorders of speech. *Int J Neurol* 4:207–214, 1964.

14. Geschwind N: *Selected Papers on Language and the Brain.* Boston, D Reidel Publishing Co, 1974.

15. Geschwind N: "Wings"—a neurologist at the theater. *N Eng J Med* 300:569–571, 1979.

16. Goodglass H, Kaplan E: *The Assessment of Aphasia and Related Disorders.* Philadelphia, Lea and Febiger, 1972.

17. Joynt RN, Goldstein MN: Minor cerebral hemisphere. *Adv Neurol* 7:147–183, 1975.

18. Levy J, Trevarthen C, Sperry RW: Perception of bilateral chimeric images following hemispheric disconnexion. *Brain* 95:61–78, 1972.

19. Milner B, Branch C, Rasmussen T: Evidence for bilateral speech representation in non-right-handers. *Trans Am Neurol Assoc* 91:306–308, 1966.

20. Mohr JP: Broca's area and Broca's aphasia, in Whitaker H, Whitaker HA (eds): *Studies in Neurolinguistics.* New York, Academic Press, 1976, vol 1, pp 201–235.

21. Mohr JP: Superficial and deep anterosuperior sylvian syndromes. *Neurol Neurocir Psyquiatr* 18(2–3 Suppl): 27–33, 1977.

22. Mohr JP, Pessin MS, Finkelstein S, Funkenstein HH, Duncan GW, Davis KR: Broca's aphasia: Pathologic and clinical. *Neurology* 28:311–324, 1978.

23. Mohr JP, Watters WC, Duncan GW: Thalamic hemorrhage and aphasia. *Brain Language* 2:3–17, 1975.

24. Naeser MA, Hayward RW: Lesion localization in aphasia with cranial

computed tomography and the Boston Diagnostic Aphasia Exam. *Neurology* 28:545–551, 1978.

25. Pines M: *The Brain Changers: Scientists and the New Mind Control.* New York, Harcourt Brace Jovanovich, 1973.
26. Reynolds AF, Harris AB, Ojemann GA, Turner PT: Aphasia and left thalamic hemorrhage. *J Neurosurg* 48:570–574, 1978.
27. Rubens AB: Transcortical motor aphasia, in Whitaker H, Whitaker HA (eds): *Studies in Neurolinguistics.* New York, Academic Press, 1976, pp 293–303.
28. Sperry RW: Cerebral organization and behavior. *Science* 133:1749–1757, 1961.
29. Vinken PJ, Bruyn GW (eds): *Handbook of Clinical Neurology: Disorders of Speech, Perception, and Symbolic Behavior.* Amsterdam, North-Holland Publishing Co, 1969, vol 4.
30. Yamadori A, Osumi Y, Masuhara S, Okubo M: Preservation of singing in Broca's aphasia. *J Neurol Neurosurg Psychiat* 40:221–224, 1977.

195. Cranial Nerve I: Olfactory Nerve

H. KENNETH WALKER, MD

Definition

Hyperosmia: increased olfactory acuity.
Hypoosmia: diminished olfactory acuity.
Anosmia: inability to recognize odors; may be unilateral or bilateral.
Dysosmia: an abnormal sense of smell.

Technique

Carry a vial of nonirritating substance in your bag: vanilla, lemon, and freshly ground coffee are good examples. If you don't have these, tobacco or scented soap will do. These odors stimulate the olfactory receptors. Do not use irritating odors such as camphor or menthol since they stimulate the trigeminal sensory receptors in addition to the olfactory receptors, potentially giving a false result.

Inform the patient that you are going to test the sense of smell. Ask the patient to place an index finger over one nostril to block it off, eg, right index finger over right nostril, and then to close the eyes. Instruct the patient to sniff repetitively and to tell you when an odor is detected, identifying the odor if recognized. Bring the test odor up to within a foot or less of the nose. Do not touch the patient when doing the test since the movement of your body will give a clue as to when the test object is being presented. Do not give any auditory clues either. Repeat the process with the other nostril. Smell is intact when the patient reports detection of an odor. Recognition of the odor involves olfactory memory, which is a higher cortical function.

Background Information

The olfactory epithelium occupies about 2.5 sq cm of area at the apex of each nostril. This patch of yellowish brown mucosa is located in a small cavity off the main nasal passage. For this reason "sniffing" provides more rapid stimulation than normal breathing. The receptors are surrounded by nasal mucous membrane and covered by a thin layer of moisture. There are two types of receptors. The first type consists of trigeminal nerve fibers which are sensitive to irritating substances and temperature; the neuroanatomy is similar to that of pain and temperature receptors elsewhere in the body.

The second type consists of olfactory nerve cells which form the principal receptor. This cell is both a receptor and a bipolar first-order neuron. Each cell has six to eight hairlike filaments, or cilia, $10–12~\mu$ in length. They project from the surface into the overlying liquid. The olfactory chemoreceptors are assumed to be on these cilia.

A molecule must be water soluble so it can penetrate the watery film overlying the receptors in order to produce an odor. The molecule also must be lipid soluble in order to penetrate the phospholipid layer of the surface membrane of the chemoreceptor. At this point the process begins that ultimately leads to recognition of the odor. Many theories have been proposed to account for odor identification; no theory is entirely satisfactory. Amoore and his group have suggested that the geometric shape and size of a molecule determine its odor. All molecules having the same shape and size would share the same primary odor, and would fit into the olfactory receptors in a "lock and key" fashion. Amoore has identified seven primary odors: camphoraceous, musky, floral, pepperminty, ethereal, pungent, and putrid. A fair amount of data supports his concept that chemicals sharing the same primary odor have similar stereochemical configurations.

Axons from the olfactory cell, grouped together as the olfactory nerve, penetrate the cribriform plate and synapse in the olfactory bulb.

The structure of the olfactory bulb is quite complex. The structural units are discrete spherical bodies, the glomeruli, about 0.2 mm in diameter. In these bodies the axons from the olfactory cell (first-order neuron) synapse with the primary dendrites of the mitral cells (second-order neuron). The number of receptors that converge on the mitral cell is very large, about 100:1. Other cell types in the bulb include the tufted cells, whose dendrites also participate in synaptic connections in the glomeruli. The olfactory bulbs apparently participate extensively in the processing of olfactory information. There are at least five feedback loops and other interconnections within the bulb. There are connections with the other olfactory bulb via the anterior commissure. Centrifugal fibers conveying impulses from the brain influence the activity of the bulb. The bulb apparently follows the neural organization of the visual and other sensory systems, in which there is an interplay of inhibitory and excitatory mechanisms acting to process incoming information under the efferent influence of the cortex.

Axons leave the olfactory bulb as the olfactory tract. Tufted cell axons mainly pass laterally to the anterior commissure and thus to the contralateral olfactory bulb. Mitral cell axons project centrally. The central areas to which the olfactory bulb projects include the anterior perforated space, the amygdaloid nucleus, and the cortex of the piriform lobe. There are secondary and tertiary connections with various other areas, including the limbic system.

Clinical Significance

Hyperosmia, or lowered threshold for odors, has been reported with Addison's disease and mucoviscidosis. Clinical perception of hyperosmia is ordinarily just about impossible either by history taking or by testing.

Hypoosmia is usually due to local processes that involve both the nasal and olfactory mucosa, such as rhinitis due to the common cold or allergy, smoking, certain industrial fumes, and intranasal polyps or carcinoma. Pernicious anemia, diabetes, and vitamin A deficiency also cause diminished olfactory acuity. Pernicious anemia can also cause anosmia. Hypoosmia occurs after total laryngectomy for reasons that are not known.

Anosmia may be bilateral or unilateral. Bilateral anosmia may be recognized by the patient, but unilateral anosmia is usually not perceived. Head trauma is probably the most frequent cause, with an incidence of 7.5% in one large series. Blows to the occiput are five times more likely to produce anosmia than blows to the forehead because of the contrecoup effect. The injury can be so trivial as to go almost unnoticed. Tumors of the floor of the anterior fossa such as meningiomas of the sphenoid ridge or olfactory groove can produce anosmia which is usually unilateral. Meningitis or abscess associated with osteomyelitis of the frontal or ethmoid bones can produce anosmia. Congenital absence of smell is present in albinos. Subarachnoid hemorrhage can cause anosmia. Hysteria is another cause for anosmia and can be identified by testing perception for coffee or vanilla which principally stimulate the olfactory cell receptors) and ammonia (which is principally a trigeminal nerve stimulator). In anosmia of organic cause the ammonia can be detected but the coffee odor cannot.

Olfactory hallucinations occur almost always for unpleasant odors such as burnt rubber. They are seen as the aura in uncinate epilepsy, in withdrawal states, and in psychiatric states.

A valuable clinical corollary is that the patient often reports hypoosmia and anosmia as a decreased or absent ability to taste food. For example, pernicious anemia is a leading possibility in an elderly patient with spastic paraparesis and anemia who complains he no longer enjoys eating because food does not taste the same.

Selected References

1.   Amoore JE, Johnson JW Jr, Rubin M: The stereochemical theory of odor. *Sci Am* 210:42–49, 1964.
2.   Doving KB: Problems in the physiology of olfaction, in Schultz HW, Day EA, Libbey LM (eds): *Symposium on Foods: The Chemistry and Physiology of Flavors.* Westport, Ct, Avi Publishing Co, 1967, chap 3, pp 52–94.
3.   Brodal A: *Neurological Anatomy,* ed 2. New York, Oxford University Press, 1969, pp 509–545.
4.   Schneider RA: The sense of smell in man: Its physiological basis. *New Eng J Med* 277(6):299–303, 1967.
5.   Sumner D: Post-traumatic anosmia. *Brain* 87:107–120, 1964.
6.   Douek E: *The Sense of Smell and Its Abnormalities.* Edinburgh and London, Churchill Livinstone, 1974.
7.   Thawley SE: Disorders of taste and smell. *South Med J* 71:267–270, 1978.

196. Cranial Nerve II: Optic Nerve
A. Visual Acuity

J. DONALD FITE, MD
H. KENNETH WALKER, MD

Definition

Normal visual acuity is 20/20 to 20/10 in each eye. 20/30 vision is considered normal below the age of 6 years.

Technique

Visual acuity is one of the measurements of macular (cone) function and is based upon the use of standardized test type. Empirically, the image of the 20/20 size test type subtends an arc of 5 minutes on the retina when placed at 20 feet (6 m) from the subject. Each component of the letter subtends 1 minute of arc. Other letters on the Snellen chart when placed at proper distances also subtend an arc of 5 minutes (Fig 154). Hence, when the 20/100 letter is placed at 100 feet (28 m) from the subject, its image is the same size on the retina as the image of the 20/20 letter placed at 20 feet (6 m). As a prerequisite for good visual acuity, the image must be focused sharply upon the retina. This is the function of the crystalline lens of the eye.

VISUAL ACUITY

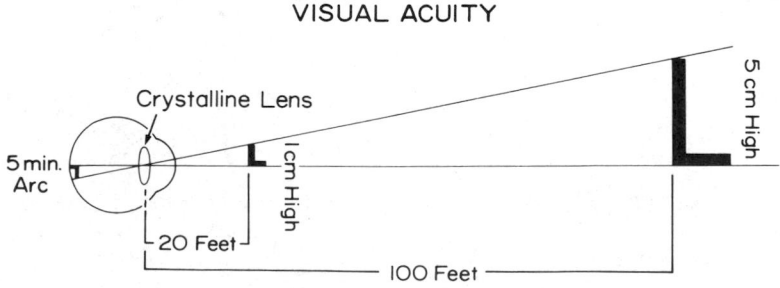

Figure 154.   The measurement of visual acuity.

With the accommodative mechanism of the eye at rest, the eye is said to be emmetropic if the image is in focus on the retina. If the image is not in focus on the retina, the eye is said to be ametropic or have a refractive error. The determination of the refractive error requires appropriate equipment and skills which are beyond the scope of this book. Fortunately, the refractive error can be corrected by a simple universal lens, the pinhole disk. To measure the visual acuity, place the patient 20 feet from a well-illuminated Snellen chart. Cover one eye and record the smallest line the patient reads with glasses or pinhole. Use Snellen notations 20/40,20/30, etc. With glasses or with the pinhole disk the patient should be able to read the 20/30 line or smaller lines. Organic disease is present if the vision cannot be improved by the pinhole disk or glasses.

If no Snellen chart is available, visual acuity may be estimated by using a reading card with letters of varying size. If the Snellen notation is not available, record the size of the letters and the distance from the patient. Remember that most patients above the age of 45 require corrective lenses for reading. If the visual acuity is markedly decreased and the patient is unable to read any letters on the Snellen chart, vision can be recorded by counting the fingers (equivalent approximately to 20/400 size letters). Record the distance the fingers are counted, that is, finger counting at 3 feet (0.9 m). Failing this the perception of hand movement or light should be recorded.

Background Information

Tests of visual acuity are primarily evaluations of pattern vision and brightness discrimination. Visual acuity may be divided into two stages. The first stage involves preretinal structures such as the pupil and lens, which are discussed in other sections of this book. The second stage includes the retinal receptors and their projections to the central nervous system. The components of this stage and analogies with the somatic sensory system are given in a scheme adapted from Cogan (Fig 155).

The structures containing the photopigment are the rods and cones. Each rod or cone is composed of an outermost segment containing the lamellated disks, and an inner ellipsoidal segment that is composed of mitochondria. The ellipsoids are larger in the cones, thus accounting for the difference in shape. The rods have greater light sensitivity, and the cones greater discriminatory ability. The center of the macula, the fovea, has only cones. Outside this area the number of cones drops and the number of rods increases, until at the periphery of the retina there are only rods and no cones.

The outermost segment of the rods and cones is composed of protein plates containing the photosensitive visual pigment: rhodopsin in the rods and three types of pigment in the cone. These compounds are de-

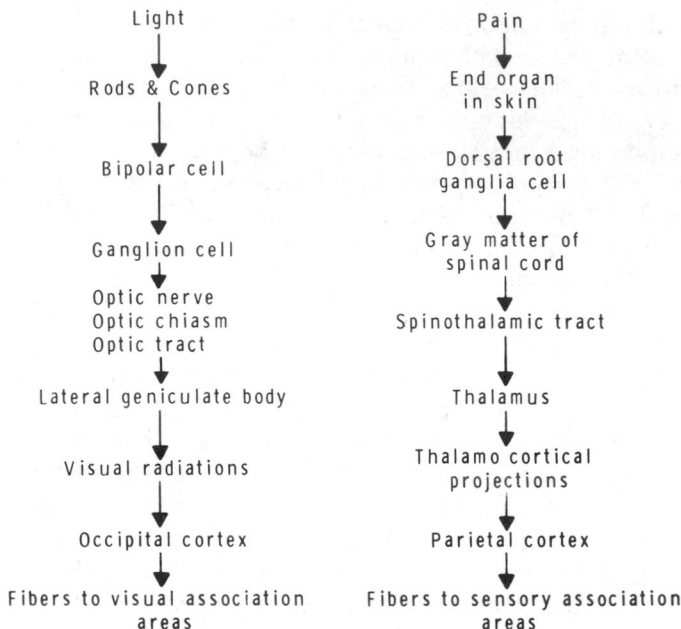

Figure 155. Analogies between the visual and somatic sensory systems. (Adapted from DG Cogan, *Neurology of the Visual System,* Charles C Thomas, 1967.)

rived from vitamin A. Light striking the pigment causes isomerization ("bleaching") of the pigment from one stereochemical configuration to another. This change in shape is presumably what causes the neural discharge.

The central nervous system utilizes receptive fields to produce the images perceived in the brain. These topographically arranged receptive fields in the retina project onto topographically arranged columns in the visual cortex in the occipital lobe.

A receptive field is roughly defined as the total area of the retina feeding into a single cell farther along the line. Consider the receptive field of one retinal ganglion cell, which is termed a "center-surround" field. There is a central area of varying size that is either excited or inhibited by a light stimulus, surrounded by an area that reacts in the opposite fashion to light (Fig 156).

There are two types of these fields:

1. "On" type. Light produces excitation of the retinal ganglion cell when the center is stimulated, and inhibition when the surround is stimulated.
2. "Off" type. Light produces an inhibition of the retinal ganglion cell when the center is stimulated, and excitation when the surround is stimulated.

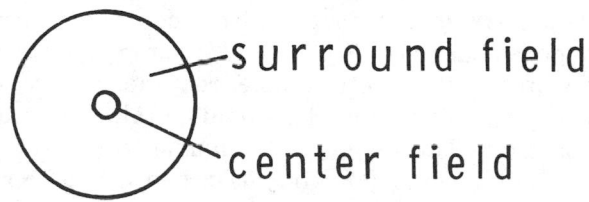

Figure 156. A center-surround receptive field.

An optimal response is obtained when a spot of light of precisely the right size is directed to the exact center of the field. Thus the retinal cell compares the amount of light striking the center of the field with the amount striking the surround, that is, there is a logarithmic system. Retinal ganglion cells vary widely in the size of their respective fields, from a few minutes of a degree in the fovea to 2° in the periphery. Visual acuity is closely related to receptive field size, and as one might expect visual acuity is greatest in the fovea where the receptive fields have the smallest area.

Receptive fields can also be analyzed with respect to color. Color is perceived only by the cones. There are three types of cone, each containing pigment responsive only to blue, green, or red. The receptive fields are of several types. The simplest has a center-surround organization, with the center having one cone type (eg, red) and the surround another cone type (eg, green). In this example red light placed in the center of the field would stimulate the cell, and green in the surround would inhibit the ganglion cell. The other types of color-receptive fields are more complex.

The lateral geniculate body is the next neuronal station after the retinal ganglion cell. An orderly topographical arrangement of the retinal projection is maintained, as outlined in the section on visual fields. Since the visual fibers have now crossed in the chiasm, each geniculate body is concerned with the contralateral half of the visual field, that is, the ipsilateral eye supplies fibers from the nasal half of its visual field, and the contralateral eye supplies fibers from the temporal half of the visual field. Thus the eyes are kept functionally separate in the geniculate bodies. Each of the six layers of the geniculate receives input from only one eye:

Layer	Eye
1	Contralateral
2	Ipsilateral
3	Ipsilateral
4	Contralateral
5	Ipsilateral
6	Contralateral

Therefore there are six separate maps of the contralateral visual field in each geniculate body. Each map is precisely superimposed and precisely in register. If one were to take a core sample from the six layers at a particular point, the resulting column of cells would all relate only to a particular area of the visual field. This concept of columnar organization, having its beginnings in the lateral geniculate body, is of overriding importance in the visual cortex.

The receptive fields of the geniculate cells seem quite similar to the receptive fields of retinal ganglion cells, except there is an increased ability of the surround field to nullify the response of the center field. Apparently each geniculate cell may receive its major input from one retinal ganglion cell, but also receive a much smaller input from numerous other retinal ganglion cells, the center of whose receptive fields lie in the periphery of the receptive field of the cell with major input. The implications and details of the processing of the visual sensory information in the geniculate bodies are little known currently.

Axons from the lateral geniculate cells project to the visual cortex of the occipital lobe, an area 2 mm thick and several square centimeters in area. The functional units of the visual cortex are vertical columns of cells that extend in a precisely perpendicular fashion from the surface of the cortex to the underlying white matter. Each column in areas 18 and 19 is composed of "simple," "complex," and "hypercomplex" cells. All cells in a single column have the same receptive field. The critical identifying characteristic of each column is the orientation of the receptive field of the column; that is, the orientation of light that produces optimal stimulation is identical for all cells in the column. For example, a slit of light with a certain orientation will stimulate all cells in one column, while a different slit orientation is necessary to stimulate cells in another column.

The geniculate axons project on simple cells located in a layer about 1 mm deep in the cortex. Axons from these simple cells then project onto complex and hypercomplex cells in layers above and below the simple cell layer. The terms "simple," "complex," and "hypercomplex" refer to the type of stimuli that provoke a response. The receptive fields of complex and hypercomplex cells are optimally stimulated by varied factors: length, width, and presence or absence of movement are critical.

The simple cells are stimulated either by the right eye or the left eye. Viewed from above, the layer containing simple cells can be divided into stripes of cells from one eye alternating with stripes from the other eye. Complex and hypercomplex cells usually get input from both eyes, with one eye being preferred over the other. In this fashion, images from the two eyes are fused into one image.

Columns in the visual cortex (area 17) project to visual association areas in area 18 and area 19. The ultimate mechanism whereby these visual areas translate patterns of light into images with forms, color, and depth is not presently known. This is an area of research that has been literally exploding in the 1960s and 1970s. See Zeki for a review of recent work.

Clinical Significance

Defective visual acuity is seen in a number of conditions. Refractive errors, perhaps the most common, can be detected during the examination by measuring the patient's vision using his glasses combined with a pinhole disk. If the vision can be improved to 20/30 or better on the Snellen chart by this method, the vision can be improved to normal by corrective lenses. Amblyopia, a condition in which the vision is poor but the examination is normal, has a variety of causes. Strabismus and a large difference in refractive error between the two eyes are the most common causes. If strabismus is not found on examination, ask about prior eye muscle surgery. In amblyopia the vision is poor from childhood, and near vision is much worse than distance vision. Defective visual acuity without structural abnormalities is seen in congenital nystagmus. Any disease process which interferes with optical transparency of the cornea, crystalline lens, or vitreous will decrease visual acuity. Corneal opacities occur with injury and inflammatory processes that scar the corneal stroma. Senile cataract is the most common cause of opacities of the crystalline lens; vitreous hemorrhage, of opacities within the vitreous. These opacities of the cornea, lens, and vitreous are seen as dark shadows against the red reflex of the retina and choroid when viewed with an ophthalmoscope.

Disorders of the retina which involve the macular region are easily recognized by ophthalmoscopic examination. Senile macular degeneration, chorioretinitis, and traumatic tears within the macula frequently cause defective visual acuity.

Lesions of the anterior visual pathways, that is, the optic nerve and optic chiasm reduce visual acuity. One should look for atrophy of the optic nerve and defective pupillary response to direct light (see section 135, The Pupil). Lesions of the visual pathway posterior to the chiasm (that is, optic tract, lateral geniculate bodies, optic radiations, and occipital cortex) do not reduce the visual acuity in the intact portions of the visual fields.

Selected References

1. Hubel DH: The visual cortex of the brain. Sci Am 209(5):54–62, 1963.
2. Wald G: Molecular basis of visual excitation. Science 162(3849):230–239, 1968.
3. Hubel DH: Effects of distortion of sensory input on the visual system of kittens. Physiologist 10:17–45, 1967.

4. Wiesel TN, Hubel DH: Ordered arrangement of orientation columns in monkeys lacking visual experience. *J Comp Neurol* 158(3):307–318, 1974.
5. Hubel DH, Wiesel TN: Sequence regularity and geometry of orientation columns in the monkey striate cortex. *J Comp Neurol* 158(3):267–294, 1974.
6. Hubel DH: *Transformation of Information in the Cat's Visual System.* Excerpta Medica International Congress Series no 49, 1962, vol 3, of the Proceedings of the International Union of Physiological Sciences, pp 160–169.
7. Wiesel TN, Hubel DH, Lam DMK: Autoradiographic demonstration of ocular-dominance columns in the monkey striate cortex by means of transneuronal transport. *Brain Res* 79:273–279, 1974.
8. Walsh FB, Hoyt WF: *Clinical Neuroophthalmology,* ed 3. Baltimore, Williams and Wilkins, 1969, vol 1, pp 1–129, 567–641.
9. Cogan DG: *Neurology of the Visual System.* Springfield, Ill, Charles C Thomas, 1967.
10. Zeki SM: Functional specialization in the visual cortex of the rhesus monkey. *Nature* 274:423–428, 1978.

196. Cranial Nerve II: Optic Nerve
B. Visual Fields

H. KENNETH WALKER, MD
J. DONALD FITE, MD

Definition

A normal visual field is an island of vision measuring 90° temporally to central fixation, 50° superiorly and nasally, and 60° inferiorly. Visual acuity increases from movement discrimination in the extreme peripheral vision to better than 20/20 in the center of vision.

Depression or absence of vision anywhere in the island of vision is abnormal.

Technique

The visual fields are examined to determine the integrity of the optic nerves and visual pathways. In essence the visual acuity is measured by exploring the island of vision with various sized test objects.

Methods of testing visual fields without special equipment include:

1. *Face confrontation.* Each eye is tested separately. An object such as a pencil eraser is moved in a plane about 2–3 cm in front of the eye into the field of vision. Position yourself directly in front of the patient and note where the object is seen by the patient in relationship to the facial outline. The patient should see the object temporally as it crosses the outline of the face, superiorly as it crosses the eyebrow, nasally as it crosses the bridge of the nose, and inferiorly just above the mouth (Figure 157).

2. *Comparison of color.* Compare the color identification in the temporal and nasal fields. Using a 0.5 cm red test object, have the patient identify the color and its intensity in the nasal and temporal fields. Compare the accuracy of color identification between the two fields. Next compare the central vision with the peripheral vision in each eye. Failure to identify the color object centrally suggests a central scotoma.

3. *Simultaneous finger counting in opposite fields of vision.* The eyes are tested singly to detect temporal or nasal field loss. If homonymous hemianopsia is suspected, both eyes can be tested at the same time. Facing the patient, rapidly present a different number of fingers in opposite fields asking the patient to add them up. Failure to call the correct number of fingers suggests loss of vision in that field. Suspected visual field loss should be confirmed by quantitative visual field testing, using the tangent screen or perimeter.

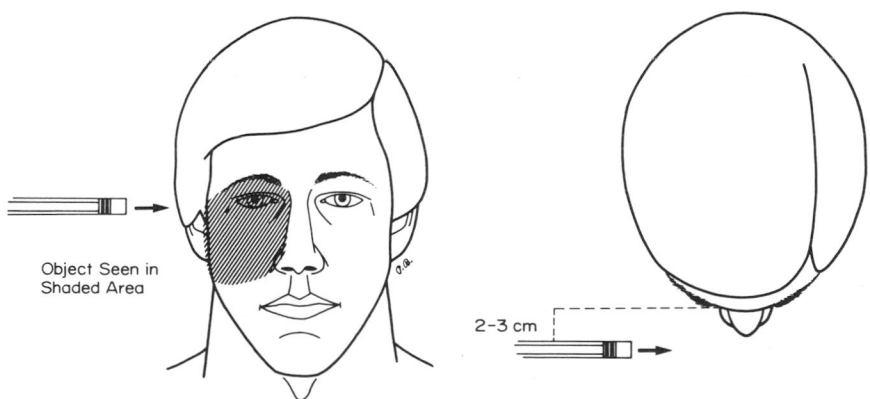

Object Seen in
Shaded Area

2–3 cm

Figure 157.   Face confrontation method of determining visual fields. Shaded area is normal visual field for this method.

4. *Description by patient.* Cover each eye separately and have the patient fixate on a distant object in the room. Ask him to describe what is seen. Pay particular attention to the temporal versus nasal fields and inferior versus superior fields.

Background Information

There is an orderly spatial arrangement of all elements of the visual sensory system from the retina to the visual cortex of the occipital lobe. This point-to-point localization should be the crucial organizing principle in your study of this system.

The area of the environment encompassed by each eye is termed the visual field. When depicted on paper, the right half of the field is oriented with respect to the patient, not the observer. The visual field of each eye is divided into the temporal half and the nasal half. A further subdivision into superior and inferior nasal and temporal quadrants is occasionally necessary for precise anatomical localization. Since the lens reverses and inverts images, it follows that:

1. The temporal half of each visual field projects onto the nasal half of each retina; consequently the visual information leaves the retina via nasal fibers.
2. The nasal half of each visual field projects onto the temporal half of each retina, and the visual information leaves the retina via temporal fibers.
3. The superior half of each visual field projects onto the lower half of each retina, and the visual information leaves the retina via inferior nasal and temporal fibers.
4. A further subdivision into quandrants may be made: eg, the superior temporal quadrant projects onto the inferior nasal quadrant of the retina.

See Fig 158 for illustration of these relationships.

Since humans have binocular vision, the visual field of each eye is precisely superimposed on the visual field of the other eye. The right half of this combined visual field is composed of the temporal half of the visual field of the right eye and the nasal half of the visual field of the left eye. All visual information in the right half of this combined visual field ultimately ends in the visual cortex of the left hemisphere, and vice versa for the left visual field. A defect in the same half of the visual field of each eye is said to be homonymous. For example, absence of vision in the right half of the visual field—the temporal field of the right eye and

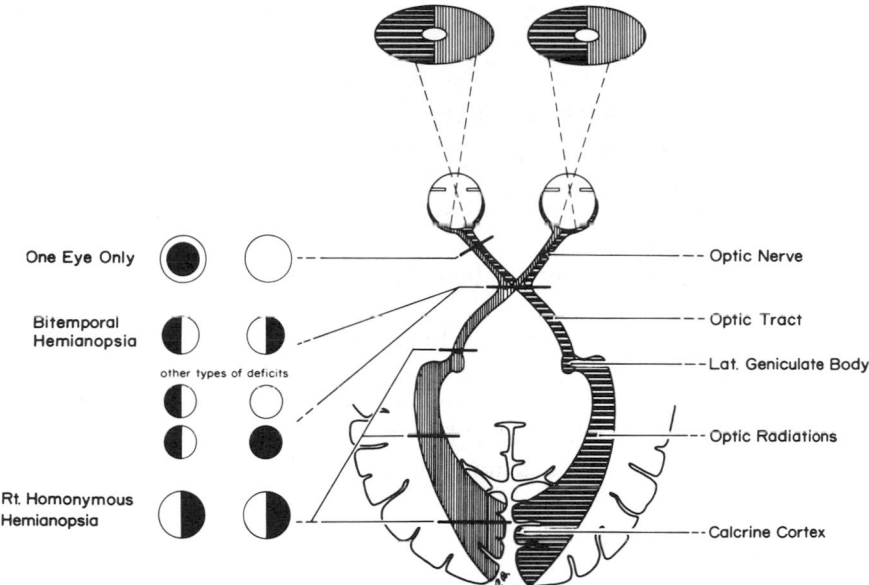

Figure 158. Anatomy of the visual fields, including some common defects.

nasal field of the left eye—is termed a right homonymous hemianopsia. Defects in opposite sides of the visual field of each eye are said to be heteronymous. Thus a heteronymous temporal hemianopsia refers to a defect in the temporal visual field of each eye, usually termed simply a bitemporal hemianopsia.

The vertical lines dividing the visual field into right-left and upper-lower halves intersect at the macula, which occupies the central 15° of the field. The blind spot corresponds to the optic disk, which is located in the nasal half of each retina and thus in the temporal half of the visual field of each eye.

As a generalization, upper retinal fibers remain upper and lower retinal fibers remain lower throughout the entire visual sensory system, except in the optic tract and lateral geniculate body. The rotation that occurs in these two structures becomes straightened out in the optic radiations.

The inner retinal layers (cells) are supplied by the ophthalmic artery, a branch of the internal carotid artery.

Axons from the retina are grouped together as the optic nerve. The upper and lower and nasal and temporal retinal fibers retain their relative positions. The optic nerve receives its blood supply from small vessels from the internal carotid, anterior cerebral, and anterior communicating arteries. Contiguous or nearby structures in close relationship to the optic nerve include:

1. Sphenoid and ethmoid sinuses
2. Carotid artery
3. Ophthalmic artery
4. Anterior communicating artery
5. Third ventricle
6. Anterior portion of circle of Willis

The next structure is the optic chiasm, where nasal fibers from each side cross to the opposite side; temporal fibers do not cross. The net effect is that all fibers from the right half of the visual field end in the left visual cortex, and vice versa for the other side. Although the fiber arrangement in the chiasm is not completely known, some useful generalizations can be made:

1. Upper and lower fibers retain their relative position.
2. Temporal fibers, all of which are uncrossed, course laterally.
3. Nasal fibers, all of which are crossed, do so beginning with the anterior lip of the chiasm.
4. Macular fibers form a "chiasm within the chiasm" since there are both crossed (nasal) and uncrossed (temporal) macular fibers. These fibers constitute 80% of all fibers in the chiasm. This large volume of crossing macular fibers forms the central core of the chiasm.

The chiasm is usually situated over the dorsum sellae; in some individuals it is anterior ("prefixed") and in others more posterior ("postfixed"). Neighboring structures are: the sella turcica and pituitary gland, the cavernous sinus, sphenoid sinus, third ventricle, circle of Willis, and the internal carotid artery. The blood supply comes from several sources, including the internal carotid, anterior cerebral, and other arteries.

The visual fibers leave the chiasm as the optic tract, which continues to the geniculate bodies. Between these two points the fibers undergo a 90° rotation, so that inferior fibers lie laterally while superior fibers lie medially in the optic tracts; macular fibers are dorsal. Fibers subserving pupillary functions peel off from the optic tract and go in the brachium of the superior colliculus to the pretectal region (see section 135, The Pupil). Related structures are: the internal carotid artery, anterior communicating artery, posterior communicating artery, and the pituitary gland. The principal blood supply is from the anterior choroidal artery.

The optic tract fibers synapse in the lateral geniculate body, a triangular "Napoleonic-hat shaped" structure that is the optic portion of the thalamus. There are six layers of cells present, each 10–20 cells thick. Each layer contains fibers from the visual field of one eye, arranged in the following fashion:

	Layer	Source of Visual Field	Visual Field Half
Medial	1	Contralateral eye	Temporal
↓	2	Ipsilateral eye	Nasal
	3	Ipsilateral eye	Nasal
	4	Contralateral eye	Temporal
	5	Ipsilateral eye	Nasal
Dorsal	6	Contralateral eye	Temporal

The maps so formed are superimposed and precisely in register, illustrating the point-to-point localization of the visual fields throughout the entire system. As a consequence of the 90° rotation of visual fibers in the optic tract, upper retinal fibers are medial and lower retinal fibers are lateral. The macular fibers occupy a large area situated dorsally in the "crown" of the Napoleonic hat. Neighboring structures include other parts of the thalamus, the pineal body, the internal capsule, and midbrain. The anterior choroidal artery supplies the lateral part of the lateral geniculate, and the posterior choroidal the medial portion; the macula area is supplied by both.

The visual fibers leave the lateral geniculate body laterally grouped as the optic peduncle, and pass in the most posterior part of the internal capsule (pars retrolenticularis), where they are contiguous to pyramidal fibers (especially those for leg and arm movements) and the thalamocortical sensory projection. This area is supplied by the anterior choroidal artery and is called the temporal isthmus: it is small (1.5 cm in diameter) and has visual, sensory, and leg motor fibers in close association. The fibers then fan out in order to circumvent the lateral ventricle. The fibers can be divided into two large groups with regard to their subsequent path to the visual cortex.

1. Upper retinal fibers from the medial aspect of the lateral geniculate body course fairly directly through the temporal and parietal lobes and project on the superior lip of the calcarine fissure.

2. Lower retinal fibers (lateral aspect of the lateral geniculate body) make a detour in the form of a forward loop into the rostral temporal lobe ("Meyer's loop") before turning backward to pass as the external sagittal stratum on the lateral wall of the temporal and occipital horns of the lateral ventricle, finally projecting onto the inferior lip of the calcarine fissure.

Note that the topographic arrangement in the optic radiation has now reverted again to upper retinal fibers coursing in the upper part of the radiations and lower retinal fibers being lower. Visual fibers from the ipsilateral eye are said to be lateral to those of the contralateral eye. Macular fibers occupy the large central portion of the radiations. Consequently, a rough generalization is that lesions of the parietal lobes cause lower visual field defects and temporal lobe lesions cause upper visual field defects. These defects are often "partial" or incomplete hemianopsias or even quadrantanopsias. Vascular supply of the optic radiation includes: the anterior choroidal artery to the temporal isthmus and anterior portions of the radiation, the middle cerebral artery to the intermediate portion, and the posterior cerebral artery to the posterior part.

The visual fibers project to the calcarine cortex (area 17) on the medial and caudal portions of the occipital lobe. The medial surface of the occipital lobe is divided by the calcarine fissure into a superior gyrus, the cuneus, and an inferior gyrus, the lingual. The fiber arrangement with respect to retinal areas and visual fields is as follows:

1. Upper retinal areas (lower visual fields): upper lip of calcarine fissure (cuneus)
2. Lower retinal areas (upper visual fields): lower lip of calcarine fissure (lingual)

The projection of central (macular) versus more peripheral visual fields, while not completely agreed upon, may be summarized as follows:

1. Central (macular) fields: the posterior tip of the calcarine region, roughly the posterior one-third of the calcarine cortex
2. Paracentral fields: medial part of calcarine cortex
3. Peripheral fields: most anterior portion of calcarine cortex

The vascular supply is from terminal vessels of the posterior cerebral artery. The macular area exists in the "watershed" zone between the posterior cerebral and middle cerebral circulation and gets its supply from both.

The final areas to which the visual fields ultimately project are areas 17, 18, and 19 and visual association areas of the adjacent parietal and temporal cortex. Area 17 sends efferent fibers to area 18. The corpus callosum connects areas 18 and 19 of one hemisphere with those areas in the opposite hemisphere. Both areas have extensive connections with other areas of the brain that will not be considered here. These areas are visual association cortex and ultimately are the portions of the brain that interpret what is seen in the visual fields, and connect "sights" with sound, smell, feel, etc. Given the present sparse knowledge of these areas, no statements can be made with respect to the projection of the visual fields upon them; in fact, projection may even be an inappropriate word.

Clinical Significance

Characteristics of the visual field defects found upon examination make it possible to divide the defects into prechiasmal, chiasmal, and postchiasmal lesions. This is helpful in recognizing the etiology of the visual field defect as well as deciding on the treatment. Prechiasmal visual field defects are characterized by defects which are limited to one eye only. Often the visual field defect crosses the vertical midline of the field and may be associated with an afferent pupillary defect, defective visual acuity, decreased color vision, and optic atrophy. In an adult tumors arising from the meninges surrounding the optic nerve in its intracranial portion or orbital portion frequently compress the optic nerve. Pituitary tumors and tumors above the chiasm such as craniopharyngiomas can compress one optic nerve. Inflammation of the optic nerve is a common finding in middle-aged adults. In young children optic nerve gliomas produce loss of vision, optic atrophy, and mild proptosis of the globe. Nutritional amblyopia, a condition seen with poor food intake and frequently large alcohol intake produces bilateral symmetrical central visual field defects that cross the midline and reduce visual acuity. Retinal lesions such as chorioretinitis produce visual field defects localized in the opposite field. That is, a retinal lesion located in the upper half of the retina will produce a visual field defect in the lower half. A lesion localized temporal to the macula will produce a nasal visual field defect. Lesions near the disk which interrupt nerve fiber bundles produce a mirror image of an arcuate defect because of interruption of the retinal fibers that extend from the disk and arc superiorly and inferiorly to the temporal retina. This arcuate field defect is characteristic of glaucomatous damage to the eye (Fig 159).

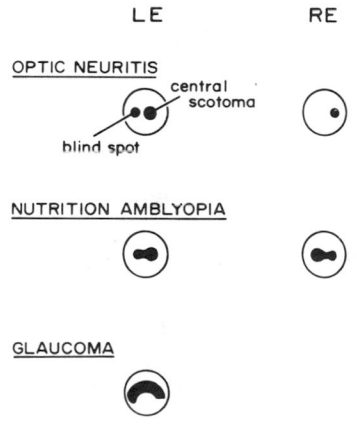

Figure 159. Typical visual field defects found in common prechiasmal visual pathway lesions.

Bitemporal hemianopsia characterizes chiasmal field defect. This localization is easily recognized when the field defects are symmetrical and extend up to the vertical meridian but do not extend into the nasal field. This type of defect is seen with total interruption of the crossing nasal fibers. Common lesions that compress the chiasm are tumors of the pituitary gland, craniopharyngiomas, aneurysms of the carotid, dilitation of the third ventricle. More difficult to recognize but no less characteristic are the visual field defects produced by small lesions which only partially interrupt the crossing nasal fibers. These lesions produce asymmetrical damage that often affects one optic nerve as well as crossing fibers. The hallmark of these early chiasmal compression defects are the presence of a temporal field defect in one eye that extends up to the vertical meridian of the field but does not extend into the nasal field. This defect can be confined to one eye only. The field and vision in the other eye may be perfectly normal or may be totally blind. Postchiasmal lesions are recognized by homonymous hemianopsia. The defects are easily recognized when the hemianopic defects are total. In this circumstance the visual field defect has lateralizing value only. That is, a right homonymous hemianopsia indicates interruption of the left visual pathways posterior to the chiasm. The lesion may be anywhere from the posterior chiasm to the occipital cortex. One must rely upon the presence of additional signs and symptoms to place the lesion in the anterior-posterior location. As an example, a right homonymous hemianopsia associated with difficulty in speaking and reading and sensory loss on the right side suggest a left parietal lobe lesion. Incomplete homonymous hemianopsias such as a superior quadrant homonymous hemianopsia is suggestive of interruption of the visual pathways in the temporal lobe. Tumors and vascular occlusions are common causes of hemispheric disease. Sudden total visual loss suggests interruption of blood flow within the basilar artery, producing bilateral calcarine cortex infarction. In this condition there is total blindness with no other neurological finding.

Selected References

1.   Walsh FB, Hoyt WF: *Clinical Neuroophthalmology,* ed 3. Baltimore, Williams and Wilkins, vol 1, pp 1–129.
2.   Brodal A: *Neurological Anatomy,* ed 2. New York, Oxford University Press, 1969, pp 462–487.
3.   Cogan DG: *Neurology of the Visual System.* Springfield, Ill, Charles C Thomas, 1966.
4.   Alexander HB: Vascular lesions affecting the visual pathways. *Arch Ophthal* 47:65–75, 1957.
5.   Hoyt WF, Luis OL: The primate chiasm. *Arch Ophthal* 70:113–129, 1963.

197. Cranial Nerves III, IV, and VI: Oculomotor, Trochlear, and Abducens Nerves
A. Conjugate Gaze

H. KENNETH WALKER, MD
J. DONALD FITE, MD

Definition

Conjugate gaze occurs when both eyes move in the same vertical or horizontal direction. It is the result of integrated supranuclear impulses which are concerned with overall function rather than movement of individual muscles.

Conjugate gaze is abnormal when either or both eyes fail to move in a horizontal or vertical direction. The symptom of diplopia is usually absent in conjugate gaze paralysis.

Technique

An excellent discussion of the methods of examination of conjugate gaze eye movements is given by Gay and Newman along with a description of the anatomical substrates for eye movement. A summary of their method of examination follows.

Eye mechanism movements to be tested include:

Fixation (position maintenance). Have the patient look at a convenient object at 2.5–3 feet (0.75–0.9 m) and if possible at 20 feet (6 m) away. Failure to hold the fixation may occur with markedly diminished vision, lack of effort, or lethargy. Fixation may be interrupted by a variety of abnormal eye movements such as nystagmus.

Pursuit movements (following or target tracking). These are slow movements mediated by the occipitomesencephalic pathways. Ask the patient to fixate on an object (eg, patient's finger) and follow the object as it is moved in the six diagnostic positions of gaze (see section 197B, Brainstem Nuclei and Peripheral Nerves, Fig 162). Diplopia (double vision) elicited in any of the six diagnostic positions of gaze is an indication of a nuclear or infranuclear lesion. Diplopia is not seen with supranuclear lesions (for discussion of diplopia, see Brainstem Nuclei and Peripheral Nerves). Do the eyes follow the objects fully and smoothly or is the movement halting and slow (cogwheeling)? Is the movement interrupted by nystagmus? If so, describe the nystagmus by noting the direction of the fast phase, that is, horizontal, left, right, up, down, or rotary (Fig 160).

Voluntary target seeking (rapid or saccadic) eye movements. These are mediated by frontomesencephalic pathways. Ask the patient to look first at one object, then another. Hold the objects 2.5–3 feet (0.75–0.9 m) in front of the patient and about 2 feet (0.6 m) apart. Repeat the procedure with the objects held vertically. Observe the rapidity and smoothness with which the eyes move. A small undershoot followed by correction is normal, but a persistent overshoot is indicative of cerebellar dysfunction (ocular dysmetria).

Compensatory movements (vestibular system). It is not necessary to routinely test the vestibular system. The principal reasons for testing are:

1. To test intactness of the end organ
2. To test intactness of brainstem mechanisms for gaze, especially in the unconscious patient
3. To separate brainstem conjugate gaze dysfunction from cortical conjugate gaze dysfunction

The structures being tested in the methods described below are: labyrinths, eighth nerve, pontine lateral gaze centers, sixth and third nuclei, medial longitudinal fasciculus, peripheral third and sixth nerves. The two

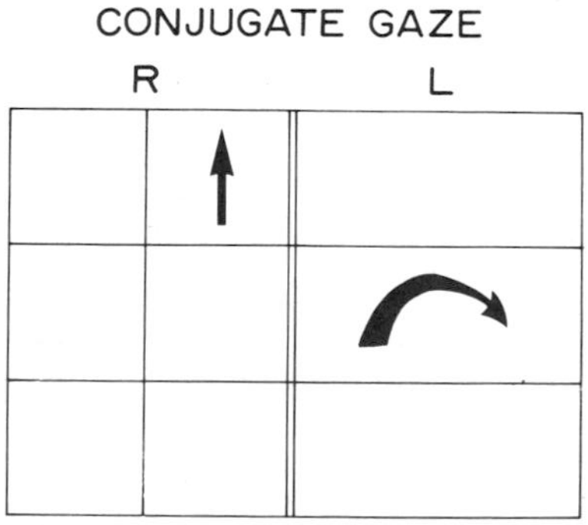

Figure 160. A simple notation for nystagmus.

tests used are the doll's head maneuver in which the patient's head is forcefully moved to the right and left, and caloric testing. In the unconscious patient start with the doll's head test. If the results are abnormal, then the caloric test must also be done because it is the stronger stimulus.

The caloric test is performed using cold or warm (44°C) water. Using cold water is usually more convenient. First inspect the tympanic membrane to make sure it is normal. Elevate the patient's head to 30° so that only the horizontal semicircular canal is stimulated. Fill an emesis basin with ice and add enough water to cover the ice. Wait a few minutes, then draw a 50-ml syringe full of the cold water. Attach a catheter to the syringe and gently inject the water into the external canal over a period of 0.5 or 1 minute. Observe the eyes for 3 minutes.

In the normal conscious patient the elicited nystagmus has a slow and fast component. The slow component is toward the side of the injection of the cold water. This is due to brainstem mechanisms. This initial slow drift is followed by a compensatory or corrective fast component—probably of higher origin—that immediately jerks the eyes back in the other direction.

In the unconscious patient with a normal brainstem and vestibular system there is no fast or corrective component with cold stimulation. Since the slow component is the only one present, there is deviation to the side of the cold stimulus. Warm water produces the opposite effect: the slow component is away from the side of stimulation and the corrective fast component toward the side of stimulation. The mnemonic for direction of the fast phase of nystagmus in the conscious patient is *COWS* (Cold Opposite Warm Same).

The test described above is a crude but easily performed method of testing the vestibular system. There are other variants that provide more subtle information.

Some principal abnormalities found on these tests are:

1. No movement in either direction: due to pontine structural lesion, or barbiturate or dilantin intoxication. The pupils are pinpoint in pontine lesions but are normal size and reactive to light with barbiturate or dilantin intoxication.

2. No movement on one side, intact on other: lesion of pontine gaze center on side of no response.

3. One eye abducts while other eye fails to adduct: internuclear ophthalmoplegia or peripheral third nerve lesion on side of failure to adduct.

4. One eye adducts while the other eye fails to abduct. Peripheral sixth nerve lesion.

Convergence (vergence) or depth-tracking movements. These are tested by having the patient fixate on an object such as a ¼-inch-high letter

Table 38. Tests of conjugate gaze.

---

1. Fixation
2. Pursuit
3. Target-seeking
4. Compensatory (vestibular)
5. Convergence
6. Opticokinetic nystagmus
7. Spontaneous or gaze-evoked nystagmus

---

printed on a tongue blade at 3 feet and slowly moving the object toward the patient's nose. The point of maximum convergence is that point at which one or both eyes lose fixation and deviate outward.

Additional test for measurement of ocular movements. Opticokinetic (OKN) or "railway" nystagmus is elicited by moving test objects slowly across the field of the patient's vision. A natural example occurs when a train passenger watches telephone poles pass by the window. It is also termed the fixation reflex. Repetitive patterns on a tape or drum are satisfactory. The eyes slowly follow the object in the direction of its movement then rapidly move in the opposite direction to pick up the next object. Both the slow (pursuit) phase and rapid (saccadic) phase are tested. Note the regularity, smoothness, and duration of the opticokinetic response.

Observe for spontaneous or gaze-evoked nystagmus. Record as shown in Fig 160. See Table 38 for a list of tests of conjugate gaze.

Background Information

The ocular motor system has five neurological control systems, each concerned with separate movements. These control systems exist for the purpose of keeping the image stationary on the retina. In order to accomplish this, the eyes must first fixate on an object of interest, then move conjugately as the object moves or as the head moves. The five primary conjugate movements and their control systems are as follows:

Movement	Control System
1. Fixation movements (position maintenance): minute eye movements ("micromovements") keep the foveae fixed on the target. They are composed of small slow movements ("microdrifts")	Occipital cortex

and small rapid movements ("microsaccades"). The mechanism of these movements is not worked out. It is assumed the supranuclear origin is the occipital cortex.

2. Target-tracking or pursuit movements (following movements): Once a target has been centered on the fovea, the purpose of these involuntary movements is to keep the fovea centered on the target. More specifically, the velocity of the eyes is matched to the velocity of the object of interest.

    Occipital cortex: areas 17, 18, 19

3. Target-seeking or saccadic movements: These voluntary movements ("movements of command") are the fastest of all eye movements. Their function is to change the fovea of the macula from one target to another. Eye movements made in examining a scene, and looking from one object of interest to several others are composed of a series of saccadic movements.

    Frontal cortex: areas 8, 6, 9.

4. Depth-tracing or vergence movements: These movements maintain fusion of the two retinal images in spite of changes in distance between the eyes and the object. The eyes must converge as the object gets closer and diverge as it recedes.

    Vergence system: areas not known for certain.

5. Compensatory movements: Keeping the fovea centered on the target in spite of movements of the head.

    Vestibular system: Labyrinths in the ear and vestibular nuclei in medulla. Proprioceptive receptors in the neck play a smaller role in these movements.

Saccadic movements originate in the frontal cortex (areas 8, 6, 9) and pursuit movements, in the occipital cortex (areas 17, 18, and 19). Unilateral stimulation of these areas produces conjugate contralateral movements. Bilateral stimulation produces conjugate vertical eye movements. Associated head and eyelid movements are also produced. The visual system depends on close cooperation between frontal and occipital areas: saccadic movements from frontal areas locate the object of interest and pursuit movements from the occipital areas keep the fovea centered on the object. This cooperation is mediated by connections between the frontal and occipital cortex (probably via the superior longitudinal fasciculus).

Convergence and divergence movements are felt to originate in the cortex, but the area(s) of origin are not clear at this time.

The exact pathways to the brainstem of supranuclear cortical fibers are unknown. They apparently pass in or around the internal capsule and eventually influence the brainstem nuclei. There is some evidence which suggests that the frontal and occipital fibers have different pathways. There is uncertainty regarding the participation of the superior colliculi in a relay between the occipital cortex and brainstem nuclei.

The vestibular system, consisting of the labyrinth and vestibular nuclei, produces compensatory movements that keep the fovea fixed on the target in spite of movement of the head. The labyrinth, embedded in the petrous bone, contains two functional components:

1. Three semicircular canals that lie at right angles to each other. The sensory receptors in the ampulla of each canal respond to linear acceleration. The anatomical arrangement in three perpendicular planes thus permits sensing angular acceleration along three axes. Each semicircular canal influences a pair of eye muscles: eg, stimulating the left horizontal canal produces a contraction of right lateral rectus muscle and left medial rectus muscle, giving conjugate right lateral gaze. There is concomitant relaxation of the antagonist muscles, in this example the right medial and left lateral recti.

2. The utricle contains otoliths, so-called because the hairs of the sensory cells stick into a gelatinous substance containing calcium carbonate crystals. The receptors respond to linear acceleration, eg, the acceleratory forces of gravity.

Central processes from the vestibular ganglion cells project topographically onto the four main vestibular nuclei in the upper lateral medulla just below the floor of the fourth ventricle. These nuclei send efferent axons in the medial longitudinal fasciculus to the brainstem nuclei of cranial nerves III, IV, and VI; these fibers are most abundant to those cranial nerve nuclei that produce horizontal and rotatory movements of the eyes.

We have now discussed briefly the contributions of the cortex and vestibular systems to ocular movements. The brainstem takes these influences and translates them into conjugate movements. Exactly where and how this integration occurs is a subject of uncertainty and discussion. The frontal and occipital pathways are probably separate.

Both frontal and occipital areas may ultimately project to the pontine paramedian reticular formation, which in turn influences the cranial nerve nuclei for lateral movements. There is considerable dispute over the existence and/or location of brainstem "centers" for conjugate gaze. Leaving these uncertainties for the future and better techniques to decide, there are some important and clinically useful anatomic correlations, especially with respect to horizontal, vertical, and convergent movements.

Horizontal movements.   Conjugate horizontal movements are produced by the frontal, occipital, and vestibular systems. Outputs from these systems probably converge on the pontine paramedian reticular formation (PPRF) somewhere in the vicinity of the abducens nucleus. The PPRF (or pontine "center" for lateral gaze) controls ipsilateral conjugate horizontal gaze by sending fibers to the ipsilateral sixth nucleus and across the midline to the contralateral medial longitudinal fasciculus (MLF). These latter fibers then ascend in the MLF and supply the portion of the contralateral third nucleus that causes the medial rectus to contract. This is summarized diagrammatically in Fig 161.

   This arrangement accounts for these observations:

   1. A lesion of the sixth nucleus causes a complete paralysis of conjugate horizontal gaze.

   2. A lesion of the MLF rostral to the sixth nucleus produces only failure of adduction of the ipsilateral eye: then the supranuclear fibers destined for the third nucleus have been interrupted.

Vertical movements.   On the basis of clinical evidence the brainstem area for conjugate vertical movements is generally felt to be in or around the superior colliculi. Stimulation has produced conjugate vertical gaze, and lesions in or around the colliculi often produce a supranuclear type paralysis of vertical gaze, that is, vertical gaze cannot be carried out by command, but can be elicited by various maneuvers such as head-tilting. In many cases there is paralysis of either upward or downward gaze, indicating the "centers" for these movements are probably anatomically separate.

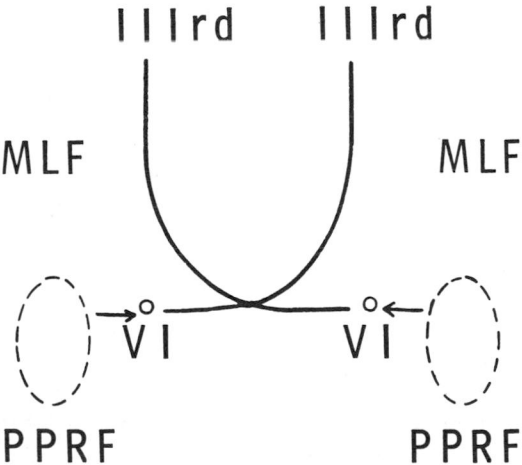

Figure 161.   Relationships among the pontine paramedian reticular formation (PPRF), sixth nerve nuclei, medial reticular longitudinal fasciculus (MLF) and third nerve nuclei.

Convergent movements. Normally accommodation is associated with convergence and pupillary constriction. These three separate functions are probably brought together in the midbrain. Lesions in the region of the superior colliculi often produce paralysis of vertical movements as described above and also paralysis of convergence, accommodation, and miosis. However the exact anatomical site is not known.

Clinical Significance

Loss of fixation occurs in congenital amblyopia and congenital chorioretinitis where vision is markedly decreased. Random conjugate movements are seen in a bilaterally blind person.

Lesions of the frontal gaze centers produce a gaze preference to one side of the body or the other. Paralysis of the left frontal gaze center produces an inability of the eyes to look to the right. If the right gaze center is intact, its action will predominate, producing conjugate deviation of the eyes to the left side of the body. This condition can be distinguished from lesions of the brainstem (which also produce conjugate gaze paralysis) by stimulating the vestibular system with the doll's head maneuver or caloric test. If the brainstem is intact, the eyes will move conjugately in all directions when one of these tests is performed. A lesion of the brainstem produces a conjugate paralysis that is not overcome by the vestibular stimulus.

Focal epileptic seizures involving, eg, the left frontal gaze center, can initially produce a forced conjugate deviation to the right side of the body. With cessation of the seizure there is often a postictal paralysis of the involved gaze center. At this time the action of the opposite gaze center, if normal, will predominate. In the example given the initial conjugate deviation to the right side of the body would be followed by conjugate deviation to the left side of the body.

Many CNS lesions can produce paralysis of the gaze centers. Common causes include all varieties of vascular lesions and neoplasms.

Lesions of the occipital center for conjugate gaze are often associated with homonoymous hemianopsias. These lesions are characterized by inability of the patient to track an object and by defects in opticokinetic nystagmus.

Cerebellar dysfunction can produce the following ocular signs:

1. Bursts of to-and-fro rapid movements of the eyes (ocular flutter)
2. Inability to change fixation from one object to another without overshooting or less commonly undershooting (ocular dysmetria)

Various ocular dysfunctions may also be present in horizontal and vertical gaze.

Lesions of the medial longitudinal fasciculus (which connects the sixth nucleus on one side with the third nucleus on the opposite side of the brainstem) produce paralysis of adduction. That is, the eye will not turn medially since the third nerve and therefore the medial rectus muscle has been disconnected from the lateral gaze center and sixth nucleus of the opposite side. There is usually nystagmus in the abducting eye as lateral conjugate gaze is attempted. This disconnection produces what is termed internuclear (between the sixth and third nuclei) ophthalmoplegia. Multiple sclerosis and vascular lesions of the pons are two common causes.

Nystagmus is seen in different disorders. It has more diagnostic value than localizing value. The following classification is simplified from Walsh and Hoyt:

1.   Nystagmus with defects of ocular fixation. Nystagmus of the blind is an example of this type.
2.   Nystagmus that occurs with gaze. Examples include drug-induced nystagmus, the nystagmus of the abducting eye seen in internuclear ophthalmoplegia, and the nystagmus seen with cerebellar lesions.
3.   Vestibular or labyrinthine nystagmus.
4.   Opticokinetic nystagmus.

Selected References

1.   Gay AJ, Newman NM: Eye movements and their disorders: An analytic evaluation, in Critchley M, O'Leary JL, Jennett B (eds): *Scientific Foundations of Neurology.* Philadelphia, FA Davis, 1972, pp 126–138.
2.   Bender MB (ed): *The Oculomotor System.* New York, Harper and Row, 1964.
3.   Bach-Y-Rita P, Collins CC (eds): *The Control of Eye Movements.* New York, Academic Press, 1971.
4.   Brodal A: *Neurological Anatomy,* ed 2. New York, Oxford University Press, 1969, pp 374–396, 429–461.
5.   Cogan DG: *Neurology of the Ocular Muscles,* ed 2. Springfield, Ill, Charles C Thomas, 1969.
6.   Zikmund V (ed): *The Oculomotor System and Brain Functions.* London, Butterworths, 1973.
7.   Walsh FB, Hoyt WF: *Clinical Neuroophthalmology,* ed 2. Baltimore, Williams and Wilkins, 1969, 1, pp 130–348.
8.   Truex RC, Carpenter MB: *Human Neuroanatomy,* ed 6. Baltimore, Williams and Wilkins, 1969, pp 360–361, 377–378, 384–390.

197. Cranial Nerves III, IV, and VI: Oculomotor, Trochlear, and Abducens Nerves
B. Brainstem Nuclei and Peripheral Nerves

J. DONALD FITE, MD
H. KENNETH WALKER, MD

Definition

Cranial nerve III

Normal:

Nerve Function and position of eye	Muscle
1. Elevation when eye is abducted	Superior rectus
2. Elevation when eye is adducted	Inferior oblique
3. Depression when eye is abducted	Inferior rectus
4. Adduction	Medial rectus
5. Lid elevation	Levator
6. Pupil constriction	Pupil sphincter

Abnormal:
1.   Total paralysis:
    a.   Eye down and out (if fourth and sixth nerves are intact).
    b.   Pupil dilated and unresponsive to any stimuli.
    c.   Ptosis: drooping eyelid.
2.   Partial paralysis: a weakness or failure of any of the functions listed under normal.

Cranial nerve IV
1.   The nerve functions to depress the eye when the eye is adducted by stimulation of the superior oblique muscle.
2.   Failure of the eye to depress is an indication of paralysis. In

an attempt to restore binocular vision, the patient often depresses the chin and tilts the head to the opposite shoulder.
Cranial nerve VI
1.   The nerve abducts the eye through stimulation of the lateral rectus muscle.
2.   Failure of abduction indicates paralysis.

Technique

Dysfunction of cranial nerves III, IV, and VI is recognized by identifying the paralysis of individual eye muscles innervated by these nerves. There are three methods commonly used to identify paralysis of the individual eye muscles.

Method 1: Observe the rotation of the eye in the fields of action of the appropriate muscle. Each eye is tested separately (Fig 162). Occlude one eye and ask the patient to fixate on a penlight or other small object. Starting with the eye in the straight ahead position, move the fixation target slowly and horizontally in the field of action of the lateral and medial rectus muscles. Observe the range and motion of the globe. The limbus should reach the outer and inner canthus. With the eye adducted move the target up into the field of action of the inferior oblique muscle and down into the field of action of the superior oblique muscle. With the eye abducted move the test object up to test the superior rectus muscle and down to test inferior rectus muscle. These are the six diagnostic positions of gaze. Note that the vertically acting oblique muscles function when the eye is adducted and the vertically acting recti muscles when the eye is abducted.

Method 2: Comparison of rotation of yoke muscles. Yoke muscles are the pair of muscles responsible for moving the eyes in a conjugate direction. For example, the left medial rectus and right lateral rectus are yoke muscles. Innervational impulses to them are equally distributed. Ask the patient to follow an object or light as it is moved in the six diagnostic fields of gaze. Failure of one eye to follow its fellow eye indicates paralysis of the appropriate muscle of that eye. Observing the light as it is reflected on the pupil is more accurate than watching the whole globe.

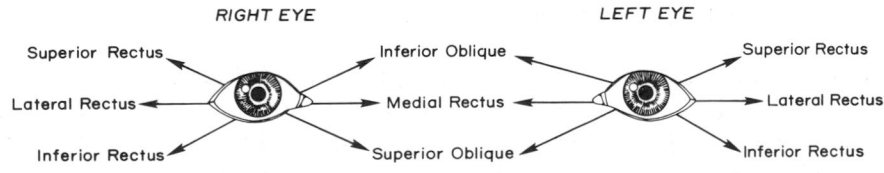

Figure 162.   Actions of the eye muscles and diagnostic positions of gaze.

The normal light reflection is displaced slightly nasal to the center of the pupil. An additional maneuver is to cover one eye and watch the corrective movement of the uncovered eye. For example, if paralysis of the right lateral rectus is suspected, cover the left eye and ask the patient to follow the light into the field of action of the right lateral rectus (right lateral gaze). When the left eye is uncovered and the right eye is covered, the left eye moves briskly outward to fixate the light. The amplitude of corrective movement will be greatest in the field of action of the paretic muscle. This procedure is useful with either eye covered but is usually enhanced by using the paralytic eye for the initial fixation. In the example above the impulses going to the right lateral rectus are equal to those going to the left medial rectus. In an attempt to move the paralyzed right lateral rectus, the impulses are increased to both eyes. The medial rectus therefore causes the left eye to move farther to the right than the partially paralyzed right eye has moved. This is known as secondary deviation.

Method 3: The red lens diplopia test. This test makes use of diplopia as a test for eye muscle weakness. The red lens over one eye enables the clinician to identify the eye to which the red image belongs. By convention the red lens is placed in front of the right eye (red is right). Hence, the red image always belongs to the right eye. A penlight and red lens are needed. Place the red lens in front of the right eye. Hold the light 2–3 feet (0.6–0.9 m) in front of the patient's eyes. Ask the patient to fixate on the light; move the light into each of the six diagnostic positions of gaze. At fixation and at each gaze position ask the patient if he sees one or two images. If the patient has diplopia, he will see two lights, one red and one white. Ask the patient to tell you how far apart the images are and to describe their horizontal (right or left) and vertical (up or down) relationships to each other in each position of gaze. Record your findings on a chart using a solid circle to represent the red light.

This test can be interpreted as follows (red lens over right eye):

1. When the patient describes the red image to the right of the white image, there is paralysis of the right or left lateral rectus muscle.
2. When the patient describes the red image to the left of the white image, there is paralysis of the right or left medial rectus muscle.
3. The image that is displaced farthest in the direction of gaze belongs to the eye with the paralyzed muscle.

The test is most valuable in interpreting horizontal diplopia.

This test can be understood by considering the relationship of the fovea to the visual field. Any image focused on the fovea occupies the center of the visual field. Thus the eyes swing conjugately to the right in order to keep an object of interest moving to the right focused on the fovea. If a muscle of one eye is weak, that eye cannot keep up with the normal eye. The normal eye keeps the object focused on its fovea and therefore in the center of its visual field. But the weak eye loses the foveal fixation, and the visual image of the object strikes the retina peripheral to the fovea. This produces two visual images, or diplopia. The distance between these two images increases as the eyes move farther into the field of action of the weak muscle since the image in the normal eye continues to be focused on the fovea. The visual image in the weak eye gets farther from the fovea.

Consider how the images are perceived by the cortex:

1. The image focused on the fovea is localized to the center of the visual field, as noted above.
2. An image focused on the retina to the left of the fovea will be localized by the cortex to the right visual field (due to the reversal of image by the lens).
3. An image focused on the retina to the right of the fovea will be localized by the cortex to the left visual field. Figures 163 and

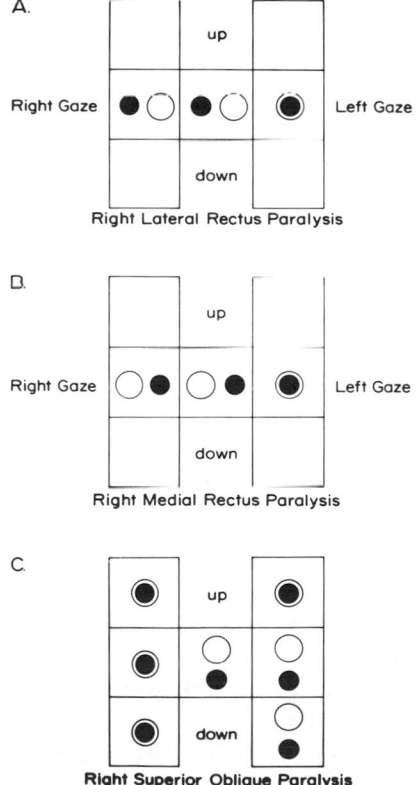

Figure 163.   Examples of red glass diplopia tests. The red lens is over the right eye and the red image is indicated by the solid circle.

NORMAL

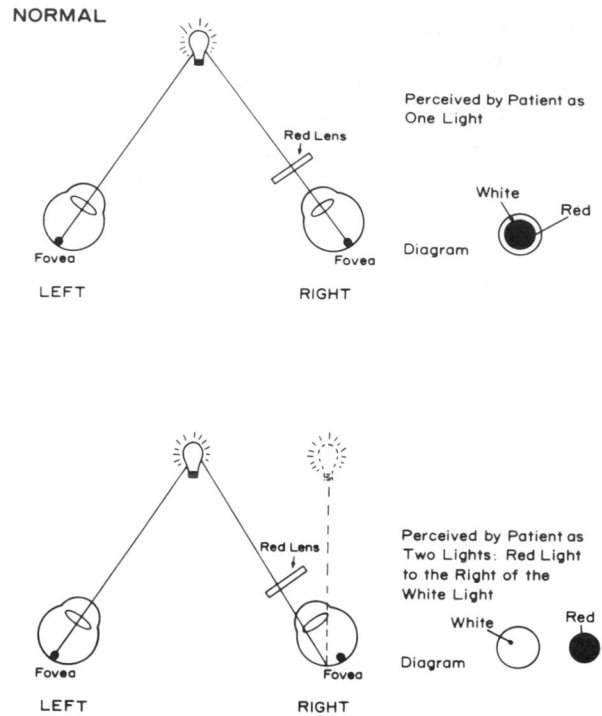

Figure 164.   Explanation of red lens diplopia test.

164 demonstrate the use of the test to detect a right lateral medial rectus paralysis and a right superior oblique paralysis.

A summary of the findings in some examples in which the red lens is over the right eye are:

1.   On right lateral gaze the red image is to the right of the white image: paralysis of the right lateral rectus. This follows the guidelines that when the red image is to the right of the white image there is paralysis of the right or left lateral rectus muscle. The right eye and, therefore, the right lateral rectus is involved since the red image is farthest in the direction of gaze.

2.   On left lateral gaze the red image is to the left of the white image: paralysis of the right medial rectus. Since the red image is to the left, one of the medial recti is involved. The right medial rectus is the culprit since the red image is farthest in the direction of gaze.

Additional tests include:

1. Head tilt test for fourth nerve paralysis. Tilt the head first to one shoulder then the other. Observe the amount of vertical separation of the eyes or of the diplopic images. The greatest separation occurs with the head tilted to the same shoulder as the side of paralysis.

2. Position of the head. Head position often gives a clue to a paretic ocular muscle. Head tilted to the shoulder and chin down are seen with superior oblique muscle paralysis opposite the direction of the tilt. The head is turned away from the side of a lateral rectus paralysis.

3. Examining the function of the superior oblique muscle in the presence of total third nerve paralysis. When the third cranial nerve is paralyzed, the eye cannot be adducted; hence, the depression of the globe in adduction (field of action of the superior oblique) cannot be performed. One should look for the secondary action of the superior oblique, which is rotation of the globe. Ask the patient to look in the direction that would normally adduct the paretic eye. Observe a conjunctival vessel nasally while asking the patient to look up and down. On down gaze the eye can be seen to rotate inward if the superior oblique is functioning.

Background Information

Nerve III: Oculomotor nerve. The nuclear groups forming the oculomotor complex lie in the midbrain underneath the aqueduct (Fig 165). The superior colliculi are above the aqueduct at this level. The medial longitudinal fasciculus lies laterally and ventrally to these nuclei and has an intimate association with them. More ventral structures include the red nucleus, midbrain reticular formation and tracts from the cortex to pons, cranial nerve nuclei, and spinal cord.

The nuclear groups are topographically arranged. The most rostral group contains the nuclei for pupillary constriction and accommodation. The central group contains the nuclei for the inferior, medial, and superior recti muscles and the inferior oblique muscle. The most caudal nuclei supply the levator muscle to the eyelids. The nuclear groups that are the most medial in the complex subserve bilateral functions (pupillary constriction and accommodation, the superior recti for vertical gaze, and the levator palpebrae muscles). The nuclei for the superior rectus muscle send their fibers across the midline to supply the contralateral muscle. The levator palpebrae muscles have a bilateral innervation.

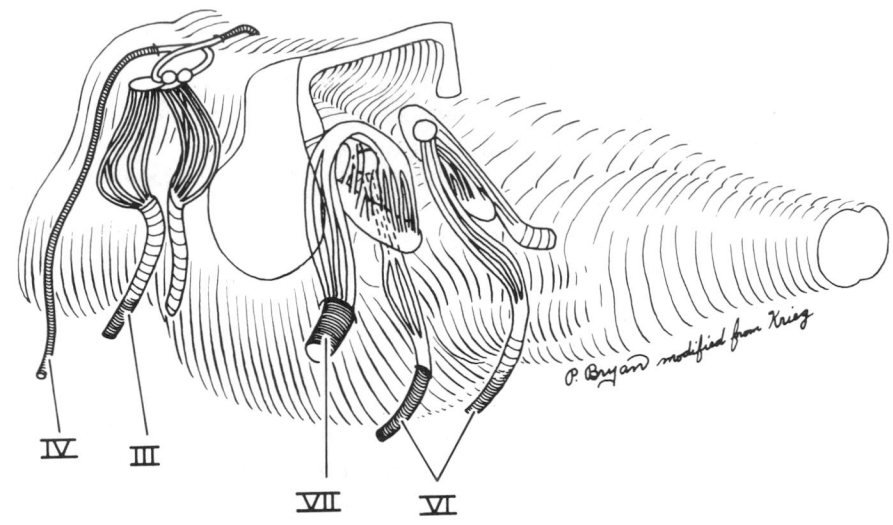

Figure 165. Brainstem nuclei of oculomotor (III), trochlear (IV), and abducens (VI) nerves. The facial (VII) nerve is shown also. (Modified from WJS Krieg, *Functional Neuroanatomy*, ed 2, Blakiston Co, 1953. Used with permission of author.)

Fibers from the nuclei course ventrally and emerge in the interpeduncular fossa.

After emerging on the ventral surface of the midbrain the third nerve passes through the tentorial incisura or "notch," the oval-shaped opening in the tentorium (Fig 166). The relationship of the third nerve to other structures in the notch is quite important clinically. The temporal lobes lie on the tentorium, and the temporal uncus bulges into the side of the notch and normally overhangs about 3–4 mm. The oculomotor nerve passes through the subarachnoid cistern in the notch, embraced above by the posterior cerebral artery and below by the superior cerebellar artery. A bit more distally the nerve lies between the posterior communicating artery medially and the overhanging edge of the temporal uncus and the tentorium laterally. In summary, in the tentorial notch the third nerve lies in close proximity to three arteries, the temporal uncus, and the tentorial edge (Fig 166). See section 193, Level of Consciousness for a discussion of uncal herniation.

The nerve proceeds anteriorly and enters the cavernous sinus. The structures closely related to the nerve here are the fourth nerve, the ophthalmic and sometimes mandibular division of the fifth nerve, and the internal carotid artery. In the cavernous sinus the third nerve is joined by sympathetic fibers from the superior cervical ganglion destined for the eye; these fibers have ascended along the internal carotid artery.

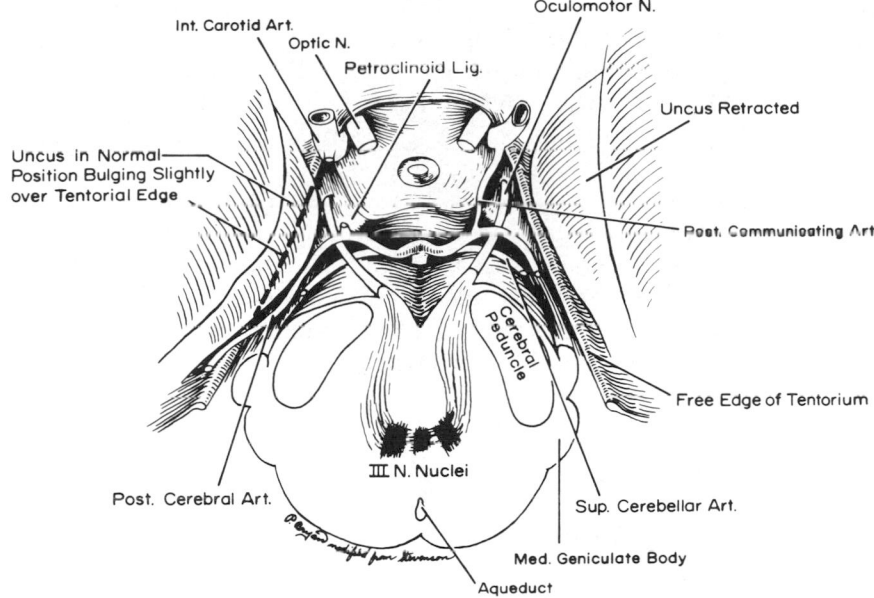

Figure 166. Relationship of structures involved in uncal herniation. (Redrawn and modified from *Clinical Neuro-Ophthalmology*, ed. 3, by FB Walsh and WF Hoyt. Copyright 1969, The Williams & Wilkins Company, Baltimore. Used with permission of author and publisher.)

An important clinical point is that the fibers for pupillary constriction are concentrated on the superior periphery of the third nerve from the emergence of the nerve at the brainstem to the middle portion of the cavernous sinus. Therefore, pressure on the nerve in the tentorial notch can involve these fibers and produce pupillary dilation before the other muscle functions are involved.

Nerve IV: Trochlear nerve.   The nucleus of the trochlear nerve is found caudad to the oculomotor nucleus, that is, in the midbrain at the level of the inferior colliculus (Fig 165). Above is the aqueduct and below is the medial longitudinal fasciculus. The course of the nerves is unique: the fibers from each nucleus curve upward, cross one another in the roof of the midbrain, and exit on the dorsal surface of the midbrain. Therefore each nucleus innervates the contralateral superior oblique muscle.

After leaving the midbrain the fourth nerve curves downward to enter the cavernous sinus, where it is related to the third nerve and other structures, as described in the preceding section on the third nerve. The nerve finally enters the superior orbital fissure and supplies the superior oblique muscle.

Nerve VI: Abducens nerve. The nuclei for the sixth nerves are in the pons beneath the floor of the fourth ventricle, just rostral to the medullary junction and the vestibular nuclei. The medial longitudinal fasciculus lies medially. Fibers from the seventh nerve loop around the sixth nucleus. Fibers from the sixth nucleus course ventrally in the pons and emerge in the groove between the pons and medulla.

The nerve then begins a long intracranial course by climbing the clivus, lying lateral to the basilar artery. It pierces the dura at the tip of the temporal bone and courses horizontally to enter the cavernous sinus where it is related to the third and fourth nerves and other structures, as described under the third nerve. It finally enters the superior orbital fissure and supplies the lateral rectus muscle.

Clinical Significance

The third cranial nerve should be known as the aneurysm nerve and the herniation nerve. Bleeding from an aneurysm at the junction of the internal carotid artery and anterior communicating artery can produce third nerve paralysis with paralysis of the pupil which is usually sudden in onset with retro-orbital pain. Paralysis of the third cranial nerve with sparing of the pupil is seen in diabetic ischemic neuropathy.

A discussion of the diagnostic importance of the third nerve in transtentorial herniation is given in section 193, Level of Consciousness.

The fourth cranial nerve is the trauma nerve. Vertex head injury is a common cause of paralysis of this nerve. This can be unilateral or bilateral. Diabetes also can produce an isolated fourth nerve paralysis.

The sixth cranial nerve is the tumor nerve. A common cause of paralysis of the sixth nerve is increased intracranial pressure.

Myasthenia gravis can mimic a neuropathy by producing isolated ocular muscle paralysis of any of the ocular muscles. The pupil is not involved in myasthenia gravis.

Selected References

1. Bender MB (ed): *The Oculomotor System.* New York, Harper and Row, 1964.
2. Bach-Y-Rita P, Collins CC (eds): *The Control of Eye Movements.* New York, Academic Press, 1971.
3. Brodal A: *Neurological Anatomy,* ed 2. New York, Oxford University Press, 1969, pp 374–396, 429–461.
4. Warwick R: Subnuclei of the oculomotor complex. *J Comp Neurol* 98:449–503, 1953.

5. Cogan DG: *Neurology of the Ocular Muscles*, ed 2. Springfield, Ill, Charles C Thomas, 1969.
6. Zikmund V (ed): *The Oculomotor System and Brain Functions*. London, Butterworths, 1973.
7. Walsh FB, Hoyt WF: *Clinical Neuroophthalmology*, ed 3. Baltimore, Williams and Wilkins, 1969, vol 1, pp 130–348.
8. Truex RC, Carpenter MB: *Human Neuroanatomy*, ed 6. Baltimore, Williams and Wilkins, 1969, pp 360–361, 377–378, 384–390.
9. Krieg WJS: *Functional Neuroanatomy*, ed 2. New York, Blakiston Co, 1953.

198. Cranial Nerve V: The Trigeminal Nerve

H. KENNETH WALKER, MD

Definition

Sensory. The sensory portion of the trigeminal supplies touch-pain-temperature to the face through its three divisions: the ophthalmic, maxillary, and mandibular nerves, as outlined in Fig 167. The innervation also includes the cornea and conjunctiva of the eye, the mucosa of the sinuses, nasal and oral cavities, and dura of the middle anterior, and part of the posterior cranial fossae. Proprioceptive impulses from the temporomandibular joint are largely carried in the motor portion of the nerve, which is incorporated into the mandibular division.

A lesion of the sensory fibers produces hypesthesia or anesthesia of the area supplied. The corneal reflex is absent when the area of supply is the eye. Proprioception for the temporomandibular joint is absent when the mandibular division of the nerve is affected.

Motor. The motor division of the nerve supplies the muscles of mastication: masseter, temporal, pterygoid, mylohyoid, and digastric. These muscles produce elevation, depression, protrusion, retraction, and side-to-side movements of the mandible. The tensor tympani and tensor palati are also supplied.

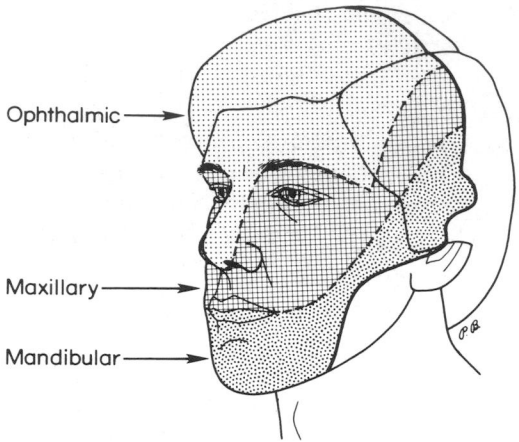

Ophthalmic

Maxillary

Mandibular

Figure 167. Areas supplied by the three sensory divisions of the trigeminal nerve.

When there is unilateral paralysis of the masticatory muscles, the mandible upon opening deviates toward the paralyzed side due to the action of the normal pterygoids on the opposite side. With bilateral paralysis, the mandible droops and no jaw movement is possible. In nuclear or infranuclear lesions, the involved muscles atrophy.

The jaw jerk is one of the deep tendon or stretch reflexes:

Normal: Tapping the mandible produces a brisk contraction.

Abnormal: With upper motor neuron lesions, there is a hyperactive or repeating reflex (clonus). With nuclear or infranuclear lesions, the reflex is absent.

Technique

Sensory. Tell the patient you are going to test his ability to feel touch or pain on the face. Request that the eyes be closed. Take a piece of cotton or the ball of your finger and lightly touch either one or both sides of each of the three divisions of the trigeminal. Ask the patient to indicate whether one or both sides of the face is touched.

Next take a safety pin and gently prick first one side of each division then the other, asking the patient to say if there is any difference in the sensation on one side compared to the other. With the patient's eyes closed touch sometimes with the sharp point of the pin and at other times with the dull guard and ask the patient to describe what he feels.

The corneal reflex is tested by telling the patient you are going to touch the eye gently in order to check the reflex. Take a wisp of cotton and twist it into a point. Ask the patient to look in the other direction, so you will not be testing the blink reflex. Then gently but firmly touch the cornea at its junction with the sclera. Sensitivity to pain increases medially from this point and decreases laterally: the junction of the cornea and sclera is a good compromise between causing pain to the patient and obtaining the reflex. Test more medially if there is no reflex at the junction. There is a rapid blink of the eye being tested and a consensual blink of the other eye. Test the integrity of the reflex by observing the consensual response of the opposite eye if there is seventh nerve weakness on the side being tested.

Motor. For motor testing:

1. Observe the skin over the temporal and masseter muscles to see if any concavity or asymmetry suggests atrophy. Look at the tip of the mandible to see if it is displaced laterally.
2. Ask the patient to clench his jaws: palpate the masseter and temporal muscles for asymmetry of volume and for tone.
3. Observe for deviation of the tip of the mandible as the jaws are opened. If there is an associated seventh nerve weakness on one side, lateral deviation of the mandible can be more easily perceived by lining up a tongue blade with the tip of the nose and the center of the mouth. Deviation is to the weak side.
4. Ask the patient to move the jaw from side to side against the resistance of your palm. The paralyzed side will not move laterally.

For the stretch reflex, demonstrate to the patient what you are going to do. Have the jaws half open and relaxed. Then place your index finger on the tip of the mandible and tap your finger gently but briskly, with a reflex hammer.

Background Information

Sensory. The three divisions of the nerve carry pain, temperature, and touch modalities from the skin of the face, the mucosa of sinuses, nose and mouth, the teeth, and portions of the dura as well as proprioceptive sensation from the teeth, hard palate, and temporomandibular joint and muscles of mastication (Fig 167). The three divisions are:

1. Ophthalmic. Upper division. Innervates forehead, upper eyelid, cornea (thus the corneal reflex), conjunctiva, dorsum of the nose, mucous membranes of certain sinuses, part of the nose,

and dura of some of the anterior cranial fossa. Leaves orbit through the superior orbital fissure, proceeds through the lateral wall of the cavernous sinus in close relation to the third, fourth, and sixth cranial nerves. Joins other two divisions to form the trigeminal (semilunar, Gasserian) ganglion.

2.   Maxillary. Supplies upper lip, lateral and posterior portions of nose, upper cheek, anterior temple, mucosa of nose, upper jaw, upper teeth, roof of mouth, and dura of part of the middle cranial fossa. The nerve leaves the pterygopalatine fossa, passes through the foramen rotundum, traverses the inferior part of the cavernous sinus, and enters the trigeminal ganglion.

3.   Mandibular. Supplies lower lip, chin, posterior cheek, and temple, external ear, mucosa of lower part of mouth, anterior two-thirds of the tongue, and portions of dura of anterior and middle cranial fossae. Proprioceptive impulses are carried largely in the motor nerve, which is incorporated into the mandibular division. It enters the cranium through the foramen ovale and goes to the trigeminal ganglion.

Sympathetic and parasympathetic fibers join the three divisions and are distributed to the pupil, to the nasal mucosa causing mucous secretion, to the lacrimal, submaxillary, and sublingual glands, to the arterioles of the face.

The trigeminal ganglion rests in Meckel's cave, a cavity on the apex of the petrous bone. In this position the ganglion is lateral to the internal carotid artery and the posterior portion of the cavernous sinus. The trigeminal ganglion contains pseudounipolar ganglion cells whose internal branches pass into the pons. These internal branches form the sensory root of the trigeminal, which is analogous to the posterior root of a spinal nerve. The root enters the lateral portion of the middle third of the pons and the branches bifurcate into ascending and descending arms or ascend or descend without bifurcating. These central processes are distributed to three sensory nuclei (Fig 168). Beginning with the lowest or most caudal they are: (1) the spinal tract nucleus, (2) the main sensory nucleus, and (3) the mesencephalic nucleus. They will be considered in that order.

1. The spinal tract nucleus (homologous to the most dorsal laminae of the dorsal horn of the spinal cord): Concerned with pain and temperature. The descending central processes of the sensory root are gathered as a bundle, the spinal tract of the trigeminal. This tract descends to the caudal medulla, where it begins to fuse with the dorsolateral tract of Lissauer in the spinal cord. The tract gives off fibers to its nucleus which lies medial. The nucleus is continuous caudally with the substantia gelatinosa of the spinal cord, and rostrally with the main sensory nucleus (see below). There is probably a topographical localization of fibers in both the tract and nucleus.

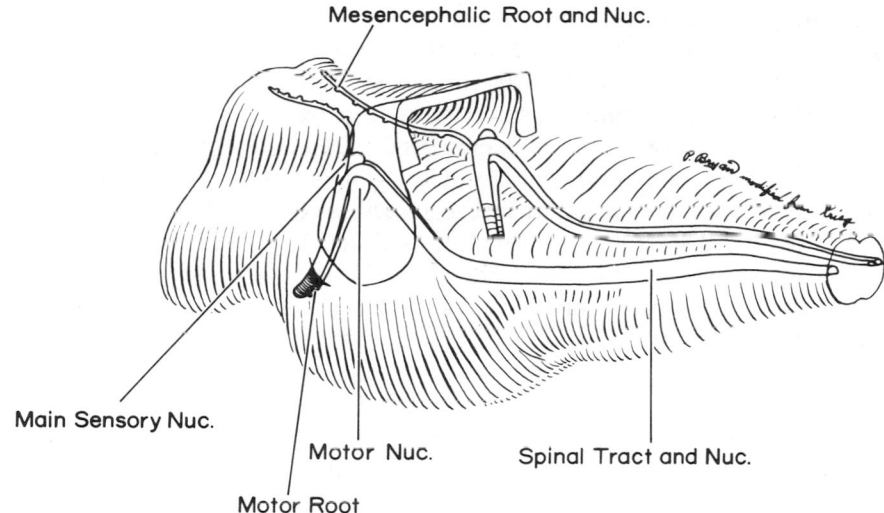

Figure 168. Trigeminal nerve. (Modified from WJS Krieg, *Functional Neuro-anatomy*, ed 2, Blakiston Co, 1953. Used with permission of author.)

The spinal tract and nucleus are generally agreed to be concerned with pain and temperature. The important clinical principle is that lesions in any of the following locations will give ipsilateral loss of pain and temperature on the face (and of course other findings depending upon location of the lesion): peripheral, nuclear, and sensory root of the trigeminal; pontine or medullary lesions involving the spinal tract and nucleus. The spinothalamic tract from the contralateral half of the body is near the trigeminal tract and nucleus. Therefore it follows that at these levels there can be contralateral loss of body pain and temperature associated with an ipsilateral loss of face pain and temperature if the lesion is sufficiently large. Vascular lesions of the lower medulla are a frequent cause of this clinical syndrome.

Secondary trigeminal fibers arise from the spinal tract nucleus, cross to the other side, form the ventral trigeminal tract, and ascend in close relationship with the contralateral medial lemniscus to the ventral posteromedial (VPM) nucleus of the thalamus.

Cortical projections from the VPM are found in the somatosensory areas of the cortex, principally the postcentral gyrus. There is a somatotopical localization.

2. The main sensory nucleus (homologous to the dorsal funiculus of the spinal cord): Concerned with tactile sensation. The ascending branches of the sensory root end in this nucleus, which lies in the pons by the entering root fibers. There is a somatotopical organization.

The large majority of ascending fibers from this nucleus cross the brainstem, travel in association with the contralateral medial lemniscus, and terminate upon the VPM of the thalamus. A smaller group of fibers does not cross but ascends near the periaqueductal gray as the dorsal trigeminal tract; this tract terminates on the ipsilateral VPM. The thalamocortical projections go to the somatosensory areas of the cortex.

3. The mesencephalic nucleus: Concerned with proprioceptive sensibility. This nucleus is located in the lateral dorsal margin of the central gray matter lying next to the fourth ventricle. Afferent impulses arise in masticatory muscles, teeth, periodontium, hard palate, and the temporomandibular joint. Most afferent fibers destined for this nucleus appear to travel with the motor root, although some fibers may be contributed by all three divisions of the nerve. The cells of origin of these fibers, unlike those described above, are not in the trigeminal ganglion; they are within the brain in the nucleus itself. This apparently represents an example of the dorsal root ganglion that exists within the substance of the central nervous system.

Most central processes of the cells of this nucleus descend as the mesencephalic tract to the motor nucleus of the fifth nerve. There are, however, other and more complex connections. Considering the source of these proprioceptive impulses and the distribution of the central processes to the motor nucleus, this nucleus may be concerned with the force of the bite.

Motor.   The supranuclear innervation originates in the lower precentral gyrus, with the contralateral contribution larger than the ipsilateral. These fibers, as part of the corticobulbar tract, descend in the genu of the internal capsule, course through the cerebral peduncles, and are distributed to the motor nuclei of the trigeminal nerve.

The motor nucleus lies in the middle of the pons medial to the main sensory nucleus. The fibers leave the pons ventral to the sensory fibers. The motor root lies against the trigeminal ganglion and is incorporated into the mandibular division of the sensory nerve.

In jaw jerk, muscle spindles are activated as the masticatory muscles are stretched suddenly by tapping on the mandible. These afferent proprioceptive impulses are largely carried in the motor portion of the nerve and end in the mesencephalic nucleus. Collaterals from this nucleus terminate on the trigeminal motor nucleus thereby setting up a two-neuron reflex arc. See section 209, Deep Tendon Reflexes.

Clinical Significance

Peripheral lesions.   Lesions involving the sensory portion of the trigeminal at any point distal to the pontine exit can produce ipsilateral pain and/or varying degrees of anesthesia. The distribution of the lesion will, of course, determine the symptoms and findings. Some of the etiologies are (from Selby et al.):

1. Peripheral lesions: craniofacial trauma, basilar skull fractures, dental trauma, maxillary sinusitis, primary or metastatic tumors, aneurysm of the internal carotid artery, cavernous sinus thrombosis, stilbamidine, trichlorethylene, lupus, scleroderma, Sjögren's syndrome, sarcoidosis, probably amyloidosis, and a fairly common benign sensory neuropathy that is at present idiopathic. Horner's syndrome can be produced by lesions of the nasociliary nerve as it runs with the ophthalmic division.
2. Lesions of the ganglion: herpes zoster infection, primary and metastatic tumors.
3. Trigeminal root lesions: adjacent tumors and vascular malformations, especially acoustic neurinoma and cholesteatomas. These lesions are prone to produce facial pain that is often misdiagnosed as tic douloureux (see below).

Central lesions. Vascular lesions, tumors, and congenital malformations (syringobulbia and syringomyelia) are the most frequent causes. Lesions of the sensory cortex will produce a raised threshold (but not anesthesia) to pain and temperature on the opposite side of the face. Thalamic lesions can produce contralateral hypesthesia and hyperpathia of the face. Midpontine lesions when unilateral produce ipsilateral decrease in tactile sensation of the face due to involvement of the main sensory nucleus, and ipsilateral paralysis of the masticatory muscles when the motor nucleus is involved. Anesthesia or hypesthesia ipsilaterally is seen if the pontine lesion involves entering sensory root fibers carrying pain and temperature modalities. Below the pons ipsilateral pain and temperature is lost if the spinal tract and nucleus are involved. When the ventral trigeminal tract carrying crossed pain-temperature fibers is involved, loss of these modalities occurs on the opposite side of the face.

Some helpful generalizations about central trigeminal lesions are given in Table 39.

Horner's syndrome can be produced due to damage of the nasociliary nerve as it runs with the ophthalmic division.

Tic douloureux or trigeminal neuralgia is a relatively frequent cause of facial pain. There is a paroxysmal pain of unbelievable intensity that involves any or all of the trigeminal division, although it is more frequent in maxillary or mandibular divisions. The pain lasts seconds to minutes and is often set off by a blast of cold or hot air, shaving, combing the hair, or similar stimulus. There are no objective findings such as anesthesia. The etiology is unknown. For years there was disagreement about whether the pain originated centrally or peripherally. Electron microscopic observations of pathologic changes in the trigeminal ganglion in

Table 39.   Location of central trigeminal lesions.

Functional Loss	Location	Structure(s)
1. Pain, temperature, touch over entire body, including face ipsilaterally	Lateral rostral pons and above	Spinothalamic and ventral trigeminal tracts contralaterally
2. Masticatory muscle paralysis and pain, temperature, touch over face ipsilaterally	Midpons	Main sensory nucleus, motor nucleus, and entering root fibers ipsilaterally
3. Pain, temperature over face ipsilaterally; pain, temperature over body and occasionally face contralaterally	Lateral inferior pons or lateral medulla	Spinal tract and spinal tract nucleus ipsilaterally; spinothalamic tract and occasionally ventral trigeminal tract contralaterally

recent years are suggestive of ganglionic origin (see also section 88, Pain and Sensory Perversions).

The motor nerve as it runs with the mandibular division can be damaged by the lesions listed above. Clinically there is atrophy and flaccid paralysis of the muscles of mastication. In unilateral paralysis as the mandible opens it will swing to the paralyzed side due to the action of the normal opposite external pterygoid. Bilateral paralysis with drooping of the mandible is very rare. Spasm of the masticatory muscles is seen with tetanus and strychnine poisoning.

Selected References

1.   Brodal A: *Neurological Anatomy,* ed 2. New York, Oxford University Press, 1969, pp 411–429.
2.   Truex RC, Carpenter MB: *Human Neuroanatomy,* ed 6. Baltimore, Williams and Wilkins, 1969, pp 364–372.
3.   DeJong RN: *The Neurologic Examination,* ed 3. New York, Harper and Row, 1967, pp 215–236.
4.   Haymaker W, Kuhlenbeck H: Disorders of the brainstem and its cranial nerves, in Baker AB, Baker LH (eds): *Clinical Neurology.* New York, Harper and Row, 1975, vol 3, chap 30.
5.   Krieg WJS: *Functional Neuroanatomy,* ed 2. New York, Blakiston Co, 1953.

6.   Haymaker W: *Bing's Local Diagnosis in Neurological Disease,* ed 15. St Louis, CV Mosby, 1969, pp 234–250.
7.   Selby G: Diseases of the fifth cranial nerve, in Dyck PF, Thomas PK, Lambert EH (eds): *Peripheral Neuropathy.* Philadelphia, WB Saunders, 1975, chap 26.

199. Cranial Nerve VII: The Facial Nerve and Taste

H. KENNETH WALKER, MD

Definition

The motor portion, or what might be called the facial nerve proper, supplies all the facial musculature. The principal muscles are the frontalis, orbicularis oculi, buccinator, orbicularis oris, platysma, the posterior belly of the digastric, and the stapedius muscle. In *nuclear* or *infranuclear* ("peripheral") lesions, there is partial to complete facial paralysis with smoothing of the brow, open eye, flat nasolabial fold, and drooping of the mouth ipsilateral to the lesion. In *supranuclear* ("central") lesions, the brow and eyelid musculature are spared; there is flattening of the nasolabial fold and drooping of the mouth contralateral to the lesion.

The sensory portion, or intermediate nerve, has the following components:

1.   Taste to the anterior two-thirds of the tongue.
2.   Secretory and vasomotor fibers to the lacrimal gland, the mucous membranes of the nose and mouth, and the submandibular and sublingual salivary glands.
3.   Cutaneous sensory impulses from the external auditory meatus and region back of the ear.

Abnormalities of taste include:

Ageusia: lack of taste
Hypogeusia: diminished taste acuity
Dysgeusia: unpleasant, obnoxious, or perverted taste

Technique

Motor. Careful and thoughtful observation is the key to discerning sub-tle signs of weakness of muscles supplied by the motor portion. Note especially the blink, nasolabial folds, and corners of the mouth. *Asym-metry* is the clue to unilateral weakness, and is best perceived during con-versation when the patient is unaware of being observed:

1. Blink: the eyelid on the affected side closes just a trace later than the other.
2. Nasolabial folds: the weak one is flatter.
3. Mouth: the affected side droops and participates manifestly less in speaking.

Ask the patient to look up or wrinkle the forehead; inspect for asym-metry. Ask him to close the eyes tightly. Look for incomplete closure or incomplete "burying" of the eyelashes on the affected side. Observe the nasolabial folds and mouth while the patient is concentrating on the eyes. As the orbicularis oculi contract tightly, there are milder associated contractions of muscles about the mouth and nose; these milder contrac-tions are better suited to displaying slight weakness than when these muscles are tested directly.

Ask the patient to smile, show you his teeth, or pull back the corners of his mouth and look for asymmetry about the mouth.

The most subtle signs of mild facial weakness are the blink reflex and incomplete lid closure. Observe the blink reflex during conversation, or tap gently on the glabella with your index finger or reflex hammer in an attempt to bring out a mild asymmetry of blink. If you strongly suspect but are having difficulty confirming a mild facial weakness, then hold the patient's head off the examining table in an inverted position. This forces the upper eyelid to work against gravity. Now ask the patient to close both eyes and inspect for incomplete closure. Tap on the glabella and note asymmetry of blink.

Taste. The four primary tastes are bitter, sweet, sour, and salty. Gross disorders of sweet or salty taste may be screened with the use of salt and sugar. With the patient's eyes closed and tongue protruded, take a tongue blade and smear a small amount of salt or sugar on the lateral surface and side of the tongue. Instruct the patient to tell you the identity of the substance. Rinse the mouth thoroughly and repeat the test on the other side, using a different substance. More detailed tests are required to assess the detection and recognition thresholds for the specific types of taste.

Background Information

The cortical fibers originate from the lower third of the motor strip, pass in the genu of the internal capsule, the middle third of the cerebral peduncle, and supply the seventh nucleus in the lower pons. The supranuclear innervation is bilateral to the muscles of the forehead and eyes but only contralateral to the muscles of the lower part of the face. This accounts for the sparing of the upper facial muscles with a contralateral cortical lesion. The anatomy of the nucleus is shown in Fig 166, section 197B.

The facial nucleus participates in the corneal reflex: corneal pain-temperature fibers go through the ophthalmic division of the fifth cranial nerve to the spinal nucleus of the fifth and thence to the ipsilateral seventh nucleus, causing the eyelid to blink. There are also central connections between the facial nucleus and the nuclei or projection systems of the second, third, fourth, sixth, and eighth cranial nerves. These connections make possible a coordination of movements among the eyelids and eyeballs and set up certain reflexes such as the blink reflex on exposure to strong light or a loud sound.

The motor fibers for the facial muscles exit from the motor nucleus, curl up and around the sixth nucleus, and descend laterally from the lower pons. At the point where the motor segment leaves the pons it is joined by the *intermediate nerve,* which is composed of contributions from three areas:

1. The superior salivary nucleus in the pons supplies secretory fibers which are distributed to (a) the lacrimal, nasal, and palatine glands (via the greater superficial petrosal nerve) and (b) the submandibular and sublingual salivary glands (via the chorda tympani nerve).
2. The gustatory (solitary) nucleus in the medulla supplies sensory fibers which are distributed to taste buds on the anterior two-thirds of the tongue (via the chorda tympani nerve).
3. The dorsal part of the trigeminal tract supplies fibers that convey cutaneous sensation from the external auditory meatus and skin back of the ear (distributed with the facial nerve proper).

First-order neurons are in the geniculate ganglion.

The facial nerve proper and intermediate nerve lie in the cerebellopontine angle with the sixth and eighth cranial nerves. The seventh, intermediate, and eighth nerves then enter the internal auditory meatus and pass through it. The facial and intermediate nerves enter the facial canal of the petrous portion of the temporal bone. The geniculate ganglion of the intermediate nerve is in this canal. The greater superficial petrosal nerve destined for the lacrimal, nasal, and palatine glands leaves just distal to the geniculate ganglion. The nerve to the stapedius muscle is given off next. The facial and intermediate nerves then descend to the stylomastoid foramen, giving off the chorda tympani at either the stylomastoid foramen or varying distances proximal to it. The chorda tympani now supplies the anterior two-thirds of the tongue and the submandibular and sublingual glands. The motor part of the facial nerve leaves the stylomastoid foramen and supplies the facial musculature. A major part of the nerve forms a plexus within the parotid gland.

Taste sensibility is composed of four qualities: sweet, salt, sour, and bitter. Taste receptors are located on the tongue, palate, pharynx, and larynx. Although all four qualities can be perceived throughout, there is considerable localization: the tongue, especially the tip and edges, is most sensitive to sweet and salt; the palate, to sour and bitter. The receptors are taste buds. Up to 8 are on each of the fungiform papillae on the anterior two-thirds of the tongue, and up to 100 on each of the circumvallate papillae on the posterior part of the tongue. The taste buds are barrel-shaped with a pore opening. Chemoreceptive taste hairs project into the barrel from neuroepithelial sensory cells. Impulses from these cells are then transmitted to the brainstem. Afferent fibers from the anterior two-thirds of the tongue travel via the lingual nerve to the chorda tympani, and then as described above to the gustatory nucleus. Taste fibers from the posterior third of the tongue, the palate, and the palatal arches travel via the glossopharyngeal nerve and the nodosal ganglion, also ending in the gustatory nucleus. There are two ascending pathways from the gustatory nucleus. One goes to the hypothalamus. The other goes to the thalamus and then to the gustatory center of the cortex, which is probably area 43 in the parietal operculum.

Clinical Significance

Motor. A lesion involving the nuclear or infranuclear portion of the facial nerve will produce a peripheral facial palsy. If all motor components are involved, there is complete paralysis of all facial muscles on the involved side. The brow is smooth, the eye does not close, the nasolabial fold is flat, and that side of the mouth droops. There is no movement at all. The paradigm of this type of involvement is Bell's palsy. This may strike at any age, often after a mild viral illness. Recovery is over a period of weeks to months and is variable. The cause is unknown. Sequelae to Bell's palsy include:

1. Interfacial synkinesis: when the eyes close the mouth will twitch. This occurs when the regenerating nerve fibers do not grow back into the proper muscles. The synkinetic movements are almost always present on the involved side.

2. Because of contractures, the face at rest may be more deeply etched on the side of the previous palsy. This can give a false impression of weakness on the opposite side.

Other causes of peripheral seventh nerve palsy include: neoplasm, trauma, middle-ear infections, parotid gland surgery, granulomatous or carcinomatous meningitis, and diabetes. The disturbance of function produced by these lesions need not be complete.

Supranuclear involvement produces contralateral paralysis of the lower facial muscles and sparing of the upper muscles due to the bilateral supranuclear innervation of the latter. Subtle weakness is often difficult to confirm. Many, perhaps even most, normal individuals have mild lower facial asymmetries, making interpretation difficult.

Anatomical localization of lesions is made by the characteristics of the dysfunction and associated structures involved. Table 40 lists some generalizations.

Taste. Patients with Addison's disease, pituitary insufficiency, or cystic fibrosis have an increased ability to detect the four primary tastes. Taste

Table 40. Facial nerve lesions.

Functional Loss	Location of Lesion
1. Paralysis of lower facial muscles with preservation of upper muscles	Above the facial nucleus; either brainstem or cortex.
2. Facial monoplegia, lateral rectus paralysis (VI), and contralateral hemiplegia (corticospinal fibers)	Ipsilateral lower pons.
3. Facial monoplegia with loss of taste on anterior two-thirds of tongue, lateral rectus palsy (VI), hearing loss (VIII), and loss of facial sensation including corneal reflex (V)	Ipsilateral cerebellopontine angle after VIIth exits from pons and before it enters internal auditory meatus; acoustic neuromas are a frequent cause of this syndrome.
4. Facial monoplegia and loss of taste to anterior two-thirds of tongue	Ipsilateral lesion between entrance of VIIth into internal auditory meatus and before departure of chorda tympani (which usually occurs somewhere in the facial canal).
5. Facial monoplegia without involvement of taste	Ipsilateral lesion after departure of chorda tympani and before bifurcation of VIIth nerve in the parotid gland.

acuity returns to normal with glucocorticoid therapy in the cases of adrenal hypofunction. Conversely, penicillamine therapy may be associated with a decreased acuity for the four primary tastes. A wide variety of conditions may cause decreased or absent taste:

1. Local lesions: lichen planus, moniliasis, infiltrative tumors, local irradiation, Sjögren's syndrome. Taste for sour and bitter is normal if the palate is not involved.

2. Palatal abnormalities: dentures that cover the palate, gonadal dysgenesis syndromes, and pseudohypoparathyroid patients with palatal abnormalities have decreased ability to detect sour and bitter while sweet and salt tastes are normal.

3. Chorda tympani: injury during stapedectomy, damage from cerebellopontine angle tumors (as acoustic neuromas), or involvement of this nerve in Bell's palsy can all produce ipsilateral loss of taste to the anterior two-thirds of the tongue.

4. Drugs other than penicillamine that can produce hypogeusia or ageusia include grisofulvin, carbimazole, thiamazole, lincomycin, clofibrate, 5-mercaptopyridoxal, tetracycline, and lithium.

5. Hypothyroid patients have decreased taste that becomes normal with thyroid replacement therapy.

6. Viral infections, especially influenza, may produce abnormalities of taste.

7. Many postoperative patients have hypogeusia or ageusia, even after minor procedures. The cause is not known.

8. Type I familial dysautonomia (Riley-Day) patients have decreased or absent taste associated with a congenital absence of taste buds. But parenteral methacholine produces normal taste acuity, raising the fascinating possibility that taste buds may not be a prerequisite for taste.

Gustatory sweating is sweating on the face associated with eating. It is seen in the following circumstances:

1. Diabetes mellitus, presumably due to the diabetic autonomic neuropathy

2. Frey's syndrome: gustatory sweating after injury, infection, or surgery of the parotid gland

3. After upper dorsal sympathectomy

4. Physiological, occurring after eating highly spiced food.

No proposed mechanism explains the occurrence of this phenomenon in all cases.

Selected References

1. Brodal A: *Neurological Anatomy,* ed 2. New York, Oxford University Press, 1969, pp 397–411.
2. DeJong RN: *The Neurologic Examination,* ed 3. New York, Harper and Row, 1967, pp 237–266.
3. Carpenter MD: *Human Neuroanatomy,* ed 7. Baltimore, Williams and Wilkins, 1976.
4. Henkin RI, Graziadei PPG, Bradley DF: The molecular basis of taste and its disorders. *Ann Intern Med* 71:791–821, 1969.
5. Henkin RI, Larson AL, Powell RD: Hypogeusia, dysgeusia, hyposmia, and dysosmia following influenza-like infection. *Ann Otol* 84:672–682, 1975.
6. Griffith IP: Abnormalities of smell and taste. *Practitioner* 217:907–913, 1976.
7. Thawley SE: Disorders of taste and smell. *South Med J* 71:267–270, 1978.
8. Pfaffman C: Neurophysiological mechanisms of taste. *Am J Clin Nutr* 31:1058–1067, 1978.
9. Rollin H: Course of the peripheral gustatory nerves. *Ann Otol* 86:251–258, 1977.
10. Stuart DD: Diabetic gustatory sweating. *Ann Intern Med* 89:223–224, 1978.
11. Kurchin A, Adar R, Zweig A, et al: Gustatory phenomena after upper dorsal sympathectomy. *Arch Neurol* 34:619–623, 1977.
12. Stroud MH, Thalmann R: A sensitive sign of facial nerve weakness. *Laryngoscope* 82:17–20, 1972.
13. May M, Hardin WB Jr: Facial palsy: Interpretation of neurologic findings. *Laryngoscope* 88:1352–1362, 1978.
14. Dastoli FR; Taste receptor proteins. *Life Sciences* 14:1417–1426, 1974.
15. Henkin RI, Schecter PJ, Hoye R, et al: Idiopathic hypogeusia with dysgeusia hyposmia, and dysmosmia. A new syndrome. *JAMA* 217:434–440, 1971.

200. Cranial Nerve VIII: The Acoustic Nerve

JOHN TURNER, MD

Definition

The Rinne and Weber hearing tests are outlined below.

WEBER

Normal. A tuning fork (usually 256 Hz) is activated and applied to the midline of the skull, the forehead, the chin, or the upper incisor teeth. There is no lateralization of the sound energy generated from the fork to either ear. (It is perceived by the patient as being in the middle of the head or on top of the head.)

Abnormal. A vibrating fork will be perceived in the ear with conductive hearing loss (drum perforation; impacted wax; middle ear fluid; stapes fixation, or otosclerosis), provided the other ear is normal.

A vibrating fork will be perceived in the ear with the best sensorineural function if some sensorineural dysfunction exists in both (aging deafness, presbycusis), ototoxicity from drugs, acoustic trauma (excess noise exposure), post-CNS infections).

RINNE

Normal. A tuning fork activated and held 1 inch from the ear and then placed on the mastoid process will be heard better (louder or more distinctly) in front of the ear than behind the ear (Fig 169). (AC > BC; air conduction better than bone conduction.)

Abnormal. A tuning fork activated and held 1 inch from the ear and then placed on the mastoid process will be heard better behind the ear. (BC > AC; bone conduction better than air conduction.)

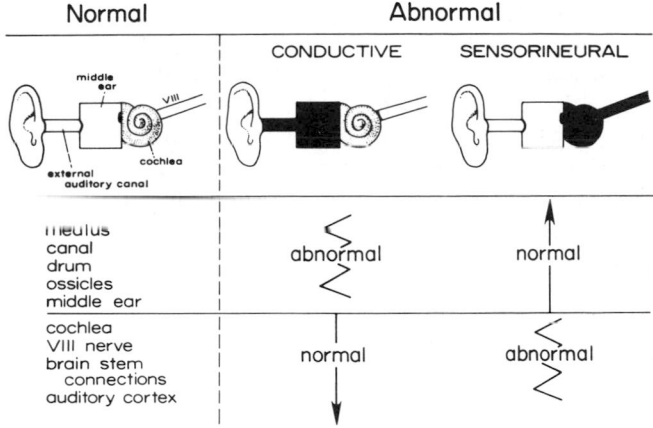

Figure 169. Site of abnormal function in conductive and sensorineural hearing loss.

Technique

The fork is struck on one tine by a rubber reflex hammer or on the examiner's elbow strongly enough to produce a sound clearly perceived by the examiner at 1 foot.

Weber (Fig 170): The fork is then held firmly on the vertex of the skull in the midline, or firmly on the forehead, the chin, or the upper incisors. The thickness of the scalp or hair will sometimes prevent ac-

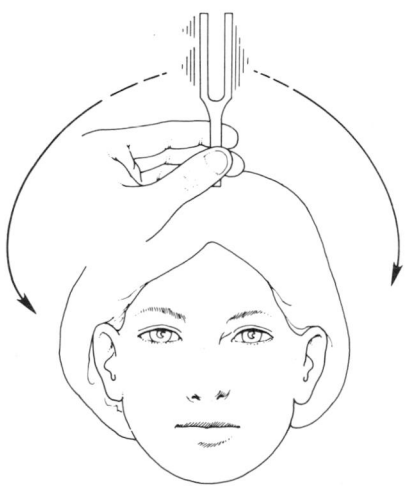

Figure 170. Midline positioning of the tuning fork for the Weber test.

curate referral response. Probably the most exact referral is from the incisor teeth. Remove false teeth and use the upper gum. Always remove wigs if using vertex. The patient is asked: Do you hear this better in the right or left ear? If the patient hesitates, then the Weber does not refer.

Rinne (Fig 171): The fork is held 1 inch from the external ear with the tines vibrating toward the external meatus. The fork is held in this position for about 5 seconds and the patient is asked: Is it louder in front? The fork is immediately shifted to the mastoid process behind the pinna and the patient is asked, "or back?" The process is repeated for the other ear.

An alternate method for the Rinne is to place the fork on the mastoid at first and then ask the patient to indicate when he stops hearing the sound. The fork is then held 1 inch from the pinna and the patient asked if he still hears the sound. If the sound is still heard, air conduction is greater than bone, AC > BC, if not, BC > AC.

Proper recording of the Rinne should be AC > BC or BC > AC for each ear.

Proper recording of the Weber should be Weber → R or Weber → L or Weber, "not referred."

Background Information

The 256-Hz fork is preferred for Weber and Rinne tests because it is of intermediate range to permit evaluation of low-tone hearing impairment without excessive vibratory sensation influencing the response. A higher-pitched fork will miss early conductive hearing losses and a lower-pitched one will test vibration predominantly.

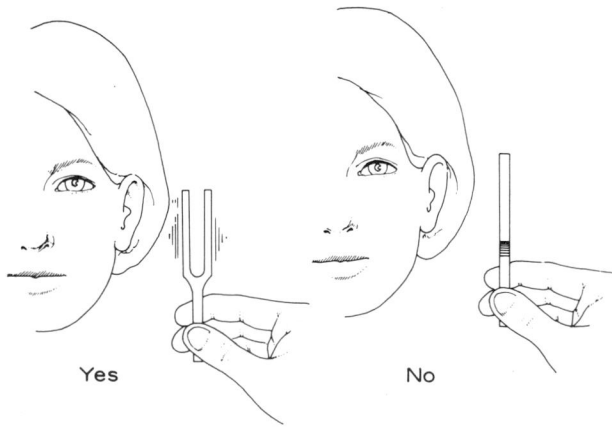

Yes   No

Figure 171.   Proper positioning of tuning fork tines for air conduction testing.

Other forks an octave apart, 512, 1024, 2048, and 4096, can be used in the same manner to evaluate losses at higher frequencies. These frequencies are also used on electronic audiometers to permit recording on an audiogram or graph of the hearing response. Accurate fork testing will permit the clinician to predict the pattern of each patient's audiogram.

Air conduction testing measures the integrity of the entire hearing apparatus from external ear to auditory cortex.

Bone conduction testing measures the integrity of the sensorineural structures (cochlea, eighth nerve, brainstem nuclei, and relays to the auditory cortex).

The combination of these two tests permits the examiner to use fundamental physiological information in categorizing the patient's hearing as being within normal limits.

Clinical Significance

All hearing loss can be categorized into conductive or sensorineural loss. Proper use of the Weber and Rinne tests combined with the clinician's knowledge of the patient's complaints and examination of the ear canal and eardrum will permit accurate classification. Some patients have combined or mixed conductive or sensorineural loss, but fork tests help define which predominates.

Weber: Certain variation to the classical abnormal findings listed above may be found.

1. A vibrating fork will be perceived in the ear with the most severe conductive loss if some conductive dysfunction exists in both (bilateral drum perforation, bilateral impacted wax, bilateral middle-ear fluid, bilateral stapes fixation).
2. In hearing loss of mixed type (both conductive and sensorineural), the rules are unpredictable and variable. Generally speaking, the Weber will refer to the ear with predominate conductive loss.

Rinne: Remember that in normal as well as in sensorineural hearing loss AC > BC. The air conduction is usually shortened in time or a louder fork is needed to allow the patient to perceive air conduction in sensorineural loss. There is nothing wrong with the patient's conductive mechanisms (external ear, canal, eardrum, middle ear, and ossicular chain). Therefore air conduction is greater than bone conduction if you get the air conduction loud enough to overcome the patient's hearing loss (threshold of hearing).

In conductive hearing loss where there is impairment of sound conduction through the canal, drum, or middle ear, the fork is heard better by bone (mastoid cortex) because sound energy is placed directly into the inner ear fluids of the cochlea and thence into the hair cells of the organ of Corti. The cochlea is thus stimulated without having to use the conductive mechanisms of the external canal, drum, and middle ear. A more detailed physiological explanation may be found in the references listed below. There is nothing wrong with the patient's sensorineural (perceptive) hearing (cochlea eighth nerve and central connections), and therefore BC > AC by the fork test. The classification of hearing loss is very important because virtually all hearing impairment can be helped. Conductive losses can be helped by surgery. Sensorineural losses can be helped with hearing aids. Unilateral sensorineural hearing loss may represent serious disease such as acoustic neuroma or brainstem tumor, and early identification is of paramount importance.

Selected References

1.   Shambaugh GE (ed): *Surgery of the Ear,* ed 2. Philadelphia, WB Saunders, 1967, chap 14, pp 369–400.
2.   Kobrak H (ed): *The Middle Ear.* Chicago, University of Chicago Press, 1969, chap 5, pp 88–108.
3.   Sataloff J (ed): *Hearing Loss.* Philadelphia, JB Lippincott, 1966, chap 3, pp 10–16.
4.   Myers D, et al: Otologic diagnosis and the treatment of deafness. *Ciba Clin Symposia* 22(2):35–69, 1970.

---

201. Cranial Nerves IX and X: The Glossopharyngeal and Vagus Nerves

H. KENNETH WALKER, MD

Definition

Glossopharyngeal nerve: lesions produce difficulty swallowing; impairment of taste over the posterior one-third of the tongue and the palate; impaired sensation over the posterior one-third of the tongue, palate, and pharynx; an absent gag reflex; and dysfunction of the parotid gland.

Vagus nerve: lesions produce palatal and pharyngeal paralysis; laryngeal paralysis; and abnormalities of esophageal motility, gastric acid secretion, gallbladder emptying, and heart rate.

Technique

Listen to the patient talk as you are taking the history. Hoarseness, whispering, nasal speech, or the complaint of aspiration or regurgitation of liquids through the nose should make you especially mindful of abnormality. Give the patient a glass of water to see if there is choking or any complaints as it is swallowed.

Have the patient open his mouth and inspect the palatal arch on each side for asymmetry. Use a tongue blade to gently depress the base of the tongue if necessary. Ask the patient to say "ahhh" as long as possible. Observe the palatal arches as they contract and the soft palate as it swings up and back in order to close off the nasopharynx from the oropharynx. Normal palatal arches will constrict and elevate and the uvula will remain in the midline as it is elevated. With paralysis there is no elevation or constriction of the affected side.

Now warn the patient that you are going to test the gag reflex. Gently touch first one then the other palatal arch, waiting each time for gagging.

Evaluation of the vocal cords is done by laryngoscopy. See section 199, Facial Nerve and Taste, for the testing of taste.

Background Information

MEDULLA NUCLEI

Motor. Two groups of motor nuclei serve these nerves:

1. Nucleus ambiguus: Located in the mid to upper medulla. Supplies the striated ("branchial") muscles of the pharynx, larynx, and upper esophagus via the ninth, tenth, and eleventh nerves. Supranuclear innervations from the lower part of the precentral gyrus are partly crossed and partly uncrossed. There are multiple connections with nuclei of neighboring brainstem nuclei for coordination of swallowing, gagging, and coughing.

2. Dorsal motor nucleus (X) and inferior salivary nucleus (IX): Located in the medulla dorsal and lateral to the twelfth nucleus. Parasympathetic fibers originating in these nuclei supply smooth muscles in pulmonary, gastrointestinal, and cardiovascular systems and are secretory to various glands of the gastrointestinal system. The principal supranuclear control is from the hypothalamus; there may be cortical innervation.

Sensory.   Two groups of sensory nuclei serve these nerves:

1. Solitary tract and nucleus, also known as the gustatory nucleus. A long nuclear column extending the length of the medulla, located lateral to the dorsal motor nucleus of the vagus. Receives sensory fibers from the ninth, tenth, and seventh (via the nervus intermedius) nerves.

The sensory fibers carried in the ninth nerve have their cell station in the superior or petrosal ganglion. They include:

    a.   Taste from posterior third of tongue. See section 199 for a discussion of taste.

    b.   Chemoreceptor and baroreceptor impulses from the carotid glomus and carotid sinus

    c.   General sensation from the posterior portion of oral cavity

The sensory fibers carried in the tenth nerve have their cell station in the nodose or jugular ganglion. They include:

    a.   Visceral sensory impulses from pulmonary, gastrointestinal, and cardiac systems

    b.   Chemoreceptor and baroreceptor impulses from aorta and carotid arteries

2. Nucleus of spinal tract of trigeminal: See section 198, The Trigeminal Nerve, for a description of this nucleus.

Pain and temperature impulses from certain parts of the ear reach this nucleus via the petrosal ganglion of the ninth and the jugular ganglion of the tenth nerve. Pain sensation from the dura of the posterior fossa also travels to this nucleus via the jugular ganglion.

PERIPHERAL COURSE

The roots of the two nerves exit together from the medulla and leave the skull through the jugular foramen in the company of the eleventh nerve.

The superior and petrosal ganglia of the ninth are in the jugular foramen. The ninth nerve descends on the side of the pharynx and then enters the pharynx. Areas supplied include the posterior third of the tongue and posterior pharynx, soft palate, the stylopharyngeus muscle, the pharyngeal plexus, secretory glandular fibers, and other areas.

After leaving the jugular foramen the vagus courses in the internal carotid sheath and ultimately ends on the stomach. With a few exceptions it supplies all the muscles of the soft palate, pharynx, and larynx, in addition to the structures in the pulmonary, gastrointestinal, and cardiovascular systems previously mentioned. The ganglia are the nodose and jugular.

Clinical Significance

For all practical purposes the ninth nerve cannot be tested separately, and isolated lesions are almost unknown. In the cerebellopontine angle, the eighth and ninth nerves can be involved by tumors. At the jugular foramen the ninth, tenth, and eleventh nerves can all be involved, eg, by a glomus tumor or other tumors. Diphtheria can cause ninth nerve paralysis. Glossopharyngeal neuralgia, similar to trigeminal neuralgia, does occur rarely. It consists of a stabbing, lancinating pain at the base of the tongue or around the palate.

The vagus nerve has many ramifications of clinical significance, as befits such a complex nerve. Only a few of those that are susceptible to historical and physical evaluation will be mentioned here.

Bilateral supranuclear denervation leads to dysphagia and dysarthria. This can be seen in a condition known as pseudobulbar palsy in which multiple small lesions in the cortex and/or brainstem interrupt the corticobulbar supply to the motor nuclei of various cranial nerves. Etiologies include multiple sclerosis, hypertensive lacunes, and other causes of bihemispheric disease.

Bilateral nuclear involvement of the vagus causes death with pharyngeal and laryngeal paralysis and cardiac arrhythmias. Unilateral nuclear or infranuclear involvement of the vagus causes ipsilateral paralysis of the soft palate, pharynx, and larynx. The voice is hoarse or nasal, the involved palatal arch is paralyzed, and liquids will enter the nasopharynx or trachea. The vocal cord on the involved side is paralyzed. Causes include: meningitis, carotid aneurysms, neoplasms, trauma, and diphtheria. Diseases that involve all peripheral nerves, such as diabetes and amyloidosis, and toxins such as lead, produce neuropathies of these nerves. Neoplasms at any point in the course of the nerve can also involve it.

Recurrent laryngeal nerve paralysis is an important condition. There is paralysis of the vocal cord ipsilaterally; the voice may be hoarse but can be normal, with the lesion discoverable only by laryngoscopy. Bilateral recurrent laryngeal paralysis produces paralysis of both cords, with a whispering voice, stridor, and even death due to tracheal obstruction by the cords. Causes of recurrent laryngeal damage include surgery or neoplasms of the thyroid, cervical adenopathy of any cause, aortic aneurysms, mediastinal tumors, and lead poisoning.

Swallow syncope, or unconsciousness produced by swallowing, is a rare complication of ninth and tenth nerve lesions. The probable mechanism is a vasovagal reflex produced by esophageal distention, with resulting cardiac inhibition. A similar syncopal syndrome has been reported also with glossopharyngeal neuralgia.

Gustatory sweating is discussed in section 199, The Facial Nerve and Taste.

Selected References

1. Aring CD: Supranuclear (pseudobulbar) palsy. *Arch Intern Med* 115: 198–199, 1965.
2. Haymaker W, Kuhlenbeck H: Disorders of the brainstem and its cranial nerves, in Baker AB, Baker LH (eds): *Clinical Neurology.* New York, Harper & Row, 1975, vol 3, chap 31.
3. Brodal A (ed): *Neurological Anatomy,* ed 2. New York, Oxford University Press, 1969, pp 363–374.
4. Davis JN, Thomas PK, Spalding JMK, et al: Diseases of the ninth, tenth and eleventh cranial nerves, in Dyck PJ, Thomas PK, Lambert EH (eds): *Peripheral Neuropathy.* Philadelphia, WB Saunders, 1975, vol 1, pp 614–627.
5. Levin B, Posner JB: Swallow syncope. *Neurology* 22:1086–1093, 1972.
6. Khero BA, Mullins CB: Cardiac syncope due to glossopharyngeal neuralgia. *Arch Intern Med* 128:806–808, 1971.

202. Cranial Nerve XI: The Spinal Accessory Nerve

H. KENNETH WALKER, MD

Definition

This nerve supplies the sternocleidomastoid and trapezius muscles, which have the following functions:

1. Rotation of head away from the side of the contracting sternocleidomastoid muscle
2. Tilting of the head toward the contracting sternocleidomastoid muscle
3. Flexion of the neck by both sternocleidomastoid muscles
4. Elevation of the shoulder by the trapezius
5. Drawing the head back so the face is upward by the trapezius muscles

With weakness or paralysis these functions are decreased or absent. When the lesion is nuclear or infranuclear, there is associated muscle atrophy and fasciculations.

Technique

Observe the volume and contour of the sternocleidomastoid muscles as the patient looks ahead. Test the right sternocleidomastoid muscle by facing the patient and placing your right palm laterally on the patient's left cheek. Ask the patient to turn his head to the left, resisting the pressure you are exerting in the opposite direction. At the same time palpate the right sternocleidomastoid with your left hand. Then reverse the procedure to test the left sternocleidomastoid.

Continue to test the sternocleidomastoid by placing your hand on the patient's forehead and pushing backward as the patient pushes forward. Observe and palpate the sternocleidomastoid muscles.

Now test the trapezius. Ask the patient to face away from you and observe the shoulder contour for hollowing, displacement, or winging of the scapula. Observe for drooping of the shoulder. Place your hands on the patient's shoulders and press down as the patient elevates or shrugs the shoulders, and then retracts the shoulders.

Background Information

The eleventh nerve has two parts. The smaller cranial part arises from cells in the nucleus ambiguus and ultimately is distributed with the vagus nerve. The main part, the spinal portion, arises from a long column of nuclei situated in the ventral part of the medulla and extending to the fourth cervical segment or lower (Fig 172). Supranuclear innervation is from the contralateral and ipsilateral areas of the precentral gyri, descending in the corticobulbar tract. As the fibers leave the cord they join together and ascend through the foramen magnum, then leave through the jugular foramen with the vagus nerve. The nerve descends in the neck near the jugular vein and supplies the sternocleidomastoid and trapezius muscles, joined by motor or sensory contributions from the upper cervical nerves.

The sternocleidomastoid muscles originate from the sternum and clavicle and insert on the mastoid process. Each one: (1) rotates the head to the opposite side of the body, that is, away from the side of the muscle; (2) tilts the head to the same side of the body. Acting together the sternocleidomastoid muscles flex the neck and bring the head forward and down.

The trapezius muscle originates on the occiput and the spinous processes of the cervical and thoracic vertebrae and inserts on the clavi-

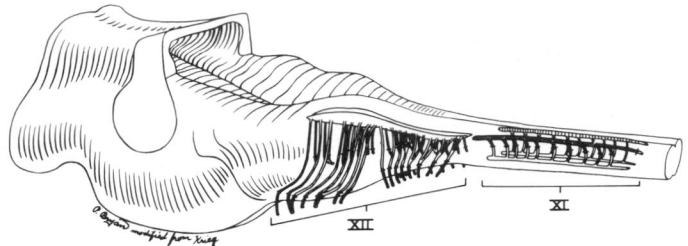

Figure 172. Elongated view depicting XI and XII. (Modified from WJS Krieg, *Functional Neuroanatomy*, ed 2, Blakiston Co, 1953. Used with permission of author.)

cle and scapula. Some controversy centers around whether all or part of the muscle is supplied by the spinal accessory nerve; many believe only its upper portion is supplied by the eleventh nerve. When the head is fixed, the trapezius elevates the shoulders. When the scapula is fixed, it draws the head ipsilaterally; jointly the trapezii pull the head back so the face is upward.

Clinical Significance

Supranuclear lesions cause moderate and often transient impairment of the sternocleidomastoid and trapezius due to the bilateral innervation. Nuclear and infranuclear lesions cause paralysis, atrophy, and fasciculations. Isolated involvement of the eleventh nerve is rarely seen; usually other nerves, such as the ninth, tenth, and twelfth, are also involved. The causes are multiple, including trauma, meningitis, and various local lesions in the neck. Spasms of the muscles, or torticollis, are seen in a large variety of conditions; they are poorly understood.

Selected References

1.   Brodal A: *Neurological Anatomy,* ed 2. New York, Oxford University Press, 1969, pp 360–363.
2.   DeJong RN: *The Neurologic Examination,* ed 3. New York, Harper and Row, 1967, pp 324–333.
3.   Krieg WJ: *Functional Neuroanatomy,* ed 2. New York, Blakiston Co, 1953.
4.   Davis JN, Thomas PK, Spalding JMK, et al: Diseases of the ninth, tenth, and eleventh cranial nerves, in Dyck PJ, Thomas PK, Lambert EH (eds): *Peripheral Neuropathy.* Philadelphia, WB Saunders, 1975, vol 1, pp 614–627.

203. Cranial Nerve XII: The Hypoglossal Nerve

H. KENNETH WALKER, MD

Definition

This nerve controls all tongue movements. Nuclear or infranuclear lesions produce paralysis, atrophy, and fasciculations of the tongue on the involved side. Supranuclear lesions produce mild to moderate contralateral weakness that may be transient. Bilateral supranuclear lesions, seen in pseudobulbar palsy, produce moderate to severe inability of the tongue to function.

Technique

Start by inspecting the tongue as it rests in the patient's mouth. Unilateral weakness or paralysis can be strongly suspected if the tongue is curled in a gentle arabesque. The tip of the tongue will point to the normal side due to unopposed normal tone in that half of the tongue. Look for atrophy and fasciculations.

Test the genioglossus by asking the patient to protrude the tongue. With unilateral weakness or paralysis the tongue will point to the affected side due to unopposed action of the normal muscle.

Background Information

The nuclei are dorsal and medial in the medulla (see Fig 172 in section 213). Supranuclear innervation is predominantly from the contralateral cortex, and descends in the corticobulbar tract. The fibers leave the medulla and pass through the hypoglossal canal. Peripherally the nerve supplies the intrinsic muscles of the tongue, the genioglossus (tongue protrusion) the hypoglossus, and the styloglossus.

Clinical Significance

Supranuclear lesions usually produce a transient mild weakness of the contralateral tongue. Nuclear and infranuclear lesions produce atrophy and fasciculations. Neoplasms, fractures, trauma, infections, and degenerative diseases can cause the latter lesions. Nuclear lesions are frequently bilateral due to the closeness of the two nuclei. Unilateral twelfth nerve involvement has been described as one of the most common cranial nerve mononeuropathies seen with metastatic tumors.

Selected References

1.   Brodal A: *Neurological Anatomy,* ed 2. New York, Oxford University Press, 1969, pp 356–360.
2.   DeJong RN: *The Neurologic Examination,* ed 2. New York, Harper and Row, 1967, pp 334–341.
3.   Davis JN, Thomas PK, Spalding JMK, Harrison MS: Diseases of the ninth, tenth and eleventh cranial nerves, in Dyck PJ, Thomas PK, Lambert EH (eds): *Peripheral Neuropathy.* Philadelphia, WB Saunders, 1975, vol 1, pp 614–627.
4.   Rubinstein MK: Cranial mononeuropathy as the first sign of intracranial metastases. *Ann Intern Med* 70:49–54, 1969.

204. Sensation

H. KENNETH WALKER, MD

Definition

I.   Exteroceptive sensation
    A.   Tactile or touch sensation:
        1.   Anesthesia: absence of touch appreciation.
        2.   Hypesthesia: decrease of touch appreciation.
        3.   Hyperesthesia: unpleasant exaggeration of touch sensation. Note that the terms above are unfortunately not specific for tactile losses. They are commonly used indiscriminately to apply to losses of all types of sensation.

B. Pain sensation:
1. Analgesia: absence of pain appreciation.
2. Hypalgesia: decrease of pain appreciation.
3. Hyperalgesia: unpleasant exaggeration of pain sensation.

C. Temperature sensation (hot or cold):
1. Thermanalgesia: absence of temperature appreciation.
2. Thermhypesthesia: decrease of temperature appreciation.
3. Thermhyperesthesia: unpleasant exaggeration of temperature sensation.

D. Sensory perversions (see section 88, Pain and Sensory Perversions:
1. Dysesthesia: painful irradiating sensation elicited by a nonpainful cutaneous stimulus such as light touch or gentle stroking. Synonyms: hyperpathia, hyperalgesia. The induced sensation often will outlast the stimulus by several seconds and frequently will generate a complaint of intense burning.
2. Paresthesia: spontaneous, abnormal sensation: tactile, painful, or thermal. It may be episodic or constant.

II. Proprioceptive sensation
A. Joint position sense: absence is described as such.
B. Vibratory sense: absence is described as such.
C. Cortical sensory functions:
1. Stereognosis: ability to identify objects by feeling them. Astereognosis is the absence of this ability.
2. Two-point discrimination: ability to separate two points on the body. Absence is described as such.
3. Sensory extinction: abnormality that occurs when an individual is able to identify only one of two identical and simultaneous stimuli. Example: light touch on each forearm elicits the perception of being touched on one side only. Visual extinction is another example.
4. Touch localization (topognosis): ability to localize stimuli to parts of the body. Topagnosis is the absence of this ability.
5. Graphesthesia: ability to recognize symbols written on the skin. Graphanesthesia is the absence of this ability.

Joint position and vibratory testing should be a part of every screening examination. Cortical sensory functions should be done only when an abnormality is suspected. Facial sensation is covered in section 198, Trigeminal Nerve.

Technique

The patient should be relaxed and in comfortable surroundings. Instructions should be detailed with frequent checks to make sure they are understood. Avoid exhausting the patient. Repetition of the examination on several different occasions will increase reproducibility of results. The results should be drawn on the patient and meticulously recorded on an outline of the body along with a description of the stimuli used.

Screening examinations on patients in whom there is no reason to suspect sensory disturbances can consist only of the testing of touch, pain, joint position, and vibratory sensibilities in a few well-chosen places. This need take only 3–5 minutes. The detailed examination must be done when disturbances are suspected or discovered on screening.

The sensory examination in its entirety is given in this section. On most occasions it is best done in a segmental fashion; eg, include the sensory testing of the upper extremities as a part of the rest of the upper extremity examination.

Exteroceptive sensation. 1. Tactile sensation. Lightly touch various areas of the face, trunk, and extremities with a wisp of cotton or using the gentlest possible touch of your finger pads. On a screening examination, it is sufficient to touch each side of the three divisions of the trigeminal, each upper extremity in three places, and the same for the trunk and lower extremities. The patient with eyes closed tells you each time and place the stimulus is applied. By testing each side of the body simultaneously, you can check also for sensory extinction (see below). Do not apply the stimuli in a rhythmic fashion but rather with an irregular rhythm. Otherwise the patient can anticipate the stimulus. If an area of sensory loss is discovered, a useful supplementary procedure is to get the patient to aid in outlining the boundaries by using his fingertips.

The method described above is quite sufficient in the majority of situations. Sekuler et al. have described a two-alternative forced-choice procedure that is more reproducible and accurate, albeit time-consuming (reference 23).

2. Pain sensation. Take a safety pin and use the point and guard in a random fashion. Use the guard as a test of the continuing attention and reliability of the patient. Test the areas described under tactile sensation when screening. The patient's eyes are closed; the response is "sharp" or "dull." Compare each side with the other, and distal with proximal. On occasion you may wish to lightly draw the point of the pin along the skin. If an area of decreased sensation is discovered, go from the area of diminished or absent sensibility to the normal area: patients can perceive the onset of a painful stimulus better than they can perceive the attenuation or cessation of the stimulus.

3. Temperature sensation. Fill one test tube with hot water and an-

other with cracked ice cubes and test various areas on the body. This is often a more sensitive test for detecting dysfunction than pain testing. An alternative method is to use a cool object such as a tuning fork. Do not ask the patient to tell you if the stimulus is hot or cold but ask to be told "what this feels like." The patient's eyes are closed during the testing.

Proprioceptive sensation. 1. Joint position sense. Always test the most distal joint first because most afflictions of proprioception involve distal joints before proximal ones. If the testing on the most distal joint is abnormal, then move successively more proximal until a normal joint is reached. If the testing on the most distal joint is normal there is rarely a need to test more proximal joints. DeMyer points out that the third and fourth digits of both upper and lower extremities have the most sparse innervation and therefore are likely to show position sense dysfunction earlier than the first, second, or fifth digits (thumb, index, and little fingers in the hand).

Grasp the joint on the lateral surfaces of the digit with your thumb and forefinger. Then take the thumb and forefinger of your other hand and move the digit up or down. It is important for you to grasp the lateral surfaces in order to separate digits you are testing from adjacent digits that might give tactile cues as the digit is moved. In addition, if you grasp the anterior-posterior (dorsal-palmar) surfaces of the digit, you may excite deep pressure receptors and not joint position receptors.

Show the patient an up or down movement and get the patient to say "up" or "down," thus making sure your instructions are understood. Then move the digit through various small excursions, randomly making up or down movements. As a generalization, the patient should be able to sense movement when your joints on the digit performing the test sense it. Sensitivity is less when the digit is in midposition (see Background Information). A normal patient will make few errors. If an abnormality in the most distal digit is discovered, test several other distal joints in other digits, then test successively more proximal joints until the test is normal.

The Romberg test is another test of position sense. Ask the patient to stand with heels together and then close the eyes. Stand close to the patient in the event of a fall. The patient will sway severely or fall if position sense is diminished or absent. This occurs because visual compensation has been removed. The Romberg test is not a test of cerebellar function; those patients sway with eyes open or closed.

2. Vibratory sense. Just as with position sense, always start with the most distal joint since disturbance will cause dysfunction earliest distally. Use a 128/second or C tuning fork as illustrated in Fig 173). The 128/second fork is better than the 256/second because there is a clearer separation of normal from abnormal.

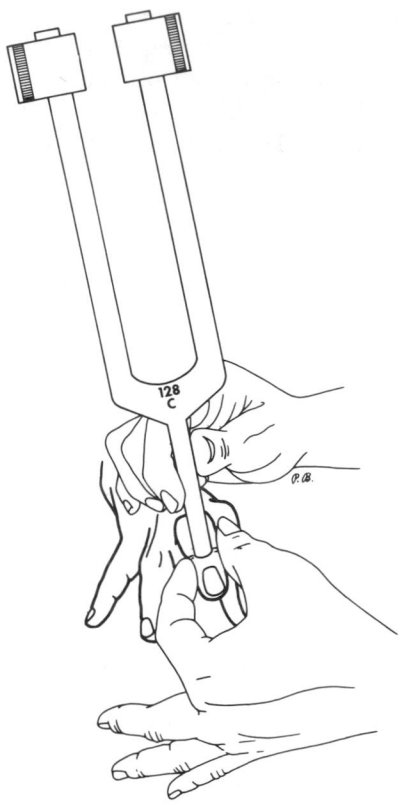

Figure 173. The timed vibratory test. The patient's hand is in heavy outline.

The timed vibratory test is the most satisfactory method to detect a mild to moderate impairment in vibratory sensation. Strike the tuning fork maximally, noting the time on the second hand of your watch. Then apply the fork to the most distal joint as illustrated. The third or fourth digits are best, as noted above. Ask the patient to describe what is felt. Usually the patient will say "a buzzing" or "like electricity." Instruct the patient to let you know instantly when the sensation stops, and note the time elapsed since the fork was struck, not since it was placed on the joint. Test both lower and upper extremities.

Normal and abnormal for this test depend upon you and your tuning fork. Do the test on normal individuals and you will rapidly get an idea of normal. Perform the test on individuals known to have peripheral neuropathy, ie, patients with diseases such as diabetes or alcoholism who have feet paresthesias, absent ankle jerks, impaired joint position sense, and impaired pain-temperature sensibilities. Once you have "standardized" the test in your hands, it will become your preferred method of vibratory testing.

Another method to determine mild to moderate impairment of vibratory sense is for the examiner to place his finger pad on the palmar or plantar surface of the joint being tested, with the tuning fork on the dorsal surface. The patient should be able to feel the vibration as long as the examiner.

If vibration is not perceived on the most distal joint, there is clearly an abnormality of vibratory sensibility. Proceed to successively more proximal joints or bony processes until vibration is perceived and note the location. Patients with diseases such as pernicious anemia can have absent vibratory sense up to the level of the sternum.

Cortical sensory functions. These can be tested only when the functions listed above are normal.

1. Stereognosis. Place an object such as a coin, knife, or comb in the patient's hand while the patient's eyes are closed and ask for a description or identification of the object. Be careful not to give auditory clues.

2. Two-point discrimination. A two-point discriminator can be bought or you can bend a paper clip and make one. Have the patient's eyes closed and ask to be told if you touch with one or two points. Do so randomly. Ordinarily only the finger pads are used, but other areas that can be tested include the lips, tongue, and palm. DeJong lists these as the normal distances that can be discriminated:

Tongue tip: 1 mm
Fingertip: 2–4 mm
Dorsum of fingers: 4–6 mm
Palm: 8–12 mm
Dorsum of hand: 20–30 mm

3. Sensory extinction. This can be done as part of tactile testing. Touch the same place on each side of the body after instructing the patient to localize the touch for you. In a random fashion touch first on one or the other side or bilaterally. Do not do so rhythmically.

4. Topognosis. This also can be part of tactile and extinction testing in that you ask the patient to tell you where each stimulus is felt.

5. Graphesthesia. Write letters or numbers on the palm or other areas as the patient's eyes are closed and ask that they be identified.

Background Information

Cutaneous sensibility is generally divided into touch (including light pressure), pain, and thermal components. The cutaneous receptors range from free nerve endings to elaborate encapsulated nerve endings such as the Pacinian corpuscle. There are many intermediate forms; examples include Merkel disks and Meissner corpuscles. For years there has been a controversy about whether there are specific cutaneous receptors for each sensory modality. An example of what is thought to be a specific receptor is the Pacinian corpuscle which records vibration. But even here agreement is not unanimous (see Sinclair, p 51). On the other hand, there are body areas, such as the ear, which have only two types of nerve endings but are sensitive to touch, pain, heat, and cold. An important point that has a bearing on this question is that sensation as perceived, interpreted, and verbally expressed by the brain involves the integration of many different impulses.

The general neuroanatomy of exteroceptive and proprioceptive sensation is as follows, starting peripherally:

1. Receptor
2. Peripheral nerve
3. Dorsal root ganglion   First neuron
4. Spinal cord neuron   Second neuron
5. Thalamic nucleus   Third neuron
6. Cerebral cortex   Fourth neuron

The tracts cross between the spinal cord and thalamus so that ultimately the right cerebral cortex receives information from the left side of the body. The site of crossing depends on the modality. Figure 174 illustrates the spinal cord structures involved in sensation.

Pain and temperature. Nerve endings that respond specifically to temperature have not been found. There are single fibers that respond to cold or hot sensations. A difference of 0.2°C in temperature causes significant discharge of these fibers.

The pain receptors are free nerve endings. Two fiber types are involved in the transmission of impulses:

1. A-delta fibers: small myelinated fibers that carry "fast" pain. This is a discrete pricking pain such as that made by the penetration of a tiny hypodermic needle.
2. C fibers: very small unmyelinated fibers that carry "slow" pain. This is an intense diffuse deeper pain that is less bearable than the fast pain.

The fibers enter the dorsal root ganglion where the first neuron is located. The impulses leave via the lateral division of the dorsal root ganglion. Most fibers then enter Lissauer's tract and ascend or descend one segment before terminating in the substantia gelatinosa. Other fibers pass directly to the substantia gelatinosa. In addition there are probably synapses on the nucleus centrodorsalis (central magnocellular nucleus)

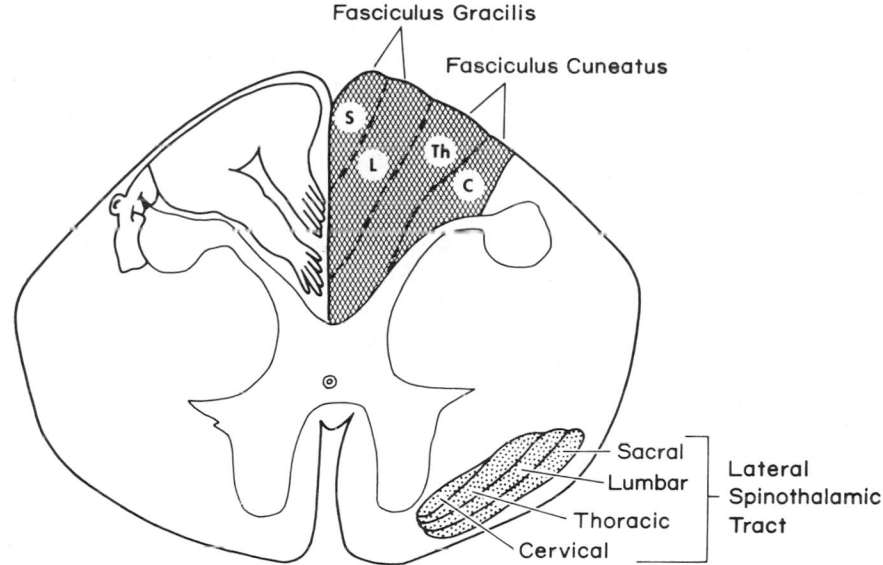

Figure 174. The posterior (dorsal) columns and lateral spinothalamic tract in the spinal cord. (Modified and used with permission of: Walker AE: *Arch Neurol Psychiat* 43:284–298, © 1940, 1976 AMA; Humphrey T: *Arch Neurol Psychiat* 73: 36–46, © 1955, 1976 AMA; Foerster O, Gagel O: *Zbl Ges Neurol Psychiat* 138: 1–92, 1932.)

of the posterior gray horn. The second-order neuron is thus in the spinal cord.

Up to this point the C fibers and delta fibers have been together. They now divide and take different routes to the third-order neuron in the thalamus.

1. A-delta fibers cross the cord in the anterior commissure and ascend in the lateral spinothalamic tract to the following areas in the thalamus:
    a. Posterior nuclei: the majority of fibers end here.
    b. Ventral posterolateral (VPL): some fibers end here.
2. C fibers also cross via the anterior commissure but ascend in the anterior spinothalamic tract and terminate in the intra-laminar and parafascicular nuclei of the thalamus. Collaterals go to the reticular formation and the hypothalamus. This system is more diffuse than the fast pain or delta fiber system.

The spinothalamic tract fibers carry impulses as follows (White et al): pain, 54% of fibers; warmth, 37% of fibers; cold, 9% of fibers. The spinothalamic tracts also carry touch and deep pressure sensations. Very little is known of the central connections with regard to temperature. What can be said is that lesions which cause disturbances in pain sensation almost invariably cause disturbances in temperature perception.

The role of the cortex in pain is complex and not well understood. There are three areas involved:

1. Somatic sensory area I: the postcentral gyrus
2. Somatic sensory area II: located at the base of the precentral and postcentral gyri, extending back into the parietal region
3. Supplementary motor area (Ms II of Woolsey): located parasagitally on the medial surface of the cortex near the representation of the foot in the precentral gyrus

See Brodal (pp 75–92) for an excellent discussion. The article by Weddell and Verrillo gives a lucid presentation of the anatomical pathways of pain.

Proprioception and vibration. Limb position information comes from three principal receptor groups: (1) stretch receptors in skeletal muscles and tendons; (2) certain skin mechanoreceptors; and (3) joint mechanoreceptors. Impulses arising from muscle spindles and tendon organs are discussed in section 209, Deep Tendon Reflexes. Receptors in the joints record various types of information. Freeman and Wyke have classified joint receptors into four types.

I: direction and speed of movement
II: acceleration receptors
III: position of the joint
IV: pain receptors

Fibers carrying these impulses go to the dorsal root ganglion (first neuron) and then to the dorsal (posterior) column of the spinal cord. Discharges from single afferent fibers are greatest during movements when the joint is in flexion or extension and least when movements are made with the joint in mid-position (Burgess and Clark). This is in accordance with clinical observations.

The receptors for vibratory sensibility are the Pacinian corpuscles. They are present in the subcutaneous connective tissue (especially fingertips, palms, toes, and soles), periosteum, around joints, and other areas. They respond to vibratory frequencies of 100–600 cps in a 1:1 fashion. Fibers from the receptors go to the dorsal root ganglion and then to the dorsal horn.

The vibratory and joint position fibers leave in the medial division of the dorsal root and enter the spinal cord. On entry they split into ascending and descending branches just like other sensory nerves. The fibers carrying impulses to the brain ascend in the dorsal column and synapse on the second-order neuron in the nucleus gracilis and nucleus cuneatus in the medulla. The ascending fibers are somatotopically arranged with the fibers from the lower part of the body most medial.

The sensibilities carried by the dorsal column are (DeMyer):

1. Position sense
2. Joint and body movements
3. Vibration sense
4. Pressure sense

Allied discriminative sensations include:

1. Texture
2. Touch localization (topagnosis)
3. Two-point discrimination
4. Weight sense
5. Graphesthesia

The organization of the second-order neurons, the nuclei gracilis and cuneatus, is complex. Spatial inhibition of the surround type has been demonstrated just as in the visual system (see section 196A, Visual Acuity). The cortex also exerts influence over the events occurring within the nuclei just as it is known to influence sensory input elsewhere (eg, the olfactory and visual systems and the muscle spindles).

Fibers from the dorsal column nuclei cross the midline in the medulla and ascend as the medial lemniscus to terminate on the third-order neuron in the VPL of the thalamus. The fibers from the medial lemniscus are restricted to the VPL. Stimulus specificity and place specificity are maintained in the VPL (Brodal). Poggio and Mountcastle studied about 1,000 single units in the VPL and reported:

42% responded only to gentle mechanical stimuli of skin receptors
32% responded to mechanical distortion of fascia or periosteum
26% responded to joint movements

All units responded only to stimulation of a localized area on the contralateral side of the body. The receptive fields of the extremities are small distally and larger proximally.

The same three areas of the cortex are involved with dorsal column sensations as noted previously for spinothalamic functions.

The traditional concept of dorsal column function is that two modality-specific spinal sensory pathways carry sensory impulses to higher centers where a complex spatiotemporal analysis is carried out:

1. Dorsal column system: vibration, proprioception, and fine touch
2. Anterolateral system (spinothalamic and spinoreticular): pain, temperature, and crude touch

Unfortunately neither human cases nor animal experiments entirely support this view.

A new view is based upon the work of Wall, Dubner, Vierck, and others. According to this concept the anterolateral system is concerned with modality analysis and the dorsal column system with spatiotemporal analysis. Thus, analysis and extraction of details regarding moving stimuli, eg, in stereognosis, is the function of the dorsal columns. See Wall, Wall, and Dubner; Azulay and Schwartz; Vierck; and Frommer et al. Clinical applications are reviewed in Ross et al (1979).

Tactile.   Several types of receptors appear to be involved with tactile sensation. These probably include Merkel's disks, Meissner's corpuscles, and free nerve endings. There is considerable difficulty in breaking tactile sensation into smaller components. Elements are carried both by the spinothalamic and dorsal column systems. Light touch appears to be carried by both. Discriminative tactile sensation, such as two-point localization, is carried by the dorsal column. Tickle is carried by the spinothalamic tracts. All components end in the VPL of the thalamus and then project to the cortex as described above.

Dermatomes.   A spinal cord segment is that part which gives rise to a pair of spinal nerves and then innervates a particular section of skin, muscles, bone, joints, and viscera. Certain features of the dermatomes are clinically important:

1.   There is overlap between contiguous dermatomes.
2.   Segmental distribution is not quite the same for touch, pain-temperature, muscles, and joints.

Clinical Significance

Peripheral neuropathy is a common cause of sensory disturbances. The degree of sensory compared to motor involvement and the distribution of impairment depends upon the nerve(s) affected and the disease. They may be classified as follows:

1.   Mononeuropathy. Involvement of one nerve.
    a.   Traumatic: eg, wrist drop (radial nerve) due to "Saturday night" palsy.
    b.   Entrapment: eg, carpal tunnel syndrome (median nerve).
    c.   Vascular: sudden onset, usually involves larger nerves, eg, third nerve palsy in diabetics.
2.   Mononeuropathy multiplex. In effect a mononeuropathy that involves several nerves over time. Usually seen in diseases prone

to cause vascular damage with nerve ischemia or infarction such as diabetes, periarteritis, rheumatoid.

3. Polyneuropathy. Symmetrical involvement beginning with the most distal nerves—usually lower extremities first—and progressing proximally. For this reason produces what is termed a "stocking" or "glove" distribution of loss. Specific diseases can be classified as to the predominance of sensory versus motor loss, although there is considerable individual variability. Good discussions can be found in Adams and Asbury; Dyck, Thomas, and Lambert; and Adams and Victor.

Conditions affecting solely the dorsal ganglia or dorsal roots are fairly rare. Tabes dorsalis is an example in which the large sensory fibers of the dorsal roots are affected. Neurosyphilis and more rarely diabetes can cause this syndrome. Herpes zoster can produce dorsal root involvement characterized by pain and skin lesions over the affected dermatome. Herniated intervertebral disks can involve one or more dorsal roots producing pain and sensory impairment; motor involvement will also be present if the ventral root is involved. Carcinomatous meningitis can predominantly involve the dorsal roots in either a focal or diffuse distribution.

Spinal cord lesions produce sensory loss also. Intramedullary lesions often produce what is termed "dissociated sensory loss": usually pain and temperature are lost, but there is sparing of touch and proprioception. Syringomyelia involving the cervical cord is a classical example of this dissociation. The syrinx, which is intramedullary, early involves the crossing of pain and temperature fibers. Touch and proprioception in the dorsal columns are not involved. The dorsal columns can be involved in diseases such as pernicious anemia and in tabes dorsalis; proprioception is impaired but pain and temperature can be normal.

Brainstem lesions can demonstrate crossed sensory disturbances, one side of the face and the other side of the body (see section 198, The Trigeminal Nerve). Thalamic lesions produce an impairment of all sensory functions on the contralateral side.

Parietal lobe involvement produces impairment of the cortical sensory functions. All lower sensory tracts must be intact before this conclusion can be reached.

Selected References

1. Adams R, Asbury A: Diseases of the peripheral nervous system, in Wintrobe MM, et al (eds): *Harrison's Principles of Internal Medicine*, ed 6. New York, McGraw-Hill, 1970, pp 1700–1713.
2. Adams RD, Victor M: *Principles of Neurology*. New York, McGraw-Hill, 1977.

3. Azulay A, Schwartz AS: The role of the dorsal funiculus of the primate in tactile discrimination. *Exp Neurol* 46:315–332, 1975.

4. Bonica J (ed): International symposium on pain. *Adv Neurol,* vol 4, 1974.

5. Brodal A: *Neurological Anatomy,* ed 2. New York, Oxford University Press, 1969, pp 31–116.

6. Burgess PR, Clark FJ: Characteristics of knee joint reception in the cat. *J Physiol London* 203:317–335, 1969.

7. Calne D, Pallis C: Vibratory sense: A critical review. *Brain* 89:723–746, 1966.

8. DeJong RN: *The Neurologic Examination,* ed 3. New York, Harper and Row, 1967, pp 57–106.

9. DeMyer W: Anatomy and clinical neurology of the spinal cord, in Baker AB, Baker LH (eds): *Clinical Neurology.* New York, Harper and Row, 1975, vol 3, chap 31.

10. DeMyer W: *Technique of the Neurological Examination: A Programmed Text,* ed 2. New York, McGraw-Hill, 1974, pp 293–323.

11. Dyck PJ, O'Brien PC, Pushek W, et al: Clinical vs. quantitative evaluation of cutaneous sensation. *Arch Neurol* 33:651–655, 1976.

12. Dyck PJ, Thomas PK, Lambert EH (eds): *Peripheral Neuropathy.* Philadelphia, WB Saunders, 1975.

13. Freeman M, Wyke B: The innervation of the knee joint: An anatomical and histological study of the cat. *J Anat* 101:505–532, 1967.

14. Frommer GP, Trefz BR, Casey KL: Somatosensory function and cortical unit activity in cats with only dorsal column fibers. *Exp Brain Res* 27:113–129, 1977.

15. Haymaker W: *Bing's Local Diagnosis in Neurological Disease,* ed 15. St Louis, CV Mosby, 1969.

16. Humphrey T: Pattern formed at upper cervical spinal cord levels by sensory fibers of spinal and cranial nerves: Relation of this pattern to associated gray matter. *Arch Neurol Psychiat* 73:36–46, 1955.

17. Hunt CC: On the nature of vibration receptors in the hind limb of the cat. *J Physiol* 155:175–186, 1961.

18. Lynn B: Somatosensory receptors and their CNS connections. *Ann Rev Physiol* 37:105–127, 1975.

19. Nathan PW: The gate-control theory of pain: A critical review. *Brain* 99:123–158, 1976.

20. Poggio GF, Mountcastle VB: The functional properties of ventrobasal thalamic neurons studied in unanesthetized monkeys. *J Neurophysiol* 26:775–806, 1963.

21. Roland PE: Astereognosis. *Arch Neurol* 33:543–550, 1976.

22. Ross ED, Kirkpatrick JB, Lastimosa ACB: Position and vibration sensations: Functions of the dorsal spinocerebellar tracts? *Ann Neurol* 5:171–176, 1979.

23. Sekuler R, Nash D, Armstrong R: Sensitive, objective procedure for evaluating response to light touch. *Neurology* 23:1282–1291, 1973.
24. Sinclair D: *Cutaneous Sensation*. New York, Oxford University Press, 1967.
25. Vierck CJ Jr: Tactile movement detection and discrimination following dorsal column lesions in monkeys. *Exp Brain Res* 20:331–346, 1974.
26. Wall PD: The sensory and motor role of impulses travelling in the dorsal columns towards cerebral cortex. *Brain* 93:505–524, 1970.
27. Wall PD, Dubner R: Somatosensory pathways. *Ann Rev Physiol* 44: 315–336, 1972.
28. Weddell G, Verrillo R: Common sensibility, in Critchley M, O'Leary J, Jennett B (eds): *Scientific Foundations of Neurology*. Philadelphia, FA Davis, 1972, pp 117–125.
29. White JC, Sweet WH, Hawkins R, et al: Anterolateral cordotomy: Results, implications, and causes of failure. *Brain* 73:346–367, 1950.

205. The Motor System

H. KENNETH WALKER, MD

Definition

I. Muscle strength
   A. Paralysis, plegia: complete loss of motor function.
   B. Weakness, paresis: less than complete loss of motor function.
   C. Monoplegia/monoparesis: paralysis/weakness of one extremity.
   D. Diplegia: paralysis of the same part on opposite sides of body (example: facial diplegia refers to bilateral facial paralysis).
   E. Hemiplegia/hemiparesis: paralysis/weakness on one side of the body.
   F. Paraplegia/paraparesis: paralysis/weakness of both legs.

    G.   Quadriplegia/quadriparesis: paralysis/weakness of all four extremities.

II. Muscle tone

    A.   Hypotonia: decreased muscle tone.

    B.   Flaccidity: absent muscle tone.

    C.   Hypertonia: increased muscle tone.

        1.   Cogwheel rigidity: a jerky yielding then holding up of muscle tone with passive movements, just as if one were pulling the limb over a ratchet.

        2.   Leadpipe rigidity: steady resistance to change by firm, tense muscles. Same degree of resistance is maintained when a new position is reached.

        3.   Gegenhalten: an increase in resistance in response to passive movement by the examiner.

        4.   Clasp-knife resistance: an increased resistance when a passive movement is begun. This resistance suddenly diminishes as the movement continues. Much like the initial resistance on opening the blade of a pocketknife, which suddenly vanishes when a certain point is reached.

        5.   Spasticity: a sustained tension in a muscle when it is passively lengthened. May be absent if the passive movement is slow.

III. Muscle volume

    A.   Atrophy: decrease in muscle volume due to lesion of peripheral nerve, ventral root, or alpha motoneuron ("lower motor neuron" lesion).

    B.   Hypertrophy: an increase in muscle volume and strength.

    C.   Pseudohypertrophy: an increase in volume associated with a decrease in strength.

IV. Muscle contraction

    A.   Fasciculations: flickering or shimmering movements of the skin over a muscle as bundles (fascicles) of muscle fibers contract. Seen in association with lower motor neuron lesion.

    B.   Myotonia: prolonged failure of relaxation.

    C.   Percussion myotonia: persistent muscle contraction after tapping the muscle with a reflex hammer.

    D.   Percussion myoedema: a local bulge surrounded by a spreading contraction occurring after tapping the muscle with a reflex hammer.

Technique

INSPECTION

Observe the patient's gait as he enters the room: equality of arm swing, sureness of foot placement, posture, distance between feet. Listen to the patient walk: scuffling, foot drop, and irregular rhythms can be picked up. Look at the patient's shoes and analyze where they are worn thin by inspecting soles, sides, and toes of both shoes.

Consider the patient's posture walking, standing, sitting, lying. Observe the relationship of the head and extremities to each other and to the trunk. Deformities of the spine, muscle spasm, localized weakness, and pain can produce significant postural changes.

Spontaneous motor activity provides clues to dysfunction that are sometimes not discovered on formal examination. Note in a rough quantitative way the number of movements made by one extremity or one side of the body as compared to the other. Observe the fine movements (or lack of them) of the hands: fingering the bedclothes or clothes, adjusting spectacles, lighting a cigarette or filling and lighting a pipe. Mild dysfunction of the corticospinal tract is often more apparent from this data than when you formally test the muscles.

With the patient undressed, inspect individual muscle contour and volume, and look for asymmetry when compared to the opposite side. Observe carefully for the presence or absence of fasciculations. This is best done with window light striking the patient at an angle.

Muscle diseases produce patterns of weakness that often are quite apparent to inspection and enable you to recognize the disease or group of muscles involved at a glance. Myotonic dystrophy is an example: the ptosis, frontal baldness, wrinkled forehead, atrophy of the masseters, curved neck, and hunched posture are unique. Each time you see weakness of a particular muscle or group of muscles you should endeavor to fix the visual memory in your mind so the next case will be recognizable. The reference by Brooke contains excellent descriptions of the appearances of weakness of individual muscles.

EXAMINATION

Palpate individual muscles, paying note to size, resilience, and consistency. Determine if the muscles are painful or tender to palpation.

Tone is evaluated by passive movement of the extremities through the full range of motion at varying speeds. The movement is carried out by the examiner with the patient completely relaxed. Tone is the degree of resistance to movement. Hypotonia, flaccidity, spasticity, and rigidity are the common disorders of tone. Descriptive terminology is given in the Definition section. Cogwheel rigidity can be brought out by stabilizing the patient's forearm with one of your hands and using the other hand to rotate the patient's hand rapidly around the wrist. At the same time the patient uses his other hand to pat repetitively on the knee. The same procedure can be carried out by rotating the forearm around the elbow joint.

Percussion is usually carried out by briskly tapping the thenar eminence with a reflex hammer. Normally there is a rapid abduction and flexion of the thumb with immediate relaxation. "Percussion myotonia" is an abnormal delay in relaxation; the contraction is sustained and persists for a number of seconds. Another method of demonstrating myotonia is to have the patient make a fist and then open and close the hand repeatedly as rapidly as possible. The third method involves the tongue. The tongue is protruded and a tongue blade placed under the tongue resting on the teeth. Be careful to have the blade between the tongue and teeth; otherwise the teeth will lacerate the tongue. Now take a reflex hammer and tap the tongue briskly but gently. If percussion myotonia is present, the tongue will mound up. "Percussion myoedema" is the term applied to the appearance of an initial depression in the muscle exactly where the tip of the reflex hammer struck the muscle. The depression spreads to the surrounding muscle much as ripples spreading from the impact of a stone thrown into a lake. The initial depression then mounds up into a tiny hill of contracting muscle; the contraction may persist for several minutes.

Examine the patient for *drift*: the patient extends the arms slightly above the horizon with wrists dorsiflexed and keeps them in that position for several minutes with eyes closed. If abnormal, there will be a drift of the affected arm and occasionally a mild drifting apart of the fingers. (Note that this is the same position used to test certain cerebellar functions and to check for abnormal movements. All of these tests may be carried out together.) Mild to moderate corticospinal dysfunction is occasionally more easily detected by this test than by testing individual muscles. At this point, the shoulder girdle can be further tested by having the patient move the outstretched arms laterally to the sides to a position of shoulder abduction. The examiner pushes down firmly while the patient resists. Observe for scapula winging when the arms are outstretched.

Fine movements of the upper extremities are tested next. Ask the patient to take the index finger and tap it against the most distal joint of the thumb of the same side (Fig 175). This should be exactly on the joint, done as rapidly as possible and without moving the hand or arm. Observe for speed, accuracy ("discretion" of movement), and ataxia. The movements will be slower with abnormality. Pay particular attention to synkinetic movements: the normal patient will move the other digits as the index finger taps, but the wrist, elbow, and shoulder remain fixed. With corticospinal dysfunction, there will often (not always) be associated or synkinetic movements of the wrist, occasionally the elbow, and on rare occasions the entire arm as the finger taps. Another test should be car-

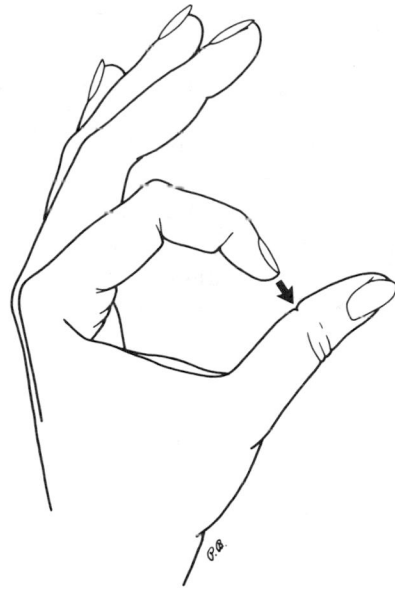

Figure 175.   The thumb tap test for fine movements.

ried out for fine movements such as buttoning or shoelace tying. Observing performance during the stereognosis test (see section 204, Sensation) is another opportunity for judging fine movements.

The lower extremities can be examined for drift. The patient lies face down on the table and flexes the knee to 45°, maintaining this position for a minute or so. Fine movements of the lower extremities are tested by asking the patient to "wiggle" the toes without moving the foot. The movements will be slower, and synkinetic movements may be present with abnormality.

Certain functional tests are extraordinarily useful in evaluating motor function—usually even more than tests of individual muscles. Gait, the most useful of these tests, has been presented under Inspection. The discussion below follows Brooke, which is an excellent source for further reading.

1. Arising from the floor. The usual complex of movement is for the patient to pull the legs under the body, place one hand on the floor for a little push, arise to a squat, then stand up with the trunk maintained in an erect position. With mild to moderate hip weakness the patient rests first on hands and knees and then straightens the knees to raise the buttocks in the air before the body: Brooke calls this the "butt first" sign of proximal lower extremity weakness. Gower's maneuver is used when the weakness is more severe: both hands are placed on the thighs, and the trunk is slowly elevated by the hands inching up the thighs.

2. Arising from a chair. The normal patient arises easily from a chair without use of the hands. With hip weakness the hands are used for support, with the amount of hand support varying with the degree of weakness.

3. Stepping onto a chair. Normally, this is done in one fluid movement without support. A very early sign of hip weakness is a pause before the movement: the patient girds his mind, then makes the movement. With more weakness the hips sag (the "hip dip") during the movement. A stool may be used if the patient feels insecure about a chair.

4. Walking on the heels. A normal individual dorsiflexes the feet and walks without any change in posture. The patient with mild anterior tibial weakness uses the trunk to counterbalance the change in weight distribution, producing stiffly held knees with the hips thrust backward.

5. Hopping or walking on the toes. A sensitive test of the plantar flexors of the feet.

6. Raising the arms above the head. The patient begins with arms by the sides of the body and then abducts them until they touch above the head. The arms are held straight during the entire maneuver. An early sign of shoulder weakness is flexing the elbows in order to give the shoulders an advantage. A sign of more severe weakness is the use of accessory muscles such as the trapezius.

Abstract motor function is tested last. This is one of the higher cortical functions, similar to speech and stereognosis. The patient's ability to carry out purposeful abstract movements and gait is tested. Disorder is termed "apraxia" (more correctly, "dyspraxia"). Unilateral and bilateral tests are described; each side must be tested:

1. Face: whistling, pursing lips as if kissing, pretending to cry, wink, shaking the head indicating yes or no.
2. Hands: making a fist, waving goodbye, playing a piano, catching a fly, pretending to comb the hair, saluting, pretending to cut a figure out of a piece of paper.
3. Trunk: turning from prone to supine position, getting into bed.
4. Legs: making a circle on the ground, kicking a ball, writing a number in the air.
5. Gait: described under Inspection.

These tests are discussed at length in Klein and Mayer-Gross.

The tests of motor function enumerated in the preceding paragraphs can easily be worked into a general screening examination. They need to be tested as a unit only when an abnormality is suspected from the history or discovered during the screening physical examination.

The tests given above (see Table 41) are arbitrarily chosen rapid screening tests for the motor system that can be worked into the general examination as each extremity is examined. A meticulous examination

Table 41. Screening motor examination.

1. Inspection
   a. Gait
   b. Posture
   c. Spontaneous motor activity
   d. Individual muscles
   e. Fasciculations
2. Palpation
3. Tone
4. Percussion
5. Drift, upper and lower extremities
6. Fine movements, upper and lower extremities
7. Functional tests
   a. Arising from floor
   b. Arising from chair
   c. Stepping onto chair
   d. Walking on heels
   c. Hopping on toes
   f. Raising arms above head
8. Abstract motor function
   a. Face
   b. Hands
   c. Trunk
   d. Legs

of individual muscles must be carried out if abnormality is suspected from the history, screening examination, or other parts of the neurological examination such as reflex or sensory examination. Excellent discussions of individual muscle testing are given in references 2, 5, 6, 11, and 18.

Background Information

Cortical fibers that influence or control voluntary muscle movement originate from several cortical areas and descend principally in the pyramidal tracts. For many years neuroanatomists felt these fibers originated solely from the large motor cells of Betz in Brodmann's area 4 of the precentral gyrus. A growing body of evidence has indicated this is not so. For example, there are about 1 million fibers in the pyramidal tracts and only about 25,000 Betz cells. It is now generally accepted the origins include:

1. The primary motor cortex (area 4 of Brodmann, the precentral gyrus). The fibers of the pyramidal tract vary considerably in diameter. The large myelinated axons arise from here. Russell

and DeMyer report that about 31% of the pyramidal fibers in the monkey originate in area 4.

2. The premotor cortex (areas 6 and 8 of Brodmann). These areas are in front of the motor cortex, the so-called motor association cortex. Russell and DeMyer found that 29% of the pyramidal fibers come from this area.

3. Primary sensory cortex of the parietal lobe (areas 3, 1, and 2 of Brodmann; first somatosensory area). Pyramidal fibers also originate in the sensory cortex; 40% in the study cited above.

4. Supplementary motor area: on the medial surface of the hemisphere in front of the leg area of the primary motor cortex.

5. Second somatosensory area: an area of parietal cortex above the Sylvian fissure.

The pyramidal tract leaves the cortex via the posterior limb of the internal capsule and the cerebral peduncles. In the brainstem corticobulbar fibers are given off to the various cranial nerve nuclei. In the medulla what is now the corticospinal fibers cross and descend as the lateral corticospinal tract. A small and variable percentage do not cross; they descend as the ventral (or anterior) corticospinal tract.

In the spinal cord the corticospinal axons have preferential sites of termination related to their cortical origins. The fibers originating in sensory cortex terminate more dorsally than those originating from motor cortex. The functional significance of this is not known. The great majority of all fibers terminate on internuncial neurons and not on alpha motoneurons. Consequently, voluntary motor activity would appear to be largely influenced by the corticospinal fibers acting on internuncial neurons which then act on the alpha motoneurons. There is anatomical and physiological evidence that a few axons from the Betz cells end directly on the alpha motoneurons. There is a definite phylogenetic progression in that the corticospinal axons in lower animals, such as the cat, have no monosynaptic connections on alpha motoneurons. The higher the animal in the evolutionary scheme, the greater the number of such connections. Electrophysiological studies suggest corticospinal fibers have a facilitatory effect on flexor muscles and an inhibitory effect on extensor muscles.

Other cortical and brainstem areas influence the activity of spinal motoneurons. These areas and their tracts include:

1. Red nucleus and rubrospinal tract
2. Vestibular nuclei and vestibulospinal tract
3. Reticular formation and reticulospinal tract

They will not be discussed here. The interested reader is referred to Brodal for what is known of their functions.

The motoneurons in the anterior horn of the spinal cord form Sherrington's "final common pathway." There are two types present:

1. Alpha motoneurons: large cells whose axons supply the voluntary muscle fibers.
2. Gamma motoneurons: small neurons which outnumber the alpha cells by about 16:1. About 30% of these supply the muscle spindles and the remainder are internuncial cells.

The alpha motoneurons have a somatotopic arrangement by column:

1. The medial columns supply the axial musculature and are more or less continuous throughout the cord.
2. The lateral columns of nuclear groups supply the extremity musculature and are principally present in the cervical and lumbosacral regions of the cord. These groups may be further subdivided (Figs 176 and 177).
   a. The most distal structures are supplied by the most lateral groups. For example, the nuclei serving the hand are more lateral than those serving the shoulder.
   b. Nuclear groups serving flexor muscles are more dorsal than those serving extensor muscles.

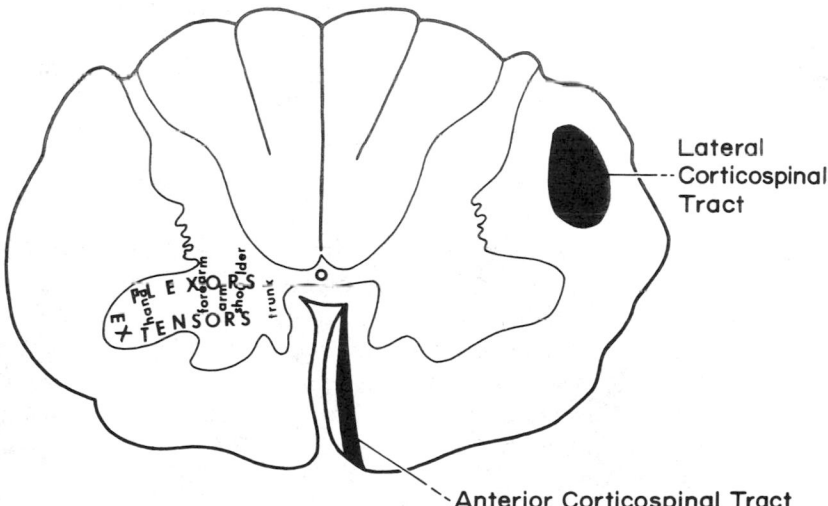

Figure 176. Arrangement of cell groups in gray matter of spinal cord (left) and position of corticospinal tracts (right). (Redrawn and modified from *Human Neuroanatomy*, ed. 7, by MB Carpenter. Copyright 1976, the Williams & Wilkins Company, Baltimore. Used with permission of publisher and author.)

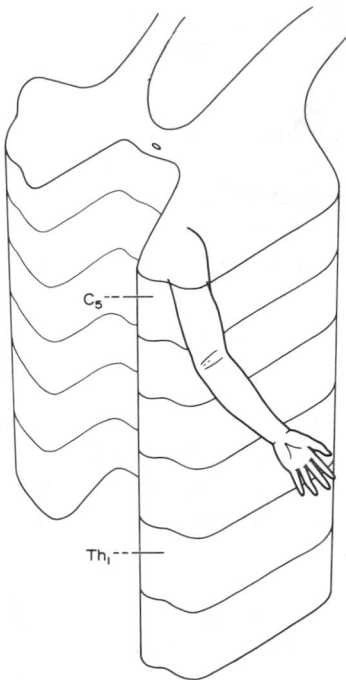

Figure 177.   Three-dimensional representation of the gray matter in the cervical cord, showing in a diagrammatic way the somatatopical arrangement of the groups of motor ventral horn cells which supply different parts of the upper extremity. The diagram does not take into account that the distal parts of the upper extremity have a far more ample motor supply (cf. small motor units) than the proximal parts. The hand, therefore, should cover a much bigger area than shown in the diagram. (Text and figure used with permission from A Brodal, MD: *Neurological Anatomy, In Relation to Clinical Medicine,* Oxford University Press, New York, 1969.)

Axons from ventral horn cells exit from the cord and synapse on muscle fibers. The synapse is called the myoneural junction. The events which occur at the synaptic cleft are of considerable importance. Acetylcholine is released from storage vesicles into the cleft where it combines with a protein receptor. The postsynaptic membrane discharges and produces the action potential in muscle. Various diseases and toxins, such as myasthenia gravis and botulism, cause their mischief by interfering with these events.

A motor unit is an alpha motoneuron, its axon, and the muscle fibers it supplies. The number of fibers supplied by each alpha motoneuron varies widely. The smallest units, and therefore the ones capable of the finest movements, are those of the extraocular muscles of the eye and the small muscles of the hand.

The ways in which the cortex is involved in voluntary movement are incompletely understood. The increase in the number of corticospinal axons that have monosynaptic contact with alpha motoneurons as there is ascent of the phylogenetic tree implies a corresponding increase in cortical control over voluntary movements. The fact that skilled movements are mostly flexor and that the corticospinal system is excitatory for flexor movements also implies a close connection between the two. The cortex also innervates the gamma motor system in the muscles (see section 209, Deep Tendon Reflexes). There is evidence that excitation of the gamma system occurs just before excitation of the alpha system, as if the former acted to "set" the muscles so the alpha motoneurons could play upon them. The contributions of the other descending system, mainly the rubrospinal and vestibulospinal, have not been discussed here, but they clearly are closely involved in voluntary movements. Brodal's conclusion with regard to the pyramidal system and motor activity is relevant to the clinician: "The anatomical and functional peculiarities of *the pyramidal tract* strongly suggest that it *plays a particular role in the central control and initiation of movements, presumably especially skilled voluntary movements of the hands and fingers"* [italics in original] (reference 3, p 243).

The brief account above largely follows the excellent discussion of Brodal.

Clinical Significance

GAIT

There are several characteristic disturbances of gait. Very good discussions are given by DeJong and Adams and Victor.

Spastic gait. This is due to upper motor neuron lesions. There are three characteristics (Victor and Adams): spastic, slow, scuffling. The involved leg is circumducted, rotated in a semicircle, with each step. The upper extremity is flexed and the lower extremity extended. The most common cause is hemiplegia due to cerebrovascular disease, but any condition that causes an upper motor neuron lesion can produce the gait.

Sensory ataxia gait. This is due to involvement of the dorsal ganglia, dorsal roots, or posterior columns of the spinal cord or, on rare occasions, higher levels. There is no knowledge of the position of the legs in space since proprioception is impaired or absent. The patient depends upon vision to take the place of position sense; consequently, the Romberg test is positive. The feet stamp as the patient walks since there is no force control. The legs are thrust forcefully in various directions. Seen in tabes dorsalis, pernicious anemia, and other conditions involving proprioceptive pathways.

Cerebellar gait. A reeling, lurching, staggering, broad-based gait much like a drunk individual. If unilateral, there is a deviation to the involved side due to hypotonia (see section 206, The Cerebellum).

Parkinsonian gait. The patient festinates, that is, walks in haste. The steps are small and shuffling. The entire body leans forward and the feet must hurry to keep up with it.

Steppage gait. This is due to foot drop. The patient lifts the foot high to avoid dragging the toe.

Apraxia of gait. As a general rule, this can be suspected when a relative says "there is something wrong with his walking" and cannot further describe what is wrong even when pressed. The motor power is present but what might be termed the "memory" of how to use the muscles to walk is lost. The steps are tiny and uncertain. Often the patient stops and has to be urged and assisted to move. Many of the associated automatic movements of gait are lost. There is difficulty in initiating gait. All of the gait movements are slow. This type of gait abnormality is seen in frontal lobe lesions or in bilateral interruption of the corticospinal tract in the internal capsule, cerebral peduncles, or high brainstem. For example, apraxia of gait often accompanies pseudobulbar palsy.

EFFECTS OF LESIONS AT VARIOUS LEVELS OF THE MOTOR SYSTEM

Motor cortex and internal capsule. The capacity to perform fine discrete movements is lost or severely impaired. Movement initiation is hesitant, and movements are slow. Weakness is marked distally and less so proximally. The ability to perform movements is lost distally, but the patient can still perform proximal movements. At the onset of the lesion muscle tone and reflexes may be lost. As reflexes return they are hyperactive, often with clonus. Muscle tone is increased and there is spasticity. The plantar reflex is extensor, that is, Babinski's sign is present (see section 210, The Plantar Reflex). There is no muscle atrophy except that due to disuse.

The changes noted above are more marked in degree when the lesion is in the internal capsule than in the motor cortex. Lesions of the motor cortex can produce more restricted paralyses than internal capsule lesions, eg, monoplegias. Associated signs and symptoms will of course depend upon the exact location of the lesion.

Brainstem. The effects are largely the same as noted above, except dysarthria (see section 194, Speech and Other Lateralizing Cortical Functions) is often quite prominent. In contrast, dysarthria can be mild or absent with higher lesions even when the facial musculature is involved.

Cranial nerve findings will depend upon the level of the lesions. The findings will often be "crossed," that is, the face will be involved on the side of the lesion and the body on the opposite side. This is because the corticospinal tract does not cross until the lower medulla.

Spinal cord.   Structures below the level of the lesion will demonstrate spasticity, hyperreflexia, and weakness as described above. At the level of the lesion, the findings will be as those described below for a lower motor neuron lesion. Autonomic motor activities may be involved depending on the extent of the lesion.

Lower motor neuron lesion.   Refers to involvement of the alpha motoneuron in the cord, the ventral root, or peripheral nerve. There are atrophy, fasciculations, flaccidity, areflexia, and paralysis.

Myoneural junction.   There is only weakness or paralysis without any other findings. The reflexes may be decreased if the weakness is severe. Caused by diseases such as myasthenia gravis and the myasthenic syndrome, and toxins such as botulism and organic phosphate.

Muscle.   Various inflammatory and metabolic diseases can produce weakness and other findings such as pain, edema, or enlargement.

Selected References

1. Adams RD, Victor M: *Principles of Neurology.* New York, McGraw-Hill, 1977, pp 71–80, 889–975.
2. *Aids to the Investigation of Peripheral Nerve Injuries: Medical Research Council.* War Memorandum no 7, ed 2, 1943 (reprinted 1975). London, Her Majesty's Stationary Office.
3. Brodal A: *Neurological Anatomy,* ed 2. New York, Oxford University Press, 1969, pp 117–254.
4. Brooke MH: Clinical examination of patients with neuromuscular disease. *Adv Neurol* 17:25–39, 1977.
5. DeJong RN: *The Neurologic Examination,* ed 3. New York, Harper and Row, 1967, pp 445–521.
6. DeMyer W: *Technique of the Neurological Examination: A Programmed Text,* ed 2. New York, McGraw-Hill, 1974, pp 177–236.
7. Granit R: *The Basis of Motor Control.* New York, Academic Press, 1970.
8. Hubbard JI: Microphysiology of vertebrate neuromuscular transmission. *Physiol Rev* 53(3):674–723, 1973.
9. Klein R, Mayer-Gross W: *The Clinical Examination of Patients with Organic Cerebral Disease.* London, Cassell and Company, 1957.

10. Liu C-N, Chambers WWL: An experimental study of the cortico-spinal system in the monkey (*Macaca Mulatta*): The spinal pathways and preterminal distribution of degenerating fibers following discrete lesions of the pre- and postcentral gyri and bulbar pyramid. *J Comp Neurol* 123:257–284, 1964.
11. Mayo Clinic, Department of Neurology and Department of Physiology and Biophysics: *Clinical Examinations in Neurology*. Philadelphia, WB Saunders, 1971.
12. Nyberg-Hansen R, Rinvik E: Some comments on the pyramidal tract, with special reference to individual variations in man. *Acta Neurol Scand* 39:1–30, 1963.
13. Rondot P: Motor function, in Vinken PJ, Bruyn GW (eds): *Handbook of Clinical Neurology*. Amsterdam, North Holland Publishing Co, 1969, vol 1, pp 147–168.
14. Rondot P: Syndromes of central motor disorder, in Vinken PJ, Bruyn GW (eds): *Handbook of Clinical Neurology*. Amsterdam, North Holland Publishing Co, 1969, vol 1, pp 169–217.
15. Rouques L: The symptomatology of affections of the peripheral motor neurons, in Vinken PJ, Bruyn GW (eds): *Handbook of Clinical Neurology*. Amsterdam, North Holland Publishing Co, 1969, vol 1, pp 218–236.
16. Russell JW, DeMeyer W: The quantitative cortical origin of pyramidal axons of macaca rhesus. *Neurology* 11:96–108, 1961.
17. Sigwald J, Raverdy P: Muscle tone, in Vinken PJ, Bruyn GW (eds): *Handbook of Clinical Neurology*. Amsterdam, North Holland Publishing Co, 1969, vol. 1, pp 257–276.
18. Walker HK: *Clinical Methods Learning System Videotapes*. Atlanta, Ga, Emory University Medical Television Network, 1978.
19. Yahr MD, Purpura DP (eds): *Neurophysiological Basis of Normal and Abnormal Motor Activities*. Hewlett, NY, Raven Press, 1967.

206. The Cerebellum

H. KENNETH WALKER, MD

Definition

The principal signs of dysfunction are:

Ataxia. Unsteadiness or incoordination of limbs, posture, and gait. A disorder of the control of force and timing of movements, leading to abnormalities of speed, range, rhythm, starting, and stopping.

Hypotonia. Normal resting muscle tension is reduced, leading to decreased muscle tone and abnormal positions of parts of the body.

Tremor. An intention tremor of the hand on purposive movement is the most common, with coarse rapid side-to-side oscillations that increase as the movement goal is approached. Resting tremors of the limbs, head, and trunk are seen; at times paroxysms of these tremors are severe enough to shake the entire bed and delude the unwary physician into suspecting seizure activity.

Gait. The station or manner of standing is abnormal: the legs are apart and there is swaying of the body. The patient staggers, reels, and lurches on walking.

Nystagmus. This is a less common manifestation of cerebellar disease, and some authorities dispute its occurrence.

Technique

Observation. Have the patient sit on the side of a bed or table. Note the position of the limbs: the hypotonia can produce bizarre positions. The head can be deviated to one side. Look for resting tremors of the limbs and trunk. At times these can be of such severity to cause the head to bob, or titubate.

Head. See if nystagmus is present by first observing the eyes in the midline position, then as they follow your finger as it moves laterally and vertically.

Speech is frequently involved. Once the characteristic changes are heard in a full-blown case, they will never be forgotten. Begin by having the patient take a deep breath and maintain "ahhh" as long as possible. This procedure basically tests the expiratory muscles and vocal cords. Listen for variations in pitch and volume, and for tremor. Now ask the patient to say "la, la, la" as long as possible. This maneuver superimposes rapid alternating movements of the tongue upon function of the expiratory muscles and vocal cords. Ask the patient to say "me, me, me" as long as possible, thus testing rapid alternating movements of the lips. Finally ask the patient to read a simple paragraph, and listen to meter, volume, pitch, and enunciation.

Upper extremities.   Passively flex and extend each arm at the elbow and assess the tone. Then have the patient extend the arm in front with elbows slightly flexed and eyes closed. Observer for tremor. Assess postural fixation and tone by observing for drift, and by tapping sharply proximally, after explaining what you are about to do. With cerebellar dysfunction there is marked wavering of the arm with the tapping and also difficulty in maintaining the posture of the trunk.

Now test rebound of the right arm by placing your right hand on the patient's right shoulder, in order to prevent the arm striking the patient's face if cerebellar dysfunction is indeed present. Grasp the patient's right wrist with your left hand. Ask the patient to sharply flex the right arm, and you suddenly let go. The patient with dysfunction will be unable to arrest the progress of the arm, and it will markedly rebound off your right arm.

Test rapid alternating movements of first one hand and then the other with the thigh-slapping test. Use the sitting position. Have the patient strike first the palm and then the dorsum of the hand upon the thigh just above the knee. Abnormalities are more likely to be brought out if you make sure that: the hand is reversed between each strike; performance is as rapid as possible; the length of the movement is about breast-high. Observe for abnormalities of force and timing, and difficulty in alternating between the palm and dorsum of the hand.

Test finger-nose-finger alternating movements by having the patient first touch the pad of your index finger with the pad of his index finger. Then the patient touches his nose with the pad of the index finger, thus requiring reversal of the hand. Have the patient do this as rapidly as possible. Observe for intention tremor, a coarse side-to-side tremor that increases as your finger or the nose is approached. There are irregularities in the control of the timing and force of the movement with cerebellar dysfunction. Abnormalities can be intensified if the position of the examiner's finger is moved each time.

An interesting little test that can be performed by some patients is to have them use their fingers to tap out a tune on the table. If there is cerebellar dysfunction there can be disturbances in timing and force of striking that will be quite apparent. This is known as arrhythmokinesis.

Lower extremities.   First the patient stands at rest. Observe whether the feet are placed fairly close together as normally, or wide apart. Normally individuals stand at rest with little or no shifting of feet or movement of the body. In cerebellar dysfunction the patient shifts about and the trunk wavers unsteadily. In many instances patients are unable to stand without support on each side.

Ask the patient to walk in the usual fashion across the room and back. With bilateral cerebellar disease there is a reeling, rolling, lurching, staggering gait that resembles drunkenness. In unilateral cerebellar disease there is deviation to the side of the lesion, probably as a result of the hypotonia.

Test tandem walking. Ask the patient to walk a straight line heel-to-toe. This is probably the most sensitive test of the vermis of the cerebellum and is the first function to be lost in alcoholic cerebellar cortical degeneration. Therefore, if you are looking for alcoholic cerebellar dysfunction, this is a reliable and rapid screening test.

Now have the patient lie face up on the bed and observe performance of the following tests:

1.   Heel-knee. The right heel taps the left knee gently, just as a hammer taps a nail. The arc of the swing should be about 2 feet. Observe for abnormalities of force and rhythm. Then test the left leg.
2.   Heel-shin. The right heel starts on the top of the left knee and, keeping it exactly on top of the shin, runs the heel down the shin to the foot. When abnormal there is a coarse side-to-side tremor as the heel goes down the shin. Start with the knee; in a few patients the abnormality is most marked about the knee, and disappears as the heel goes on down the shin. Also insist that the heel be placed exactly on top of the shin since this makes the dysfunction more prominent.

Background Information

The field of cerebellar anatomy and physiology is one of the most complex and rapidly advancing areas in the neurosciences. In the following section we will give only the briefest background information, focusing primarily on some clinical correlations.

Anatomically (Fig 178) the cerebellum can be divided transversely into three lobes, anterior, posterior, and flocculonodular, and longitudinally into a midline vermis and two lateral hemispheres (Larsell's nomen-

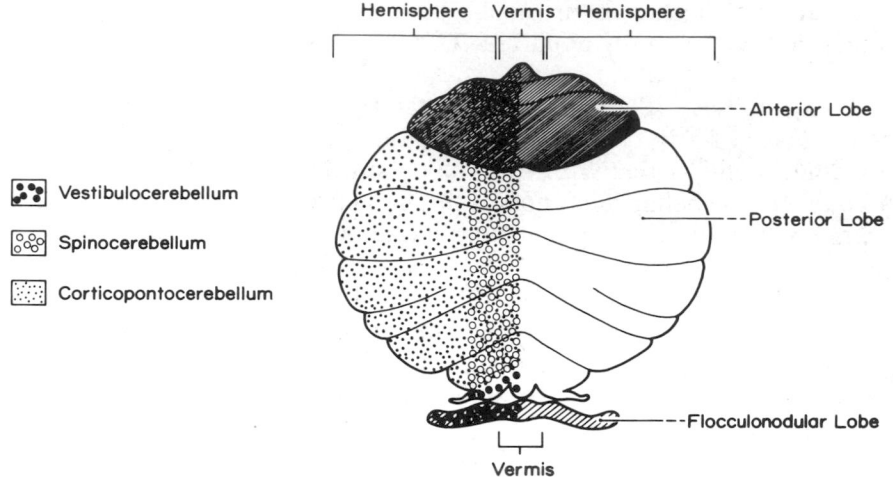

Figure 178. Anatomy and organization of the cerebellum. (Modified from W DeMyer, *Technique of the Neurological Examination: A Programmed Text,* ed 2, McGraw-Hill, 1974, and A Brodal, *Neurological Anatomy,* ed 2, Oxford University Press, 1969, using O Larsell's nomenclature, in J Jansen (ed), *Comparative Anatomy and Histology of the Cerebellum from Myxinoids Through Birds,* University of Minnesota Press, 1967)

clature). The following simplified scheme of cerebellar organization given in Table 42, is modified from DeMeyer. There are exceptions to some of the generalizations.

The cerebellum can be divided into three longitudinal zones on the basis of afferent connections:

1. Vestibulocerebellum: afferents from vestibular nuclei
2. Spinocerebellum: afferents from the spinal cord
3. Pontocerebellum or corticocerebellum: afferents from cerebral cortex via pontine nuclei

These divisions project onto the cerebellar nuclei and have efferent connections as outlined in the scheme. These three subdivisions do not exactly correspond to the anatomical divisions; there is considerable overlap.

DeMyer has put the function of the cerebellum very lucidly by pointing out that the cerebellum probably evolved out of the vestibular nuclei. Using information provided by the vestibular system the cerebellum equilibrates the contractions of axial musculature, so that the eyes and head are properly positioned. In higher animals the cerebellum takes on the additional role of seeing to the smooth performance of voluntary movements by the limbs, working closely with the cerebrum. Thus the

Table 42. A simplified scheme of cerebellar anatomy.

Lobe	Phylogenetic Subdivision	Afferent and Efferent Cerebellar Peduncle	Midline Nucleus
Anterior	Paleocerebellum (spinocerebellum)	Superior	Interpositus (emboliform and globose)
Posterior	Neocerebellum (cortico- or pontocerebellum)	Middle	Dentate
Flocculo-nodular	Archicerebellum (vestibulocerebellum)	Inferior	Fastigial

cerebellum, "sitting astride the vestibular nuclei," receives on the one hand information from the proprioceptive system, and on the other, information about commands that the cerebral cortex is sending to muscles. The cerebellum sees to it that the movements are performed in a smooth coordinated fashion, receiving constant feedback about what is actually happening.

Information as to what is happening in the muscles comes from muscle spindles, tendon organs, touch and pressure receptors, and from the labyrinth. These afferent impulses converge on the Purkinje cells of the spinocerebellar and vestibulocerebellar portions of the cerebellar cortex (Fig 178), either directly or after synapse on granule cells. Efferent output from the Purkinje cells goes to the cerebellar nuclei (dentate, fastigial, and interpositus) and thence to the spinal cord (and therefore the lower motor neurons), vestibular nuclei, or cerebral cortex.

The interrelationships with the cerebral cortex are complex. Basically each area of the cerebral cortex that sends efferents to the cerebellum in turn gets efferents from that area of the cerebellum. The pathways from the cerebral cortex to the cerebellum can be divided into two groups (Brodal):

1. Routes via the inferior olive, pontine nuclei, and red nucleus which show a precise topical organization.
2. Routes via the reticular nuclei principally. These nuclei are diffusely organized and thus can integrate impulses from many different sources before they reach the cerebellum.

Cerebellar efferents to the cortex go from the dentate nucleus mostly to the nucleus ventralis lateralis of the thalamus, thence to the cortex.

Efferents from the cerebral cortex to the cerebellum go to the contralateral cerebellar hemisphere. Thus the right cerebellar hemisphere ultimately receives afferents from the right side of the body and the left cerebral cortex, and sends efferents to the same locations.

The cerebellum probably ultimately exerts its influence on motor activity via the cerebral cortex. It also directly influences the gamma fiber systems at the spinal cord level, thus influencing postural tone and reflexes. The nature of the cerebellar influence is still incompletely understood.

There are many problems with localization of cerebellar symptoms. The following generalizations are crude but helpful:

Disturbance	*Localization*
Limb ataxia (especially upper limbs) and hypotonia	Lateral lobes
Disturbed equilibrium—truncal ataxia: drunken gait, titubation of head and trunk	Flocculonodular lobe
Gait ataxia: inability to do tandem walking	Anterior lobe

Clinical Significance

The cerebellum can be involved in a large variety of systemic diseases, in addition to mass lesions and congenital afflictions. Alcoholism and remote cancer produce a cerebellar syndrome that at least initially begins within the anterior lobe and produces ataxia. Lead, mercury, dilantin, and other toxic or therapeutic agents can cause cerebellar degeneration. Various viral infections and hypoxia can produce prominent cerebellar involvement. Vascular disease can produce involvement of the cerebellum directly or by involvement of the cerebellar peduncles in the brainstem. Examples include the posterior inferior artery syndrome, the superior cerebellar artery syndrome, and the anterior inferior cerebellar artery syndrome. Common neoplasms include metastases, astrocytoma, medulloblastoma, angioblastoma, and acoustic neuroma.

Note that this section has not been concerned with ataxia due to involvement of the posterior columns of the spinal cord, the functions of which must be tested before considering ataxia to be of cerebellar origin.

Selected References

1. Holmes G: The cerebellum of man. *Brain* 62:1–30, 1939.
2. Eccles, J, Ito M, Szentagothai J: *The Cerebellum as a Neuronal Machine.* New York, Springer-Verlag, 1967.

3. Dow R, Moruzzi G: *The Physiology and Pathology of the Cerebellum.* Minneapolis, University of Minnesota Press, 1958.
4. Brodal A: *Neurological Anatomy,* ed 2. New York, Oxford University Press, 1969, pp 255–303.
5. Nyberg-Hansen R, Horn J: Functional aspects of cerebellar signs in clinical neurology. *Acta Neurol Scand* (suppl) 51:219–245, 1972.
6. Brown JR: Diseases of the cerebellum, in Baker AB, Baker LH (eds): *Clinical Neurology.* New York, Harper & Row, 1975, vol 2, chap 29.
7. DeMyer W: *Technique of the Neurological Examination: A Programmed Text,* ed 2. New York, McGraw-Hill, 1974, pp 237–258.
8. Victor M, Adams R, Mancall E: A restricted form of cerebellar cortical degeneration occurring in alcoholic patients. *Arch Neurol* 1:579–688, 1959.
9. Brennan RW, Bergland RM: Acute cerebellar hemorrhage. *Neurology* 27:527–532, 1977.
10. Adams RD, Victor M: *Principles of Neurology.* New York, McGraw-Hill, 1977, pp 52–61.

207. Involuntary Movements: Tremor, Chorea, Athetosis, Myoclonus, Asterixis

H. KENNETH WALKER, MD

Definition

The principal signs of dysfunction are:

Tremor. Purposeless involuntary movements resulting from the alternating contractions of opposing muscle groups.

1. Tremor at rest occurs when muscles are at rest, for example, pill-rolling tremor of parkinsonism.
2. Postural tremor occurs when muscles maintain a posture such as outstretched arms, eg, fine tremor of hyperthyroidism.
3. Action tremor (intention tremor) occurs near the end of a goal-directed movement, for example, coarse side-to-side tremor of cerebellar disease seen as the finger-nose test is done.

Chorea. Brief, jerky, explosive movements, "fidgeting"; eg, Sydenham's chorea seen in rheumatic fever.

Athetosis. Writhing, sinuous movements, especially marked in the digits and extremities, eg, as seen in hepatic encephalopathy.

Myoclonus. Sudden brief twitches or jerks of groups of muscles or a single muscle, eg, as seen in metabolic encephalopathies such as uremic encephalopathy.

Asterixis. "Liver flap." An intermittency of sustained posture, illustrated by "flapping" of hands when arms are outstretched and wrists dorsiflexed, eg, as seen in hepatic encephalopathy. A "foot flap" is seen in many patients with asterixis of the hands.

Technique

When abnormal movements are present they often can be observed when taking the history or performing other parts of the physical. If such movements are observed or suspected, they can be studied more carefully by inspecting the patient (1) at rest, (2) while maintaining a posture such as erect with outstretched arms, and (3) performing goal-directed movements such as the finger-nose-finger test.

Systematically inspect the resting patient with the face then proceeding with upper extremities, trunk, and lower extremities. Chorea produces sudden grimaces about the face; the patient is unable to maintain tongue protrusion—it darts in and out. Inspect the tongue as it rests inside the mouth as certain types of tremor can involve the tongue. Myoclonic twitches can be seen quite well about the shoulders and distal upper extremities. Restless fidgeting or purposeless movements of the arms are among the earliest signs of chorea. Sinuous twistings of the hand are seen with athetosis.

Have the patient maintain a posture by standing with arms outstretched, slightly flexed at the elbow, and with hands extended at the wrist, as though the patient were halting traffic.

Asterixis.   The hands "flap," that is, flex briefly at the wrist, then immediately snap back into the extended position. A foot flap can often be brought out by having the patient dorsiflex the feet and maintain them in that position. The flap is identical to that seen in the hands.

Chorea, athetosis, and myoclonus.   This posture is well suited to bringing out the abnormalities produced by these movements, since they all will produce changes in the position of the limb.

Tremor. Certain tremors are provoked by sustained posture:

1. Hands. Observe carefully for distal postural tremors, such as the fine rapid tremor of the hands seen in hyperthyroidism.
2. Shoulders, neck. Tremors involving these structures produce head bobbing when the neck is affected and coarse tremors of the entire arm when the shoulder girdle is involved.

Observe voluntary goal-directed movements. Ask the patient to perform the finger-nose-finger test (see section 207, The Cerebellum), and watch for tremors that usually occur maximally just before the goal is reached. Note whether the involved segments are distal (wrist, fingers) or proximal (shoulder), as this helps in neuroanatomical localization. A coarse side-to-side tremor is characteristic of cerebellar disease. Chorea is manifested as a break or interruption in the performance of what is intended to be a smooth voluntary movement.

The following information should be recorded on all abnormal movements:

1. Structures or segments involved
2. State of muscles when they occur: at rest, maintaining posture, or during goal-directed movements
3. Description of movement(s) including the pattern of involvement of various segments, duration and frequency
4. Factors which increase or decrease movements: rest, exercise, anxiety, alcohol

The progress and influence of treatment on tremors that involve the hands can be followed by having the patient write the same sentence and draw an Archimedes' spiral each visit.

Background Information

The mechanisms underlying these abnormal movements are very poorly understood. The extrapyramidal motor system is clearly involved in certain tremors, chorea, and athetosis. This system refers anatomically to the basal ganglia (caudate, putamen, globus pallidus, and amygdala) and related brainstem reticular formation. Experimental evidence also suggests that the ventral lateral nucleus of the thalamus and the cerebral cortex are involved. References 1, 2, and 3 present further details.

Disease of the cerebellum or its brainstem connections produces a coarse action tremor. Experimentally this tremor has been reproduced by lesions of the dentate nucleus or the brachium conjunctivum which contains a large number of projection fibers from the dentate nucleus. Clinically lesions of the cerebellum or brachium conjunctivum prior to its decussation produce ipsilateral tremor.

Myoclonus is seen in a wide variety of disturbances. An important form occurs in multiple muscle groups in association with metabolic encephalopathy, especially uremic or carbon dioxide encephalopathy. In these circumstances myoclonus presumably indicates neuronal injury. However, the specific pathophysiology is unknown.

Asterixis was described by Adams and Foley in 1949; it is seen in many of the metabolic encephalopathies. Physiologically the electromyogram shows a lapse of electrical activity in the muscle as the wrist flaps down, followed by a compensatory muscle contraction that jerks the hand up again. The neurophysiology is not known.

Clinical Significance

Tremor. The pill-rolling tremor of parkinsonism is present at rest. This is a coarse, regular movement involving the thumb and index finger. Although the tremor predominantly involves the distal upper extremity, the face and tongue may be involved also. Sleep decreases the tremor, and emotion makes it worse. The tremor often increases as the patient walks.

Other causes of tremor at rest are rarer. They include drug-induced tremors (principally phenothiazines), severe cases of essential tremor (benign familial tremor), Wilson's disease, chronic acquired hepatocerebral degeneration, mercury poisoning, general paresis.

As a generalization proximal tremors, that is, those involving shoulder, pelvic girdle, or neck, are produced by lesions of the cerebellum and its brainstem connections. They are usually coarse and slow. Distal postural tremors, involving wrists and finger joints, result from midbrain or basal ganglia problems. Many of these are fine and rapid. However, there are exceptions to these generalizations, and in many cases the site of neurological dysfunction is not really known.

1. Anxiety and fatigue tremors: fine rapid tremors involving the fingers. The injection of epinephrine into normal individuals produces tremors identical to those seen in anxiety or with fatigue.
2. Thyrotoxicosis: a fine rapid tremor of the fingers identical to the tremors listed above.
3. Essential (benign familial) tremor: a coarse irregular tremor that usually starts in the hands and fingers and eventually involves the voice, head, and neck. Usually becomes worse with goal-directed movements. Difficulty with handwriting, piano playing, typing, or drinking coffee is often the most prominent com-

plaint. Drinking alcohol diminishes the tremor. There is a strong heritable tendency. Onset is in early adult life. Treatment with propranolol is efficacious in some patients. See reference 3.

4.   Cerebellar tremor: coarse irregular tremor involving the shoulder girdle and neck, seen in patients with diseases of the cerebellum; a prime example is alcoholic cerebellar cortical degeneration. When quite severe it can be present at rest also.

5.   Lithium tremor: seen in individuals being treated with lithium. Quite similar to essential tremor.

Postural tremors are also seen in Wilson's disease, acquired hepatocerebral degeneration, and certain poisons, especially mercury. Mercury poisoning was known as the "hatters' shakes" because workers involved in the manufacture of felt hats were exposed to mercury.

Action (intention) tremors: seen during voluntary activity, usually being most prominent near the end of goal-directed movement. The same generalizations about localization apply as given for postural tremors. A good example is the coarse side-to-side tremor seen in cerebellar disease as the finger approaches the nose. Note that although we speak here of the finger, the actual origin of the tremor is in the elbow or shoulder joint.

The statements made above about tremors are generalizations to which there are numerous exceptions. However, they form a useful bedside approach to the analysis of tremor disorders. The final diagnosis is made upon this analysis in addition to a meticulous history and physical examination.

Chorea and athetosis.   Sydenham's chorea is seen in children and adolescents and is often associated with rheumatic fever. Huntington's chorea is an autosomal dominant whose characteristics appear usually in adulthood. Chorea gravidarum is seen in pregnancy. Chorea has been reported in a large variety of other conditions, especially diseases such as lupus erythematosus in which there is a cerebral arteritis.

Athetosis occurring during childhood involves both sides of the body ("double athetosis") and is felt to be due to neonatal cerebral hypoxia. In adults it usually involves only one side of the body and is seen most often with strokes.

Myoclonus and asterixis.   Myoclonus involving multiple muscle groups is seen most often in patients with metabolic encephalopathies, such as those produced by uremia, carbon dioxide, or hypoxia.

Asterixis was first described in hepatic encephalopathy. It is also seen in other metabolic disorders such as uremia, hypokalemia, carbon dioxide narcosis due to chronic pulmonary disease, dialysis dementia, hypoxia, and hypomagnesemia. Asterixis has been caused by the following drugs: dilantin, phenobarbital, carbamozepine, prinidone, and perhaps with diazepam and flurazepam. Structural lesions producing asterixis, even unilateral asterixis, have been located in the midbrain and thalamus.

The combination of myoclonus and asterixis in a patient with stupor is strongly suggestive of a metabolic encephalopathy as the etiology of the stupor rather than a structural brain lesion.

Selected References

1.   Adams RD, Foley J: Neurological changes in more common types of severe liver disease. *Trans Am Neurol Assoc* 74:217–219, 1949.
2.   Carpenter MB: Brain stem and infratentorial neuraxis in experimental dyskinesia. *Arch Neurol* 5:504–524, 1961.
3.   Critchley E: Clinical manifestations of essential tremor. *J. Neurol Neurosurg Psychiat* 35:365–372, 1972.
4.   Curzon G: The biochemistry of dyskinesias. *Int Rev Neurobiol* 10: 323–370, 1967.
5.   Duvoisin R: Clinical diagnosis of the dyskinesias. *Med Clin N Am* 56(6):1321–1341, 1972.
6.   Fahn S: Differential diagnosis of tremors. *Med Clin N. Am* 56(6): 1363–1375, 1972.
7.   Halliday AM: The clinical incidence of myoclonus, in Williams D: *Modern Trends in Neurology.* New York, Appleton-Century-Crofts, 1967, vol 4, pp 69–105.
8.   Leavitt S, Tyler HR: Studies in asterixis. *Arch Neurol* 10:360–368, 1964.
9.   Marshall J: Tremor, in Vinken PJ, Bruyn GW (eds): *Handbook of Clinical Neurology: Diseases of the Basal Ganglia.* Amsterdam, North-Holland Publishing Co, 1968, vol 6, chap 31, pp 809–825.
10.   McDowell F, Lee JE: Extrapyramidal diseases, in Baker AB, Baker LH (eds): *Clinical Neurology.* New York, Harper and Row, 1975, vol 2, chap 26.
11.   Niedermeyer E, Bauer G, Burnite R, Reichenbach D: Selective stimulus-sensitive myoclonus in acute cerebral anoxia. *Arch Neurol* 34: 365–368, 1977.
12.   Shuttleworth E, Wise G, Paulson G: Choreoathetosis and dilantin intoxication. *JAMA* 230:1170–1171, 1974.
13.   Swanson PD, Luttrell CN, Magladery JW: Myoclonus: A report of 67 cases and review of the literature. *Medicine* 41:339–356, 1962.
14.   Tarsy D, Lieberman B, Chirico-Post J, Benson DF: Unilateral asterixis associated with a mesencephalic syndrome. *Arch Neurol* 34:446–447, 1977.
15.   Truex RC, Carpenter MB: *Human Neuroanatomy,* ed 6. Baltimore, Williams and Wilkins, 1969, pp 498–517.

16. Wolf P: Periodic synchronous and stereotyped myoclonus with post-anoxic coma. *J Neurol* 215:39–47, 1977.
17. Yahr MD: Involuntary movements, in Critchley M, O'Leary J, Jennett B (eds): *Scientific Foundations of Neurology.* Philadelphia, FA Davis, 1972, pp 83–88.

208. Suck, Snout, and Grasp Reflexes

H. KENNETH WALKER, MD

Definition

The following reflexes are covered:

Suck reflex: sucking movements by the lips when the lips are stroked or touched. Normal only in infants up to age 1 year.

Snout reflex: puckering or protrusion of the lips upon percussion. Normal only in infants up to age 1 year.

Grasp reflex: flexion or "grasping" of the hand with stimulation of the palmar surface. A similar phenomenon can occur in the foot. Normal only in infants up to age 1 year.

Technique

The suck and snout reflexes are tested by stroking, touching, and percussing the lips at the angles on each side. The response can usually be obtained on both sides. The stimulation should be gentle.

To obtain the grasp reflex the examiner's hand is gently inserted into the patient's hand as conversation is occurring. The palmar surface is touched or stroked. The flexor surfaces of the fingers may be stimulated also as the examiner's hand lies in the palm. The stimulus should be in a distal direction. With a positive response the patient grasps the examiner's hand with variable strength and continues to grasp as the examiner's hand is removed. Ability to voluntarily release the grip depends on the activity of the reflex: some patients can do so readily, others can even be lifted off the bed due to the strength of the grip. A variant is for only the flexor surfaces of the fingers to be stimulated by stroking. In positive responses, the fingers will curve much like a bird's claw and hook the examiner's fingers or hand. Some clinicians maintain that the reflex is brought out more easily if the patient is lying on the side with the hand to be tested uppermost.

A foot grasp reflex can be elicited by gently stroking the plantar surface medially with a blunt object. The lateral surfaces of the foot bend as if to make a cup out of the plantar surface. The toes adduct, there is hollowing of the sole with some wrinkling of the skin. If the toes also flex, this is called the tonic foot response (reference 7). In patients who also have the Babinski reflex, the Babinski can usually be elicited more laterally than the grasp.

Background Information

Lesions of the supplementary motor area and perhaps its corticofugal projection fibers are felt to be responsible for the grasp reflex after age 1 year. It is always abnormal then. The reflex may therefore be characterized as a "release phenomenon." The supplementary motor area is located on the medial surface of the frontal lobe, just in front of the leg area of the primary motor cortex. Stimulation of this area produces postural type movements predominantly. The grasp reflex is influenced experimentally by postural changes.

The suck and snout reflexes are felt to be due to similar release phenomena since they generally appear under the same conditions as the grasp.

Very little is known of the neurophysiology of these reflexes.

Clinical Significance

These three reflexes are seen in bilateral frontal lobe disease and, at least in the case of the suck and snout, also in corticobulbar lesions. On rare occasions, they can occur unilaterally. Neoplasms can cause them. They can be seen in decreased levels of consciousness in a host of conditions: metabolic encephalopathies, infection, head trauma. Diseases which cause multiple CNS lesions, such as multiple sclerosis and the hypertensive lacunar state, can also produce them.

Selected References

1.   Adie WJ, Critchley M: Forced grasping and groping. *Brain* 50:142–170, 1927.
2.   Seyffarth H, Denny-Brown D: The grasp reflex and the instinctive grasp reaction. *Brain* 71:109–183, 1948.

3. Pollack S: The grasp response in the neonate. *Arch Neurol* 3:574–581, 1960.
4. DeJong RN: *The Neurologic Examination*, ed 3. New York, Harper and Row, 1967, pp 245–317, 616.
5. Brodal A: *Neurological Anatomy*, ed 2. New York, Oxford University Press, 1969, p 199.
6. Paulson GW: Some lesser-known reflexes in neurology. *Ohio State Med J* 69:515–516, 1973.
7. Botez MI, Bogen JE: The grasp reflex of the foot and related phenomena in the absence of other reflex abnormalities following cerebral commisurotomy. *Acta Neurol Scand* 54:453–463, 1976.
8. Brain WR, Curran RD: The grasp reflex of the foot. *Brain* 55:347–356, 1932.
9. Magee KR: Clinical analysis of reflexes, in Vinken PJ, Bruyn GW (eds): *Handbook of Clinical Neurology*. Amsterdam, North Holland Publishing Co, 1969, vol 1, pp 237–256.

209. Deep Tendon Reflexes

H. KENNETH WALKER, MD

Definition

Normal. When a muscle tendon is tapped briskly the muscle immediately contracts due to a two-neuron reflex arc involving the spinal or brainstem segment that innervates the muscle. The afferent neuron whose cell body lies in a dorsal root ganglion innervates the muscle spindle or Golgi tendon organ associated with the muscles; the efferent neuron is an alpha motoneuron in the anterior horn of the cord. The cerebral cortex and a number of brainstem nuclei exert influence over the sensory input of the muscle spindles by means of the gamma motoneurons that are located in the anterior horn; these neurons supply a set of muscle fibers that control the length of the muscle spindle itself.

Hyporeflexia. Absent or greatly diminished response to tapping, which usually indicates a disease that involves one or more of the components of the two-neuron reflex arc itself.

Hyperreflexia. Hyperactive or repeating (clonic) reflexes usually indicate an interruption of corticospinal and other descending pathways that influence the reflex arc, due to a suprasegmental lesion, that is, a lesion above the level of the spinal reflex pathways.

By convention the deep tendon reflexes are graded as follows:

0   = No response; always abnormal
1+ = A slight but definitely present response; may or may not be normal
2+ = A brisk response; normal
3+ = A very brisk response; may or may not be normal
4+ = A tap elicits a repeating reflex (clonus); always abnormal.

Whether the 1+ and 3+ responses are normal depends on:

1.   What they were previously, that is, the patient's reflex history
2.   What the other reflexes are
3.   Analysis of associated findings, such as muscle tone, muscle strength, or other evidence of disease

Asymmetry of reflexes suggests abnormality.

Technique

All of the commonly used deep tendon reflexes are presented here in a group. In a screening examination you will usually find it more convenient to integrate the reflex examination into the rest of the examination of that part of the body: that is, do the upper extremity reflexes when examining the rest of the upper extremity. However, when an abnormality of the reflexes is suspected or discovered, the reflexes should be examined as a group with careful attention paid to the technique of the examination.

Valid test results are best obtained when the patient is relaxed and not thinking about what you are doing. After a general explanation, mingle the specific instructions with questions or comments designed to get the patient to speak at some length about some other topic. If you cannot get any response with a specific reflex—ankle jerks are usually the most difficult—then try the following:

1.   Several different positions of the limb.
2.   Get the patient to put slight tension on the muscle being tested. One method of achieving this is to have the patient strongly contract a muscle not being tested.

3.   In the upper extremity have the patient make a fist with one hand while the opposite extremity is being tested.

4.   If the reflex being tested is the knee jerk or ankle jerk, have the patient perform the "Jendrassik maneuver," a reinforcement of the reflex (see reference 6). The patient's fingers of each hand are hooked together so each arm can forcefully pull against the other. The split second before you are ready to tap the tendon, say "pull."

5.   In general, any way to distract the patient from what you are doing will enhance the chances of obtaining the reflex. Having the patient count or give the names of children are examples.

The best position is for the patient to be sitting on the side of the bed or examining table. The Babinski reflex hammer (Fig 179) is very good. Use a brisk but not painful tap. Use your wrist for the action, not the arm. In an extremity a useful maneuver is to elicit the reflex from several different positions, rapidly shifting the limb and performing the test. Use varying force and note any variance in response.

Note the following features of the reflex response:

1.   Amount of hammer force necessary to obtain contraction.
2.   Velocity of contraction.
3.   Strength of contraction.
4.   Duration of contraction.
5.   Duration of relaxation phase.
6.   Response of other muscles that were not tested. When a reflex is hyperactive, that muscle often will respond to the stretch of a nearby muscle. A good example is reflex activity of a hyperactive biceps or finger reflex when the brachioradialis tendon is tapped. This is termed "overflowing" of a reflex.

After obtaining the reflex on one side, always go immediately to the opposite side for the same reflex so that you can compare them.

Jaw jerk. Place the tip of your index finger on a relaxed jaw, one that is about one-third open. Tap briskly on your index finger and note the speed as the mandible is flexed (see section 198, The Trigeminal Nerve).

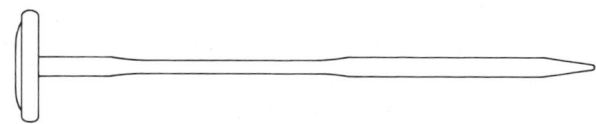

Figure 179.   The Babinski reflex hammer.

Biceps reflex. The forearm should be supported, either resting on the patient's thighs, or resting on the forearm of the examiner. The arm is midway between flexion and extension. Place your thumb firmly over the biceps tendon, with your fingers curling around the elbow, and tap briskly. The forearm will flex at the elbow.

Triceps reflex. Support the patient's forearm by cradling it with yours or by placing it on the thigh, with the arm midway between flexion and extension. Identify the triceps tendon at its insertion on the olecranon, and tap just above the insertion. There is extension of the forearm.

Brachioradialis reflex. The patient's arm should be supported. Identify the brachioradialis tendon at the wrist. It inserts at the base of the styloid process of the radius, usually about 1 cm lateral to the radial artery. If in doubt, ask the patient to hold the arm as if in a sling—flexed at the elbow and halfway between pronation and supination—and then flex the forearm at the elbow against resistance from you. The brachioradialis and its tendon will then stand out.

Place the thumb of the hand supporting the patient's elbow on the biceps tendon while tapping the brachioradialis tendon with the other hand. Observe three potential reflexes as you tap.

1. Brachioradialis reflex: flexion and supination of the forearm.
2. Biceps reflex: flexion of the forearm. You will feel the biceps tendon contract if the biceps reflex is stimulated by the tap on the brachioradialis tendon.
3. Finger jerk: flexion of the fingers.

The usual pattern is for only the brachioradialis reflex to be stimulated. But in the presence of a hyperactive biceps or finger jerk reflex, these reflexes may be stimulated also.

Finger jerk. Have the patient gently curl his fingers over your index finger, much as a bird curls its claws around the branch of a tree. Then raise your hand, with the patient's hand now being supported by the curled fingers. Tap briskly on your fingers, so the force will be transmitted to the patient's curled fingers. The response is a flexion of the patient's fingers.

Knee jerk. Let the knees swing free by the side of the bed, and place one hand on the quadriceps so you can feel its contraction. If the patient is in bed, slightly flex the knee by placing your forearm under both knees and lifting them slightly off the bed. Tap the patella tendon. There will be contraction of the quadriceps with extension of the lower leg. If the reflex is hyperactive there is sometimes concomitant adduction of the ipsilateral thigh. Adduction of the opposite thigh and extension of the opposite lower leg also can occur simultaneously if those reflexes are hyperactive. Note that this so-called crossed thigh adduction or leg extension tells you that the reflexes in the opposite leg are hyperactive. They tell you nothing about the state of the reflex in the leg being tested. Use the Jendrassik maneuver if there is no response.

Ankle jerk. With the patient sitting, place one hand underneath the sole and dorsiflex the foot slightly. Then tap on the Achilles tendon just above its insertion on the calcaneus. If the patient is in bed, flex the knee and invert or evert the foot somewhat, cradling the foot and lower leg in your arm. Then tap on the tendon.

If no response is obtained have the patient face a chair and kneel on it, with the knees resting against the back of the chair, the elbows on the top of the back, and the feet projecting over the seat. First dorsiflex the foot slightly and tap on the tendon. Use the Jendrassik maneuver if this doesn't work. This position is well suited to observing the relaxation phase of the reflex in patients with suspected thyroid disease.

See DeJong for a description of numerous other reflexes that are useful in certain situations.

Background Information

A stretch reflex is the contraction of a muscle in response to stretching of muscle spindles, which are receptors that lie in parallel with extrafusal muscle fibers. The reflex is composed of a two-neuron arc: the afferent neuron, whose cell body is in a sensory ganglion, innervates the spindle. When the muscle spindle is stretched, this neuron fires and monosynaptically excites alpha motoneurons in the anterior horn of the spinal cord. This alpha motoneuron is the second neuron; it supplies the muscle that is being tapped or transiently stretched. The detailed mechanisms underlying the operation of the spindle are quite complex, but considerable knowledge about them is now available in the literature, and new details are added constantly. The muscle spindle is a slender, spindle-shaped structure that is intermingled with the usual muscle fibers. Each spindle is composed of two types of elongated, poorly staining fibers: nuclear bag fibers and nuclear chain fibers. Each contains multiple nuclei. Six to ten of these fibers lie within the spindle's connective tissue sheath. They are called "intrafusal" muscle fibers, since they lie inside the fusiform structure, in contrast to the surrounding "extrafusal" fibers that make up the contractile element of muscle.

Afferent sensory terminals that innervate the spindle fibers are of two types: primary and secondary (Fig 180). The spindles fire according to the velocity and amount of stretch that is placed upon the central nuclear regions of the intrafusal fibers. The degree of stretch that is communicated to the central portion of the fibers is determined by two factors:

Muscle Receptors	Fiber types	Pathways	Sensory endings	Gamma Motoneurons (efferents to spindles)
Muscle spindle	Nuclear bag fiber	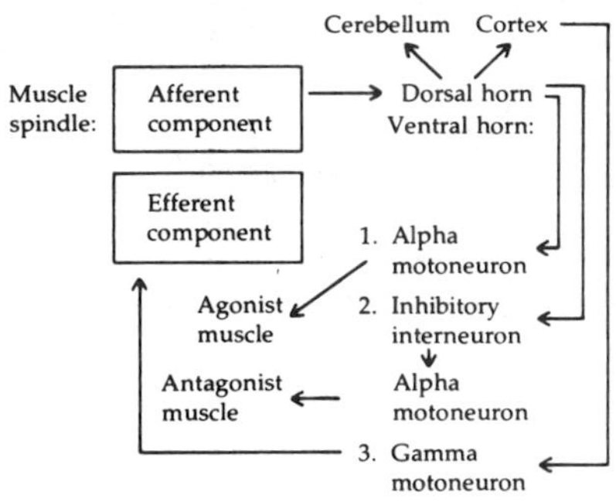 Muscle spindle: Afferent component → Cerebellum Cortex; → Dorsal horn; Ventral horn: 1. Alpha motoneuron 2. Inhibitory interneuron → Alpha motoneuron 3. Gamma motoneuron. Efferent component → Agonist muscle; Antagonist muscle	Lie in parallel with extrafusal fibers. Sensory endings: Group 1a "primary ending" Synonym: annulospiral ending. Gives information about length and velocity of extension of muscle: Dynamic firing: spindle firing is greatest while muscle is lengthening; firing ceases with contraction and is reduced with steady lengths below that seen during the stretching process.	Small anterior horn motoneurons that receive descending cortical impulses and then send efferent axons to the muscle spindles (see diagram under Pathways). As they fire there is a contraction of the intrafusal fibers of the muscle spindle. This causes a stretching of the central part of the spindle where the sensory fibers are, and consequently the sensory fibers fire. This setup probably allows supraspinal structures to regulate the sensitivity of the muscle spindles, or their background firing levels. Gamma dynamic motoneurons supply group 1 primary endings and increase their responsiveness to velocity of spindle elongation. Gamma static motoneurons supply group 1 and group 2 endings and increase their levels of firing in response to steady stretches.
	Nuclear chain fiber	As above, with the exception that the excitatory reflex pathway may involve one or more interneurons.	Lie in parallel with extrafusal fibers. Sensory endings: Group 1a as above Group II "secondary ending" Synonym: flower-spray ending. Gives information about length and velocity of extension of muscle: Static firing: response greatest when stretch is constant after contraction has ceased.	
Golgi tendon organ		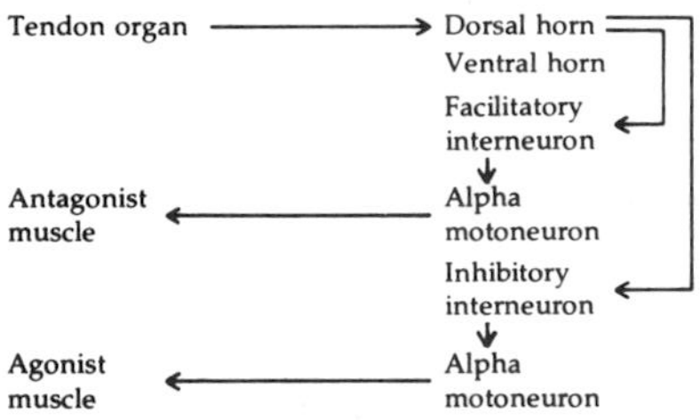 Tendon organ → Dorsal horn; Ventral horn: Facilitatory interneuron → Alpha motoneuron → Antagonist muscle; Inhibitory interneuron → Alpha motoneuron → Agonist muscle	Lie in series with extrafusal fibers, since they are attached to tendons. Sensory endings: Group 1b. Gives information about muscle tension: fires briskly during contraction, but little during passive elongation of the muscle.	

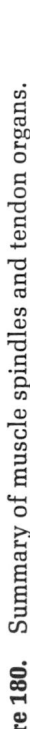

Figure 180.   Summary of muscle spindles and tendon organs.

1. The length and change in length of the surrounding extrafusal fibers (see Fig 180).
2. The degree of contraction of the intrafusal fibers (see below).

Impulses from the spindle receptors enter the dorsal horn where the information takes four routes:

1. To the cortex.
2. To directly synapse on an alpha motoneuron that causes immediate contraction of the muscle innervated by the spindle, the agonist.
3. To synapse on an inhibitory neuron that in turn synapses on an alpha motoneuron that goes to a muscle antagonistic to the one innervated by the spindle. Thus there is concomitant relaxation of the antagonist as the agonist contracts.
4. To the cerebellum via the dorsal spinocerebellar tracts.

The previous paragraph describes the course taken by the afferent impulses from the sensory nuclei of the muscle spindles. Recall now that the second component of the spindle was a contractile element, the intrafusal fibers. The firing of the spindle afferents is dependent upon the length of the extrafusal fibers (as outlined above), and the length of the intrafusal fibers. The contraction of the ends of intrafusal fibers and thus the strength of the central portions is controlled by gamma motoneurons: these small neurons are located in the anterior horn and are influenced by the cerebellum, cortex, and various brainstem nuclei. The probable function of this motor innervation of a sensory structure is to enable these supraspinal structures to "set" and thus ultimately regulate the sensitivity of the spindle. The higher centers and, in particular, the cortex thereby get sensory information from the muscle spindles and, in turn, through the gamma motoneuron, control the amount and quality of information received.

The Golgi tendon organ, which is the second major muscle receptor, is attached between the extrafusal fibers and the tendon. Thus the tendon organ is in series with the extrafusal fibers and will fire as the muscle contracts. The spindles, in contrast, are parallel with (that is, alongside) the extrafusal fibers and so fire when the extrafusal fibers relax (that is, are stretched). The impulses from the tendon organ go through the dorsal horn and synapse on an inhibitory interneuron which in turn synapses on an alpha motoneuron that goes to the agonist. Therefore the tendon organ ultimately causes relaxation of the agonist and, by way of interneurons, a facilitation of the antagonist. Information is also conveyed from these receptors to the cerebellum and cortex.

The spinal reflexes that are set up by the mechanisms described above serve the function of keeping the muscle fibers adjusted to a certain length and to a certain tension, thereby maintaining muscle tone and ultimately limb posture.

Clinical Significance

Absent stretch reflexes indicate a lesion in the reflex arc itself. Associated symptoms and signs usually make localization possible:

1. Absent reflexes and sensory loss in the distribution of the nerve supplying the reflex: lesion involves afferent arc of the reflex—nerve or dorsal horn.
2. Absent reflex with paralysis, muscle atrophy, and fasciculations: lesion involves efferent arc—anterior horn cells or efferent nerve, or both.

Peripheral neuropathy is today the most common cause of absent reflexes. The causes include diseases such as diabetes, alcoholism, amyloidosis, uremia; vitamin deficiencies such as pellagra, beriberi, pernicious anemia; remote cancer; toxins including lead, arsenic isoniazid, vincristine, diphenylhydantoin. Neuropathies can be predominantly sensory, motor, or mixed and therefore can affect any or all components of the reflex arc (see Adams and Asbury for a good discussion). Muscle diseases do not produce a disturbance of the stretch reflex unless the muscle is rendered too weak to contract. This occasionally occurs in diseases such as polymyositis and muscular dystrophy.

Hyperactive stretch reflexes are seen when there is interruption of the cortical supply to the lower motor neuron, an "upper motor neuron lesion." The interruption can be anywhere above the segment of the reflex arc. Analysis of associated findings enable localization of the lesion.

The stretch reflexes can provide excellent clues to the level of lesions along the neuraxis. Table 43 lists the segmental innervation of the common stretch reflexes. For example, if the biceps and brachioradialis reflexes are normal, the triceps absent, and all lower reflexes (finger jerk, knee jerk, ankle jerk) hyperactive, the lesion would be located at the C6–C7 level, the level of the triceps reflex. The reflex arcs above (biceps, brachioradialis, jaw jerk) are functioning normally, while the lower reflexes give evidence of absence of upper motor neuron innervation.

The laterality of reflexes is also helpful. For example, if all the reflexes on the left side of the body are hyperactive, and those on the right side normal, then a lesion is interrupting the corticospinal pathways to that side somewhere above the level of the highest reflex that is hyperactive.

Individual nerve and root lesions can be identified by using information about the reflexes along with sensory and motor findings. *Aids to*

Table 43. Segmental innervation of stretch reflexes.

Reflex	Nerve or Root
Jaw jerk	Trigeminal nerve
Biceps	C5–C6
Brachioradialis	C5–C6
Triceps	C6–C7
Finger jerk	C8–T1
Knee jerk	L3–L4
Ankle jerk	S1

the Investigation of Peripheral Nerve Injuries is a valuable pamphlet to carry in your bag to help in testing and analyzing muscles with respect to their innervation.

Selected References

1. Brodal A: *Neurological Anatomy,* ed 2. New York, Oxford University Press, 1969, pp 125–150.
2. Matthews PBC (ed): *Mammalian Muscle Receptors and Their Central Actions.* London, E Arnold, 1972.
3. DeMyer W: *Technique of the Neurological Examination: A Programmed Text,* ed 2. New York, McGraw-Hill, 1974, pp 189–210.
4. Adams RD, Asbury AK: Diseases of the peripheral nervous system, in Wintrobe MM, et al (eds): *Harrison's Principles of Internal Medicine,* ed 6. New York, McGraw-Hill, 1970, chap 354, pp 1700–1713.
5. *Aids to the Investigation of Peripheral Nerve Injuries.* Medical Research Council, War Memorandum no 7, ed 2, 1943 (reprinted 1975). London, Her Majesty's Stationery Office.
6. Gassel MM, Diamantopoulos E: The Jendrassik maneuver. *Neurology* 14:555–560, 640–642, 1964.
7. Bussel B, Morin C, Pierrot-Deseilligny E: Mechanism of monosynaptic reflex reinforcement during Jendrassik manoeuvre in man. *J Neurol Neurosurg Psychiat* 41:40–44, 1978.
8. DeJong RN: *The Neurologic Examination,* ed 3. New York, Harper and Row, 1967, pp 589–607.
9. Henneman E: Peripheral mechanism involved in the control of muscle, in Mountcastle V (ed): *Medical Physiology,* ed 13. St. Louis, CV Mosby, 1974, pp 617–635.
10. Paulson GW: Some lesser-known reflexes in neurology. *Ohio State Med J* 69:515–516, 1973.

11. Garnit R: The functional role of the muscle spindles: Facts and hypotheses. *Brain* 98:531–556, 1975.
12. Magee KR: Clinical analysis of reflexes, in Vinken PJ, Bruyn GW (eds): *Handbook of Clinical Neurology.* Amsterdam, North Holland Publishing Co, 1969, vol 1, pp 237–256.

---

210. The Plantar Reflex

H. KENNETH WALKER, MD

Definition

Normal. Stroking the lateral part of the sole of the foot with a fairly sharp object produces plantar flexion of the big toe; often there is also flexion and adduction of the other toes. Termed the flexor plantar reflex.

Abnormal (the Babinski reflex). Stroking the sole produces extension (dorsiflexion) of the big toe, often with extension and abduction ("fanning") of the other toes. Termed the extensor plantar reflex, or Babinski reflex.

Technique

Place the patient in a supine position and tell him you are going to scratch the foot, first gently and then more vigorously, in order to test a certain reflex. Fixate the foot by grasping the ankle or medial surface with the examiner's hand that will be closest to the midline of the patient: examiner's left hand when the patient's left foot is being tested, and vice versa with the right foot. Begin with light stroking, using your finger; then use a blunt object such as the point of a key. Finally, if no abnormal response has been obtained, take a tongue blade and break it in half longitudinally and use the sharp point. The reason for the graded stimuli is twofold: first, light touch, as with a finger, frequently obtains the reflex without causing the massive withdrawal response that on occasion makes interpretation of the response difficult. Second, one cannot conclude the response is normal until a noxious stimulus is indeed used, since the reflex is a cutaneous nociceptive reflex.

The first line to be stroked begins a few centimeters distal to the heel and is situated at the junction of the dorsal and plantar surfaces of the foot (Fig 181). The line extends to a point just behind the toes and then turns medially across the transverse arch of the foot. Stroke slowly, taking 5–6 seconds to complete the motion. Do not dig into the sole, but stroke.

Successive lines are stroked, each about 1 cm medial to the preceding stroke, until the examiner is stroking the midline of the foot. The reason for beginning laterally is that in some cases the response is abnormal laterally and then becomes normal as the midline is approached. The occurrence of the extensor response on any of these lines is abnormal, even if the response is flexor on another line of stroking. This variation relates to variability in the receptive field of the reflex, undoubtedly due to the extent of corticospinal involvement as well as individual differences.

The reflex is normal if the abnormal response is not obtained from any of the stroke lines using all of the stimuli described.

A good habit is to describe whatever response is obtained in addition to noting whether in your opinion the response is normal or abnormal.

Background Information

The neurophysiology of this reflex has not been completely elucidated. The account given here follows the suggestions made by Kugelberg, Eklund, and Grimby and is the result of their electromyographic studies. Each area of the skin of the body appears to have a specific reflex response to noxious stimuli. The purpose of the reflex is to cause the with-

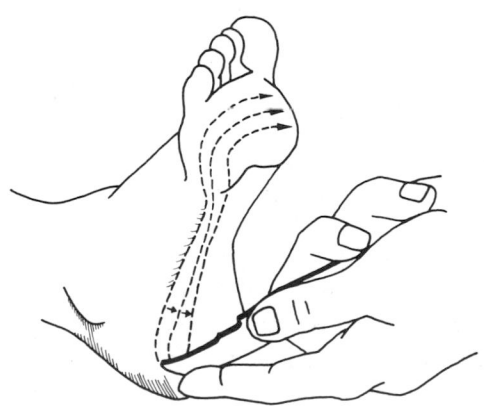

Figure 181. Testing the plantar reflex.

drawal of the area of the skin from the stimulus. This reflex is mediated by the spinal cord, but influenced by higher centers. The area of skin from which the reflex can be obtained is known as the receptive field of the reflex. To be more specific, a noxious stimulus to the sole of the foot, which is the receptive field, causes immediate flexion of the toes, ankle, knee, and hip joints with attendant withdrawal of the foot from the stimulus. The reader is invited to remember his own experiences with this reflex, an example being stepping on a sharp object while barefoot. There is an instant involuntary flexion of all joints with withdrawal. Another reflex in the normal individual is the great toe reflex: stimulation of the ball of the toe, which is the receptive field, causes extension (dorsiflexion) of the toe with flexion at ankle, knee, and hip joints. The two differences between these two reflexes are in the receptive fields and the fact that the great toe is flexed in one and extended in the other. The reason for the extension in the toe reflex is to remove the toe from the stimulus.

The abnormal plantar reflex, or Babinski reflex, is the elicitation of toe extension from the "wrong" receptive field, that is, the sole of the foot. Thus a noxious stimulus to the sole of the foot produces extension of the great toe instead of the normal flexion response. The essential phenomenon appears to be recruitment of the extensor hallucis longus, with consequent overpowering of the toe flexors (reference 3). The movements at the other joints remain the same.

The corticospinal tract influences the segmental reflex in the spinal cord. When the corticospinal tract is not functioning properly, the result is that the receptive field of the normal toe extensor reflex enlarges at the expense of the receptive field for toe flexion so that toe extension can be elicited from what is normally the receptive field for toe flexion. The maintenance of territorial integrity of the receptive fields is apparently one way in which the cortex exerts its influence under normal conditions.

Clinical Significance

The clinical significance of the plantar reflex, a nociceptive segmental spinal reflex that serves the purpose of protecting the sole of the foot, lies in the fact that the abnormal response reliably indicates that there is a metabolic or structural abnormality somewhere in the corticospinal system upstream from the segmental reflex. Thus the extensor reflex has been observed in structural lesions such as hemorrhage, brain and spinal cord tumors, and multiple sclerosis, and in abnormal metabolic states such as hypoglycemia, hypoxia, and anesthesia.

There is disagreement about whether the response is plantar flexion or dorsiflexion in the majority of newborns (see references 7 and 10). In all cases, however, the response does become flexor by the 6th to 12th month of life.

On rare occasions the extensor reflex has been reported in individuals who were otherwise normal; however, there is no long-term follow-up of these cases reported in the literature. In summary, there is widespread agreement among neurologists that an extensor plantar response after the 6th to 12th month of life indicates structural or metabolic dysfunction of the corticospinal system.

The receptive field for the extensor plantar response can be quite extensive. On occasion the extensor reflex has been elicited by stimulating as high as the face. Even in the same individual there is often shrinkage in the receptive field as time passes after the occurrence of the lesion.

The reflex response is on occasion equivocal. For example, there may be flexion of the toes before extension. Landau has addressed very nicely this question of an initial flexor movement of the toe followed by extension:

> But even when the abnormal response is maximally developed, as in our illustrated case of paraplegia, early flexion may occur, especially with threshold stimulation. What these observations amount to practically is that competent clinical judgment of this peculiar behavior, God's gift to the neurologist, has more validity than an arbitrary rule concerning the initial direction of hallux movement (reference 8).

On other occasions the reflex may be unequivocally flexor on one side and the toe remains neutral without movement on the other side. Under these circumstances remember the question is whether there is evidence of corticospinal tract dysfunction and not whether the response is flexor or extensor. This question can often be answered by looking for other evidence of corticospinal dysfunction such as repeating deep tendon reflexes, or withdrawal of the big toe after a painful stimulus such as a pin (Bing's sign). This latter sign is on occasion quite helpful, being unequivocally positive when the toe reflex is uncertain or negative. All indications are that Babinski's sign and Bing's sign are equivalent in meaning.

Selected References

1. Babinski JF, in Wilkins RH, Brody IA (eds): Babinski's sign. *Arch Neurol* 17:441–446, 1967.
2. Walshe F: The Babinski plantar response: Its form and its physiological and pathological significance. *Brain* 79(4):529–556, 1956.
3. Landau WM, Clare MH: The plantar reflex in man with special refer-

ence to some conditions where the extensor response is unexpectedly absent. *Brain* 82:321–355, 1959.

4. Kugelberg E, Eklund K, Grimby L: An electromyographic study of the nociceptive reflexes of the lower limb: Mechanism of the plantar responses. *Brain* 83:394–410, 1960.

5. Brain R, Wilkinson M: Observations on the extensor plantar reflex and its relationship to the functions of the pyramidal tract. *Brain* 82(3):297–320, 1959.

6. Brodal A: *Neurological Anatomy in Relation to Clinical Medicine,* ed 2. New York, Oxford University Press, 1969, pp 236–240.

7. Hogan GR, Milligan JE: The plantar reflex of the newborn. *N Eng J Med* 285:502–503, 1971.

8. Landau W: Clinical definition of the extensor plantar reflex (Letter). *N Eng J Med* 285:1149–1150, 1971.

9. Dohrmann GJ, Nowack WJ: The upgoing great toe: Optimal method of elicitation. *Lancet* 1:339–341, 1973.

10. Ross ED, Velez-Borras J, Rosman NP: The significance of the Babinski sign in the newborn: A reappraisal. *Pediatrics* 57:13–15, 1976.

CHAPTER EIGHT

Clinical Methods for the Pediatric Patient

ALBERT RAUBER, MD

This chapter, written for the examiner not yet experienced with children, is not designed to be a description of a comprehensive pediatric evaluation. The hints offered here suggest a basic attitude of approach and serve as examples of subtle skills each examiner should strive to develop.

The gathering of clinical data in pediatrics requires a special approach. The rapid changes due to growth require assorted sizes of equipment. Ear specula, sphygmomanometer cuffs, and stethoscopes should be available in several sizes to achieve good results. Even more important is the physician-patient relationship that must be established. The human being is innately programmed to respond favorably to a smiling face. Smile at the patient and the parent and introduce yourself. A friendly smile conveys the clinician's confidence, indicates that no harm is intended, and reduces the patient's anxiety. Use of the patient's name emphasizes that you are dealing with a person, not a case. Recognize all members of the patient constellation in establishing the doctor-patient relationship. Include the parents in your concept of "the patient."

Subjective information is often difficult to obtain from the child. The younger the child, the more completely the history is obtained from others. Hence, the information may be more objective about the child, but more subjective about the informer (what are the fears and anticipations of the informer?). Be aware of the "hidden agenda." In as many as 30% of clinic visits, the real reason for bringing the child to the doctor is not disclosed at once and may only be revealed later by good interviewing on the part of the clinician. Worthwhile information can be obtained from a small child by one who knows how children think and talk and act at different ages. The limitation of vocabulary must always be considered.

Pediatrics has been compared to veterinary medicine with good reason. Like a small animal, a child will react warily and become defensive or evasive if the examiner takes a too forward approach. Begin with simple, nonthreatening maneuvers; end with those examinations requiring bright lights or discomfort. The physical examination should start at a distance of 10 feet. Draw some conclusions at that point. You may modify them as you get closer, but you should start with a general view. Look for specific data. Don't forget that the normal finding may be the important item. Observe the color, breathing, spontaneous motor functions, affect, cranial nerve signs, neck stiffness (which may be difficult to assess later if the child resists), body size and shape, and other indicators of general physiological status. Often prognosis, and hence disposition, will hinge more immediately on these observations than on a diagnosis not yet completed. Make these general observations a habit in every case.

An early touch by warm, clean hands is helpful. Begin with parent-like activity such as assisting in undressing. This makes use of an adult-child relationship that is familiar and acceptable to the child. With small children, the examination should be introduced while the child is still on the parent's lap. Use the examining table as you would a surgical instrument! Manipulations of areas of the body that cannot be seen by the patient produce more anxiety and must be done very gently and with explanation. Like a magician, you should develop a distracting patter to accompany your act.

There is little place for formality in pediatrics. Children are unimpressed with pomposity. Children are also expert at detecting insincerity. Thus, a frank, honest approach is best. Speak with a child on his or her terms without becoming childish yourself. You and your patient can then accept each other with mutual respect.

The foregoing comments suggest that you cannot expect to conduct the examination in the sequential head-to-toe manner often done with adults. Examine what is offered first. Undress and examine succeeding parts gradually. Leave genitalia and bottoms covered at all times except when examining that area. With young infants, listen to the heart and palpate the abdomen early since crying may later hinder the evaluation. Auscultation of the lungs is facilitated by vigorous ventilation during crying, although fine, detailed hearing may be impaired. Little children have problems in controlling acts that are usually reflex. To ask a four-year-old child to take a deep breath will almost certainly cause breathing to stop. Raising the arms overhead, by fixing the shoulder girdle and compelling diaphragmatic breathing, is a more effective way of causing the lower lobes to be ventilated.

There are certain areas of trouble you should be aware of. One of these is the ticklish tummy. Surprisingly, this is most often encountered in the teenage boy. A trick useful in overcoming this is to include the child's hand in the examination. In a larger child, interweave the patient's fingers with yours; if the child's hand is too small to do this, place it under yours as you palpate the abdomen. Flexing the hips assists in relaxing the abdominal musculature. For small babies it may be necessary to fold their thighs upon the abdomen with one hand as you palpate with the other. Light, gentle pressure reveals more than heavy palpation, which tends to push masses and viscera away.

Little boys have very active cremaster reflexes, so much so that just removing their underpants may cause the testicles to retract completely out of the scrotum. Block the external inguinal rings with a thumb and forefinger prior to handling the scrotum and its contents to prevent a testis from running away from you.

When examining the genitalia of little girls, it sometimes helps to ask them to close their eyes. This tends to overcome modesty. Both sexes are very modest at an early age.

Most of the neurologic examination can be done by alert observation as you examine other parts. For example, is the face symmetrical when the child cries? If so, the seventh cranial nerve is intact. Did he bite the tongue blade when you examined the throat? If so, the motor division of the fifth nerve is intact. When he stuck his tongue out, did it deviate from the midline? There is information about the twelfth nerve. If he accurately grabbed the otoscope as you tried to insert it, information has been gained about proprioception and cerebellar function. Assess gait and equilibrium as you watch the child walk in. Children often inhibit tendon reflexes. Here is where distracting conversation and game playing can be useful. In testing sensation instead of asking, "Did you feel that?" ask the child to count to the next higher number each time you touch.

Examination of the eyes, ears, nose, and throat is usually the most difficult because these are sensitive parts of the body, and much frightening instrumentation is unveiled. Most children will open their mouths if they believe you will not stick anything into it. Therefore, begin by placing one hand on the child's head to steady and move it as desired; use the other hand to wield your flashlight. The child knows you do not have a third hand ready with the universally hated tongue blade. If you stand above, have the child look upward (neck extension will open the throat) as you look downward into the throat. You will see most of the structures. When the tongue blade is used, begin by using it to lift the lips and cheeks away from the gingiva as you inspect the oral mucosa, gingiva, and teeth. Only at the very end should the tongue blade touch the tongue, and then only to push it aside or to draw it out. Avoid pushing the tongue back into the throat. If you can get the child to pant "like a hot puppy dog," this causes continuous air movement through the larynx and inhibits the gag reflex. To open an absolutely recalcitrant mouth, place the tongue blade in the gingivolabial sulcus holding it in the vertical plane. Gently but firmly push it straight back toward the temporal-mandibular joint. This almost reflexly opens the mouth. Seizing the moment, slip the tongue blade vertically between the upper and lower molar teeth. The mouth is thus propped open for inspection.

Precede the ear examination by a manipulation of the pinna to assure that there is no tender lesion in the external ear. Most errors result from a failure to appreciate that the largest speculum that can comfortably enter the ear will not reveal the entire tympanic membrane. This leads to reliance on single criteria such as the light reflex, redness, or mobility for diagnosis. The novice may never see some of the important bony landmarks for failure to incline the speculum at the often extreme angle necessary to bring these into view. Usually the anterior-inferior quadrant is seen first. Here the light reflex is found. Follow it superiorly and posteriorly toward the center of the drum, the umbo. This is the inferior end of the attachment of the drum to the malleus. Follow the malleus superiorly and anteriorly until the short process of the malleus comes into view as a little white knob. You will learn to judge from the degree of prominence of this bony landmark whether the drum is retracted or distended under tympanic pressure. Shrapnell's membrane lies above the short process and is the first part of the drum to yield to pressure in the tympanum. Thickness of the drum is judged by its transparency and varies with age, usually being greater in early infancy. Hypertransparency may indicate the presence of clear fluid behind the drum. Although pneumatoscopy can be useful, there may be difficulty obtaining the necessary airtight seal, and one should be aware that the canal of an infant's ear may also yield to pressure, thus affecting the reliability of pneumatoscopy.

Difficulty is often encountered in examining the eyes because the child may not fix his gaze as you desire. Have an attractive object for him to look at. If none is at hand, enlist the parent, who can stand where you wish and command the patient's attention by talking. The disparity of size between the examiner and the patient also creates a problem. With the child seated on the edge of the examining table you will probably find yourself bending over such that some part of your head is in front of both of the patient's eyes. This obstruction may make it impossible for the child to fix his gaze on anything.

Rapid change in growth and development is an essential characteristic of a child. No examination is complete without assessment of growth and development. Here the essential instruments are pieces of paper, ie, standard charts of growth and development. The accurate and sequential plotting of data on these charts will indicate deviations from normal that may escape even a practiced eye. Skill in their use must be cultivated as much as for any other diagnostic instrument.

Although nothing will replace experience, remember that repeating the same errors is not experience. Observe yourself as well as the patient.

Modify your techniques and observe again. Be scientific in evaluation and improvement of your skills since you will be your own teacher most of your professional life.

Selected References

1. Korsch BM: Practical techniques in observing, interviewing and advising parents in pediatric practice as demonstrated in an attitude study project. *Pediatrics* 18:467–490, 1956.
2. Korsch BM, Negrete VF: Doctor-patient communication. *Sci Am* 227:66–74, 1972.
3. Kempe CH, Silver HK, O'Brien D: *Current Pediatric Diagnosis and Treatment,* ed 5. Los Altos, Calif, Lange Medical Publications, 1978.
4. Barness LA: *Manual of Pediatric Physical Diagnosis,* ed 4. Chicago, Year Book Medical Publishers, 1972.
5. Green M, Richmond J: *Pediatric Diagnosis: Interpretation of Signs and Symptoms in Different Age Periods,* ed 2. Philadelphia, WB Saunders, 1962.

PART FIVE

The Laboratory

CHAPTER NINE

Introduction to the Laboratory

DAVID H. VROON, MD
W. DALLAS HALL, MD

The laboratory tests discussed in this text are predetermined and represent a part of the Defined Data Base collected on patients hospitalized at Grady Memorial Hospital. A total of 30 individual laboratory items are performed at the time of the initial patient profile, history, and physical examination. These 30 laboratory tests can be divided into the following categories: hematologic tests (5), urinalysis tests (6), blood chemistries (18), and VDRL or RPR (1).

These tests were chosen with regard to the principles of selecting any data base items, discussed in Chapter 2, "The Medical Record." The admission laboratory data recorded on consecutive hospital admissions to the internal medicine service of Grady Memorial Hospital was used to determine the prevalence of abnormal admission laboratory parameters. Table 44 indicates the results for a few of these selected tests. The relatively high prevalence of abnormalities reflects both the severity and multiplicity of medical problems in the particular population served. The selection of this multitest data base is not intended as a disease screening effort, but rather is an attempt to define the nature and severity of specific diseases in a highly symptomatic population. The inclusion of specific tests is based on an effectiveness that presumes that test results are meaningful, cost justifiable, and lead to some definitive positive or negative action as to the presence, risk, or prognosis of a specific disease. The predictive value model illustrated below is most pertinent to test effectiveness and implies that the selection of laboratory data base items must be tailored to disease prevalence in the population studied. Less extensive laboratory testing might be appropriate for asymptomatic or healthier patient groups.

Table 44. Representative admission laboratory abnormalities in 600 patients hospitalized on the Internal Medicine Service of Grady Memorial Hospital.

Test	Value	Emergency Medical Admissions (%)	Elective Medical Admissions (%)
Hematocrit	>55 vol %	2.3	0.0
	<36 vol %	43.2	32.1
	<20 vol %	6.5	0.6
Blood glucose (random)	>500 mg/dl	4.2	0.9
	>110 mg/dl	59.6	36.7
	<60 mg/dl	1.5	1.1
Blood urea nitrogen	>100 mg/dl	3.2	0.2
	>20 mg/dl	38.4	20.0
	<5 mg/dl	2.3	1.1
Serum sodium	<120 mEq/liter	1.5	0.0
	<135 mEq/liter	30.2	8.3
	>145 mEq/liter	10.6	7.3
	>160 mEq/liter	0.8	0.0
Serum potassium	<3.0 mEq/liter	2.7	0.4
	<3.5 mEq/liter	14.5	6.6
	>5.5 mEq/liter	6.6	2.1
	>7.0 mEq/liter	1.2	0.0
Serum total CO_2 content	<10 mEq/liter	6.2	0.2
	<20 mEq/liter	25.7	5.1
	>30 mEq/liter	6.5	3.4

Physicians are increasingly dependent on laboratory data for the identification and management of patient diseases. This dependency is fostered by the availability of instruments which provide reliable measures of multiple test parameters on single specimens, and on the availability of new analytical methods capable of specifically quantitating substances occurring in biological fluids at low concentration levels. However, the proliferation and availability of laboratory tests presents the clinician with new problems. It is clearly easier to produce test results than it is to understand and apply them clinically. Cost containment efforts must accompany the proliferation of laboratory services. Basic guidelines to the cost-effective utilization and clinical application of laboratory services are presented in this chapter. Subsequent sections describe each of the 30 selected tests with regard to pertinent basic science information and clinical significance.

Cost-effective utilization of laboratory services must be based on an awareness that the clinical laboratory is a finite resource. This applies to the volume and frequency of tests requested and more specifically to the priority of services demanded. Cost justification for measuring multiple tests on single specimens is primarily based on the economy of automated chemical analyses with batch processing and does not extend to other areas of testing. A general understanding of laboratory instrument design is required to appreciate this important concept.

Laboratory instruments can be categorized generally as "multiphasic," "discrete" or "batch processing." The cost-effectiveness of measuring multiple test parameters on single specimens is largely restricted to scheduled batch processing on fully automated instruments utilizing the continuous flow principle. Sequential Multiple Analyzer (SMA) systems are by far the most comon batch analyzers utilized for chemical determinations; they are multiphasic in that multiple parameters are measured simultaneously. Specimen samples are sequentially aspirated and split into a predetermined number (SMA 6, SMA 12, SMA 18) of analytical modules, each with "continuously flowing" reagents and reaction-detection systems appropriate to the specific analytes. Operational cost is proportional to the duration of the run regardless of the number of specimens and tests processed. Cost per test is therefore minimal when batches of specimens are processed at maximum throughout; however, these instruments cannot be cost-effectively employed for emergency or unscheduled analyses.

The second group of laboratory systems include a larger number of manual methods and automated instruments categorized as "discrete." These are designed primarily for performance of selected tests on individual specimens. The Automated Clinical Analyzer (ACA) is the most popular instrument in this group. These systems support a variety of testing modes, including emergency and unscheduled processing. However, operational cost is considerably higher and directly related to the number of tests performed. It is often possible to perform 18 to 20 tests on continuous flow instrumentation at the same cost of performing 1 or 2 tests by discrete methods; clinicians should be aware of this differential when unscheduled, priority test processing is considered. The difference is pennies rather than dollars per test.

Intelligent interpretation of laboratory data must consider nondisease variables that may alter laboratory tests results; these factors are summarized in Table 45. Therapeutic agents may alter the concentration of body fluid constituents. Drugs and their metabolites may cause analytical interference by reacting chemically as analytes, by accelerating or inhibiting chemical reactions, or by spectral interferene if light absorbance of the drug is similar to that of the reaction end point. The potential for drug interference therefore varies with the specific analytical method.

Table 45. Nondisease factors that affect laboratory test results.

Factor	Variable
Drugs and other therapies	Metabolic effect
	Direct analytical interference (chemical or photometric)
Specimen matrix characteristics	Analytical interference
	Photometric interference
Specimen collection and preprocessing	Specimen type (arterial, venous, etc.)
	Serum contamination by intracellular constituents; presence of anticoagulant or preservatives; temperature and duration of storage; duration of venous occlusion
Physiological	Age, sex, weight
	Dietary state
	Time of day
	Physical state: ambulatory vs. supine

Since most laboratories employ multiple methods to measure each test parameter under different circumstances, analytical interferences may not be constant even for the same test.

Specimen matrix characteristics may cause analytical interferences, particularly with methods which depend on photometric detection. The presence of colored substances, such as hemoglobin or bilirubin, and the presence of turbidity due to hypertriglyceridemia are commonly encountered specimen characteristics which affect those photometric methods which employ shorter wavelengths of the visible spectrum (400–600 nm) as illustrated in Fig 182. Endogenous metabolites are an additional source of both chemical and photometric error. Methods selected for multiphasic testing are often not chemically specific due to instrument limitations or cost considerations. Although these methods yield reliable measurements in the normal specimen, the presence of abnormal endogenous metabolites or exogenous therapeutic agents may cause spurious results when clinical specimens are analyzed.

Photometric interferences are effectively minimized on SMA systems by specimen or reaction product dialysis which excludes larger molecules. For nondialyzable analytes, they are minimized by the use of specimen blanks. Direct chemical or photometric interference by dialyzable endogenous or exogenous substances is difficult to remove. Discrete analyzers use reaction-rate monitoring, improved chemical specificity, and variations of specimen blanking to minimize interference; photometric interference is often more significant than chemical. For example, the Coulter S provides no mechanism for excluding specimen matrix effects and therefore overestimates hemoglobin in the presence of lipemia.

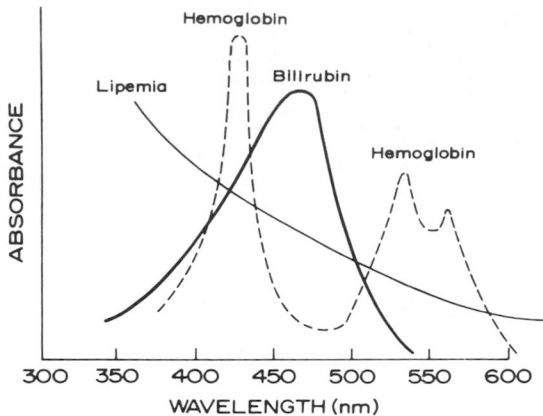

Figure 182. Absorbance characteristics of compounds that may produce photometric interference.

The effects of improper specimen collection and preprocessing on laboratory results are often overlooked. Hemolysis, in addition to photometric problems related to the presence of serum hemoglobin, invalidates certain serum or plasma determinations through release of erythrocyte contents (eg, lactate dehydrogenase, acid phosphatase, potassium, iron, and magnesium). The threshold of visibility for hemoglobin in serum or plasma is approximately 50 mg/dl and can be noted and reported at this level. However, certain substances (notably potassium, iron, and lactate dehydrogenase) may significantly contaminate serum and cause spurious elevations in the absence of visible hemolysis in the specimen. Careful collection and separation of serum or plasma from cells within one hour are critical to obtaining the most reliable results.

Physiological effects on laboratory test results are often acknowledged but not fully considered in interpreting test results. For example, a transfer of extravascular fluid to the intravascular space occurs in the supine position and may alter levels of nondiffused substances such as hemoglobin, hematocrit, protein, and lipoproteins. The variation is usually no more than 10% but may be significantly greater in the presence of edematous states. Laboratory test reference values are traditionally defined on ambulatory subjects; patients at bed rest have lower normal values for a number of laboratory tests.

The clinical application of laboratory data requires understanding of test characteristics as well as correlation with clinical findings. Laboratory tests, even when accurately performed, may lack the specificity and sensitivity required for decision making in the management of many clinical problems. The *specificity* of a test defines the incidence of true negative (or normal) results in subjects without a specific disorder. Hence, a test which is 90% specific has a 10% incidence of false positive results. The *sensitivity* of a test defines the incidence of true positive (or abnormal) results when applied to subjects with a specific disease. A test which is 90% sensitive is expected to detect 90% of subjects with a disease and yield a 10% incidence of false negative results. The sensitivity and specificity of tests are directly related to the reference value used to distinguish positive and negative test results. The occurrence of an overlap of results in healthy and diseased subjects is characteristic of virtually all laboratory tests. Therefore, the selection of a single reference value implies a trade-off between maximum sensitivity and maximum specificity. The traditional statistically derived "normal range" reference does not consider the distribution of test results in disease states or the relevant sensitivity and specificity characteristics of the test. An optimal definition of reference values would include consideration of sensitivity and specificity required for specific clinical decisions.

The ability of a test to predict the presence or absence of a specific disorder is dependent on the prevalence of the disease as well as the specificity and sensitivity of the test. This concept is particularly pertinent to the selection and interpretation of laboratory test data such as those obtained with multiphasic testing. The relationship of test sensitivity, specificity, and predictive value is illustrated in Table 46. Even a test characterized by a high degree of sensitivity and specificity will have poor diagnostic value if applied to a mixed population who have a low prevalence of the clinical problem studied. Diagnostic value is enhanced when the patient population is prescreened in some manner to isolate high disease prevalence groups for more definitive testing. Four methods are used intuitively by clinicians to accomplish this goal: selective testing based on observed clinical problems, restriction of multiphasic testing to

Table 46. Test sensitivity, specificity, and diagnostic value.

Test Characteristics (%)		Disease Prevalence (%)	Frequency of Positive Tests per 1,000 Subjects		Predictive Value of Positive Test* (%)
Sensitivity	Specificity		True Positive	False Positive	
95	80	0.1	9.5	198	4.6
95	95	0.1	9.5	49.5	16
95	80	50	475	100	83
95	95	50	475	25	95

* Percentage of positive results that are true positives.

hospitalized patients with high disease prevalence, observation of primary and secondary tests for the same clinical problem, and consideration of the quantitative nature (ie, degree of abnormality) of the test result. These approaches have not yet been fully developed in the clinical laboratory. However, the advent and availability of new automated data processing systems now makes it possible to quantitatively define the diagnostic value of a test or test group based on the level of measurement. Until this becomes further developed, clinicians must continue to interpret and apply laboratory data with an awareness of test characteristics related to disease prevalence.

Selected References

1. Collen MF, Feldman R, Siegelaub AB, et al: Dollar cost per positive test for automated multiphasic screening. *N Eng J Med* 283:459–463, 1970.
2. Griner PF, Liptzin B: Use of the laboratory in a teaching hospital. *Ann Intern Med* 75:157–163, 1971.
3. Leonard PJ, Smith DH, Cope JT, et al: Laboratory tests in health screening: Their feasibility and usefulness in a general practice. *J R Coll Gen Practit* 21:714–718, 1971.
4. Grams RR, Johnson EA, Benson ES: Laboratory data analysis system. Section III, Multivariate normality. *Am J Clin Pathol* 58:188–200, 1972.
5. Schneiderman LJ, DeSalvo L, Baylor S, et al: The "abnormal" screening laboratory result. Its effect on physician and patient. *Arch Intern Med* 129:88–90, 1972.
6. Hall WD: A defined laboratory data base, in Walker HK, Hurst JW, Wood MF (eds): *Applying the Problem-Oriented System.* New York, Medcom, 1973, pp 407–411.
7. Young DS, Pestaner LC, Gibberman V: Effects of drugs on clinical laboratory tests. *Clin Chem* 21:1–432, 1975.
8. Krieg AF, Gambino R, Galen RS: Why are clinical laboratory tests performed? When are they valid? *JAMA* 233:76–78, 1975.
9. Ransohoff DF, Feinstein AR: Problems of spectrum and bias in evaluating the efficacy of diagnostic tests. *N Eng J Med* 299:926–930, 1978.

HEMATOLOGY

211. Hematocrit

HERBERT KANN, MD

Definition

The hematocrit is a measure of the volume of packed red blood cells, expressed as a percentage of whole blood volume. For an adult, normal values are generally accepted to be in the range of 40–54 (men) and 37–47 (women). Anemia is present when the hematocrit is below normal; erythrocytosis, when the hematocrit is above normal. Different normal values apply in pregnancy and in the newborn.

Technique

Ordinarily the hematocrit will be supplied as a printed value obtained from an automated cell counter. The automated cell counter does not directly measure the hematocrit; it computes a value which is a product of red cell count times average cell size. For direct determination of hematocrit, the technique is as follows:

1. Fill two microhematocrit tubes two-thirds full. When using blood obtained by a finger stick or heel stick, heparinized tubes are used. When using blood obtained by venipuncture and anticoagulated in EDTA, heparinized microhematocrit tubes need not be used.

2. Seal one end by plunging the end of the tube into a bed of clay; when the tube is withdrawn a 2–3-mm plug of clay remains inside the capillary, providing a seal. If the clay is not available the capillary can be sealed by heating one end over a Bunsen burner.

3. The sample is spun 5 minutes in a centrifuge designed to accommodate capillary tubes.

4. The hematocrit is then read using a hematocrit reader; these differ in design and ordinarily will display simple instructions for use. The value can be obtained without a reader by measuring the height of the column

of packed cells and the height of the column of cells plus plasma; the hematocrit is then calculated:

$$\frac{\text{Height of column of packed cells}}{\text{Height of column of packed cells plus plasma}} \times 100$$

Background Information

The hematocrit is used to evaluate the adequacy of a patient's red cell mass. In general this evaluation could as well be made from the hemoglobin concentration or the RBC count. Before the development of the automated cell counter, the hematocrit was easiest to measure and was therefore used more often than the hemoglobin or RBC count; now many hospital laboratories measure all these parameters with equal ease using the automated cell counter. Slightly different information is obtained from each parameter. For instance, an anemic individual may have a normal red cell count but a low hemoglobin and hematocrit if the red cells are abnormally small and have a low hemoglobin content.

While it is usually true that the hematocrit is a valid indicator of red cell mass, some exceptions should be borne in mind. For example, after acute blood loss there may be no appreciable change in hematocrit for several hours, in spite of a significant decrease in red cell mass. The fall in hematocrit will only occur when the plasma volume begins to increase toward normal. Even when the red cell is stable, the hematocrit fluctuates with changes in plasma volume; thus, in a patient who is dehydrated, the red cell mass will be overestimated from the hematocrit simply because the plasma volume is decreased; and in a patient whose plasma volume is increased (as in pregnancy), the hematocrit will fall, even when there has been no decrease in red cell mass.

Clinical Significance

A very low hematocrit may be associated with symptoms of weakness, easy fatigability, or dyspnea on exertion, and with signs of pallor, tachycardia, or postural hypotension. When the hematocrit is closer to a normal value, there may be no symptoms or signs of anemia. A high hematocrit ordinarily produces no symptoms, and no signs other than a ruddy complexion. Any hematocrit outside the normal range requires investigation, particularly since an abnormal hematocrit is often a clue to the presence of serious underlying disease.

An early step in the diagnostic evaluation of anemia should be assessment of the rate of erythrocyte production. If production is low, the evaluation is directed toward definition of the factor(s) limiting erythropoiesis, of which iron deficiency is by far the most common. If, on the other hand, production is high, evaluation is directed toward definition of the factor(s) responsible for accelerated loss of RBCs. Accelerated loss could be due either to bleeding or to hemolysis. The early broad categorization of anemia—decreased production versus accelerated loss—helps determine the subsequent steps in diagnostic evaluation. In particular, this categorization eliminates from consideration certain diagnostic procedures that might otherwise be considered. For example, the patient whose anemia is characterized by accelerated loss of RBCs with increased erythrocyte production is ordinarily not a candidate for a bone marrow examination; that particular diagnostic study would be useful primarily in evaluating anemias associated with decreased RBC production.

The rate of production of erythrocytes is easily assessed from the reticulocyte count. Reticulocytes are newly formed RBCs. These cells have special staining properties as a result of the lingering presence of small amounts of RNA. Reticulocytes will be increased in number in patients whose anemia is due to excessive loss but not in patients whose anemia is due to decreased production. For a logical, concise description of red cell physiology and pathophysiology, together with a systematic approach to the diagnosis of red cell abnormalities, the reader is referred to reference 2.

Selected References

1. Schwartz E, Gill FM: Hematology of the newborn, in Williams WJ, Beutler E, Erslev AJ, et al (eds): *Hematology*, ed 2. New York, McGraw-Hill, 1977, pp 37–48.
2. Hillman RS, Finch CA: *Red Cell Manual*, ed 4. Philadelphia, FA Davis, 1974, pp 23–81.

212. White Blood Cell Count

HERBERT KANN, MD

Definition

The white blood cell count (WBC) is the number of white blood cells per cubic millimeter of whole blood. In most white adults the generally accepted range of normal is 5,000–10,000/cu mm; in blacks the lower limit of normal is 3,600/cu mm. In newborns the range of normal values is higher.

Technique

As with the hematocrit, this information is ordinarily obtained as a printed value from an automated cell counter. When the count is done by hand, the blood is first diluted in a solution that lyses erythrocytes and stains lightly the nuclei of leukocytes. The diluted blood is then counted in a hemocytometer chamber, in which each large square is 1 mm on a side; since the depth of the chamber is 0.1 mm, the number of cells in 10 squares is equal to the number of cells in a volume of 1 cu mm. Since the blood is diluted prior to counting, a correction for dilution (ordinarily 20×) must be made in order to calculate the number of WBC/cu mm of whole blood.

Background Information

A working assumption is that the production of WBCs is under hormonal control in a fashion similar to erythropoietin control of red cell production; but to date no equivalent substance for control of white cell production has been identified. Under ordinary circumstances most of the WBCs will be granulocytes. Approximately one-half of all circulating granulocytes are marginated along the walls of blood vessels. These marginated cells are not collected when blood is sampled, and therefore they are not enumerated. However, under some circumstances, these granulocytes will detach themselves from the vessel walls, and if the blood is sampled at such a time, the WBC may be elevated by about a factor of two. Granulocytes will shift from the marginated pool into the circulating pool during severe pain or severe emotional stress and following a seizure or strenuous exercise. In each of these situations, the factor responsible for the shift in granulocytes from the marginated into the circulating pool may be an increase in the circulating level of adrenergic steroid. Epinephrine injections can also induce the same sort of shift. The important point is that leukocytosis occurring under these special circumstances be recognized as a normal event and not interpreted as evidence indicating an underlying problem such as bacterial infection.

Clinical Significance

An increased WBC is often taken as evidence of infection. Although considering the possibility of infection in anyone with leukocytosis is appropriate, emphasis should be placed on the uncertainty of direct correlation. On the one hand, leukocytosis can be seen in patients who are not infected, eg, in association with severe pain, emotional stress, after vigorous exercise, or with primary hematologic problems such as leukemia or polycythemia rubra vera. On the other hand, patients who have viral infections or overwhelming bacterial infections may not have leukocytosis.

A decreased WBC (leukopenia) is less common than leukocytosis. Leukopenia may be associated with several chemical compounds, with collagen vascular disease, especially systemic lupus erythematosus, and with primary hematologic disease. For a concise review of white cell physiology and pathophysiology see reference 2.

Selected References

1. Orfanakis NG, Ostlund RE, Bishop CR, et al: Normal blood leukocyte concentration values. *Am J Clin Pathol* 53:647–651, 1970.
2. Boggs DR, Winkelstein A: *White Cell Manual,* ed 3. Philadelphia, FA Davis, 1975.
3. Broun GO Jr, Herbig FK, Hamilton JR: Leukopenia in Negroes. *N Eng J Med* 275:1410–1413, 1966.

213. White Blood Cell Differential

HERBERT KANN, MD

Definition

The differential is a listing of the various types of white blood cells present in the peripheral blood. One-hundred white cells are enumerated and the number of cells of each type expressed as a percentage value. The distinctions between normal and abnormal values are not sharp. The limits of normal given below are approximate and are intended to serve only as general guidelines.

Neutrophils (polymorphonuclear leukocytes, polys, and segs)	50–60%
Lymphocytes	25–30%
Monocytes	3–7%
Eosinophils	1–3%
Basophils	0–1%
Juvenile forms (bands, stabs)	0–5%

More accurate limits of normal can be established when the absolute number of cells of each type is calculated. In terms of cells per cubic millimeter, those limits are approximately as follows:

Neutrophils (polys, segs)	1,100–6,050
Lymphocytes	1,500–4,000
Monocytes	200–950
Eosinophils	0–700
Basophils	0–150
Juveniles	100–2,100

When the number of cells of a certain type exceeds the upper limit of normal, the descriptive term applied depends on the cell type involved; there may be neutrophilia, eosinophilia, basophilia, lymphocytosis, or monocytosis. An abnormally low number of cells of a certain type would be recognized by terms such as neutropenia or lymphocytopenia. For example, a white blood cell count of 5,000/cu mm with 70% lymphocytes and 20% neutrophils reflects a neutropenia (1,000) rather than a lymphocytosis (3,500).

Technique

This information will usually be presented to the clinician in numerical form, having been collected and tabulated by a laboratory technician. The proper performance of a white blood cell differential is a skill that requires practice. The steps in the procedure are given below.

Preparation of a sample for staining requires spreading blood cells in a film of the proper thickness on a glass slide. Slides must be cleaned by soaking in 70% alcohol, then buffing dry with a lint-free cloth. A drop of blood from a finger stick or an EDTA-anticoagulated sample is placed near one end of a glass slide. The bottom edge of a second slide is used to spread the drop of blood in the following way: the upper slide is tilted so that the lower edge of its narrow end touches the lower slide at about its midpoint; that edge is dragged back until it touches the drop of blood, then advanced forward, spreading the drop of blood in a film which becomes progressively thinner. In a few seconds the blood airdries and is ready for staining.

Either Wright's or Giemsa's stain is commonly used. Just enough stain is added to cover the slide. After 1–2 minutes, the stain is diluted with water or buffer added dropwise until the solution is just about to overflow the slide. The diluted stain is left on for 3–5 minutes; during this time stain and water are mixed by blowing over the surface of the slide. Stain is then flushed from the slide under tap water, the bottom of the slide buffed dry, and the slide left at a vertical tilt for the top surface to dry by drainage and evaporation.

For microscopic examination, find a proper area of the slide for evaluation by beginning at the end of the slide where the film of cells is thinnest, opposite the end to which the drop of blood was applied. Locate the feathered edge where the thin film of blood cells ends, move back one or two microscopic fields to an area where the cells are close together but not quite touching, and begin the cell enumeration.

One hundred leukocytes are counted; the percentage of each cell type is recorded. By multiplying the total leukocyte count by the percentage of each cell type, the absolute number of cells of each type can be calculated.

Neutrophils have cytoplasmic granules that stain lightly with a very faint purple hue against a pink cytoplasmic background. The nucleus of a mature neutrophil is lobulated, usually having three or four bulky clumps of chromatin connected by thin strands of nuclear material. Juvenile forms resemble mature neutrophils, except that their nucleus exists as a single strip or band of material that has not matured into the lobulated, segmented configuration of a mature cell. Lymphocytes usually have no cytoplasmic granules. Their cytoplasm stains light blue; their nucleus is round and stains a much darker blue. Monocytes are slightly larger than neutrophils and contain cytoplasmic granules that stain lightly. The color of the cytoplasmic granules is variable, usually tan, but sometimes pink or pink purple. The monocyte nucleus is large and is composed of chromatin that is loosely compacted. The shape of the nucleus is not an especially helpful identifying feature: it may be round, oval, kidney-shaped, or in some other less easily described configuration. Particularly for the inexperienced observer, some monocytes may be difficult to distinguish from metamyelocytes, and other monocytes may be hard to distinguish from large lymphocytes. Eosinophils have large cytoplasmic granules that stain red or red orange. Their nuclei are segmented, but usually have no more than two or three lobes, fewer lobes than are seen in neutrophils. Basophils are the most readily recognized white cell; their distinctive feature is the blue black color of their cytoplasmic granules. Atypical lymphocytes have very large nuclei and an abundant amount of cytoplasm; a morphologic feature that may be especially helpful in identifying these cells is a darkening of the pale blue cytoplasm around the outer margin of the cell. Other leukocytes are seen in the peripheral blood only under abnormal circumstances; these may include metamyelocytes, myelocytes, promyelocytes, myeloblasts, and plasma cells.

Background Information

Host defense mechanisms are dependent on normally functioning white blood cells. Neutrophils and eosinophils are phagocytic. Lymphocytes carry out one or another function, depending on whether they are B (bone-marrow-derived) or T (thymus-derived) lymphocytes. The B lymphocytes are responsible for antibody production, the T lymphocytes for cell-mediated immunity. These two classes of lymphocytes cannot be distinguished from each other by the ordinary light microscopy employed in performing a white blood cell differential count. Monocytes are phagocytic and they also perform certain steps in "processing" of antigenic materials. Basophils contain large amounts of histamine, which is released in allergic reactions.

Clinical Significance

Neutrophilia is commonly seen as a consequence of bacterial infection. Neutropenia is often drug induced but may be a consequence of either marrow damage or an enlarged spleen. In a neutropenic patient with no history of drug ingestion and no splenomegaly, a reasonable next step in evaluation would be a bone-marrow examination for assessment of granulocyte production.

Lymphocytosis is often seen in association with viral infections, including infectious mononucleosis. The presence of atypical lymphocytes is good evidence in support of a viral etiology for the lymphocytosis. For a more complete list of causes of lymphocytosis see reference 0.

A diagnosis of chronic lymphocytic leukemia may be entertained only when lymphocytosis is sustained; chronic lymphocytic leukemia is not a disease of children, and is rarely seen in young adults. Acute lymphocytic leukemia, which occurs in children as well as in adults, is characterized by the presence in the peripheral blood of lymphoblasts, cells which differ morphologically from normal lymphocytes. The blasts tend to be large cells with only a thin rim of cytoplasm, with nucleoli and, in some cases, cleft nuclei. Lymphocytopenia is a comparatively infrequent laboratory finding. Lymphocytopenia may be caused by decreased production of lymphocytes, as is often seen after radiation therapy or chemotherapy of neoplasia; by excessive loss of lymphocytes, as in intestinal lymphangiectasia; or by less readily understandable mechanisms.

Monocytosis is seen in association with some infections, eg, tuberculosis and primary hematologic abnormalities (see reference 8 for a listing of causes of monocytosis). Frequent causes of eosinophilia are infections by parasites, allergic conditions, and dermatologic disorders. Basophilia is occasionally a clue to the presence of either chronic myelocytic leukemia or one of the other myeloproliferative disorders.

The presence of immature white cells in the peripheral blood generally indicates a serious medical problem. Juvenile forms, metamyelocytes, and some myelocytes may appear in a patient with a severe bacterial infection. In the absence of an infection, the presence of immature myeloid elements in the peripheral blood is a useful clue to the possible presence of an important abnormality of the bone marrow; attention should be directed to disorders such as myelofibrosis, tumor metastases to the marrow, or acute or chronic myelocytic leukemia. In acute myelocytic leukemia, expect to see predominantly the most immature forms (blasts and promyelocytes) without appreciable numbers of cells at the later levels of maturation (myelocytes and metamyelocytes). In chronic myelocytic leukemia, expect to see cells from the entire spectrum of myeloid maturation, with a predominance of the more mature forms.

Selected References

1. Orfanakis NG, Ostlund RE, Bishop CR, et al: Normal blood leukocyte concentration values. *Am J Clin Path* 53:647–651, 1970.
2. Williams WJ: Examination of the bone marrow, in Williams WJ,

Beutler E, Erslev AJ, et al (eds): *Hematology*, ed 2. New York, McGraw-Hill, 1977, pp 25–32.

3. Boggs DR, Winkelstein A: *White Cell Manual*, ed 3. Philadelphia, FA Davis, 1975.

4. Finch SC: Granulocytosis, in Williams WJ, Beutler E, Erslev AJ, et al (eds): *Hematology*, ed 2. New York, McGraw-Hill, 1977, pp 746–755.

5. Finch SC: Granulocytopenia, in Williams WJ, Beutler E, Erslev AJ, et al (eds): *Hematology*, ed 2. New York, McGraw-Hill, 1977, pp 717–746.

6. Cassileth P: Lymphocytosis, in Williams WJ, Beutler E, Erslev AJ, et al (eds): *Hematology*, ed 2. New York, McGraw-Hill, 1977, pp 968–972.

7. Cassileth P: Lymphocytopenia, in Williams WJ, Beutler E, Erslev AJ, et al (eds): *Hematology*, ed 2. New York, McGraw-Hill, 1977, pp 972–974.

8. Cassileth P: Monocytosis, in Williams WJ, Beutler E, Erslev AJ, et al (eds): *Hematology*, ed 2. New York, McGraw-Hill, 1977, pp 974–977.

214. Platelets

HERBERT KANN, MD

Definition

There is considerable variability from one clinical laboratory to the next in the accepted range of normal for platelet counts. A general range of normal would be 250,000 ± 50,000/cu mm.

Technique

Quantitative platelet counts are ordinarily done only by experienced medical technologists, and only on special request. Under usual circumstances platelet number is estimated during examination of the stained peripheral blood film. An easy way of estimating platelet number in a patient who is not anemic is to compare the number of platelets and red cells in a microscopic field. Since the normal platelet count is 250,000/ cu mm and the normal RBC count 5 million/cu mm, the ratio of platelets to RBCs should be about 1:20. A typical oil-immersion microscopic field would contain about 200 red cells and 8–10 platelets.

Background Information

More than any other cells in the peripheral blood, platelets are pooled in the spleen. Whenever there is splenomegaly, thrombocytopenia may occur. Other causes of thrombocytopenia are shortened platelet survival and decreased production. Survival below the normal period of 10 days may be predicated on altered immunity, as in idiopathic thrombocytopenic purpura, systemic lupus erythematosus, or a side effect of a drug, quinidine being the most frequent offender; abnormal endothelial surfaces as in thrombotic thrombocytopenic purpura or Rocky Mountain spotted fever; or disseminated intravascular coagulation. A decrease in the rate of platelet production occurs as a consequence of marrow damage. For an excellent comprehensive discussion of platelet physiology and pathophysiology see reference 1.

Clinical Significance

When the platelet count rises above 1 million/cu mm, the risk of thrombosis increases by an appreciable degree. Paradoxically, the risk of hemorrhage is also increased in these patients. Such degrees of thrombocytosis are not infrequent in patients with polycythemia vera or following splenectomy.

In patients with platelet counts below 20,000, the probability of hemorrhage is quite high; however, factors other than the platelet count itself are important determinants of hemostasis. Thus in a patient with neoplasia complicated by infection, hemorrhage may occur when the platelet count is 25,000; whereas in an otherwise healthy patient with aplastic anemia, a platelet count of 25,000 may provide adequate hemostasis. Whenever the onset of thrombocytopenia is abrupt, hemorrhage can occur with platelet counts as high as 50,000 or more.

Platelets are usually consistently depressed in cases of disseminated intravascular coagulation and are characteristically the last coagulation abnormality to return to normal with successful therapy. For a logical approach to the diagnosis of platelet abnormalities see reference 2.

Selected References

1.   Harker LA: *Hemostasis Manual*, ed 2. Philadelphia, FA Davis, 1974, chap 2, pp 5–19.
2.   Harker LA: *Hemostasis Manual*, ed 2. Philadelphia, FA Davis, 1974, pp 42–46.

215. Red Blood Cell Morphology

HERBERT KANN, MD

Definition

The normal red blood cell (RBC) is 6–9 μ in diameter and has an area of central pallor the diameter of which is one-third the total diameter of the cell. Normal RBCs are round, tan, and contain no inclusions. In a blood film from a normal person, only a few cells will have characteristics different from these.

When the red cells on a peripheral blood film appear normal, the morphology is described as normochromic and normocytic. Abnormally small RBCs are described as microcytic; large RBCs are described as macrocytic. Anisocytosis is the term used to denote variability in cell size.

When the area of central pallor is greater than one-third of the total diameter of the cell, hypochromia is present. The area of central pallor may be completely lost in some cells such as schistocytes, which come in a whole variety of bizarre shapes, and spherocytes, which are perfectly round.

A target cell is an erythrocyte that has a portion of its hemoglobin trapped in a dimple in the middle of the cell, forming what looks like a bull's-eye.

Abnormal RBC shapes include oblong cells with blunt ends (elliptocytes); oblong cells with sharp ends (sickle cells); cells in which the area of central pallor is slitlike rather than round (stomatocytes); cells shaped like teardrops (teardrops); cells with irregular, thorny surface projections (acanthocytes or spur cells); and cells with regularly scalloped margins (crenated cells). When there are many different cell shapes, the appropriate descriptive term is poikilocytosis.

Often a few of the RBCs will stain gray or blue gray rather than the usual tan. This is referred to as polychromatophilia, and the cells are called shift cells.

Various types of RBC inclusions may be recognized in a routinely prepared peripheral blood film. Basophilic stippling is the term used to describe multiple, small, dark blue inclusions. Depending on the size of the dark blue particles, basophilic stippling is described as coarse, which is abnormal, or fine, which may be of little significance. A different sort of RBC inclusion is the Howell-Jolly body. Howell-Jolly bodies are larger than the inclusions of basophilic stippling and fewer in number. Howell-Jolly bodies stain a purple or pink purple color. Cabot rings and malaria parasites are inclusion bodies which can be seen in peripheral blood films stained in the usual manner. They are seldom encountered. Other sorts of RBC inclusions, such as Heinz bodies, are not visible in peripheral blood films prepared and stained in the usual manner. They can be demonstrated only when the cells are prepared and stained by special techniques.

A variety of types and shapes of abnormal erythrocytes are shown in Fig 183.

Technique

RBC morphology is assessed during microscopic examination of the peripheral blood film. Evaluate RBC morphology only in an area of proper thickness on the slide: when the film is too thin (near the feathered edge), RBC morphology is distorted artifactually; when the film is too thick, the RBCs will be piled on top of one another, preventing an adequate assessment of the morphology of individual cells. Cell size can be measured directly if there is a micrometer in the eyepiece of the microscope. When there is no micrometer in the eyepiece, size can be roughly estimated by comparing the size of RBCs and small lymphocytes: a normal RBC should be slightly smaller than a small lymphocyte.

Background Information

The size and shape of the normal red cell allow it to move easily through the microcirculation and to exchange oxygen and carbon dioxide across its cellular membrane. Some abnormalities of red cell morphology can be understood to interfere with normal function. For example, sickled

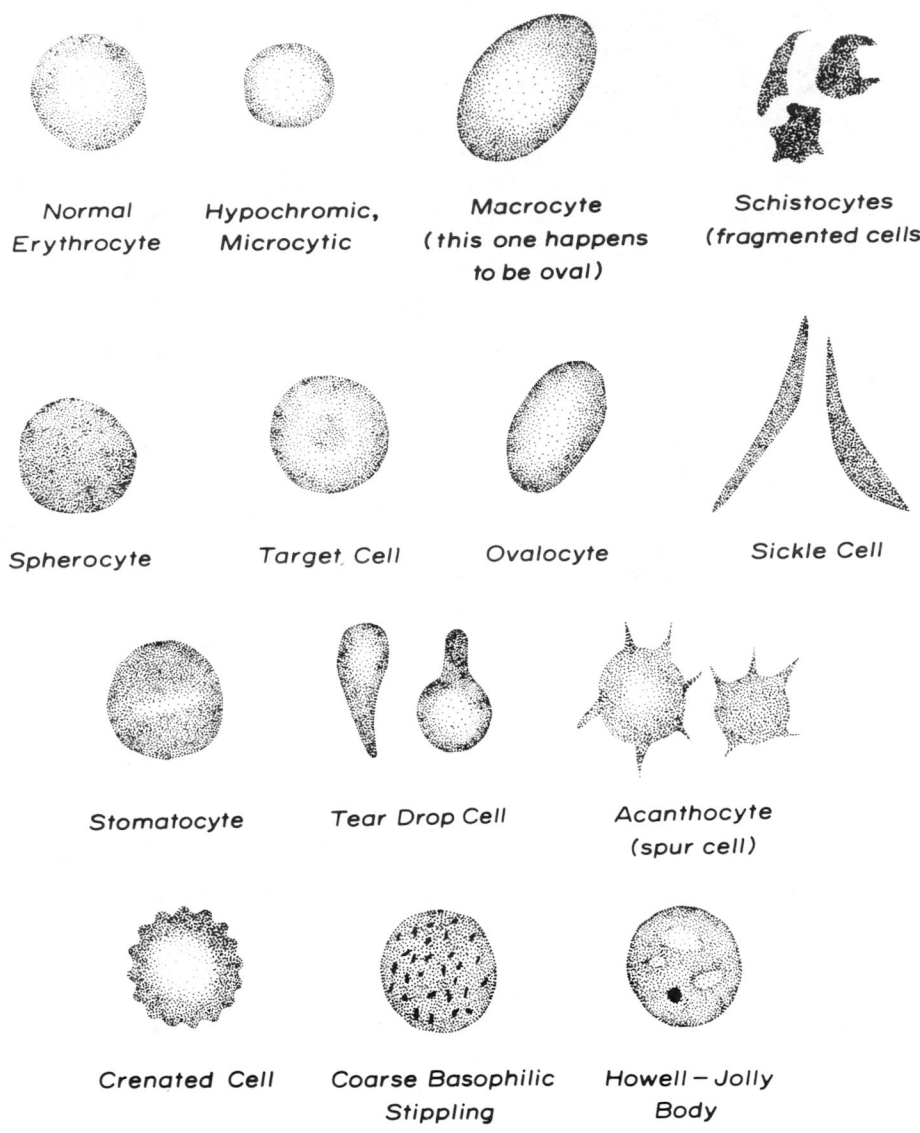

Figure 183.   Types and shapes of abnormal erythrocytes.

erythrocytes, which are not deformable, may not pass normally through the microcirculation.

The normal, mature RBC, whose cytoplasm is full of hemoglobin, will look tan in a stained peripheral blood film. A less mature RBC will contain in its cytoplasm both hemoglobin and ribonucleic acid. Since RNA stains blue, the cytoplasm of such a cell will be either blue or gray, depending on the amount of RNA remaining in the cytoplasm. An RBC with homogeneous blue- or gray-staining cytoplasm would normally remain in the marrow until its maturation was completed, but under certain circumstances it may be delivered prematurely into the peripheral blood as a shift cell. A shift cell is an immature erythrocyte that has been shifted prematurely from its rightful place in the bone marrow into the peripheral blood. Shift cells are visible in a normally stained peripheral blood film. For a thorough discussion of abnormalities of RBC morphology see reference 1.

Clinical Significance

Small, pale RBCs are seen with iron deficiency and other conditions in which hemoglobin synthesis is impaired, including the thalassemias (globin synthesis abnormalities) and pyridoxine-responsive anemia (a heme synthesis abnormality).

Young RBCs are larger than normal, and therefore macrocytosis is to be expected when the reticulocyte count is high. Other causes of macrocytosis are liver disease, characterized by macrocytic target ells, and megaloblastic anemia, characterized by oval macrocytes.

Spherocytes are seen with hereditary spherocytosis and with immune hemolytic anemias.

Large numbers of target cells are seen with thalassemia (microcytic target cells), liver disease (macrocytic target cells) and with either heterozygous or homozygous hemoglobin C disease.

Ovalocytes are seen in hereditary ovalocytosis and in small numbers in normal people. Sickle cells are seen in patients who are homozygous for the sickle hemoglobin gene and in patients with sickle hemoglobin plus certain other abnormal hemoglobins. They are not found in the peripheral smear of patients with sickle trait (hemoglobin SA). Stomatocytes occur in hereditary stomatocytosis and also in alcoholics with liver disease. Burr cells are seen in patients with advanced renal failure. Spur cells or acanthocytes occur in a few patients with hepatic failure and in a rare hereditary abnormality of lipid metabolism, abetalipoproteinemia. Poikilocytes may occur in severe anemia of nearly any sort but should especially call to mind possibilities such as megaloblastic anemia, myelofibrosis, or metastatic tumor in the marrow. Fragmented RBCs (schistocytes) are produced when erythrocytes are destroyed mechanically in the circulation; some settings in which this may occur are malfunctioning prosthetic heart valves, vasculitis, thrombotic thrombocytopenic purpura, and disseminated intravascular coagulation.

The presence of shift cells in the peripheral blood implies at least two things of importance regarding the erythropoietic mechanism. First, there is an increased erythropoietin stimulation of the marrow. Thus chronic renal failure is not a prominent possibility for the etiology. Second, there is an ability of the marrow to respond, at least in part, to erythropoietin.

Inclusion bodies may be a nonspecific finding (fine basophilic stippling); a clue to the presence of lead poisoning (coarse basophilic stippling); or a point in favor of megaloblastic anemia, hemolytic anemia, or prior splenectomy (Howell-Jolly bodies). For an excellent review of the clinical significance of morphologic abnormalities of RBCs see reference 1.

In general, RBC morphologic abnormalities are sought as useful clues to the etiology of an anemia. However, abnormalities of RBC morphology can also provide clinically useful information in nonanemic patients. An extreme example from my own experience involved a patient who became ill on the last leg of an around-the-world trip. Symptoms were fever and sore throat. The only prominent physical finding was an erythematous pharynx with a pustular exudate. This patient appeared to have an exudative pharyngitis. She was not anemic. However, assessment of her problem changed dramatically when the peripheral blood film was examined, and her RBCs were found to be loaded with malaria parasites. In spite of prompt initiation of appropriate antimalarial therapy, her clinical course was very difficult, with complications of severe intravascular hemolysis, disseminated intravascular coagulation, and acute renal failure. This particular case is cited as an example of a situation in which initial diagnosis and management would have been inappropriate if RBC morphology had not been evaluated in a nonanemic patient. This point can be made using less dramatic examples. Consider the patient with a compensated hemolytic process who has spherocytes in the peripheral blood: a proper evaluation of the cause of spherocytosis could lead to a diagnosis of an immune hemolytic process, which might be the earliest manifestation of a serious underlying illness. Erythrocyte fragments in the peripheral blood film of a nonanemic patient may imply the presence of abnormalities of the microvasculature or the possibility of disseminated intravascular coagulation. Additional examples could be cited, but by now the point should be clear that examination of RBC morphology may provide information of fundamental importance in nonanemic patients.

Selected Reference

1.   Lessin LS, Bessis M: Morphology of the erythron, in Williams WJ, Beutler E, Erslev AJ, et al (eds): *Hematology*, ed 2. New York, McGraw-Hill, 1977, pp 103–134.

216. Urinalysis: Color and Odor

BARRY J. ROSENBAUM, MD

Definition

Urinalysis is the analytical testing of the urine for certain biochemical and histopathological abnormalities. Normal, concentrated urine has a deep yellow or amber color and may be either clear or cloudy. Normal dilute urine may be completely colorless. Abnormal urine pigments range from black to red depending on the abnormality present. Normal urine has a pungent odor slightly suggestive of ammonia. Abnormal urine odors range from sweet to vinegary.

Taste was once included in the qualitative analysis of the urine. Indeed, diabetes mellitus was once diagnosed by the presence of a sweet urine taste. Today, we forego this unaesthetic test since more precise methods can detect sugar in the urine.

Technique

In 1827, Bright demonstrated the importance of urinalysis. At that time the technique was cumbersome and time-consuming. Now a careful urinalysis can be done in 2–5 minutes excluding time necessary for centrifugation. The potential information is so key that the urinalysis is one of the laboratory tests that the physician ought to do. The following comments concern proper collection and processing of the specimen in order that any abnormalities may be validly detected. The clean-catch technique maximizes the potential information gain and minimizes the amount of extraneous material, contamination, and biochemical changes involved in an improperly handled specimen. A clean-catch specimen is necessary to provide uncontaminated urine for possible culture and to exclude such items as hair, smegma, urethral cells, or skin bacteria from interfering with microscopic examination. The optimal sample is a first morning specimen because the urine is usually most concentrated after overnight fasting. Many diseases first manifest themselves by causing a loss of the concentrating ability of the kidney, and a first morning dilute specimen may be an early clue. Chemical tests measure concentration of substances. A dilute specimen may therefore lead to false negative results. The urine specimen should be examined within 30 minutes, as formed elements will begin to break down and certain chemical reactions begin to take place that will render the analysis inaccurate. If the examination cannot be accomplished until a later time, the freshly passed specimen may be immediately put into a refrigerator at standard temperature. This will keep the urine reasonably unchanged for 8 to 12 hours. There have been methods described for keeping urine specimens preserved for longer periods of time, but these methods are uniformly unsatisfactory.

The patient is given a clean urine container and damp paper towels (or equivalent wipes) and is instructed to:

Male patient

1. Pull back the foreskin if uncircumsized.
2. Clean the end of the glans with the damp towel, stroking away from the urethral orifice.
3. Initially pass a small portion of urine into the urinal or toilet.
4. Obtain a 20–50 ml specimen by putting the receptacle into the stream.
5. Let the rest of the urine go into the urinal or toilet.

Female patient

1. Squat or stand astride the toilet bowl.
2. Separate the labia minora with the fingers, exposing the urethral meatus.
3. Cleanse the area around the meatus by stroking away from the orifice.
4. Forcibly void, keeping the labia separated and allowing the initial portion of the stream to go into the toilet.
5. Place the urine receptacle into the stream and collect 20–50 ml of urine.
6. Release the labia and allow the rest of the urine to go into the toilet.

The female patient may have to be given a funnel or utilize a special collecting-toilet cover in order to adequately catch a specimen. Clean-catch specimens free of all red blood cells are difficult to obtain during active menstruation.

Ten to 15 ml of urine are then placed into a conical centrifuge tube and gently centrifuged. Half-speed for 10 to 15 minutes is safe and adequate for most table-top centrifuges. If the urine is clear and not abnormally pigmented, all studies except the microscopic analysis may then be done on another aliquot from the specimen container while the initial portion is being centrifuged. If the urine is unclear or contains abnormal pigments, the rest of the testing should be done only on the supernatant of the centrifuged sample. This obviates interference with the refractive index and with the biochemical color reactions on various types of reagent strips.

The tube of urine should be placed against the sleeve of a white lab coat or against a white piece of paper and observed for color and clarity before centrifugation. Air may then be brushed across the top of the tube toward one's nostrils and any abnormal smell recorded. Color and clarity are again observed after centrifugation.

Background Information

The characteristic yellow color of urine is due to variable concentrations of urochrome pigments. Normally excreted compounds such as phosphates, sulfates, and urates may be present in high concentrations and come out of solution, especially in cold or refrigerated samples, causing a cloudy appearance. Therefore a cloudy urine is not necessarily abnormal.

The smell of the urine normally comes from the excretion of aromatic organic compounds. Ammonium-containing compounds may emit ammonia gas and contribute to the odor. Certain foods such as asparagus have aromatic metabolic products that are passed in the urine, imparting a unique odor.

Clinical Significance

The color of the urine may be affected by a multitude of abnormalities. Blood, hemoglobin, or myoglobin may impart colors ranging from red to black; bilirubin, from deep yellow to green; porphyrins, from purple to brown. Drugs like methylene blue impart a blue green color; certain proprietary compounds (eg, DeWitt's pills) or blood-borne pseudomonas pigments produce a green urine; phenazopyridine and certain intravenous vitamin preparations may cause an orange color; phenolphthalein imparts a red or bluish green color depending on the urine pH. Diseases such as melanoma and alcaptonuria may cause black urine. Pigmenturia may also result from percutaneous absorption of certain hair dyes.

The opaqueness of urine may be due to abnormalities other than pigmentation. Large amounts of epithelial cells may be present from such disorders as cystitis, vaginitis, and urethritis and may impart an opalescent color despite efforts at obtaining a good clean-catch. Upper urinary tract infections and pyelonephritis may cause excretion of large amounts of pus cells, also clouding the urine.

Certain diseases affect urine odor. Large amounts of ketone bodies will give the urine a sweet smell; urine with certain branch-chain keto-acids may smell like maple syrup and may be associated with a disease of the same name. Finally, urine infected with urea-splitting organisms such as *Proteus* species may have a very pungent ammoniacal smell because of the presence of large amounts of ammonia.

Selected References

1. Kark RM, Lawrence JR, Pollak VE, et al: *A Primer of Urinalysis,* ed 2. New York, Harper and Row, 1963.
2. Block LH, Lamy PP: These drugs discolor the feces or urine. *Res Physician,* 15:47–53, 1969.
3. Stone HH: The green urine syndrome: An ominous manifestation of pseudomonas toxemia. *Bull Emory Univ Clinic* 3:81–86, 1964.
4. Marshall, Palmer WS: Dark urine after hair coloring. *JAMA* 226:1010, 1973.

217. Urinalysis: Specific Gravity

BARRY J. ROSENBAUM, MD

Definition

Both specific gravity and refractive index measure the content of urine solute relative to the volume of solvent. These serve as fairly accurate indicators of the body's fluid and osmolar balance, a major physiological function of the kidney. Most refractometers are scaled in terms of specific gravity, and these are the units used. The refractive index is a function of the amount of dissolved solids in a solution. The specific gravity is an index of weight per unit volume.

A first morning urine specimen of a person who has fasted 8–12 hours should be concentrated and have a refractive index of 1.018 or higher. No further tests of concentrating ability are necessary if the value exceeds this figure. Indexes lower than 1.018 may indicate malfunction of the renal concentrating mechanism and need to be investigated with more sophisticated tests.

Technique

A drop or two of the supernatant from the centrifuged sample is placed in the cleaned chamber of a refractometer. The index is read directly by viewing where the horizontal line made by the junction of the light and dark areas intersects the scale. The refractometer is now found in virtually every urinalysis laboratory in place of the older and less reliable hydrometer.

Background Information

The ability of the kidney to concentrate and dilute urine is primarily a function of the antidiuretic hormone (ADH) system. This endocrine system closely regulates the osmolar concentration of the body by two major mechanisms. One allows back diffusion of solute-free water from the distal portion of the nephron and the collecting duct into the medullary circulation of the kidney. The other allows dilute urine to proceed through the collecting system of the kidney without water reabsorption.

The renal tubular aspects of this feedback system depend on three factors:

1. The integrity of countercurrent multiplier dynamics to maintain a hypertonic renal medulla.
2. The biochemical state of the tubular cells of the collecting ducts allowing them to react appropriately to the presence of antidiuretic hormone.
3. The maintenance of a functioning, ascending limb of the loop of Henle to generate a dilute urine filtrate.

This biofeedback system is normally so sensitive that a change in serum osmolality of only 1–2% is enough to cause a change in the renal excretion of solute-free water. An increase in serum osmolality normally leads to stimulation of ADH release and water retention; a decrease in serum osmolality normally leads to inhibition of ADH release and water excretion. In summary, the measurement of urine refractive index is a reflection of the kidney's ability to control the osmolar state of the body by reabsorbing or excreting solute-free water.

Clinical Significance

The refractive index of urine from healthy kidneys reflects the state of hydration of the patient. An index of 1.028 or higher may imply dehydration. Indexes of 1.005 or lower may imply antidiuretic hormone deficiency diseases, inability of the renal tubule to react to the hormone, or excessive water intake such as with compulsive water drinking.

Diseases affecting the renal parenchyma may directly impair the nephron's ability to form concentrated urine or may cause biochemical changes in the tubular cells rendering them unresponsive to ADH. Examples of the former include interstitial diseases such as pyelonephritis, medullary cystic disease, hypertension, gout, amyloidosis, and analgesic abuse; examples of the latter include metabolic disturbances such as prolonged potassium deficiency and hypercalcemia. In these cases the urine remains isotonic with a glomerular ultrafiltrate of plasma of approximately 1.010.

Since the refractive index measures total solids per unit of volume of solvent, solutes with large molecular weights and sizes may cause abnormally high urinary indexes. Indexes greater than 1.040 are usually due to the presence of these substances. Glucose, protein, and radiographic dyes all elevate the refractive index of the urine, the latter as high as 1.060 to 1.070. When these substances are present in the urine, direct measurement of the urine osmolality should be performed since this test reflects the pressure exerted by individual particles in solution rather than the molecular size or weight of the particles.

Selected References

1. Harrington JT, Cohen JJ: Clinical disorders of urine concentration and dilution. *Arch Intern Med* 131:810–825, 1973.
2. Schrier RW, Berl T: Nonosmolar factors affecting renal water excretion. *N Eng J Med* 292:81–88, 141–145, 1975.
3. Jamison RL, Maffly RH: The urinary concentrating mechanism. *N Eng J Med* 295:1059–1067, 1976.

218. Proteinuria

W. DALLAS HALL, MD

Definition

Proteinuria is the excretion of protein into the urine. The normal adult excretes less than 150 mg per/day. This quantity, delivered into a daily urine volume of 1,000–2,000 ml, results in a urine protein concentration of 5–15 mg/dl, undetectable by most tests designed to screen for proteinuria.

Technique

Urine dipstick techniques often combine a chemical reagent with an indicator dye. The reagent usually detects free amino groups, and the indicator has a pH optimum. An example is tetrabromphenol blue which reacts with free amino groups to generate a green color change in an acid medium. Albumin has a relatively large number of free amino groups and reacts well. Globulins in general, and light chains in particular, react more weakly than albumin. Thus, patients with light chain-uria, such as from multiple myeloma or active lupus nephritis, may have negative or minimal reactions with dipstick indicators, yet manifest considerable turbidity when the urine is tested with a few drops of sulfosalicylic acid.

"Trace," and "1+, 2+, 3+, 4+" are ordinal estimates of the magnitude of proteinuria based on the degree of color change in the dipstick indicator. These estimates have been chemically quantitated and correspond to protein values of approximately 15, 30, 100, 300, and 1,000 mg/dl, respectively. Since most color reactions are shades of green, recognition may be difficult for the 1–3% of normal persons who have some degree of red green color blindness.

Normal urine which is very concentrated and of low volume may show trace or 1+ protein reactions. Conversely, abnormal urine which is very dilute and of high volume may show negative reactions. Urine with a pH of 7.0–8.0 may show trace or 1+ false positive reactions in the absence of proteinuria.

Background Information

The normal adult has proteinuria in the amount of 70–90 mg/per day. This consists primarily of low-molecular-weight serum proteins. Albumin is the predominant serum protein leaked through the normal glomerulus. In addition, the renal tubules secrete a high-molecular-weight protein into the urine. This is known as Tamm-Horsfall protein and provides the matrix for urinary casts.

There are glomerular and tubular types of proteinuria. The majority of proteinuric states are glomerular, reflecting an exaggerated loss of serum proteins through a damaged or excessively permeable glomerular capillary membrane. Albumin typically comprises 60–80% of the urinary protein, the remainder consisting of assorted globulins such as transferrin. The relative loss of higher-molecular-weight proteins is known as non-selective proteinuria and can be assessed by measurement of specific urinary proteins of varying molecular weights. Urine protein electrophoresis is unfortunately of little or no value in assessing selectivity or nonselectivity. Tubular proteinuria refers to the relative excess of urinary proteins with molecular weights below that of albumin (69,000). Such low-molecular-weight proteins include lysozyme, light chains, ribonuclease, and beta-2-microglobulin. Tubular proteinuria is characteristic of diseases with predominant tubular and minimal glomerular damage.

Persistent proteinuria of 1+ or greater should be quantitated by submitting a timed urine collection for chemical measurement. The absolute level of protein excretion is influenced physiologically by factors such as the serum protein concentration, the glomerular filtration rate, and the mean glomerular capillary hydrostatic pressure. Two of these factors are considered by expressing the magnitude of proteinuria as the permeability index (PI). The PI is the ratio of protein clearance to creatinine clearance according to the equation:

$$PI = \frac{\text{Urinary protein (gm/liter)*}}{\text{Serum albumin (gm/dl)}} \times \frac{\text{Serum creatinine (mg/dl)}}{\text{Urine creatinine (mg/dl)}} \times 10$$

Use of the PI will help avoid fallacious thinking engendered by considering proteinuria only in absolute terms such as 1.0 or 2.0 gm per day. Under normal circumstances, the PI should be less than 0.01, reflecting the normal minimal urinary loss of protein relative to glomerular filtration rate. PI values of 0.05 or greater indicate high-grade proteinuria consistent with any glomerular disease known to be associated with clinical manifestations such as the nephrotic syndrome. Many patients with serious glomerular disease have a PI $\geq$ 0.05 when the absolute level of proteinuria may be only 0.5–2.0 gm per day.

* Note that this denominator must be converted from g/total volume or mg/dl to g/liter.

Clinical Significance

High-grade proteinuria with a calculated PI $\geq$ 0.05 has major significance as an indicator of serious glomerular disease. Persistent 3+ or 4+
proteinuria is usually confirmed to have a PI of 0.05 or greater. Examples
include patients with lupus erythematosus, diabetes mellitus, renal vein
thrombosis, amyloidosis, and various types of glomerulonephritis. Diabetic patients with persistent proteinuria have a considerable decrease in
life span relative to diabetic patients without proteinuria. High-grade
proteinuria is the most common indication for percutaneous renal biopsy.

Low-grade proteinuria (PI $<$ 0.05) may be associated with transient
physiological abnormalities, mild glomerular disease, or interstitial forms
of renal disease with tubular proteinuria. Examples include patients with
benign orthostatic proteinuria, febrile proteinuria, and various interstitial
renal diseases such as pyelonephritis.

Selected References

1. Manuel Y, Revillard JP, Betuel H (eds): *Proteins in Normal and Path-
    ological Urine.* Baltimore, University Park Press, 1970.
2. Heinemann HO, Maack TM, Sherman RL: Proteinuria. *Am J Med*
    56:71–82, 1974.
3. Rennie IDB, Keen H: Evaluation of clinical methods for detecting
    proteinuria. *Lancet* 2:489–492, 1967.
4. Pollak VE: Proteinuria. I, Mechanisms. *Hosp Pract* 6:49–56, 1971.

219. Glucosuria and Ketonuria

JOHN K. DAVIDSON, MD
HARRY K. DELCHER, MD
W. DALLAS HALL, MD

Definition

Glucosuria occurs in all normal individuals. Normal urine glucose
concentrations range 3–25 mg/dl. Levels above 25 mg/dl in randomly
collected fresh urine (or above 100 mg/dl during a glucose tolerance test)

are abnormal. However, many semiquantitative techniques do not detect glucosuria until the level reaches 50–250 mg/dl.

Ketonuria refers to the presence of abnormal amounts of ketone bodies in the urine. The ketone bodies are acetoacetic acid (a ketoacid), acetone (a ketone), and beta-hydroxybutyric acid (neither a ketone nor a ketoacid) (Fig 184).

Technique

Fehling's, Benedict's, and Clinitest are methods for detecting glucosuria. They are based on reduction of copper sulfate and are not specific for glucose. Positive tests are thus produced by any reducing substance including glucose (glucosuria), fructose (hereditary fructosuria), lactose (pregnancy lactosuria), pentose (xylulosuria or plum ingestion), galactose (galactosemia), homogentistic acid (alcaptonuria), ascorbic acid, and various conjugated therapeutic compounds.

Enzyme methods are specific for glucose. Semiquantitative enzyme methods are used in commercially available test strips such as Testape, Clinistix, Uristix, and Labstix. The reagent strip is coated with glucose oxidase, and the formed hydrogen peroxide oxidizes orthotoluidine to a blue or purple color. Reagent strips are considerably more sensitive than Clinitest tablets, usually detecting glucose concentrations of 50 mg/dl or more and occasionally detecting concentrations as low as 15 mg/dl. Large amounts of substances such as ascorbic acid may interfere with the enzymatic reaction and give false negative results. A quantitative method for measuring urine glucose is the oxygen rate method glucose autoanalyzer. This method provides sensitivity down to 3 mg/dl urine glucose and can be performed in one minute.

Ketonuria is usually estimated semiquantitatively by Acetest tablets, Labstix, Ketostix, or Acetone Test—"Denco." These are usually based on a crude reaction with nitroprusside which detects acetoacetate, and to a much lesser degree, acetone. Substances such as L-dopa can produce false positive nitroprusside tests. Unfortunately, beta-hydroxybutyric acid

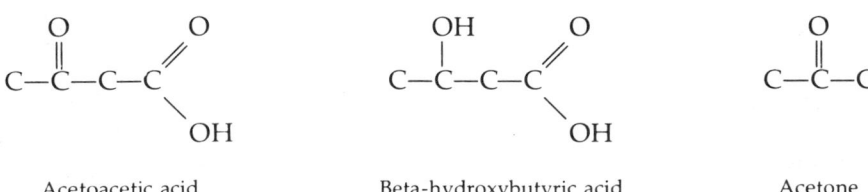

Acetoacetic acid   Beta-hydroxybutyric acid   Acetone

Figure 184.   Structural configurations of ketone bodies.

does not react in these tests. The reference method is quantitative specific enzymatic analysis of acetoacetate or beta-hydroxybutyrate. These enzymatic methods are not generally available.

Background Information

The escape of glucose into the urine is a function of the plasma glucose level, the glomerular filtration rate, and the capacity of the renal tubules to reabsorb glucose. Assuming normal glomerular filtration rate and glucose reabsorption, a plasma glucose value of 170–180 mg/dl (range, 130–300 mg/dl) is usually associated with the appearance of glucosuria ("threshold"). If glomerular filtration rate is decreased, as from diabetic nephropathy or nephrosclerosis, the plasma glucose value may rise markedly above the usual threshold without glucosuria. If the renal tubules manifest impaired capacity to absorb glucose, as with pregnancy, Fanconi syndromes, and acute tubular necrosis, glucosuria may occur with normal plasma glucose levels.

The breakdown of adipose tissue (lipolysis) releases free fatty acids into the blood. Lipolysis is enhanced by alcohol, catecholamines, growth hormone, and glucagon. Lipolysis is inhibited by insulin and glucose. Plasma free fatty acids are transported to the liver where they are oxidized to two carbon fragments. These two carbon fragments participate in the formation of acetoacetic acid. Some of the acetoacetic acid is spontaneously decarboxylated to acetone, which vaporizes and is excreted in expired air. Most of the residual acetoacetic acid is reduced to beta-hydroxybutyric acid, depending on the availability of reduced nicotinamide adenine dinucleotide (NADH). Circulating acetoacetate and beta-hydroxybutyrate are peripherally utilized by tissues such as muscle. Peripheral utilization is evidenced by the typically higher ketone levels in arterial versus venous blood samples. The nonutilized plasma ketones are then excreted into the urine depending on their glomerular clearance rate, that is, approximately 4–41 ml, 10–48 ml, and 10–14 ml per minute for acetoacetate, beta-hydroxybutyrate, and acetone, respectively. Ketonemia is a necessary precursor of ketonuria. Patients with impaired glomerular filtration may have ketonemia without ketonuria; conversely, ketonuria may become more apparent (in a ketonemic patient) with improvement of glomerular filtration rate.

Clinical Significance

Glucosuria implies either that plasma glucose is elevated or that the renal tubules have an impaired capacity to reabsorb glucose. The former is common in patients with diabetes mellitus; the latter is relatively rare and may occur with pregnancy, acute tubular injury, hereditary renal glucosuria, and disorders of proximal tubule function such as the Fanconi syndromes. Renal glucosuria can be readily detected and specifically defined with the advent of more sensitive methods of quantitating urine glucose.

Rapid determinations of plasma glucose are now usually available such that there is less dependence on urine glucose values. Multiple plasma glucose measurements are clearly preferable to "sliding scale" urine glucose schemes of monitoring insulin therapy. Measurement of urine glucose remains a valuable and relatively inexpensive method for following outpatient diabetic control. It is also useful for screening large patient populations for the presence of diabetes mellitus. Values above 25 mg/dl (quantitative oxygen rate method) are abnormal and indicate further evaluation. Approximately 28% of persons with urine glucose concentrations of 26–100 mg/dl will have diabetes or suspect diabetes by glucose tolerance testing. These relatively low levels of urine glucose are readily detected by glucose oxygen consumption methods. Quantitative urine glucose screening may prove more practical and valid for detection of diabetes than screening of fasting or two-hour postprandial plasma glucose values.

Ketonuria is presently limited to the detection of acetoacetic aciduria. This ketoacid may be produced in excess whenever there is lipolysis with liberation of excess free fatty acid substrates. The classic examples are diabetic ketoacidosis and starvation ketosis. Ketoacidosis may also be produced by isovaleric acidemia, maple syrup urine disease, and various intoxicants such as isopropyl alcohol, paraldehyde, jet bead berry ingestion, and milk sickness due to ingestion of milk or meat from animals that have been poisoned with snakeroot, richweed, or rayless goldenrod.

Diabetic ketoacidosis is usually associated with overproduction of both acetoacetic and beta-hydroxybutyric acids. The ratio of beta-hydroxybutyrate to acetoacetate changes with the severity of the acidosis, ranging from 1 in untreated mild cases to 6 in severe cases. As acidosis is corrected with appropriate therapy, there is a fall in total ketones, but the amount of acetoacetate may rise relative to the amount of beta-hydroxybutyrate. Semiquantitative estimates of only acetoacetate may thus give a misleading impression of transient acceleration of the ketosis.

Alcoholic ketoacidosis is a condition where metabolic acidosis is due predominantly to an excess of beta-hydroxybutyric acid. Routine tests for ketonuria or ketonemia may thus be deceptively normal. Starvation ketoacidosis, diabetic ketoacidosis, and "alcoholic" ketoacidosis may be admixed in a single patient. Initial plasma glucoses above 150–200 mg/dl are considered indicative of a diabetic component to the ketoacidosis.

Selected References

1. Bradley GM, Benson ES: Examination of the urine, in Davidsohn I, Henry JB (eds): *Todd-Sanford Clinical Diagnosis by Laboratory Methods,* ed 15. Philadelphia, WB Saunders, 1974, chap 2.

2. Werk EE Jr, Knowles HC Jr: The blood ketone and plasma free fatty acid concentration in diabetic and normal subjects. *Diabetes* 10:22–32, 1961.

3. James RC, Chase GR: Evaluation of some commonly used semiquantitative methods for urine glucose and ketone determination. *Diabetes* 23:474–479, 1974.

4. Kadish AH, Sternberg JC: Determination of urine glucose by measurement of oxygen consumption. *Diabetes* 18:467–470, 1969.

5. Levy LJ, Duga J, Girgis M, et al: Ketoacidosis associated with alcoholism in nondiabetic subjects. *Ann Intern Med* 78:213–219, 1973.

6. Cooperman MT, Davidoff F, Spark R, et al: Clinical studies of alcoholic ketoacidosis. *Diabetes* 23:433–439, 1974.

7. Hadden JW, Metzner RJ: Pseudoketosis and hyperacetaldehydemia in paraldehyde acidosis. *Am J Med* 47:642–647, 1969.

8. Budd MA, Tanaka K, Holmes LB, et al: Isovaleric acidemia: Clinical features of a new genetic defect of leucine metabolism. *N Eng J Med* 277:321–327, 1967.

9. Felts PW: *Current Concepts: Coma in the Diabetic.* Kalamazoo, Mich, The Upjohn Co, 1974, pp 14–17.

10. Davidson JK, Reuben D, Sternberg JC, Ryan WT: Diabetes screening using a quantitative urine glucose method. *Diabetes* 27:810–816, 1978.

11. Shah JH, Wongsurawat N, Aran PP: Effect of ethanol on stimulus-induced insulin secretion and glucose tolerance. *Diabetes* 26:271–277, 1977.

220. Urine Sediment

W. DALLAS HALL, MD

Definition

The urine sediment refers to the formed elements of the urine in a centrifuged specimen. These include red blood cells, white blood cells, epithelial cells, casts, crystals, bacteria, and fungi.

A normal high-power field (hpf) of a fresh, centrifuged clean-catch urine contains less than 5 red blood cells, less than 10 white blood cells, a few epithelial cells, occasional hyaline casts, occasional crystals, and no bacteria or fungi.

Technique

Centrifuge 10 ml of urine at 2,000 rpm for five minutes. Then pour off all of the supernatant, leaving a volume of no more than 0.5 ml. Flick the bottom of the tube with one finger to disperse the formed elements. Place one drop on a slide and affix with a coverslip.

Grossly cloudy urines should be evaluated with one drop of unspun urine adjacent to the drop of spun urine. Grossly bloody urine should have a few drops of white cell diluting fluid (acetic acid) added prior to centrifugation. In each of these two circumstances, centrifugation time need not exceed 30–60 seconds.

First peruse the area under the coverslip using a low-power microscope objective. Suspicious cellular or hematin casts may thus be identified, especially along the margins of the coverslip preparation. Constantly adjust the light intensity to assist in locating various types of casts. Formed elements under low power should be further identified under high power.

Background Information

Hematuria.   The daily urinary excretion of approximately 200,000 red blood cells is diluted into a urine volume of 1,000–2,000 ml. This results in approximately 100–200 RBCs/ml of urine. When centrifuged, concentrated into various final volumes and expressed as RBC/hpf, usually none or only one RBC appears in a random hpf, and no more than 5 RBCs/hpf should appear in the most concentrated area. These RBCs may arise from the urethra, seminal vesicles, prostate, bladder, ureter, renal pelvis, or renal parenchyma. Ultimately they derive from the circulation; thus, excretion may be enhanced under physiological circumstances (fever, exercise) leading to accelerated renal blood flow.

Pyuria.   The daily urinary excretion of approximately 750,000 white blood cells is also diluted into a urine volume of 1,000–2,000 ml. This results in approximately 375–750 WBCs/ml of urine. Under the above conditions of centrifugation and dilution, there are usually less than 2 WBCs in a random hpf, and no more than 10 WBCs/hpf in the most concentrated area. The white cells reaching the urine arise from the same anatomical structures as the red cells. In addition, epithelial cells and leukocytes from vaginal discharge often contaminate the routinely collected urine specimen. Normal leukocyte excretion rate is approximately four times higher in women than in men. Leukocytes in the urine are usually of the neutrophilic series and reflect the same stages of maturation as do circulating neutrophils. Lymphocyturia may be noted with renal transplant rejections, and plasmacyturia has been noted in patients with multiple myeloma. Epithelial cells usually derive from the vagina, bladder, or renal tubules.

The daily urinary excretion of approximately 5,000 casts accounts for 2 to 5 casts per ml of normal urine. These are usually hyaline casts, the matrix of which is Tamm-Horsfall mucoprotein secreted by the renal tubules. The number of casts in the urine bears an inverse relationship to the urine pH.

Fine and coarse granular casts consist of antigenic protein granules contained within the Tamm-Horsfall matrix. These protein granules appear to represent fragments of parent serum proteins (albumin, transferrin, haptoglobin, IgG). It follows that fine and coarse granular casts are seen more commonly in proteinuric patients. The width of these and other casts reflects the width of the tubule where they originated. Hence, multiple broad casts imply a disease process with dilated tubules.

Red cell casts indicate primary glomerular disease. These casts usually contain 10–50 well-defined red cells and should be differentiated from hyaline casts which contain only 1–2 RBCs or WBCs. Red cell casts must also be differentiated from casts containing fat droplets or *Candida* organisms. Fatty casts are refractile and have a wide variation of particle size; associated findings may include doubly refractile fat bodies and Maltese crosses seen under polarized light, and oval fat bodies seen under routine microscopy. Oval fat bodies are orange yellow structures about twice the size of white cells and contain 10–100 particles that have the appearance of tiny eggs. *Candida* casts are usually suspected when free yeast forms exist in other areas of the sediment.

White cell casts indicate inflammatory renal parenchymal disease and are most commonly noted in bacterial pyelonephritis. Nonbacterial inflammation of the kidney may also produce white cell casts. Examples include any exudative glomerulonephritis, periarteritis nodosa, and renal infarction. White cell casts should be differentiated from renal tubular epithelial cell casts that slough in conditions such as acute renal tubular injury.

Hematin casts do not usually contain definable red cells. They are often present when the spun sediment has a tan or brown button. Under the microscope they appear as dark brown, brownish orange, or brownish black structures. They usually indicate acute renal tubular injury but may occasionally be seen in patients with severe jaundice, analgesic nephropathy, chronic renal failure, and profound dehydration.

The three most common crystals seen in the urine sediment are urates, phosphates, and oxalates. The interested reader should review reference 3 for an excellent series of photographs of these various crystal forms. Urate crystals occur predominantly in acid urine and may be suspected if the spun sediment button is pink or if the microscopic hue of the crystals is light yellow. Phosphate crystals occur in alkaline urine and may be suspected if the spun sediment button is white and multiple tiny amorphous black particles are present on microscopic examination. These crystals dissolve when a few drops of acid are added to the urine. Oxalate crystals occur more frequently in acid urines and often reflect intake of oxalate-containing foods such as spinach, cabbage, tomatoes, apples, or grapes. Cystine crystals are hexagonal and occur in acid urines. Sulfa crystals appear like bound haystacks. In general, crystalluria occurs more as a result of extremes of urine pH than increased excretion of the parent substance. Crystal formation is temperature dependent such that clinical implications should be made only on fresh urine at body temperature. Consider the heavy crystal sediment that occurs when normal urine is refrigerated. Bacteria are normally absent in bladder urine and in freshly voided urine.

Clinical Significance

Hematuria can result from prerenal, renal, or postrenal etiologies. Prerenal causes are unusual but include coagulation abnormalities. Hematuria from coagulation defects other than hemophilia implies an underlying renal or genitourinary defect that predisposes to bleeding.

Renal causes of hematuria include glomerulonephritis, tumor, and tissue injury such as from nephrolithiasis, papillary necrosis, or renal infarction. Patients with sickle trait often present with relatively painless gross hematuria. Hematuria from glomerular disease is usually associated with granular casts, proteinuria, and hypertension.

Postrenal etiologies are the most frequent causes of hematuria. Examples include hemorrhagic cystitis, bladder neoplasm, and prostatitis. Hematuria in the absence of an immediately obvious cause demands intravenous pyelography or cystoscopy, or both.

Pyuria indicates renal or genitourinary inflammation unless there is contamination of the specimen. Pyuria commonly occurs without significant urinary tract infection, and significant urinary tract infection commonly occurs without pyuria. It follows that the number of white cells in the urine is an insensitive guide for detecting infection. Urine culture and examination of the unspun sediment are preferable. When bacteria are seen in a drop of unspun fresh urine, a colony count of 100,000 or more is implied with 85% confidence. The presence of these bacteria is the quickest and most economical way of screening for significant urinary tract infection. Therapy can be instituted in a symptomatic patient pending identification of the organism. Conversely, the absence of bacteria in the urinary sediment of a symptomatic patient suggests other causes of dysuria or pyuria. The most important implication of pyuria and bacteriuria is that either may lead to discovery of a correctable abnormality of the urinary tract.

Red cell casts strongly indicate primary glomerular disease such as glomerulonephritis or lupus nephritis. Parenchymal disease is also implied by the presence of multiple fine and coarse granular casts in patients with otherwise unexplained gross or microscopic hematuria. White cell casts mean upper tract inflammation and may be the only sign of pyelonephritis in patients who have no other clinical or roentgenographic evidence of renal parenchymal disease. Hematin casts usually indicate acute renal tubular injury and are danger signals which announce a need for radical changes in patient management. Bacterial casts occur only with upper urinary tract inflammation. Candida casts imply that the fungal infection is systemic or has involved the renal parenchyma. Fatty casts, oval fat bodies, doubly refractile fat bodies, and Maltese crosses indicate hyperlipoproteinuria and glomerular proteinuria, as with the nephrotic syndrome.

Urate, oxalate, and phosphate crystalluria may be of no clinical significance in patients who have aberrations of urine pH. On occasion, however, persistently alkaline urine may cause enough crystalluria to give rise to dysuria. The patient may then be discovered to have renal tubular acidosis or idiopathic hypercalciuria rather than infection. Patients with ethylene glycol intoxication may have an excessive number of urine oxalate crystals. Hexagonal cystine crystals may indicate that unexplained hematuria or nephrolithiasis is caused by cystinuria. Sulfa crystals should be routinely sought in patients who are receiving sulfa therapy in conjunction with chronic renal failure or nocardiosis.

Selected References

1. Addis T: The number of formed elements in the urine sediment of normal individuals. *J Clin Invest* 2:409–415, 1926.
2. Relman AS, Levinski NG: Clinical examination of renal function, in Strauss MB, Welt LG (eds): *Diseases of the Kidney*, ed 2. Boston, Little, Brown, 1971, pp 96–106.
3. Berman LB: The art of urinalysis. *Gen Pract* 34:94–108, 1966.
4. Winkel P, Statland BE, Jorgenson K: Urine microscopy: An ill-defined method examined by a multifactorial technique. *Clin Chem* 20:436–439, 1974.
5. Burton JR, Rowe JW, Hill RN: Quantitation of casts in urine sediment (Letter). *Ann Intern Med* 83:518–519, 1975.
6. Rutecki GJ, Goldsmith C, Schreiner GE: Characterization of proteins in urinary casts: Fluorescent-antibody identification of Tamm-Horsfall mucoprotein in matrix and serum proteins in granules. *N Eng J Med* 284:1049–1052, 1971.
7. Prescott LF: The normal urinary excretion of renal tubular cells, leukocytes and red blood cells. *Clin Sci* 31:425–435, 1966.

221. Blood Urea Nitrogen

W. DALLAS HALL, MD
DAVID H. VROON, MD

Definition

Urea is the principal nitrogenous end product of protein metabolism and amino acid degradation. It has a molecular weight of 60 and is distributed throughout total body water. Concentration of blood urea is approximately twice (60/28) that of blood urea nitrogen since urea contains two nitrogen atoms; in the United States the concentration of urea is often expressed as urea nitrogen; in European countries, as urea.

The normal range of urea nitrogen in blood, serum, or plasma is 5–20 mg/dl, but this varies widely with protein intake, protein catabolism, hepatic urea synthesis, and renal urea excretion. For example, an average BUN might be 8 mg/dl for individuals with a 35 gm daily protein intake and 20 mg/dl for individuals with a 140 gm daily protein intake.

Technique

Two groups of methods are commonly used to determine urea nitrogen: enzymatic substrate assays utilizing urease, and methods based on reaction with diacetylmonoxime (Fearon reaction) or substituted diketone compounds. Sequential Multiple Analyzer (SMA) systems use a modified Fearon reaction in which diacetyl reacts with urea in the presence of acidic ferric ions and produces a yellow chromogen:

$$\text{Urea} + \text{Diacetyl} \longrightarrow \text{Yellow chromagen}$$
$$\text{(absorbs at 520 nm)}$$

This method provides a clinically reliable measurement of urea; reaction with dibasic amino acids and other peptides is usually insignificant due to the low concentration of these substances in biological fluids. Spurious elevations have been observed with ingestion of sulfonyl urea compounds.

Enzymatic methods are based on the hydrolysis of urea (by urease) into ammonia and carbonic acid with either reaction product measured in a second step; the quantitation of the reaction products is proportional to urea concentration.

$$\text{Urea} + \text{H}_2\text{O} \xrightarrow{\text{urease}} 2\,\text{NH}_3 + \text{CO}_2$$

An enzymatic method using the Berthelot reaction with hypochloride and phenol to quantitate ammonia is available on SMA systems but not widely used. Urease procedures are often employed on discrete analyzers such as the Dupont ACA and Beckman Analyzers. Ammonia on the ACA is quantitated by reductive amination of alpha-ketoglutarate by the enzyme glutamate dehydrogenase with simultaneous oxidation of reduced nicotinamide adenine dinucleotide. The Beckman instrument quantitatively detects the rate of conductivity change produced by enzymatic hydrolysis of urea.

Chemical specificity is generally enhanced by enzymatic substrate assay; however, the infrequency and minor degree of interference observed with the colorimetric SMA method may not warrant use of more

expensive and chemically specific methods. Furthermore, urease procedures are in themselves susceptible to various interferences.

Background Information

Urea is formed exclusively via the urea cycle in the liver (Fig 185).
The level of the blood urea nitrogen represents a balance between the
rate of urea synthesis by the liver and the rate of urea excretion by the
kidney. Production of urea is increased whenever more amino acid substrates are delivered to the liver (high dietary protein, blood protein in
the gastrointestinal tract, catabolic tissue breakdown, or inhibition of
anabolism by corticosteroid therapy). Production of urea is decreased
whenever substrate delivery to the liver is limited (malnutrition, starvation) or when there is diminution of key urea cycle enzyme activity such
as from destruction of hepatic parenchymal cells.

Normal excretion of urea nitrogen by the kidney is massive, amount-
ing to over 10,000 mg per day in the usual adult. Normally, 40–60% of
filtered urea is reabsorbed. Minor changes in reabsorption can make major changes in blood urea nitrogen levels.

Reabsorption of urea is enhanced by slow urine flow, volume contraction, depressed glomerular filtration, and depressed renal plasma flow
(as from low cardiac output). Reabsorption of urea is decreased by urine
flow rates in excess of 2 ml per minute, volume expansion, increased
glomerular filtration rate, and increased renal plasma flow.

Clinical Significance

The serum creatinine is a more specific test than the BUN to assess
the adequacy of renal function. The BUN, however, is useful as a screening test for renal dysfunction. In addition, the BUN often helps clinicians

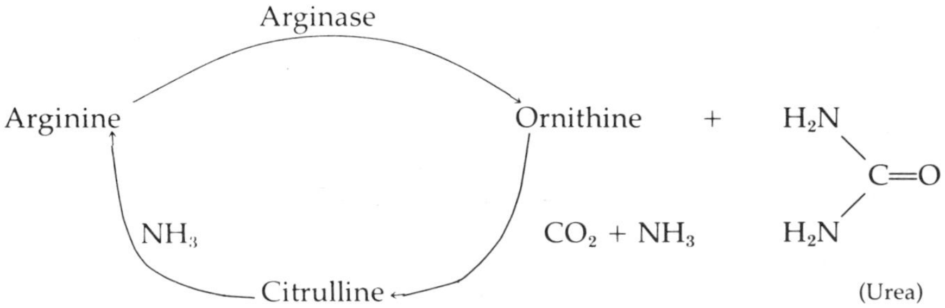

Figure 185.   Urea cycle.

identify dietary and physiologic derangements that are independent of renal function. An elevated BUN (azotemia) can be interpreted properly only by knowing the serum creatinine level. The creatinine helps approximate what proportion of the azotemia is due to renal disease and what proportion is due to prerenal physiologic factors.

Calculate the ratio of BUN to creatinine (BUN/Cr ratio). The ratio is approximately 10 in a patient with adequate dietary intake, normal protein metabolism, and normal circulatory status. For example, a patient with renal failure and a BUN of 46 mg/dl would be expected to have a creatinine of 4–5 mg/dl if the patient is eating normally, has a normal volume status, normal cardiac output, and good hepatic function.

BUN/Cr ratios in excess of 15 imply either a primary or complicating prerenal disorder (prerenal azotemia). A patient with a BUN of 60 mg/dl and a creatinine of 2 mg/dl (BUN/Cr = 30) has some prerenal factor, such as volume depletion, high protein feedings, marked protein catabolism, blood in the gastrointestinal tract, poor renal plasma flow, corticosteroid therapy, or some combination of the above. The section on creatinine discusses how to assess whether primary renal disease may also be present in such a patient.

BUN/Cr ratios below 8 generally imply either inadequate protein intake, defective urea synthesis, marked renal urea excretion, or accelerated creatinine production. Thus, a patient with a BUN of 28 mg/dl and a creatinine of 4 mg/dl (BUN/Cr = 7) is likely to have low protein intake, severe liver disease, or rhabdomyolysis. Low BUN/Cr ratios are also typical of patients on chronic hemodialysis since ultrafiltration of urea greatly exceeds that of creatinine.

As mentioned earlier, the diagnostic value of the BUN for assessment of renal function is limited relative to knowing the level of serum creatinine. Patients may have serious renal disease with a BUN of 17 mg/dl, or no renal disease with a BUN of 35 mg/dl. Complications of renal failure such as altered mental status, seizures, pericarditis, and bleeding tendency correlate poorly with BUN levels between 50–150 mg/dl.

Selected References

1. Automated and manual direct methods for the determination of blood urea. *Clin Chem* 11:624–627, 1965.
2. Kassirer JP: Clinical evaluation of kidney function: Glomerular filtration. *N Eng J Med* 285:385–389, 1971.
3. Gallagher JC, Seligson D: Significance of abnormally low blood urea levels. *N Eng J Med* 266:492–495, 1962.
4. Dosseter JB: Creatininemia versus uremia. *Ann Intern Med* 65:1287–1299, 1966.

5.   Rickers H, Brochner-Mortensen J, Rodbro P: The diagnostic value of plasma urea for assessment of renal function. *Scand J Urol Nephrol* 12:39–44, 1978.

222. Plasma Glucose

JOHN K. DAVIDSON, MD
HARRY K. DELCHER, MD
W. DALLAS HALL, MD

Definition

Glucose is a six-carbon (hexose) monosaccharide with a molecular weight of 180. The range of normal in a fasting plasma sample is often given as approximately 60–100 mg/dl. However, the mean plasma glucose level in normal humans fasted overnight is 92 mg/dl with a range of 78–115 mg/dl. Nonfasting or random plasma glucose levels above 150 mg/dl are not generally seen in patients with normal carbohydrate tolerance. Random plasma glucose levels above 150 mg/dl thus require further evaluation.

Technique

The specimen should be collected into an antiglycolytic agent such as sodium fluoride or iodoacetate. Plasma glucose values fall at a rate of approximately 5% per hour in the absence of antiglycolytic agents or without immediate separation of the clot. This in vitro artifact is referred to as "desk-top" hypoglycemia.

Methods which measure reducing substances are based on the ability of glucose to reduce metal ions such as Cu^{++} (cupric-neocuprine method) or FE^{+++} (ferricyanide method) to lower oxidation states that form colored complexes. Despite lessening of interference by dialysis or by adding substances such as sodium carbonate, these methods also detect nonglucose-reducing substances. The positive bias is approximately 5–15 mg/dl in the usual specimen and considerably greater in patients with uremia and diabetic ketoacidosis. In uremia the true glucose averages 30 mg/dl (range, 0–80 mg/dl) lower than the value determined by reducing methods.

Methods that measure true glucose employ either aromatic amines (orthotoludine method) or enzymes such as glucose oxidase or hexokinase. Hexokinase is an enzyme which catalyzes the phosphorylation of D-glucose to glucose-6-phosphate in the presence of ATP and magnesium ions. NADPII-2 (formerly TPNH) is formed and absorbs strongly at 340 nm.

Background Information

Diabetes mellitus is a disorder of carbohydrate metabolism related to either an absolute deficiency in insulin or a relative lack of insulin effect in target tissues. Relative lack of insulin effect is associated with obesity and a deficiency or defect in cellular insulin receptors. The prevalence of diabetes mellitus in the United States population is approximately 4–5%.

Several different terms have appeared in the literature to describe demographic, clinical, laboratory, or genetic features of diabetes mellitus. These include prediabetes, juvenile diabetes, adult or maturity onset diabetes, chemical or latent diabetes, gestational or pregnancy diabetes, and lipodystrophic diabetes.

Juvenile diabetes is often used to describe the patient whose disease onset is prior to age 20. These patients classically have less than 1% of the normal pancreatic insulin content. They exhibit low fasting serum insulin levels which stimulate poorly or not at all following glucose challenge. They typically have a high incidence of end-organ damage. Control of blood glucose almost always requires insulin and is difficult in 85–90% of patients.

Adult or maturity onset diabetes usually has its onset after the age of 30. Ninety-seven percent of cases have body weight in excess of ideal body weight (see section on body size). There is usually some component of insulin resistance. Blood insulin levels may be within the normal range but respond subnormally following glucose challenge. Complications are variable. Regulation of the plasma glucose can be accomplished in 60–80% of patients by intensive dietary therapy alone.

Chemical or latent diabetes refers to carbohydrate intolerance without associated signs or symptoms. Common presentations include adult onset patients, or patients tested because of a strong family history of diabetes. Fasting or random plasma glucose measurements are commonly within the range of normal. Abnormal glucose tolerance to cortisone stress once indicated patients with chemical or latent diabetes, but it is now recognized that perfectly normal patients may manifest "elevated" glucose levels under the conditions of stress simulated by administration of corticosteroids.

Gestational or pregnancy diabetes refers to the temporary appearance of glucosuria or abnormal carbohydrate tolerance during pregnancy. Caution must be exercised that the techniques employed specifically measure glucose rather than other reducing substances such as lactose. Most glucose tolerance test (GTT) point criteria are different in the presence of pregnancy.

Lipodystrophic diabetes refers to a group of disorders usually characterized by some visible abnormality of body fat combined with an unusual degree of insulin resistance but a rare development of ketoacidosis. Many forms have relatively specific physical or biochemical features.

Prediabetes is the most controversial term used in characterizing diabetic patients. The term once referred to patients who had completely normal glucose measurements but were destined to be diabetic. Examples included the mate of an identical twin diabetic or the offspring of bilateral diabetic parents. The assumption of diabetes in each of these latter two categories is now open to question since longer-term follow-up is unrevealing in a significant number. In addition, there are semantic difficulties in labeling a disease "pre" if it is presumed present.

There are exceptions to almost every statement in the preceding paragraphs describing clinical types of diabetes mellitus. We strongly recommend categorization of patients into a simpler scheme based on objective standards. This classification states that the patient has "definite diabetes mellitus," "suspect diabetes mellitus," or "no diabetes mellitus." Three extensively studied sets of criteria assist in this classification and are defined in the following section.

Clinical Significance

A sufficient amount of unequivocal data should support the diagnosis of diabetes. An erroneous diagnosis of diabetes can result in anxiety, unwarranted restrictions in employability, driving automobiles or flying airplanes, uninsurability or access to "rated" insurance only, unnecessary dietary restrictions, and potentially hazardous treatment with insulin.

In contrast, a valid diagnosis of diabetes mellitus implies an increased risk for hyperlipidemia, coronary disease, cerebrovascular disease, pregnancy complications, peripheral neuropathy, kidney disease, unexplained pruritus or edema, hypertension, cataracts, glaucoma, blindness, *Candida* infections, Dupuytren's contracture, peripheral vascular disease, tuberculosis, mucormycosis, periodontal disease, skin abscesses, gallstones, amyotrophic lateral sclerosis, hypoaldosteronism, and chondrocalcinosis.

A diagnosis of diabetes mellitus can be established in one of two ways: three fasting venous plasma glucose levels of 150 mg/dl or higher or an abnormal GTT in a properly prepared patient who has no other acute or chronic illnesses known to be associated with abnormal carbohydrate tolerance.

The reference test for establishing the diagnosis of diabetes is the oral glucose tolerance test in the properly prepared individual. It is more sensitive and specific than fasting or random blood samples, or semi-quantitative urine tests. Unfortunately, the reproducibility of the GTT leaves much to be desired because age, diet, activity, various medications, and nondiabetic illnesses may significantly modify the results. The significance of a moderately abnormal or borderline test for subsequent development of the diabetic syndrome is debatable, which is why the "diabetes suspect" category is recommended unless all three methods of classification are positive or negative. Whether a patient is classified as diabetic or nondiabetic depends on the sets of criteria used in assessment of the GTT results (Table 47).

Proper preparation for a glucose tolerance test includes an adequate intake of carbohydrate (approximately 300 gm per day) for three days and discontinuation of hormones such as oral contraceptives or other medications such as thiazide diuretics for approximately one week prior to testing. The recommended intervals for GTT sample collection are fasting (0), 60, 90, 120, and 180 minutes following a 100-gm oral glucose load. Patients clinically suspected of having reactive hypoglycemia should have additional samples collected at 240, 300, and 360 minutes. The GTT is contraindicated in patients with fasting or random plasma glucose levels above 200 and 300 mg/dl, respectively, since hyperglycemic hyperosmolar coma may be precipitated. Table 47 contains three sets of standard criteria recommended as a guide to suspect or confirm diabetes mellitus from the GTT results.

Hypoglycemia may be categorized as reactive hypoglycemia, hypoglycemia caused by exogenous factors, and fasting hypoglycemia. Examples of reactive hypoglycemia include early diabetes mellitus, dumping syndromes, leucine sensitivity, and fructose intolerance. Exogenous hypoglycemia may be associated with insulin or sulfonylurea therapy and ingestion of ethanol, various toxins, and a wide variety of drugs. Examples of fasting hypoglycemia include insulinoma or other neoplasms, pituitary or adrenal insufficiency, and liver diseases such as hepatitis.

Some patients are symptomatic with a plasma glucose value of 50 mg/dl, whereas others are asymptomatic with a value as low as 30 mg/dl. Beta blockade will mask the catecholamine-related tachycardia of hypoglycemia. Worsening of carbohydrate tolerance has also been reported with certain beta blockers.

Since prolonged or repeated hypoglycemic episodes can result in permanent brain damage and death, all patients with measured plasma glucose levels <50 mg/dl should be regarded as having hypoglycemia

Table 47.   GTT criteria for diagnosis of diabetes mellitus.*

A.   U.S. Public Health Service (Wilkerson Point) criteria

Nonpregnant	Pregnant
Fasting > 130 mg/dl = 1 point	Fasting > 105 mg/dl
60′ > 195 mg/dl = ½ point	60′ > 190 mg/dl
120′ > 140 mg/dl = ½ point	120′ > 165 mg/dl
180′ > 130 mg/dl = 1 point	180′ > 145 mg/dl
Definite diabetes = 2–3 points	Definite diabetes = 2 or more abov▼
Suspect diabetes = ½–1½ points	Suspect diabetes = 1 above
No diabetes = zero points	No diabetes = 0 above

B.   Fajan-Conn criteria

60′	185 mg/dl
90′	165 mg/dl
120′	140 mg/dl

Definite diabetes = all 3
Suspect diabetes = 1–2
No diabetes = none

C.   Revised UGDP [†] summation criteria

Fasting + 60′ + 120′ + 180′
Diabetes = >700 summation
Suspect diabetes = 500–700
No diabetes = <500

Example (nonpregnant)

Time	Value (mg/dl)	Criteria
F =	106	A = ½ point (suspect diabetes)
60′ =	150	B = 2 points (suspect diabetes)
90′ =	168	C = 498 (no diabetes)
120′ =	142	
180′ =	100	

---

   * All based on true glucose levels rather than commonly employed reducing substance methods (see comments under Technique).
   † The UGDP summation criteria actually state diabetes >600 and no diabetes <600. This additional modification is recommended and based on experience in using these criteria.

until proved otherwise. If asymptomatic, they should be classified as hypoglycemia suspects and carefully studied to determine whether symptomatic hypoglycemia develops after either fasting or glucose loading.

   Early therapy of hypoglycemia completely reverses the presenting signs and symptoms. Thus, all comatose patients should be considered hypoglycemic until proved otherwise, regardless of any seemingly apparent primary etiology of the comatose state.

Symptoms and signs similar to those of hypoglycemia frequently occur in emotionally disturbed patients. Thus a diagnosis of symptomatic hypoglycemia cannot be confirmed unless the timing of symptoms and signs coincides with low plasma glucose levels.

Selected References

1. Mager M, Farese G: What is "true" blood glucose? A comparison of three procedures. *Am J Clin Pathol* 44:104–108, 1965.
2. Davidson JK: Diabetes in socioeconomically deprived neighborhoods, in Fajans SS, Sussman KE (eds): *Diabetes Mellitus: Diagnosis and Treatment.* New York, American Diabetes Association, 1971, vol 3, pp 207–210.
3. Davidson JK: Diabetes mellitus in adults, in Conn HF (ed): *Current Therapy.* Philadelphia, WB Saunders, 1974, pp 386–409.
4. Cooper GR: *Diagnosis and Detection Methods of Diabetes: Syllabus for Sixth Annual American Diabetes Association Allied Health Postgraduate Course.* Atlanta, Ga, Emory University School of Medicine, Diabetes Unit, 1974, pp 11–22.
5. Davidson JK: Hypoglycemia, in Schwartz GR, Safar P, Stone JH, et al (eds): *Principles and Practice of Emergency Medicine.* Philadelphia, WB Saunders, 1978, pp 1075–1078.
6. Seltzer H: Drug-induced hypoglycemia. *Diabetes* 21:955–966, 1972.
7. Waal-Manning HJ: Metabolic effects of β-adrenoreceptor blockade. *Drugs* 2:121–126, 1976.
8. Siperstein MD: The glucose tolerance test: A pitfall in the diagnosis of diabetes mellitus. *Adv Intern Med* 20:297–323, 1975.
9. Olefsky J, Farquhar JW, Raven GM: Do oral and intravenous glucose tolerance tests provide similar diagnostic information in patients with chemical diabetes mellitus? *Diabetes* 22:202–209, 1973.
10. Davidson JK, Reuben D, Sternberg JC, Ryan WT: Diabetes screening using a quantitative urine glucose method. *Diabetes* 27:810–816, 1978.

223. Serum Sodium

W. DALLAS HALL, MD
DAVID H. VROON, MD

Definition

Sodium is present in body fluids as a metallic inorganic cation. It has an atomic weight of 23 and is distributed largely (50–60%) in the plasma and interstitial spaces of the extracellular fluid compartment.

The normal range for serum sodium concentration is 135–145 mEq/liter serum. Since serum is 93% water, this could also be stated as 145–155 mEq/liter of serum water. The latter accounts for the difference in the sodium concentration considered to be isotonic in serum (140 mEq sodium per liter serum) and the sodium concentration contained in "normal" saline (154 mEq sodium per liter water).

Technique

Plasma or serum sodium is most commonly measured by flame emission photometry based on the principle that atoms of certain metallic elements, given sufficient energy such as heat, will emit this energy at specific wavelengths characteristic for the element. The intensity of emitted light at the characteristic wavelength is proportional to the concentration of the element. Sodium emits energy primarily at 589 nm (yellow), potassium at 768 nm (violet), and lithium at 671 nm (red). Sodium and potassium are usually measured simultaneously with two photodetection systems; lithium is usually employed as an internal standard to compensate for variations in atomization rates and flame stability.

Flame emission photometry provides a very accurate and precise technique for quantitation of sodium and potassium in biological fluids and, until recent years has been virtually the only method utilized on both discrete and multiphasic systems, including SMA equipment. Newer instruments, including the SMAC, SMA 2, and Beckman Astra 8 systems, utilize ion specific electrodes to measure sodium and potassium. Other than technical considerations, potentiometric methods offer no advantages over flame photometry for plasma serum or urine. Both approaches are prone to error secondary to displacement of plasma mater by lipemia or rarely by hyperproteinemia.

However, the use of ion specific electrodes on discrete analyzers designed to directly measure electrolytes on whole blood specimens offers the advantage of speed of analysis since no centrifugation is required and the instrument can be transported to the bedside. In addition, direct potentiometric determination of sodium on whole blood specimens does not appear to be subject to significant volume displacement error by lipemia or hyperproteinemia, presumably because no sample dilution is required.

Background Information

Sodium is the major extracellular fluid cation and (along with attendant anions) provides the source for more than 90% of the effective osmotic pressure of plasma. Serum or plasma osmolality can be estimated as follows:

$$\text{Estimated osmolality} = 1.86\,[\text{Na}] + \frac{\text{Glucose}}{18} + \frac{\text{BUN}}{2.8}$$

In the absence of elevated glucose, urea, mannitol, alcohol, or other abnormal osmotically active substances, serum osmolality is directly related to serum sodium.

The concentration of sodium in serum is dependent not only on the amount of exchangeable body sodium (approximately 60 mEq/kg) but also on the amount of exchangeable body potassium (approximately 50 mEq/kg) and the total body water content (approximately 0.6 liter/kg). These three variables are related because Na^+ is the major solute in the extracellular water, K^+ is the major solute in the intracellular water, and H_2O is freely diffusible between the two compartments. This relationship is mathematically expressed in the Edelman formula:

$$\text{Serum }[Na^+] = \frac{\text{Total exchangeable }Na^+\text{ and Total exchangeable }K^+}{\text{Total body water}}$$

Hence, serum sodium concentration is a reflection of all the factors that control body water, body sodium, and body potassium.

Clinical Significance

Abnormalities of serum Na^+ are most often due to water abnormalities rather than sodium or potassium abnormalities. In part, this is because sodium gain or loss is frequently isotonic, in which case the concentration of serum Na^+ remains within normal limits. Failure to appreciate this leads to erroneous statements such as, "The sodium is 141 so the patient must not be dehydrated," or "The sodium is low so the patient must be salt depleted."

Let us consider a serum Na^+ concentration of 120 mEq/liter. Five questions must be answered:

1. Is the measurement analytically correct? Check that the anion gap, $(Na + K) - (Cl + HCO_3)$, is greater than eight. For example,

Na^+	120 mEq/liter
K^+	4.0 mEq/liter
Cl^-	100 mEq/liter
HCO_3	19 mEq/liter

Then the anion gap, $(120 + 4) - (100 + 19) = 5$, and the sodium measurement could be in error.

2. Is there reason to suspect pseudohyponatremia due to displacement of plasma water? Significant artifactual depression of measured serum sodium concentration due to water displacement occurs only with marked hypertriglyceridemia (more than 1,500 mg/dl) manifest by grossly turbid serum. In this situation, the serum water displacement affects cations and anions equally such that the anion gap is not altered; however, the calculated osmolality will be considerably lower than the measured osmolality, since the latter is a direct measure of solute particles per kilogram of water.

Water displacement by hyperproteinemia is rarely a cause of spurious hyponatremia; however, serum viscosity changes associated with paraproteinemias may induce analytical errors in sodium determination, particularly on SMA systems. These errors, in contrast to lipoprotein water displacement, are suggested by low anion gaps regardless of measured sodium concentration. It should be noted, however, that low anion gaps may also occur (in the absence of erroneous sodium measurements) in paraproteinemic states as a result of the presence of additional anions that accompany the cationic paraproteins.

Hyponatremia associated with a normal serum osmolality (285–300 mOsm/kg serum) is of significance only in suggesting analytical error or the presence of significant water displacement by lipid protein or some other serum solute such as glucose, mannitol, or alcohol.

3. Does the patient have a relative excess of serum water? This is the most common cause of hyponatremia and results from dilution of the extracellular Na^+ content. Try to document evidence of volume expansion (congestive heart failure, inappropriate antidiuretic hormone activity), excessive plasma osmotically active solutes other than sodium (glucose, mannitol), or hypotonic fluid intake (excessive water drinking). Dilutional hyponatremia is common when a patient with an impaired

ability to excrete water (eg, cirrhosis, congestive heart failure) is placed on oral or parenteral sodium restriction without a proportionate reduction in water intake.

4. Is the patient salt depleted? Salt depletion is a relatively infrequent cause of hyponatremia because salt loss is commonly accompanied by equivalent water loss. Salt depletion severe enough to lower the serum sodium to 120 mEq/liter would be easily detected by the usual clinical parameters of volume depletion indicated in Table 48.

If a patient has a serum sodium below 125 mEq/liter and most of the above-mentioned clinical parameters are inconclusive, then one may be confident that the problem is not simply one of salt depletion.

If dehydration is confirmed and the etiology is not apparent, determine if the sodium loss is renal or extrarenal by measuring the urinary sodium concentration prior to therapy.

5. Has sodium shifted from the extracellular to the intracellular compartment? As mentioned under Background Information, total body K^+ is a determinant of the serum Na^+ concentration. It is thus possible, as in some cases of diuretic-induced hypokalemia, to have total body K^+ depletion and a shift of Na^+ from the extracellular to the intracellular compartment.

Hypernatremia is invariably associated with hyperosmolality and is most commonly related to a deficit in water (although most of these patients also have a sodium deficit). Determine why the patient may have had an inadequate water intake (stupor, depressed thirst mechanism) or why there has been excessive water loss or excretion. Renal causes of excess water loss include osmotic diuresis and insufficient amount or effect of antidiuretic hormone.

Extreme or rapid changes in osmolality may cause neurological manifestations including stupor, coma, and focal or generalized seizure activity. These neurological changes may also be primary manifestations of

Table 48. Objective signs of volume depletion.

---

1. Weight loss
2. Poor skin turgor
3. Flat neck veins in the supine position
4. Standing drop in mean arterial blood pressure more than 10 mm Hg
5. Standing rise in heart rate more than 20 beats per minute
6. Relative elevation in laboratory values (hematocrit, total protein, albumin, BUN, uric acid, urine specific gravity)
7. Low measurements of central venous pressure or pulmonary capillary wedge pressure
8. Low measurement of plasma or total blood volume
9. High urinary osmolality

---

some other disorder. Hence, they should be attributed to the high or low osmolality only when they are proved to reverse after return of the osmolality to normal. Complete reversal of neurological signs may be delayed for days following correction of the osmolality. This time lag can be wisely spent in carefully considering underlying etiologies such as cerebrovascular accident, primary or metastatic brain tumor, encephalitis or meningitis, subdural hematoma, drug overdose, and others.

Selected References

1. Earley LE: Sodium metabolism, in Maxwell MH, Kleeman CR (eds) *Clinical Disorders of Fluid and Electrolyte Metabolism.* New York, McGraw-Hill, 1972, pp 95–119.
2. Edelman IS, Liebman J, O'Meara MP, et al: Interrelations between serum sodium concentration, serum osmolality, total exchangeable potassium and total body water. *J Clin Invest* 37:1236–1256, 1958.
3. Leaf A: The clinical and physiologic significance of the serum sodium concentration. *N Eng J Med* 267:22–30, 77–84, 1962.
4. Bartter FC, Schwartz WB: The syndrome of inappropriate secretion of antidiuretic hormone. *Am J Med* 42:790–806, 1967.
5. Fichman MP, Vorherr H, Kleeman CR, et al: Diuretic-induced hyponatremia. *Ann Intern Med* 75:853–863, 1971.
6. Moses AM, Miller M: Drug-induced dilutional hyponatremia. *N Eng J Med* 291:1234–1241, 1974.

224. Serum Potassium

W. DALLAS HALL, MD
DAVID H. VROON, MD

Definition

Potassium is a metallic inorganic cation. It has an atomic weight of 39 and is distributed primarily in the intracellular fluid compartment. The normal range for serum potassium concentration is 3.5–5.2 mEq/liter serum. Values are approximately 0.5 mEq/liter lower in samples collected as plasma rather than serum.

Technique

Methodology for the potassium measurement is discussed in the previous section, Serum Sodium. Since more than 95% of total body potassium occurs in the intracellular compartment, special considerations are warranted when determinations are made on extracellular fluids. The contribution of intracellular platelet potassium accounts for the usual 0.3–0.5 mEq/liter higher serum than plasma potassium concentration. Significantly greater increments may occur during the clotting process when thrombocytosis, leukocytosis, or fragile leukocytes are present. The in vitro contribution of erythrocytes is an additional factor since red blood cell potassium concentration exceeds 100 mEq/liter and erythrocyte membrane disruption causes artifactually elevated extracellular potassium concentration. Although in vitro erythrocyte destruction is commonly detected by the presence of visible hemoglobin, changes may occur in the absence of visible hemolysis. Active transport (associated with absorption and phosphorylation of glucose) normally counteracts the twenty-fold concentration gradient for potassium across the erythrocyte membrane. The direction of potassium shift with prolonged exposure of serum or plasma to erythrocytes is determined by these opposing forces. For example, in vitro absorption of glucose by cellular elements may be associated with spuriously low extracellular potassium concentrations, whereas inhibition of phosphorylation by low temperature, glucose depletion or fluoride favors increased extracellular potassium concentration. Consistently reliable potassium determinations are therefore obtainable only on plasma specimens collected carefully and separated expeditiously (within 30–60 minutes). Failure to consider these specimen factors is perhaps a more significant cause of misleading potassium results than analytical errors. Unfortunately, single specimen multiphasic testing as provided by SMA systems does not support optimal potassium measurement because serum is usually the only specimen acceptable for all test measurements.

Background Information

Potassium is the major intracellular cation and provides the source for most of the effective osmotic pressure within cells. The ratio of potassium concentration inside and outside the cell membrane is an important determinant of nerve tissue excitation and the force of muscle contraction. Resting membrane potential is proportional, in part, to the logarithm of the ratio of intracellular to extracellular K^+. Potassium is also a determinant of protein synthesis, carbohydrate metabolism, and the transport of hydrogen and chloride ions in gastric and renal tubular cells. Hypokalemia exerts a suppressive effect on gastrointestinal smooth muscle activity, the release of insulin from the pancreas, and the synthesis of aldosterone in the adrenal gland. Hypokalemia stimulates renin release from the kidney.

The total exchangeable body potassium content is approximately 50 mEq/kg, over 95% of which is within cells. Less than 1% of the total body K^+ is in serum. This intracellular distribution of K^+ implies that minor compartmental shifts can make major changes in the serum level. Such is the case with extracellular acidosis where each 0.1 unit blood pH fall leads to a rise of 0.4 to 1 mEq/liter serum K^+ (and vice versa with alkalosis). Compartmental K^+ shift occurs during infusion of glucose and insulin where K^+ and phosphate are shifted intracellularly into liver and muscle glycogen stores. In severe muscle injury, large amounts of intracellular K^+ may be suddenly released into serum.

Clinical Significance

Hypokalemia and hyperkalemia demand clinical attention because either can be associated with fatal cardiac arrhythmias or total muscle paralysis, or both.

Interpretation of any absolute level of serum K^+ must be in context of the clinical setting. For example, a serum K^+ of 5.9 mEq/liter in a patient with diabetic ketoacidosis (blood pH of 7.10) likely represents total body K^+ depletion and danger of hypokalemia upon correction of the acidosis. Conversely, a serum K^+ of 5.9 mEq/liter in a patient with acute oliguric renal failure may be early warning of impending hyperkalemic cardiac arrest if therapy is not instituted.

Hypokalemia is usually associated with some degree of total body K^+ depletion. Patients with serum K^+ levels below 3.5 mEq/liter should be carefully evaluated for cardiac arrhythmias because myocardial irritability is accentuated, moreso in the presence of digitalis therapy. Proximal muscle strength and deep tendon reflexes should also be carefully evaluated, although both are often deceptively normal in a hypokalemic patient complaining of weakness. Adynamic ileus, gastric atony, and polyuria are additional reversible clinical consequences of severe or prolonged hypokalemia.

Hypokalemia is more often due to body K^+ losses than to intracellular shifts. Provided the hypokalemia is known to be of at least three to five days duration, measurement of urinary K^+ content prior to therapy will help determine whether the origin of K^+ loss is renal or extrarenal. Chronic extrarenal K^+ loss is usually associated with relatively low urinary K^+ excretion (<30–40 mEq per day), whereas renal potassium-losing syndromes will usually have a significant amount of urine K^+ excretion (>30–40 mEq per day) despite the presence of hypokalemia. Documentation of renal-K^+-wasting may represent the first clinical hint of excessive mineralocorticoid activity or primary renal tubular disorders.

Hyperkalemia may be associated with low, normal, or occasionally high total body K^+ content. Any patient with a serum K^+ exceeding 6.4 mEq/liter should have rapid and careful evaluation of the electrocardiogram for evidence of hyperkalemic cardiac toxicity. Specific data should be sought from the history, physical, and laboratory examinations. A sample checklist would include:

1. Renal disease. The serum creatinine will help determine the presence or absence of renal failure as a contributing cause.
2. Spironolactone (Aldactone), triamterene (Dyrenium), or oral supplemental K^+ therapy.
3. Excessive dietary K^+ intake, especially juices, oranges, peaches, bananas, tomatoes, or special high-protein feedings.
4. Areas of tissue necrosis or muscle trauma.
5. Occult blood in the thigh, gastrointestinal tract, retroperitoneal, or pleural space that might be hemolyzing and releasing large amounts of K^+ into the serum.
6. A low serum bicarbonate level. This may indicate the presence of acidosis with shift of K^+ into the serum. Measurement of blood pH is frequently indicated in patients with hyperkalemia.
7. Signs of Addison's disease.
8. Evidence of isolated hypoaldosteronism.
9. White counts in excess of 100,000/cu mm or platelet counts in excess of 1 million/cu mm. This may indicate that K^+ is being released from the cells during the in vitro clotting process. Under these circumstances, serum K^+ is high, heparinized plasma K^+ is normal, and there are no hyperkalemic changes on the electrocardiogram.

Selected References

1. Black DAK: Potassium metabolism, in Maxwell MH, Kleeman CR (eds): *Clinical Disorders of Fluid and Electrolyte Metabolism.* New York, McGraw-Hill, chap 4, 1972.
2. Surawicz B: Relationship between electrocardiogram and electrolytes. *Am Heart J* 75:814–834, 1967.
3. Schwartz WB, Relman AS: Effects of electrolyte disorders on renal structure and function. *N Eng J Med* 276:383–388, 1967.
4. Kaplan N: Hypokalemia in the hypertensive patient with observations on the incidence of primary aldosteronism. *Ann Intern Med* 66:1079–1090, 1967.
5. Kassirer JP, Harrington JT: Diuretics and potassium metabolism: A

reassessment of the need, effectiveness and safety of potassium therapy. *Kidney Int* 11:505–515, 1977.

6. Hall WD, Wollam GL: The etiology and management of hypokalemia. *Week Update Cardiol* 1(12):2–7, 1979.

---

225. Serum Chloride

W. DALLAS HALL, MD
DAVID H. VROON, MD

Definition

Chloride is an inorganic anionic halogen with an atomic weight of 35.5. It is distributed almost exclusively within the extracellular space, as is bromide ("bromide space"). Chloride is neither a hydrogen ion donor (acid) nor a significant hydrogen ion acceptor (base) according to Bronsted theory. Normal serum chloride levels range 96–106 mEq/liter.

Technique

A variety of techniques for determination of chloride depend on the formation of undissociated complexes with silver or mercury. In the colorimetric SMA and ACA methods, chloride displaces thiocyanate from mercuric thiocyanate, and the thiocyanate released then reacts with ferric ions to yield a colored complex, ferric thiocyanate:

$$2Cl^- + Hg(SCN)_2 \longrightarrow HgCl_2 + (SCN)^-$$

$$3(SCN)^- + Fe^{3+} \longrightarrow Fe(SCN)_3$$
$$\text{(absorbs at 480 nm)}$$

Commonly used mercurimetric techniques are based on titration of Cl^- with a standard solution of mercuric ions forming undissociated $HgCl_2$; the end point is detected colorimetrically when excess Hg^{2+} forms a colored complex with an indicator dye, diphenylcarbazone. Electrometric techniques measure Cl^- by titration with silver ions, with Ag^+ detected amperometrically at the end point. More recently ion-specific electrodes have been used to measure chloride potentiometrically in both serum and sweat.

All of the methods involving reaction with silver or mercuric ions are susceptible to interference by bromide, other halogens and sulfhydryl ions. Specific ion electrodes are presumably not susceptible to bromide interference. Br⁻ is an anionic halide which displaces Cl⁻ in biological fluids; erroneous quantitation of bromide on a milliequivalent for milliequivalent basis may result in artifactual elevation of chloride concentration as measured with methods using silver or mercuric ions. The SMA colorimetric method is reportedly more sensitive to Br⁻ than Cl⁻ and therefore overestimates chloride; this error may be reflected in a low anion gap which has been widely publicized as a marker for bromide intoxication.

Background Information

Chloride is the major anionic element of the extracellular fluid. Along with the bicarbonate anion, it is reabsorbed more readily by the renal tubules (in conjunction with sodium) than other anions such as phosphate, sulfate, and organic acids. Sodium reabsorption is thus accompanied by chloride reabsorption; it is also accompanied by hydrogen ion secretion and bicarbonate reabsorption. Chloride depletion usually occurs in association with salt and water depletion. In the volume-contracted state, renal sodium reabsorption, hydrogen ion secretion, and bicarbonate reabsorption all become accelerated. The kidney has a limited capacity to excrete bicarbonate under these circumstances. This enhanced renal bicarbonate reabsorption accounts for the relatively persistent metabolic alkalosis in patients who are volume depleted or chloride depleted, or both.

Salt and water depletion activates the renin-angiotensin-aldosterone system. Excessive aldosterone leads to accelerated renal loss of potassium whenever sodium bicarbonate is delivered to distal tubular sites. The kidney has a limited capacity to conserve potassium under these circumstances. This accounts for the relatively persistent hypokalemia in the volume- and chloride-depleted alkalotic state. In each of the above states, chloride would be virtually absent from the urine.

In volume-expanded states associated with a primary excess of mineralocorticoid activity, chloride would be abundant in the urine. Further addition of volume and chloride by administration of NaCl would not be expected to improve the metabolic alkalosis. This setting is referred to as saline-resistant metabolic alkalosis and is typical of patients with excessive mineralocorticoid activity.

Clinical Significance

Abnormalities of serum chloride should be considered relative to the serum sodium concentration. For instance, a 10% dilution of serum sodium from 140 to 126 mEq/liter would be expected to be associated with a 10% dilution of serum chloride from 100 to 90 mEq/liter. Hypochloremia no more implies chloride depletion than hyponatremia implies sodium depletion.

Hyperchloremia is commonly seen in water-depleted states or clinical settings where excessive saline has been administered. A 10% concentration of serum sodium from 140 to 154 mEq/liter would be expected to be associated with a 10% concentration of serum chloride from 100 to 110 mEq/liter. Thus, hyperchloremia no more implies chloride excess than hypernatremia implies sodium excess. The reader should refer to the section, Serum Sodium, for additional comments on this important point.

The absolute level of a low serum chloride (in a volume-depleted patient) provides clues concerning how the patient may have developed the hypochloremia. Most clinical volume depletion is isotonic with respect to extracellular fluid composition after expected compensatory mechanisms. The concentration of serum sodium and chloride is thus typically normal. Severe vomiting, however, leads to disproportionate chloride loss because gastric chloride content is 1.5–3 times greater than gastric sodium content. Electrolyte values in a patient who has been vomiting might include a serum sodium concentration of 133 mEq/liter (5% depressed) and a serum chloride concentration of 85 mEq/liter (15% depressed). Extremely low serum chloride levels in the range of 45–70 mEq/liter are most often associated with gastric outlet obstruction, protracted vomiting in alcoholics, or self-induced vomiting. Disproportionate loss of chloride relative to sodium is also characteristic of therapy with loop diuretics.

As previously mentioned, chloride depletion may account for persistence of either metabolic alkalosis or hypokalemia. Clinically, this is often encountered in patients with chronic obstructive pulmonary disease who have been placed on diuretics and salt restriction, and in patients who require prolonged nasogastric suction. Repletion of volume and chloride are necessary for maintenance of appropriate serum potassium and blood pH levels in these patients. Chloride may be administered as sodium chloride, potassium chloride, calcium chloride, lysine monochloride, arginine monochloride, ammonium chloride, or hydrochloric acid, depending on other clinical considerations.

Elevated levels of serum chloride relative to sodium occur in respiratory alkalosis and in hyperchloremic varieties of metabolic acidosis. Typical of the hyperchloremia of respiratory alkalosis would be the woman in normal third trimester pregnancy who presents with a serum bicarbonate level of 19 mEq/liter and a serum chloride of 109 mEq/liter.

These values should never be assumed to represent a metabolic acidosis without either an arterial or a venous estimate of blood pH.

Most metabolic acidoses are not associated with elevated chloride levels. The presence of hyperchloremic (normal anion gap) metabolic acidosis thus limits the diagnostic possibilities. Hyperchloremic acidosis occurs whenever the kidney is unable to conserve bicarbonate relative to chloride. Common causes include interstitial renal diseases such as obstruction, pyelonephritis, gout, or analgesic abuse. Hyperchloremic acidosis may also be seen with gastrointestinal bicarbonate loss, acetazolamide-induced carbonic anhydrase inhibition, or, occasionally, extrarenal influences such as excessive parathyroid hormone activity.

A spurious elevation of chloride measurement may also be observed in bromide intoxication. The usual clinical clues include an altered mental status and a value of (Na + K) − (total CO₂ content + chloride) below 8 mEq/liter.

Selected References

1. Skeggs LT Jr, Hochstrasser H: Multiple automatic sequential analysis. *Clin Chem* 10:918–936, 1964.
2. Seldin DW, Rector FC Jr: The generation and maintenance of metabolic alkalosis. *Kidney Int* 1:306–321, 1972.
3. Schwartz WB, van Ypersele de Strihou C, Kassirer JP: Role of anions in metabolic alkalosis and potassium deficiency. *N Eng J Med* 279: 630–639, 1968.

226. Serum Total CO₂ Content

W. DALLAS HALL, MD

Definition

Bicarbonate is an inorganic anion with a molecular weight of 61. Total CO₂ content of serum is the test most commonly offered by clinical laboratories as an estimate of bicarbonate. True total CO₂ content is 2–3 mEq/liter greater than bicarbonate concentration because it includes measurement of dissolved CO_2 and carbonic acid. The total CO_2 content should not be confused with PCO_2, which is the partial pressure of CO_2 gas in blood expressed in mm Hg (or expressed in Torr where 1 Torr is the pressure generated by 1 mm Hg at sea level).

The normal range for total CO_2 content is 23–30 mEq/liter serum of plasma in venous samples; values are approximately 2 mEq/liter lower in serum or plasma from arterial blood.

Technique

Total CO_2 content is most commonly determined by specimen acidification, which converts all forms of carbonate to dissolved CO_2 with subsequent measurement of CO_2 by volumetric, manometric, colorimetric, or specific electrode technics. SMA systems absorb the CO_2 released by serum acidification into an alkaline buffer containing the pH indicator dye, cresol red. The color change is detected photometrically and is related proportionally to total CO_2 content.

Reliable determination of total CO_2 content must include measures to avoid loss of the volatile CO_2 component. Exposure of specimens to room air results in immediate loss of volatile CO_2 because of the pressure differential. Since the ratio of nonvolatile bicarbonate to volatile carbonic acid is normally 20:1, this loss usually does not exceed 1–3 mEq/L and is proportional to PCO_2. Significantly greater changes occur when the original sample has a high PCO_2 content or when serum has prolonged in vitro exposure to metabolically active cellular elements. A major disadvantage of SMA systems is the fact that the specimen is in open cups waiting for sampling. CO_2 loss can be minimized by immediate specimen alkalinization because, at pH 8.6, plasma PCO_2 approximates that of room air. However, prior specimen treatment is technically cumbersome and compromises the concept of total automation; it is therefore not routine. Artifactual CO_2 loss can be minimized with methods that use discrete automated or manual systems.

Background Information

Maintenance of acid-base balance in the body is largely a function of various compounds capable of buffering acids and bases. In the human the best buffers are those weak acids and their conjugate bases which have a pKa (negative logarithm of the dissociation constant) close to that of body fluid pH. Maximal acid or base loads can thus be captured with minimal perturbations of pH. The major buffers in the blood are the carbonic acid system (pKa = 6.1), the imidazole radicals of hemoglobin (pKa = 6.0), the phosphate system (pKa = 6.8), and the free amino (pKa =

9.5) and carboxyl (pKa = 4.5) groups of basic or acidic amino acids. The total buffer contribution of these substances is also a function of their availability. For instance, phosphate is an optimal body buffer (pKa of 6.8 for the second ionization), but there are less than 2 mEq/liter in serum as compared with more than 20 mEq/liter of bicarbonate. This explains why plasma bicarbonate and red cell hemoglobin provide the most important contributions to the total buffer capacity of whole blood (46–53 mEq/liter). Hemoglobin is, of course, absent from the serum or plasma sample in which total CO_2 content is measured.

Carbonic acid has a dissociation constant of 7.95×10^{-7}. The negative logarithm of this dissociation constant, pKa, is 6.10 for plasma carbonic acid, which is in equilibrium with CO_2:

$$CO_2 + H_2O \rightleftharpoons H_2CO_3 \rightleftharpoons H^+ + HCO_3^-$$

The blood pH of 7.40 is above the carbonic acid pKa of 6.10. Hence, the predominant form of carbonic acid becomes ionized and exists in the serum as bicarbonate ion.

Bicarbonate and hydrogen ions are continually generated from the 700 gm of CO_2 formed daily from the oxidative processes of active tissue cells. Most of this CO_2 is excreted by the lungs. A minor amount combines with ammonia as the sole carbon source in the hepatic synthesis of urea (see the section, Blood Urea Nitrogen). Approximately 40–60 mEq per day of formed hydrogen ions are excreted by the kidney after combining with either ammonia (NH_3) or titratable buffers ("titratable acidity") such as phosphate and creatinine. Bicarbonate is steadily utilized as a buffer for those H^+ ions which enter the extracellular fluid. Bicarbonate which is filtered through the glomerulus is reclaimed by tubular reabsorption such that less than 5 mEq per day escapes into the urine of normal individuals. Hence, the normal urine pH is below 6.1. Physiological factors that enhance renal tubular bicarbonate reabsorption include volume contraction, hypochloremia, hypokalemia, elevated PCO_2, excess mineralocorticoids, and carbonic anhydrase activity. Physiological factors that inhibit renal tubular bicarbonate reabsorption include volume expansion, hyperchloremia, decreased PCO_2, mineralocorticoid deficiency, carbonic anhydrase blockers and excessive parathyroid hormone activity.

All charged particles in serum are electrolytes in that they will move toward the cathode or anode in a solution through which an electric current is passed. Cationic electrolytes include Na^+, K^+, Ca^{++}, Mg^{++}, Zn^{++}, and so forth: anionic electrolytes include HCO_3^-, Cl^-, $PO_4^=$, $SO_4^=$, lactate$^-$, beta-hydroxybutyrate$^-$, acetoacetate$^-$, protein, and so forth. In any solution, the sum of positively charged particles equals the sum of negatively charged particles. The arbitrary designation of Na^+, K^+, HCO_3^-, and Cl^- as the four electrolytes to be commonly measured was based on prominent physiological roles for these ions. However, the selection process chose more cations ($Na^+ = 140$ mEq/liter plus $K^+ = 4$ mEq/liter for a total of 144 mEq/liter) than anions (HCO_3^- of 25 mEq/liter plus Cl^- of 100 mEq/liter for a total of only 125 mEq/liter). The difference between the sum of the Na^+ and K^+, and the sum of the HCO_3^- and Cl^- is referred to as the "anion gap" and represents the excess mEq/liter of other anions present normally (phosphate, lactate, weak organic acids) but not ordinarily quantitated in the measurement of electrolytes. The normal anion gap (d) is approximately 16 mEq/liter with a range of 9–21 mEq/liter when calculated according to the formula:

$$d = (Na + K) - (HCO_3 + Cl)$$

Changes in the calculated anion gap occur whenever the pool of unmeasured cations or anions is disproportionately altered. Clinical conditions which result in an increased unmeasured anion pool are relatively common and are reflected in an increased anion gap since measured anions are displaced relative to measured cations. The increased anion gap may provide a marker to the presence of these conditions. Conditions that cause significantly decreased unmeasured anions or increased unmeasured cations are reflected in a decreased anion gap. Thus, a decreased anion gap could occur with the presence of cationic paraproteins, lithium toxicity, marked hypoproteinemia, hypercalcemia, and hypermagnesemia. Since these clinical conditions are relatively uncommon, a low anionic gap more often suggests an error in electrolyte measurement, particularly sodium.

Metabolic acidosis due to accumulation of endogenous acid may be associated with an increased anion gap since unmeasured anions (lactate, acetoacetate, beta-hydroxybutyrate, formate) are dissociated from buffered H^+ ions. The occurrence of increased anion gaps in azotemia is related to decreased excretion of unmeasured anionic metabolites. Increased anion gaps may also occur (in the absence of acid-base disturbance) as a result of therapeutic administration of anionic salts such as carbenicillin.

Clinical Significance

For clinical purposes, the total CO_2 content of serum can be considered to represent the bicarbonate concentration. Before blood pH and PCO_2 measurements were readily accessible, bicarbonate measurements were the best estimate of the acid-base status of a patient. Arterial or venous blood pH measurements are now used to confirm estimates of acid-base balance made from bicarbonate levels.

Bicarbonate levels below 10 mEq/liter almost always indicate a metabolic acidosis; a pH measurement may be indicated to gauge the severity. Bicarbonate levels above 40 mEq/liter almost always indicate a metabolic alkalosis; a pH measurement may be indicated to gauge the severity. Bicarbonate levels between 10 and 40 mEq/liter may occur in the presence of acidemia (pH $\leq$ 7.35) or alkalemia (pH $\geq$ 7.45), or neither; a pH measurement is necessary to more precisely characterize the acid-base status of the patient. The limitations on clinical interpretation of bicarbonate levels of 10–40 mEq/liter are exemplified by the following three statements:

A patient can have clinically significant respiratory acidosis and a blood pH of 7.20 (acidemic) with a serum bicarbonate which is 18, 25, or 30 mEq/liter.

A patient can have clinically significant respiratory alkalosis and a blood pH of 7.58 (alkalemic) with a serum bicarbonate which is 18, 25, or 30 mEq/liter.

A serum bicarbonate level of 15 mEq/liter may be associated with a pH which is 7.5 (alkalemic), 7.4 (normal), or 7.3 (acidemic).

Observations such as these are often explained by the presence of mixed acid-base disorders. They illustrate the need for determining blood pH whenever an acid-base disturbance is suspected and the bicarbonate level is between 10 and 40 mEq/liter.

The calculation of anion gap is most useful in evaluating acid-base disorders when the anion gap is wide (ie, >21 mEq/liter). This implies that the patient has a disorder (metabolic acidosis) creating additional amounts of unmeasured anions such as lactate, beta-hydroxybutyrate, acetoacetate, salicylate, formate, or sulfate. The blood pH will be reduced below 7.40 if the acid-base disturbance is not complicated by a second acid-base disturbance in the same patient (ie, if the patient does not have a mixed acid-base disorder). In the presence of mixed disorders, a wide anion gap (metabolic acidosis) may exist when the blood pH is low (acidemia), normal, or high (alkalemia).

Although a wide anion gap is indicative of metabolic acidosis, there are varieties of metabolic acidosis that are associated with a normal anion gap. These are collectively known as hyperchloremic acidosis and generally indicate the presence of interstitial varieties of renal disease with impairment of hydrogen ion secretion or bicarbonate reabsorption, or both.

An excellent review of the concept of the anion gap, including the differential diagnosis of both wide and narrow gaps, is contained in reference 3.

Selected References

1. Report of the ad hoc committee of the New York Academy of Sciences Conference: Statement of acid-base terminology. *Ann Intern Med* 63:885–889, 1965.
2. Elkinton JR: Clinical disorders of acid-base regulation: A survey of seventeen years' diagnostic experience. *Med Clin N Am* 50:1325–1350, 1966.

3. Emmett ME, Narins RG: Clinical use of the anion gap. *Medicine* 56: 38–54, 1977.
4. Seldin DW, Rector FC: The generation and maintenance of metabolic alkalosis. *Kidney Int* 1:306–321, 1972.
5. Kassirer JP: Serious acid-base disorders. *N Eng J Med* 291:773–776, 1974.
6. Oh MS, Carroll HJ: The anion gap. *N Eng J Med* 297:814–817, 1977.
7. Rose BD: *Clinical Physiology of Acid-Base and Electrolyte Disorders.* New York, McGraw-Hill, 1977, pp 295–376.

227. Serum Glutamate-Oxaloacetate Transaminase

W. DALLAS HALL, MD
DAVID H. VROON, MD

Definition

The transaminase group of enzymes catalyzes the interconversion of amino acids and alpha-ketoacids by transfer of amino acid groups. Hence, they link amino acid and carbohydrate metabolic pathways. GOT (glutamic oxaloacetate transaminase) is an intracellular enzyme that catalyzes the transfer of an amino group from aspartate to alpha-ketoglutarate, producing oxaloacetate and glutamate, that is:

$$
\begin{array}{ccccccc}
\text{COO}^- & & \text{COO}^- & & \text{COO}^- & & \text{COO}^- \\
| & & | & \text{GOT} & | & & | \\
\text{HC—NH}_2 & + & \text{C=O} & \longleftrightarrow & \text{C=O} & + & \text{HC—NH}_2 \\
| & & | & & | & & | \\
\text{CH}_2 & & \text{CH}_2 & & \text{COO}^- & & \text{CH}_2 \\
| & & | & & & & | \\
\text{COO}^- & & \text{CH}_2 & & & & \text{COO}^- \\
& & | & & & & \\
& & \text{COO}^- & & & & \\
\end{array}
$$

Aspartate   Ketoglutarate   Oxaloacetate   Glutamate

Preferred nomenclature for the enzyme is aspartate amino-transferase (AAT). Normal adult levels are less than 45 mIU/ml.

Technique

Measurement of SGOT activity by ultraviolet spectrophotometry is preferred and commonly used on SMA and other automated and manual systems. Since the primary reaction does not provide a directly detectable product or substrate, a coupled enzymatic reaction employing malic dehydrogenase (MDH) is used:

$$\text{Aspartate} + \text{alpha-ketoglutarate} \xrightarrow{\text{GOT}} \text{glutamate} + \text{oxaloacetate}$$

$$\text{Oxaloacetate} + \text{NADH} + \text{H}^+ \xrightarrow{\text{MDH}} \text{malic acid} + \text{NAD}^+$$

(absorbs at 340 nm)   (nonabsorbing at 340 nm)

The decrease in absorbance at 340 nm due to the oxidation of nicotinamide adenine dinucleotide phosphate (NADH) per unit time is a measure of the rate of transamination.

SGOT is a relatively stable enzyme under a variety of storage conditions. Red cell concentrations are approximately 10 to 15 times normal serum levels; hemolysis and prolonged exposure of serum to cells must be avoided.

Background Information

Transaminase reactions are involved in both amino acid catabolism and gluconeogenesis. GOT is present in high activity in tissues such as the heart, liver, muscle, and kidney; lesser activities are found in the pancreas, spleen, lung, brain, and erythrocytes. When tissue injury occurs, necrosis or increased cellular permeability, or both, result in the release of intracellular enzyme into the extracellular fluid and circulation. Serum enzyme levels may become increased, depending on the rate of release and rate of disappearance of the enzyme. The serum GOT activity is a relatively nonspecific measure of cellular injury. Isoenzymes of SGOT exist, but their measurement has not found clinical application.

Clinical Significance

The highest and most frequently observed serum elevations of GOT are associated with various liver diseases, disorders of muscles, and myocardial infarction.

The serum GOT level is classically elevated within 18 hours of an acute myocardial infarction, the peak often occurring during the second day with a return to normal within three to five days. Reinfarction may result in a second increase in serum enzyme activity. Patients with acute myocardial infarction may have normal serial measurements of GOT activity, either because the total mass of the infarcted tissue is relatively small or because the sampling interval is not appropriate to detect the rise. A more sensitive enzymatic indicator of myocardial infarction is the serum creatine phosphokinase (CPK). In most but not all cases, the level of serum CPK activity rises within 6–8 hours of myocardial infarction, and peaks earlier than the SGOT. Specificity is enhanced by fractionation of the total CPK into those components which derive primarily from myocardial muscle (MB isoenzyme) versus those which derive primarily from skeletal muscle (MM isoenzyme). The availability of these more sensitive and specific CPK isoenzyme analyses has displaced measurement of SGOT in the diagnosis of acute myocardial injury.

Liver conditions with cell necrosis or altered cell permeability may give rise to increased serum GOT levels. Greatest elevations occur in acute hepatitis, where the increase in GOT level follows a time course similar to that of bilirubin. Elevations usually appear during the 1st week, peak during the 2nd week, and return to normal by the 8th to 10th week. A few cases have persistent elevations of GOT for one year or longer with or without biopsy evidence of activity or chronic disease.

The absolute height of serum GOT in liver conditions is not a valid indicator of the disease severity since many serious chronic liver diseases have GOT values below 100 mμ/ml. Serum GOT levels are below 400 mμ/ml in 90% of cases of isolated extrahepatic biliary obstruction.

Liver congestion commonly occurs in patients with right-sided heart failure. Elevation of hepatic GOT will usually accompany such cases. Measurement of other enzymes may be helpful to identify hepatic origin of the GOT. For example, serum glutamic pyruvate transaminase (SGPT, or alanine aminotransferase) and gamma glutamyl transferase (GGT) derive primarily from the liver.

Muscle disorders associated with striking elevation of serum GOT include crush injuries, polymyositis, and rhabdomyolysis. Lesser elevations may be seen in the muscular dystrophies. GOT levels are usually normal with disorders such as myasthenia gravis and primary anterior horn cell diseases. Other conditions which may contribute to serum GOT levels include intensive and prolonged muscle exercise, electroshock, and intramuscular injection of irritating substances.

Selected References

1. Meyers F, Evans JM: The serum transaminase (SGOT) and electrocardiogram in autopsy-confirmed acute myocardial infarction. *Am Heart J* 67:15–17, 1964.

2. Mosley JW, Galambos JT: Viral hepatitis, in Schiff L (ed): *Diseases of the Liver*, cd 4. Philadelphia, JB Lippincott, 1975, chap 18.

3. Schmidt E: Strategy and evaluation of enzyme determinations in serum in diseases of the liver and the biliary system, in Demers LM, Shaw LW (eds): *Evaluation of Liver Function: A Multifaceted Approach to Clinical Diagnosis*. Baltimore-Munich, Urban and Schwarzenberg, 1978, p 79.

228. Lactate Dehydrogenase

DAVID H. VROON, MD

W. DALLAS HALL, MD

Definition

Lactate dehydrogenase (LDH) is an intracellular enzyme found in all human tissues capable of glycolysis. It catalyzes the reversible oxidation of lactate to pyruvate. The enzyme has a molecular weight of 140,000 and is a tetramer of two different subunits, the H monomer (abundant in heart) and the M monomer (abundant in liver). This tetramer structure permits the formation of five isoenzymes which are identifiable by electrophoretic migration: H_4 or LDH_1, H_3M or LDH_2, H_2M_2 or LDH_3, HM_3 or LDH_4, and M_4 or LDH_5. This numbering system is currently used in both Europe and America; however, older literature still reflects the original American numbering system, which is reversed.

LDH is ubiquitous, occurring in virtually every body cell. The normal range for serum LDH activity as determined by the SMA method is 100–225 U/liter. This activity probably reflects normal cellular turnover. The relative proportion of isoenzymes is: $LDH_2 > LDH_1 > LDH_3 > LDH_4 > LDH_5$.

Technique

The most popular methods for assaying LDH activity are based on the rate of increase or decrease in absorbance of nicotinamide adenine dinucleotide phosphate (NADH) in the reversible reaction between lactate and pyruvate:

$$\underset{\text{Lactate}}{\overset{\displaystyle CH_3}{\underset{\displaystyle COO^-}{\overset{\displaystyle |}{\underset{\displaystyle |}{HCOH}}}}} \quad + \quad \underset{\substack{\text{(nonabsorbing at}\\ \text{340 nm)}}}{NAD} \quad \underset{\xleftarrow{\hspace{1.5cm}}}{\overset{LDH}{\xrightarrow{\hspace{1.5cm}}}} \quad \underset{\text{Pyruvate}}{\overset{\displaystyle CH_3}{\underset{\displaystyle COO^-}{\overset{\displaystyle |}{\underset{\displaystyle |}{C{=}O}}}}} \quad + \quad NADH \quad + H^+$$

$$\text{(absorbs at 340 nm)}$$

SMA as well as most other systems use the forward, or lactate-to-pyruvate, reaction; the reverse reaction is used less frequently but offers some advantages. Results vary depending on the direction of reaction and specific reaction conditions.

The most common cause of spurious elevations of serum LDH is in vitro release of enzyme from erythrocytes which contain 100 times normal serum activity per unit volume. Spurious and significant elevations occur prior to visible threshold of hemoglobin; erythrocyte enrichment is mainly from the fast migrating LDH_1 and LDH_2 components. Careful collection and prompt separation of serum and cells is mandatory for reliable assay and isoenzyme study.

Serum is preferred since anticoagulants may inhibit enzyme activity. The presence of substances such as chloroquine and furosemide which absorb at 340 nm are potentially interfering; however, interference is eliminated with rate-reaction monitoring methods and minimized with a specimen blank on SMA systems. The stability of LDH varies with different isoenzymes. The cathodal tetramers, LDH_4 and LDH_5, are unstable at refrigerator and freezer temperatures, whereas LDH_1 and LDH_2 are stable over a wide range of temperatures.

As with other enzyme assays involving a mixture of isoenzymes, selecting reaction conditions with optimal sensitivity for all components is problematic. Conditions are often optimized for normal specimens but are not necessarily optimal for all isoenzyme distributions in various clinical states. Since LDH_1 and LDH_2 are dominant, methods may be less sensitive to serum enrichment by hepatic LDH_5; this is the case with the SMA method.

Background Information

The reduction of pyruvate is the final step in anaerobic glycolysis. Further oxidation of pyruvate, with the production of adenosine triphosphate (ATP), occurs in the aerobic citric acid cycle. Tissues with limited aerobic capacity relative to their energy demands, eg, striated muscle, convert pyruvate to lactate quite effectively. The NADH produced in this final glycolytic reaction is used to further stimulate glycolysis. The formed lactate diffuses out of these tissues and can be oxidized by tissues with greater aerobic capacity.

The occurrence of elevated LDH reflects serum enrichment secondary to cellular injury. Techniques for determining the relative isoenzyme distribution in clinical specimens are well defined and readily available; interpretation of observed patterns is difficult because of the ubiquitous nature of LDH isoenzymes and because of the overlapping patterns observed in different organ systems. The fact that organ specific patterns are superimposed on normal serum patterns presents additional interpretive problems. Consequently, the effective clinical use of LDH isoenzyme study is mostly confined to assisting in the differential diagnosis of myocardial infarction. The finding of increased LDH_1 in excess of LDH_2 is highly specific for myocardial necrosis when hemolysis and renal infarction are excluded. The sensitivity of using LDH isoenzymes is less than that of creatine phosphokinase isoenzymes. However, LDH isoenzymes may be the only relevant serum enzymatic test in patients presenting more than 48 hours after the onset of myocardial infarction.

The concentration of LDH relative to other intracellular enzymes in different tissue cells may enhance interpretation of serum levels. For example, the erythrocyte contains 10 times more LDH than SGOT; hemolysis is therefore manifested by a proportionally higher serum LDH than SGOT. Hepatic cells are rich in both LDH and SGOT: however, LDH_5 has a relatively short half-life and is not assayed with maximal sensitivity by most methods. Thus, except for acute hepatocellular injury, dramatic elevations of LDH relative to SGOT are not typically observed. Serum levels of creatine phosphokinase (CPK) provide further assistance with interpretation of LDH due to the sensitivity of CPK for skeletal muscle injury and its absence in erythrocytes and hepatic cells.

LDH is also capable of reducing other alpha-keto and alpha-gamma-diketo acids; the more anodic isoenzymes, LDH_1 and LDH_2, show differential affinity for alpha-hydroxybutyric acid. Use of this substrate as a biochemical rather than electrophoretic assessment of LDH isoenzymes has been popularized by certain automated systems; the measured enzyme activity is referred to as alpha-hydroxybutyric dehydrogenase (HBD). It is not specific for myocardial LDH isoenzymes and does not enhance diagnostic discrimination; electrophoretic methods are preferred.

Clinical Significance

Because of the general utility of glycolysis as an energy-producing pathway, LDH is found in significant amounts in all tissues. Thus, an elevation of the enzyme may be observed whenever cellular injury occurs in virtually any organ. Elevations of total enzyme activity must therefore be interpreted in conjunction with other clinical information. Since LDH is nonspecific and insensitive to many disease states relative to other tests, its isolated measurement does not usually contribute significantly to diagnosis. Its inclusion on chemistry profiles is justified only by the enhanced tissue specificity of concurrently observing multiple enzymes. LDH has also been referred to as a "biochemical sedimentation rate," serving as a nonspecific but sensitive indicator of cell injury or death.

High normal or a slightly elevated level of LDH activity (ie, 200–249 U/liter) is one of the most frequent abnormalities noted on automated chemistry reports. In part, this relates to the ubiquity of the enzyme in various tissues and the minimal amount of insult necessary to cause release of LDH from these tissues. The clinician must neither overinterpret nor underinterpret these levels. Consider the level in context of all of the patient's clinical abnormalities as well as the associated laboratory values to best decide how vigorously to pursue a level of, say, 230 U/liter. An expensive diagnostic evaluation is not indicated in an otherwise asymptomatic patient whose associated laboratory values are normal and who has recently fallen and bruised the thigh or hip. Conversely, malignancy may be uncovered in a patient with an LDH of 240 U/liter in conjunction with recent weight loss and several other laboratory values (alkaline phosphatase, hematocrit, uric acid, platelet count, calcium) which hover in the high normal or borderline range.

The highest levels of total serum LDH are usually seen with disorders involving necrosis of a large mass of LDH-containing tissue, eg, alcoholic rhabdomyolysis or disorders such as organic phosphorus poisoning, where multiple body organs are simultaneously involved. High levels of LDH are invariable in megaloblastic and hemolytic anemias. Disseminated malignant neoplasms may also be associated with very high levels of serum LDH.

Selected References

1. Wolf PL, Williams D, Von Der Muehll E: *Practical Clinical Enzymology and Biochemical Profiling.* John Wiley and Sons, 1973.
2. Posen S: Turnover of circulating enzymes. *Clin Chem* 16:71–84, 1970.
3. Wilkinson JH: Serum isoenzymes. *Crit Rev Clin Lab Sci* 1:599–637, 1970.
4. Van Dijk YM, Eylath U, Czackeo E, Abraham AS: Differential diagnosis of chest pain: Use of isoenzyme LDH_1 level as a criterion. *Postgrad Med* 65:189–192, 1979.

229. Alkaline Phosphatase

DAVID H. VROON, MD

Definition

Alkaline phosphatases are a group of enzymes (isoenzymes) that nonspecifically hydrolyze phosphate esters at an alkaline pH. Most laboratories now express enzyme activity in the International Unit (IU or U), the amount of enzyme that catalyzes the conversion of one micromole of substrate per minute under defined reaction conditions. Using the SMA method, the normal range observed in an adult population is 35–125 U/liter. Intraindividual enzyme activity has been shown to vary considerably less than the interindividual variation included in the normal range. Therefore, comparison with preestablished values in an individual may be particularly useful.

Technique

A variety of methods employing different substrates and reaction conditions are used on automated and manual systems to measure alkaline phosphatase activity. Methods based on enzyme-substrate reactions are preferred since they yield directly detectable products. Older procedures such as the Bodansky and Kind-King, which use beta-glycero-phosphate and phenylphosphate substrates, respectively, are technically impractical.

Methods employing the Bessey-Lowry substrate, para-nitrophenyl-phosphate (PNPP), are popular. The presence of amino alcohol buffers enhances sensitivity and reproducibility. The SMA method is based on enzymatic hydrolysis of PNPP under alkaline conditions, producing p-nitrophenol and inorganic phosphate. Para-nitrophenol is a yellow chromogen in alkaline solution and is detected spectrophotometrically after dialysis to remove other serum pigments such as bilirubin. The reaction proceeds at a temperature of 37.5°C and a pH of 10.25:

$$\text{Para-nitrophenyl phosphate} \xrightarrow[\text{Mg}^{2+}]{\text{alkaline phosphatase}}$$
$$\text{(colorless)}$$

$$\text{Para-nitrophenol} + \text{H}_3\text{PO}_4 + \text{H}_2$$
$$\text{(absorbs at 410 nm)}$$

As with other enzyme assays, reaction conditions must be carefully controlled to avoid analytical variation. Enzyme activity may be inhibited by the presence of fluorides, arsenates, cyanide, and high concentrations of phosphate; chelating anticoagulants interfere by removing the activavator Mg^{2+}. Bromsulfophthalein absorbs at 410 nm and causes an apparent increase in activity with nonkinetic methods. Alkaline phosphatase uniquely and variably increases in activity when unbuffered serum specimens are stored for 12 to 24 hours at room or refrigerator temperatures.

Background Information

Alkaline phosphatase activity is present in many tissues; activity in normal adult serum is derived predominantly from hepatic, osseous, reticuloendothelial, and vascular sources. Physiologic bone growth in growing children increases serum activity to 2–5 times the levels observed in adults. Pregnancy is another physiologic cause for 2- to 3-fold elevations of serum alkaline phosphatase. The rise is due primarily to placental alkaline phosphatase and is observed in the second and third trimesters with return to normal in the first postpartum month. Intravenous infusion of commercial albumin preparations which have been derived from human placental tissue are associated with prominent elevations in serum alkaline phosphatase. Methods sensitive to the intestinal isoenzyme may show elevations after a fatty meal, particularly in individuals with blood groups B or O.

Serum elevations of alkaline phosphatase are due to release of intracellular alkaline phosphatase isoenzymes from altered cell wall permeability or from increased production of alkaline phosphatase. Alkaline phosphatase elevations may thus be due to isoenzymes of placental, hepatobiliary, gastrointestinal, bone, or vascular endothelial origin. These isoenzymes can be studied by differential chemical inhibition, heat inactivation, immunologic methods or electrophoretic migration. Electrophoretic techniques and thermal stability are most commonly applied. The placental isoenzyme is characterized by heat stability and beta electrophoretic migration; its presence correlates with maturity of the cytotrophoblast of the microvilli. Isoenzymes of hepatobiliary origin are of intermediate heat stability and migrate in the alpha-1 and alpha-2 zones; elevations are observed in a variety of hepatobiliary disorders. The isoenzyme derived from gastrointestinal mucosa migrates in the beta-gamma region; serum elevations occur with destructive mucosal lesions, but may also be observed in chronic liver disease. The isoenzyme of bone origin is characterized by heat lability and electrophoretic mobility slightly cathodal to the alpha-2 liver fraction; serum elevations are related to osteogenesis. The isoenzyme of vascular endothelial origin is heat labile with migration similar to the bone fraction. Serum elevations of vascular endothelial origin are most often related to angioblastic proliferation occurring with the reparative process following tissue destruction, such as myocardial, pulmonary, or renal infarction.

The sensitivity of different assay methods for isoenzymes varies; therefore, even when methods produce comparable results in normal specimens, variations may occur in abnormal specimens.

Clinical Significance

The majority of elevated alkaline phosphatase levels are associated with diseases of the liver or bone, or both. Therefore, these organ systems are of prime consideration in the differential diagnosis.

A variety of primary and secondary hepatic conditions may be associated with elevated serum levels with contribution from hepatic cells, bile duct epithelium, intestinal mucosa, vascular endothelium, or all. Since alkaline phosphatase production is particularly increased in response to cholestatic lesions, serum levels may provide a sensitive indicator for obstructive and space-occupying (neoplastic) or infiltrative (sarcoidosis, tuberculosis) lesions. The biliary isoenzyme may be observed in serum prior to elevation of total alkaline phosphatase activity. Bilirubin excretion is compromised only with more extensive cholestasis or hepatic cell disruption; therefore, differential elevations of bilirubin and alkaline phosphatase are of diagnostic acid. Hepatic cell lesions may be manifested by hyperbilirubinemia and dominant elevations of parenchymal enzymes, such as SGOT or SGPT; alkaline phosphatase elevations may be only minimal. Partial biliary obstruction or infiltrative lesions often result in dramatic serum alkaline phosphatase increases with minimal compromise of bilirubin excretion. More complete biliary obstruction is manifested by increases in both bilirubin and alkaline phosphatase. The pattern will not differentiate extrahepatic from intrahepatic cholestasis; however, the presence of the intestinal isoenzyme suggests intrahepatic disease. The occurrence of this isoenzyme in hepatic disease is apparently related to a compromised conversion to a hepatic isoenzyme.

Diseases of bone associated with elevated serum alkaline phosphatase levels are largely restricted to the presence of osteoblastic activity. Elevations are generally detectable prior to roentgenographic abnormalities. Neoplastic disease involving bone can be associated with marked increase in alkaline phosphatase levels when the lesion incites an osteoblastic reaction, such as metastatic adenocarcinoma of the prostate. Conversely, osteolytic lesions such as occur with multiple myeloma are not associated with serum elevations. Metabolic diseases which are usually associated with serum enrichment by the bone isoenzyme include rickets, osteomalacia, and Paget's disease. Levels are usually normal in osteoporosis. Elevated serum alkaline phosphatase levels are a late manifestation of primary or secondary hyperparathyroidism, and normal levels are found in the majority of cases. Increased bone alkaline phosphatase is observed after bone fractures, rising after 1 week and persisting for 6 to 12 weeks.

Changes in serum alkaline phosphatase occurring with neoplastic disease may be due to hepatic metastases, bone metastases, or direct contribution by neoplastic cells. Isoenzymes with physicochemical characteristics similar to the placental enzyme have been attributed to ectopic production by a variety of neoplasms. This group includes Regan's (carcinoplacental isoenzyme) and the variant Nagao's isoenzyme. These isoenzymes may be of value in monitoring cancer therapy.

A significant occurrence of clinically obscure elevations has been noted when multiphasic testing is applied to hospital populations. Because of the ubiquitous nature of alkaline phosphatase, increased serum activity may be caused by a wide variety of lesions involving multiple organs. Attempts to define organ source by isoenzyme study may be met with limited success due to technical limitations and the overlapping physicochemical characteristics of the various isoenzymes.

Evaluation of the relative tissue contributions to an elevation of total alkaline phosphatase should include the following:

1. Exclude physiologic or spurious causes. Was the assay performed on a freshly collected specimen?
2. Observe for the presence of clinical or biochemical clues to the origin of increased enzyme activity. Associated SGOT elevation suggests hepatic origin because significant SGOT does not exist in bone. Disproportionate elevation of LDH relative to SGOT suggests a nonhepatic origin or multi-organ system disease. The association of elevated LDH, hypercalcemia, and hyperuricemia suggests malignancy.
3. Is the elevation transient such as that observed in various tissue reparative processes or passive congestion of the liver? Transient elevations have also been reported with glucose hyperalimentation and uncontrolled diabetes mellitus.
4. Electrophoretic isoenzyme studies may distinguish bone and hepatobiliary origins. They may also identify an abnormal band. However, studies are often definitive only with dramatic elevations of total serum activity. The qualitative nature of the procedure limits its ability to determine relative tissue contributions in borderline elevations of alkaline phosphatase unless an abnormal band is present.
5. Measurement of other enzymes such as leucine aminopeptidase (LAP), 5'-nucleotidase, or gamma-glutamyl transferase (GGPT) may assist with identifying the hepatobiliary system as the source of elevated alkaline phosphatase. However, these enzymes also have different tissue distribution and specificity/

sensitivity characteristics for hepatobiliary disease; interpretation related to defining the source of an obscure alkaline phosphatase elevation is therefore limited.

Selected References

1. Massry SG, Coburn JW, Popoutzer MM, et al: Secondary hyperparathyroidism in chronic renal failure. *Arch Intern Med* 124:431–441, 1969.
2. Kaplan MM: Alkaline phosphatase. *Gastroenterology* 62:452–468, 1972.
3. Wolf PL: Clinical significance of an increased or decreased serum alkaline phosphatase level. *Arch Pathol Lab Med* 102:497–501, 1978.

230. Serum Bilirubin

DAVID H. VROON, MD
W. DALLAS HALL, MD

Definition

Bilirubin is a yellow compound with a molecular weight of 523. It is formed in the reticuloendothelial system as a breakdown product of heme. The concentration of total bilirubin in normal subjects does not usually exceed 1 mg/dl; however, values as high as 1.5–2.0 mg/dl are occasionally observed in the absence of disease. In normal subjects, virtually all serum bilirubin is in the unconjugated form. Conjugated serum bilirubin normally occurs in negligible amounts, if at all; stated normal ranges such as 0–0.5 mg/dl are more a reflection of analytical error than the actual presence of conjugated bilirubin. Jaundice, a yellow discoloration of the skin and mucous membranes, is usually evident when total serum bilirubin exceeds 2.5 mg/dl.

Technique

Bilirubin, a yellow pigment with an absorption peak at 460 nm, can be detected directly by spectrophotometric techniques; other yellow pigments (lipochromes, carotenoids, and medications) may interfere. Direct spectrophotometry is used only in neonates when other pigments can be ignored.

Most methods for determination of bilirubin are based on the diazo reaction in which bilirubin is reacted with diazotized sulfanilic acid to produce azobilirubin which acts as an indicator. Participation of unconjugated bilirubin in the reaction requires the addition of a solubilizing substance such as alcohol in the Malloy-Evelyn procedure or caffeine-sodium benzoate in the Jendrassik-Grof modification. This reaction is relatively specific for bilirubin; however, analytical errors are common due to inadequate standardization and specimen characteristics.

SMA systems use the preferred Jendrassik-Grof method; other automated or manual systems use this method or a modification of the Malloy-Evelyn procedure. Direct reacting or conjugated bilirubin is assayed in the absence of a solubilizing agent; total (conjugated plus unconjugated bilirubin) is determined in the presence of a solubilizing agent.

The qualitative detection of bilirubin in urine using either the Ictotest or dipstick is also based on the diazo reaction. Because unconjugated bilirubin is nonpolar and tightly bound to albumin, it is not filtered at the glomerulus. Conjugated bilirubin is only partially protein bound and is filtered and detectable in urine by the diazo reaction. Detectable bilirubinuria usually occurs at serum conjugated bilirubin levels of 1 mg/dl.

The reliability of bilirubin determinations is compromised by the lack of stable standards, particularly for conjugated bilirubin. Additional difficulty is encountered with hemolyzed specimens; hemoglobin, in addition to interfering spectrophotometrically, specifically suppresses the color intensity of azobilirubin and may cause spuriously low bilirubin levels (especially the conjugated fraction). Finally, bilirubin is an unstable compound which is readily oxidized to biliverdin which does not participate in the diazo reaction. Reliable determinations on biological specimens depend on immediate assay or adequate preservation, including protection from light.

Background Information

Knowledge of bilirubin metabolism is essential to understanding hepatic disease and the differential diagnosis of jaundice. A brief description of bilirubin metabolism is presented here. The student is referred to reference 2 for a more complete review.

Bilirubin is formed in the reticuloendothelial system by catabolism of heme-containing proteins, predominantly hemoglobin. Normal bilirubin load is derived primarily from senescent erythrocytes; as much as 20% is produced by catabolism of hemoglobin and other heme-containing proteins in the bone marrow. Bilirubin is tightly bound to albumin and transported in blood to the liver where it is dissociated from its protein carrier and transported from sinusoidal blood to the hepatocyte. Uptake by the hepatocyte depends on complex mechanisms that are not well defined.

In the hepatocyte, bilirubin is made soluble by conjugation with glucuronic acid, a process catalyzed by glucuronyl transferase. (The liver of newborns, particularly prematures, has a less than adequate glucuronyl transferase system for about two weeks.) Soluble or conjugated bilirubin is then excreted into the duodenum via bile; excretion is the rate-limiting step in eliminating bilirubin from the body. Intestinal bacteria enzymatically convert bilirubin to several related compounds collectively termed "urobilinogen." Approximately 10% of urobilinogen is reabsorbed into portal blood and reexcreted by the liver and then the kidney; the remainder is excreted in feces.

When bilirubin excretion is impaired, conjugated bilirubin is "regurgitated" into the bloodstream. Since conjugated bilirubin is polar and poorly reabsorbed following glomerular filtration, it is excreted (bilirubinuria) whenever plasma levels exceed 0.4–1.0 mg/dl and renal function is normal. When complete biliary obstruction occurs, renal excretion generally maintains the plasma total bilirubin level below 30–40 mg/dl, despite continued production.

Clinical Significance

Jaundice may result from an abnormality in any one of the steps involved in bilirubin metabolism, excretion, or both. Hemolysis results in excessive production of bilirubin, and if the production exceeds hepatic uptake, the levels of serum unconjugated bilirubin may reach 3–6 mg/dl. Unconjugated hyperbilirubinemia in the range of 1–6 mg/dl is usually due to some variety of hemolytic anemia or to defects in conjugation such as Gilbert's syndrome. Levels of unconjugated bilirubin above 6 mg/dl in adults are almost always associated with primary or complicating liver disease. However, the clinician must realize that patients may have active hemolytic anemia with normal levels of unconjugated bilirubin when the production rate is modest and liver function is good.

Hepatocellular diseases such as hepatitis or cirrhosis are commonly associated with impairment of both uptake and hepatic excretion of bilirubin; the ability to conjugate bilirubin may be relatively intact. Elevated levels of both conjugated and unconjugated bilirubin are present in the serum, and total bilirubin levels may become markedly elevated. The fraction of conjugated to total bilirubin does not usually help differentiate between extrahepatic cholestasis and intrahepatic cholestasis, since appreciable amounts of conjugated bilirubin are found in the plasma in both cases. The ability of a damaged liver to preserve bilirubin metabolism is remarkable. Serum bilirubin is therefore a relatively insensitive liver test. For instance, the majority of patients with hepatitis or cirrhosis have serum bilirubin levels that are within normal limits.

Complete extrahepatic biliary obstruction results in retention of conjugated bilirubin which is refluxed into the bloodstream, distributed throughout albumin-containing compartments, and excreted through the kidneys. However, partial obstruction of the extrahepatic bile ducts or obstruction of only a portion of the intrahepatic bile ducts can be readily compensated by the residual bile ducts. Significant intrahepatic or extrahepatic obstruction can therefore exist with normal serum bilirubin levels. Hyperbilirubinemia or jaundice occurs only when the degree of obstruction advances, when bilirubin production is accentuated by some other process, or when renal excretion becomes impaired.

Selected References

1. Schmid R: Bilirubin metabolism in man. *New Eng J Med* 287:703–709, 1972.
2. Dusol M, Schiff ER: Clinical approach to jaundice. *Postgrad Med* 57:118–124, 1975.

231. Uric Acid

W. DALLAS HALL, MD
DAVID H. VROON, MD

Definition

Uric acid is a weak organic acid end product of purine metabolism. It has a molecular weight of approximately 169 and a pKa of 5.75. The latter accounts for almost total ionization (98%) at the normal blood or joint pH of 7.40, where it exists primarily as a complex with sodium (monosodium urate) with a solubility near 120 mg/dl. In more acidic body fluids, such as urine, more of the uric acid form is nonionized and the solubility may be as low as 6 mg/dl. The ionized and nonionized forms of uric acid are shown in Fig 186.

A liberal normal range for uric acid in men is 4–8 mg/dl, but this varies widely with the method used and the population studied. Premenopausal women have levels approximately 1 mg/dl lower than men.

Technique

Uric acid is measured on protein-free filtrates of blood, urine, or body fluids by either colorimetric or enzymatic methods. Colorimetric techniques are commonly employed on SMA systems and depend on the ability of urate to reduce phosphotungstic acid to a detectable colored product, tungsten blue. This is a nonspecific reaction and is therefore subject to positive bias in the presence of other strong reducing substances. Artifactual elevations of uric acid measured by colorimetric methods are common and have been reported with marked hyperglycemia, serum salicylate levels above 13 mg/dl, ascorbic acid therapy, and excessive intake of xanthines. For a listing of over 200 compounds which may induce artifactual increases or decreases in serum uric acid, see reference 2. Uric acid results obtained by SMA colorimetric methodology are usually 1 mg/dl higher than the true serum uric acid concentration; bias may be significantly greater in the presence of an unusual specimen matrix occurring in some clinical states such as uremia.

Uric acid is specifically measured by enzymatic methods, such as employed on the Dupont ACA instrument. Uric acid is converted to allantoin and CO_2 by uricase and measured by differential absorbance at 293 nm:

$$\text{Uric Acid} + 2\ H_2O + O_2 \xrightarrow{\text{uricase}} \text{allantoin} + H_2O_2 + CO_2$$

Uric Acid $+ 2\ H_2O + O_2$ (absorbs at 293 nm) → allantoin $+ H_2O_2 + CO_2$ (nonabsorbing at 293 nm)

Enzymatic methods are highly specific but considerably more expensive due to reagent cost and the need for detection devices capable of

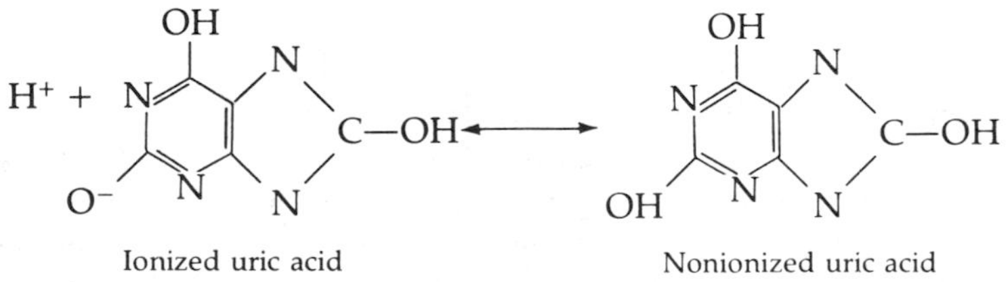

Ionized uric acid   Nonionized uric acid

Figure 186. Ionized and nonionized forms of uric acid.

reading in the ultraviolet range. Specific methods utilizing uricase are also available on SMA systems and are replacing the older colorimetric methods.

Background Information

Phosphoribosylpyrophosphate (PRPP), glutamine, glycine, and aspartic acid act as substrates for the formation of the parent purine, inosinic acid. Inosinic, adenylic, and guanylic acid react to form hypoxanthine with the assistance of key enzymes such as hypoxanthine-guanine phosphoribosyl transferase (HG-PRTase). Hypoxanthine is converted to xanthine then to uric acid with the assistance of another enzyme, xanthine oxidase. Hypoxanthine and xanthine are oxypurines.

The usual rate of production of uric acid is about 10 mg per day. The adult body pool is about 1,200 mg, distributed through approximately 50% of total body water. A small amount (1–2 mg/dl) of uric acid may be bound to serum globulins. Production of uric acid is increased in most clinical conditions associated with increased nucleic acid synthesis and breakdown.

Uric acid is removed from the body by two major routes: excretion through the kidney (75%) and bacterial uricase-mediated catabolism in the gut (25%). The kidneys filter uric acid at the glomerular level. Almost all of the glomerular filtrate is then proximally reabsorbed. Excretion of filtered uric acid is thus largely a function of subsequent proximal secretion plus some back diffusion into the tubular lumen.

Major regulatory factors acting to increase renal excretion of uric acid include volume expansion (such as with saline loading or osmotic diuresis) and vasoconstriction (such as with angiotensin or norepinephrine infusions). In contrast, volume contraction (as with dehydration or most diuretics) decreases excretion of uric acid. In addition, an important regulatory effect is exerted by the presence of many weak organic acids which are handled by the kidney in a fashion similar to uric acid. These acids may compete to either inhibit or enhance uric acid excretion according to whether they are present in high or low concentrations.

Examples of weak organic acids which typically inhibit renal uric acid excretion and result in a rise in serum uric acid include:

1. Ketoacids such as acetoacetic acid, beta-hydroxybutyric acid, and branch-chain isoleucine and leucine forms found in clinical ketosis due to diabetes, alcoholism, starvation, isopropyl alcohol intoxication, or maple syrup urine disease.
2. Lactic acid found in excessive amounts in clinical settings such as lactic acidosis, acute alcoholism, glucose-6-phosphatase deficiency, glycogen storage disease, and essential hypertension.

3. Acetylsalicylic acid in doses below approximately 2.5 gm per day.

Examples of weak organic acids which typically accelerate renal uric acid excretion ("uricosuric") and result in a fall in serum uric acid include:

1. Pyrazinoic acid (Pyrazinamide)
2. Propylsulfamyl benzoic acid (Benemid), a clinical uricosuric agent
3. Acetylsalicylic acid in doses above approximately 2.5 gm per day
4. Iopanoic acid (Telepaque), a dye for gallbladder studies
5. Mefenamic acid (Ponstel), an analgesic
6. Tienilic acid (Ticrynafen), a uricosuric diuretic

Clinical Significance

Even when uric acid is measured with a high degree of chemical specificity and statistical data defining the usually encountered values by age and sex are available, clinical interpretation is complicated by a variety of physiologic and pathophysiologic factors. An elevated uric acid level is a relatively common abnormality found on chemical profiles; in most cases it is a secondary rather than a primary disorder. Hyperuricemia may occur either when production exceeds the normal capacity for elimination, or when excretory routes are unable to eliminate even a normal uric acid load.

The following thought process may be helpful in the evaluation of hyperuricemia, eg, 11 mg/dl:

1. Is the value really 11 mg/dl, or does the patient have renal failure with retention of interfering chromogens such that the true uric acid determined by uricase methods may be 7–10 mg/dl? Is there any reason to suspect artifact from nonuric acid compounds retained in the serum of this particular patient? Have all of the patient's current medications been considered with regard to artifactual elevations?
2. Is there suppressed renal excretion of uric acid because of dehydration, thiazide diuretics, vasopressor substances, alcohol, or the presence of weak organic acids such as ketoacids, lactic acid, or low-dose acetylsalicylic acid?
3. Is there increased nucleic acid turnover and accelerated production of uric acid, such as with tissue trauma, acute leukemia, psoriasis, or malignancy?

In patients with acute illness, hyperuricemia is often transient and related to one or several of the above pathophysiologic mechanisms. Hyperuricemia may thus be treated by rehydration, clearing ketosis, and withholding alcohol, thiazides, or low-dose aspirin. Improvement of the underlying catabolic disorder can also be expected to improve the hyperuricemia.

More specific measures such as alkalinizing the urine and blocking uric acid production may be indicated to reduce the risk of renal failure if the course of patient therapy is projected to accelerate rather than reduce uric acid production. An example would be instituting chemotherapy for acute leukemia. Another example would be patients who have acute renal failure when there is clear evidence (urinary tract obstruction from urates, bladder full of uric acid crystals, and so forth) that the acute renal failure is related to hyperuricemia rather than other causes.

Chronic hyperuricemia is most often found in asymptomatic patients. These patients have an accelerated risk of developing an attack of gout within 4–12 years, but to date there is no convincing evidence that they are more likely than normouricemic patients to develop heart disease, uric acid stones, urinary tract infections, or deterioration of renal function. In patients with gout, however, the risk of stone formation is clearly greater with higher levels of urinary uric acid excretion, particularly above 900 mg per day.

Hyperuricemia is so common that it is of limited diagnostic value in the setting of acute arthritis. Although approximately 90% of patients with acute gout have hyperuricemia, so do about 25% of patients with acute nongouty arthritis. Special procedures such as joint x-rays and examination of the joint fluid crystals are more specific.

Hypouricemia (uric acid less than 2 mg/dl) is most often transiently noted in patients taking high-dose salicylates, receiving intravenous saline loads, or returning from a gallbladder series. Chronic hypouricemia may be seen in conjunction with a variety of systemic diseases. Hypouricemia may provide a clue to the presence of primary diseases such as proximal renal tubular disorders, Wilson's disease or hereditary xanthine oxidase deficiency.

Selected References

1.   Wyngaarden JB, Kelley WN: Gout, in Stanbury JB, Wyngaarden JB, Frederickson DS (eds): *The Metabolic Basis of Inherited Disease,* ed 4. New York, McGraw-Hill, 1978, pp 916–1010.
2.   Young DS, Pestaner LC, Gibberman V: Effects of drugs on clinical laboratory tests. *Clin Chem* 21:1–432, 1975.
3.   Steele TH, Oppenheimer S: Factors affecting urate excretion following diuretic administration in man. *Am J Med* 47:564–574, 1969.
4.   Goldfinger S, Klinenberg JR, Seegmiller JE: Renal retention of uric

acid induced by infusion of beta-hydroxybutyrate and acetoacetate. *N Eng J Med* 272:351–355, 1965.

5.	Yu TF, Sirota JH, Berger L, et al: Effect of sodium lactate infusion on urate clearance in man. *Proc Soc Exp Biol Med* 96:809–813, 1957.
6.	Fessel WJ, Siegelaub AB, Johnson ES: Correlates and consequences of asymptomatic hyperuricemia. *Arch Intern Med* 132:44–54, 1973.
7.	Liang MH, Fries JF: Asymptomatic hyperuricemia: The case for conservative management. *Ann Intern Med* 00:666 670, 1978.
8.	Dwosh JL, Roncari DAK, Marliss E, et al: Hypouricemia in disease: Study of different mechanisms. *J Lab Clin Med* 90:153–161, 1977.

232. Serum Creatinine

W. DALLAS HALL, MD
DAVID H. VROON, MD

Definition

Creatinine is a nitrogenous organic acid catabolite of muscle creatine. It has a molecular weight of 113, pKa of 4.7, and is distributed throughout total body water. The normal range is usually stated to be 0.5–1.4 mg/dl, but this varies widely with the individual's body muscle mass. For example, 1.3 mg/dl would likely be abnormal in a 3-year-old child or a 70-year-old woman, whereas 1.5 mg/dl would likely be normal for a muscular 25-year-old man. During third trimester pregnancy, the range of normal for serum creatinine is lower (0.4–1.0 mg/dl). The evaluation of borderline elevations of serum creatinine is accomplished by obtaining a creatinine clearance and correcting the results to 1.73 sq m.

Technique

Virtually all commonly used methods for creatinine determination are based on the reaction described by Jaffé in which creatinine reacts with picric acid in alkaline solution to produce an organ-red complex.

$$\text{Creatinine} + \text{picrate} \xrightarrow{\text{NaOH}} \text{red chromogen (absorbs at 510 nm)}$$

This reaction is nonspecific and is therefore susceptible to positive interference from noncreatinine, Jaffé-positive substances. The most notable interfering substances are acetone, acetoacetate, pyruvate, ascorbic acid, glucose, barbiturates, and protein, which produce side reactions with alkaline picrate and may result in artifactual increases in serum creatinine.

Several modifications of the Jaffé reaction are intended to reduce sources of error. SMA systems depend on dialysis to eliminate protein, protein-bound, and other larger noncreatinine chromogens; however, artifactual increases may still be observed in patients with ketoacidosis or in patients receiving high doses of ascorbic acid. Determination of urine creatinine is more accurate since noncreatinine chromogens occur at relatively low concentration. Kinetic variations, as utilized on the Dupont ACA, minimize interference by noncreatinine chromogens by differential reaction rates. Measurement of true creatinine is performed by manual methods that use Lloyd's reagent, an aluminum silicate which selectively absorbs creatinine prior to the Jaffé reaction.

Background Information

Creatine is formed in the liver and pancreas primarily from the reaction of arginine and glycine amino acid substrates with the enzyme arginine transamidinase. The formed creatine diffuses into the blood and is absorbed by muscle tissue where it is phosphorylated (ATP) to creatine phosphate, a reaction catalyzed by the enzyme creatine phosphokinase (CPK). Creatine phosphate and, to a lesser extent, creatine spontaneously decompose to creatinine at a rate of 1–2% per day. The formed creatinine is cleared by glomerular filtration into the tubules where, unlike urea, it is not reabsorbed. There is slight tubular secretion of creatinine into the urine and final excretion occurs at a relatively steady rate of 15–20 mg/kg per day.

The chemical reactions described are shown in Fig 187.

The creatinine clearance is a better indicator of glomerular filtration rate than is the serum creatinine level. This is particularly true in non-steady state circumstances such as acute renal failure when the serum creatinine may have risen to only 2–3 mg/dl yet the creatinine clearance is extremely low, often below 10 ml per minute per 1.73 sq m. However, timed urine collections are notoriously invalid because of imprecise timing, inexact measurements of urine volume, missed voidings, or spillage. It thus behooves the clinician to make clinical decisions from the creatinine clearance only when he is assured of adequacy of the sample. Two methods can be used to improve the adequacy and reliability of the sample. One method is to collect short-term samples when the patient is known to have voided at a certain time (such as 4:17 PM) and all urine is collected until the next voiding four or more hours later (such as 9:28 PM, or 5 hours and 11 minutes, or 311 minutes). The second method is a calculation of total 24-hour urinary creatinine content:

$$\text{mg/dl urinary creatinine} \times \frac{\text{ml urine}}{100} \times \frac{1{,}440 \text{ minutes}}{\text{minutes of collection,}}$$

divided by the patient's weight in kilograms. This is known as the creatinine coefficient. Creatinine coefficients below 10 mg/kg (in the absence of acute renal failure) indicate invalid urine collections and tell the clinician that the calculated creatinine clearance will be artifactually low. A normal creatinine clearance is generally above 80 ml per minute per 1.73 sq m. Examples of calculating the creatinine coefficient and creatinine clearance are given below:

	Example A	Example B
Time	1,440 minutes (24 hours)	311 minutes
Urine volume	2,000 ml	216 ml
Urine creatinine	90 mg/dl	75 mg/dl
Serum creatinine	2.0 mg/dl	1.0 mg/dl
Weight	100 kg	50 kg
Surface Area	2.20 sq m	1.10 sq m

Creatinine coefficient

$$90 \times \frac{2{,}000}{100} \times \frac{1{,}440}{1{,}440} \times \frac{1}{100} \qquad 75 \times \frac{216}{100} \times \frac{1{,}440}{311} \times \frac{1}{50}$$
$$= 18 \text{ mg/kg/day} \qquad\qquad = 15 \text{ mg/kg/day}$$

Creatinine clearance

$$\frac{90}{2.0} \times \frac{2{,}000}{1{,}440} \qquad\qquad \frac{75}{1.6} \times \frac{216}{311}$$
$$= 62.5 \text{ ml/min} \qquad\qquad = 32.6 \text{ ml/min}$$

Creatinine clearance/1.73 sq m

$$\frac{2.20}{1.73} = \frac{62.5}{x} \qquad\qquad \frac{1.10}{1.73} = \frac{32.6}{x}$$

where x = 49.2 ml/min/1.73 sq m   where x = 51.3 ml/min/1.73 sq m

Clinical Significance

The level of serum creatinine is an excellent screening test of renal function. Creatinine levels, however, may remain within the range of normal limits in patients with only one kidney (agenesis, transplant donor), particularly if there is compensatory hypertrophy of the remaining normal kidney. This implies that at least a 50% reduction in renal function must occur before the level of serum creatinine rises above the usual normal range. Since creatinine levels reflect glomerular filtration of creatinine, pa-

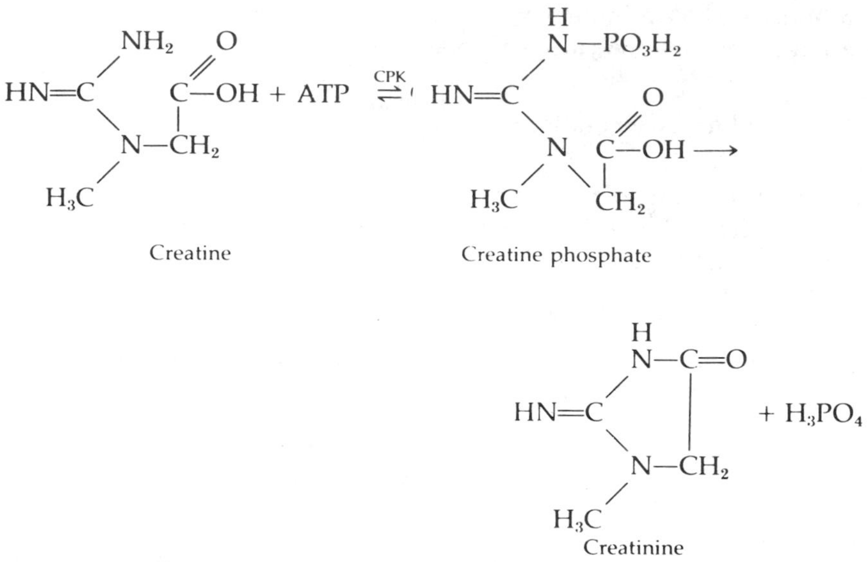

Figure 187.   The production of creatinine.

tients may have normal levels despite clinically significant tubular or interstitial disease (pyelonephritis, renal tubular acidosis).

Creatinine levels are more valuable than BUN levels for assessment of the severity of renal disease. This is because dietary and physiological parameters alter the BUN but have minimal effects on the creatinine. For example, dehydration or low cardiac output states will usually be associated with some decrease in glomerular filtration rate but marked increases in the rate of urea reabsorption. The consequence is that serum creatinine may rise to the 1.5–3 mg/dl range, whereas the BUN in these same circumstances may rise above 100 mg/dl. Creatinine levels above 3 mg/dl are only rarely caused by prerenal factors alone, and in such cases, the clinician is obligated to establish the integrity of parenchymal renal function. Data that help establish the integrity of parenchymal renal function would include a normal urinalysis, negative urine culture, and an ability of the tubules to conserve sodium and concentrate the urine to at least 1.020 specific gravity or 700 mOsm/liter.

In patients with known kidney disease, creatinine levels chronically in the range of 2.5–4.9 mg/dl imply severe reduction in renal function; levels 5–9.9 mg/dl imply extremely severe renal disease, and levels above 10 mg/dl (or creatinine clearances below 5 ml per minute per 1.73 sqm) usually mean it is time (or past time) to evaluate the patient for chronic replacement therapy in the form of chronic dialysis or kidney transplantation.

Selected References

1. Doolan PD, Alpen EL, Theil GB: A clinical appraisal of the plasma concentration and endogenous clearance of creatinine. *Am J Med* 32:65–79, 1962.
2. Henry JB: *Clinical Chemistry: Clinical Diagnosis by Laboratory Methods.* Philadelphia, WB Saunders, 1974.
3. Brøchner-Mortensen J, Jensen S, Rodbro P. Assessment of renal func tion from plasma creatinine in adult patients. *Scand J Urol Nephrol* 11:263–270, 1977.

233. Serum Calcium

JAMES O. WELLS, JR., MD
W. DALLAS HALL, MD
DAVID H. VROON, MD

Definition

Calcium is a divalent cation with an atomic weight of 40. Serum calcium is normally maintained within a narrow range approximately 8.5–10.8 mg/dl, but the limits of normal for different methods and populations can vary as much as 0.5 mg/dl. Since calcium is divalent (valence of 2), a total serum calcium level of 10 mg/dl represents 2.5 mM/liter or 5 mEq/liter.

Technique

Serum is the preferred specimen for determination of calcium since most plasma anticoagulants are chelating agents which result in spuriously low values. Samples should be collected in the fasting and resting state without prolonged venous stasis since hemoconcentration elevates the protein-bound fraction.

Total calcium is most commonly measured colorimetrically on SMA and other automated or manual systems. Cresolphthalein complexone, a metal complexing dye, forms a purple complex with calcium in alkaline solution. Magnesium and other heavy metal interferences are minimized by the addition of 8-hydroxy-quinoline and potassium cyanide. Protein-bound calcium is released by acidification of the serum sample prior to reaction:

$$Ca^{2+} + CPC \qquad \text{Ca-CPC complex (absorbs at 570 nm)}$$
$$Mg^{2+} + \text{8-quinolinol} \qquad \text{Mg-quinolinate (nonabsorbing at 570 nm)}$$

Atomic absorption spectrophotometry is the reference method for serum calcium determinations. It provides greater chemical specificity but is not routinely employed due to technical considerations and the lack of automation. The colorimetric SMA method provides adequate chemical specificity with the usually encountered specimen matrix characteristics; however, day-to-day precision may be as high as 6% (95% confidence limits). This implies that the 95% confidence limits for an isolated calcium measurement of 10.0 mg/dl are 9.4 and 10.6 mg/dl, a range which spans more than 50% of the usual normal range (8.5–10.8 mg/dl). Confidence limits can be improved by repetitive determinations with the coefficient of variation inversely related to the square root of the number of repetitions. For example, when the average of four determinations is 10 mg/dl, the coefficient of variation is decreased to 1.5% and the result can be interpreted with 95% confidence that the true calcium is between 9.7 and 10.3 mg/dl.

Background Information

Total serum calcium exists in three physiochemical states:

1. Ionized ("free"). This is the only physiologically active form of serum calcium and represents approximately 60% of the normal total serum calcium level. It also forms the vast majority of the ultrafiltrable calcium, the remainder consisting of complexed calcium.

2. Protein-bound ("nondiffusable," "nonfiltrable"). This fraction represents approximately 40% of the normal total serum calcium level. The calcium is reversibly bound predominantly to albumin (80%) and to various globulins (20%). This fraction is poorly diffusible, not ultrafiltrable, and absent from most interstitial fluids unless considerable amounts of protein are present such as in lymph.

3. Complex-bound ("complexed"). This fraction represents approximately 6% of the normal serum calcium and is usually less than 1 mg/dl. It is the portion of ionized calcium which has formed relatively soluble (and ultrafiltrable) complexes with circulating anions, depending on the relative concentration of the anion and the pH of the serum. This calcium fraction is complexed primarily with bicarbonate, citrate, and phosphate,

respectively; significant binding to anionic sulfate may also occur with sulfate retention in chronic renal failure.

Because only the ionized or free form is physiologically active and controlled, significant changes in total measured calcium may occur with variations in protein concentration in the absence of disordered calcium homeostasis. Techniques for specifically measuring ionized calcium are currently available but not widely used because of the requirements for expensive instrumentation and rapid analysis of anaerobic specimens. Consequently, a variety of formulas are available for correcting total calcium or for estimating ionized calcium. The most commonly used formula corrects the measured calcium to a normal albumin concentration (4.0 gm/dl) assuming a normal in vivo pH and an average binding coefficient:

Corrected serum calcium
$$= 0.7(4.0 - \text{measured albumin}) + \text{measured calcium}$$

Interpretation of total calcium levels is often misleading unless allowance is made for protein concentration. Formulas which use total protein to estimate ionized calcium are less reliable, particularly in hypoalbuminemic states, which are often associated with hyperglobulinemia. It should be emphasized that calculated values for "ionized calcium" are important as a screening procedure, but are not a substitute for direct measurement of ionized calcium when clinically indicated.

Approximately 99% of total body calcium is contained within the mineralization collagen matrix of bone as an insoluble salt of phosphate and, to a lesser degree, carbonate; a small fraction of this bone calcium is in equilibrium with the extracellular fluid. Bone crystal lattice formation is usually in the form of hydroxyapatite (calcium phosphate combined with calcium hydroxide) with lesser amounts of apatite (calcium phosphate combined with fluoride) and a relatively small amount of calcium carbonate. The concentration of calcium within tissues other than bone is very small; for example, erythrocytes contain almost no calcium.

Extracellular fluid calcium is predominantly regulated by three factors: flux between bone and plasma calcium, variable absorption of calcium from the small intestine, and reabsorption of filtered calcium by the kidney. These three processes are regulated mainly by parathyroid hormone (PTH), thyrocalcitonin (TCT), and vitamin D as indicated in Fig 188.

PTH release is stimulated by a fall in ionized calcium and suppressed by a rise in ionized calcium; it activates adenylcyclase in kidney and bone cells. The major clinical effects of PTH are to accelerate calcium and phosphate release from bone, decrease renal phosphate reabsorption, increase renal calcium reabsorption and assist the kidney in conversion of 25-HCC to the more active vitamin D metabolite (1,25-DHCC) capable of increasing small intestine transport of calcium. The net effect of administration of PTH is to elevate serum calcium and reduce serum phosphate levels.

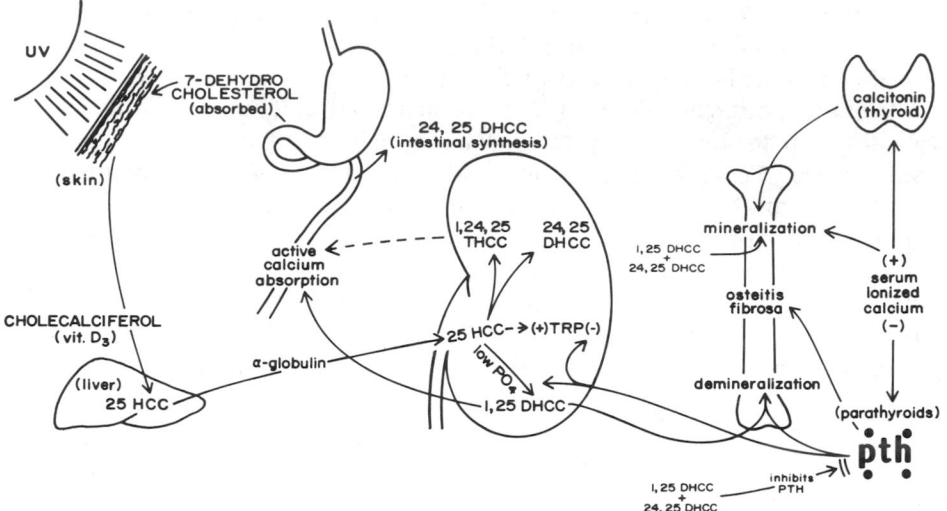

Figure 188. Regulation of calcium balance by parathyroid hormone (PTH), thyrocalcitonin (TCT), and vitamin D metabolites.

Thyrocalcitonin release is stimulated by a rise in ionized calcium; it is suppressed by a fall in ionized calcium. The major effect of TCT is to inhibit bone mobilization of calcium; additional effects include enhancement of renal phosphate excretion and stimulation of gastrin and gastric acid secretion. The net effect of administration of TCT is to reduce both serum calcium and serum phosphate levels.

7-Dehydrocholesterol (DHC) is a substrate for vitamin D synthesis. DHC is activated in skin by ultraviolet light where it is converted to cholecalciferol (CC), known as vitamin D_3. The liver hydroxylates CC to 25-HCC which is carried to the kidney by an alpha-globulin transport protein. 25-HCC undergoes 1-hydroxylation (to 1,25 DHCC) exclusively in the kidney, a reaction which occurs in direct proportion to the level of PTH and (to a lesser extent) in inverse proportion to the cellular phosphate content. 1,25-DHCC elevates calcium in two ways: (1) it stimulates the synthesis of calcium-binding protein in the small intestine, thus causing an increase in active intestinal transport of calcium, and (2) it exerts a permissive effect on the action of PTH to mobilize bone calcium. In large quantities, it may independently mobilize bone calcium and phosphate. The roles of other less potent metabolites of vitamin D are not yet clearly defined. 1,24,25-THCC appears to increase gut calcium absorption and to have no action on bone; it may be a metabolite of 1,25-DHCC. 24,25-DHCC is abundant in anephric serum, is synthesized in the intestine as well as the kidney, and appears to be required along with 1,25-DHCC to recalcify demineralized bone in uremic patients and to inhibit parathyroid hormone release. Vitamin D does not exert an appreciable influence on renal phosphate handling, although 25-DHCC has been demonstrated to increase phosphate reabsorption in experimental animals.

Several vitamin D preparations are commercially available. Ergocalciferol (vitamin D_2) must be activated in the liver and kidney prior to any effect on intestinal calcium transport; it has a very slow onset of action and a half-life of approximately 40 days. Dihydrotachysterol (Hytakerol) has a more rapid onset of action with a therapeutic effect usually apparent within 10–14 days; it has a hydroxyl group at the 3 position which, because of its steric configuration, may confer an action similar to but weaker than 1,25-DHCC. Calcitrol (Rocaltrol) is the synthetic form of 1,25-DHCC; it is very potent with an onset of action within 1–2 days.

Calcium is a very important extracellular fluid cation since it reduces the permeability of biological membranes and inhibits key enzymes concerned with intermediate metabolism and various types of ionic transport. These properties may account for the necessity of ionized calcium for muscle contraction, nerve conduction, pancreatic insulin release, and gastric H^+ secretion.

Clinical Significance

Hypercalcemia occurs in a variety of disorders. A partial list of etiologies illustrates various pathophysiologies.

1. Excessive bone resorption due to PTH (primary hyperparathyroidism) or PTH-like substances (some nonmetastatic malignancies)
2. Excessive nonhormonal bone demineralization (metastatic bone lesions, Paget's disease)
3. Excessive intestinal calcium reabsorption (sarcoidosis, milk-alkali, vitamin D intoxication)
4. Excessive exogenous calcium infusion (high calcium hemodialysis)
5. Excessive serum protein concentrations (artifacts and some dysproteinemias)
6. Excessive renal calcium reabsorption (thiazide-induced, possibly volume contraction)

Extremely high levels of ionized calcium are particularly dangerous because of the risk of psychosis or coma, subacute renal failure, nephrocalcinosis, muscle ischemic necrosis, or enhanced arrhythmogenic potential of digitalis. Moderately elevated levels often produce nausea, arthralgias, or subtle organic confusion; underlying hypertension may be aggravated because of a direct effect of calcium to increase vascular tone.

Borderline or intermittently elevated levels of calcium in a relatively asymptomatic patient create a classic management dilemma in medicine. On the one hand, normocalcemic or intermittently hypercalcemic primary hyperparathyroidism is well documented. On the other hand, there are innumerable factors that may cause true or artifactually small and transient elevations in the measured calcium level. Consider the following factors in evaluating borderline elevations of serum calcium:

1. Common methods of determining total serum calcium are imprecise relative to the range observed in normal individuals; additional significant changes occur with variation in serum protein concentration.

2. Tourniquet-induced venous stasis for two minutes causes a rise in plasma proteins and an increment of up to 1 mg/dl in measured total calcium. This is best suspected when there is a relatively high level of serum albumin. Serum albumin levels of 5 gm/dl or greater are frequently associated with "hypercalcemia."

3. Total calcium levels are transiently increased by 0.2–0.4 mg/dl following a meal. Borderline elevated nonfasting calcium levels should be repeated in the fasting state. The difference may be likened to "random" versus "fasting" plasma glucose elevations, though in a more subtle sense.

4. Vigorous hyperventilation or exercise may raise the total calcium level an average of 0.4 and 0.6 mg/dl, respectively.

5. Hypercalcemia may be noted in approximately 2% of patients receiving thiazide diuretics. The cause of the hypercalcemia may either be entirely related to the thiazides or may be caused by an underlying disorder that becomes apparent or is unmasked during thiazide therapy. Several possible mechanisms may be responsible. First, thiazides reduce plasma volume such that weight loss and modest elevations in the serum albumin level may be associated with mild transient and reversible rises (below 12 mg/dl range) in the serum calcium level. Thiazides also enhance renal calcium reabsorption which accounts for their benefit in the treatment of idiopathic hypercalciuria; they may also enhance the action of PTH in bone calcium mobilization. In contrast, furosemide accelerates urine calcium loss. Hypercalcemia due solely to thiazide diuretics should be associated with normal or low levels of PTH relative to the serum calcium level. In the absence of other causes of hypercalcemia, the serum calcium level should return to within the normal range upon discontinuation of the thiazide diuretic with or without substitution of furosemide. Causes of hypercalcemia such as primary hyperparathyroidism should be suspected if the PTH level is inappropriately elevated during thiazide-induced hypercalcemia or if elevated calcium levels persist four weeks or more after discontinuing thiazide diuretics.

Decreased total calcium (hypocalcemia) is often of no direct consequence since it is usually associated with a decreased level of albumin with no decrease in the physiologically active ionized calcium fraction.

The total calcium level of a hypoalbuminemic patient can be best interpreted by adding approximately 0.7 mg/dl for each 1 gm/dl reduction in albumin below 4 according to the formula given under Background Information. It should be reiterated that these types of calculations are highly dependent on many patient variables and are no substitute for direct measurement of the actual level of serum ionized calcium.

The most striking manifestations of true hypocalcemia are tingling and tetany (occasionally seizures). These occur because nerve and muscle condition and contraction are no longer under the usual inhibitory effect of ionized calcium. Myocardial contractility and digitalis effect may be reduced in the presence of low levels of serum ionized calcium. Marked hypocalcemia is sometimes asymptomatic until symptoms are precipitated by alkalinization such as with intravenous bicarbonate therapy or during hyperventilation (eg, atelectasis or pulmonary emboli following subtotal parathyroidectomy). The effect of alkalinization is to reduce the ionized component of the total calcium concentration.

True hypocalcemia is most commonly noted in chronic renal failure, in primary forms of hypoparathyroidism, or transiently following parathyroidectomy. Less frequent causes include severe magnesium deficiency (with suppressed release of PTH), pseudohypoparathyroidism, malabsorption, massive muscle necrosis with tissue calcium deposition, metastatic osteoblastic bone lesions, chronic anticonvulsant therapy, and thyrocalcitonin excess from medullary thyroid or other carcinomas.

Selected References

1. McLean F, Hastings AB: The state of calcium in the fluids of the body. I, The conditions affecting the ionization of calcium. *J Biol Chem* 108:285–322, 1935.
2. Boonstra CE, Jackson CE: Hyperparathyroidism detected by routine serum calcium analysis. *Ann Intern Med* 63:468–474, 1965.
3. Wills MR, Pak CYC, Hammond WG, et al: Normocalcemic primary hyperparathyroidism. *Am J Med* 47:384–391, 1969.
4. DeLuca HF: The kidney as an endocrine organ for the production of 1,25-dihydroxyvitamin D_3, a calcium-mobilizing hormone. *N Eng J Med* 289:359–365, 1973.
5. Christensson T, Hellström K, Wengle B: Hypercalcemia and primary hyperparathyroidism: Prevalence in patients receiving thiazides as detected in a health screen. *Arch Intern Med* 137:1138–1142, 1977.
6. Boris A: Structure-activity relationships of vitamin D analogues. *Am J Med* 62:543–544, 1977.
7. DeLuca HF: The kidney as an endocrine organ involved in the function of vitamin D. *Am J Med* 58:39–47, 1975.

8. David DS: Clinical studies of vitamin D analogues in renal failure. *Am J Med* 62:544–546, 1977.
9. Payne RB, Carven ME, Morgan DB: Interpretation of serum total calcium: Effects of adjustment for albumin concentration on frequency of abnormal values and on detection of change in the individual. *J Clin Pathol* 32:56–60, 1979.

234. Serum Inorganic Phosphate

W. DALLAS HALL, MD
DAVID H. VROON, MD

Definition

The total blood phosphorus consists of phospholipids, inorganic phosphates, and organic phosphates. Virtually all inorganic phosphate occurs in the extracellular fluid. The intracellular content of total phosphorus greatly exceeds the extracellular phosphorus content because of the high intracellular concentration of organic phosphates and phospholipids. In fact, organic phosphates are the predominant intracellular anions in the body (100 mM/liter cell water). For clinical purposes, only the inorganic phosphate fraction is measured in the usual clinical chemistry request.

Serum inorganic phosphorus refers to ionized HPO_4^{--} and $H_2PO_4^{-}$ and does not include the previously mentioned and more abundant organic phosphate esters. At the serum pH of 7.4, the equilibrium ratio of $HPO_4^{--}:H_2PO_4^{-}$ is about 4:1. Both forms contribute to the serum total inorganic phosphorus measurement; the concentration of free PO_4^{---} ion and of phosphoric acid (H_3PO_4) in serum is negligible. Unlike calcium, inorganic phosphate is minimally (10–20%) protein bound.

Normal adult levels are approximately 2.5–4.5 mg/dl. Higher levels are characteristic of newborns and periods of active growth such as puberty. Serum levels expressed in milligrams per deciliter can be converted to millimoles per liter by multiplying by 0.323. Concentration expressed as milliequivalents per liter will depend on pH but will be approximately 0.5 times the concentration in milligrams per deciliter.

Technique

A variety of colorimetric methods are used to measure inorganic phosphorus in serum; these methods depend on the formation and selective reduction of phosphomolybdic acid to molybdenum blue by a suitable reducing agent:

$$\text{acid pH}$$

$$PO_4^{---} + MoO_4^{--} \xrightarrow{\hspace{3cm}} \text{phosphomolybdate}$$
$$\text{(molybdate)}$$

$$\text{Phosphomolybdate} + \text{stannous chloride} \xrightarrow{\hspace{2cm}} \text{molybdenum blue}$$
$$\text{(reducing agent)} \qquad\qquad \text{(absorbs at 660 nm)}$$

Prolonged exposure of serum to cells prior to analysis may result in esterification of inorganic to organic phosphate; conversely, cellular leakage with serum enrichment by organic phosphates and subsequent hydrolysis may cause positive errors. Prompt separation of serum and avoidance of hemolysis are mandatory prerequisites to reliable inorganic phosphate determinations. Serum inorganic phosphate may be lowered after high-carbohydrate meals or increased after high-protein meals. The level of serum phosphate has diurnal variation, and serum samples are optimally collected in the morning after an overnight fast.

Background Information

Extracellular inorganic phosphate is necessary as a supply system for synthesis of nucleotides, phospholipids, and high-energy phosphates such as adenosine triphosphate (ATP). ATP is formed in the red cell chiefly by glycolysis from glucose, inorganic phosphate, and adenosine diphosphate (ADP). ATP is continually utilized for energy-requiring processes such as the sodium-potassium pump, resulting in the formation of ADP and liberation of inorganic phosphate. When the rate of glycolysis exceeds energy demands, eg, glucose loading during a glucose tolerance test, serum inorganic phosphate is decreased. When the in vivo rate of glycolysis is decreased and energy demands persist, inorganic phosphate increases. Concentrations of red cell ATP and 2,3-diphosphoglycerate (2,3-DPG) are often depressed whenever serum inorganic phosphate is below 1 mg/dl.

The influence of pH on glycolysis is partially responsible for the increased levels of phosphate seen in acidosis and the decreased levels of phosphate seen in alkalosis. Acidosis tends to slow glycolysis and raise serum phosphate levels; alkalosis tends to accelerate glycolysis and lower serum phosphate levels. For example, hyperphosphatemia commonly accompanies lactic acidosis.

The serum phosphate level is not a primary regulator of parathyroid hormone (PTH) synthesis or release except as changes in serum phosphate may indirectly alter the level of ionized calcium. Phosphate is a necessary ingredient of bone matrix.

Clinical Significance

Elevated levels of serum phosphate are most commonly encountered in chronic renal failure when glomerular filtration rate (creatinine clearance) is reduced below 25 ml per minute and elevated levels of PTH can no longer induce enough extra urinary phosphate excretion ("phosphaturia") to maintain the serum phosphate levels in the normal range. High levels of phosphate also complex and reduce the serum ionized calcium such that PTH is further stimulated, a positive feedback loop is created, and bone disease worsens. In addition, a chronically elevated calcium and phosphorus product ($Ca \times PO_4$) above 60–80 may be associated with vascular, muscle, myocardial, or kidney deposits of calcium phosphate. These deposits interfere with normal tissue physiology and metabolism and can result in gangrene, myopathy, heart block, or progressive renal failure. They may, however, be resolved to a considerable extent if the ion product is reduced. Phosphate levels above 5 mg/dl in patients with chronic renal failure are thus usually treated with phosphate-binding antacids, reduction in phosphate intake, or both.

Elevated phosphate levels may also result from muscle necrosis; for instance, a rise in phosphate disproportionate to blood urea nitrogen was used in the Korean War as a clue to devitalized muscle and the need for tissue debridement. Increased phosphate levels are also typical of hypoparathyroidism, are indicative of disease activity in acromegaly, and are commonly found in assorted acidotic states.

Low levels of serum phosphate occur in over 50% of cases of primary hyperparathyroidism but are more commonly seen in conjunction with intravenous glucose therapy, acute alcoholism or cirrhosis, gram-negative septicemia, chronic antacid therapy, and in association with various causes of respiratory alkalosis and, to a lesser degree, metabolic alkalosis. Low levels may also be noted in renal phosphate-wasting disorders (vitamin D–resistant rickets, Fanconi syndromes).

Phosphate levels below 1.5 mg/dl are generally considered undesirable because of the following considerations:

1.   Bone pain and osteomalacia (unmineralized bone matrix) with fractures can result from chronic phosphate depletion.
2.   A phosphate-depletion syndrome of marked weakness and debility has been described and may be associated with depletion of ATP as an energy source.

3. Severe phosphate depletion may be associated with depletion of red cell ATP and acquired hemolytic anemia.
4. Articular manifestations mimicking ankylosing spondylitis have been described with chronic phosphate depletion.
5. Reversible neurological disturbances such as ballismus, electroencephalographic abnormalities, and possible psychological derangements have been noted with phosphate depletion.
6. Hypophosphatemia has been reported to cause increased myocardial stroke work; contractile force improved following phosphate repletion. Darsee and Nutter noted three cases of cardiomyopathy which reversed after correction of severe hypophosphatemia.

Selected References

1. Betro MG, Pain RW: Hypophosphatemia and hyperphosphatemia in a hospital population. *Br Med J* 1:273–275, 1972.
2. Knochel JP: The pathophysiology and clinical characteristics of severe hypophosphatemia. *Arch Intern Med* 137:203–220, 1977.
3. Fitzgerald F: Clinical hypophosphatemia. *Ann Rev Med* 29:177–189, 1978.
4. Territo MC, Tanaka KR: Hypophosphatemia in chronic alcoholism. *Arch Intern Med* 134:445–447, 1974.
5. Lotz M, Zisman E, Bartter FC: Evidence for a phosphorus-depletion syndrome in man. *N Eng J Med* 278:409–415, 1968.
6. Mostellar ME, Tuttle EP Jr: Effects of alkalosis on plasma concentration and urinary excretion of inorganic phosphate in man. *J Clin Invest* 43:138–149, 1964.
7. Moser CR, Fessel WJ: Rheumatic manifestations of hypophosphatemia. *Arch Intern Med* 134:674–678, 1974.
8. Lotz M, Ney R, Bartter FC: Osteomalacia and debility resulting from phosphorus depletion. *Trans Assoc Am Physicians* 77:281–295, 1964.
9. O'Connor LR, Wheeler WS, Bethune JE: Effect of hypophosphatemia on myocardial performance in man. *N Eng J Med* 297:901–903, 1977.
10. Darsee JR, Nutter DO: Reversible severe congestive cardiomyopathy in three cases of hypophosphatemia. *Ann Intern Med* 89:867–870, 1978.

235. Cholesterol

MARIO DIGIROLAMO, MD

Definition

Cholesterol and triglycerides are lipids normally found in human blood in association with the plasma lipoproteins. Table 49 shows ranges of plasma cholesterol and triglyceride which may be considered desirable, borderline abnormal, and definitely abnormal in adults. This arbitrary classification into three subgroups may not adequately represent the continuity of the association between plasma lipid levels and the atherogenic risk, but it provides practical ways of separating the normal from the abnormal levels for diagnostic and therapeutic purposes.

Technique

Blood should be collected in the morning after an overnight fast with abstention from alcohol for at least 24 and preferably 48 hours. Patients should have a steady weight (ie, not on weight-reducing diets) and be free of stresses such as acute infection or myocardial infarction. Either serum or plasma can be collected and analyzed for cholesterol and triglycerides. Serum is preferred since various anticoagulants (with the exception of heparin) produce artificial lowering of both cholesterol and triglyceride levels (versine up to 4%, oxalate up to 9%, citrate up to 14%, and fluoride up to 18%). The standard reference method for cholesterol determination is the manual Abell-Kendall method, which can be semi-

Table 49. Plasma lipid levels (mg/dl).

	Desirable	Borderline Abnormal	Abnormal
Cholesterol	<200	200–280	>280
Triglyceride	<100	100–200	>200

automated. An enzymatic method using cholesterol-oxidase is available and appears reliable, although earlier problems existed with enzyme stability and impurities. Completely automated methods, such as the SMA, give less accurate results and are subject to a number of limitations; the imprecision of these automated methods, however, does not substantially affect utility of the cholesterol value for clinical judgment. Triglyceride concentration is usually measured by an enzymatic determination of glycerol after hydrolysis of the triglyceride. Serum cholesterol values exceeding 240 mg/dl or triglyceride values exceeding 150 mg/dl for a repeated determination within two to three weeks. If the hypercholesterolemia or hypertriglyceridemia is confirmed, request lipoprotein electrophoresis.

A simple additional test which can be run at the bedside is the so-called chylomicron test (see Fig 189). When the plasma from a fasting patient is stored in the refrigerator at 4°C for 12 hours, its appearance can provide clues to the underlying lipid and lipoprotein abnormality. A clear appearance can represent normal or a type II hyperlipoproteinemia; a creamy layer with clear infranatant is typical of type I; a cloudy plasma throughout is typical of type IV; a creamy layer and cloudy infranatant is seen in types III and V. The creamy layer derives from chylomicra; the cloudy or milky appearance, from triglycerides. Cholesterol produces no turbidity.

Background Information

The plasma lipids consist mainly of cholesterol, triglyceride, phospholipid, and free fatty acids. They are insoluble in water and therefore require a vehicle or carrier to circulate from one tissue to another. These vehicles, the lipoproteins, are compounds formed of a protein and a lipid component. The four major classes of lipoprotein are chylomicra, very low-density lipoproteins (VLDL or pre-beta), low-density lipoproteins (LDL or beta), and high-density lipoproteins (HDL or alpha). A fifth class is occasionally referred to as the free fatty acid–albumin complex. Each of the four major lipoprotein classes contains varying proportions of cholesterol, triglyceride, phospholipid, and protein. Indeed, the different chemical and physical structures of these protein-lipid aggregates allow separation of the different classes on the basis of lipoprotein density by ultracentrifugation and on the basis of different molecular charges by paper or agarose-gel electrophoresis. Since all four lipoproteins contain cholesterol, triglyceride, and phospholipid, an increase in total cholesterol or triglycerides above normal limits could derive from the increase in concentration of one or more of the lipoproteins. A marked hypercholesterolemia would derive more readily from an elevation of the LDL (beta-lipoprotein) since it is the richest in cholesterol.

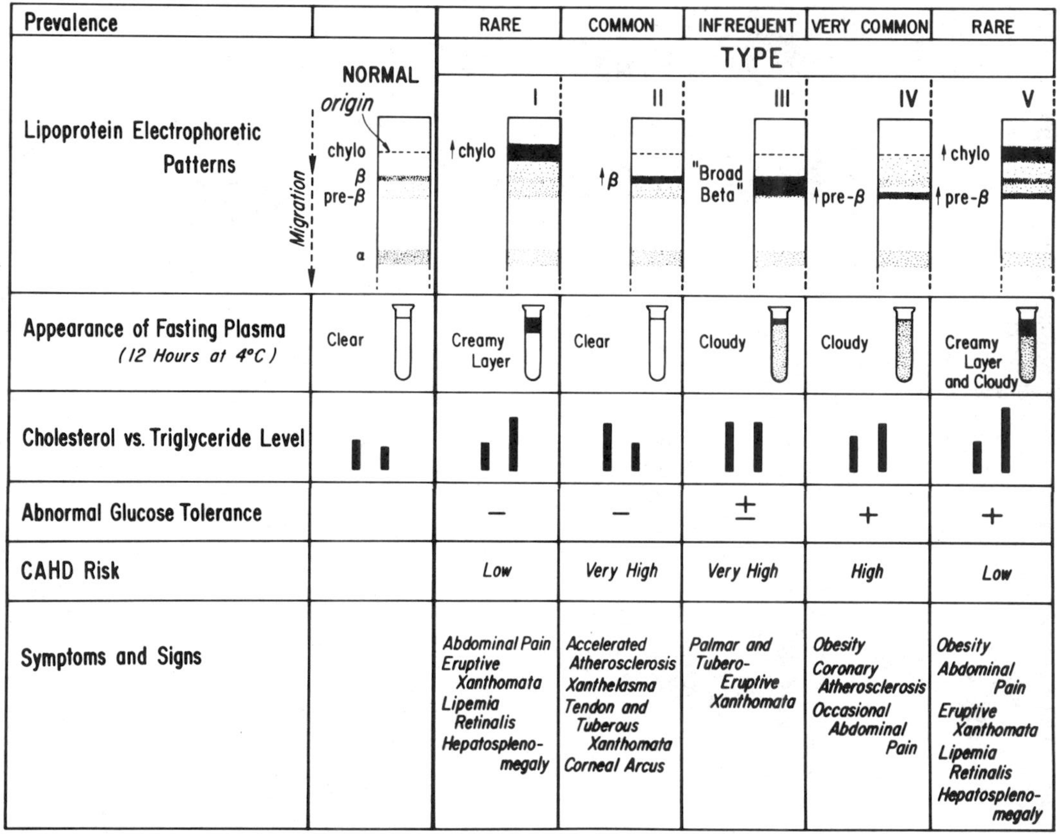

Figure 189.   Some clinical and laboratory characteristics of the five major types of hyperlipoproteinemia.

Recent studies have clarified the origin, metabolism, and fate of the lipoproteins. Thus, the classification of a lipid disorder in terms of the specific abnormal lipoprotein type provides useful clues to the pathophysiology, prognosis, and therapy of the underlying metabolic disorder. Fig 189 shows some clinical and laboratory aspects of the five major types of hyperlipoproteinemias.

The chylomicron is a lipoprotein of intestinal origin. Following hydrolysis and absorption of dietary lipid, chylomicra originate from reconstituted triglyceride of dietary origin and small proportions of cholesterol, phospholipid, and protein. Chylomicra impart a visible milky or lactescent hue to the plasma for one to five hours following a meal. This occurs as soon as they reach the peripheral circulation via the lymphatic system and thoracic duct. Chylomicra carry the exogenous triglycerides and are acted upon by a group of enzymes called lipoprotein lipase (LPL). Lipoprotein lipase, which can be activated by heparin, dissociates the triglyceride from the chylomicra. The resulting free fatty acids mobilize to adipose tissue, heart, skeletal muscle, and other tissues. The liver primarily removes the residual glycerol.

The VLDL, or pre-beta-lipoproteins, are synthesized mainly in the liver. The triglyceride that makes up the bulk of these pre-beta-lipoproteins derives from precursors such as carbohydrate and from circulating free fatty acids mostly mobilized from adipose tissue. These endogenous triglycerides circulate in association with the other lipid and protein components of VLDL; they impart a milky appearance to the plasma and undergo a fate similar to the exogenous triglyceride of chylomicra.

The LDL, or beta-lipoproteins, carry the greatest portion of plasma cholesterol. This lipoprotein, which normally has a half-life of three days, appears to be a remnant of VLDL metabolism after this latter lipoprotein has unloaded the endogenous triglyceride. Beta-lipoprotein has the greatest atherogenic potential. Both familial and acquired instances of hyperbeta-lipoproteinemia are known to occur.

The HDL, or alpha-lipoproteins, carry considerable phospholipid and modest amounts of cholesterol, but the greatest proportion of protein. Alpha-lipoproteins and chylomicra appear to have the least atherogenic potential of any of the plasma lipid classes. Actually, the HDL have recently assumed a protective role in atherogenesis, in part because of their capacity to remove cholesterol from tissues.

A large portion of the circulating cholesterol originates from the diet, but it can also be synthesized by liver, skin, and other organs. Cholesterol is essential to the structure of every cell. In particular, cholesterol is the precursor of adrenal steroids, gonadal steroids, and bile acids. The structural integrity of the brain and nervous system depends in part on the presence of cholesterol. Foods of animal origin contain the most dietary cholesterol. Particularly rich are liver and animal meats, eggs, and certain seafoods such as shrimp and lobster.

Cholesterol levels in the plasma are relatively stable during a 24-hour period. In contrast, triglyceride levels fluctuate and are highest between 1 and 4 hours after meals. Excessive cholesterol intake, age, and overweight tend to be associated with higher cholesterol levels. Excessive dietary fat can lead to elevation of exogenous triglycerides; in some individuals, excessive carbohydrate intake can lead to elevation of endogenous triglycerides. Poor nutrition, particularly limitation of animal fats and dairy products, and underweight are associated with lower cholesterol levels.

Clinical Significance

Marked deviations of cholesterol levels (below 150 or above 280 mg/dl) usually receive attention in modern medical practice. Although no causative role for cholesterol per se has been proved, considerable epidemiologic and experimental evidence links high cholesterol levels to premature and excessive atherosclerosis. Epidemiologic studies have shown higher cholesterol levels and associated higher risk of atherosclerotic lesions in overweight and sedentary individuals who eat excessive amounts of calories, oils, animal fat, and dairy products. The modern practice of medicine emphasizes disease prevention and directs clinicians to pay due attention to patients with lipid levels in the borderline as well as definitely abnormal range.

Visible accumulations of cholesterol and other lipids occur in xanthelasma, xanthomas, and arcus corneae. Accumulation of cholesterol and other lipids also manifests as fatty streaks or atheromatous plaques in the intima and media of medium- and large-size arteries. Lipid deposition, thrombosis, ulceration, calcification, and loss of elasticity of the affected vessels are all part of the atherosclerotic process.

Both congenital and acquired conditions may lead to elevated cholesterol levels. Among the congenital conditions, a great deal of attention has recently been directed, for its atherogenicity, to familial hypercholesterolemia (type II hyperbetalipoproteinemia of Fredrickson), seen in offspring of type II patients. These offspring may have cholesterol levels above "normal" in umbilical cord blood and during infancy. In addition, they develop premature atherosclerosis and often manifest acute myocardial infarction prior to 30 years of age.

Acquired causes of hypercholesterolemia include hypothyroidism, diabetes mellitus, nephrotic syndrome, hyperadrenocorticism, certain liver diseases, glycogen storage disease type I, alcohol ingestion, lipodystrophy, and use of certain types of contraceptive steroids. The acquired hypercholesterolemia is frequently reversible with reversal of the primary disease state.

Abnormal levels of triglycerides have also been implicated as risk factors for coronary atherosclerotic heart disease (CAHD) and atherosclerosis in general, but this association is somewhat weaker and more questionable than that for abnormal levels of cholesterol and CAHD.

Marked elevations of plasma triglycerides are seen in patients with type I hyperlipoproteinemia and congenitally deficient lipoprotein lipase activity, in patients with obesity and type IV hyperlipoproteinemia, occasionally in patients with type III, and in diabetic patients. The elevated triglyceride levels of insulin-dependent diabetic patients may reflect poor control of blood sugar and represent the contribution of several factors, including increased lipid mobilization from adipose tissue, increased triglyceride synthesis in the liver, reduced clearance by impaired LPL activity (an insulin-dependent enzyme), and possibly others. Severe hypertriglyceridemia may be associated with dramatic symptoms and signs, such as acute abdominal pain, hepatosplenomegaly, neuromuscular abnormalities, and eruptive xanthomatosis.

Almost paradoxically, recent studies have indicated that not "all cholesterol is bad." Increased serum levels of HDL, the high-density lipoproteins carrying one-third to one-fifth of the total plasma cholesterol, may protect against atherosclerosis; decreased levels of HDL may predispose to atherosclerosis. The strong inverse correlation between plasma levels of HDL and mortality from cardiovascular disease has led to a reassessment of the value of simple cholesterol determination and to the desirability of a high HDL cholesterol–total cholesterol ratio.

There are three rare genetically determined disorders in which one or more of the lipoprotein classes in the plasma are very low or absent, and cholesterol levels are consequently very low. These are:

1. *Abetalipoproteinemia.* Chylomicra, very low-density lipoproteins, and low-density lipoproteins are missing. Major manifestations of this disorder include malabsorption of fat, thorny appearance of erythrocytes (acanthocytosis), atypical retinitis pigmentosa, and degenerative changes in the nervous system.

2. *Hypobetalipoproteinemia (LDL deficiency).* The lipoprotein concentration is markedly below normal. Patients frequently appear well, but acanthocytosis and nervous system dysfunction may be present.

3. *Tangier disease, or HDL deficiency.* High-density lipoproteins circulate in small amounts and present abnormalities in the apolipoprotein composition. Patients with this disorder present with orange tonsils, often have neurologic abnormalities, and have increased storage of cholesterol esters in most tissues of the body.

Selected References

1. Abell LL, Levy BB, Brodie BB, et al: A simplified method for the estimation of total cholesterol in serum and demonstration of its specificity. *J Biol Chem* 195:357–366, 1952.

2. Fredrickson DS, Levy RI, Lees RS: Fat transport in lipoproteins: An integrated approach to mechanisms and disorders. *N Eng J Med* 276:34–44, 94–103, 148–156, 215–225, 273–281, 1967.

3. Fredrickson DS, Levy RI: Familial hyperlipoproteinemia, in Stanbury JB, Wyngaarden JB, Fredrickson DS (eds): *The Metabolic Basis of Inherited Disease.* New York, McGraw-Hill, 1972, chap 28.

4. Fredrickson DS, Gotto AM, Levy RI: Familial lipoprotein deficiency (abetalipoproteinemia, hypobetalipoproteinemia, and Tangier disease), in Stanbury JB, Wyngaarden JB, Fredrickson DA (eds): *The Metabolic Basis of Inherited Disease.* New York, McGraw-Hill, 1972, chap 26.

5. DiGirolamo M, Schlant RC: Etiology of coronary atherosclerosis, in Hurst JW (ed-in-chief), Logue RB, Schlant RC, Wenger NK (eds): *The Heart,* ed 4. New York, McGraw-Hill, 1978, chap 62B.

6. Schlant RC, DiGirolamo M: Modification of risk factors in the prevention and management of coronary atherosclerotic heart disease, in Hurst JW (ed-in-chief), Logue RB, Schlant RC, Wenger NK (eds): *The Heart,* ed 4. New York, McGraw-Hill, 1978, chap 62H.

7. Tzagournis M: Triglycerides in clinical medicine: A review. *Am J Clin Nutr* 31:1437–1452, 1978.

8. Miller GJ, Miller NE: Plasma-high-density-lipoprotein concentration and development of ischaemic heart-disease. *Lancet* 1:16–19, 1975.

236. Serum Total Protein: Albumin and Globulin

W. DALLAS HALL, MD
DAVID H. VROON, MD

Definition

The total serum proteins include enzymes, transport proteins, antibodies, and coagulation factors. They are grouped as albumin and globulins according to solubility features. Fibrinogen protein is not included in the total serum protein measurement because it is consumed in the conversion of plasma to serum.

The normal range of serum total protein content is approximately 6–8 gm/dl. Of this, albumin comprises 3.5–5 gm/dl; the residual represents the total globulins, approximately 2–4.5 gm/dl.

Technique

The biuret procedure is by far the most popular clinical method for measurement of total serum protein. It is used on SMA and most other automated systems. This method is based on the reaction of cupric ion with peptide linkages of protein in basic solution to yield a blue copper–protein complex.

$$Cu^{2+} + protein \xrightarrow{OH^-} \text{colored complex}$$
$$\text{(absorbs at 540 nm)}$$

The biuret reaction is specific for proteins in biological fluids; interferences are most often photometric and related to inadequate blank correction for specimen color or turbidity.

Refractometry is a rapid, manual technique occasionally used to measure total serum, particularly in association with electrophoretic fractionation. The reliability of refractometry is dependent on the presence of clear sera and the absence of normal amounts of nonprotein substances such as glucose, urea, bilirubin, and lipids which contribute significantly to the refractive index.

Techniques for clinical measurement of the albumin fraction of total serum protein include dye-binding methods, electrophoresis, and immunoprecipitation. Dye-binding procedures are employed in most automated systems; they are based on the proportional change of color when albumin is mixed with buffered solutions of pH indicator dyes. This spectral shift, a phenomenon known as the "protein error" of pH indicators is related to dye-anion protein binding. Bromcresol green (BCG) is the preferred and most widely used indicator dye.

$$\text{Albumin + BCG dye} \xrightarrow{\text{pH 4.2}} \text{albumin-BCG complex}$$
$$\text{(nonabsorbing at 600 nm)} \qquad \text{(absorbs at 600 nm)}$$

In contrast to other methods such as 2-(4'-hydroxyazobenzene) benzoic acid (HABA), BCG methods are not very susceptible to photometric interference or binding displacement by heparin, salicylates, or bilirubin. A disadvantage is incomplete specificity of bromcresol green for albumin since alpha and beta globulins react to some extent. The BCG method may produce significant positive errors in clinical conditions associated with low serum albumin and high alpha and beta globulins (ie, nephrosis or hepatic failure).

Electrophoretic fractionation of serum proteins is often and mistakenly regarded as the most reliable method for the measurement of serum albumin. Accurate measurement by electrophoresis is limited by variation in staining, the type of densitometer scanner used and the accuracy of the total protein determination. However, when overestimation of serum albumin by dye-binding methods is suggested clinically, electrophoresis is a preferred method and offers the added feature of measuring individual globulin fractions.

Background Information

Albumin is a very negatively charged water-soluble protein molecule with a molecular weight of approximately 65,000, isoelectric point of 4.7, and sedimentation constant of 4.5 Svedberg units. Albumin is synthesized by hepatocytes and has a half-life of approximately three weeks. The serum level of albumin does not appear to regulate hepatic albumin synthesis.

Albumin provides approximately 80% of the intravascular colloid osmotic pressure (oncotic pressure), the residual generated by globulins of higher molecular weight. Since proteins are of relatively high molecular weight, they contribute only minimally to total osmotic pressure. The oncotic pressure, however, assumes a major role in body fluid distribution. For instance, serum albumin is present in a concentration of 3.5–

5 gm/dl, or 35–50 gm/liter. Almost half of the total body albumin pool is located in the relatively small intravascular compartment. As such, volume is held within the vascular tree against the extravasating force of capillary hydrostatic pressure. A fall in serum oncotic pressure leads to unopposed hydrostatic capillary pressure. Hypoalbuminemia thus enhances the tendency to edema with disproportionate distribution of volume into the extravascular compartment. The concentration of serum albumin is critical for maintenance of adequate intravascular volume.

Albumin also functions as a carrier protein for transport of compounds such as fatty acids, amino acids, certain metals, and hormones. In addition, the majority of drugs are bound to serum albumin. The degree of binding is variable and susceptible to change, such as may occur with competitive displacement by other therapeutic compounds. Albumin-bound compounds generally exert no physiological or pharmacological activity.

Proteins can be characterized by their mobility through transport media (liquid, filter paper, agarose gel, cellulose acetate, starch block, acrylamide gel) in a charged field. This is known as electrophoresis. If antibody is incorporated into the media, the process is known as immunoelectrophoresis. Hundreds of serum proteins thus migrate into different zones referred to as gamma, phi (fibrinogen), beta, alpha-2, alpha-1, and alpha-0 (albumin) from slowest to fastest movement toward the anode. Fibrinogen (phi) protein and the beta band of hemoglobin protein are absent since electrophoresis is usually performed on serum which has been separated from the whole blood.

Alpha-1 globulins include predominantly alpha-1 antitrypsin and alpha-1 acid glycoprotein (orosomucoid) with a minor contribution from cortisol binding globulin (CBG). Alpha-2 globulins include predominantly alpha-2 macroglobulin and haptoglobin with lesser contributions from HS glycoprotein and ceruloplasmin. Beta globulins consist mainly of transferrin, C3, C4, and hemopexin. Transferrin is an example of a serum protein that falls rather than rises in response to acute and chronic inflammation. Gamma globulins are essentially all immunoglobulin (antibody) proteins such as IgG, IgA, and IgM, with minor amounts of IgD and IgE. Although most gamma globulins are immunoglobulins, many immunoglobulins are not gamma globulins because immunoglobulins may migrate in the beta, alpha-2, or gamma zones.

Clinical Significance

The ratio of albumin to globulin was once used as an expression of serum protein abnormalities. Since the advent of methods for identification and quantitation of specific proteins, this ratio is no longer of clinical use.

An elevated level of either total serum protein or total globulin is usually related to either dehydration or an increase in one of the globulin fractions. Serum electrophoresis is indicated to determine which globulin zone may be elevated. Most commonly this will be the gamma globulins, distorted in either a broad-based (polyclonal) pattern or a spiked (monoclonal) pattern. Cirrhosis, collagen disease, and diffuse skin disorders are common causes of polyclonal gammopathy. Multiple myeloma, malignancy, and macroglobulinemia are common causes of monoclonal gammopathy. Immunoelectrophoresis is indicated for any monoclonal peak. It must be appreciated that total serum protein, albumin, and globulin measurements are an inadequate screen for suspected disorders such as multiple myeloma. Bone marrow aspiration and examination of the urine for light chains may offer the only diagnostic clues. Bence-Jones proteins are light chains with specific thermal characteristics.

A low level of total serum protein most commonly occurs when both the albumin and gamma globulins are depressed (ie, nephrotic syndrome or protein-calorie malnutrition). An elevated level of serum albumin is found only in association with intravascular volume depletion or laboratory artifact.

A low level of serum albumin (hypoalbuminemia) may result from an expanded plasma volume at a time when the total body albumin pool is normal. Such is the case in normal third-trimester pregnancy and in some patients with congestive heart failure. Hypoalbuminemia is a classic finding of advanced liver disease, nephrotic syndrome, protein-losing enteropathies, and protein-calorie malnutrition.

Patients with hypoalbuminemia often have difficulty in maintaining an effective circulating blood volume. Their extracellular fluid volume may pool into spaces such as the alveoli, pleura, peritoneum, or retroperitoneum. They may have reduced transport of substrate fatty acids and amino acids, exaggerated or toxic responses to seemingly normal doses of protein-bound pharmacological agents, and hypotensive circulatory responses if intravascular volume is further reduced by diuretic therapy.

Selected References

1.   Rothschild MA, Oratz M, Schreibner SS: Albumin synthesis. *N Eng J Med* 286:748–757, 816–821, 1972.
2.   Wall RL: The use of serum protein electrophoresis in clinical medicine. *Arch Intern Med* 102:618–658, 1958.
3.   Leonardy JG: Serum protein electrophoresis in office practice. *S Med J* 64:129–137, 1971.
4.   Dayton PG, Israili AH, Perel JM: Influence of binding on drug metabolism and distribution. *Ann NY Acad Sci* 226:172–194, 1973.

5.   Koch-Weser J, Sellers EM: Binding of drugs to serum albumin. *New Eng J Med* 294:311–316, 526–531, 1976.
6.   Alper CA: Plasma protein measurements as a diagnostic aid. *N Eng J Med* 291:287–290, 1974.
7.   Speicher CE, Widish JR, Gaudot FJ, Hepler BR: An evaluation of the overestimation of serum albumin by bromcresol green. *Am J Clin Pathol* 69:347–350, 1978.

237. PPD Tuberculin Skin Test

JOHN E. MCGOWAN, JR., MD

Definition

A diagnostic study in which a killed extract called purified protein derivative (PPD) from *Mycobacterium tuberculosis* organisms is injected intradermally in an attempt to determine whether the subject has previously been infected by *M. tuberculosis*. If such infection has occurred, the intradermal injection of this extract results in production of a localized inflammatory response.

Technique

PPD tuberculin should be used at a strength of 5 tuberculin units, a measure standardized by biological assay. This preparation is frequently called "intermediate strength PPD." A detergent such as Tween-80 is added to the preparation to reduce adsorption of the PPD to glass. One-tenth milliliter of this solution is introduced into the skin with a short small-gauge (usually 25–27 gauge) needle connected to a syringe calibrated for tuberculin. The injection is usually made on the volar (or dorsal) surface of the forearm and should be made just beneath the surface of the skin by angling the needle with bevel upward to a point at which the bevel has just disappeared beneath the skin's surface. A discrete elevation of the skin (wheal) should appear during intracutaneous injection of the full 0.1-ml dose. No blood should appear when the needle is withdrawn.

The site of injection should be inspected 48 to 72 hours after the injection and the presence or absence of induration determined by both inspection and palpation with the fingertip. Erythema without induration is not a positive reaction. Readings should be made in a good light, with the forearm slightly flexed at the elbow. A ball-point pen may be used to define the limits of induration (see reference 4). Once the margins of induration are ascertained, the widest diameter of the indurated area should be measured by holding a ruler perpendicular to the long axis of the forearm. This diameter, in millimeters, should be recorded as the result of the PPD test.

The test should be recorded as positive, doubtful, or negative according to the following criteria:

> Greater than or equal to 10 mm of induration equals positive reaction: past or present infection with M. tuberculosis.
>
> From 5 to 9 mm of induration equals doubtful reaction: this degree of induration can result from infection with either M. tuberculosis (the causative agent of clinical tuberculosis) or from infection with atypical mycobacteria.
>
> Less than or equal to 4 mm of induration equals negative reaction: lack of infection with M. tuberculosis.

The interpretation of results should be explained to the patient.

Background Information

PPD is a mixture of low-molecular-weight proteins, nucleic acids, and polysaccharides. It is extracted from autoclaved cultures of M. tuberculosis by precipitation with trichloroacetic acid or neutral ammonium sulfate. As such, it represents a purified, but not entirely pure, extract of the organism. In patients who have been infected with M. tuberculosis, intradermal injection of the PPD stimulates a population of T lymphocytes sensitized to tubercle bacilli to produce a variety of mediators that cause other cells to evoke a characteristic localized inflammatory response at the site of injection. The reaction of the PPD tuberculin skin test tends to persist throughout life, although the response may diminish with increasing age.

Response to tuberculin in infected populations approximates a normal distribution with a mean of 18 mm and a standard deviation of 5 mm. The dose of 5 tuberculin units has been chosen as the standard test dose because epidemiologic studies suggest that the fewest number of false positive and false negative reactions occur when this dosage is used for testing. Both false positive and false negative reactions do occur: the

5-tuberculin-unit PPD skin test best separates infected from noninfected patients but is not infallible.

Response to PPD tuberculin skin testing may decrease or disappear during any severe or febrile illness, measles or other viral infections, immunization with live virus vaccines, Hodgkin's disease, sarcoidosis, overwhelming miliary or pulmonary tuberculosis, administration of adrenal corticosteroids, or therapy with other immunosuppressive drugs. Thus, a negative reaction to PPD does not exclude the diagnosis of tuberculosis. In patients who do not react to tuberculin, the functioning of the delayed hypersensitivity (cellular) reaction mechanism may be evaluated by intradermal testing with one or more antigens to which most persons have been sensitized; for example, *Candida*, streptokinase and streptodornase (SKSD), mumps, or trichophyton. Pregnancy does not appear to affect the response to PPD.

Clinical Significance

A positive reaction to the tuberculin skin test indicates the presence of infection with *M. tuberculosis* but does not signify that disease is present. Thus, the probability of *M. tuberculosis* infection increases with increasing diameter of induration, but a "huge" reaction does not necessarily indicate the presence of clinical disease due to *M. tuberculosis*. However, most individuals who develop clinical tuberculosis have been infected with *M. tuberculosis* much earlier than the time at which symptoms appear. Since the early stages often are asymptomatic, response to the PPD skin test may be the only way of detecting a patient who has been infected with the tubercle bacillus. Conversely, a negative PPD skin test, in the absence of the factors mentioned above that interfere with the test, can help the clinician to exclude tuberculosis.

Selected References

1. *The Tuberculin Skin Test.* New York, American Lung Association, 1974.
2. MacLean RA: Tuberculin testing antigens and techniques. *Chest* 68(suppl):455–459, 1975.
3. Rooney JJ, Crocco JA, Kramer S, Lyons HA: Further observations on tuberculin reactions in active tuberculosis. *Am J Med* 60:517–522, 1976.
4. Sokal JE: Measurement of delayed skin-test responses. *N Eng J Med* 293:501–502, 1975.
5. Freedman S, Kongshavn PL: Immunobiology of tuberculin hypersensitivity. *Chest* 68(suppl):470–474, 1975.

238. Serologic Testing for Syphilis

SUMNER E. THOMPSON III, MD, MPH

Definition

Treponema pallidum, the bacterium responsible for causing syphilis, produces a brisk, sustained antibody response in the human host. These antibodies can be easily measured and quantitated; they form the basis for confirming the clinical diagnosis and measuring the response to treatment.

Technique

All testing can be performed on serum. No special methods of collection or storage of specimens are necessary. A single test such as the VDRL is inexpensive and requires less than 1 ml of serum to perform. Most state laboratories will perform serologic testing free of charge.

Background Information

Modern serologic tests are divided into two groups:

1. Nonspecific, nontreponemal, or reagin tests. These measure the ability of serum to react with an artificial antigen, usually a cardiolipin-lecithin compound. This antibody is termed *reagin* (this should not be confused with the skin-sensitizing IgE which has the same name) and is present transiently after a variety of conditions such as immunizations and febrile illnesses, or permanently in such conditions as collagen-vascular diseases, leprosy, and drug addiction. Such patients are said to have acute or chronic biological false positive (BFP) tests. Treponemal tests can aid in differentiating these sera from those of syphilitics.

The advantages of these tests are that they are simple to perform, thus useful for screening purposes; they are widely available, cheap, and easily reproducible; they can be quantitated to follow disease response to therapy; and they are useful for assessing the probability of reinfection. In addition, they may be performed on spinal fluid. The drawbacks are that they are not specific for syphilis, and they are relatively insensitive in very early or very late syphilis (see Table 50). Tests in common use today are:

VDRL (Venereal Disease Research Laboratory) slide test. At present this is the standard nontreponemal test used in the United States. Heated serum is used to flocculate the cardiolipin-lecithin antigen. This is the test of choice for quantitation and for testing cerebrospinal fluid.

RPR (rapid plasma reagin). This test can be done at the bedside if necessary. It comes as a commercially available kit. Results are comparable generally with the VDRL.

2. *Specific or treponemal tests.* These detect antibody (primarily IgG) directed against *T. pallidum* itself. Tests in use today are:

TPI (Nelson test) (Treponema pallidum immobilization). This is the original specific test. It is falling into disuse because it is relatively insensitive when compared with other specific tests and is extremely difficult to perform reliably.

FTA-ABS (fluorescent treponemal antibody-absorbed). This test has been in use since 1964. Presently it is the most commonly employed specific test. Interpretation is subjective and requires a high degree of skill to ensure accurate results.

MHA-TP (microhemagglutination-Treponema pallidum). This test has been in use since 1970. It is a simpler, more reproducible test than the FTA-ABS and in the future may become the standard specific test.

The advantages of these tests are high sensitivity and specificity (sensitivity is the percentage of positive results in a series of specimens taken from patients who have the disease; specificity is the percentage of negative results in a series of specimens taken from normal subjects who do not have the disease); and they are useful for distinguishing between biological false positive reactions and true syphilis.

The disadvantages of these tests are that they are technically difficult to perform; interlaboratory reproducibility fluctuates; they are relatively

Table 50. Reactivity of tests for syphilis.

Test	Stage of Disease (%)			
	Primary	Secondary	Latent	Late
VDRL	72	100	73	77
FTA-ABS	91	100	97	100
TPI	46	98	95	95
MHA-TP	79	100	98	100

expensive; they tend to remain positive for life, limiting their usefulness for following response to therapy; and they are not standardized for use on cerebrospinal fluid.

Clinical Significance

In clinical practice there is no need to use more than one type of reagin test and one type of treponemal (specific) test. It is necessary to have a rough idea of the reactivity of the various tests in the various stages of syphilis in order to interpret results correctly.

The following examples of serologic reactions illustrate the range of possible interpretations:

1. VDRL (+); FTA-ABS (−)
   a. Syphilis not present. Patient is a "false positive reactor." Quantitative VDRL would be helpful since BFPs are seldom greater than 1:32 and usually are lower (1:4, 1:8).
   b. Repeat FTA-ABS since a laboratory error could have occurred resulting in a false negative in a patient who has syphilis.
2. VDRL(−); FTA-ABS (+). This pattern can occur in the presence or absence of active syphilis.
   a. Active syphilis present. In both primary and late syphilis the FTA-ABS is more sensitive than the VDRL (see Table 50).
   b. Active syphilis not present. This pattern can be seen in adequately treated syphilis since the FTA-ABS tends to remain positive for life, and the VDRL often reverts to negative within 6 to 18 months after treatment, depending on how long it has been reactive.
3. VDRL (−); FTA-ABS (−)
   a. Any patient without syphilis.
   b. Syphilis present. In incubating syphilis soon after infection with the spirochete, by definition there are no signs or symptoms. Repeat serologies within 3 months in those suspected of having the disease.
4. VDRL persistently (+). This can be seen in untreated or inadequately treated disease, but can also be found in a small percentage of adequately treated patients. These "serofast" individuals should have periodic quantitative VDRLs, since a twofold or greater rise may indicate reinfection. Serofast patients with FTA-ABS (−) are likely to be chronic BFP reactors and should be evaluated for conditions associated with this.
5. FTA-ABS "borderline (+)." A single report does not indicate

syphilis. All patients with this reaction should be retested. Persistent borderline tests probably do not indicate syphilis. The true significance of this finding is not known.

In a patient with syphilis the physician must decide if a lumbar puncture is indicated. If so, what are the appropriate serologies?

Not all patients with syphilis require a CSF examination. It may not be necessary to examine spinal fluid on patients with primary or secondary syphilis, or early latent syphilis (known to be of less than 2 years duration). During early syphilis the CSF is frequently abnormal (elevated protein or cell count, or reactive serology). This invariably returns to normal after adequate penicillin therapy. In contrast, it is probably advisable to examine spinal fluid on the following types of patients:

1. Any patient with latent syphilis of greater than 2 years duration, or of unknown duration (this is the most frequent finding in the hospitalized patient when serologies are done routinely during admission).
2. Any patient beyond early stages of the disease who has unexplained neurologic findings. The clinical presentations of neurosyphilis are so varied that a reactive CSF serology may be necessary to arrive at a correct diagnosis.
3. Any patient treated for primary, secondary, or latent syphilis with any antibiotic other than penicillin. This should be done within a year of diagnosis and treatment since the efficacy of any drug except penicillin in treating neurosyphilis is not known.

At the present time the quantitative VDRL slide test is the CSF serology of choice for diagnosing neurosyphilis. However, this test is not ideal for following response to treatment in the CSF. Titers may drift down to nonreactive status only after years. No other serologic test can be recommended at this time.

Selected References

1. Drusin LM: The diagnosis and treatment of infectious and latent syphilis. *Med Clin N Am* 56:1161–1174, 1972.
2. Jaffe HW: The laboratory diagnosis of syphilis: New concepts. *Ann Intern Med* 83:846–859, 1975.
3. Sparling PF: Diagnosis and treatment of syphilis. *N Eng J Med* 284: 642–653, 1971.
4. Center for Disease Control: Syphilis: Recommended treatment schedules, 1976. Recommendations established by the Venereal Disease Control Advisory Committee. *Ann Intern Med* 85:94–96, 1976.

239. The Electrocardiogram

JOHN R. DARSEE, MD
J. WILLIS HURST, MD

Definition

The electrocardiogram (ECG, or EKG) is a clinical tool which measures the quantity or quality of electrical impulses traversing the cardiac conduction system and myocardium. Only a small quantity of electrical current is generated by the heart and considerable amplification must be employed since the ECG detects only the final sum of currents. The usual ECG is also referred to as a scalar electrocardiogram and contrasts with the vectorcardiogram (VCG) which detects and represents the path of electrical impulses in three dimensions. The VCG will not be discussed in this section.

The sinus node, atrioventricular node, and bundle branches are important components of ventricular activation but do not have a direct representation on the electrocardiogram. Their activation must be deduced by inference. Atrial depolarization, ventricular depolarization, and ventricular repolarization are imaged on the electrocardiogram by the P wave, the QRS complex and the T wave, respectively.

Six waves, one segment, and three intervals characterize the basic features of the electrocardiogram (Fig 190).

1. P wave: in sinus rhythm, the first deflection from the baseline, and usually a positive wave. The P wave represents the depolarization (electrical activation) of the atria and is usually no taller and no wider than 2 to 2.5 mm.
2. Q wave: the first negative (downward) deflection after the P wave, provided that it precedes the R wave. The Q wave may represent either normal initial ventricular activation (usually of the upper interventricular septum) or an electrical "dead zone," particularly if it is deep, wide, or of new onset.
3. R wave: the first positive (upward) deflection after the P wave. The R wave usually represents depolarization of the bulk of ventricular myocardium.

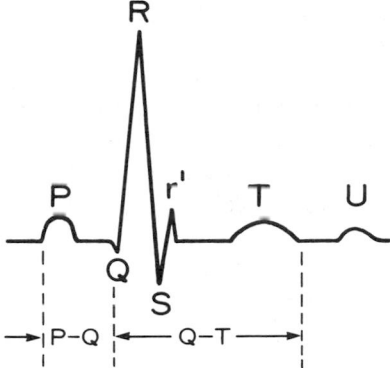

Figure 190. The P-QRS-T complex consists of six waves, one segment and three intervals.

4. S wave: the negative deflection following the R wave. The S wave is not usually present in every lead. It represents the depolarization of the ventricle that is opposite in direction from the view obtained from a particular ECG lead. For example, when the sum of electrical activity is moving toward lead I, a positive deflection is recorded; when the sum of electrical activity is moving away from lead I, a negative deflection (such as as the S wave) is recorded.

5. T wave: the next positive or negative deflection following the QRS complex. The T wave represents ventricular repolarization and is usually the same polarity (+ or −) as the R wave. There are no absolute measurements for the T wave; however, the area under the T wave should theoretically approximate the area under the R wave.

6. U wave: a small wave which follows the T wave and is generally in the same direction. The U wave is probably an afterpotential, thought to be due to the repolarization of Purkinje fibers. The U wave is more easily recognized in bradycardiac patients, or whenever the T wave is smaller than usual.

7. S-T segment: the horizontal (or near horizontal) line connecting the end of the S wave (or the end of the R wave if no S wave is present) and the beginning of the T wave. The length of the S-T segment is not usually important. Rather, the elevation above or depression below the baseline is indicative of an abnormality of epicardial or myocardial origin, often related clinically to ischemia or inflammation.

8. P-Q and P-R intervals: the interval from the beginning of the P wave to the beginning of the Q wave (P-Q) or the R wave (P-R).

These intervals represent the time required for atrial depolarization plus the time for current to traverse the atrioventricular node and bundle branches prior to depolarization of the interventricular septum. The normal P-Q interval is from 0.11 second to 0.19 second. When it is 0.10 second or less, the impulse may be originating from a low atrial focus, or a "rapid transit" bypass tract may be conducting the impulse around the atrioventricular node. A P-Q interval of 0.20 second or greater is called first-degree heart block and is usually (but not always) due to slowed conduction within the atrioventricular node.

9.   QRS interval: the interval from the beginning of the Q wave to the end of the S wave. The usual QRS interval is less than 0.10 second.

10.   Q-T interval: the interval from the beginning of the Q wave (or beginning of the R wave in the absence of a Q wave) to the end of the T wave. This represents the time required for ventricular depolarization and repolarization. The normal Q-T interval depends on the heart rate, but in general should not be greater than one-half the time between two successive R wave peaks (ie, the R-R interval). The Q-T interval may be corrected for heart rate (QTc) according to Bazett's formula:

$$QTc = \frac{QT\ interval}{\sqrt{RR\ interval}}$$

The normal QTc is less than 0.425. The QTc interval is abnormal in certain electrolyte disturbances, in patients taking antidepressant and antipsychotic medications, and in a variety of myocardial abnormalities. Measurement of the interval from the beginning of the Q wave to the beginning of the T wave may also be useful. This particular measurement is referred to as the Q-T$_o$ interval.

A grid is provided on the ECG paper for purposes of measurement and timing of the electrical forces. The grid allows units of voltage to be assigned in the vertical direction and units of time to be assigned in the horizontal direction (Fig 191). The vertical and horizontal lines are 1 mm apart. Every fifth horizontal line is more heavily inscribed for easier identification of 5-mm increments. The intervals on the horizontal scale represent 0.04 second; those between the heavier lines represent 0.20 second. If the rhythm is regular, the heart rate may be determined by dividing the number of large squares (including any fractional part of a square) between two successive R waves into 300. The intervals and the method of calculating heart rate are only true if the paper speed is the usual 25 mm/second.

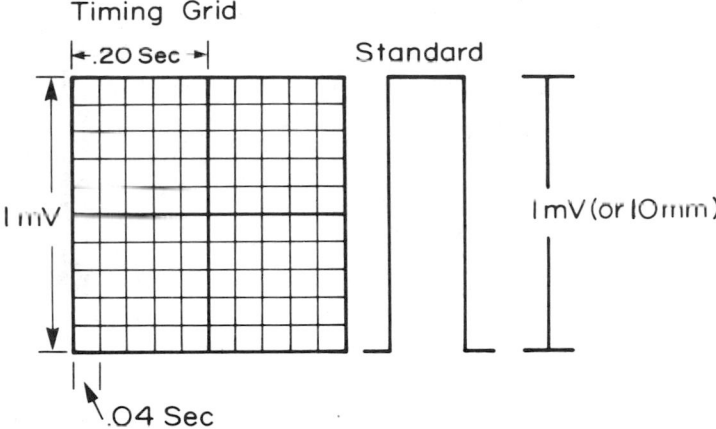

Figure 191. On the voltage-timing grid, units of voltage are measured in the vertical direction and units of time in the horizontal direction. The voltage standard should measure 1 mV (or 10 mm). Reproduced from Hurst JW, Myerburg RJ: *Introduction to Electrocardiography*, ed 2. New York, McGraw-Hill Book Company with permission of the authors and publisher.

On the vertical scale, a 1-mv impulse deflects the galvanometer 10 mm. If the amplitude of the tracing is too large to be confined to the paper, the standardization may be reduced by one-half, and an appropriate notation (½ standard) made on the tracing.

Technique

Recording the electrocardiogram. The patient should be placed in the supine position, told that there is no expected discomfort from the test, and asked to lie as quietly as possible. When applying the electrodes to the limbs and chest, skin resistance may be reduced by briskly rubbing the skin until an erythema is produced and by interposing an electrode jelly between the skin and the electrode.

One electrode is attached to each of the four limbs according to the label on the electrode. The color codes are: white (right arm), black (left arm), green (right leg), and red (left leg). The fact that black and white leads are used on the arms can be easily remembered since a black and white newspaper is held by the arms.

Some electrocardiographs have a chest electrode that is moved across the chest for recording each of the precordial leads; others have six separate electrodes that can be positioned simultaneously. In either case, they are located as diagrammed in Fig 192.

During the recording, the patient should be reminded not to move,

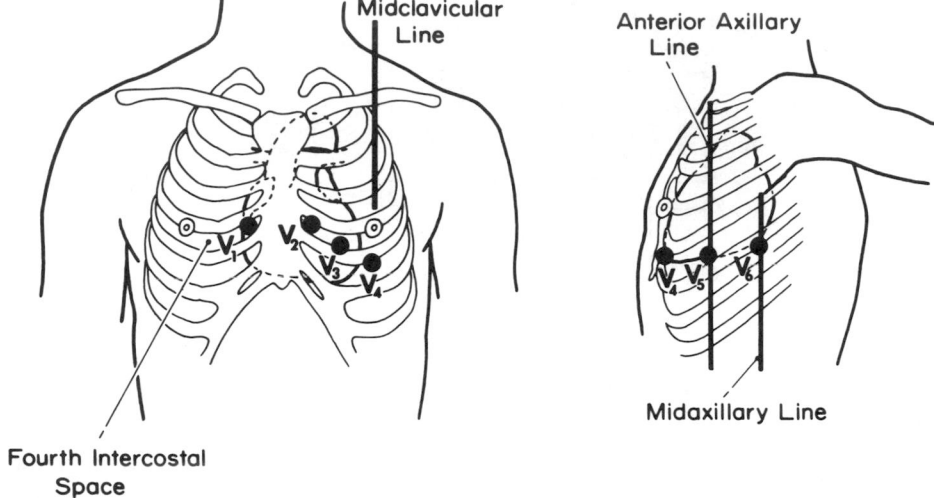

Figure 192. Proper placement of the precordial leads.

and to breathe quietly. After recording all twelve standard leads, the tracing must be properly labeled with the patient's full name as well as the year, month, day, and hour of recording.

Reading and interpreting the electrocardiogram. A systematic approach for interpreting the electrocardiogram will help prevent omissions. This approach can be viewed as a series of questions:

1. Is the tracing properly labeled?
2. Were the limb leads placed correctly?
3. Is the tracing properly standardized?
4. What is the heart rate? _____/minute
5. What are the following three intervals?
   P-R interval _____ sec
   QRS interval _____ sec
   Q-T interval _____ sec
6. What is the angle of the following six ECG vectors: mean P vector, mean QRS vector, initial 0.04 QRS vector, terminal 0.04 QRS vector, mean T vector, and mean ST vector (if present)?
7. Are the intervals and vectors all within normal limits? If not, what might be the altered cardiac anatomy or physiology responsible for the abnormality?
8. How does the clinical information correlate with the conceived alteration in cardiac anatomy or physiology?
9. Has the electrocardiographic interpretation made more conclu-

sions than the actual data should allow? For example, be cautious about diagnoses inferred from small Q waves. Q waves do not always mean myocardial infarction. For example, small Q waves in leads II, III, and aV$_F$ are not infrequent and may be normal. Clinical correlation and previous tracings are required for proper interpretation.

Background Information

Brief history of electrocardiography.   One of the first electrocardiograph-like machines was made by Einthoven around 1900, utilizing a string galvanometer. This instrument was heavy and cumbersome and filled a large portion of a room. The tracing was made while two hands and one foot of the patient were in buckets of water. Subsequent methods of amplification used coil galvanometers with more inertia than Einthoven's sensitive quartz string galvanometer.

The standard limb leads were the first leads used by Einthoven and are still used today. Lead I was recorded by connecting the galvanometer to the left and right arms and measuring the potential difference (voltage) between them as it changed instantaneously throughout the cardiac cycle. Leads II and III measure the instantaneous potential difference between the right arm and left leg, and the left arm and left leg, respectively. The limbs represented their respective anatomical sides of the heart (Fig 193).

Wilson developed the precordial leads in an attempt to obtain additional information by recording closer to the heart. Each limb was connected to a central point through a 5,000 ohm resistance. The junction of the three wires was used as an indifferent electrode (the "central

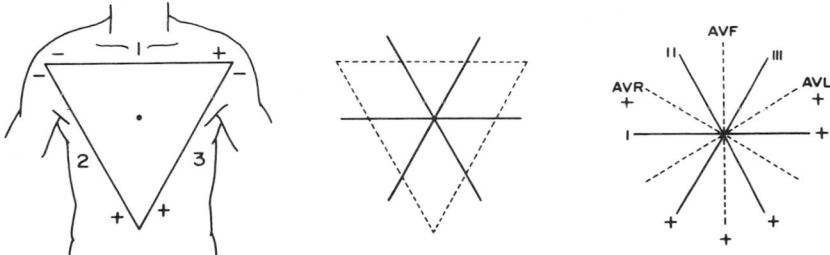

Figure 193. Einthoven's triangle is a representation of the three leads that Einthoven used in the early twentieth century. The leads have been relocated so that they join at their midpoints. This was the beginning of the frontal plane reference circle (or lead graph) that we use today. Reproduced from Hurst JW, Myerburg RJ: Introduction to Electrocardiography, ed 2. New York, McGraw-Hill Book Company, 1973, with permission from the authors and publisher.

terminal") with a constant potential near zero. The exploring electrode was placed (more or less arbitrarily) on six different points on the precordium that corresponded generally to the long axis of the heart (Fig 192).

Shortly after Wilson's development of the central terminal came the augmented unipolar limb lead concept of Goldberger. The potential of each extremity was augmented by disconnecting the resistor from one limb at a time. These three leads were designated aV_R, aV_L, and aV_F, which stood for *augmented voltage* to the *right*, *left*, and *foot*.

Indications for ordering an electrocardiogram.   Although not every clinician would agree on all the indications for an ECG, there are several clinical situations in which the electrocardiogram is particularly useful:

1. Baseline tracing. As a part of the clinician's data base on each patient, the ECG serves as a comparison if abnormalities are noted in future tracings during a clinical illness.

2. Loss of consciousness. One of the important differential diagnoses in patients with a history of loss of consciousness is a cardiac dysrhythmia. Evidence of a dysrhythmia and/or conduction disturbance is sometimes apparent from the standard 12-lead electrocardiogram.

3. Clinical evidence of dysrhythmia. This is often perceived by the patient as palpitation or an awareness of the heart beat.

4. Chest pain. *A normal ECG never rules out angina pectoris, myocardial ischemia, or myocardial infarction.* However, an abnormality in the ST segment, T wave, or the initial 0.04 second ("initial forces") of ventricular depolarization provides information crucial to subsequent patient evaluation and management.

5. Evaluation of cardiovascular disease. A careful analysis of the electrocardiogram in patients with suspected cardiac disease will often provide immediate clues to the presence of certain varieties of heart disease.

6. Determination of cardiac manifestations of systemic diseases or metabolic abnormalities. Many diseases have important cardiovascular manifestations which may be reflected in the electrocardiogram. Severe metabolic derangements (such as hyperkalemia, hypokalemia, hypercalcemia, hypocalcemia) are often reflected in the ECG and may suggest immediate courses of action (eg, intravenous calcium or bicarbonate for severe hyperkalemia). The ECG often suggests the diagnosis before laboratory results are available.

Limitations of the electrocardiogram.   Although the standard 12-lead ECG is useful, several important limitations may be enumerated:

1. It is frequently normal in patients with heart disease, particularly coronary atherosclerotic heart disease.

2. It may be abnormal in patients without heart disease.

3. If the exact position of each of the precordial leads is not marked (with temporary dye, for example) in patients with serial tracings, changes in the ECG ("poor anterior forces," "slow R wave progression") may be due only to a change in lead position.

4. The variability of the relationship between the long axis of the heart and the thorax (particularly in patients who are obese, emphysematous, pregnant, or megalomastic) may lead to an unusual or even bizarre pattern in the precordial leads when the heart itself is normal.

5. The ECG cannot be used to diagnose the presence or absence of congestive heart failure.

6. In the presence of conduction disturbances (particularly left bundle branch block and complete heart block), epicardial injury currents and electrical dead zones are often occult or undetectable. For example, a patient with preexisting left bundle branch block (LBBB) may reveal no additional initial force abnormalities in a setting of acute myocardial infarction. A vectorcardiogram may be more helpful in these situations.

7. Multiple disorders may cause similar changes in the electrocardiogram. For example, a casual observer may interpret the ST segment changes of "digitalis effect" as myocardial ischemia if close attention is not paid to the QRS-ST gradient.

8. Right and left ventricular hypertrophy may be more difficult or even impossible to diagnose from the ECG in the presence of bundle branch block, left pleural effusion, pneumothorax, pericardial effusion, coexistent ventricular dilatation, emphysema, a large electrical dead zone, or extreme obesity. An analysis of QRS, T, and ST vectors and their components is often useful in these cases. Left ventricular hypertrophy is diagnosed by one of several methods; some rely primarily on the voltage of R and S waves, and other criteria utilize additional features such as the P-wave configuration, or the duration of the QRS complex measured from the onset of depolarization to the peak of the R wave. As these criteria become more sensitive (detect more cases), they become less specific (detect more false positives) and include individuals with a thin chest wall but a normal heart, and other nonpathological conditions. The diagnosis of right ventricular hypertrophy is even more difficult by any of the criteria available.

9. ST segment changes, T wave inversion, and even Q waves may disappear in patients with a previous myocardial infarction. Hence, patients with previous myocardial infarction may have a normal ECG.

10. The typical sequential ECG changes of acute myocardial infarction occur less often when there is electrocardiographic evidence of previous myocardial damage.

Importance and utility of the vector method. As the excitation wave proceeds through the atrial and ventricular myocardium, the electrical forces generated vary in magnitude and direction from instant to instant during a single cardiac cycle (Fig 194). These electrical forces of the heart can be considered as vectors. Vectors may be represented on paper by arrows with both a length and a direction in three dimensions. This variation in magnitude and direction of electrical forces (represented by arrows) is due to the distribution of the conduction system, the varying thicknesses of heart muscle, and the fact that instantaneous vectors pointing in opposite directions may cancel each other.

The flow of electrical forces is a result of individual myocardial cells "depolarizing" at slightly different times, but in a particular order. A

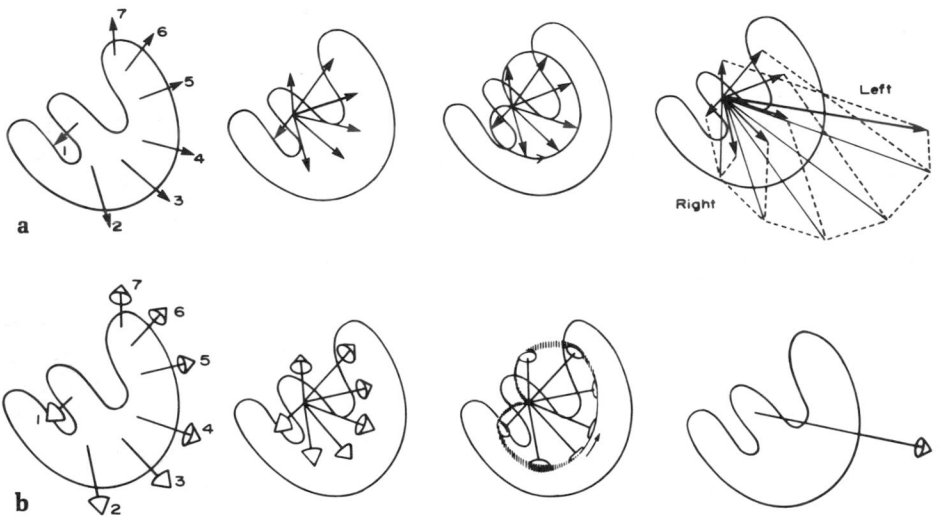

Figure 194.   *A,* Diagram illustrating the depolarization of the ventricular muscle as viewed in two dimensions (looking at the front of the heart). The numbered arrows indicate the general sequence in which instantaneous electrical forces are generated during a single QRS cycle. In the second portion of the figure, the vectors have been drawn as if all forces arise at a common origin in the upper interventricular septum. If a line is drawn through the tips of each of these instantaneous vectors, we can reconstruct the general shape of what is called the "QRS loop." The "mean QRS vector" is produced by vector summation of all the instantaneous vector arrows (this is purely diagrammatical to illustrate the point since, in practice, we cannot "sum up" these vectors in this way). (Adapted from *Introduction to Electrocardiography,* by JW Hurst and RJ Myerburg, with permission from the authors and publisher.) *B,* Diagram illustrating the depolarization of the ventricles if viewed in three-dimensional space. Note that each instantaneous vector and the final "mean QRS vector" also have frontward-backward direction as well as their direction in two dimensions as shown in *A.* The diagrams represent three-dimensional pictures of what was seen in *A.* (Adapted from *Introduction to Electrocardiography* ed 2, by JW Hurst and RJ Myerburg, New York, McGraw-Hill Book Company, 1973 with permission from the authors and publisher.)

single muscle cell has a cell membrane with a series of positive and negative charges (dipoles) in equilibrium with each other. At rest, the cell is in the polarized state. The electrically impervious myocardial cell membrane prevents any flow of current or neutralization of the positive and negative charges until external forces (electrons) change the membrane potential, neutralize successive dipoles, and produce an electromotive force. This process is called depolarization. The reverse process, which occurs milliseconds later, is called repolarization and is actually a return to the baseline state. The sequential changes in the voltage inside one cell (resulting from depolarization and repolarization) are represented by the "action potential" (Fig 195).

The sequential, orderly "summing up" of all the separate action potentials represents the successive depolarization of each myocardial cell and is detected on the scalar ECG as the P, QRS, and T waves (Fig 196). This P-QRS-T complex represents the direction, magnitude, and velocity of successive depolarizations.

The P-QRS-T complex is a representation of changing electrical forces as perceived from only *one* lead position. For example, lead 1 "views the heart" as if it were standing just outside the lateral left ventricular wall, looking at the heart, and observing the electrical changes from this one vantage point. Lead aV$_F$ views the heart and its electrical charges from the underside, diaphragmatic border. A completely different

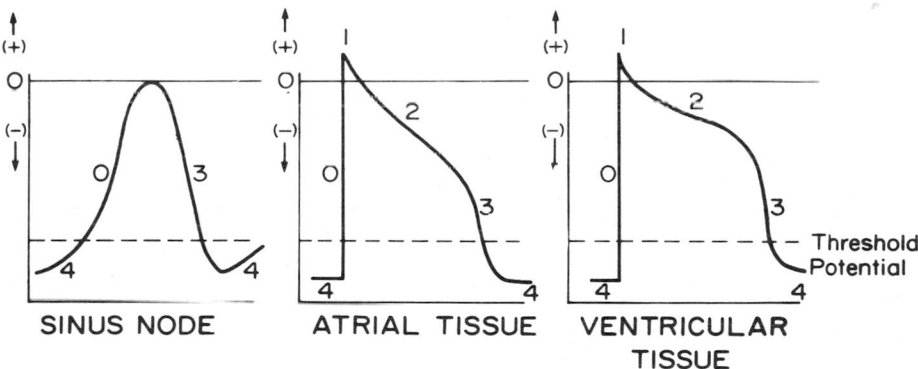

SINUS NODE	ATRIAL TISSUE	VENTRICULAR TISSUE

Figure 195.   Action potentials from different types of cells in the heart. Note that the action potential from one cell (or any cell) in the sinus node lacks the "overshoot" of phase 1 and yet has spontaneous phase 4 depolarization, making it a pacemaker cell. Note that the shape of the sinus node action potential differs from that of the atrial and ventricular action potential in that phase 4 moves spontaneously back up toward the threshold potential. This is called "spontaneous phase 4 diastolic depolarization" and identifies the sinus node as pacemaker tissue. Pacemaker cells can be found in the very distal part of the A-V node, and a few in the atria and ventricles.

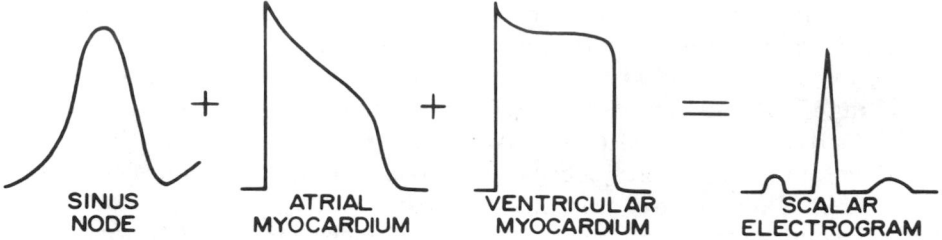

Figure 196.   The combined action potentials from cells throughout the heart make up the standard P, QRS, and T waves of the scalar electro-cardiogram.

picture is painted by the ECG in these two leads (Fig 197). Hence, the scalar ECG can only "view the heart" one lead at a time. What actually happens with each electrical systole and diastole is represented by three different loops: the P loop, the QRS loop, and the T loop. The P loop and T loop can be constructed diagrammatically in the same manner as was the QRS loop in Fig 194. The P loop represents the sequence of de-polarization of the atrial myocardium; the T loop represents repolariza-tion of ventricular muscle.

Figure 198 is an illustration of how the depolarization and repolar-ization sequence would be seen if one viewed the heart and thorax as three-dimensional objects. The scalar ECG depicts these three loops from 12 isolated vantage points, the 12 standard ECG leads.

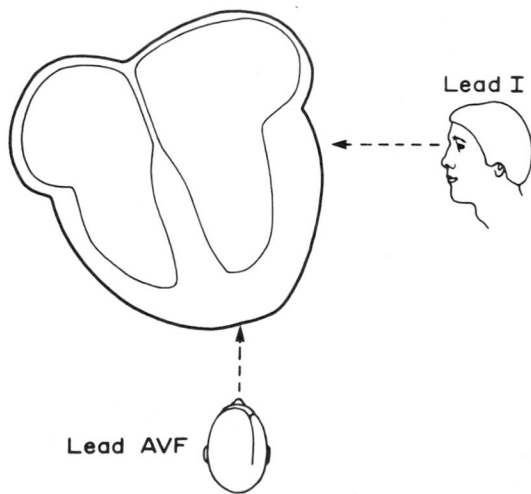

Figure 197.   Each lead "views" the sequence of electrical changes that occur with each electrical systole and diastole from a different vantage point.

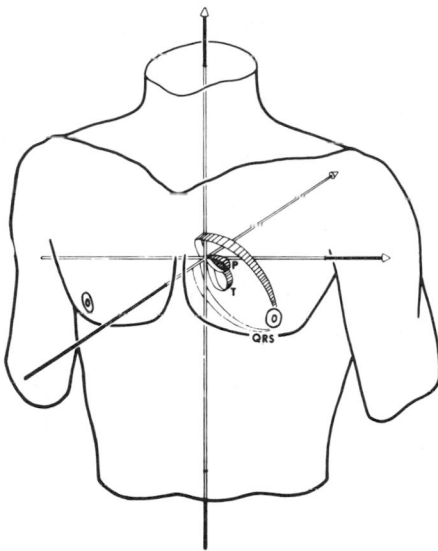

Figure 198.   The P, QRS, and T loops as seen in three dimensions.

Construction of the major cardiac vectors.   The mean P, QRS, and T vectors represent a straight line drawn from the origin of the vector loop to the point of maximum excursion from the origin. In general, about 50% of the area of the loop is contained within the loop on either side of this line. The mean vectors depict the general direction and size of their respective loops. What follows is a simple method of determining the direction and magnitude of these vectors from the scalar ECG and drawing them on paper as arrows in three-dimensional space.

The mean QRS vector.   Choose the two leads from I, II, and III which have the largest R waves (area underneath the R wave) (Fig 199A). In the more unusual case, in which the S waves are larger than the R waves, choose the two leads with the largest S waves. Then, remembering that the area of a triangle is equal to 0.5 (base × height), estimate the area underneath the R waves in the two leads (Fig 199B). If Q or S waves are present in the two selected leads, estimate their areas and subtract any Q or S wave area from the R wave area in that lead. On the lead graph (Fig 200) mark off in millimeters the numbers you have just calculated (on the two leads to which they belong), making sure to mark on the (+) side of the lead if the resultant area number is positive and on the (−) side of the lead if the resultant area number is negative (Fig 199C). Construct a perpendicular line from these two points (Fig 199D). The point where these two lines cross should be used as the tip of the arrow for the mean QRS vector in *two* dimensions. Once the vector has been constructed for

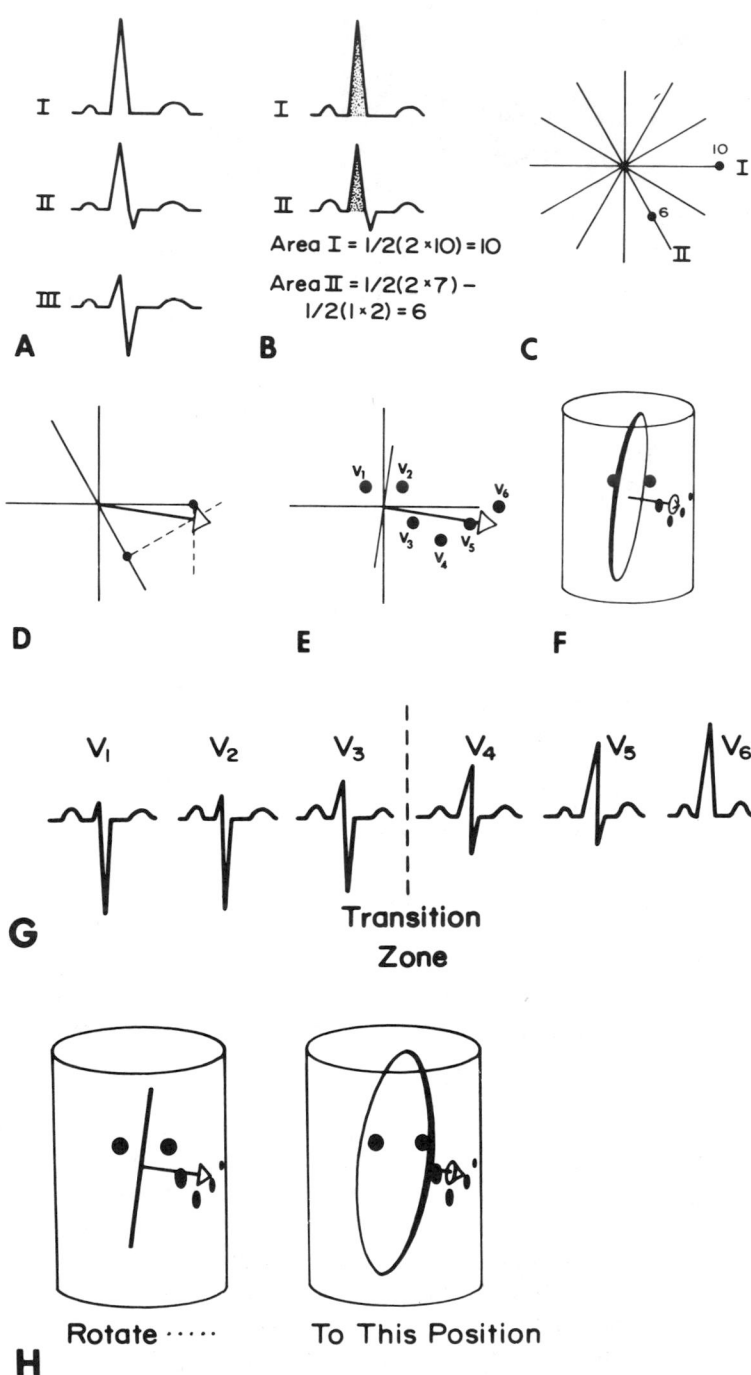

Figure 199. Determination of the mean QRS vector in three dimensions (for details, see text).

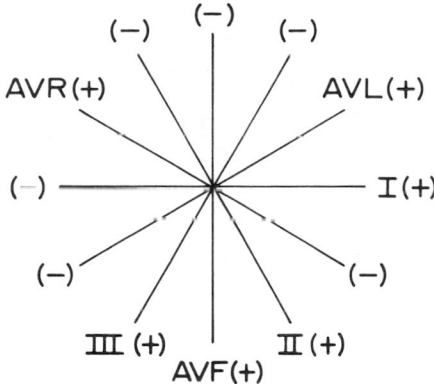

Figure 200. The lead-graph of the hexaxial system. Each lead is separated from the next by 30°. This is a graph which should be used for plotting vectors in two dimensions (ie, the "frontal plane").

the two-dimensional frontal plane (that is, looking at the heart from the front only), draw the precordial leads on the lead-graph as if you were viewing the front of the patient with the six chest leads in place (Fig 199E).

What this two-dimensional drawing represents is the six leads painted on a cylinder (roughly approximating the human thorax). Next, draw a perpendicular to your frontal plane vector (Fig 199E). This perpendicular line on the paper represents the edge of a circular plane sitting inside the cylinder (Fig 199F). Inspect the QRS complexes from the precordial leads (V_1-V_6) and decide at what point the QRS complex becomes more positive than negative (that is, where the area beneath the R becomes greater than the area beneath the S) (Fig 199G). The vector arrow attached to the center of the circular plane moves more posteriorly as the front of the plane moves from the V_1-V_2 interspace to the V_3-V_4 interspace. The front of the circular plane may move in any direction to intersect the transition zone. This three-dimensional concept can be represented on paper by drawing an ellipse around the tip of the line drawn perpendicular to the vector arrow, and intersecting the transition zone. Then draw a similar (but smaller) ellipse around the end of the vector arrow (Fig 201). Anterior and posterior vectors are drawn as shown in Fig 202. You have now constructed the mean QRS vector in three-dimensional space!

The mean T vector. The T vector can be constructed using precisely the same method (step-by-step) that was used for the mean QRS vector (Fig 203).

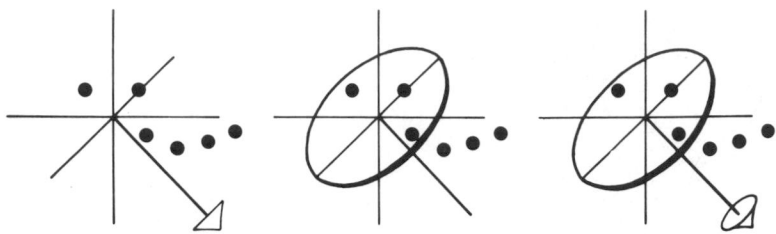

Figure 201. An easy method for drawing the conceptualized mean QRS vector in its anterior-posterior orientation. Note that the ellipse at the base of the arrowhead is a miniature version of the ellipse encompassing the perpendicular line at the base of the vector.

Anterior Vectors Posterior Vectors

Figure 202. Examples of several anterior and posterior vectors.

The mean P vector, initial 1/2 and terminal 1/2 P vectors. The mean P vector can be constructed in exactly the same manner as the mean QRS and mean T vectors. The initial-1/2-P vector is constructed in a similar manner, but uses only the area underneath the first 50% of each P wave. The terminal-1/2-P vector uses only the last 50% of each P wave. The initial-1/2-P vector and terminal-1/2-P vector correspond roughly to right and left atrial depolarization, respectively.

The initial 0.04 second QRS vector. The same method is employed as in the determination of the mean QRS vector; however, only the first 0.04 seconds (the first "small block") of the QRS area is considered. The initial 0.04 QRS vector yields information regarding the magnitude and direction of the initial depolarization of the ventricle. The initial depolarization is most often disturbed as a result of an electrical dead zone. Myocardial infarction may produce an electrical dead zone manifested as Q waves or loss of R wave force. An electrical dead zone can also result from the fibrosis of cardiomyopathy or from infiltrative myocardial processes such as amyloidosis, hemochromatosis, granulomas, and metastatic cancer.

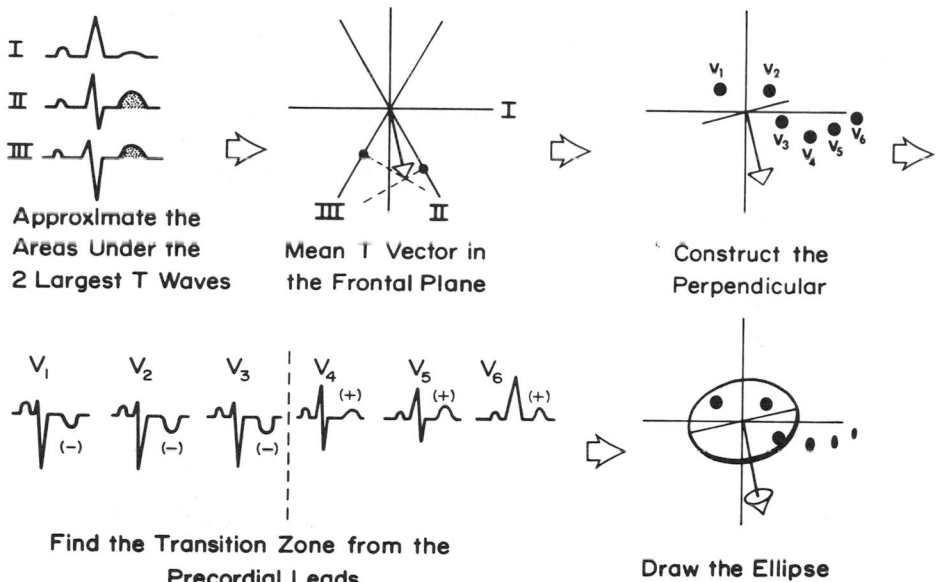

Figure 203. Determination of the mean T vector in three dimensions (the procedure is exactly the same as those used for the mean QRS vector, except the area under the T wave is used).

Said in another way, Q waves (directional changes in initial ventricular depolarization) are not specific for myocardial infarction.

The anatomical region of the heart having the electrical dead zone can be determined by plotting the initial 0.04 QRS vector in three dimensions, imaging the shape of the heart as it lies in the thorax, and ascribing the dead zone to the region which is anatomically 180° away from the direction of the vector (Fig 204).

The terminal 0.04 second QRS vector. The terminal 0.04 second QRS vector is constructed utilizing only the area underneath the last 0.04 second (one small block) of each QRS complex. When the QRS complex is abnormally wide (>0.10 second duration), the terminal 0.04 QRS vector is useful in determining the anatomical region of the heart in which there is slowing of conduction velocity, or even bundle branch block. When the terminal 0.04 QRS vector is drawn in three dimensions, it points toward the area of slowed conduction, or bundle branch block (Fig 205).

The ST segment vector. In many patients, the ST segment is not above or below the baseline (the T-P segment), and it will be difficult, if not impossible, to draw an ST segment vector. In patients with ST segment

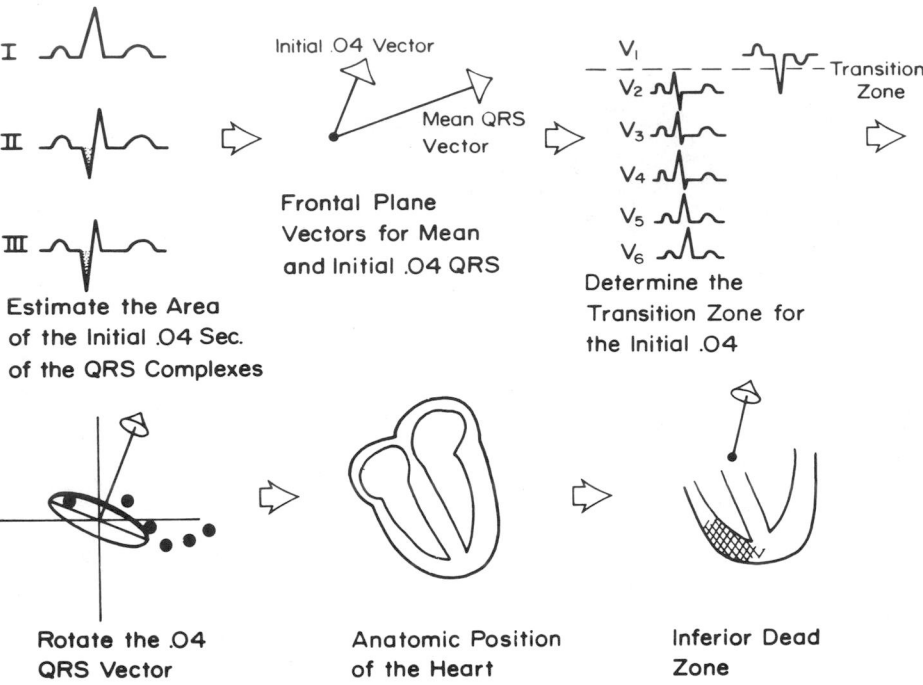

Figure 204. Determination of the initial 0.04-second QRS vector (the procedure is the same as those used for the mean QRS vector, except that only the first 0.04 second of the QRS is used). This vector points 180° away from an electrical dead zone.

elevation or depression, the area underneath (if the ST segment is elevated) or above (if the ST segment is depressed) the ST segment can be used to plot a three-dimensional ST vector using the same method as described for the mean QRS vector. In patients with early myocardial infarction (epicardial injury), the ST segment vector points at the area of anatomical injury (Fig 206).

A rather large ST vector may be encountered in some normal persons. The normal mean ST vector is usually parallel with the mean T vector, which may also be quite large. A normal ST vector can be differentiated from the ST vector of pericarditis, subendocardial ischemia or potassium effect by its stability on serial tracings and by the absence of associated abnormalities.

The ventricular gradient. In later paragraphs, examples of normal and abnormal QRS, ST, T, P, initial 0.04 QRS, and terminal 0.04 QRS vectors will be shown. A very useful concept that is the foundation for many of the examples is the "ventricular gradient." The ventricular gradient helps

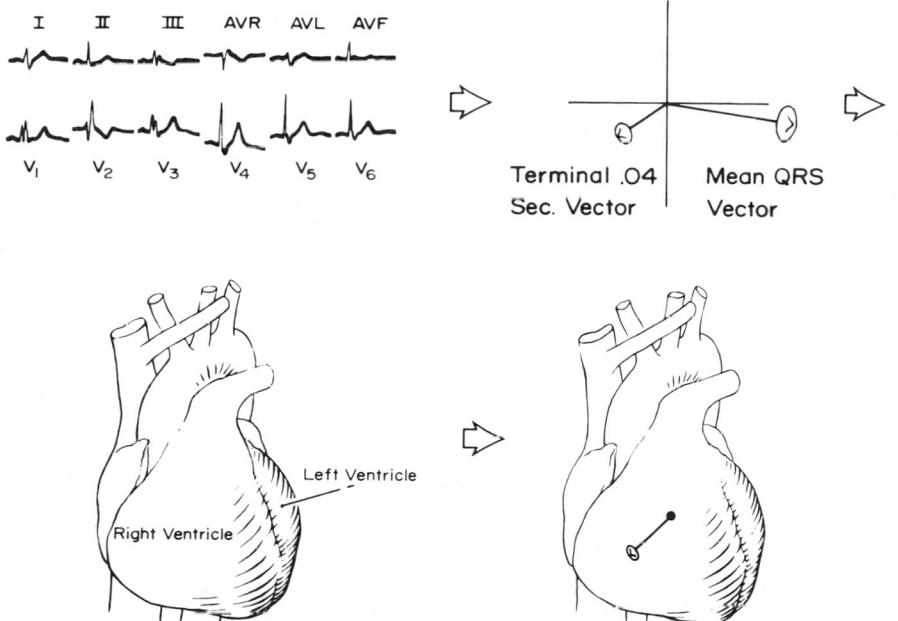

**Right Ventricle is Anterior,
Left Ventricle is Posterior**

**Terminal .04 Vector is Directed
Toward the Right Ventricle, ∴ RBBB**

Figure 205. When there is a conduction delay in one ventricle or bundle branch block, the terminal 0.04 QRS vector points toward the area or ventricle in which the delay or block occurs.

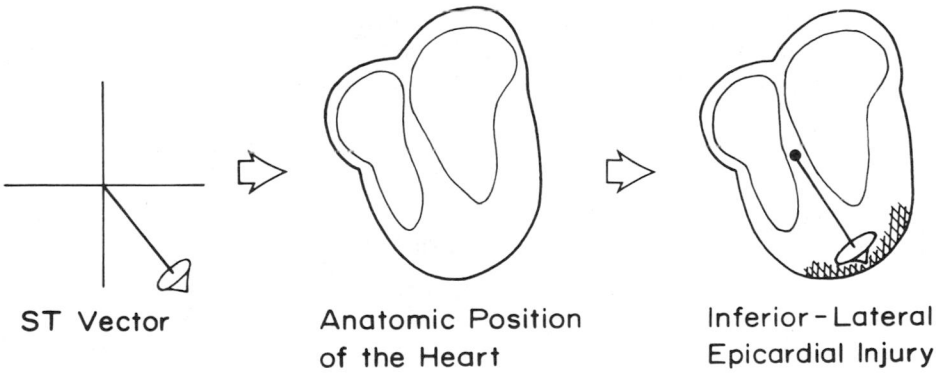

ST Vector

**Anatomic Position
of the Heart**

**Inferior - Lateral
Epicardial Injury**

Figure 206. The ST vector (determined by using the area beneath the ST segment and plotted in a manner similar to that used for the QRS) points toward the anatomical area of injury.

to determine whether abnormal T waves (repolarization) are secondary to an abnormality of the QRS (depolarization), or whether they are a primary manifestation of ventricular disease. Secondary T wave changes occur largely from hypertrophy or conduction disturbances. Primary T wave changes occur primarily as a manifestation of epicardial injury or myocardial ischemia but may occur as a result of electrolyte imbalance, quinidine and digitalis therapy, hypothyroidism, and other disorders. There are, of course, exceptions to these generalizations.

The ventricular gradient (gradient vector) can be determined from the mean QRS and the mean T vector (Fig 207).

1. First draw the mean QRS and mean T vector in three-dimensional space.
2. Complete the parallelogram that is bound on two sides by these two vectors.
3. Draw the gradient vector originating from the point of origin of the QRS and T vectors; draw the arrowhead in the opposite corner of the parallelogram.
4. Two basic rules apply:
   a. A normal gradient vector lies within about 30° of either side of the mean QRS vector.
   b. A normal gradient vector lies within the 0° to +90° lead quadrant (lower right quadrant) and is usually between +10° and +80°.
5. If the ventricular gradient is normal, there are either no "T wave changes" on the scalar ECG, or the patient has secondary T wave changes which are due to some alteration in the time sequence of onset of depolarization and therefore repolarization throughout the heart muscle, as in ventricular hypertrophy or bundle branch block. If the ventricular gradient is abnormal, the patient has *primary* T wave changes that reflect a change in the duration of the excited state in some region of the heart muscle, as in myocardial ischemia or injury.

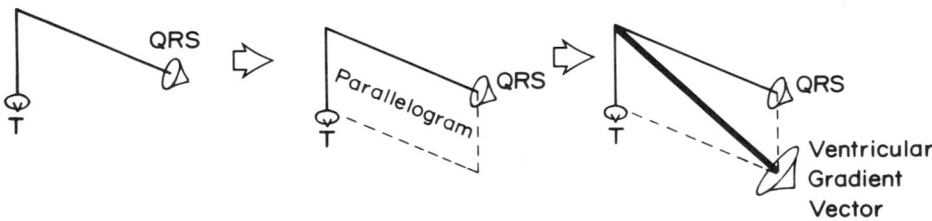

Figure 207.   The ventricular gradient vector is the diagonal of the parallelogram bounded on two sides by the mean QRS and mean T vectors as they are plotted in three dimensions.

Although the ventricular gradient is an extremely useful concept, the method used to determine the ventricular gradient partially limits its clinical usefulness. This is true primarily because the manual measurements and calculations used to derive the mean QRS and mean T vectors depend on the inertia of the pen recorder in the ECG machine, the thickness of the lines, and the absolute size of QRS and T waves. When the QRS vector loop resembles a circle, it may even be difficult to construct the mean QRS vector in the frontal plane (Fig 208).

Examples of normal and abnormal vectors. Figure 209 shows three important P vectors. Fig 210A-E represents normal mean QRS and T vectors. If the ventricular gradient were constructed for each of the examples in Fig 210A-E, it would be normal.

Mean QRS vectors with secondary ST or T vectors. Note in Fig 210F-J, that the ST vector is directed in the same general direction as the T

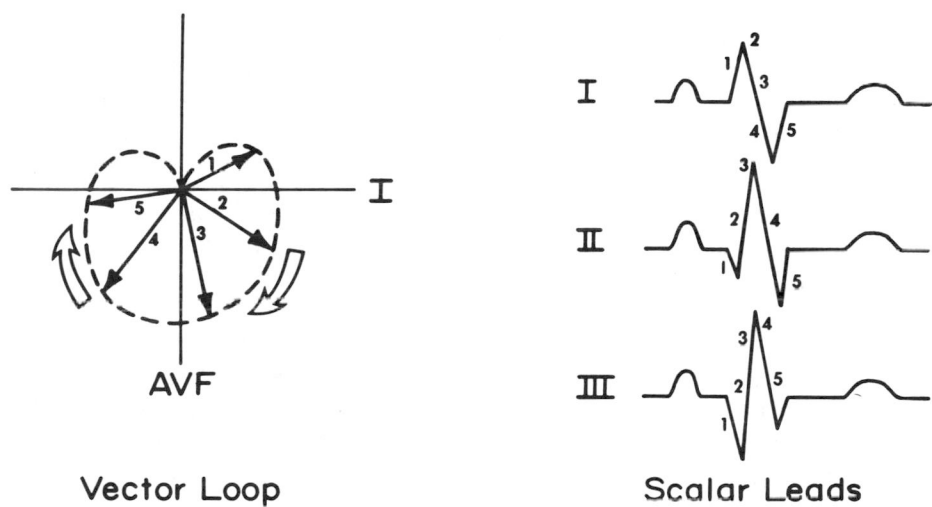

| Vector Loop | Scalar Leads |

Figure 208. A mean QRS vector may be difficult to determine from the scalar leads when the vector loop approximates a circle.

Normal Mean
P Vector

Left Atrial Abnormality
(Terminal -1/2- P Vector)

Right Atrial Abnormality
(Initial -1/2- P Vector)

Figure 209. The three most useful P vectors.

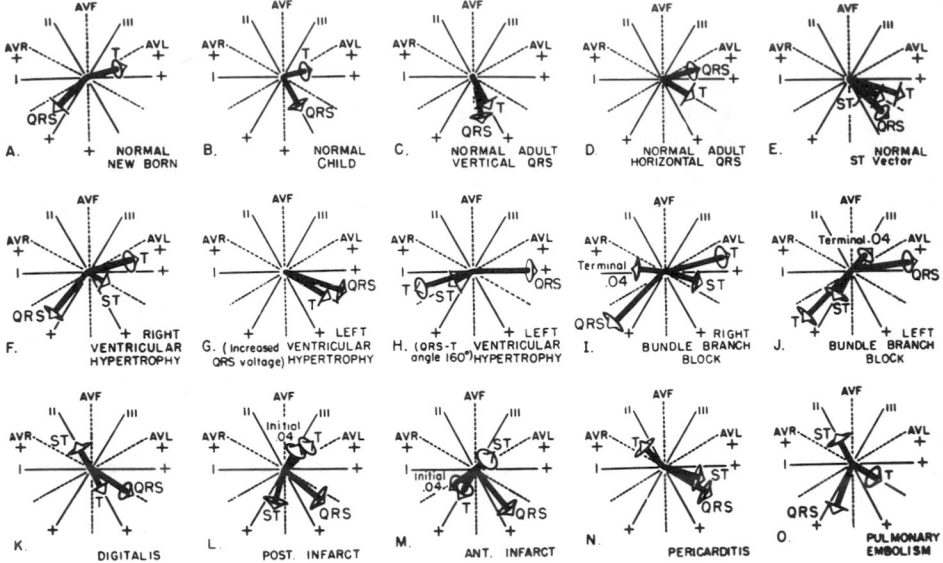

Figure 210. The diagrams above illustrate the spatial vector arrangements for most of the electrocardiographic syndromes commonly observed in clinical practice. Reproduced from Hurst JW, Meyerburg RJ: *Introduction to Electrocardiography,* ed 2. New York, McGraw-Hill Book Company, 1973, with permission of the author and publisher.

vector. The ventricular gradient is normal in these five examples. In right and left bundle branch block, the terminal 0.04 second QRS vectors point to the right and left, respectively.

Mean QRS vectors with primary ST or T vectors. Except in the case of digitalis, the ventricular gradient is abnormal in Fig 210K-O. In the two examples of myocardial infarction, note that the initial 0.04 second QRS vectors point 180° away from the area of infarct if a three dimensional heart is superimposed on the lead graph.

Examples of usefulness of the vector method include:

> *Left ventricular hypertrophy with secondary ST and T wave changes.* On initial inspection of Fig 211A, the depressed ST segments and inverted T waves might suggest myocardial ischemia to some observers. However, by plotting the mean QRS, ST, and T vectors and then determining the ventricular gradient, the ST and T wave changes are categorized as secondary to the left ventricular hypertrophy (Fig 211B).
>
> *Left bundle branch block with previous lateral myocardial infarction.* A casual examiner might call Fig 212A isolated left bundle

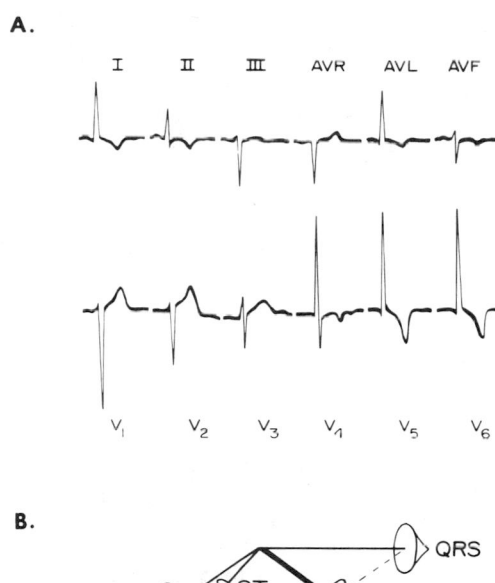

Figure 211.   A, An electrocardiogram from a patient with left ventricular hypertrophy. B, The direction of the gradient vector determines that the inverted T waves are "secondary" to an abnormality of repolarization, and not due to ischemia or infarction.

branch block. However, the initial 0.04 QRS vector suggests there is an electrical dead zone in the lateral wall of the left ventricle (Fig 212B). Left bundle branch block, per se, usually eliminates even the small "normal" Q waves that may occur in leads I and aV$_L$.

Early repolarization. The ST segment elevation in Fig 213A might be misinterpreted as evidence of epicardial injury. However, by plotting the QRS, ST and T vectors (Fig 213B), the mean ST segment vector is noted to be directed in the same general direction as the mean QRS vector.

Dysrhythmias.   There are several basic electrophysiologic mechanisms on which most of the dysrhythmias encountered in clinical practice are based. Recall that the changes in intracellular and extracellular concentrations of electrolytes such as sodium, potassium, chloride, and calcium account for the depolarization and repolarization of myocardial cells. These ion fluxes also change the charges on the inside of the cell as they move across the myocardial cell membrane. During one electrical systole and diastole, the change in the charge can be represented by a diagram of the instantaneous intracellular voltage (Fig 214).

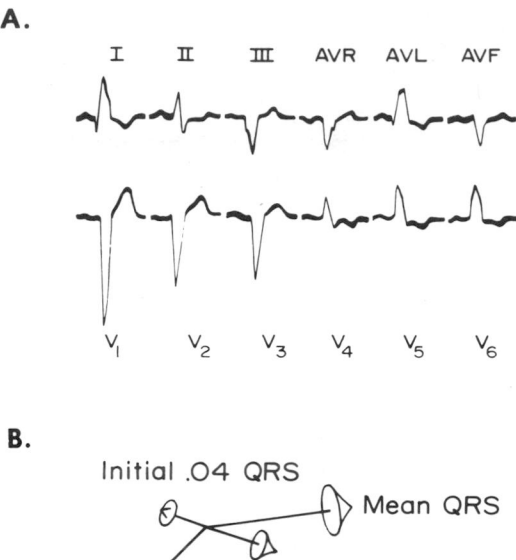

Figure 212. *A*, The electrocardiogram shows left bundle branch block with small Q waves in leads I and aV_L. *B*, The initial 0.04-second QRS vector suggests there is an electrical dead zone in the lateral wall of the left ventricle (180° opposite from the direction of this vector).

Alterations in the action potential account for the four basic electrophysiologic properties of the heart: (1) automaticity, (2) excitability, (3) refractoriness, and (4) conductivity. The effect of each of these properties on the action potential is diagrammed in Fig 215.

Cardiac cells can be divided into two basic types: pacemaker cells (specialized cardiac fibers) and nonpacemaker cells (contractile muscle fibers). Looking again at the shape of the action potentials in Fig 205, note that the sinus node action potential shows it is "automatic;" that is, the negativity attained at the end of phase 3 is not maintained during the subsequent diastole; the membrane potential slowly declines (moves upwards) toward the level of the threshold potential. This is called spontaneous phase 4 diastolic depolarization and is present only in pacemaker fibers. Therefore, diastolic depolarization is the potential change responsible for the property of *automaticity*. There are both *actual* and *latent* pacemakers: in an actual pacemaker the diastolic depolarization is gradual; in a latent pacemaker, the diastolic depolarization moves more abruptly toward threshold potential.

Dysrhythmias may occur as a result of altered automaticity either from: (1) an increase or decrease in the function of pacemaker fibers, or

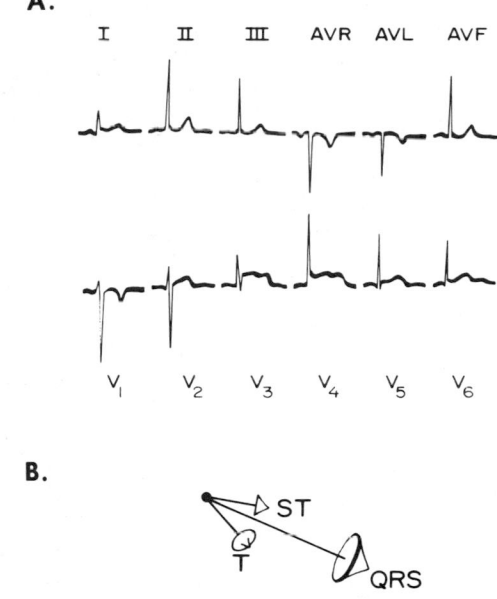

Figure 213. *A,* The electrocardiogram shows an elevation of the ST segment in leads I, V_2, V_3, V_4, V_5 and V_6. *B,* The QRS, ST, and T vectors point in the same general direction, suggesting the "early repolarization" syndrome.

CARDIAC ACTION POTENTIAL

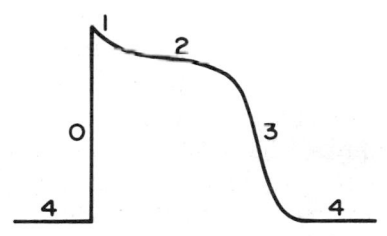

Phase	Ion	Direction
O	Na^+	Into Cell
I	Cl^-	Into Cell
	K^+	Out of Cell
2	Ca^{++}	Into Cell
	K^+	Out of Cell
3	K^+	Out of Cell

Figure 214. The cardiac action potential is a result of the movement of several ions across the myocardial cell membrane during the different phases of the action potential.

(2) injury to a nonpacemaker fiber causing it to act like a pacemaker fiber. The rate of a pacemaker can be changed by altering the rate of diastolic depolarization, the maximum diastolic potential (end of phase 3), or the threshold potential.

The other basic mechanism responsible for dysrhythmias is reentry. Reentry probably results from nonuniformity of cardiac tissue with re-

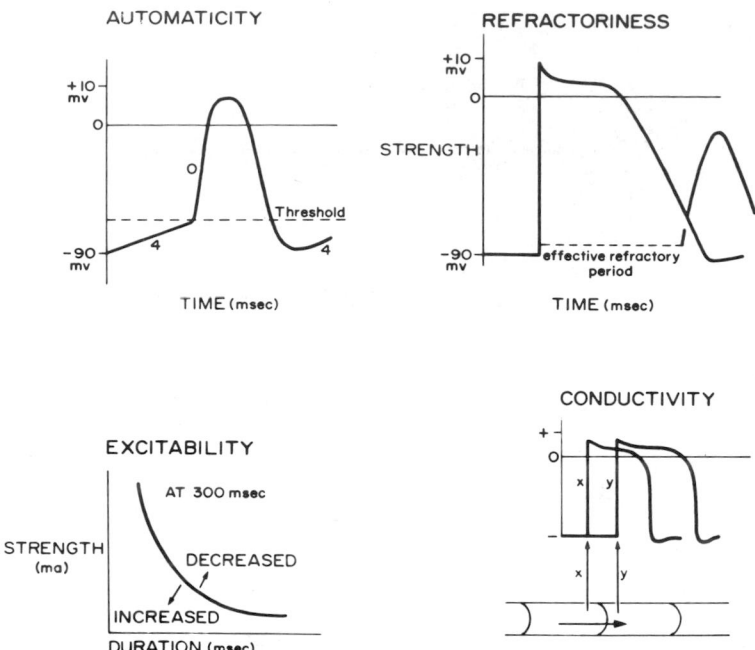

Figure 215.   The four basic electrophysiologic properties of the heart (for definitions see text).

spect to its ability to be excited (*excitability*) and its ability to conduct an impulse (*impulse conductivity*). There are two types of reentry: (1) *focal* reexcitation resulting from adjacent fibers with different excitability and (2) *circus* reentry. Focal reexcitation is reentry without the development of a circus movement; if adjacent fibers repolarize at different rates, the faster ones may be reexcited by the slower fibers which have not yet completely repolarized. Circus reentry is the propagation of an impulse in a circular path; this requires a region of tissue which initially fails to respond to a wave of excitation (ie, it is refractory) in one direction, but is excited slightly later by the same impulse returning in the opposite direction.

Clinical Significance

Recognition of dysrhythmias.   Three primary factors which account for the initiation and maintenance of most cardiac dysrhythmias are altered automaticity, reentry, and temporal dispersion of the refractory period. Although an isolated factor cannot always be identified, try to determine the mechanism of any dysrhythmias since the most effective therapy will be directed toward the correction of the specific electrophysiologic abnormalities.

The clinical recognition of cardiac rhythm disorders is often classified by anatomical site of origin (sinus node, atrial, junctional, ventricular). The problem that some readers face when trying to analyze and identify a particular rhythm disorder is not knowing which chapter or section to read since the anatomical site of origin is not clear. We would like to present this discussion of dysrhythmias by classifying them into five easily recognized categories. The categories are based on heart rate, and subdivided with respect to the width of the QRS complex and the presence or absence of P waves. The five categories are: normocardias, tachycardias, bradycardias, abnormal beats, and abnormal P-R intervals. Related dysrhythmias within each category are defined in Tables 51–55.

Clinical settings in which dysrhythmias occur. Several clinical settings predispose patients to dysrhythmias through the mechanisms previously discussed. These are outlined below.

1. Patients with ischemic myocardium. Myocardial tissue which has been rendered ischemic may have areas in which the velocity of conduction is slowed. This can cause the depolarization wave to be delayed long enough in these ischemic areas that the surrounding tissue completely or incompletely repolarizes, allowing the slowed depolarization wave to reenter the surrounding repolarized tissue. This reentry may lead to a premature ventricular complex or multiple sequential ventricular complexes in certain situations. Ischemic tissue may also allow the temporary transformation of nonpacemaker ventricular

Table 51.   Normocardias (rate usually 60–100 beats/minute; rhythm regular unless stated otherwise).

A.   Normal QRS complex ($\leq$ 0.10 sec)
  1.   Sinus rhythm. Preceding P waves are present.
  2.   Sinus dysrhythmia. Preceding P waves are present, rhythm slightly irregular.
  3.   Nonparoxysmal junctional tachycardia. P waves are absent or are inverted in II, III, aV_F.

B.   Wide QRS complex (> 0.10 sec)
  1.   Accelerated idioventricular rhythm. P waves are absent or inverted in II, III, aV_F.
  2.   Bundle branch block. P waves precede each QRS complex.
  3.   Wolff-Parkinson-White syndrome.

Table 52. Tachycardias (rate > 100 beats/minute; rhythm regular unless stated otherwise).

A.   Normal QRS complex (≤ 0.10 sec)
1.   Sinus tachycardia. Preceding P waves are present; rate is usually <180/minute; sinus tachycardia is not a primary rhythm disorder but is secondary to other systemic disturbances.
2.   Atrial tachycardia. Preceding P waves are often hidden but precede QRS; atrial rate ranges from 180 to 240 beats/minute; QRS rate varies depending on the presence or absence of AV block; the rhythm may or may not begin suddenly; P waves are often large or bizarre (Fig 216).
3.   Atrial flutter. The P waves appear "sawtoothed" and usually occur at rates near 300/minute; QRS rate about 150, 100 or 75 beats/minute depending on the degree of AV block; "sawtoothed" P waves (flutter waves) best recognized in II, III, aV$_F$ (Fig 217).
4.   Atrial fibrillation. No P waves; baseline flat or "wiggly"; QRS complexes appear at unpredictable intervals although the QRS rate is usually <200/minute (Fig 218).

B.   Wide QRS complex (>0.10 sec)
1.   Sinus tachycardia, atrial tachycardia, atrial flutter, or atrial fibrillation associated with bundle branch block or "aberrant conduction."
2.   Ventricular tachycardia. P waves are either absent, inverted in II, III, aV$_F$ if conducted retrograde, or upright and at a different rate from the QRS indicating A-V dissociation. QRS complexes usually occur faster than 120/minute [Fig 219].
3.   Ventricular flutter. P waves are absent; regular undulating waves of ventricular activity occur between 180 and 260/minute.
4.   Wolff-Parkinson-White. Associated preceding P waves with a short P-R interval; QRS may or may not be wide; if the QRS is wide, a delta wave may mark the premature ventricular depolarization as a slur on the upstroke of the QRS.

C.   No recognizable QRS complex
1.   Monitoring leads are loose.
2.   Ventricular fibrillation. Coarse or fine, irregular, undulations of baseline (Fig 220).
3.   Ventricular standstill. Straight line.

---

tissue into pacemaker tissue with spontaneous phase 4 depolarization and an action potential which resembles that of pacemaker tissue.
2.   Patients with infarcted myocardium. Myocardial tissue which has undergone necrosis may conduct electrical impulses abnormally, or not at all. This may cause an abnormal direction

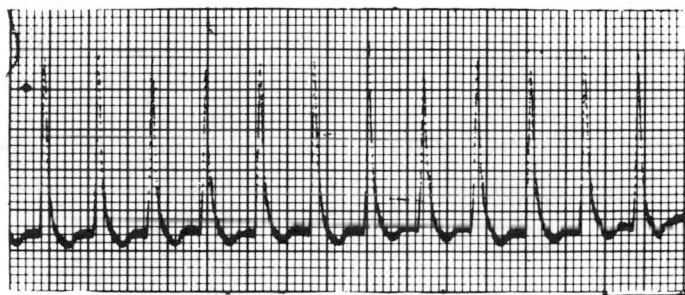

Figure 216. Paroxysmal atrial tachycardia. A short strip obtained during an attack of paroxysmal atrial tachycardia, demonstrating a heart rate of 222 beats/min (R-R interval = 0.27 sec). The P waves cannot be discerned because of the extremely rapid rate. Reproduced from Hurst JW, Meyerburg RJ: *Introduction to Electrocardiography,* ed 2. New York, McGraw-Hill Book Company, 1973, with permission of the author and publisher.

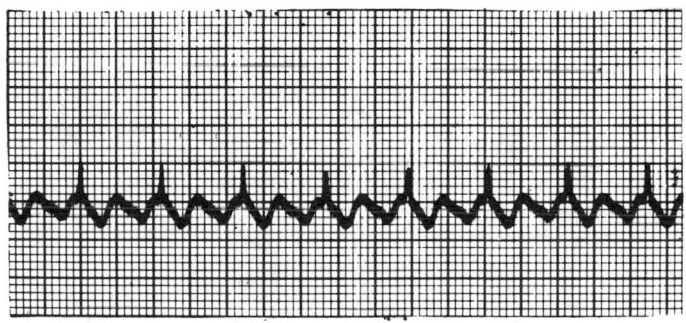

Figure 217. Atrial flutter with 2:1 A-V conduction. The atrial flutter rate is 272/min (P-P interval = 0.22 sec), and the ventricular rate is 136/min (R-R interval = 0.44 sec). Sawtooth flutter waves may be less obvious in the presence of the more rapid ventricular response. As the atrial flutter rate increases and/or the ventricular response increases, atrial flutter becomes more difficult to recognize. Reproduced from Hurst JW, Myerburg RJ: *Introduction to Electrocardiography,* ed 2. New York, McGraw-Hill Book Company, 1973, with permission of the author and publisher.

of the propagation wave and a delay in ventricular depolarization or repolarization, leading to a prolonged duration of the QRS complex, and a temporal dispersion of the refractory period in some myocardial cells.

3. Elderly patients. As the heart ages, degeneration and calcification of the conduction tissue is not an unusual occurrence. These processes often lead to clinical entities such as the bradycardia-tachycardia syndrome (alteration in sinus node function and atrial automaticity), A-V delay and block, and

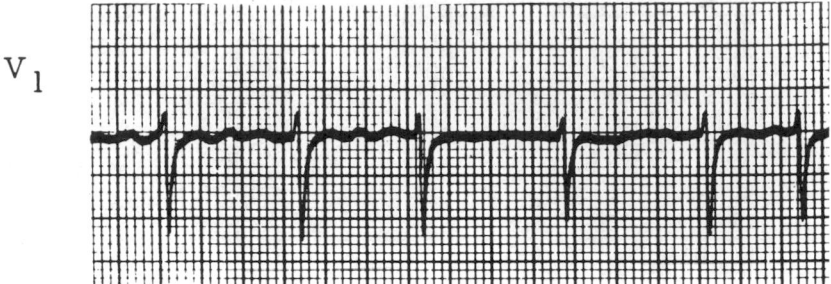

Figure 218. Atrial fibrillation. There is a grossly irregular ventricular response, with R-R intervals varying from 0.76 to 0.45 sec. The baseline shows fibrillatory wave activity with some variation in the depth of the waves. Reproduced from Hurst JW, Meyerburg RJ: *Introduction to Electrocardiography*, ed 2. New York, McGraw-Hill Book Company, 1973, with permission of the author and publisher.

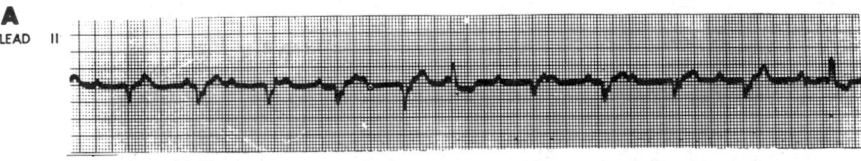

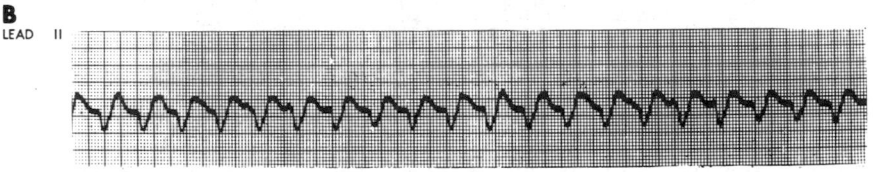

Figure 219. Ventricular tachycardia. *A*, Complete heart block is present, as manifested by the absence of any relationship between the P waves and QRS complexes and an idioventricular rhythm. The rate of the idioventricular rhythm, however, is much more rapid than the normal escape rate of a ventricular pacemaker (P-R interval of basic rhythm = 0.86 sec, rate = 70/min). Therefore, even though the rate does not conform to the usual definition of tachycardia (rate = 100), it is an abnormal rate for this pacemaker and is therefore called an accelerated ventricular rhythm. Note, too, the irregular extrasystolic activity present. *B*, Ventricular tachycardia with a rate of 136/min is present. Complete heart block is still present and a number of the P waves are easily seen. Since the P-P intervals are quite constant, the presence of the other P waves is inferred. The P waves and QRS complexes are completely independent of each other because of the complete heart block. Reproduced from Hurst JW, Meyerburg RJ: *Introduction to Electrocardiography*, ed 2. New York, McGraw-Hill Book Company, 1973, with permission of the author and publisher.

bundle branch block, which may require either pacemaker therapy or pharmacologic intervention.

4. Drug related problems. Patients taking drugs such as digitalis, quinidine, propranolol, tricyclic antidepressants, phenothiazines, diuretics, and ethanol are predisposed to dysrhythmias, particularly if taking toxic doses. The mechanisms underlying these dysrhythmias are briefly described below.

   a. Digitalis. The rhythm disturbances which result from digitalis excess are secondary to the following electrophysiologic phenomena: enhanced automaticity in the sinus node and in the His-Purkinje system, increased vagal tone, increased conduction velocity in the atrioventricular node (conduction delay or block), junctional or ventricular tachyarrhythmias, and premature ventricular complexes.

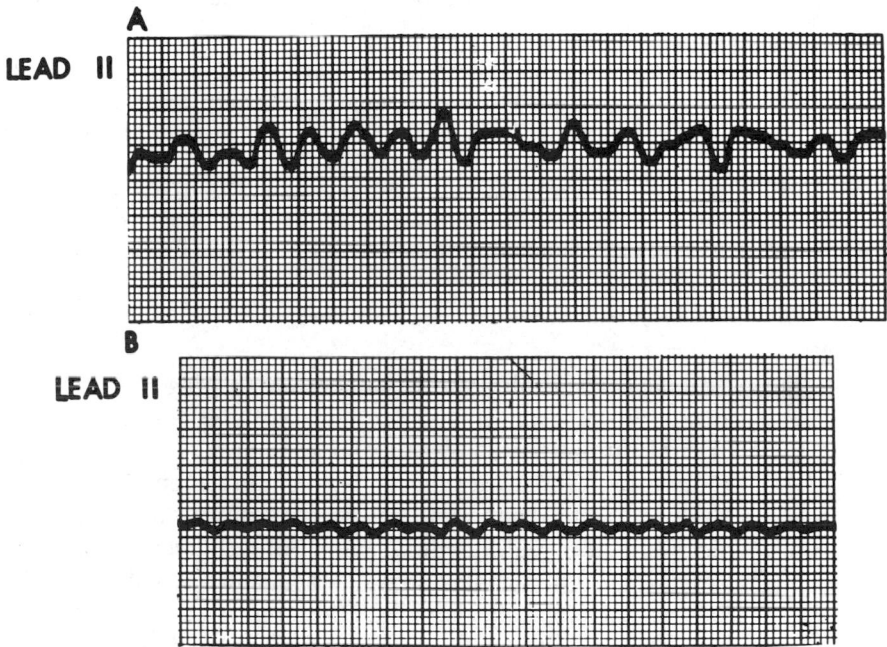

Figure 220. Ventricular fibrillation. This rhythm is incompatible with life since it represents uncoordinated ventricular activity with no cardiac output. It is, however, frequently treatable, the success of treatment depending on the setting in which it occurs. A, Coarse ventricular fibrillation. Note the irregular waveform activity. B, Fine ventricular fibrillation. This type of pattern frequently precedes the complete cessation of electrical activity at the time of biological death of the heart and is very difficult to defibrillate. Reproduced from Hurst JW, Meyerburg RJ: *Introduction to Electrocardiography*, ed 2. New York, McGraw-Hill Book Company, 1973, with permission of the author and publisher.

Table 53. Bradycardias (rate < 60 beats/minute; rhythm regular unless stated otherwise).

A. Normal QRS complex (≤ 0.10 sec)

    1. Sinus bradycardia. Preceding P waves are present.

    2. Sinus pause. The P waves occur late but the QRS and the T are unchanged and follow each P wave.

    3. Sinus exit block. Interval from P wave to P wave doubles, triples, or quadruples; the sinus node fires but atrial depolarization does not occur; the QRS and T are unchanged and follow each P wave.

    4. Multiple nonconducted premature P waves. Early atrial depolarization finds the A-V node or ventricle refractory; the P waves are often hidden somewhere within the Q-T intervals of the preceding beat.

    5. Junctional escape rhythm. The P waves are absent or inverted in II, III, aV_F; the QRS rate is often between 40 and 60/minute.

B. Wide QRS complex (> 0.10 sec)

    1. Sinus bradycardia or junctional rhythm associated with bundle branch block or "aberrantly conducted" QRS complexes.

    2. Idioventricular rhythm. The P waves are usually absent but if present are inverted in II, III, aV_F.

    3. Severe hyperkalemia. No P waves; the QRS is wide and may become similar to a "sine wave" in the most severe cases.

    4. Dying heart. Isolated, bizarre QRS complexes (also called agonal rhythm).

Digitalis is probably the most commonly prescribed cardiac drug, so the manifestations of digitalis excess are extremely important to learn and recognize.

b. Quinidine. This drug may depress intraventricular conduction, allowing reentry dysrhythmias to occur; or decrease the resting membrane potential, enhancing automaticity. Quinidine excess is associated with widening of the QRS complex and lengthening of the Q-T interval. Cardiac toxicity may lead to atrioventricular and intraventricular block, ventricular tachyarrhythmias and depression of myocardial contractility. "Quinidine syncope" is an uncommon but important complication of quinidine therapy. It is characterized by ventricular tachycardia or fibrillation, which may be irreversible.

c. Procainamide. The electrophysiological effects of this drug include: decreased cardiac excitability and increased electrical threshold for stimulation, increased refractory period of all cardiac cells, decreased spontaneous diastolic pace-

Table 54.   Abnormal beats.

A. QRS complexes occurring prematurely (ie, earlier than expected from the preceding R-R intervals)
1. Normal QRS ($\leq$ 0.10 sec)
   a. Atrial premature complex. The P wave is early and usually has a different shape; followed by normal QRS and T waves (Fig 221). Also called PAC.
   b. Junctional premature complex. Early QRS complex associated with no P waves or inverted P waves in II, III, aV$_F$ (Fig 222).
2. Wide QRS ($>$ 0.10 sec)
   a. Atrial or junction premature complex associated with bundle branch block or aberrantly conducted QRS complex.
   b. Ventricular premature complex. P waves are absent or inverted in II, III, aV$_F$; T wave is usually opposite in polarity from QRS (Fig 223). Also called PVC or VPC.

B. QRS complexes occurring late (ie, later than expected from the preceding R-R intervals)
1. Normal QRS ($\leq$ 0.10 sec)
   a. Atrial escape beat. Late P wave following by QRS and T.
   b. Junctional escape beat. Late QRS associated with either no P waves or with inverted P waves in II, III, aV$_F$.
2. Wide QRS ($>$ 0.10 sec)
   a. Atrial or junctional escape beat associated with bundle branch block or aberrantly conducted QRS complex.
   b. Ventricular escape beat. No P waves or inverted P waves in II, III, aV$_F$.

C. Extra or bizarre QRS complexes occurring at regular intervals
1. Normal QRS ($\leq$ 0.10 sec)
   a. Atrial bigeminy. Atrial premature complexes occurring every other beat.
   b. Junctional bigeminy. Junctional premature complexes occurring every other beat.
   c. Atrial parasystole. Atrial beats (P wave followed by QRS-T) occur at regular intervals (or multiples) from each other, not related or coupled to the basic rhythm.
   d. Junctional parasystole. Junctional beats (QRS-T without preceding P wave sometimes QRS-P-T) occur at regular intervals (or multiples) from each other; not related or coupled to the basic rhythm.
   e. Electrical alternans. Every other QRS complex changes polarity to some degree, but occurs on time.
2. Wide QRS ($>$ 0.10 sec)
   a. Ventricular bigeminy. Ventricular premature complexes occur every other beat; trigeminy if every third beat or

Table 54.   Abnormal beats. (continued)

        if two out of three beats; quadrigeminy if every fourth beat.

  b.   Ventricular parasystole. Ventricular beats (QRS-T) occurring at regular intervals (or multiples) from each other, not related or coupled to the basic rhythm.

  c.   Bidirectional ventricular tachycardia. QRS rate > 100, polarity of QRS complexes changes (often in alternating beats).

---

        maker activity, widened QRS complex (often a sign of toxicity), and prolonged Q-T interval. Cardiac toxicity may be manifested as progressive QRS widening, ventricular ectopic complexes, ventricular fibrillation, or electrical asystole.

  d.   Propranolol. Toxic cardiac reactions to propranolol include cardiac failure, sinus bradycardia, various degrees of sinoatrial and atrioventricular block, and electrical asystole. No pathognomonic electrocardiographic manifestation of propranolol toxicity has been described; however, sinus

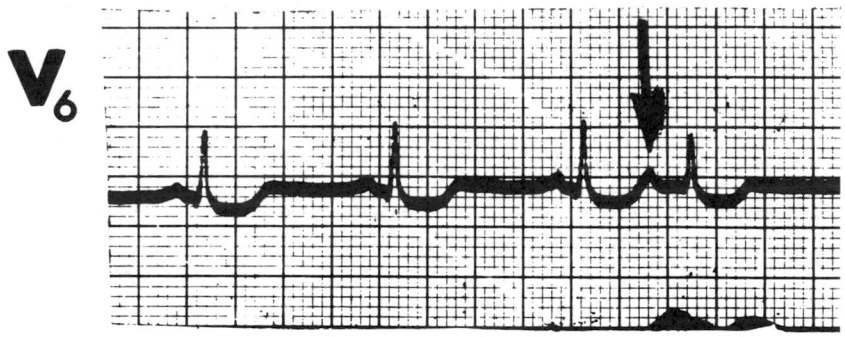

Figure 221.   Premature atrial contraction. The fourth QRS is early and of the same configuration as the other complexes. The differential diagnosis lies between premature atrial beat and premature A-V nodal beat. There is an abrupt upward deflection at the end of the T wave of the complex preceding the premature beat. This deflection is not present in the T waves of the other complexes on the tracing and is the representation of the superimposed P wave of the premature atrial beat. The pause following the premature beat is noncompensatory (< two full cycle lengths from the P wave before the early P wave to the P wave after it, see text), which is characteristic of premature atrial beats. The P-R interval of the premature complex is prolonged because of residual refractoriness in parts of the A-V conduction system at the time of the early beat. Reproduced from Hurst JW, Meyerburg RJ: *Introduction to Electrocardiography*, ed 2. New York, McGraw-Hill Book Company, 1973, with permission of the author and publisher.

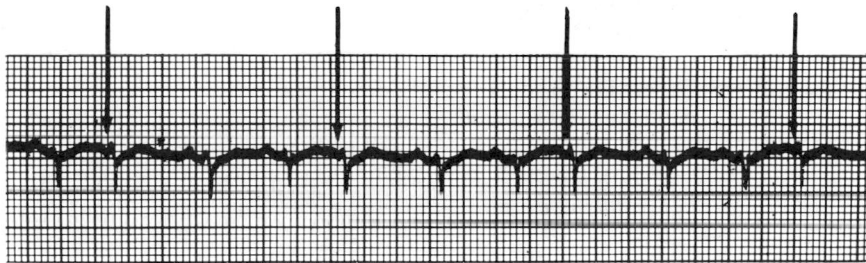

Figure 222. Junctional premature beats with fixed coupling intervals. Every third beat is a premature beat (the third, sixth, ninth, and twelfth complexes). These beats occur early and have the same configuration of the QRS complexes of the sinus beats. In addition, the premature beats are preceded by inverted P waves (arrows) beginning 0.04 sec before the QRS. Since the P-R interval is less than 0.12 sec, it may be concluded that the P waves are conducted retrograde from the focus of the junctional pacemaker. Since the P wave precedes the QRS, the site of the pacemaker is probably high in the A-V junction. The P-R intervals of the sinus beats are constant at 0.14 sec, and the premature junctional beats are followed by a fully compensatory pause.

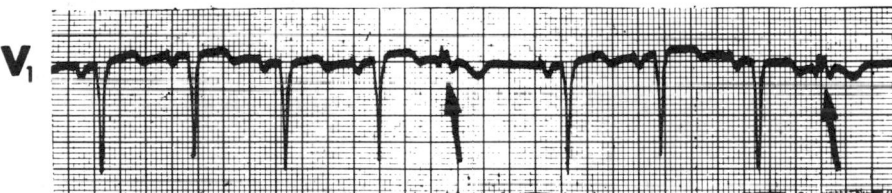

Figure 223. Premature ventricular contractions. There is a normal sinus rhythm, with the fifth and ninth beats (arrows) occurring early and having a markedly different configuration from that of the normal sinus beats. They have a QRS duration in excess of 0.12 sec and are not preceded by discernible P waves. Both premature beats are followed by a fully compensatory pause; that is, the two sinus cycles from the second to the fourth beat measure 0.143 sec and the two cycles from the fourth to the sixth beat (which includes the abnormal fifth beat) measure 1.44 sec. All these characteristics favor the diagnosis of premature ventricular beats. Finally, it can be positively demonstrated that the sinus node cycle is not interrupted. The P-P interval of the cycle preceding the first premature beat measures 0.72 sec in duration. If one measures 0.72 sec from the P wave of the fourth beat, it is seen to coincide with the inverted wave at the beginning of the ST segment of the premature beat, which exactly matches the configuration of the normal P waves in this lead. Thus, the P wave originates in the sinus node and discharges the atria but is not conducted to the ventricles. Finally, measuring from the P wave at the end of the premature beat to the next P wave demonstrates the expected 0.72 sec length of the cycle. Reproduced from Hurst JW, Meyerburg RJ: *Introduction to Electrocardiography,* ed 2. New York, McGraw-Hill Book Company, 1973, with permission of the author and publisher.

Table 55.   Abnormal P-R intervals.

A.   Atrioventricular dissociation (A-V dissociation)
1.   Secondary to usurpation. If the independent QRS rate is faster than the P wave rate, or at least fast enough that the P wave does not conduct completely through the AV node, the QRS (ventricle) *usurps* the power to pace the heart from the sinus node.
2.   Secondary to block. If the AV node is diseased or affected by drugs to the extent that sinoatrial impulses fail to traverse the AV node (decremental conduction), dissociation of atrial (P waves) and ventricular (QRS) activity may occur as a result of *block* (see C below).
3.   Secondary to escape. If normal sinoatrial pacing does not occur, narrow or wide QRS complexes may follow as a protective escape mechanism, which paces the heart at a slower than normal rate. In this case, P waves may not be seen (Fig 224).

B.   Short P-R intervals
1.   Bypass tract around the A-V node allowing more rapid conduction from atria to ventricles. The P waves are usually upright in II, III, and aV$_F$.
2.   Low atrial pacing focus. The P waves are usually inverted in II, III, and aV$_F$.

C.   Long P-R intervals (atrioventricular block)
1.   First-degree heart block. P-R interval is usually $\geq$ 0.20 sec (Fig 225).
2.   Second-degree heart block.
a.   Mobitz I. Repetitive cycles in which the P-R interval lengthens with each beat until a P wave is not followed by a QRS complex, thus ending the cycle (Fig 226).
b.   Mobitz II. The P-R interval is usually normal; the P waves do not lose cadence but one or more P waves are not followed by a QRS complex; the QRS complexes are often prolonged and drop out unpredictably. A sudden increase in vagal tone (Valsalva, cough, bowel movement) may mimic this conduction disturbance (Fig 227).
3.   Third-degree heart block. Atrioventricular dissociation with a QRS rate between 20 and 40/minute. If a few P waves conduct to a QRS complex, and/or if the QRS rate > 40, it is called "incomplete or high grade" AV block.

D.   Subnodal conduction delay
The several types of atrioventricular block can be mimicked electrocardiographically by conduction delay in both bundle branches or Purkinje fibers from both ventricles.

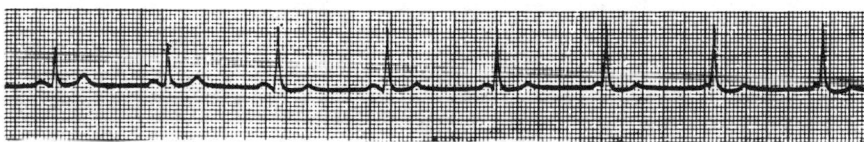

Figure 224.   A-V dissociation due to sinus bradycardia and junctional escape. The first three complexes are normal sinus beats with normal A-V conduction. The heart rate is just below 60 beats/min. The fourth beat is a junctional escape beat with a slightly different QRS morphology and shorter interval between the onset of the P wave and the onset of the QRS complex than the preceding sinus beats. The sinus node rate slows a little more during the next few cycles and the junction escape rate remains relatively constant, perpetuating the A-V dissociation. As the sinus rate then increases, the P waves emerge from the QRS complexes and finally recapture the ventricles (last two complexes). The atrial (higher) pacemaker is slower than the junctional (lower) pacemaker during the period of dissociation, permitting the A-V dissociation to occur. Reproduced from Hurst JW, Meyerburg RJ: *Introduction to Electrocardiography*, ed 2. New York, McGraw-Hill Book Company, 1973, with permission of the author and publisher.

> bradycardia and prolongation of the P-R interval are the most common abnormalities.
>
> e.   Phenothiazines and tricyclic antidepressants. Both groups of drugs may cause a prolongation of the Q-T interval, ventricular dysrhythmias, a form of ventricular tachycardia in which the polarity of the QRS complex changes (called "torsade de pointes"), and syncope.

5.   Metabolic problems. Hypokalemia, hyperkalemia, hypocalcemia, hypomagnesemia, hypoxemia, acidosis, and alkalosis may predispose patients to problems with cardiac rhythm. The mechanisms for dysrhythmias in these cases are based primarily on changes in the shape or duration of the action potential.

V_1

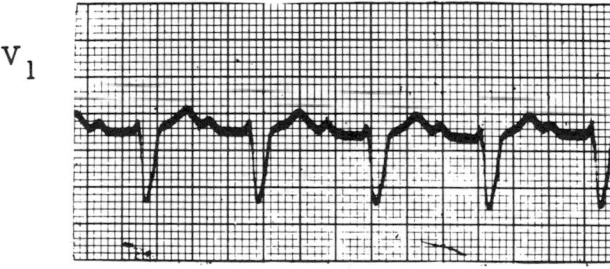

Figure 225.   First-degree A-V block. The P-R interval is constant and prolonged to 0.27 sec. When the heart rate is rapid in the presence of first-degree heart block, the P waves may be buried in the T waves of the preceding complexes. In this situation, the recognition of the pacemaker site may be difficult and carotid sinus pressure may aid in diagnosis.

LEAD II

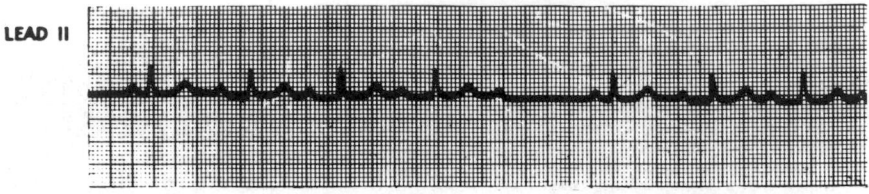

Figure 226. Second-degree heart block, type I (the Wenckebach phenomenon). The characteristics of a Wenckebach phenomenon are (1) progressively increasing P-R intervals with (2) progressively decreasing R-R intervals and (3) a pause due to a dropped beat, the pause being less than twice the length of the last R-R interval (usually the shortest) in the period. The greatest increment of P-R interval occurs between the first and second complexes of any period, and the increment progressively decreases through the period. Thus, in the first Wenckebach period on the electrocardiogram, the first P-R interval is 0.20 sec and the second P-R interval is 0.30 sec, giving an increment of 0.30-0.20 = 0.10 sec; the next increment is 0.33-0.30 = 0.03 sec; and the last increment is 0.35-0.33 = 0.02 sec. The R-R intervals decrease from 0.92 to 0.84 sec. Then the last R-R interval before the pause should also decrease but does not do so in this case because of the presence of the concomitant sinus rate variation. The duration of the pause due to the dropped beat is 1.63 sec, which is less than twice the R-R interval of the last cycle of the period (0.85 × 2 = 1.70).

    a.   In patients with hypokalemia, there is an increase in the magnitude of the resting potential except in severe hypokalemia in which there may be a paradoxical decrease in the resting membrane potential. A second effect of hypokalemia is to prolong the myocardial cell action potential. Slowing of the rate of repolarization increases the likelihood of dysrhythmias since the action potential may not have returned to baseline prior to the next depolarization wave. Hypokalemia may also induce a delay or block in

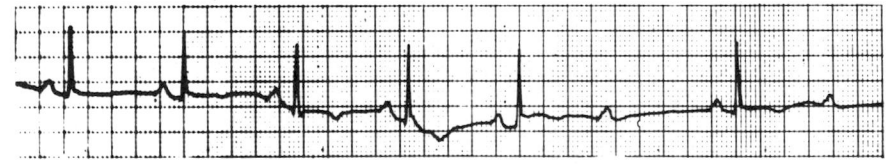

Figure 227. Second-degree heart block, type II. The first five complexes on the tracing represent normal sinus rhythm at a rate of approximately 65/min. The sixth atrial beat (P wave) is abruptly blocked, and the seventh is conducted with a normal P-R interval. The patient then continues in 2:1 block to the end of the strip. Note that the P-R intervals prior to the first dropped beat are constant, as opposed to the progressive prolongation prior to the dropped beat in type I block (the Wenckebach phenomenon).

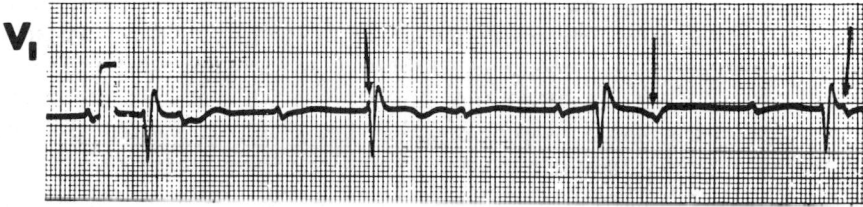

Figure 228. Complete heart block. The ventricular rate is 32 beats/min and the ventricular rhythm is regular. There is no fixed relationship between the P waves and QRS complexes. The arrows indicate some of the P waves that fall within the QRS complexes or T waves and may be difficult to discern. There is some variation in the P-P intervals. The P wave irregularity has a definite pattern; namely, the P-P interval tends to be shorter when a QRS complex falls between the two P waves and to be longer when the two P waves fall between two QRS complexes. Thus, the P-P intervals between the first and second, sixth and seventh, and eighth and ninth P waves are 0.75, 0.76, and 0.77 sec, respectively; and the P-P intervals between the second and third, fifth and sixth, and seventh and eighth P waves are 0.82, 0.79, and 0.82 sec, respectively. This phenomenon is called ventriculophasic sinus arrhythmia, a common finding in complete heart block with normal atrial activity.

atrioventricular conduction in experimental animals: however, prolongation of the P-R interval in the clinical setting is rare. The T wave is small and the U wave appears to be larger (probably representing a change in Purkinje fiber repolarization).

b. Hyperkalemia lowers the cardiac resting membrane potential, and reduces the rate of rise and the amplitude of the action potential. Hyperkalemia, therefore, can slow conduction velocity, produce decremental conduction, and contribute to the genesis of lethal rhythms. In patients with mild hyperkalemia (serum levels of 6.0 to 6.5 mEq/liter), atrioventricular conduction is actually accelerated, which may improve conduction in sinus rhythm with A-V block. At potassium levels of 7.0–7.5 mEq/liter or greater, conduction is depressed. Potassium-induced depression of conduction may lead to ventricular ectopy via the mechanism of reentry, and may cause junctional tachycardia from increased automaticity. Hyperkalemia also accelerates repolarization and shortens the plateau phase of the action potential. The characteristic tall, peaked T waves on the electrocardiogram are caused by the acceleration in repolarization.

c. Hypocalcemia prolongs the cardiac action potential and causes the amplitude to be reduced. This may increase the tendency to decremental conduction and, along with nonuniform prolongation of the relative refractory period, may lead to dysrhythmias. Hypocalcemia has little or no effect on either the magnitude of the resting potential or the slope of phase 4 depolarization in ranges of ionized calcium encountered clinically. The duration of the QRS complex may be decreased. The Q-T interval is prolonged, especially the Q-T$_o$ interval.

d. Hypercalcemia shortens the duration of the cardiac action potential while increasing the extent of depolarization. In patients with extreme elevation of serum calcium, shortening of the Q-T interval prolongation of the P-R interval, degrees of atrioventricular block, and prolongation of the QRS have been reported. Elevated calcium levels also enhance the arrhythmogenic potential of digitalis.

e. In the absence of hypocalcemia and hypokalemia, the concentration of magnesium within the range encountered in clinical situations has little or no effect on the ventricular action potential. The effects of hypocalcemia may be exaggerated by hypomagnesemia. Although there is very little evidence that "spontaneous" hypomagnesemia gives rise to clinical dysrhythmias, it appears that digitalis-toxic dysrhythmias may occur after less digitalis in the presence of hypomagnesemia. Elevation of the extracellular Mg^{++} concentration to 3–5 nM/liter depresses atrioventricular conduction. This is probably due to slowing of the upstroke velocity of phase O, which is similar to the effect of hyperkalemia. It is not certain that elevations of serum magnesium to levels encountered clinically have any recognizable effect on the electrocardiogram.

f. Acidosis and alkalosis are usually associated with alterations in the concentration of potassium and ionized calcium. Changes in pH per se probably have little "primary" effects on the electrical activity of the heart. However, abrupt changes in pH disrupt the ionic equilibrium of the myocardial cell. A rise in the extracellular concentration of hydrogen ion (acidosis) results in the movement of hydrogen ion into cells and potassium ion out of cells; the opposite is true for a decrease in extracellular hydrogen ion concentration (alkalosis). During metabolic alkalosis, ionized calcium is often decreased, leading to a prolongation of the Q-T interval.

g. Hypoxia is an important cause of many rhythm disorders. Cardiac excitability is most vulnerable to hypoxia, and is usually decreased within 20 minutes or less of acute hypoxia. Following respiratory arrest with hypoxia, the force of cardiac contraction falls within minutes, long before electrical activity disappears. As the contractility of the hypoxic heart fails, the myocardial tissue and specialized conduction fibers become more prone to rhythm disorders and conduction block through an increase in automaticity and a decrease in excitability and conductivity. The absolute level of pAO_2 (partial pressure of oxygen in the blood) that is associated with dysrhythmias is highly variable since myocardial oxygenation is dependent not only on arterial oxygen concentration, but also on coronary blood flow, ventricular wall tension, and a number of other factors.

In summary, a patient may have serious and life-threatening heart disease and the ECG may be normal. For example, severe coronary atherosclerotic heart disease may be present in a patient whose ECG is normal. On the other hand, the ECG may be abnormal and have no significance as far as the patient's prognosis is concerned. Numerous ST-T wave abnormalities are in this category. Finally, a certain electrocardiographic abnormality may be caused by several disease processes. The ECG is the best method to use in an effort to identify the nature of a cardiac dysrhythmia, but it does not always answer all the problems related to the condition. The seriousness of most dysrhythmias is determined by the clinical context in which they are found.

Selected References

1. Hurst JW, Myerburg RJ: *Introduction to Electrocardiography,* ed 2. New York, McGraw-Hill, 1973.
2. Hoffman BF, Cranefield PF: *Electrophysiology of the Heart.* Mount Kisco, NY, Futura Publishing Co, 1976.
3. Bayley RH: *Biophysical Principles of Electrocardiography.* New York, Paul B. Hueber, 1958.
4. Han J (ed): *Cardiac Arrhythmias: A Symposium.* Springfield, Ill, Charles C Thomas, 1972.
5. Antonaccio MJ (ed): *Cardiovascular Pharmacology.* New York, Raven Press, 1977.

240. The Chest X-Ray

STEWART R. ROBERTS, JR., MD

Definition

The chest x-ray is the most frequently requested radiographic procedure, constituting 25–40% of all radiographic examinations. Some physicians and insurance carriers question the routine use of the chest radiograph in the young patient with no chest symptoms.

Technique

The standard chest x-ray is obtained in a frontal (PA film) and a lateral projection. The frontal film is exposed with the patient standing upright facing the film holder (cassette), the x-ray beam coming from an x-ray tube 6 feet behind the patient. Because the beam travels from a posterior to anterior direction in regard to the patient, it is termed a "PA" film (Fig 229). The lateral film is exposed with the patient erect with his left side against the cassette, because the heart is a prominent left-sided structure and its magnification is diminished by placing the patient's left side nearer the cassette. If the patient is too ill to be radiographed in a standing position, an AP supine film may be obtained. This film is exposed with the patient lying on his back, the x-ray beam entering the chest anteriorly from an overhead tube 40 inches away, exposing the film underneath the patient's back. Because the beam travels from an anterior to posterior direction in regard to the patient, it is termed an "AP" supine examination of the chest (Fig 230). The film may also be obtained with the patient semi-erect or sitting. This film is often obtained with portable bedside equipment and is generally a less satisfactory examination than the erect PA film. This is because the portable x-ray unit is smaller, its x-ray beam is less powerful, and the film quality is compromised.

Detecting whether a chest x-ray was made in the PA or AP projection is simple. The differences are outlined in Table 56. For a PA film, the patient stands erect, faces the film cassette, elevates his chin, rolls the shoulders forward while holding the hands behind the back, then takes

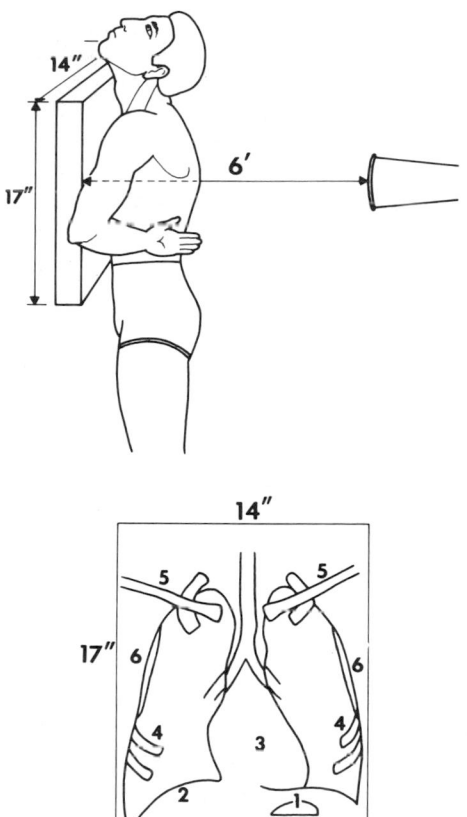

Figure 229. PA upright chest film technique: The x-ray beam passes through the patient in a posterior to anterior direction, coming from an x-ray source 6 feet away from the film cassette, exposing a radiograph 14 × 17 inches. Because the patient is erect, an air-fluid (1) level is present in the stomach. The diaphragms (2) are low. Anterior structures, the heart (3), anterior ribs (4), and clavicles (5), are close to the film and are not magnified. The shoulders are rotated forward so that the scapulae (6) do not project significantly over the lungs. A 6-foot 3-inch, 200-lb male subject is easily filmed on the 14-×-17-inch radiograph (see Table 56 for comparison of the PA upright and AP supine chest x-rays).

a deep breath and holds it. Consider the effect of this position on the PA film: the erect position may cause an air-fluid level to be found in the stomach, the diaphragms are lower because the abdominal viscera fall and inspiration depresses the diaphragms, and rolling the shoulders forward serves to move the scapulae laterally such that they do not project significantly over the underlying lung. Since the anterior thorax is placed against the cassette, there is very little magnification of anterior struc-

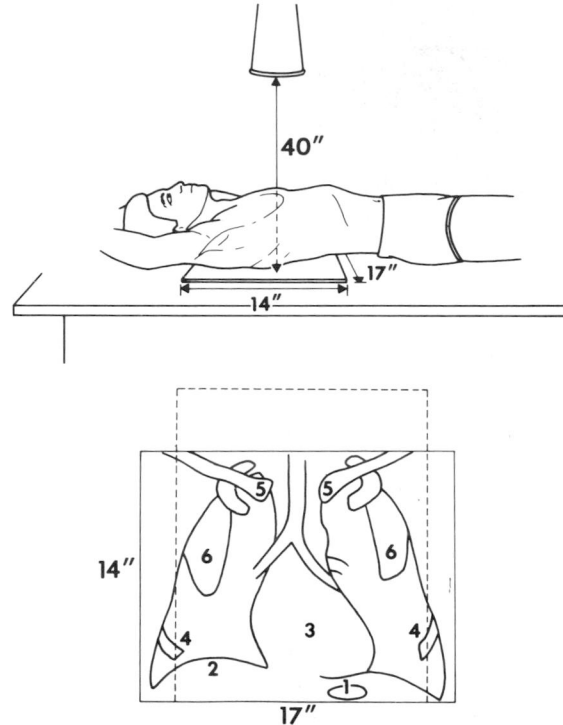

Figure 230. AP supine chest film technique: The x-ray beam passes through the same subject from an anterior to posterior direction, coming from an x-ray source 40 inches away. Because of the shorter tube-film distance (40 inches AP as opposed to 6 feet PA), there is greater beam divergence and magnification of the subject. Thus, the 14-×-17-inch cassette has been turned on its long side to encompass this large subject. The subject is supine; thus, a gastric air bubble (1), not an air-fluid level, is present. Because the patient is supine, the effect of gravity on lowering the abdominal viscera is lost, and the diaphragms (2) are approximately one interspace higher. The anterior thoracic structures, the heart (3), the anterior ribs (4), and the clavicles (5), are further away from the film, are relatively magnified, and appear larger than on the PA film. The scapulae (6) lie beneath the patient and project medially over the lungs (see Table 56).

tures such as the clavicles, anterior ribs, and cardiac silhouette. On the other hand, the gastric air bubble is not well seen on the AP supine chest examination. The abdominal viscera do not fall away from the diaphragm so the diaphragms tend to be relatively higher. The anterior thoracic structures are further away from the cassette and are magnified. Thus, the clavicles, anterior ribs, and cardiac silhouette appear larger. Also, the film is made with the patient lying on his scapulae, such that the scapulae project more medially over the lungs. Many radiologists find that the

Table 56. Comparison of the PA upright and AP supine chest x-ray.

PA Upright Chest	Item	AP Supine Chest
Air-fluid level	Gastric air bubble	Usually absent
Lower	Diaphragms	Higher
Not magnified	Anterior structures (heart, anterior ribs, and clavicles)	Magnified
More lateral	Scapulae	More medial
Short	Exposure time	Long
Less (25 mr)*	Radiation exposure	More (75 mr)
More satisfactory	Film quality	Less satisfactory

* mr = milliroentgen.

quick identification of an air-fluid level in the stomach and the more lateral position of the scapulae are two quick and easy check points helpfull in identifying the PA film.

Magnification on the AP supine chest film is largely attributable to the shorter distance between the x-ray tube source and the film. This shorter tube-film distance leads to greater divergence of the x-ray beam with resultant greater magnification of the object, especially the anterior thorax which is furthest from the film.

PA and lateral films exposed in the radiology department utilize a powerful kilovoltage technique that minimizes patient radiation by exposing the film in a matter of milliseconds. During this brief time, respiration is suspended. Portable AP films are exposed by smaller and less powerful mobile units which require more prolonged patient exposure. Thus, respiration in a dyspneic or obtunded patient more frequently blurs pulmonary vascular detail or shows diaphragmatic motion. Because many very ill patients require various catheters and tubes, the AP supine chest is often deliberately slightly overexposed so that these tubes may be identified within the mediastinum, and infiltrates behind the heart can be better visualized.

Phototiming is increasingly used for PA and lateral chest films. A radiosensitive feedback device is located in the film holder apparatus: when the x-ray beam passes through the subject, it strikes a sensitive plate and when an optimal level of exposure is obtained, a feedback mechanism automatically cuts off the current. So whether the patient is a skinny marathon runner or a jovial Santa Claus, relatively consistent film exposure can be obtained.

Background Information

The radiologist has an experienced concept of the normal, the normal variant, and the abnormal chest x-ray in ages ranging from infancy to old age. The radiologist studies the radiograph much as a pathologist evaluates a surgical specimen. First, he notes and describes the morphology depicted on the film (analogous to the gross specimen). Then he concentrates on the subtleties of the morphology (analogous to the microscopic). Finally, he renders his opinion or impression based on the pattern of shades of black and white on the film. The radiologist has a gamut of differential diagnoses for these varying patterns.

The radiologist also relates to the clinician who views the radiograph as part of his laboratory profile following completion of the history and physical examination. The clinician's approach tends to be both subjective and objective. Most often the thought processes of radiologist and clinician coincide. Occasionally, however, some radiographic patterns will virtually exclude some clinical impressions. Conversely, clinical data often color and narrow the differential diagnoses of the radiologist. The clinical history is as important to the radiologist as the chest film is to the clinician.

When an abnormality is detected, the radiologist will frequently suggest additional studies useful for elucidation of the problem. Consultation and review of the films with the radiologist best determines the most appropriate next procedure for maximal benefit at a minimal cost and radiation exposure. Additional studies suggested on the basis of the chest examination are listed in Table 57. A brief technical description of each examination, its appropriate use, an estimate of the radiation exposure, approximate cost, and appropriate comments are provided. Questions raised by a current examination are often resolved by comparison with previous films. At other times a simple follow-up examination will suffice.

Three questions should routinely be asked prior to interpretation of a chest x-ray:

1.   Is the film technically satisfactory?
2.   Is the patient position acceptable?
3.   Is the requested study the most appropriate examination for the problem at hand?

Examination of the film is then begun by a series of scanning random eye movements. This is followed by pattern eye movements following a checklist of items for completeness. This process helps avoid being misled by the presence of some gross abnormality. A suggested checklist would include, in order:

1. Subdiaphragmatic tissues
2. Diaphragm and pleura
3. Lungs and pulmonary vasculature
4. Heart and aorta
5. Mediastinum
6. Bony thorax
7. Soft tissues

The following section outlines the clinical significance of carefully evaluating each of these areas. Features of the normal PA and lateral chest x-ray are outlined in Figs 231 and 232.

Clinical Significance

1. *Subdiaphragmatic tissues*
   a. Gastric air bubble. Identify the air outlining the fundus of the stomach. Ask yourself three questions: Is the mucosal pattern normal? Is an intraluminal mass present? Is there evidence of extrinsic compression from an enlarged liver or spleen? If no gastric air bubble is identified, obstructing esophageal lesions such as achalasia, carcinoma, or stricture warrant consideration. The gastric air bubble is sometimes not visualized normally.
   b. Liver and spleen size. The upper borders of the liver and spleen are included on the chest film. These organs may occasionally be outlined entirely. Do they appear normal in size? Are abnormal calcifications present? Is there free air beneath the diaphragm? Is ascites present?
   c. Gas in the large bowel is a normal finding. Often the splenic and hepatic flexures are outlined by air which ascends to these more superior portions. Are the flexures in normal position or are they displaced by organ enlargement or masses?

2. *Diaphragm and pleura.* Normally the right diaphragm is higher than the left because the heart sits on the left diaphragm and depresses it when the patient is upright. Normally the dome of the right diaphragm on inspiration is below the level of the sixth anterior rib. Ask yourself if the diaphragms are depressed from asthma or pulmonary overinflation. Are they elevated from obesity, suboptimal inspiratory effort, or restrictive lung disease? Are the diaphragms blurred by respiratory motion? Are the costophrenic angles sharp? The pleura envelopes the lungs such that the peripheral portions of the lungs should be searched for abnormal pleural densities. Be certain to look specifically for a tiny apical pneumothorax.

3. *Lungs and pulmonary vasculature.* The lungs are filled with air and show up black on the chest x-ray. Only the arteries and veins are

Table 57. Comparison chart of various roentgenographic examinations of the thorax.

Examination	Technique	Use	Exposure (mr)*	Approximate Cost†	Comment
1. PA chest Lateral chest	Patient standing, full inspiration, 6-foot tube-film distance	Standard examination	25 70	PA only: $18 PA and lat: $27	Standard chest examinations in x-ray department.
2. PA chest (high KVP) Lateral chest (high KVP)	See above	Becoming standard	20 45	$27	
3. AP chest supine	Patient supine	Portable examination	75	$26	Patient cannot be transported to x-ray department.
4. AP bucky chest	Patient supine	Greater detail, especially for large patients	325	$18	Bucky grid reduces scatter radiation and gives sharper film detail.
5. Expiratory PA chest	Patient standing	Question of pneumothorax, air trapping	30	$18	Potentiates appearance of pneumothorax; in unilateral check-valve bronchial obstruction, the ipsilateral diaphragm does not elevate normally and the mediastinum is shifted to the contralateral side.
6. Rib views (2 of each side of thorax)	AP supine and oblique	Question of rib fractures	650 unilateral examination	$31 unilateral examination	2 films: unilateral ribs; 4 films: bilateral ribs; films are exposed with low KVP to bring out bone detail.
7. Oblique views (2)	Bilateral oblique films with patient 45°-angle to film	Question of pulmonary infiltrate	270	$27	Often uncovers suspicious pulmonary infiltrate because of obliquity of patient.

	Position	Indication		Cost	Comments
8. Bilateral decubitus views (2)	Patient lies on one side, then the other; x-ray beam horizontal	Detection of free pleural effusion	50	$27	Frequently requested by clinician when simple follow-up PA examination several days later would suffice; comparison with previous films helpful.
9. Apical lordotic	Patient erect and lordotic; leans with back against film	Question of apical infiltrate underlying clavicle or first rib	40	$18	Not indicated for "apical pleural thickening"; frequently requested inappropriately; the lordotic view elevates the clavicle and anterior ribs, uncovering the underlying apical lung for better evaluation; often shows suspicious right middle lobe lingular infiltrate to good advantage.
10. Cardiac series (4)	PA, lateral, left and right obliques	Cardiac evaluation	275	$38	Most often adds little to careful evaluation of PA and lateral chest; barium-outlined esophagus may aid in evaluating left atrial enlargement.
11. Screening pulmonary tomograms (9 cuts)	Patient supine	Identification of possible mass or metastatic disease	1,700	$76	Usually not indicated when PA and lateral chest films show no suspicious lesion.
12. Focal pulmonary tomograms (6 cuts)	Patient supine	Evaluation of known pulmonary mass	1,500	$64	For better definition of mass: does mass contain calcium, cavity, abnormal vessels? Often adds little to careful evaluation of PA and lateral chest; be certain to compare current with previous chest x-rays.

Table 57. (continued)

Examination	Technique	Use	Exposure (mr)*	Approximate Cost†	Comment
13. Mediastinal tomograms (6 cuts)	Patient supine	Evaluation of hilar and mediastinal masses	3,100	$64	Question of hilar adenopathy, calcification or fat in mediastinal mass; often of little value in simple contour abnormalities of the mediastinum; fluoroscopy and barium swallow may be helpful.
14. Thoracic spine (2)	AP supine lateral	Detail of vertebral bodies	AP: 825 Lat: 2,450 Total: 3,300	$30	Highest radiation exposure of any two film examinations of thorax; equivalent to 1.4 min of chest fluoroscopy.
15. Cardiac fluoroscopy (3 min)	Patient standing and turning in different projections	Question of abnormal pulsations such as aneurysm, prominent pulmonary artery pulsations, cardiac calcification	5,200	$22	Cardiac calcification best seen at fluoroscopy rather than on plain film.
16. Chest fluoroscopy (3 min)	See above	Question of lung lesion, diaphragmatic paralysis mediastinal mass vs tortuous vessel, air trapping, vascular lung lesion, ie, arteriovenous malformation, pulmonary varix	5,200	$22	Brief fluoroscopy often solves problems better than tomograms, and often may be accomplished in less than 1 min exposure; provides a dynamic study of pulsations, influence of respiration; spot films of pulmonary nodule may show calcification not identifiable on plain film.

	Technique	Indication	Radiation exposure*	Cost†	Comments
17. Perfusion lung scan	Technesium[99] administered IV	Question of pulmonary emboli	Lung: 400–1,000 whole body: 10	$135	Helps exclude clinically significant pulmonary emboli; compare patient irradiation and cost with that of pulmonary arteriogram.
18. Ventilation lung scan	Xenon[133] inhaled	Evaluation of perfusion defects: emboli vs chronic obstructive pulmonary disease	Lung: 250–500 whole body: 1–2	$140	Little radiation exposure to whole body, for gas is exhaled.
19. Pulmonary arteriogram (2 runs)	Fluoro for catheter positioning; serial films after contrast injected	Question of pulmonary emboli	25,000	$200	Demonstrates filling defects in pulmonary arteries.
20. Thoracic aorta arteriogram (1 run)	See above	Question of aortic dissection	15,000	$203	Provides anatomical localization of abnormality.
21. Computerized tomography of the thorax		Excellent for evaluation of mediastinal and hilar lesions; pleural lesions seen to good advantage	3,000	$275	More sensitive in detection of pulmonary nodules than linear tomography; however, less sensitive in detection of calcification within the nodule.

* Radiation exposure is skin dose at entry calculated in milliroentgens.
† Cost of medical care may vary regionally. Listed are charges of radiographic examinations rendered by Emory University Hospital in 1979, rounded to the nearest dollar.

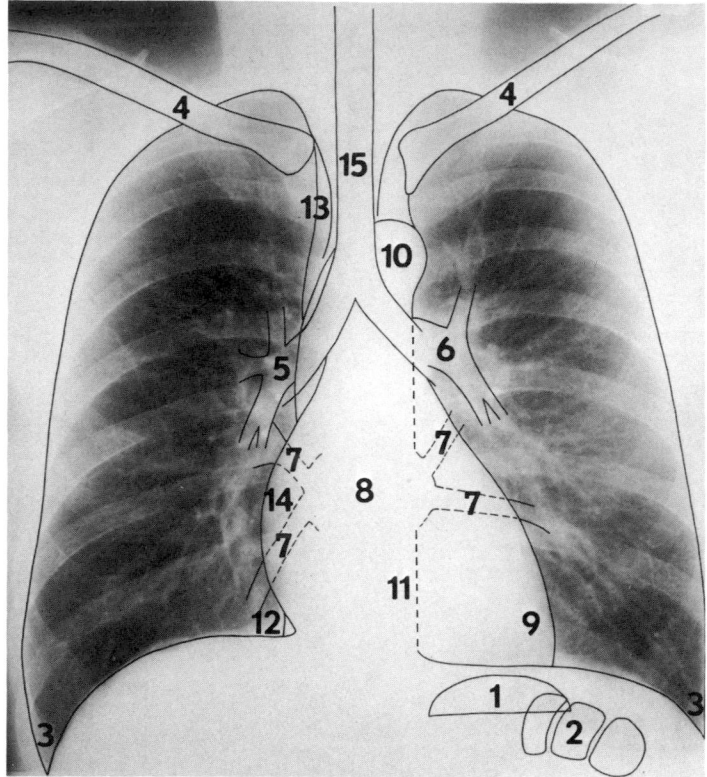

Figure 231. PA chest x-ray. (1) Gastric air-fluid level, (2) air in splenic flexure of colon, (3) costophrenic angles, (4) clavicles, (5) right pulmonary artery, (6) left pulmonary artery (higher than right), (7) pulmonary veins, (8) left atrium, (9) left ventricle at cardiac apex, (10) arch of aorta (aortic knob), (11) descending aorta seen through cardiac silhouette, (12) inferior vena cava, (13) superior vena cava, (14) right atrium, (15) trachea.

normally visualized. The pulmonary arteries leave the main pulmonary trunk and divide into right and left branches, constituting the principal components of the hilar shadow. They then permeate each lung and taper distally. In the upright position, gravity causes the circulation to the lung bases to predominate over that of the upper lung by a ratio varying from 3:1 to 10:1. This predominant vascular distribution to the lower lung zones is apparent on the upright but not the supine chest examination.

The pulmonary veins drain the lung and enter the left atrium slightly below the hilum. The right lung is divided into three lobes and 10 segments, and the left lung into two lobes and eight segments. Use the fissures to help identify these various lobes and segments. Search the lung

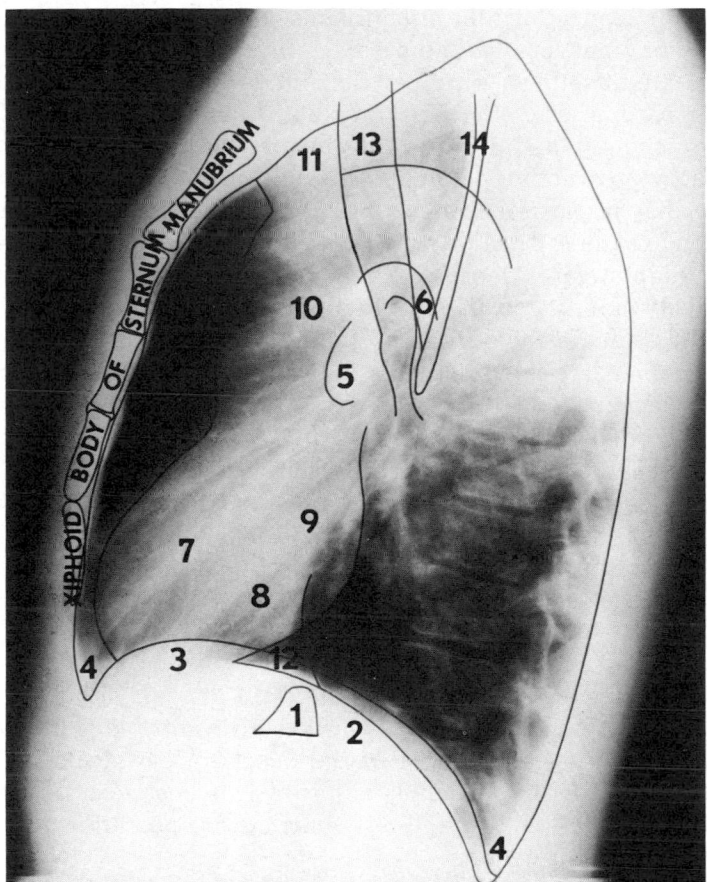

Figure 232. Lateral chest x-ray. (1) Gastric air-fluid level, (2) left diaphragm (anterior portion obliterated by the heart), (3) right diaphragm, (4) costophrenic angles, (5) right pulmonary artery, (6) left pulmonary artery (higher than right), (7) right ventricle (anterior), (8) left ventricle (posterior), (9) left atrium (posterior), (10) ascending aorta, (11) brachiocephalic vessels, (12) inferior vena cava, (13) trachea, (14) scapula.

for infiltrates. Locate the infiltrate by lobe and segment. Ask yourself where you might hear rales on auscultation. Classify the infiltrate. Does it occupy the air spaces (alveolar infiltrate) or does it simply impart a loss of clarity to the pulmonary vessels (interstitial infiltrate). The pulmonary vessels course in the interstitial tissues; therefore, an infiltrate in the pulmonary interstitium blurs the normal vessel outlines.

4. *Heart and aorta.* It is necessary to have a good inspiratory film to judge cardiac size. In a normal subject a film exposed in inspiration will show a heart of normal size. If the same subject has a chest film ex-

posed in full expiration, the diaphragms are elevated, the heart is elevated and lies transversely, and cardiac enlargement and even pulmonary edema are simulated. So a proper film made in inspiration is important in judging cardiac size. Certain body builds and disease states such as obesity, pregnancy, and ascites will elevate the diaphragm. Others such as asthma or obstructive pulmonary disease will depress the diaphragm. When the diaphragm is elevated, the mediastinum will appear relatively widened and the heart will lie transversely and appear relatively enlarged. When the diaphragm is depressed, the mediastinum will appear elongated and relatively skinny and the heart will appear more vertical. If the heart is enlarged, evaluate the aortic and pulmonary outflow tracts to help determine whether left-sided or right-sided chambers contribute principally to the enlargement.

On a normal chest film taken during adequate inspiration, the diaphragmatic dome should be at or below the sixth anterior rib. The transverse diameter of the heart should not exceed 50% of the transverse diameter of the thorax measured from inner rib border to inner rib border at the level of the right dome of the diaphragm. This is known as the cardiothoracic ratio. Measurements from the PA and lateral chest film can also be used to calculate the cardiac volume, an improved quantitative index of cardiomegaly.

The right border of the heart is the right atrium. The right ventricle is anterior, overlying the more posterior left ventricle. Both ventricles constitute the soft tissue density of the heart as it projects into the left thorax. Since the right ventricle is anterior, it is best seen on lateral projection. Since the left atrium and left ventricle are posterior, they are also best seen on lateral projection.

The ascending, transverse, and descending portions of the aorta should be studied in both projections. In the young, the aorta is elastic and "coiled." With age or hypertensive vascular disease the aorta becomes less tightly coiled (uncoiled, elongated, or tortuous aorta).

5. *Mediastinum.* The mediastinum extends from the thoracic inlet to the diaphragm. Its lateral borders are enclosed by the parietal pleura. Anteriorly it extends from the sternum and posteriorly to the anterior border of the thoracic vertebrae. The principal components of the mediastinum are the heart and great vessels, the trachea, esophagus, and various nerves and lymphatics. Mediastinal masses are identified by their displacement of adjacent lung (because of the difference in the soft-tissue density of the mass and the air density of the lung); by their displacement of other mediastinal structures such as the tracheal air column or barium-filled esophagus; or by a difference in radiodensity of the mediastinal mass itself (fat or calcium). First, identify the tracheal air column. Note its bifurcation into right and left main-stem bronchi. The soft-tissue density anterior to the trachea on the lateral film represents the brachiocephalic vessels. The normal esophagus is not visualized on the chest

x-ray, for unlike the rigid collagenous walls of the trachea, the walls of the esophagus are soft and collapsible.

In lateral projection the mediastinum is divided into three compartments: anterior, middle, and posterior. The anterior mediastinum is the retrosternal clear space which lies anterior to the heart, ascending aorta, and brachiocephalic vessels. The middle mediastinum contains the heart and great vessels, the trachea and main bronchi, and various lymphatics and nerves. The mediastinum is bordered posteriorly by the anterior margins of the thoracic vertebral bodies. The posterior mediastinum contains the esophagus, descending aorta, thoracic duct, the azygos veins, nerves, and lymphatics. Tumors of nerve-root origin occur here.

One must be familiar with the anatomical contents of these various mediastinal compartments since this forms the basis for the differential diagnosis of mediastinal masses. Thus, an anterior mediastinal mass may be a teratoma or thymoma; a middle mediastinal mass may be a lymphoma or other hilar lymphadenopathy; and a posterior mediastinal mass may be a tumor of neurogenic origin.

6. *Bony thorax.* Each rib should be followed individually from its posterior origin as it courses anteriorly to end in the costal cartilage. The lateral rib margin is best studied in the frontal projection since there is no overlying lung and the bony cortex and trabecular pattern are more clearly outlined. Blunting of the costophrenic angle may give a clue to a recent rib fracture with an associated hemorrhagic pleural effusion, or it may represent pleural reaction from an old rib fracture or pleurisy.

The thoracic vertebrae are best seen in lateral projection and are barely visible through the mediastinal silhouette on a technically satisfactory chest examination. On a well-centered chest examination the clavicles are symmetrical in their relationship to the manubrium. Examine each component of the shoulder girdle: the clavicle, scapulae, glenoid fossae, and proximal humeri.

7. *Soft tissues.* Is the patient obese or emaciated, or are the soft tissues of normal thickness? Both breasts should be visibly present and symmetrical in adult women. Is one absent from a previous mastectomy? Is there a diminution in soft tissue above one clavicle from previous radical neck surgery? Is there a pulmonary nodule which could represent a skin mole? The nipples are seen as symmetrical densities usually projecting within the fifth anterior interspace. Be certain that a nodule in the fifth anterior interspace is not within the lung parenchyma and is in the same position as the nipple on the other side. Do not be confused by axillary skinfolds on the lateral film.

Selected References

1. Felson B: *Chest Roentgenology*. Philadelphia, WB Saunders, 1977.
2. Fraser RG, Pare JAP: *Diagnosis of Diseases of the Chest: An Integrated Study Based on the Abnormal Roentgenogram*. Philadelphia, WB Saunders, 1970.
3. Heitzman ER: *The Lung: Radiologic-Pathologic Correlations*. St Louis, CV Mosby, 1973.
4. Heitzman ER, Proto AV, Goldwin RL: The role of computerized tomography in the diagnosis of diseases of the thorax. *JAMA* 241:933–936, 1979.
5. Meschan I: *An Atlas of Normal Radiographic Anatomy*. Philadelphia, WB Saunders, 1959.
6. Meschan I: *Analysis of Roentgen Signs in General Radiology*. Philadelphia, WB Saunders, 1973, vol 2.
7. Paul LW, Juhl JH: *The Essentials of Roentgen Interpretation*. Hagerstown, Md, Harper and Row, 1972.
8. Sagel SS, Evens RG, Forrest JV, et al: Efficacy of routine screening and lateral chest radiographs in a hospital-based population. *N Eng J Med* 291:1001–1004, 1974.
9. Squire LF, Colaice WM, Strutynsky N: *Exercises in Diagnostic Radiology: The Chest*. Philadelphia, WB Saunders, 1970.
10. Wittenborg MH, Aviad I: Organ influence on the normal posture of the diaphragm: A radiological study of inversions and heterotaxies. *Br J Radiol* 36:280–288, 1963.

241. Approach to the Radiographic Examination of the Abdomen

STEWART R. ROBERTS, JR., MD

Radiographic examinations of the abdomen are not recommended as routine screening tests for most patient populations. However, these examinations are frequently requested, the examinations available are numerous, the sequence of the examination is important, and the expense of the examinations is significant. This chapter is included for those reasons.

The word *abdomen* derives from the Latin, *abdere,* "to hide." Pathology within the abdomen may certainly be hidden. In no other part of human anatomy is the physician so relatively dependent on the radiographic examinations. Proper utilization of this radiographic armamentarium requires the appropriate selection of that examination likely to yield the greatest and most prompt diagnostic information at least cost to the patient.

Six categories of examinations include: (1) plain film examinations; (2) nonvascular contrast studies; (3) vascular contrast studies (arteriograms); (4) ultrasound; (5) computerized tomography; and (6) nuclear medicine. Patient preparation instruction for the appropriate radiographic examination is often available at the nurses' station on hospital patient care areas. A brief discussion of each category follows.

The Plain Film Examinations of the Abdomen

No contrast agent is involved in these studies; thus, they are termed "plain film" examinations. Several varieties of plain film studies of the abdomen are available and represent radiographs exposed with the patient in different positions. There are supine, upright, oblique, lateral decubitus, and cross-table lateral films of the abdomen. The varying patient positions and the relationship of the x-ray beam source and film are depicted in Fig 233.

The KUB film of the abdomen is not recommended for all patients since it cannot be consistently shown to be cost-effective as a routine procedure, especially in patients without abdominal symptoms. KUB stands for "kidneys, ureters, bladder" and represents the main areas of interest on an abdominal film in the earlier days of radiology. It is an AP supine film of the abdomen since the x-ray beam comes from a source anterior to the patient and exposes a film posterior to the supine patient (Fig 233A). The AP supine film is the most often requested plain film examination of the abdomen. It is also the "scout film" for an intravenous pyelogram (IVP) examination. The combination of the AP supine and upright film of the abdomen is the initial study usually requested for suspected intestinal obstruction. The upright abdominal film (Fig 233B) or an upright chest film may reveal subdiaphragmatic free air in cases of perforated abdominal viscus.

If the patient is too ill to stand, a left lateral decubitus film may be requested. There is much confusion about lateral decubitus films. The left lateral decubitus position simply means the patient lies on the left side, the x-ray beam is projected across the table, and the film exposed (Fig 233D). Thus, the patient's right side is up and free air would collect

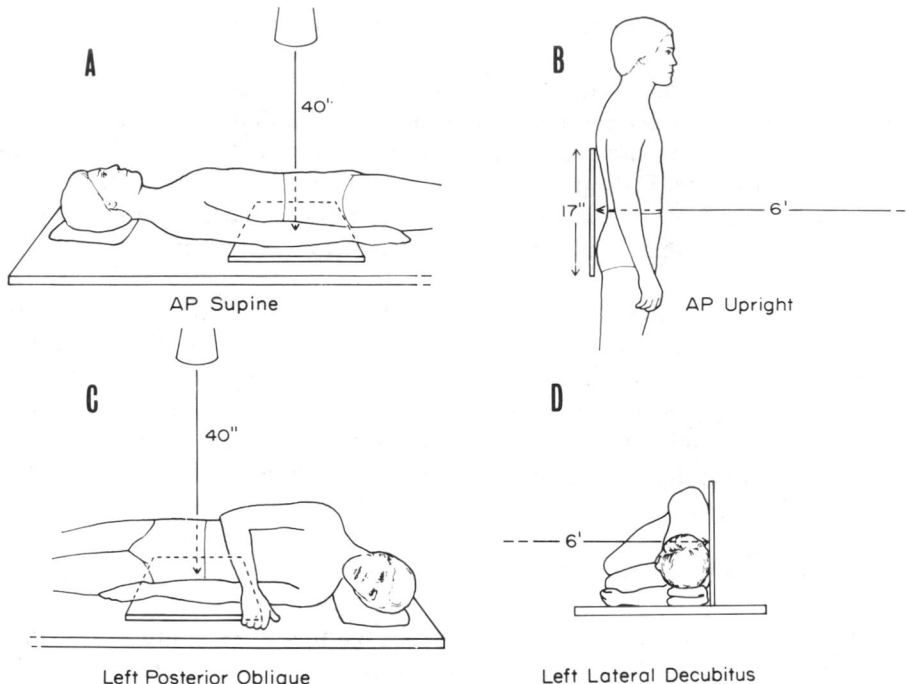

Figure 233. Plain film of the abdomen. *A*, AP supine: The patient lies supine on the radiographic table. The x-ray beam source is anterior to the patient, 40 inches from the film which is posterior to the patient. *B*, AP upright: The patient is erect. The x-ray beam source is anterior to the patient, 6 feet from the film which is posterior to the patient. *C*, Left posterior oblique: The patient lies on the left side of the back at 45° (half way between lying on the side and lying on the back). The x-ray beam source is 40 inches above the table top. *D*, Left lateral decubitus: The patient lies on the left side. The x-ray beam source is 6 feet away and parallel to the table top. It exposes a film posterior to the patient.

above the lateral surface of the liver. A helpful aid in determining patient position on the lateral decubitus film is to locate the gastric air-fluid level: the dependent position of the gastric fluid level would indicate that the patient is in the left lateral decubitus position.

Oblique films of the abdomen are included in the IVP examination, often 15 minutes after dye injection. A left posterior oblique film is also used in the evaluation of a suspected aneurysm of the lumbar aorta (the lumbar aorta is just to the left of the midline, so the left posterior oblique position rotates the aorta off the spine and shows it to best advantage (see Fig 233C).

Portable examinations of the abdomen are not ideal studies since the portable x-ray unit is not as powerful as larger stationary units which emit a higher kilovoltage peak (kVp) beam in a shorter period of time. The portable abdominal x-ray is often unsatisfactory in the obese patient. One should not expect the quality of examination from a portable study as one expects from the same examination performed in the x-ray department. Because the x-ray unit must be taken to the bedside, a portable film of the abdomen is more expensive and costs approximately $27. A supine film of the abdomen in the x-ray department costs approximately $18. A two-film study such as an AP supine and upright abdomen costs approximately $35.

Barium in the gastrointestinal tract will obscure most of the abdomen and the bony structures of the lumbar spine and pelvis. Generally one should obtain plain film studies of the abdomen, pelvis, and lumbar spine prior to barium contrast studies. Otherwise renal calculi, lumbar compression fractures, or lytic metastasis to the bony pelvis may be obscured. Repeat examinations necessitated by poor planning are expensive and time-consuming as well as an unnecessary burden and risk to the ill patient.

Nonvascular Contrast Examinations

When both a barium enema (BE) and an upper gastrointestinal series (UGI) are to be done, the BE should be scheduled first. This is because the barium for an UGI will become mixed with fecal content as it reaches the colon and will lose its value as a contrast agent. When an obstructing lesion of the colon is a possibility, administration of barium for upper gastrointestinal studies is undesirable. Also note that sigmoidoscopy the morning of a scheduled BE introduces a great deal of air into the colon and complicates the BE examination such that it may be a suboptimal study. Commonly requested contrast examinations of the abdomen and their costs are listed in Table 58.

Vascular Contrast Examinations

These invasive studies (a catheter is passed into an artery or vein) must be obtained prior to barium contrast examinations unless sufficient time is allowed for the complete evacuation of barium, a matter of several days. Commonly requested vascular studies of the abdomen are listed in Table 58.

Table 58.   Commonly requested contrast examinations of the abdomen.*

Examination	Cost ($)
UGI	61
BE	61
Air contrast BE	71
Oral cholecystogram	42
Small-bowel follow-through	61
Barium swallow	39
IVP	61

* Cost of medical care may vary between institutions, states, and regions. Listed are approximate charges of radiographic examinations rendered by Emory University Hospital in 1979.

Ultrasound

The sonar beam was developed in oceanography since sound travels rapidly through water, but slowly through air. Ultrasound of the abdomen is useful in the evaluation of solid structures, but the sonar beam is impeded by intestinal gas. The barium filled intestine also obscures the sonar beam, so ultrasound studies should often be ordered prior to barium contrast examinations. Commonly requested ultrasound examinations of the abdomen are tabulated in Table 60.

Computerized Tomography (CT)

This expensive examination provides excellent delineation of abdominal organs and spaces. It is particularly helpful in the evaluation of the pancreas and retroperitoneal masses. Unlike arteriography it has the advantage of being noninvasive. Again, barium in the gastrointestinal tract interferes with CT, so when CT is indicated it should be done first. Water-

Table 59.   Commonly requested abdominal arteriograms.

Examination	Cost ($)
Lumbar aorta and femoral artery runoff	428
Celiac axis	410
Bilateral renal arteries	519

Table 60.   Commonly requested ultrasound examinations of the abdomen.

Examination	Cost ($)
Obstetrics	80
Abdomen survey	95
Gall bladder	75
Pancreas	90
Pelvic	90
Lumbar aorta	80

soluble contrast is often administered orally to the patient during this examination to help in outlining the stomach and bowel contours. Commonly requested abdominal CT examinations are listed in Table 61.

Nuclear Medicine

Radioisotopic examination of the abdominal organs or study of intra-abdominal abscess by the radioisotope laboratory is impaired by the presence of barium in the gastrointestinal tract. Hence, when indicated, these examinations should generally be ordered prior to barium examinations. Commonly requested nuclear medicine studies of the abdomen are listed in Table 62.

Sequence of Radiographic Abdominal Examination

The least expensive examination likely to yield the most diagnostic information should be selected in appropriate sequence. Duplication is to be avoided. Demonstration of the same pathology by ultrasound, CT, and arteriography is a luxury not to be afforded in the interest of academic pursuit. Table 63 provides the optimal sequence of radiographic abdominal procedures when more than one procedure is anticipated.

Table 61.   Commonly requested CT examinations of the abdomen.

Examination	Cost ($)
Total abdomen	275
Pancreas (10–12 cuts)	225
Retroperitoneum	275
Tumor follow-up	275

Table 62.   Commonly requested nuclear medicine examinations of the abdomen.

Examination	Approximate Cost ($)
Liver-spleen scan	120
Renal flow and function studies with computer analysis	182
Whole body gallium scan (for abscess, etc.)	173
Liver-lung scan for subphrenic abscess	175

Table 63.   The optimal radiographic sequence when multiple radiographic studies of the abdomen are anticipated.

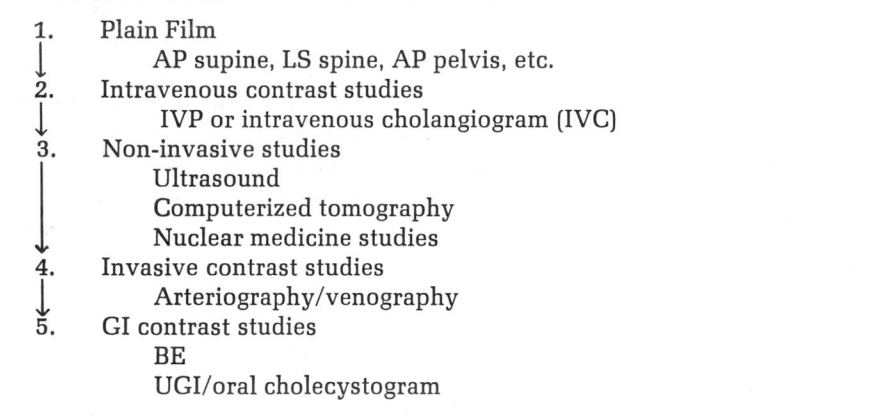

1. Plain Film
        AP supine, LS spine, AP pelvis, etc.
2. Intravenous contrast studies
        IVP or intravenous cholangiogram (IVC)
3. Non-invasive studies
        Ultrasound
        Computerized tomography
        Nuclear medicine studies
4. Invasive contrast studies
        Arteriography/venography
5. GI contrast studies
        BE
        UGI/oral cholecystogram

Selected References

1.   Alfidi RJ (ed): Whole body computer tomography. *Rad Clin N Am* 15:349–456, 1977.
2.   Felson B (ed): The acute abdomen. I, Bowel obstruction. *Semin Roentgenol* 8:265–340, 1973.
3.   Felson B (ed): The acute abdomen. II, Inflammatory diseases. *Semin Roentgenol* 8:361–466, 1973.
4.   Felson B (ed): A primer of sonography. *Semin Roentgenol* 15:247–328, 1975.
5.   Paul LW, Juhl JH: *Essentials of Roentgen Interpretation,* ed 3. New York, Harper and Row, 1972.
6.   Sheedy PF II, Stephens DH, Hattery RR, et al: Computed tomography of the pancreas. *Rad Clin N Am* 15:349–366,1977.

MARI: The Medical Aggregate Record Inquiry System

VLADIMIR SLAMECKA, DLS
HENRY N. CAMP, BA
ALBERT N. BADRE, PhD
W. DALLAS HALL, MD

Introduction

In 1972, following a number of years of cooperative activities, the School of Information and Computer Science of Georgia Institute of Technology and Emory University School of Medicine established a joint education program in biomedical information and computer science. The principal orientation accrued from the interest of both institutions in the design of information systems for medicine and health care. The central theme of the research components of the program has been that of biomedical knowledge and its effective utilization. Biomedical knowledge exists in a variety of forms and repositories, and the joint research program has gradually focused on the medical record as a repository of valuable information about the clinical experience in health care.

The potential of computerized medical records for the practice of health care goes well beyond the capability of storing individual records into the computer and retrieving them from a computer console. Basically, the extended use of the medical record bank is related to the ability of the computer to swiftly carry out analyses across the data base of records; these analyses are generically known as "aggregate analyses." Accordingly, the first phase of the interinstitutional program, conducted between 1974 and 1978 under the partial support of the National'Library of Medicine, was devoted to the establishment of a computerized bank of medical records, and to the development and demonstration of an extensive software system for the exploration and aggregate analysis of data contained within these records. This system is known as MARI, the Medical Aggregate Record Inquiry system.

The Data Base of Medical Records

Although in theory the ideal data base of medical records should contain the greatest wealth of data and cover the broadest possible patient population, this is not a realistic goal at the present time. At best we can hope to capture the most comprehensive medical data bank which can feasibly be collected in medical practice.

The medical record designated and implemented by Emory University School of Medicine and affiliated hospitals is exemplary of this goal. Emory University School of Medicine adopted the problem-oriented medical record system in 1969, and has since systematically revised key components at regular intervals. At Grady Memorial Hospital in Atlanta, the largest teaching hospital of Emory University School of Medicine, this problem-oriented medical record has been fully adopted and its use is monitored and supervised. The selection of this medical record as the basis of the computerized data base was thus natural.

The medical record bank consists of medical records derived from patients who have common diagnostic and therapeutic problems in internal medicine. The information processed on each patient consists of four documents. The first is the admission Defined Data Base which includes over 200 items of history and physical examination and 30 items of laboratory data. The second document is the Initial Plans of the clinician; it enumerates the data base criteria justifying the diagnosis and indicates the initial diagnostic tests, special diagnostic procedures, and selected drugs or other therapies. The third document is the Complete Problem List which indexes all medical diagnoses (and problems) of the patient and is linked to the Defined Data Base and Initial Plans form by a common problem number. The final document is the Discharge Summary which is programmed to provide a tabular listing for the results of diagnostic tests, procedures, and therapies during the course of hospitalization. The data base currently includes extensive data on more than 600 consecutive patients electively admitted to the internal medicine diagnostic area of Grady Memorial Hospital since February 1, 1978.

The information gathered in these four documents contains the following data types:

1. Keywords: key medical phrases from the Problem List and Initial Plans documents (eg, pneumonia, sputum culture, penicillin).

2. Qualitative responses: the physician's assessment of some items, such as headaches, dizziness or ECG. Qualitative responses may have the following values: normal or no, abnormal or yes, not applicable, unknown, and incomplete.

3. Numeric data: actual numeric values such as laboratory results, weight, blood pressure, heart rate, physician's ID, etc.

4. Supporting data number: the combinations of item numbers (from the Defined Data Base) that the clinician indicates as supportive of the Problem Statement. Abnormal as well as normal item values can be supportive.

5. Matches: data items with unique value, such as male or female.

6. Free text: narrative comment entered by the clinician in the patient's four documents.

The MARI System Functions

Most of the different uses of the information contained in the source documents can be categorized into one or more of three main areas: (1) retrieval of a single patient record or portions thereof; (2) retrieval of a single parameter (a diagnosis, a text, a drug, a symptom) from multiple records, and (3) analysis of various relationships between and among multiple parameters in multiple records. MARI offers six primary functions, combinations of which provide the necessary power to support these three basic capabilities. The six functions, whose names are actual computer commands, are described below.

How Many. "How many" is the primary search strategy of MARI; it finds and counts all patient records that satisfy the conditions specified. The following interaction illustrates the manner in which MARI prompts a user to combine commands for a "how many" type of question. The terminal keys necessary for the user to select during entry are underlined.

How many patient records have qualitative response for d56 (history of hypertension) of abnormal, and have numeric values for d127 (diastolic blood pressure) in the range of (units are mm Hg) 105–114 and have keywords for Rx of digoxin?

Questions concerning any of the more than 200 items of history, physical, or laboratory examination can be formulated by referring to the respective data item number, preceded by a d (for data base number).

What are the statistics? This function gives the count of records, the mean, the maximum, the minimum, and the standard deviation of numeric data items such as those contained in either the physical examination or the laboratory. The following interaction illustrates a type of "what are the statistics" question.

> What are the statistics for d225 (glucose) for all records that have keywords for final problems of diabetes and do not have keywords for Rx of insulin?

Display. This function retrieves a single element of a patient record (such as current medications), a range of elements (such as all laboratory results), or an entire document (such as the Defined Data Base, Complete Problem List, and Initial Plans). The function also allows the user to peruse details (such as the narrative chief complaint and present illness) of all patient records that satisfy specific search criteria. The following interaction illustrates a type of "display" question.

> Display d242–d242e (ECG intervals and interpretation) for all records that have matches for dsex equal to F (female) and have keywords for initial problems of coronary artery disease.

List the most frequent. This function provides a list of data items, sorted according to the frequency of occurrence. For example, MARI will allow construction of the following command to determine the most-often prescribed drugs for patients with single or multiple disease processes:

> List the most frequent keywords for Rx for all records that have keywords for initial problems of peptic ulcer disease and have keywords for initial problems of nephrotic syndrome.

By use of negatives, the user can also build questions that exclude certain items; eg:

> List the most frequent keywords for Rx for all records that have keywords for final problems of hypertension and do not have keywords for final problems of diabetes.

Similar command formulations can search for the most prevalent patient diagnoses and the most frequent special diagnostic tests requested for specific problems.

Show the usage. This function produces an alphabetized listing of the occurrences of various types of data within the clinical databank. The function can produce histograms of problem statements, drugs, tests, numeric values for lab tests, and the patterns of signs and symptoms used by physicians to arrive at certain diagnoses.

The following interaction represents a type of "show the usage" question. Note that the example illustrates a method for determining which Defined Data Base items are considered most relevant in diagnostic decision making.

> Show the usage for clinician's abnormal supporting data numbers for all patients that have active problems of angina pectoris.

We might anticipate responses such as chest pain, smoking history, high cholesterol, and abnormal ECG. Changes in patterns of decision making over time would, in part, reflect the impact on new knowledge.

Compute the costs. This function calculates the costs of initial diagnostic testing for all records in a specified group. For example:

> Compute the costs of diagnostic testing for all records that have keywords for active problems of hypertension; end.

This will produce a table showing the initial cost of evaluating hypertension. The table shows the number of patients with active hypertension, the total number of tests ordered, and the maximum, the minimum, and the mean number of tests per patient, costs per patient, and costs per test. As with all other functions, any amount of qualifying on the group may be done. In addition to the costs table, a breakdown of individual test costs can be requested.

The six primary MARI functions permit a flexible examination of the correlations among virtually all non-narrative data elements in the computerized clinical data bank. Furthermore, in combination they allow relatively sophisticated aggregate analyses of medical data.

The MARI query language is a modified menu approach designed to help overcome some of the traditional problems confronting a user when he interfaces with the computer terminal. The limited number of menus are short English language phrases that represent primitive operations commands. The sequence of presentation of these menus is determined automatically according to the user's information-seeking purpose. As demonstrated in the previous examples, the query is built gradually on the terminal screen by concatenating the selected commands into an English sentence. To select an item from the menu, the user is required only to type in the first character of the phrase. This technique allows the user to build highly complex questions, exploring an almost unlimited number of relationships among the data categories and types. See the example given at the end of this Appendix.

The Hardware and Software

The MARI system was developed on a Digital Equipment Corporation PDP-11/45 with 256k bytes (128k words) of core memory, memory management hardware, a floating point processor, 16-line multiplexer, and a Telefile dual spindle disk with a capacity of 113 megabytes per spindle, or a total of 226 megabytes of disk on-line, with an average access time of 44 milliseconds. The system supports 9 terminals on-line, including 6 Beehive Medical Electronics B200 CRTs, a Lear-Seigler ADM-3, a Diablo printer, and a General Electric Terminet 1200 printer.

The system communicates with three cathode ray terminals (CRTs) and a printer located at Grady Memorial Hospital via Vadic modems on three leased lines at 1200 baud asynchronous. They interface to a DZ-11 multiplexer which is asynchronous and self-programmable; therefore, services range from 110 to 9600 baud under program control. The MARI system is also able to communicate with a PDP 11/70 computer and a Prime 400 computer over 9600 baud communication links. The system is developed under the Unix operating system in the C programming language, both products of Bell Laboratories.

System and Data Security

Extensive procedures have been implemented to protect the security, confidentiality, and privacy of patient information contained within the computerized data bank. A password, different for each security-cleared user, is required for entry into the system. Any item of data from an individual patient record requires reentry and revalidation of the user password. Three failures (erroneous password entry) causes the program to terminate automatically with a printout of warnings at certain control terminals. Different users have different levels of clearance for the medical record information. The clearance levels exist down to individual data items. Entry, storage and retrieval of patient information has been reviewed and approved by the Emory University Human Investigations Committee as well as the legal authorities representing Grady Memorial Hospital. The official hospital Medical Record Committee periodically reviews the project with regard to record content and health care delivery. Each MARI project employee with any level of entrance into the system is required to review and sign a formal document concerning confidentiality of patient information.

Keyword Indices and Programs

Keywords are a data type in the MARI system which represent key medical phrases from the narrative of patient records, specifically from the Problem List and the Initial Plans. They are nomenclatural in value and represent a pragmatic attempt at solving the problem of the clinician wishing to search on information contained in free text. Because the current state of the art of natural language processing of medical record text is still in the research stage, the intermediate but practical solution is to capture the free text as written, and to display it verbatim upon request.

For purposes of aggregate analysis, however, the data entry clerk enters not only the full free text, but also its key medical terms. For example, the free-text phrase "s/p pneumonia × 3 in '65" is entered in full; then, at MARI's request, the keyword "pneumonia" is also entered. The computer screens the appropriate (diagnosis, test, drug) index of medical phrases where a corresponding numeric code is identified and stored in an attribute list of keywords for that patient.

MARI uses indices of medical phrases for diagnoses, drug names, and diagnostic tests and procedures. The diagnosis or problem statement index includes only those terms (or synonyms) that occur in actual usage in the medical records entered. The drug index contains the drug list used at Grady Memorial Hospital including the generic and trade names of each drug. The diagnostic tests and procedure index is also derived from the list of all possible diagnostic tests provided by the hospital.

The MARI keyword indices are designed to automatically grow as the system is used. Whenever the data entry clerk enters a term not contained in one of the indices, a new file is written. It includes the term or phrase, the patient number, the medical problem, the term type, and the date and time of entry. The file is processed weekly by an off-line program which generates a report of all new terms entered in the system and assigns them tentative new index numbers. This list of physician-generated nomenclatures and abbreviations is evaluated by one physician. Only obvious phrases or terms are allowed to exist as alternate terms, thus avoiding judgments which could be controversial, even among medical experts.

In this way the system adapts to the new environment of different hospitals or wards in that it captures the majority of terms actually used in those environments. MARI, while designed to use the nomenclature of medical "dialects" indigenous to local environments, can of course be made compatible with those terms which match with more generalized terminological authorities such as the newly approved standard nomenclature (ICDA-9 or ICDA-9-CM).

Implementation of the Pilot Testing Phase

The problem-oriented style for manually recording patient data is used throughout the medicine services of all hospitals of Emory University School of Medicine. It is now also taught and used in the majority of the 120 medical schools in the United States. This homogeneity of medical record structure makes possible the application of advances in computer technology designed for medical information systems.

The pilot patient project began February 1, 1978, on one of the nine

Internal Medicine inpatient areas of Grady Memorial Hospital. This area was selected since patients are electively admitted for diagnostic problems in all represented specialties of internal medicine. The average age of the study patients is 51.3 years and approximately half are above the age of 40.

Certain aspects of the data collection system merit emphasis. First, the history and physical form (Defined Data Base) is extremely detailed and represents considerably more data than primary care physicians usually collect on either hospitalized or office patients. We began with this volume of patient data because a lesser amount of information would tend to reduce the chance of identifying potentially relevant medical knowledge embedded within the data bank. Experience with the MARI system may allow constriction of the current data base for low-yield items and expansion for high yield items. A second important aspect of the data collection system is the absence of abstraction of any medical record information. The data entered is exactly what the clinician has recorded. The diagnostic nomenclature is clinician generated and represents the day-to-day "lingo" of medical practice, including standard and nonstandard abbreviations as well as misspellings.

During the first year of operation, more than 600 patient records were entered. Each record contains approximately 16,000 bytes of information, providing total system storage of nearly 10^7 bytes of medical data. Approximately one hour per record is required for efficient data entry.

MARI indexes contain 1,913 clinician-generated nomenclature terms for diagnoses (or problems), 1,150 diagnostic test terms, and 1,296 separate medications (brand and generic names synonymous). Each special diagnostic test is linked to the indication for requesting the test. Each drug is linked to the indication for ordering the drug. With the "compute the costs" function, the cost for each special diagnostic test ordered is tabulated. Hence, the student or clinician may consider the possible yield of the test in context of the dollar cost of tests considered for an individual problem, or for a set of problems in a given patient.

MARI Information Uses

The following are a few examples of MARI outputs which have been generated at the request of clinicians or administrative personnel.

Display of the Complete Problem List or Entire Patient Record. Certain patients entered originally into the computer have reappeared under emergency circumstances. MARI may provide timely patient information when the usual patient chart cannot be immediately located.

Frequency listing of abnormality in the history and physical examination. This type of frequency listing has been applied classically to cost-benefit analyses of laboratory data. It is unique to have the capability to assess the yield of over 200 individual items of patient history and physical examination data. Although results are dependent on the study population and have utility primarily for that population, such data is rarely available for any population of patients. Yet data from the history and physical examination forms the matrix for most medical decision-making.

The 8 most frequently abnormal data base items in the study group of hospitalized patients are:

1. History of present illness (100%)
2. History of past disease/hospitalizations (88%)
3. History of current medications (87%)
4. Physical exam of teeth and gums (74%)
5. History of smoking (62%)
6. History of hypertension (60%)
7. History of weight change (57%)
8. History of dyspnea (56%)

In contrast is a listing of the 8 least frequently abnormal data base items:

1. History of hemospermia (0.0%)
2. Physical exam of cranial nerve I (0.3%)
3. History of disturbance of vegetative function (0.6%)
4. Physical exam of venous hum (0.6%)
5. Physical exam of pulsus alternans (0.6%)
6. History of breast pain (1.3%)
7. History of nipple discharge (1.3%)
8. Physical exam of ears (1.9%)

These types of data make it possible to relate yield of abnormality and time or dollar cost to the decision-making utility of the data items. Such objective information has generally been lacking in the traditional evolution of the patient history and physical examination.

Frequency listing of decision-making utility of collected data. During the pilot study, the normal or abnormal items of data which support the diagnostic statement are indicated by the clinician on the top portion of the problem-oriented Initial Plans document (see Fig A1). It thus became possible to compare the clinical utility of medical data with the yield of abnormality for a data item. Below are listed the 8 most frequently used items of abnormal patient data which were indicated by the clinicians as supporting the diagnoses made in the study population. (Note that the utility list differs appreciably from the yield list.)

1. History of present illness (90%)
2. Physical exam of blood pressure (67%)
3. History of weight change (66%)

4.   History of chest pain (56%)
5.   History of current medications (55%)
6.   History of inadequate exercise (55%)
7.   History of cardiac medications (55%)
8.   History of palpitations (50%)

A similar listing can be made for the utility of normal patient data in the decision-making process. Data such as these describe basic ingredients of the usual decision-making processes in clinical medicine.

Frequency listings of diagnoses, diagnostic tests, and drug orders. Listed below are the 10 most frequent diagnoses in the study population:

1.   Hypertension
2.   Chest pain/coronary disease
3.   Diabetes mellitus
4.   Anemia
5.   Undiagnosed symptom cluster
6.   Abnormal chest x-ray
7.   Weight loss
8.   Abdominal pain
9.   Obesity
10.   Melena

Listed below are the 10 most frequent special diagnostic tests (ie, not routinely done) initially ordered in the study population:

1.   Serum iron studies
2.   Cardiac catheterization
3.   Upper GI series
4.   Barium enema
5.   Prothrombin time
6.   Stool guaiac
7.   Reticulocyte count
8.   Urine fractionals
9.   Platelet count
10.   AFB culture

Listed below are the 10 most frequent drugs initially ordered in the study population:

1.   No medication
2.   Thiazide diuretic
3.   Potassium salts
4.   Digoxin

5. Nitroglycerine
6. Acetaminophen
7. Aluminum hydroxide
8. Propranolol
9. Flurazepam
10. Furosemide

These types of listings provide a basis for didactic instruction such as medical schools or postgraduate education courses. The focus may be placed on common patient problems, frequently ordered tests, or commonly used medications. The listings also provide data relevant to hospital standards and accreditation.

Descriptive statistics. The patient data is empirical and there is no specific study design with regard to patient selection. Hence, the statistical programs are primarily descriptive. Following is a display of the plasma glucose levels in patients *not* known to have diabetes.

Number	354 patients
Mean plasma glucose	101.0 mg/dl
Minimum	40.0
Maximum	297.0
Standard deviation	25.9
Variance	674.5

Note that one patient has the abnormal value of 297 mg/dl yet is not currently diagnosed as diabetic. We may proceed to print this patient's record, telephone number, and primary physician.

Relationships among documents or items within documents. One of the most powerful functions of MARI is the ability to create complex searches relating hundreds of data items which may initially appear unrelated to each other. Recall that MARI stores the decision-making data of all past clinicians confronted with a specific problem. MARI allows the user to capture this previous decision-making knowledge. The example given is a search on the data most frequently used in decision making for the problem of diabetes mellitus. Note that the 10 items, listed in order of usage, differ from the traditional textbook description of diagnostic criteria for diabetes mellitus (ie, polydipsia, polyuria, polyphagia, hyperglycemia, and glucosuria):

1. Positive family history
2. Weight change
3. Hyperglycemia
4. Eye examination

5. Urinary frequency
6. Visual dysfunction
7. Glucosuria
8. Nocturia
9. Sensory perversions
10. Sensory exam of the lower extremities

Unknown data clusters and sign-symptom complexes. Patients frequently manifest a cluster of signs and symptoms which are almost certainly related (temporal profile, etc.), yet which the clinician is unable to further refine to the level of a diagnosis. These clusters are often referred to as syndromes or sign-symptom complexes. MARI allows the user to ask the computer what diagnoses were (or were not) identified by other clinicians confronted with patients manifesting these same sign and symptom clusters. Detailed exploration of the knowledge contained within the data bank may add additional signs or symptoms to what are now recognized as relatively defined diseases. Similarly, MARI may identify groups of patients with clusters of specific signs and symptoms which are not currently recognized as defined diseases.

Future Plans for MARI

It is anticipated that several years will be required to introduce the potential of interfacing with this relatively novel way of viewing medical knowledge. The products generated by MARI have thus far been more than helpful in the initial interface. During the initial pilot phase, 58 fourth-year medical students, 75 physician houseofficers, and 18 full-time faculty interacted with the system. In addition, the first Emory University School of Medicine Medical Grand Rounds on MARI was held on December 7, 1978, and was attended by more than 200 medical and administrative participants. A videotape of the conference has been edited for distribution to educational medical television subscribers across the country. The analytical power and potential applications of the MARI system are barely explored at this point in time. We welcome innovative suggestions from the reader interested in medical knowledge.

We wish to acknowledge the major contributions, dedication, and competence of Wanda Buchheit, PA; Karen Reynolds, MARI senior programmer, and Win Strickland, MARI systems programmer. Others associated with earlier phases of the effort include L.J. Gallaher, A.P. Jensen, Stephen Newell, and Leah Williams. The development of the MARI system was supported in part by NIH grant LM-02211 from the National Library of Medicine.

Doe, Martin
(SAMPLE)

INITIAL PLANS DOCUMENT

GRADY MEMORIAL HOSPITAL
ATLANTA, GEORGIA

PATIENT IDENTIFICATION

PROBLEM #____2____ : *Fever, Cough, Chills*
Directly Supporting Data (Circle is abnormal; mark "X" if normal but clearly related
to the above problem)
S: 1 2 ③ 4 5 6 7 8 9 10 11 12 13 14 15 16 17 18 19 20 21 22 23 24 25 26 27 28 29 30
     31 32 33 34 35 36 37 ㊳ 39 40 41 42 43 44 45 46 47 48 49 50 51 52 53 54 55 56 57
     58 59 60 61 62 63 64 65 66 67 68 69 70 71 72 73 74 75 76 77 78 79 80 81 82 83 84
     85 86 87 88 89 90 91 92 93 94 95 96 97 98 99 100 101 102 103 104 105 106 107 108
     109 110 111 112 113 114 115 116
     123 124 125 126 127 128 129 130 131 132 133 134 135 136 137 138 139 140 141 142
     143 144 145 146 147 148 149 150 151 152 153 154 155 156 157 158 159 160 161 162
     163 164 165 166 �X67 168 169 170 171 172 173 174 175 176 177 178 179 180 181 182
     183 184 185 186 187 188 189 190 191 192 193 194 195 196 197 198 199 200 201 202
     203 204 205 206 207 208 209 210 211 212 213 214 ㉕ 216 217 218 219 220 221 222
     223 224 225 226 227 228 229 230 231 232 233 234 235 236 237 238 239 240 241 242
     ⟨243⟩
Other Directly Supporting Normal or Abnormal Data not covered by the 243 above numbered
items   *Pa O2 = 67 mm Hg*_____,_____,_____,_____,
_____,_____,_____,_____,

A: *Most likely bacterial pneumonia in previously healthy 48 year old male;*

     little evidence for pulmonary emboli. Needs antibiotic coverage; not Pcn allergic

P: Diagnostic: Test or Procedure:
   R/O Bacterial   *Sputum culture*
   _____   *Sputum Gram Stain*

   R/O Tuberculosis   *AFB Stain and Culture*
   R/O Cancer   *Sputum cytology*

   Therapeutic:
 * *Penicillin G. 1.2 million units IM q 12 h*

   Educational:

* orders by physician   SIGNATURE: ___*J.W. Bridges (Sample), MD*___
                                                        #3-407
                                  COUNTERSIGNATURE: _____

Figure A1.   Initial Plans document.

Example: The Process of Formulating Questions

Posing questions to computers usually requires the user to know and observe certain rules, some of which may be complicated. MARI does not make such a demand; the system is designed to be used by individuals with minimal or no computer experience. MARI accomplishes this by guiding the user step by step in the process of composing the question, making sure that, regardless of its complexity, the resulting command is logical and can be executed by the computer.

The gradual composition of the question is accomplished as follows. MARI presents the user with short, bracketed lists (called menus) of words or phrases; from each such menu the user selects one phrase, and types in its first letter only, followed by pressing the RETURN key. MARI acknowledges the choice by deleting the bracketed list and replacing it with the phrase selected. MARI then immediately displays the next menu. The process continues until the user question is complete. To close the query, the user types in "e" (for "end"). This signals the computer to begin executing the command.

This technique allows the user to build highly complex searches, exploring an almost unlimited number of relationships among any of the data categories and types. An example of the following simple interaction illustrates the manner in which MARI guides, and responds to, a user interested in learning how many patients had hypertension as a final problem:

MARI: Patient group desired is all. (How many, What are the statistics, Display, List the most frequent, Show the usage, Compute the costs)

User: H

MARI: Patient group desired is all. How many records have (Qualitative responses, Numeric data, Keywords, Clinicians' decision-supporting data numbers, Matches)

User: K

MARI: Patient group desired is all. How many records have keywords for problems of (keyword)

User: Hypertension

MARI: Patient group desired is all. How many records have keywords for problems of hypertension (And, End)

User: E

MARI: Patient group desired is all. How many records have keywords for problems of hypertension; end.

Selected References

1. Hall WD, Camp HN, Reynolds KD, Slamecka V: Clinical decision-making: Applications of the MARI system, in Dunn RA (ed): Proc. 3rd Computer Application in Medical Care, New York, IEEE, October 1979, pp 77–80.
2. Slamecka V, Camp HN, Badre AN, et al: MARIS: A knowledge system for internal medicine. *Informat Processing Management* 13: 273–276, 1977.
3. Hall WD, Slamecka V, Camp HN: MARI: *Innovations in Computerized Medicine* (videotape 78-70). Atlanta, Georgia Regional Medical Television Network of Emory University School of Medicine, 1978.
4. Camp HN, Reynolds KD, Strickland WE: *Software Design of the MARI Medical Information System*. Atlanta, Georgia Institute of Technology School of Information and Computer Science, July 1979, working paper.
5. Badre AN, Slamecka V: Problem solving approaches to clinical decision processing. *Biosci Commun* 2:269–281, 1976.

Index

Abdomen
  auscultation of, 753–755
  inspection of, 748–752
  mass in, 759–760, 761–762
  palpation of, 756–762
  swelling of, 116–119
  x-rays of, 1176–1182
Abdominal aorta, 742–743
Abdominal fluid wave, testing for, 763–764
Abdominal pain, 109–115, 143, 758–759, 760–761
  causes of, 113–115
  and tenderness, 756–761
Abducens nerve, 897–914
Abetalipoproteinemia, 1109
Abortion, 257, 258 (See also Fertility control)
Absenteeism, 469
Abstinence, sexual, 254
Abstraction, 825–828 (See also Mental status)
ACA laboratory system, 1006
Acalculia, 853
Acanthocytes, 1025
Accelerated drug reactions, 441
Accessory muscles, respiratory, 502, 633
Acetone test, 1036
Acetylsalicylic acid, 1087
Achalasia
  associated with dysphagia, 101
  LRI associated with, 171
Aching, 200 (See also Pain)
Acidosis
  and EKG, 1160
  metabolic, 1068, 1069
  renal tubular (RTA), 251
Acoustic nerve, 930–934
Acoustic neuroma, 88
  and tinnitus, 72, 74, 75
Acropachy, 730–733
Actinic keratosis, 333, 334
Activity
  diet and, 481
  social, 418–419
  usual day's, 472–474
Addiction (see Alcoholism; Drugs)
Addison's disease, 129

Adenomas
  parathyroid, 58
  rectal, 129
Adenosis, of female breast, 650
Adie's syndrome, 582
Adipose tissue, 522 (See also Fat; Obesity)
Adnexa, 784
Adult kwashiorkor, 526
Aerophagia, 104
Affect, of patient, 812, 813–816 (See also Mental status)
Ageusia, 923
Aging
  constipation associated with, 133–134
  and hearing loss, 70
Agnosia, 853
Agraphia, 870
Albumin
  in serum, 1111–1115
  in urine, 1033–1034
Alcohol
  dependence on, 439–440, 468
  ethanol content of, 149–150
  and homocidal tendencies, 431
  metabolism of, 149
  palpitations associated with, 192, 193
  questioning about, 437–438
  seizures associated with, 346
Alcoholic intake, history of, 148–151
Alcoholic ketoacidosis, 1038
Alcoholics Anonymous, 440
Alcoholism
  chronic, 501
  impotence associated with, 249, 302
  and Korsakoff's syndrome, 821
  pancreatitis associated with, 144
  parotid enlargement associated with, 608
Alexia, 871, 873, 875
Alkaline phosphatase, 1077–1081
  elevated, 1079–1080
Alkalosis, and EKG, 1160
Allergy, drug, history of, 441–444
Alopecia, 532
Alopecia areata, 534
Alport's syndrome, 251
Alzheimer's dementia, 842
Amaurotic pupil, 578

"Amaurosis fugax," 350
Amebiasis, 124
Amblyopia, 887
  congenital, 904
  nutritional, 895
Amnesia
  and Korsakoff's syndrome, 843
  retrograde, 842
  traumatic, 842
Ampicillin, allergic reaction to, 443
Analgesia, 943
Anaphylactic drug reactions, 441, 443
Anemia
  and bruits, 551
  causes of, 391–393
  cyanosis associated with, 734
  diagnostic approach to, 1012–1013
  and hematemesis, 95
  hemolytic, 399
  history of, 390–393
  hypersplenic, 392
  hypoproliferative, 391
  iron deficiency, 98
  in medullary cystic disease, 251
  "milk," 395
  pernicious, 597
  sickle cell, 396–400
Anemic crisis, associated with sickle cell
    disease, 399
Anesthesia, 942
Aneurysms
  of abdominal aorta, 762
  berry, 373, 376
  Charcot-Bouchard, 373
  congenital, 373
  of internal carotid artery, 582
  saccular, 373
Angina pectoris
  and chest pain, 187, 188
  and EKG, 1128
  and third heart sound, 699
  therapy for, 476
Angiography, 41
  for occult bleeding, 795
Angiokeratoma corporis diffusum, 251
Ankle, examination of, 804
Ankle jerk, 987, 991
Anomia, 870, 874
Anorexia, 34
Anorgasmia 306–309
Anoscope, 788, 790
Anosmia, 880–881
Anterior inferior cerebellar artery, and
    dizziness, 49–50
Anthrax, 177
Antibiotics
  allergic reactions to, 443
  for cholecystitis, 142
  diarrhea associated with, 128
  vaginitis associated with, 264
Antidepressants, tricyclic, 1154
Antidiuretic hormone system, 1031
Antipyretics, 38–39

Antitoxins, 445, 449
Anus
  examination of, 788–790
  lump in, 137 (See also Rectum)
Anxiety, 422–424
Aorta, abdominal, 742–743
  on x-ray, 1173–1174
Aortic aneurysm, and chest pain, 190
Aortic distensibility, 518
Apex impulse, 669–676
Aphasia
  anomic, 861, 871, 872
  anterior, 868
  Broca's, 868, 872
  bucco-facial, 868
  conduction, 869–870, 872
  fluent, 870
  motor, 868
  nonfluent, 868
  posterior, 870
  receptive, 870
  sensory, 870
  transcortical, 870–871, 872
  Wernicke's, 870–871, 872
Aplastic crisis of sickle cell disease, 399
Apneustic respiration, 846
Appearance of patient, 499–501, 812–813,
    816
Appendicitis, pain of, 115, 226, 759
Appetite, associated with psychological
    disturbances, 435
Apraxia, 862, 960
  buccofacial, 870, 874
  constructional, 864, 865
  dressing, 866
  limb, 870
Areola, examination of, 651–653 (See also
    Breast; Nipple)
Argylle-Robertson pupils, 582
Arm muscle circumference, 524
Arrhenoblastoma, 531
Arrhythmia
  and abnormal beats, 1153–1155
  and chest pain, 191
  drug use associated with, 1151–1154
  stroke associated with, 370–371
  syncope associated with, 196–197 (See
      also Heart disease)
Arrhythmokinesis, 171
Arsenic, as a cause of cancer, 333
Arterial blood pressure, mean, 517–518
Arterial bruits, 551
Arterial pulse tracing, 513, 514
Arteries, "hardening of," (see Athero-
    sclerosis)
Arteriography
  of abdomen, 1181, 1182
  carotid, 613
  coronary, 187, 188
  for hematuria diagnosis, 230
  pelvic, 276
  pulmonary, 1171
  thoracic, 1171

Arteriovenous malformations, 551
Arthritis
    gonoccocal, 409
    history of, 410–420
    Jaccoud's, 410
    joint stiffness of, 402–403
    rheumatoid, 408, 409
    septic, 409
Articulation, testing patient's, 854, 855
Ascending reticular activating system,
    849, 851
Aschoff bodies, 208, 209
Ascites, 762–765
    associated with abdominal swelling, 118
    bile, 764
    bloody, 765
    chylous, 765
    pancreatic, 764
Aspirin, 458, 460
    wheezing associated with, 162–163
Associations of thought, 831–833
Association areas, 860
Association cortex, 860
Astereognosis, 943
Asterixis, 850, 976, 978, 979–980
Asthma
    cardiac, 184
    causes of, 162–163
    history of, 161–163
    Monday, 177
Ataxia, 969
Ataxic breathing, 846
Atherosclerosis
    bruits associated with, 551
    claudication associated with, 202
    smoking associated with, 174
    stroke associated with, 371–372
    and thrombosis, 375
    TIA's associated with, 350
Athetosis, 976, 979
Atopy, history of, 161
Atrial fibrillation, 510, 511, 660, 1148–1149
Atrial flutter, 509, 511, 1148, 1149
Atrial gallops, 701–704
Atrial tachycardia, 509, 511, 1148, 1149
Atrioventricular (A-V) block, EKG for,
    1156, 1157
Atrophy, 956
Attention span, of patient, 820–822 (See
    also Mental status)
Auditory canal, external, 552, 553, 556, 557
Auscultation
    of abdomen, 753–755
    of arteries, 743–747
    for bowel sounds, 753–755
    for bruits, 746–747, 753–755
    cardiac, 685, 689, 703
    of carotid artery, 741
    chest, 634–638
    of femoral artery, 743–744
    of heart sounds, 681–682
    of liver, 766–768
    of popliteal artery, 744

    for rubs, 753–755
    of spleen, 774, 775
"Auscultatory gap," 515
Autoimmune disorders, and fever, 38
Autonomic neuropathy, and sweating, 44
Autosomal dominant traits, 453, 454
Autosomal recessive traits, 453, 454
A wave, of jugular venous pulsations,
    657–660
Axilla, palpation of, 646
Axillary nodes, 626, 650

Babinski reflex, 992, 993
Babinski reflex hammer, 985
Bacteremia, 387, 400
Bacteriuria, 224
Barbiturate abstinence syndrome, 439
Barbiturates
    questioning about, 437–438
    seizures associated with, 346 (See also
        Drugs)
Barium enema, 1179, 1180
    for pelvic mass, 276
Barium studies, 1179–1180
Barlow click-murmur syndrome, 713
Bartholin gland
    abscess of, 276
    examination of, 782
    inflammation of, 268
Basal cell carcinoma, 330
Basal cell epithelioma (BCE), 332, 333–
    334, 335
Basilar artery occlusion, and dizziness,
    49
Basophils, 1016
Beau's lines, 543–544
Bedwetting (see Enuresis)
Behavior (see Mental status examina-
    tion)
Belching, 103
Bell's palsy, 926, 928
Benign-fibroadenoma, of female breast,
    650
Benign positional vertigo, 49, 88
Benign prostatic hypertrophy, 791, 792
Bernstein test, 108
Berry aneurysms, 551
Bessey-Lowry units, 1077
Bicarbonate, in serum, 1065–1069
Bigeminy, 510, 1153–1154
Bilirubin
    metabolism of, 121–122
    in serum, 1080–1084
Bing's sign, 995
Biologic false positive (BFP) results, 241,
    1118
Biopsy, marrow, 40–41
Biot's breathing, 503, 506
Birth control, 253–259
Biferiens pulse, 668
Bitemporal hemianopsia, 896
Bladder
    function, related to psychiatric dis-

turbances, 436
irritability of, 221, 222
neuropathic disturbances of, 236
"shy," 235
Bleeding
abnormal, 385–390
causes of, 388–389
after dental extractions, 386
excessive, 385–390
gastrointestinal, 380, 388
generalized spontaneous, 386, 389
menstrual, 269–274
nasal, 386, 388
with sexual intercourse, 269, 271, 385
related to surgery, 386, 389
related to trauma, 386, 389
urinary, 386, 389
vaginal, 269–274, 385–386, 388
Blindness
fleeting, 350
monocular, 350
pure word, 871, 875
transient, 348–350
Blink, 848
Blood
in diarrhea, 124
expectoration from lungs, 158
in stool, 123, 124, 793–795
Blood cells (see Red blood cells; White
blood cells)
Blood glucose, 1005
Blood pressure, 513–531
elevated (see Hypertension)
measurement of, 514–516
normal in adults, 513
Blood urea nitrogen (BUN), 1005, 1044–
1048, 1055
Body density, 523
Body habitus, 528–532
Body size, 500 (See also Appearance)
Bones, examination of, 797 (See also
Joints)
Bony thorax, on x-ray, 1175
Borborygmi, 754
Borrelia, 40, 241
Bowel
related to psychiatric disturbances, 436
sounds, auscultation of, 753–755
on x-ray, 1167
Brachial artery pulse, 741–742
Bradycardia-tachycardia syndrome, 1151
Bradycardias, 1152
definition of, 508
relative, 40
sinus, 511, 512, 1152
Breast
benign cyst of, 649
cancer of, 315–316, 318, 320
examination of, 641–656
glandular tissue of, 648–649
lump in, 314–316, 641
mass in, 641
nipple discharge from, 319–321
pain in, 316–319

tumor of, 641, 649–651
Breathing
Biot's, 503, 506
Cheyne-Stokes, 502–503, 506, 846
obstruction of, 603
Breathlessness, 152–154
Breath sounds, 634–638
Bright's disease, 250
Broca's area, 860, 861, 862
Bronchiectasis, 159, 171, 184
Bronchitis, 159, 171, 174, 184
Bronchospasm, and cardiac asthma, 184
Bruising, 385–390
Bruits
abdominal, 746–747, 753–755
arterial, 551
carotid, 612–614
cranial, 548–552
hepatic arterial, 766, 767–768
orbital, 548–552
peripheral, 740–748
splenic, 774
thyroid, 619
Budd-Chiari syndrome, 765
Buerger's disease, smoking associated
with, 174
BUN (see Blood urea nitrogen)
Bundle branch block
and EKG, 1147
left, 1129, 1142–1144
right, 687
Burning, 200 (See also Pain)
Bursitis, 409

Calcium
in serum, 1093–1100
total body, 1094–1096
Calculation, testing patient's ability, 857
Calf circumference, measuring, 727
Caloric need, 480, 481
Caloric requirement chart, 481
Caloric stimulation, for vertigo, 88
Caloric test, 899
Cancer
arsenic in, 333
breast, 315–316
of oropharynx, 587, 588
skin, 332–335
squamous cell, of mouth, 603
thyroid, 60–61 (See also Carcinoma)
Candida, in vaginal discharge, 266, 268
Cannabanoids, 438–439
Cannon wave, of jugular venous pulsations, 659, 662
Carbon dioxide, laboratory tests for, 1065–
1070
Carcinoid syndrome, wheezing associated
with, 163
Carcinoma
basal cell, 330, 594
and hematemesis, 96
medullary, 58
oral, 588, 593, 594
ovarian, 261

Carcinoma (*continued*)
 penile, 780
 smoking associated with, 174
Cardiac alternans, 735–736, 739
Cardiac asthma, 184
Cardiac disorders, syncope associated
 with, 196
Cardiac fluoroscopy, 1170
Cardiac output, 517
Cardiac series, x-ray, 1169
Cardiomyopathy, associated with chest
 pain, 190
Cardiovascular disease
 and EKG, 1128
 family history of, 214–219
 morbidity/mortality from, 519–520
 weight gain associated with, 34
Carditis, and rheumatic fever, 207
Carey-Coombs murmur, 209
Caries, examination for, 589–590
Carotene, 120, 328
Carotenoid pigments, 120, 328
Carotid artery, 626
 bruits of, 612–614
 pulse of, 663–669, 741
Carotid sinus hypersensitivity, 198
Cataplexy, 380
Cataract, history of, 64–65
Catheterization
 and UTI, 221
 and x-rays, 1179–1180
CAT scan, 1171
Celiac disease, 130
Centrencephalic seizures, 342–343, 346
Cerebellar hemorrhage, and dizziness, 50
Cerebellopontine tumors, dizziness with,
 50
Cerebellum, 969–975
 anatomy and organization of, 972–974
Cerebral embolism, 371, 372, 375
Cerebral hemorrhage, 371, 373
Cerebral thrombosis, 371, 374
 causes of, 372
Cerebral vascular disease, and syncope,
 197 (*See also* Syncope)
Cervical nodes, 626
Cervical spine, examination of, 801–802
Cervix, examination of, 783
Chalazion, 569
"Charley horse," 362, 364
Chest
 auscultation of, 634–638
 discomfort of, 185–191
 examination of, 628–641
 fluoroscopy of, 1170
 motion of, 631–634
 percussion of, 639–641
 structure, 628–631
 x-ray of, 640, 1162–1176
Chest pain, 185–191
 CAD associated with, 187, 188
 cardiomyopathy associated with, 190
 causes of, 188
 and EKG, 1128

 and history of heart disease, 213
Cheyne-Stokes breathing, 502–503, 506,
 846
Chiari-Frommel syndrome, 320
Chief complaint, in medical record, 28–32
Children
 and asthma, 162–163
 ear examination of, 552, 1000
 examination of, 997–1001
 enuresis in, 236
 epistaxis in, 77
 eye examination of, 1000
 genital examination of, 999
 heart murmur in, 712, 716
 hematochezia in, 124
 immunizations for, 445–446
 pica in, 395
 suicide of, 428
 third heart sound in, 696–697
 throat examination of, 999–1000
 urinary stream of, 234–235
Chills, 38–41
Chloride, in serum, 1062–1065
Choking, 100–101, 441
Cholecystectomy, indications for, 142, 147
Cholecystitis
 associated with gallstone disease, 142
 associated with pancreatitis, 145
 renal pain associated with, 226
Cholera, immunization for, 447
Cholestasis, 122, 1084
Cholestatic jaundice, 122
Cholesterol, 484, 1104–1110
Choluria, 120
Chorea, 976, 979
 and rheumatic fever, 207
 Sydenham's 210
Choroiditis, 576
Chromosome anomalies, 454–455
"Chuckle," 754
Cirrhosis, 1083
 ascites associated with, 764
 and low serum phosphate levels, 1102
Claudication, 200–203
 causes of, 202–203
 intermittent, 201–202
Clicks
 diastolic, 705, 707
 examination for, 705–708
 systolic, 705–707
Clinical methods
 the course at Emory, 15, 17–20
 for pediatric patient, 997–1001
 teaching and learning, 13–20
 videotapes of, 18, 19
Clinitest methods, 1036
Clitoris, 782
Clothing, patient's, 500 (*See also* Appearance)
Clubbing, 730–733
 of nails, 544
Cluster migraine, 339
Cocaine, questioning about, 437–438, 439
Coffee ground vomitus, 92, 93, 94

Coin lesions, and previous chest x-rays, 169
Coitus
frequency of, 287–290
marital, 288–290
Coitus interruptus, 254 (See also Fertility control)
Cold intolerance, 52–54
Colic, renal, 226–227
Colitis
diarrhea associated with, 129
ulcerative, 124
Colon, pain originating in, 115
Coma, 844
examination during, 845
Compensatory movements, eye, 898–899, 901
Complete Problem List, of medical record, 7–9, 10, 15, 22
Compliance, with drug use, 464
Computerized medical records, 1183–1197
"Concordant" alternans, 736
Concussion, 360
Condoms, 254 (See also Fertility control)
Conductive hearing loss, 68, 69
Confabulation, 821, 838
Congenital heart disease, 215–219
Congestion
nasal, 81
pelvic, 292
pulmonary, PND associated with, 183–184
Congestive heart failure (see Heart failure)
Conjugate gaze, 897
testing, 900
Conjunctivitis, 66, 567, 569
Consciousness
level of, 844–852
loss of, 1128 (See also Syncope)
organic disorders of, 810–811
Consensual response, of pupil, 577, 578
Constipation
causes of, 133–134
hemorrhoids associated with, 137
history for, 131–134
and menstruation, 262
Construction, testing patient's ability, 857
Contraception, risks of, 258–259
Contraceptives
oral, 256–257
types of, 254–258 (See also Fertility control)
Contracture, 364
Convergence, eye, 899–900, 904
Convulsion, 340 (See also Seizures)
Cooper's ligaments, 649
Cords, of thrombosed veins, 727
Corneal reflex, testing, 916–917
Coronary artery disease
and chest pain, 187, 188
smoking associated with, 174
therapy for, 476
Corpus callosmum, 866–868

Cortical sensory functions, 947
Corynebacterium vaginale, 264, 265, 266
Costovertebral joint motion, 803
Costs
of laboratory tests, 1005–1006
medical, 490–492
of x-ray examinations, 1168–1171, 1179, 1180–1182
Cough, 155–158
causes of, 157
mechanisms of, 156
Courvoisier's sign, 761
Crackles, 635, 636, 637
Cramp syndromes, 368
Cranial bruits, 548–552
Cranial nerves
(I) Olfactory, 878–881
(II) Optic, 882–896
(III) Oculomotor, 897–914
(IV) Trochlear, 897–914
(V) Trigeminal, 915–923
and trigeminal neuralgia, 355
(VI) Abducens, 897–914
(VII) Facial, 923–929
(VIII) Acoustic, 930–934
acoustic neuroma associated with, 72–74
(IX) Glossopharyngeal, 934–938
(X) Vagus, 934–938
(XI) Spinal Accessory, 938–940
(XII) Hypoglossal, 941–942
Creatinine
excretion of, 524–525
in serum, 1089–1093
Crohn's disease, 148
associated with diarrhea, 129
Cruveilhier-Baumgarten disease, 767
Cryptomenorrhea, 262
Cryptorchism, 244
Crystalluria, 1042–1043
Cullen's sign, 751
Culture
cervical, 267
rectal, 267
Curet, for removing earwax, 554
Cushing's syndrome, 531
CVA pain, 225–227
causes of, 226
C wave, of jugular venous pulsations, 657, 658, 659, 661
Cyanosis, 733–735
central, 734
and occupation, 471
peripheral, 734
Cystic disease, 251
Cystic fibrosis, sinus complications of, 82
Cystinosis, 251
Cystinuria, 1044
Cystitis, 221, 223, 224
Cystocele, and urinary incontinence, 236
Cysts
Bartholin gland, 275, 312
brachial, 626
in breasts, 649

Cysts (*continued*)
  dermoid, 626
  hydatid, 771
  mucous retention, 329
  of neck, 611
  ovarian, 276
  sebaceous, 626
  thyroglossal, 611, 619–620
  thyroid, 610–611
Cytology smear, cervical, 782

Daily activities, of patient, 472–474
Data Base
  comprehensive care, 5
  computerized, 1183–1197
  defined, 5–12, 15, 16–17, 18, 19, 20, 1184–1185
  problem-specific, 5
  specialty, 5
Deafness, 67–71
  and dizziness, 49–50
  pure word, 871, 873
Death summary, 10
Deep tendon reflexes, 983–992
Deep vein thrombophlebitis, 729
Defecation
  hemorrhoids associated with, 137
  reflex, 133
Defense mechanisms, 423
Defined Data Base, 5–12, 15, 16–17, 18, 19, 20, 1184–1185
  types of, 5
Dehydration, 724
  skin, 326
Delayed allergic drug reactions, 441, 442
Del Castillo syndrome, 320
Delirium, 829
Delphian node, 620
Delusions, 828–831 (*See also* Mental status)
Dementia, senile, 842
Denco, 1036
Densitometry, body, 523
Dentures, 586
Depression
  biochemical changes associated with, 426
  and clinical appearance, 813–814
  history for, 425–429
  insomnia associated with, 379, 381
  questioning about, 413–414, 425–426
  and substance abuse, 438
  weight loss and, 36
Dermatofibroma, 330
Dermatological history, 321–324
Dermatomes, 952
Dermatoses, 326
"Devil's pinches," 389
Diabetes mellitus, 62–63
  adult onset, 1049
  and blood glucose, 1049–1053
  chemical, 1049
  clinical indicators of, 62–64
  diarrhea associated with, 129
  and diet, 478, 483–484

dizziness associated with, 49
dysphagia associated with, 101
family history of, 62–63
gestational, 1050
GTT criteria for diagnosis, 1052
impotence associated with, 249
ketoacidosis in, 1038
latent, 1049
lipodystrophic, 1050
parotid enlargement associated with, 608
prediabetes, 1050
and pregnancy, 1050
vaginitis associated with, 263
vomiting associated with, 92
weight gain associated with, 34
Diaphragm
  as a method of birth control, 255
  on x-ray, 1167
Diarrhea
  anxiety associated with, 436
  bloody, 124
  causes of, 126–130
  exudative, 127
  history for, 125–130
  osmotic, 126
Diastolic blood pressure, definition of, 513
Diet
  average American, 480
  and liver disease, 484
  for renal failure, 484–485
  therapeutic, 483–485
Dietary recall, and nutritional history, 477, 480
Digitalis, 1151–1152
Dilatation
  cardiac, 694
  gastric, 117
Diplegia, 955
Diplopia, 65, 898
  and neurological symptoms, 348, 349
Diphtheria, immunization for, 446, 447
Direct response, of pupil, 578
Disability, 469
Discharge
  nipple, 319–321
  urethral, 237–239
  vaginal, 263–269
Discharge summary, 10, 1084
"Discordant" alternans, 736
Discrimination, two-point, 947
Disorientation
  spatial, 865
Distention, gastric, 112, 118
Diuretics
  thiazide, 1098
  and urinary frequency, 221
Diverticulum
  Meckel's, 124
  pharyngeal, 157
  urethral, 236
Dizziness, 44–51
  associated with cerebrovascular disease, 49–50
  associated with diabetes, 49

associated with epilepsy, 45, 50
associated with TIA's, 47, 50
causes of, 48–51
and psychiatric disorders, 46
questionnaire for, 85
Dominant hemisphere, 859–864
Dorsalis pedis artery pulse, 744–745
Dorsiflexion sign, 727
Double-peaked pulse, 667
Down's syndrome, 216
DPT vaccine, 446, 447
Drawer sign, 806
Drawing, testing patient's ability, 857
Dressing
and right hemisphere of brain, 866
testing patient's ability, 857
Drift, 958
Drinking (see Alcohol, Alcoholism)
"Dropsy," 723
Drugs
abuse of, 437–440
adverse reactions to, 463–464
allergy to, 327, 441–444
antidepressant, 426, 1154
antithyroid, 57
constipation associated with, 133
dependency on, 379, 381
and dysrhythmias, 1150–1154
and hearing loss, 70
and homicidal tendencies, 431
history for use, 457–465
interaction, 460–463
nonprescription, 460, 461
prescription, 460
side effects of, 90
syncope associated with, 195
thrombophlebitis associated with, 729
and tinnitus, 72
vertigo associated with, 88
Drumstick finger, clubbing, 731
"Dry heaves," 89
Duodenal ulcer
abdominal pain associated with, 114
history for, 138–139
Dysarthria, and basilar artery occlusion, 49
Dysesthesia, 325, 351, 352, 943
Dysgeusia, 923
Dysgraphia, 870
Dysmenorrhea, 261–262
Dyspareunia, 261, 310–314
"Dyspepsia," 103
Dysphagia, 99–102
Dyspnea
causes of, 154
history for, 152–154
and occupation, 471
paroxysmal nocturnal (PND), 182–185
Dyspraxia, 960
Dysrhythmias, 1143–1161
associated with drug use, 1150–1154
sinus and EKG, 1147 (See also Arrhythmias)
Dyssomnias, 378, 379, 382
Dystrophy

muscular, 171, 217
myotonic, 217, 957
Dysuria, 220–223, 224

Ear
examination of, 552–558
ringing in (see Tinnitus)
Eardrum, 552, 553, 555–558
Ebstein's anomaly, 707
ECG (see Electrocardiogram)
Edema
history of, 723–724, 725
joint stiffness associated with, 402
nocturia and, 228
pulmonary, 183, 184
Edinger-Westphal nucleus, 580, 581, 582
Education, of patient, 486–489
Effusion
joint, 407–408
pleural, 640
Ehlers-Danlers syndrome, 218
Eighth cranial nerve, 930–934
Einthoven triangle, 1127
Eisenmenger's syndrome, 694
Ejaculation, 247
premature, 294–297
Ejaculatory incompetence, 297–298
EKG (see Electrocardiogram)
Elbow, examination of, 800 (See also Joints)
"Electrical" alternans, 736, 1153
Electrocardiogram, 1122–1161
abnormal beats on, 1153–1155
AV block on, 1156, 1157
Bazett's formula, 1124
delta waves, 1148–1149
depolarization, 1131–1132
extremity leads, 1127–1128
history of, 1127–1128
indications for, 1128
interpreting, 1126
limitations of, 1128–1129
precordial leads, 1126
P-Q and P-R intervals of, 1123–1124
QRS interval, 1124
QT interval, 1124–1126
recording, 1125–1126
repolarization, 1131–1132, 1143
scalar, 1122, 1132
S-T segment of, 1123
technique for performing, 1125–1126
and vector method, 1129–1143
ventricular fibrillation on, 1148, 1151
ventricular gradient, 1138–1141
waves of, 1122–1124
Ellis-Van Creveld syndrome, 218
Embolism
atherosclerotic, 613
cerebral, 371, 372, 375
pulmonary, 500, 729
Embolus, pulmonary, 190, 691
Emotions
and dyspnea, 154
and indigestion, 105
and interpersonal relationships, 416–422

Emotions (*continued*)
  and vegetative function, 433–436
  and WBC, 1015 (*See also* Psychiatric
    examination)
Emphysema
  bullous, 640
  smoking associated with, 174
Encephalitis, Herpes simplex, 841–842
Encephalogram, ECHO, 376
Endometriosis, 262, 274, 313
Energy requirements, of activities, 180
Enuresis, 235, 236, 379, 382
Environmental inhalation, 175–178
Eosinophils, 1016
Epicritic, component of cutaneous sensa-
    tion, 352
Epididymitis, 780–781
Epigastric hernia, 135
Epilepsies
  generalized, 345–346
  international classification of, 345–346
Epilepsy, 340–347
  akinetic, associated with syncope, 197
  aura ictus, 341
  dizziness associated with, 45, 50
  focal, 341, 343
  grand mal, 346
  petit mal, 346
  and seizures, 340–347, 348
  tinnitus associated with, 75
Epiphera, 567
Epispadias, 780
Epistaxis, 76–78
  causes of, 77–78
  hematemesis associated with, 95
  melena associated with, 98
Epitrochlear node, 622, 626–627
Equipment, for performing physical ex-
    amination, 496
Erection, penile, 247
  difficulty with (*see* Impotence)
Erythema marginatum, 207–208, 210
Escherichia coli, 126, 128
Esophageal ulcer, 139
Esophagitis
  chest pain associated with, 188
  hernia associated with, 136
  reflux, 106–108
Esophagus
  carcinoma of, 626
  inflammation of, 106, 108
  motor disorders, and dysphagia, 100–
    101
Estrogens
  and body habitus, 530–531
  and nipple pigmentation, 652
Ethanol, content of alcohol, 149–150
Ethmoid sinus, 561, 562
Eustachian tube, obstruction of, 557
Exercise level, 178–181
Exophthalmos, 66, 569
Expiration, examination of, 632, 633–634
    (*See also* Respiration)

Exposure
  to asbestos, 177
  to radiation, 1168–1171
  to ultraviolet light, 334 (*See also* En-
    vironmental inhalation)
Exteroceptive sensation, 944, 948–
    952
Extremity ratios, 530
  abnormal prportions of, 531
Eye chart, Snellen, 563
Eyes
  alignment of, 565, 566
  examination of, 563–570
  far-sighted, 575
  history of dysfunction, 64–66
  light reflex, 571–572
  movements of, 900–904
  near-sighted, 575
  physiology of, 882–887

Fabry's disease 218, 251
Face
  features of, 501 (*See also* Appearance)
  pain, 80
  and parotid enlargement, 606, 607
  recognition, testing patient's ability,
    857, 866
  synkinetic movements of, 926–927
Facial nerve, 923–929
  lesions of, 927–928
"Factitious fever," 40
Faint
  common, 196, 197
  prank, 196
Familial dysautonomia (*see* Riley-Day
    Syndrome)
Family history
  of heart disease, 214–219
  and heritable disease potential, 450–
    455
  of musculoskeletal disease, 410–412
  of renal disease, 250–252
  of sickle cell gene inheritance, 396–
    400
Family relationships, 416–417
Fasciculations, 956
Fat
  definition of, 522
  in diet, 484
  subconjunctival, 120 (*See also* Obesity)
Fatigue
  low hematocrit associated with, 1012
  tremors of, 978
Fear vs. anxiety, 422 (*See also* Anxiety)
Feces, daily weight of, 126 (*See also*
    Stools)
Feculent vomitus, 94
Feet (*see* Foot)
Fehling's methods, 1036
Females
  ideal body weight for, 521
  sexual function, history of, 279–287
Female escutcheon, 530
Female genitalia (*see* Genitalia, female)

Feminization, 529–530
  clinical significance of, 531
Femoral artery pulse, 743–744
Femoral hernia, 135
Femoral nodes, 622
Fertility control, methods of, 254–258
Fever
  "factitious," 40
  and hearing loss, 70
  history of, 38–41
  hypersensitivity, pneumonitides associated with, 177
  relapsing, 40
  rheumatic, 206–211
  of undetermined origin (FUO), 40–41
Fibrillation
  atrial, 1148, 1149
  ventricular, 1151
Fibroadenomas, 650
Fibrocystic disease, 315, 318
Fibrous hyperplasia, 650
Final common pathway, 963
Finances, of patient, 489–493
Finger identification, 857
Finger jerk, 986, 991
First heart sound, 681–688
Fissures, anal, 125
Fistulas
  aortointestinal, 96
  arteriovenous, 716–717
  oral-antral, 594
  oral-nasal, 594
  urethrovaginal, 236
  vesicovaginal, 236
Fitz-Hugh-Curtis syndrome, 768
Fixation, eye, 897
Flaccidity, 956
Flank pain, 225–227
Flatulence, 103
Fluorescein, and jaundice, 120
Fluorescein string test, 795
Fluorescent Theponemal Antibody-
    absorbed Test, 1119
Fluoroscopy
  cardiac, 1170
  chest, 1170
Flutter
  atrial, 1148, 1149
  ocular, 904
  ventricular, 1148
Follicle-stimulating hormone (FSH), 273,
    274
Food
  and emotional disorders, 433–436
  and nutritional history, 477–485
Food-drug interactions, 483
Foot, examination of, 804
Forbes-Albright syndrome, 320
Fourth heart sound, 700–704
Fovea, 573
Fractures, skull, 361
Freckles, 330
Free T4, 56
Frequency, urinary, 220–223, 224

Freud, Sigmund, 414
Frey's syndrome, 44, 928
Friedreich's ataxia, 217
Frigidity, 303–305
Frontal sinus, 560, 561, 562
Funduscopic examination, 571–577
Fungal infection
  and hair loss, 534
  of nails, 546
FUO (see Fever, of undetermined origin)

Gag reflex, 935
Gait, 957, 965–966, 969
  apraxia of, 966
  cerebellar, 966
  observation of, 806–807
  Parkinsonian, 966
  sensory ataxia, 965
  spastic, 965
  steppage, 966
Gallbladder
  disease of, 141–143
  pain of, 114, 141
  pancreatitis associated with, 145
Gallop
  atrial, 701–704
  description of, 697
  summation, 704
  ventricular, 696–699, 703
Gallstones, 141–142
  pancreatitis associated with, 145
Gamma globulins (see Globulin)
Gaseousness, and indigestion, 103
Gastric air bubble, and chest x-ray, 1167
Gastric emptying, 104
Gastric obstruction, pain with, 114
Gastric ulcer, history of, 138, 139
Gastrointestinal bleeding, 386, 388
  hemorrhage, causes of, 96
  and melena, 98
  and ulcers, 140
Gastrointestinal gas, 104
Gastrointestinal (GI) series, 276, 454
Gastrointestinal surgery, history of, 146–
    148
Gastroscopy, 98
Geneology, symbols for, 451
Genetic counseling, 252
Genitalia, female
  examination of, 781–787
Genitalia, male
  examination of, 779–781
  lesions of, 243–244
German measles, 446 (See also Rubella)
Gerstmann's syndrome, 875
GI (see Gastrointestinal)
Giemsa's stain, 1017
Gilbert's syndrome, 122, 1083
Gingiva (see Gums)
Glands
  Bartholin, 268, 276, 782
  of female breast, 648–649
  lacrimal, 567
  mammary, 652

Glands (continued)
  Montgomery's, 652
  salivary, 605, 608, 609
  sebaceous, 652
  sweat, 652
  urethral, 238
Glaucoma, 568, 576
  angle closure, 568, 571
  cupping of, 574
  detection of, 568, 570
  history for, 65, 66
  open angle, 568
Globulin, in serum, 1111–1115
Glomerular disease, 1035
Glomerulonephritis, acute hemorrhagic, 725
Glossopharyngeal nerve, 934–938
Gluconeogenesis, 1071
Glucose, 1055
  in plasma, 1048–1053
Glucose tolerance test (GTT), 1050–1052
Glucosuria, 1035–1039
Glutamic oxaloacetate transaminase (GOT), 1071–1072
Glycogen storage diseases, 367, 412
Goiter, 54
  history for, 54–58
  removal of, 57
Golgi tendon organ, 989
Gonadotrophin-releasing hormone (GnRH), 273
Gonococcus, 264
Gonorrhea
  urethral discharge associated with, 238–239
  in vaginal discharge, 267, 268
Goodpasture's syndrome, 160
Gout, 409
  familial, 411
  hyperuricemia associated with, 1088
  joint pain associated with, 404
Gouty tophi, 409
Grand mal seizure, 346
Granulocytes, 1014–1015
Granulomatosis, Wegener's, 160
Graphesthesia, 947
Grasp reflex, 981–982
Graves' disease, 57, 58
Graves speculum, 783
Gray-Turner sign, 751
Guaiac, stool, 793–796
Guillain-Barre syndrome, 359
Gumma formation, 242
Gums, examination of, 585–596
Gustatory sweating, 43
Gynecologic history, 259–260
Gynecomastia, 530, 531
Gyri
  angular, 861
  supramarginal, 861

Habitus, body, 528–532
Hair
  dye abuse, 535

examination of, 532–535
growth of, 533
loss of, 534
sulfur content of, 533
Hallucinations, 828–831
  hypnogogic, 380
  olfactory, 881
Handedness, 858, 862
Hands
  examination of, 799–800
  tremors of, 977
Hashimoto's thyroiditis, 58, 61, 620
"Hawking," 157
Head, trauma to, 360–362
Headache, 336–340, 375
  due to brain tumor, 338
  mechanisms of, 337–338
  migraine, 338, 339, 348, 842
Hearing loss, 67, 68
  causes of, 69–71
  conductive, 68, 69
  sensorineural, 68–69, 70
Heart
  abnormal beats, 1153–1155
  electrophysiologic properties, 1144–1146
  murmur, 213 (See also Murmurs)
  on x-ray, 1173–1174 (See also Electrocardiogram)
Heart block
  complete, 1159
  first-degree, 1124
  second-degree, 1156, 1158
  third-degree, 1156
Heartburn, 103, 106–108
Heart disease
  congenital, 215–219
  family history of, 214–219
  previous, 211–214
  rheumatic, 206
Heart failure
  alcoholism associated with, 151
  congestive, 675, 691
  hemorrhoids associated with, 137, 138
  history for, 213
  orthopnea associated with, 184–185
  PND associated with, 184–185
Heart sounds
  1st, 681–688
  2nd, 688–695
  3rd, 695–700
  4th, 700–794
  vs. pulmonary artery pulsation, 680
Heat intolerance, 52–54
Heerfordt syndromes, 608
Height, 521–528
Hematemesis, 94–97
  causes of, 96
  and ulcers, 140
Hematobilia associated with GI hemorrhage, 96
Hematochezia, 123–125
Hematocrit, 1005, 1011–1013

Hematuria, 229, 1041, 1042–1043
  causes of, 230–231
  associated with stones, 232
Hemianesthesia, 376
Hemianopsia, 896
Hemidiaphragm, 169
Hemiparesis, 955
Hemiplegia, 376, 955
Hemisphere
  dominant, 859–864
  nondominant, 864–866
Hemoccult, 793–794
Hemoglobin, 1007
  sickle, 397
Hemolytic anemia, associated with
    sickle cell disease, 399
Hemophilia, 387–388
Hemoptysis, 158–160
  causes of, 159–160
  and melena, 98
Hemorrhage
  cerebral, 371, 373
  gastrointestinal, 96
  hypertensive intracerebral, 375, 376
  in joints, 408
  retinal, 576
  splinter, 545
  subarachnoid, 376 (See also Bleeding)
Hemorrhoids
  examination of (see Rectal examination)
  history for, 136–138
Hemosiderin, 328
Hemostasis, mechanisms for, 387–388
Hepatic adenomas, 761
Hepatic arterial bruit, 766, 767–768
Hepatic friction rub, 766, 767–768
Hepatitis, 1083
  alcoholic, 768, 771
  immunization for, 448
Hepatocellular jaundice, 122 (See also
    Jaundice)
Hepatomegaly, 771
Hereditary (see Inheritance)
Hering-Breuer reflex, 504
Hernia
  diaphramatic, 135
  epigastric, 135
  examining for, 777
  femoral, 776
  hiatal, 135, 136
  history for, 134–136
  incisional, 135
  incarcerated, 136, 778
  paraesophageal, 135
  sliding, 135
  strangulated, 136, 778
  umbilical, 135, 136
  uncal, 850, 913
Herniation, central, 851
Heroin, questioning about, 437, 439
Herpes simplex encephalitis, 841–842
Herpes zoster, 953
Hesitancy, 234–237
Hesselbach's triangle, 135

High density lipoproteins (HDL), 1105,
    1107, 1109
Hip, examination of, 806–807
Hippocampus, lesions of, 839
Hirschprung's disease, 133
Hirsutism, 532
Histoplasmosis, 177
History, 26–27
Hoarseness, history for, 78–79
Hobbies, patient's, 474–476
Hodgkin's disease
  and night sweats, 43
  and PPD test, 1117
  pruritis associated with, 326
Hollenhorst crystals, 613
Holt-Oram syndrome, 218
Homan's test, 727
Homocidal tendency, 430–433
Homocystinuria, 218
Homosexuality, history for, 281–283
Hordeolum, 569
Horizontal movements, eye, 903
Hormones
  diarrhea associated with, 128–129
  enterogastrone, 104
  estrogen, 530
  follicle-stimulating (FSH), 273, 274
  GnRH, 273
  luteinizing, 273
  thyroid, 52–53, 55–57
Horner's histamine cephalgia, 339
Horner's syndrome, 583, 921
  and sweating, 43
Hospitalizations
  history of, 456–457
  for psychiatric problems, 413–415
Howell-Jolly bodies, 1023
Hums
  abdominal venous, 766, 767, 768
  cervical venous, 614–616, 766
  venous, 549
Hunger, and weight gain, 35
Hydroceles, 780
Hymenectomy, 313
Hypalgesia, 943
Hyperalgesia, 943
Hyperalimentation, 482
Hyperbilirubinemia (see Jaundice)
Hypercalcemia, 1097–1098
  and EKG, 1160
  and pancreatitis, 145
Hypercalciuria, 232–233
Hypercapnia, 153
Hyperchloremia, 1062–1064
Hypercholesterolemia, 1108
Hyperesthesia, 942
Hyperimmune globulin to hepatitis B
    (HBIG), 448
Hyperinflation, detection of, 640
Hyperkalemia, 1060–1061
  arrhythmias associated with, 1158–1159
Hyperkinetic pulse, 665–666, 672
Hyperlipoproteinemia, 1106
  and pancreatitis, 145

Hypermagnesemia, 1160
Hypermenorrhea, 272
Hyperosmia, 880
Hyperparathyroidism, and pancreatitis, 145
Hyperpigmentation, 329
Hyperreflexia, 984
Hypersomnias, 378, 379, 380
Hypersplenism, 775
Hypertension
  borderline, 520 (See also Blood pressure)
  history for, 203–205
  physiology of, 516–519
  portal vein, 766
  pulmonary, 691
  stroke associated with, 374
Hyperthyroidism, 53, 57, 620
  and cervical venous hums, 616
Hypertonia, 956
Hypertrophic osteoarthropathy, 731
Hypertrophy, 956
  left ventricular, 1142
  prostatic, 791
Hyperuricemia, 1087–1088
Hyperventilation, central neurogenic, 846
Hyperventilation syndrome, 49, 198–199
Hypervitaminosis-A, 482
Hypesthesia, 942
Hypnosis, 420
Hypnotics, questioning about, 437–440
Hypoalbuminemia, 764, 1114
Hypobetalipoproteinemia, 1109
Hypocalcemia, 1098–1099
  and EKG, 1159
Hypocholeremia, 1064
Hypogeusia, 923
Hypoglossal nerve, 941–942
Hypoglycemia, 199, 1051
Hypokalemia, 1059–1061, 1157–1158
Hypokinetic pulse, 665
Hypomagnesemia, 1160
Hypomenorrhea, 272
Hypoosmia, 880
Hyporeflexia, 983
Hypospadias, 780
Hypotension, orthostatic, 195
Hypothalmic disease, 58
Hypothyroidism, 53, 57, 531, 620
Hypotonia, 956, 969
Hypouricemia, 1088
Hypovolemia, 655
Hypoxanthine-guanine phosphoribosyl transferase (HG-PRTase), 1086
Hypoxemia, 153
  and arrhythmias, 1160

Ichthyosis, 540
Icterus, 120 (See also Jaundice)
Idiopathic hypertrophic subaortic stenosis (IHSS), 668, 702, 713
Idioventricular rhythm, and EKG, 1147
Ileus, paralytic, 754–755
Illusions, examining for, 828–831

Immune Serum Globulin (ISG), 448
Immunizations, 445–449
Immunizing agents, 447
Immunoglobulin (IG), 448
Impotence, 246
  causes of, 248, 301–302
  and ejaculatory incompetence, 297
  history for, 299–302
  medications associated with, 300
  primary, 299
  questioning about, 278, 299–300
  secondary, 299, 301–302
Impulse
  apex, 669–676
  parasternal, 677–679
  visual, 859
  xiphisternal, 678
Inclusion bodies, 1025–1026
Income, median household, 849
Incontinence, urinary
  history for, 234–237
  overflow, 235–236
  "stress," 235–236
  total, 236
Index
  cardiac, 517
  Quetelet, 523–524
  resistance, 517–519
Indigestion, history for, 102–105
Infarction
  cerebral, 39
  lacunar, 374
  myocardial, 189–190, 664, 1128, 1148, 1150
  pulmonary, 159
  renal, 226
Infection
  Borrelia, 40, 241
  and fever, 38–39, 40
  fungal, 534, 546
  gonorrheal, 264
  renal, 226
  respiratory, 170–172
  sinus, 80
  Staphlococcus aureus, 224
  streptococcal, 206, 210
  urinary tract, 223–225
  vaginal, 263
  and WBC, 1015
Infectious mononucleosis, lymphadeno-pathy associated with, 626
Inflammation
  of joints, 404, 405
  renal, 226
  synovial, 409 (See also Edema)
Influenza, immunizations for, 447
Inguinal canal, examination of, 776–779
Inguinal hernia, 134–135
Inguinal nodes, 622
Inhalation, environmental, 175–178
Inheritance
  of abnormal bleeding, 386–387, 389
  and cardiovascular disease, 214–219
  of disease, 450–455

Mendelian patterns of, 453, 454
and metabolic problems, 359
of musculoskeletal disease, 410–412
of renal disease, 250–252 (See also Family history)
Initial Plans, in medical records, 9, 11, 15, 18, 1188, 1191
Injury (see Trauma)
Insect bites, 326
Insomnias, 378 379, 381, 382
Inspiration, examination of, 632, 633–634
Insurance, national health, 491
Intellectual function, testing, 817–819
Intercourse, sexual, 287–290
bleeding with, 269, 271, 385
frequency of, 287–290
pain with, 310–314
Interfacial synkinesis, 926–927
Intermittency, 234–237
Interpersonal relationships, 416–422
Interview
initial, 28
physician-patient, 28–31
Intolerance
fatty food, 141
lactose, 118, 485
Intoxication
arsenic, 547
barbiturate, 899
dilantin, 899 (See also Alcoholism)
Intraocular pressure, 565, 567
in detecting glaucoma, 568
Intrauterine devices (IUD's), 255 (See also Fertility control)
Intravenous pyelogram (IVP), 1177, 1178, 1182
Iodides, and thyroid disease, 58
Iopanoic acid, 1087
IQ test, 818–819
Iron deficiency, 99, 395, 597
Irradiation
to the neck, 59–61
and thyroid cancer, 59 (See also Radiation therapy)
Ischemia
headache associated with, 338
myocardial, 189–190
Isoenzymes, 1078–1079
Itching, history for, 325–327

Jacksonian march, 343
Jaffe reaction, 1090
Jaundice, 147–148
and bilirubin metabolism, 1082–1084
causes of, 122
cholestatic, 122
hepatocellular, 122
history for, 119–123
testing for, 1081–1082
Jaw jerk, 916, 985, 991
Jaws, examination of, 592–593
"Jelling," 402
Jendrassik maneuver, 985, 987

Joint
edema of, 402
effusion, 407–408
examination of, 798–799
pain, 403–406
position sense, 945
stiffness in, 401–403
swelling of, 406–410 (See also Musculoskeletal system, examination of)
Jones criteria, for rheumatic fever, 206–207, 210
Joule, 480
Judgement, examination of, 822–825
Jugular venous pressure, examination of, 653–655
Jugular venous pulsations, examination of, 656–662
Juvenile forms of white cells, 1016

Kassowitz' law, 242
Keratoses, 329, 330
Ketoacidemia, 412
Ketoacidosis, 1038
Ketogenesis, 150
Ketone bodies, in urine, 1036–1038
Ketonuria, 1035–1039
Ketostix, 1036
Kidney
pain associated with, 115
polycystic disease, 251–252 (See also Renal disease)
Kiesselbach's triangle, 77
Kilocalories, 480
Kilograms, 522
Knee
drawer sign of, 806
examination of, 804–806
Knee jerk, 986–987, 991
Koch-Weser formula, 520
Koilonychia, 544
Korotkoff sound, 515, 516, 736
Korsakoff's psychosis, 840
Korsakoff's syndrome
amnesiac, 843
confabulation associated with, 821
related to mental illness, 420 (See also Wernicke-Korsakoff syndrome)
Kussmaul breathing, 502
Kyphosis, 802

Labia majora, 782
Labia minora, 782
La belle indifference, 815
Lability of affect, 815
Laboratory tests, introduction to, 1004–1010 (See also specific tests)
Labstix, for urine tests, 1036
Lacrimal glands, 567
Lactase deficiency, 485
Lactate dehydrogenase (LDH), 1073–1076
Lactation, 320 (See also Breast)
Lactic acid, 1086

Lacunar infarction, 374
Language, and brain, 863
Laparotomy, 41, 795
Laryngitis, 78
Lateral medullary syndrome, and dizziness, 50
Laurence-Moon-Biedl-Bardet syndrome, 218
Lawrence's sign, 727
Laxatives, diarrhea associated with, 128
Lean body mass, 523
Learning, of clinical methods, 13–20
Leatham's classification, of murmur, 711
Lentigo, 330
Lentigo malignant melanoma, 331
Leptospira, 241
Le Riche syndrome, 248
Lesions
    auditory nerve, 74
    brainstem, 953, 966–967
    breast, 641, 649–651
    cardiac, 208–209
    coin, 169
    facial nerve, 927–928
    lip, 592
    male genital, 243–244
    malignant, growth of, 169
    of motor system, 966–967
    of mouth, 594
    muscle, 967
    perineal, 264
    precancerous, 594
    skin, 539–540
    spinal cord, 967
    temporal lobe, 88
    thalamic, 953
    of trigeminal nerve, 921, 922
    valvular, 209 (*See also* Cancer, Mass, Tumor)
Lethargy, 844
Leukemia
    chronic lymphocytic, 1019
    joint swelling associated with, 409
    myelocytic, 1019
    and WBC, 1015
Leukocytopenia, 1016
Leukocytosis, 1015
Leukopenia, 1015
Leukoplakia, 594
Leydig cell hyperplasia, 531
Libido, 293, 300
Lifestyle, history of, 472–476
Lindsay's nails, 542
Lipidosis, glycolipid, 251
Lipolysis, 1037
Lipoproteins, 1105, 1107, 1109
Lips
    cancer of, 594
    examination of, 592
Liver
    auscultation of, 766–768
    size and shape of, 769–771
    on x-ray, 1167
"Logorrhea," 870

Long-acting thyroid stimulator (LATS), 57–58
Loss of control, 430–433
Loudness, measurement of, 69
Lowenburg cuff test, 727
LRI (*see* Infection, respiratory)
Lumbar spine, 802–803
Lung abscess, and night sweats, 43
Lung disease, dyspnea associated with, 154
Lungs
    scan, 1171
    on x-ray, 1167, 1172–1173
Lunula, 542
Lupus erythematosus, systemic
    and thrombophlebitis, 729
Luteinizing hormone (LH), 273
Lymphadenopathy, 621–628
Lymphangiectasia, 765
Lymphocytes, 1016
Lymphocytopenia, 1019
Lymphocytosis, 1019
Lymph nodes
    cervical, 609
    examination of, 621–628
Lymphomas
    and LDH levels, 1075–1076
    LRI associated with, 171

Macrocytosis, 1025
Macroglossia, 598
Macula, examination of, 573
Malabsorption syndrome
    cause of, 129–130
    diarrhea caused by, 127
Males
    genitalia, examination of, 779–781
    ideal body weight for, 521
    sexual history of, 276–302
Malignancy, occult, and thrombophlebitis, 729
Mallory-Weiss syndrome, 94
Malnutrition, 482
    definition of, 477
    protein-energy, 524, 526–527
    associated with weight loss, 34
Mandible, deviation of, 594
Marasmus, 524, 526
Marcus-Gunn pupillary sign, 578, 579
Marfan's syndrome, 707
MARI (*see* Medical Aggregate Record Inquiry system)
Marital coitus, 288–289
Masses
    abdominal, 759–760, 761–762
    breast, 641
    groin, 776–777
    pelvic, 275–276
    scrotal, 779, 780–781
    testicular, 245–246
Mastication, muscles of, 590–591
Masturbation, history of, 290–293
Maxillary sinus, 560, 561, 562
McArdle's disease, 363

Measles
  German, 626 (See also Rubella)
  immunization for, 447
Mediastinum
  masses of, 1175
  on x-ray, 1174–1175
Medical Aggregate Record Inquiry
  system (MARI), 1183–1197
Medical records
  computerized, 1103–1197
  data base for, 5–12, 15, 16–17, 18, 19, 20
  history, 26–27
  problem-oriented (POMR), 4–12
  source-oriented, 4
Medications
  and emotional problems, 415
  history for use, 457–465
  questioning about, 457–458
Medullary thyroid carcinoma, 58
Medullary cystic disease, 251
Mees' lines, 542–543, 547
Mefenamic acid, 1087
Megacolon, 117, 133
Megaloblastic crisis, 399
Mclanomas, 329, 331, 332
Melena
  history of, 97–99
  ulcers associated with, 140
Memory, examination of, 837, 844 (See
  also Mental status)
Menarche, 272, 273
Mendelian traits, 453, 454
Meniere's disease, 88
  tinnitus associated with, 74, 75
  vertigo with, 50
Meningitis, 70
Meningococcal vaccine, 446
Menopause, 272
  breast changes during, 649, 652
  endocrine control of, 274
  and nipple discharge, 320
Menorrhagia, 272
Menstruation, 258, 262, 271
  abnormal, 274
  and breast pain, 316–317
  changes in, 260–261
  characteristics of, 272–273
  and emotional disorders, 434–435
  endocrine control of, 273–274
  excess, 271
  history of, 269–274
  normal, 273–274
  painful, 260–262
  pelvic examination during, 787
Mental illness, etiologies of, 419–421
Mental status, examination of, 810–843
MET, 179
Metabolism changes, 52
Methadone, 439
Methemoglobinemia, 734
Metrorrhagia, 272
Microhemagglutination-Treponema Pallidum Test, 1119
Midbrain, herniation of, 851

Migraine headache, 338, 339, 348, 842
  cluster, 339
Mitral regurgitation, rheumatic, 714–715
Mitral stenosis
  and first heart sound, 686–687
  and pulmonary artery pulsation, 680
  murmur of, 720
Mitral valve prolapse, 707, 713
  and chest pain, 190
Mole, change in, 327–332
Monday asthma, 177
Monocytes, 1016
Monocytosis, 1019
Mononeuropathy, 952–953
Mononucleosis, infectious, 626
Monoplegia, 955
Morphine, questioning about, 437–440
Moses' test, 727
Motor behavior, 812, 815, 816
Motor examination, screening, 961
Motor function, abstract, 960
Motor performance, of patient, 858
Motor persistence, 866
Mouth (See specific structure)
Movements, involuntary, 975–980
Mucopolysaccharides, 218, 219
Mucosa
  buccal, 586–587
  oral, 585–596
Muehrcke's lines, 543
Multifactorial disorders, 454
Multiple sclerosis
  and vertigo, 88
Mumps, immunization for, 447
Murmurs, heart, 214
  Carey-Coombs, 209
  classification of, 711
  diastolic, 719–722
  examination for, 708–722
  holosystolic, 711, 713–714
  innocent, 712
  midsystolic, 712
  organic, 708
  Still's, 712
  systolic, 708–718
Muscles
  accessory in respiration, 502, 503
  contraction of, 956
  cramps in, 362–369
  examination of, 797–798
  lesions of, 967
  of mastication, 590–591
  pain in, 200–203
  sternocleidomastoid, 938–940
  strength of, 955–956
  tone of, 956, 957–958
  trapezius, 938–940
  volume, 956
Muscular dystrophy, 171, 217
Musculoskeletal system
  common problems of, 808
  examination of, 796–809
  hereditary diseases of, 410–412
Myasthenia, 357

Myasthenia gravis, 171
Myelocytes, 1019
Myeloma, 171, 408
Myocardial disease, 208–209
 familial, 217
Myocardial infarction, 189–190, 664, 1128, 1148, 1150
Myoclonus, examining for, 976, 978, 979–980
Myomata, uterine, 274, 276
Myoneural junction, lesions of, 967
Myopathy
 ocular, 217
 weakness associated with, 357

Nail matrix, 541
Nail-patella syndrome, 251
Nails
 clubbing of, 544
 examination of, 541–548
 half-and-half, 542
 Lindsay's, 542
 postmetabolic changes of, 546–547
 shell, 546
 spoon, 544
 Terry's, 542
 yellow, 546
Narcolepsy-cataplexy syndrome, 379
Narcotics, 439
Nasal bleeding, 386, 388
Nasal septum, 560
Nasopharynx, 599
Nausea
 flank pain associated with, 226
 history for, 89–91
 pancreatitis associated with, 144
 and vomiting, 91–94
Neck
 basal cell epithelioma of, 335
 examination of, 609–612
 irradiation to, 59–61
 lymph nodes in, 603, 623
 surgery, history of, 59–61
 tremors of, 977
Nelson test, 1119
Neoplasm
 and fever, 38
 thyroid, 620
Nephritis, 250
Nephrosclerosis, 205
Nerve
 chorda tympani, 925
 cranial (see Cranial nerves)
 intermediate, 925
Nervous tension
 and indigestion, 103, 105
 questioning about, 413–414
Neuralgia
 postherpetic, 354
 trigeminal, 355
Neurological symptoms, episodic, 348–350
Neuroma, acoustic, 72–74

Neuropathy
 peripheral, 952–953, 990
 retrobulbar, 151
 and weakness, 357, 359
Neurosis, 823–824
Neutropenia, 1016, 1018–1019
Neutrophilia, 1018
Neutrophils, 1016, 1017–1018
Nevus, 327
 cells, 328, 329
 pigmented, 330
Nicking, arteriovenous, 574, 575
Nicotine adenine dinucleotide phosphate (NADH), 1073–1076
Night cramps, 200–201
Nightmares, 382–383
Night sweats, 41–44
Night terrors, 379, 384
Nipple
 discharge from, 319–321
 examination of, 651–653
Nocturia, 227–228
 differential diagnosis of, 226
Nodes
 axillary, 626, 650
 enlarged, examining for, 622
 epitrochlear, 622
 femoral, 622
 inguinal, 622
 lymph, 623
 popliteal, 622
 supraclavicular, 651
Nodules
 rheumatoid, 409
 subcutaneous, 208
Noise exposure, tinnitus associated with, 74
nonrapid eye movement sleep, 383, 384
Noonan's syndrome, 218
Normocardias, 1147 (See also Arrhythmia)
Nose
 discharge from, 82, 83
 epistaxis, 76–78
 examination of, 558–562
 obstruction of, 82, 83
 physiology of, 82, 83
Nutrition
 definition of, 477
 history, 477–486
 inadequte, and weight loss, 36
Nystagmus, 66, 905, 969
 opticokinetic, 900

Obesity, 482, 485
 childhood, 524
 dietary counseling for, 526
 history for, 35–36
 organic causes of, 525–526
 vs. overweight, 523
 risks of, 525
 sociological consequences of, 525
Occlusion, 595

Occupation
  and inhalational exposure, 175–176
  and patient profile, 468–471
Ocular flutter, 904
Oculomotor nerve, examination of, 897–914
Odynophagia, 101
Olfactory nerve, examination of, 878–881
Olfactory hallucinations, 881
Oligomenorrhea, 272, 274
Onanism (see Masturbation)
Onychogryphosis, 546
Onycholysis, 544
Onychomycosis, 546
Ophthalmoscope, 571–573
Opioids, 437–440
Optic atrophy, 573
Optic disc
  cup, 573
  examination of, 572
Optic nerve, examination of, 882–896
Oral cavity
  cancer of, 587, 588, 593, 594, 603
  examination of, 585–596
Oral contraceptives, 256–258, 483
Oral mucosa, examination of, 585–596
Orbital bruits, 548–552
Orgasm
  male, 307–308
  and masturbation, 290–293
  and premature ejaculation, 294, 296
  in women, 307–309
Orientation, examination for, 834–836
Orthopnea
  dyspnea associated with, 154
  history for, 182–185
  mechanisms for, 183–184
Orthostatic hypotension, 195
Osler, Sir William, 13, 241, 500, 592
Osler-Weber-Rendu disease, 78
Osmolality, urine, 1030–1032
Ossicular chain, 556
Osteoarthritis, 402–403, 409
Osteoarthropathy, hypertrophic, 731–732
Osteogenesis imperfecta, 66, 218, 219
Osteomyelitis
  sickle cell disease associated with, 400
  sinus complications of, 83
Osteoonychodystrophy, hereditary
  (HOOD), 251
Otoscope, 554
Ovalocytes, 1025
Ovarian carcinoma, 261
"Overbite," 590
"Overjet," 590
Overweight vs. obesity, 523
Owane's sign, 727
Oxalates, in urine sediment, 1042
Oxygen, maximal consumption of, 179

Pachydermoperiostosis, 731
Pack-years, cigarettes, 173
Paget's disease, 653, 666, 1079

Pain, 351–356
  abdominal, 109–115, 143, 756–759, 760–761
  of angina pectoris, 187, 188–189
  associated with muscle contraction, 362–369
  associated with sickle cell disease, 399
  in breast, 316–319
  chest, 185–191
  claudication, 200–203
  CVA, 225–227
  with exercise, 200–203
  expression of, 798
  in eye, 65
  facial, 80
  flank, 225–227
  gallbladder, 114, 141
  groin, 776–778
  growing, 210
  head, 336–340
  with intercourse, 310–314
  in joints, 403–406
  kidney, 115
  menstrual, 261–262
  in muscles, 200–203
  pancreatic, 114
  pelvic, 260–262
  of peptic ulcer, 139
  periodontal, 592
  periumbilical, 115
  sensation, 943, 944, 948–950
  sinus, 81–82
  somatic, 110–111
  spleen, 115
  while swallowing, 101
  testicular, 245–246
  on urination, 220–221, 222
  visceral, 110
Pallor, 119–120, 1012
Palpation
  of abdomen, 756–762
  bimanual, 783–784
  of carotid pulse, 663
  of scrotum, 779–780
  of spleen, 772–773, 775
  of thyroid, 617–619
  of uterus, 783–784
Palpebral fissures, 848
Palpitations, 192–193
  causes of, 193
  mechanisms of, 192
Palsy
  facial, 926
  pseudobulbar, 937, 941
Pancreatitis, 761
  and alcohol intake, 151
  causes of, 145
  associated with gallstones, 145
  history of, 143
  pain with, 114
  pathophysiology of, 144–145
  vomiting associated with, 93
Papillae, on tongue, 597
Papilledema, 574, 575–576

Papillomatosis, 650
Pap smear, 783, 787
Paralysis, 955
    facial, 926, 927
    of masticatory muscles, 915–916
    postictal, 342
    stroke associated with, 370
    Todd's, 342
    of vocal cords, 937
Paralytic ileus, 754–755
Paranasal sinuses, 81–82
Paranoia, 431
Paraphasia, 870, 874
Paraplegia, 955
Parasternal impulse, 677–679
Parathyroid adenomas, 58, 61
Parathyroid hormone, 1095–1096
Parenchymal disease, 1042
Paresis, 955
Paresthesia, 351, 354, 943
Parinaud's syndrome, 582
Parkinson's disease, gait of, 966
Parotid enlargement, 605–609
    associated with alcoholism, 608
    associated with diabetes, 608
    detection of, 605
    and facial appearance, 606, 607
Paroxysmal nocturnal dyspnea (PND),
    182–185
Patient education, 487–488
Patient presentation, 21–24
Patients
    dietary history of, 477–486
    education of, 486–488
    finances of, 488–493
    hobbies of, 474–476
    occupation of, 468–471
    physician's interview with, 28–31
    profile of, 468–493
    usual day activities, 472–474
Pediatrics examination, 997–1001
Pedigree, family, 450, 451, 452, 453, 455
Pellagra, 597, 990
Pelvic disease, 262
    inflammatory (PID), 261, 262, 268, 274,
    313
Pelvic examination, 781–787
Pelvic mass, 275–276
Pelvic pain, 260–262
Pendred's syndrome, 55
Penicillin
    allergic reaction to, 442–443
    prolonged use of, 598
Penile erection, 247
Peptic ulcer disease
    history for, 138–140
    operations for, 147
    pain with, 139
    symptoms of, 114
Percussion
    of chest, 639–641
    of muscles, 958
    of spleen, 773–774
Percussion myoedema, 956
Percussion myotonia, 956

Periarteritis, and syphilis, 242
Pericarditis
    and chest pain, 189–190
    constrictive, 660, 661, 662, 665, 691, 699
Perineal body, 782
Periodontal disease, 595
Peripheral circulatory failure, 195–196
Peripheral neuropathy, 952–953, 990
Peripheral pulses, 740–748
Peripheral vestibular disorders, 48
    and dizziness, 50
Peristalsis, 754
Peritoneum and abdominal pain, 112–113
Periumbilical pain, 115
Permeability index (PI), 1034–1035
Pertussis, immunization for, 447
Perversions, sensory, 351–356
Petit mal seizures, 346
Peutz-Jegher's syndrome, 546
Peyronie's disease, 780
Phantom pain, 354
Pharmacists, 459
Pharynx, examination of, 599–604
Phenothiazines, 1154
Pheochromocytomas, 58
    sweating associated with, 43
Phimosis, 780
Phonation, 854, 855
Phosphate
    in serum 1100–1103
    in urine sediment, 1042
Photosensitivity, 539
Physical activity (see Exercise level)
Physical examination
    equipment for performing, 496
    example sequence, 497
    introduction to, 496–499
    style for, 498
Physician-patient relationship, 28–31
    and pediatric patient, 997
Piaget, Jean, 819
Pica, 393–396
Pickwickian syndrome, 525
Pigmentation
    changes in, 328
    normal, 328 (See also Skin)
Piles, 136, 137
Pinguecula, 569
Pinnae, examination of, 552, 556
Pituitary disease, 57, 58
Plantar reflex, examination of, 992–996
Plaque, 594
Plasma glucose, 1048–1053
Plasma lipid levels, in blood, 1104
Platelets, 1020–1022
Plegia, 955
Pleura, on x-ray, 1167
PND (see Paroxysmal Nocturnal
    Dyspnea)
Pneumococcal vaccine, 446
Pneumonia
    bacterial, 171, 172
    history for, 170–172
    Klebsiella, 157
    mycoplasma, 40, 172

necrotizing, 159
recurrent, 172
sickle cell disease associated with, 400
viral, 172, 241
Pneumonitides, hypersensitivity, 177
Pneumothorax, 640, 676
Pohl's sign, 534
Poikilocytes, 1025
Poiseuille's law, 517
Poisoning
arsenic, 547
lead, 1025–1026
and level of consciousness, 850
mercury, 978
Poliomyelitis vaccine, 447
Polyarthritis, and rheumatic fever, 207, 209–210
Polyneuropathy, 953
Polyps, rectal, 124
POMR (see Problem-Oriented Medical Record)
Pontine paramedian reticular formation (PPRF), 903
Popliteal artery, pulse of, 744
Popliteal nodes, 622
Posterior tibial artery, pulse of, 744
Postnasal drip, 80, 104
Postural reflexes, 848
Potassium, in serum, 1058–1062
Poverty, definition of, 489
PPD Tuberculin Skin Test, 166–168, 1115–1117
P-Q interval, EKG, 1123–1124
Precordial leads, placement of, 1126
Pregnancy
breast changes during, 649, 652
diabetes during, 1050
hemorrhoids associated with, 137
pickle pica of, 395
risks of, 258
toxemic, 205
and UTI, 224
vomiting associated with, 93
Premature ejaculation, 294–297, 302
Present illness, in medical record, 28–32
P-R interval, EKG, 1123–1124
Problem-Oriented Medical Record (POMR), 4–12
Procainamide, 1152
Proctitis, gonorrheal, 124
"Profile sign," clubbing, 730
Progesterone injections, 257
Progress notes, in medical records, 9, 11, 15, 18
Projection, 423
Prolapse, of mitral valve, 707, 713
Propranolol, 665, 1152, 1154
Proprioceptive sensation, 943, 945–947, 948–952
Propylsulfamy benzoic acid, 1087
Prostatitis, 221, 791
Prostate
cancer of, 791–792
examination of, 790–792
hypertrophy of, 791

nodules in, 791
Protein, serum total, 1111–1115
Proteinuria, 1033–1035
Proverbs, in mental status examination, 826–827
Pruritis, 325–327
Pseudocysts, 145, 761
Pseudohypertrophy, 956
Pseudoinsomnia, 382
Psoriasis
and nails, 545
Psychiatric disorders
and dizziness, 46
history for, 413–415
and vegetative function, 433–436
Psychiatric examination (see Mental status examination)
Psychogenic disorders, and vertigo, 85
Psychosis
and homocidal tendency, 431
and judgement, 823–825
Korsakoff's, 840
organic, 830
and suicide, 429
Pterygium, 569
Puberty
and body habitus, 530–531
breast development during, 649
and clubbing, 732
Pulmonary artery pulsation, 679–680
Pulmonary edema, and PND, 183, 184
Pulmonary embolism, and thrombophlebitis, 729
Pulmonary embolus, and chest pain, 190
Pulmonary hypertension, chest pain related to, 190–191
Pulmonary vasculature, on x-ray, 1167, 1172–1173
Pulsation
jugular venous, 656–662
pulmonary artery, 679–680
Pulse
amplitude, 507
deficit, 507
rate and rhythm, 507–513
Pulses
brachial, 741–742
carotid, 663–668, 741
diminished, 747
dorsalis pedis, 744–745
femoral artery, 743–744
intensity of, 745–746
peripheral, 740–748
popliteal artery, 744
posterior tibial, 744
radial, 742
"water-hammer," 747
Pulsus alternans, 510, 735–740
Pulsus paradoxus, 512, 516
"Pulsus parvus et tardus," 666–667
Pupils, 567–568
Argylle–Robertson, 582
dilating, 571
examination of, 577–584
Marcus–Gunn, 578–579

Pupils (*continued*)
  tests for function, 578
  tonic, 582
Pursuit movements, of eye, 897–898, 901
P wave, 1122, 1149, 1152
Pyelography (*see* Intravenous pyelogram)
Pyloric muscle, 105
Pylorospasm, 105
Pyorrhea, 595
Pyranzinoic acid, 1087
Pyuria, 1041, 1043

QRS complex, 1122–1124
QRS vector, 1126
Quadraplegia, 956
Questionnaire
  dizziness, 85
  for vertigo, 87
Questions, during patient interviews, 28–32
Quetelet index, 523–524
Quinidine, dysrhythmia associated with, 1151–1152
"Quinidine syncope," 1151–1152
Q wave, 1122–1124, 1127

Rabies, immunizing for, 447
Radial artery pulse, 742
Radiation exposure, of chest x-rays, 1168–1171
Radiation therapy, history of, 59–61
Radiography
  abdomen, 1176–1182
  chest, 168–169, 640, 1162–1176
Rales, 638
Range of motion
  of digits, 799
  of hip, 806–807
  of radiohumeral joints, 800
  of shoulder, 800
  for TM joint, 801
  of toes, 804
  of wrists, 799–800
Rapid eye movement sleep, 383
Rapid Plasma Reagin Test, 1119
Rash
  history for, (*see* Dermatological history)
  and rheumatic fever, 207–208, 210 (*See also* Skin)
Rationalization, 423
Raynaud's phenomenon, 734, 747
Reaction formation, 423
Recreation, questioning about, 474–476
Rectum
  bleeding from, 123–125
  examination of, 788–790
  pain in, 115
  villous adenomas of, 129
Red blood cells
  hematocrit test for, 1011–1013
  morphology of, 1022–1026
  in urine, 1041–1044

Red lens diplopia test, 908–910
Red light test, 578
Reed's syndrome, 707
Reflex
  Babinski, 992, 993
  biceps, 986, 991
  branchioradialis, 986, 991
  corneal, 916–917, 925
  deep tendon, 983–992
  gag, 935
  grasp, 981–982
  plantar, 992–996
  snout, 981–982
  stretch, 987, 990
  suck, 981–982
  triceps, 986, 991
Reflex hammer, Babinski, 985
Reflux esophagitis, 106–108
Refractive index, in urinalysis, 1030–1032
"Refractory period," in males, 289, 293, 298
Refsum's disease, 217
Regurgitation
  aortic, 666, 667, 721
  mitral, 665, 674, 679, 699
  pulmonic, 691, 721
  rheumatic mitral, 714–715
  tricuspid, 660, 661, 715
Relationships
  interpersonal, 416–422
  physician-patient, 28–31
  religious, 418–419
  social, 418
"Relative bradycardia," 40
Renal colic, 226, 232
Renal disease
  causes, related to family history, 252
  hereditary, 250–252
  and serum creatinine level, 1091–1092
  vomiting associated with, 93
Renal function, testing, 1046–1047
Renal infarction, 226
Renal infection, 226
Renal tubular acidosis (RTA), 251
Repression, 423
Residential history, and inhalational exposure, 176
Respiration, rate and rhythm of, 502–506
Respiratory patterns, and level of consciousness, 846
Retching
  history of, 89–91
  and vomiting, 92
Retina
  diseases of, 65
  hemorrhage, 576
  vessels, 572–573
Retraction phenomena, of breast, 650
Retrocochlear lesions, 68–69
Retroperitoneal area, and abdominal pain, 113
Rheumatic fever
  history for, 206–211

hospitalization associated with, 457
Rheumatoid diseases, genetic transmission of, 411
Rheumatoid nodules, 409
Rhinitis, 83
Rhinorrhea, 81 (See also Nose)
Rhonchi, 638
Ribs, on x-ray, 1175
Right-left orientation, 857
Rigidity, cogwheel, 956
Riley-Day syndrome, and sweating, 43
Rinne test, 72, 930–934
Romberg test, 945
Rotatory sensations, 50 (See also Dizziness, Vertigo)
Roth spot, 576
Rubella
    immunization for, 446
    lymphadenopathy associated with, 626
    maternal, 215
Rubs
    abdominal, 753–755
    hepatic friction, 766, 767, 768
    pericardial, 717
Rumbles, 722
R wave, 1122–1124

Saccadic movements, of eye, 901–912
Sacroiliac joints, examination of, 803
St. Vitus' dance, 210
Salivary glands, 605, 609
    tumors of, 608
Salmonella
    diarrhea caused by, 128
    sickle cell disease associated with, 400
Scabies, 326
Scalar electrocardiogram, 1122, 1132
Scars
    burn, 334
    facial, 501
    incisional, 749
Schatzki ring, 101
Schistocytes, 1025
Schizophrenia, 831–833
Sclerae, yellow, 501
Scleroderma, and dysphagia, 101
Scoliosis, 802
Scrotum
    examination of, 779–781
    masses in, 779, 780–781
    palpation of, 779–780
Seborrheic keratosis, 330
Sedatives, questioning about, 437–440
Sediment, urine, 1040–1044
Seizures, 340, 350
    aura ictus, 341
    centrencephalic, 342–343
    epileptic, 340–349
    focal, 341, 342, 344
    generalized, 345, 346
    grand mal, 341–342
    international classification of, 345–346
    partial, 345

petit mal, 346
posttraumatic, 361
Seminal vesicles, 791
Senile dementia, 842
Sensation, examination of, 942
Sensorineural hearing loss, 68–69, 70
Sensory extinction, 943, 947
Sensory perversions, 351–356
Septal defect
    atrial, 661, 678, 691, 693
    ventricular, 665, 678, 693, 715
Septicemia, 227
    and thrombophlebitis, 729
Serologic test for syphilis, 1118–1121
Serology, positive, 240
Serum acid phosphatase, 792
Serum alkaline phosphotase, 1077–1081
Serum bilirubin, 1081–1084
Serum calcium, 1093–1100
Serum chloride, 1062–1065
Serum cholesterol, 1104–1110
Serum creatine phosphokinase, 1072
Serum creatinine, 1089–1093
Serum glutamate-oxaloacetate transaminase (SGOT), 1070–1072
Serum inorganic phosphate, 1100–1103
Serum lactate dehydrogenase, 1073–1076
Serum potassium, 1005, 1058–1062
Serum sodium, 1005, 1054–1058
Serum total CO_2 content, 1005, 1065–1070
Serum total protein, 1111–1115
Sexual history, 276–287
Sexual intercourse
    associated with psychological disturbances, 436
    and UTI, 224
Sexual relationships, 419
Sexual words, 278–280
Shift cells, 1025
Shigella, diarrhea caused by, 128
"Shin splints," 210
Shocks, 95
Shortness of breath
    history of, 152–154
    associated with physical exertion, 179
    in recumbent position, 182–185
Shoulder, examination of, 800
Sickle cell disease
    crisis of, 399
    family history of, 396–400
    and hematuria, 231
    pathophysiology of, 397–398
Sinus arrhythmia, 508
Sinus bradycardia, 508–509, 511, 512, 1152
Sinus dysrhythmia, and EKG, 1147
Sinus exit block, 1152
Sinus pause, 1152
Sinus rhythm, normal, 510
Sinus tachycardia, 509, 511, 512
Sinuses
    diseases of, 82–84
    paranasal, 81–82
    sinusitis, 80–84
    transillumination of, 560

Skin
  and breast mass, 650
  cancer of, 332–335
  cyanosis of, 733–735
  disease, prevalence of, 540
  examination of, 536–540
  lesions, 330–331, 539–540
  pigmentary changes in, 328
  turgor, 538
Skinfold thickness, 524
Sleep
  apnea, 378, 379, 381
  associated with psychological distur-
    bances, 435
  disorders, 378–385
  paralysis, 380
Sleepwalking, 382
SMA laboratory system, 1006, 1045–1046,
  1062–1063, 1066
Smallpox, immunization for, 447
Smoking
  and cancer, 174
  and heart disease, 213
  hemoptysis associated with, 160
  history for, 173–175
Snellen chart, 563
Snout reflex, 981–982
Social relationships, 418
Sodium, in serum, 1054–1058
Sodium restriction, dietary, 484
Soft tissues, on x-ray, 1175
Somatic pain, 110–111
Somnambulism, 379, 382
Somnolence syndrome, 525
Sound, measurement of, 69
Spasm
  bronchospasm, 184, 441
  esophageal, 99
  visceral, 112
Spatial orientation, 865
Speculum
  for ear examination, 553–555
  for nasal examination, 559
  for pelvic examination, 783
Speech, 970
  audible spectrum of, 69
  examination of, 854
Spermatoceles, 781
Sphenoid sinuses, 562
Spherocytes, 1025
Sphygmomanometer, 514
Spinal accessory nerve, examination of,
  938–940
Spine
  cervical, 801–802
  on chest x-ray, 1170
  lumbar, 802–803
  thoracic, 802–803
Spleen
  examination of, 772–775
  hypersplenism, 775
  pain associated with, 115
  on x-ray, 1167
Splenic percussion sign, 773–774

Splenomegaly, 761
  causes of, 775
Splinter hemorrhages, 545
"Split brains," testing of, 865
Spondylitis, ankylosing, 405
Sputum
  color of, 157–158
Squamous cell carcinoma, 332, 333, 334,
  335
S-T segment, EKG, 1123
Staphlococci, in GI infections, 126
Staphlococcus aureus infections, 224
Starling's Law, 724
Stature, 500 (*See also* Appearance)
Steatorrhea, 127, 129
Stein-Leventhal syndrome, 531
Stenosis
  aortic, 660, 665
  mitral, 720
  pulmonic, 660, 665, 691
  pyloric, 105
  tricuspid, 660, 661, 665
Stensen's duct, 600, 606
Stereagnosis, 943, 947
Sterilization, 257
Sternocleidomastoid muscle, 938–940
Steroids, 534
Stillbirth, 240, 242
Still's murmur, 712
Stimulants, questioning about, 437–440
Stimuli, graded, 847
Stippling, basophilic, 1023
Stoke-Adams syncope, 198
Stomach, carcinoma of, 98
Stomatitis, 598
Stomatocytes, 1022
Stones
  bilirubin, 142
  gallstones, 141–142
  history of, 231–233
  kidney, 250
  ureteral, 245
Stools
  black tarry, 97
  blood in, 123, 124, 793–795
  formation, of, 132
  guaiac test of, 793–795 (*See also* Diar-
    rhea)
Strabismus, 568
"Straight back syndrome," 630
Straight leg raising test, 803
Stress
  emotional (*see* Emotions)
  testing for, 181
  urinary incontinence, 235–236
Stretch reflex, 987, 990
Stroke, history of, 369–378
Stupor, 844
Stye, 569
Subarachnoid hemorrhage, 376
Subcutaneous nodules, and rheumatic
  fever, 208, 210
Sublingual space, 588, 594, 605
Submaxillary gland, 605

Substance abuse, 437–440
Suck reflex, 981–982
Suicide
and depression, 426, 427–429
prevention of, 426
questioning about, 427–429
Sulfhemoglobin, 734
Surface area, of body, 523
Surgery
bleeding associated with, 386, 389
gastrointestinal, 140–140
to the neck, 59–61
Swallowing
difficulty in, 99–192
mechanisms for, 100–101
and syncope, 197
S wave, 1123–1124
Sweat glands, 42, 652
Sweating, gustatory, 928
Swelling
abdominal, 116–119
in joints, 406–410
periarticular, 408
scrotal, 779, 780–781
Swimmer's ear, 557
Swinging light test, 578, 579
Sydenham's chorea, 210
Syncope, 348
associated with chest pain, 198
effort, 196
history for, 194–199
micturition, 196
"quinidine," 1151–1152
tussive, 196
vasodepresser, 195, 197
Synkinesis, interfacial, 926–927
Synovitis, 409, 805
Syphillis
Argylle Robertson pupil of, 582
associated with emotional state, 420
cardiovascular, 242
CNS, 242
congenital, 242–243
history for, 239–244
infectiousness of, 242
late complications of, 242
serologic test for, 240, 1118–1121
Systolic clicks, 190
Systolic hypertension, 520
Systolic pressure, definition of, 513

Tabes dorsalis, 953
Tachycardia, 703, 1148–1152
atrial, 509, 1148, 1149
bradycardia-tachycardia syndrome, 1151
definition of, 509
junctional, 509, 1147
ventricular, 1148, 1150, 1151
Tactile sensation, 942, 944, 952
Tamm-Horsfall protein, 1034
Tamponade
cardiac, 665
pericardial, 676

Tandem walking, 971
Tangier disease, 1109
Target cells, 1025
Taste, 934, 936
altered sensations of, 527
and facial nerve, 923, 924, 926, 927
Teaching clinical methods, 13–20
Teeth
abnormal, 589
examination of, 588–590
normal, 588
Telangiectasias
hemoptysis associated with, 160
hereditary hemorrhagic, 387
Telogen, 533
Temperature, body
control of, 52–53
recording of, 38–39
rectal, 42
sensation, 943, 944–945, 948–950
Temporal lobe, lesions of, 88, 841
Temporomandibular joint, 590–591, 801
Temporomandibular syndrome, 595
Tenderness, abdominal, 756–761 (See also Abdomen)
Tendons, physiology of, 987–990
Tenosynovitis, 408
Tension headaches, 339
Terry's nails, 542
Testes, undescended, 779
Testicle, examination of, 779–780
mass in, 245–246
pain in, 245–246
Tests
for abstract thought, 825–826
blood (See specific test)
caloric, 899
of conjugate gaze, 900
finger-nose-finger, 970
fluorescein string, 795
glucose tolerance (GTT), 1050–1052
hearing, 930–934
heel-knee, 971
heel-shin, 971
Homan's, 727
IQ, 818–819
laboratory, introduction to, 1004–1010
(See also specific tests)
Lowenburg cuff, 727
Moses', 727
of position sense, 945
for prostatitis, 791
psychological, 818
red lens diplopia, 908–910
red light, 578
Romberg, 945
Rinne, 930–934
straight leg raising, 803
swinging light, 578, 579
for syphilis, 1118–1121
thigh-slapping, 970
thumb tap, 959
timed vibratory, 946
Weber, 930–934

Tetanus, immunization for, 367, 369
Tetany, 90
T4, 55–56
Thalamus, ventral posteromedial nucleus of, 919–920
Thalassemia, 1025
Therapeutic diets, 483–485
Therapy, radiation, 59–61
Thermanalgesia, 943
Thermhyperesthesia, 943
Thoracic spine, 802–803
  on x-ray, 1170
Thorax, roentgenographic examinations of, 1168–1171
Three-glass test, for chronic prostatitis, 791
"Thrill," 746–747
Thrombocytopenia, idiopathic immunologic, 387
Thrombophlebitis
  deep vein, 729
  examination for, 726–730
  Homan's, 727
  Lawrence's, 727
  Lowenberg cuff, 727
  Moses', 727
  Owane's, 727
  suspicious clinical settings, 728–729
Thrombosis, cerebral, 371, 372, 374
Thumb tap test, 959
Thyrocalcitonin (TCT), 1095–1096
Thyroglossal cysts, 619–620
Thyroid autoantibodies, 57
Thyroid bruit, 619
Thyroidectomy, 60
Thyroid gland, 609, 610
  cancer of, 59
  disorders of, 54–59
  examination of, 617–621
  irradiation to, 59–61
  nodules of, 610
  surgery of, 57, 59–61
Thyroid hormones, 55–57
  and heat/cold intolerance, 52–53
Thyroiditis
  autoimmune, 58
  Hashimoto's, 58, 61, 620
  subacute, 620
Thyrotoxicosis, 978
  and carotid pulse, 666
  and first heart sound, 686
  and fourth heart sound, 703
  onchyolysis associated with, 544
  palpitation associated with, 193
Thyroxine (T4), 55–56
TIA's (see Transient Ischemic Attacks)
Tibial artery pulse, 744
Tic douloureux, 355, 921
Tics, 210
Tindall effect, 328
Tinea capitis, 534
Tinnitus, 549
  acoustic, 72

  causes of, 72
  and dizziness, 50
  history for, 71–76
Todd's paralysis, 342
Tomograms
  mediastinal, 1170
  pulmonary, 1169
Tongue
  coat, 597
  examination of, 587, 596–599
Tonometer, 565, 567
Tonsil fossa, 601
Tonsils, examination of, 599–604
Tophi, gouty, 409
Topognosis, 943, 947
Topographic ability, testing, 857
Torticollis, 940
Touch, testing sensation of, 942, 944, 952
Toxicity
  coumadin, 389
  digitalis, 65 (See also Medications; Poisoning)
Toynbee maneuver, 555
Trace elements, 481
Trachea, 610
Tragus, 552
Tranquilizers, 415 (See also Drugs; Medications)
Transient ischemic attacks, 348, 349, 374
  atherosclerotic emboli associated with, 613
  and dizziness, 47, 50
Transillumination
  of scrotum, 777
  of sinuses, 560
Trapezius muscle, 938–940
Trauma
  bleeding associated with, 386, 389
  head, 360–362
  and joint pain, 404
Tremors, 969, 975, 977, 978–979
Treponema pallidum, 1118–1121
Triceps reflex, 986, 991
Trichomonas, 265–266, 268
Trichorrhexis, 535
Tricuspid valve, abnormalities of, 660–661
Trigeminal nerve
  examination of, 915, 923
  lesions of, 921, 922
  neuralgia, 921
Triglycerides, 1104–1110
Triiodothyronine (T3), 55
Trochlear nerve, examination of, 897–905, 906–914
Tropical spure, 130
T3, 55
Tubal ligation, 257
Tuberculosis
  hemoptysis associated with, 159
  history for, 164–166
  and night sweats, 43
  postprimary pulmonary, 165

skin test for, 1115–1117
Tumor
    abdominal, 118
    bladder, 230
    breast, 641, 649–651
    optic, 581
    ovarian, 531
    parotid, 608
    pituitary, 895
    testicular, 245–240
    thyroid, 61
    vascular, 551
Tumor plop, 699
Tuning fork, for hearing tests, 930–934
Turgor, of skin, 538
Turner's syndrome, 218
T vector, 1126
T wave, 1123–1124
Two point discrimination, 943, 947
Typhoid fever, immunizations for, 447

Ulcers
    duodenal, 138, 139
    esophageal, 139
    gastric, 138, 139
    marginal, 140
    peptic, 138–140
Ultrasonography, 1180
Ultraviolet light, 334
Umbilical hernia, 135, 136
Uncal herniation, 580, 582, 913
Unconsciousness, 348, 990
Urates, in urine sediment, 1042, 1043
Urea, blood, 1044–1048
Uremia, 387
Urethral discharge, 237–239 (See also
    Vagina, discharge from)
Urethritis
    dysuria associated with, 222–223
    nongonococcal, 238–239
Urethroscopy, 239
Urgency
    causes of, 221, 222
    dysuria associated with, 222
    history of, 220–223
URI (see Infection, respiratory)
Uric acid, in serum, 1084–1089
Urinalysis
    color and odor, 1027–1030
    for flank pain, 221, 224
    specific gravity, 1030–1032
Urinary bleeding, 389
Urinary frequency, 220–223
Urinary incontinence, stress, 235–236
Urinary stream flow abnormality, 234–
    237
Urinary tract infections, 223–225
Urine
    blood in, 229, 1041, 1042–1043
    concentrated, 120
    glucose concentrations of, 1035–1039
    ketone bodies in, 1035–1039
    laboratory test of, 1027–1032

    protein in, 1033–1035
    RBC in, 1041, 1044
    refractive index of, 1030–1032
    sediment of, 1040–1044
    specific gravity of, 1030–1032
    WBC in, 1041–1042
Urobilinogen, 121–122
Urography, for flank pain, 226
Urticaria, 210, 326, 441
Uterus
    frontal section of, 786
    palpation of, 783–784
U wave, 1123

Vaccines, 445–449
Vagina
    bleeding from, 269–274, 385–386
    discharge from, 263–269
    examination of, 784
    infection in, 263
Vaginismus, 310, 313
Vaginitis
    atrophic, 263, 311
    corynebacterium vaginale, 264, 265, 266
    examination for, 254–265
    nonspecific, 267
Vagus nerve, examination of, 934–938
Valsalva maneuver
    and cardiac auscultation, 692
    and ear examination, 555
Varicella-Zoster Immune Globulin
    (VZIG), 448
Varicoceles, 780
Vascular disease, cerebellar disease
    associated with, 974
Vascular insufficiency, and vertigo, 88
Vascular system, familial diseases of,
    218
Vascular tumors, and bruits, 551
Vasculitis, 387
Vas deferens, 780
Vasectomy, 257
Vectorcardiogram, 1122
Vector method, EKG, 1129–1135
Vegetative function, psychological dis-
    turbances associated with, 433–436
Venereal disease, 264
    granulomatous, 275
    history for, 239–244
Venereal Disease Research Laboratory
    Slide Test, 1119–1120
Venous hums, 549
    abdominal, 766, 767, 768
    cervical, 614–616, 766
Ventilatory system (see Respiration)
Ventricular fibrillation, 1148, 1151
Ventricular flutter, 1148, 1150
Ventricular gallops, 696–699, 703
Venticular gradient, 1139–1143
Ventricular tachycardia, 509–510, 511,
    1148, 1150, 1151
Vergence movements, eye, 901
Vertebral artery, and dizziness, 50
Vertical movement, eye, 903

Vertigo, 44–45, 47, 50, 69
  benign positional, 49
  causes of, 86–87
  history of, 84–89
  questionnaire for, 87 (See also Dizziness)
Very low-density lipoproteins (VLDL), 1105, 1107
Vestibular neuronitis, 88
Vestibular nuclei, and vertigo, 87
Vestibular system, 85–86
Vibratory sensation, testing, 945–947
Videotapes, in clinical methods, 28, 29
Violence, potential for, 430–433
Virchow's nodes, 626
Virilism, 529
Virilization, 529
  clinical signs of, 531
  hirsutism associated with, 535
Visceral pain, 110
Vision
  central, 563
  dysfunction of, 64–66
  peripheral, 563
  physiology of, 890–894
Visual acuity, 564, 566–567, 569
Visual fields, 888–896
  testing, 563, 564, 569
Vitamin D, 482
Vitamin deficiency, 597–598 (See also Diet)
Vitamins
  fat soluble, 481
  water soluble, 481
Vocal cords
  examination of, 935
Voiding, frequent, 220
Vomiting
  of blood, 94–97
  causes of, 93–94
  flank pain associated with, 226
  history for, 91–94
  and nausea, 91–94
  pancreatitis associated with, 144
  ulcers associated with, 140
Vomitus
  coffee ground, 92, 93, 94
  feculent, 94
Vulvovaginitis, 221
V wave, of jugular venous pulsations, 657, 658–659, 661

Waldeyer's ring, 599
Walking, tandem, 971 (See also Gait)
Waveforms, of jugular venous pulse, 656–662

Wax removal, from ears, 553, 554–555
Weakness
  and hematocrit, 1012
  history for, 357–360
  neurological symptoms associated with, 349
  stroke associated with, 370
  and vertigo, 87
Weber hearing test, 72, 930–934
Weed, Dr. Lawrence, 4, 5
Weight, body, 521–528
  change in, 33–37
  gain in, 34, 35, 37
  ideal, 521
  loss of, 33, 34, 36–37
  reduction, 485
Wenchebach phenomenon, 1158
Wenchebach Type I AV block, 511
Werner's syndrome, 217
Wernicke-Korsakoff's syndrome, 838, 839, 841
Wernicke's area, 860, 861
"Wet dreams," 307
Wharton's duct, 600
Wheezing
  causes of, 162–163
  history of, 161–163
  and PND, 184–185
White blood cell count, 1014–1015
White blood cell differential, 1016–1020
White blood cells, in urine, 1041–1042
White, Dr. Paul Dudley, 26
Wilson's disease, 546, 978, 979
Windkessel effect, 516
Wolff-Parkinson-White syndrome, 193, 1147, 1148
Work relationships, 418 (See also Patients, occupation of)
Wright's stain, 1017
Wrists, examination of, 799–800
Writing, testing, 856–857

Xanthelasma, 569
Xeroderma pigmentosa, 335
Xiphisternal impulse, 678
X-linked traits, 453, 454
X-ray chest, 640, 1162–1176 (See also Radiographs)
X wave, of jugular venous pulsations, 657, 658–659, 661, 662

Y wave, of jugular venous pulsations, 657, 658–659, 661, 662

Zollinger-Ellison syndrome, 128–129, 140